The New Laser Therapy Handbook

A guide for research scientists, doctors, dentists, veterinarians and other interested parties within the medical field.

By

Jan Tunér and Lars Hode

Prima Books AB

2010

Copyright 2010:
Prima Books AB
Spjutvägen 11
772 32 Grängesberg
Sweden
Fax +46 240 23037
info@prima-books.com
www.prima-books.com

ISBN-13 978-91-976478-2-3

Cover illustrations: Some applications for LPT as documented in randomized clinical trials. Their PubMed identification numbers (PMID) are as follows:
20001318, 15966876, 18269665, 19892282, 17463313, 20116702, 19484402, 17069496, 16806710, 18341417, 12973834, 18817474, 17508839, 17725472 , 14677160, 16371497, 19841862, 15389743 , 15165387, 17352635, 17975958, 18087899, 16262574, 10423050, 10469307, 17625032

Book editing and design by Anders Nobel - anders.nobel@irradia.se
Cover front photo
Chandra/Hubble/Spitzer X-ray/Visible/Infrared Image of M82
Credit: NASA, ESA, CXC, and JPL-Caltech
Printed by UP Print, Tallinn, Estonia

Preface

This is the 5th book in English by the authors since 1996. We have seen an important development during this period. Laser phototherapy has not yet become mainstream medicine but the amount of qualified research has increased considerably and the previous incredulity has rather changed into curiosity. The treatment modality is at the moment in the difficult transition period between animal or small clinical studies. 40 years without full recognition may seem as a very long period, but on the other hand it took some 100 years for steam power to become widely used and just about as much for electricity.

Our ambition has been to present an entirely new book, containing all the important new studies. However, time has not been sufficient and when the 2004 edition of The Laser Therapy Handbook was almost sold out, we decided to use the old manuscript but still update it considerably. The basic manuscript comes from "Low level laser therapy - clinical practice and scientific background", published in 2002. In the paperback from 2004 several updates were included. However, the majority of the high quality studies in the field of laser therapy have been published during the last five years. From a tiny number around 25 studies on PubMed in 2000, the annual number of papers there has been around 250 in recent years. Fortunately, most of these papers have verified our previous statements. In Pubmed. there are now around 6000 scientific articles about LPT and the Pedro database of controlled clinical trials contains 136 hits. In the last two years, the amount of scientific evidence for laser therapy in clinical conditions has reached a level similar or above that of painkiller drugs in some musculoskeletal disorders.

Critics of laser phototherapy sometimes claim that the method is not well enough documented. This is not entirely wrong; the literature is not crystal clear and the number of studies for many particular indications is low. But looking over the entire field, we can see that a therapy that works "from top to toe", in animals and in laboratory monolayers cannot be entirely wrong. With more than 130 randomised clinical trials, LPT in itself has more documentation than several traditionally performed therapies. And we do not have to understand all about the very complicated photobiological processes before we start to apply a method. After all, Finsen was awarded the Nobel Prize in medicine in 1903 for his light therapy of lupus vulgaris, and it took 100 years before the actual mechanism was explained in a scientific way (1).

Photomedicine is of a very complex nature. To fully understand the subject a person should be an expert in physics, medicine, cell biology and scientific methodology. Lack of understanding of the complex nature has led to numerous mistakes in therapy, research set up and, not least, in the evaluation of phototherapy research. While negative studies can give useful clues to non working parameters, a negative outcome can also be the result of improper parameters. On the other hand, positive studies now and then give too little information about the parameters to make a definite evaluation possible. We have endeavored to analyse negative as well as positive studies and to give recommendations for suitable parameters in the clinic as well as in the laboratory.

The literature is the key to a better understanding of phototherapy. We have therefore emphasised the listing of old and new literature and to present most of these as small mini-abstracts. References to old and possibly less relevant literature have been maintained, since these references are difficult to find and may be of interest to readers. The focus is on the positive studies, not neglecting the negative ones. The reason is that we sometimes feel that the critics are updated on the minority of negative reports but less updated on the vast majority of positive reports.

Phototherapy is a field for researchers and different categories of users within mainstream as well as in paramedical medicine. It is not possible to compile a book that meets the needs of all these categories. Researchers would rather have more about mechanisms and clinicians more about the actual treatment parameters. We have tried to give a little to everybody and you are welcome to pick whatever you need from this Swedish "smorgasbord".

Many readers of our previous books have asked for more detailed treatment parameters. However, we do not favour the "cookbook" approach since there are so many parameters at work and every laser user must adapt to the characteristics of the laser/lasers available and the type of condition treated. This is one of the reasons why we have chosen to present many mini-abstracts from the literature, rather than to make standard recommendations or statements.

Pharmaceuticals have greatly contributed to the improved global health situation but have also generated serious adverse effects; not only to the patients but also to the environment. Laser phototherapy has been used for 40 years and no serious adverse effects have been documented. Phototherapy can be used in combination with traditional therapies to reduce the need of pharmaceuticals or, sometimes, in its own right as a monotherapy, without the serious adverse effects often caused by pharmaceuticals. We firmly believe that laser phototherapy has a great potential in health care and that this therapeutic modality merits more attention. It is our aspiration that this book will contribute to a better understanding of a promising therapeutic opportunity.

Jan Tunér and Lars Hode

1.　Moller KI, Kongshoj B, Philipsen PA, Thomsen VO, Wulf HC. How Finsen's light cured lupus vulgaris. Photodermatol Photoimmunol Photomed. 2005; 21 (3): 118-124.

Terminology in this book

The therapeutic lasers used today are mainly below 500 mW. However, many lasers used for surgery can be defocused and arranged to give energy densities of the same values as the former. Thus, a therapeutic laser could be defined as a laser using energy densities below the threshold where irreversible changes in cells occur.

We have slightly changed the title to "The New Laser Therapy Handbook" to underline the fact that this is not an entirely new book. However, we now favour the term *Laser phototherapy (LPT)* which is an emerging terminology. An advantage of this term is that it offers a good description of the therapy and an option to define various phototherapies by using "LED phototherapy", "Broadband polarised light phototherapy" etc. And they are all part of *Photomedicine*.

The term "soft laser" was originally used to differentiate therapeutic lasers from "hard lasers", i.e. surgical lasers. Several different designations then emerged, such as "MID laser" and "Medical laser". "Biostimulating laser" is another term, with the disadvantage that one can also give inhibiting doses. The term "bioregulating laser" has thus been proposed. One of the most frequent terms, "low-power laser", is misleading, since high-power lasers, too, are used for laser therapy.

An unsuitable name is "low-energy laser". The energy transferred to tissue is the product of laser output power and treatment time, which is why a "low-energy laser", over a long period of time, can actually emit a large amount of energy.

Regarding the laser instrument itself, we have chosen to use the term *therapeutic laser* rather than "Low-Level Laser", since high-level lasers are also used for laser therapy. Another reason is that many of the traditional laser types today are not really Low Level anymore and the commercial trend, at least, is towards higher output power. The MeSH definition is as follows:

- *Treatment using irradiation with light at low power intensities and with wavelengths in the range 540nm-830nm. The effects are thought to be mediated by a photochemical reaction that alters CELL MEMBRANE PERMEABILITY, leading to increased mRNA synthesis and CELL PROLIFERATION. The effects are not due to heat, as in LASER SURGERY. Low-level laser therapy has been used in general medicine, veterinary medicine, and dentistry for a wide variety of conditions, but most frequently for wound healing and pain control.*
- *Year introduced: 2002.*

It is obvious that the nanometre range used by MeSH in inappropriate and should be changed, at least to 540-1064 nm. LPT effects have been observed for much higher ranges such as Er:YAG and even CO_2, but the photobiology of these wavelengths is less explored.

It is obvious that the question of nomenclature is far from solved. This is because there is a lack of full agreement internationally, and the names proposed thus far have been rather unwieldy. The degree of confusion is illustrated in scientific journals, even the specialised ones, where different terms are sometimes used in the same issue and, indeed, even in one and the same paper.

Although we are using the term LPT in this book, we are aware of the fact that this term is not yet accepted by MeSH. As key words in scientific papers we will still have to adhere to the accepted MeSH terms.

MeSH key words in PubMed search: LLLT/Laser Biostimulation/ Laser Irradiation, Low-Power/Laser Therapy, Low-Power/ Low-Level Laser Therapy/ Low-Power Laser Irradiation/ Low-Power Laser Therapy.

References - why make it easy?

There are many systems for giving references in a scientific paper or in a scientific book. In fact, there are too many. In this book we have chosen the following system:

Smith B T, Jones S. The effect of laser therapy on aphte. J Laser Sci. 2009; 14 (2): 12-19.

Here we have the name of the authors, the title of the paper, the abbreviated name of the journal, the year, the volume, the issue and the pages. This is very straightforward. Looking back, we wish we had deleted some space, like between initials and volumes. But to change this, we would have to change all the references from the 1998 book, so we have kept the system. References have a number, and the number is given within brackets in the running text, from 1 and onwards. But there are many other systems. Some will give the name of the authors in the running text and either have the references in the time as they appear, or alphabetically. Some list all authors of a paper, others only the first six and then "et al." should be added.

There are many other ways to complicate the writing of references. The name of the authors could be given with full name or just initials of the first name(s). The name of the journal could be abbreviated or written in full, in italics or not and the ways to put full stops and commas also offer a lot to complicate things. Look at this:

Smith, B. T. & Jones, S. (2009) The effect of laser therapy on aphte. Journal of Laser Science **14**, 12-19.

Here italics are used for the journal and bold for the volume (omitting the useful information about the issue). And introducing as many dots and commas as possible. And a little "&" to the menu.

There are computer programmes to handle these things for the professionals. Good for them. But it would be even better if the scientific world could find some consensus. The therapy described in this book has many names and there is no consensus about the nomenclature. We are not alone!

Contents

Chapter 1 Some basic laser physics ... 1

1.1 Energy ... 2
1.1.1 Electromagnetical radiation ... 2
1.1.2 Wavelength and frequency ... 2
1.1.3 Photon energy ... 3
1.1.4 The electomagnetic spectrum ... 3
1.1.5 The optical field ... 3
1.1.6 Radiation risks ... 4
1.1.7 Can electromagnetic radiation cause cancer? ... 5
1.1.8 Protective mechanisms ... 5

1.2 Various sources of radiation ... 5
1.2.1 Natural sources of radiation ... 5
1.2.2 Man-made sources of radiation ... 6
1.2.3 The light-emitting diode (LED) ... 6
1.2.4 The laser ... 8
1.2.5 Laser design ... 8
1.2.6 The properties of laser light ... 12
1.2.7 Coherence ... 12
1.2.8 Polarisation ... 16
1.2.9 Output power ... 16
1.2.10 Continuous and pulsed lasers ... 16
1.2.11 The pulse peak power ... 17
1.2.12 Average power output ... 17
1.2.13 Power density ... 18
1.2.14 Collimation ... 20
1.2.15 Risk of eye injury ... 20
1.2.16 Decisive in the risk of eye injury ... 23

1.3 Laser types in medicine and surgery ... 28

1.4 The surgical lasers ... 29
1.4.1 The carbon dioxide laser (CO_2-laser) ... 30
1.4.1.1 Carbon dioxide lasers in surgery ... 31
1.4.1.2 Carbon dioxide lasers in dental applications ... 34
1.4.2 The Nd:YAG laser ... 36
1.4.2.1 Nd:YAG lasers in surgery ... 36
1.4.2.2 Nd:YAG lasers in dentistry ... 36
1.4.3 Ho:YAG lasers ... 38
1.4.4 Er:YAG lasers ... 38
1.4.5 Argon laser ... 40
1.4.6 Copper vapour laser ... 40
1.4.7 KTP/532-laser (frequency doubled Nd:YAG laser) ... 40
1.4.8 Ruby laser ... 41
1.4.9 Alexandrite ... 42
1.4.10 High power semiconductor lasers ... 42
1.4.11 Dye laser ... 42
1.4.12 Excimer laser ... 42

1.5	Thearpeutic lasers	43
1.5.1	The Helium-Neon laser (HeNe)	43
1.5.2	Indium-Gallium-Aluminium-Phosphide lasers (InGaAlP)	44
1.5.3	Gallium-Aluminium-Arsenide lasers (GaAlAs)	45
1.5.4	The Gallium-Arsenide laser (GaAs)	45
1.5.5	The defocused strong lasers	46
1.5.6	Some "exotic lasers"	47
1.5.7	The krypton laser	47
1.5.8	The nitrogen laser	47

Chapter 2 Therapeutic instruments 49

2.1	A customer's guide	50
2.1.1	History	50
2.1.2	What will tomorrow's lasers look like	51
2.1.3	Handheld laser and automatic devices	52
2.1.4	Which type of laser is best suited for which task?	53
2.1.4.1	HeNe laser and InGaAlP laser	53
2.1.4.2	GaAs laser	53
2.1.4.3	GaAlAs lasers	54
2.1.4.4	Combination probes	55
2.1.4.5	Therapeutic CO_2-lasers	56
2.1.5	Which laser should I buy?	56
2.1.6	Stronger = better?	57
2.1.7	How much should a laser cost?	60
2.1.8	Is a therapeutic laser really worth the money?	60
2.1.9	Do you need to update your laser?	61
2.1.10	Microcomputer features	61
2.2	Ten points to consider when choosing an instrument	61
2.3	How do I maintain my laser?	64

Chapter 3 Biostimulation 67

3.1	History	68
3.2	A few words on mechanisms	71
3.2.1	Photoreceptors	74
3.3	What parameters to use	76
3.3.1	Laser parameters	76
3.3.1.1	Which wavelength?	76
3.3.1.2	Output power	77
3.3.1.3	Average output power	77
3.3.1.4	Power density	77
3.3.1.5	Energy density	78
3.3.1.6	Treatment dose	78
3.3.1.7	Calculation of doses	78
3.3.1.8	Dose ranges	80
3.3.1.9	Calculation of treatment time for a desired dose	82
3.3.1.10	"Ready reckoner"	83
3.3.1.11	Dose per point	85

3.3.1.12	Pulsed or continuous light	86
3.3.1.16	Pulse repetition rate (PRR)	86
3.3.2	Patient parameters	90
3.3.2.1	Treatment area	90
3.3.2.2	Treatment intervals	91
3.3.2.3	Pre- or postoperative treatment?	94
3.3.3	Treatment method parameters	95
3.3.3.1	Local treatment	96
3.3.3.1.1	Shallow problems	96
3.3.3.1.2	Deeper problems	96
3.3.3.1.3	Treating inside the body	97
3.3.3.2	Systemic treatments	97
3.3.3.2.1	Acupuncture.	97
3.3.3.2.2	Trigger points	109
3.3.3.2.3	Spinal processes	109
3.3.3.2.4	Dermatome	109
3.3.3.2.5	Blood irradiation	110
3.3.3.2.6	Irradiation of lymph nodes	114
3.3.3.2.7	Irradiation of ganglions	114
3.3.4	Combination treatment	114
3.3.5	Interaction with medication	115
3.4	**Other considerations**	**118**
3.4.1	What about collimation?	118
3.4.2	Depth of penetration, greatest active depth	118
3.4.2.1	Factors that reduce penetration	120
3.4.2.2	Tissue compression	121
3.4.2.3	How deep does the light penetrate?	121
3.4.3	Laser light irradiation through clothes	123
3.4.4	The importance of the tissue and cell condition	123
3.4.5	The importance of ambient light	125
3.4.6	In vitro/in vivo	126
3.5	**Laser Therapy with high output lasers**	**126**
3.5.1	Laser therapy with carbon dioxide lasers	126
3.5.2	Laser therapy with Nd:YAG lasers	128
3.5.3	Laser therapy with ruby lasers	129
3.5.4	Laser therapy with Er:YAG lasers	130
3.5.5	Laser therapy with surgical diode lasers	130
3.6	**Risks and side effects**	**131**
3.6.1	The importance of a correct diagnose	131
3.6.2	Cancer	131
3.6.3	Cytogenetic effects?	132
3.6.4	A false picture of health	132
3.6.5	Tiredness	132
3.6.6	Pain reaction	132
3.6.7	Do high doses of laser therapy damage tissue?	133
3.6.8	Is it only an effect of temperature?	134
3.6.9	Protection against radiation injury	136

3.7		**How to measure effects of laser therapy**	**138**
3.7.1		Thermography	138
3.7.2		Magnetic resonance imaging	139
3.7.3		High resolution digitised ultrasound B-scan	139
3.7.4		Tensile strength	139
3.7.5		Other objective methods	140
3.8		**"Is laser therapy effective?"**	**140**
3.8.1		Does laser therapy really work?	141
3.8.2		Why the controversy?	142
3.8.3		Does it have to be a laser?	143
3.8.4		FDA (Food and Drug Administration)	143
3.8.5		How well documented?	145
3.8.6		Confused?	146
3.8.7		Experience and attitudes	146
3.8.8		The funding of research	147

Chapter 4 Medical indications 149

4.1		**Who and what can be treated?**	**150**
4.1.1		Acne	150
4.1.2		Allergy	152
4.1.3		Arteriosclerosis	153
4.1.4		Arthritis.	153
4.1.5		Asthma	170
4.1.6		Blood preservation	172
4.1.7		Blood pressure	173
4.1.8		Bone and cartilage regeneration	174
4.1.9		Cancer	190
4.1.10		Cardiac conditions	203
4.1.11		Carpal tunnel syndrome	208
4.1.12		Cell transplants	212
4.1.13		Cerebral palsy	214
4.1.14		Crural and venous ulcers	214
4.1.15		Delayed onset muscular soreness (DOMS)	218
4.1.16		Depression, psychosomatic problems	222
4.1.17		Diabetes	223
4.1.18		Duodenal/gastric ulcer	229
4.1.19		Epicondylitis	230
4.1.20		Erythema multiforme major	234
4.1.21		Fibrositis/fibromyalgia	235
4.1.22		Gynaecologic indications	236
4.1.23		Headache/Migraine	238
4.1.24		Haemorrhoids	239
4.1.25		Hair loss	239
4.1.26		Herpes simplex	242
4.1.27		Immune system modulation	246
4.1.28		Inflammation	248
4.1.29		Inner ear conditions	256
4.1.30		Laryngitis	256
4.1.31		Lichen	256

4.1.32	Low back pain	257
4.1.33	Microcirculation	259
4.1.34	Morbus Sluder	265
4.1.35	Mucositis	266
4.1.36	Muscle regeneration	266
4.1.37	Mycosis	270
4.1.38	Nerve conduction	271
4.1.39	Nerve regeneration and function	272
4.1.40	Oedema	285
4.1.41	Ophthalmic problems	289
4.1.42	Pain	293
4.1.43	Plantar fasciitis	304
4.1.44	Salivary glands	305
4.1.45	Sinuitis	309
4.1.46	Spinal cord injuries	310
4.1.47	Snake bites	311
4.1.48	Sports injuries	313
4.1.49	Stem cells	315
4.1.50	Stroke - irradiation of the brain	318
4.1.51	Tendinopathies	322
4.1.52	Tinnitus, vertigo, Ménière´s disease	330
4.1.53	Tonsillitis	342
4.1.54	Trigeminal neuralgia	342
4.1.55	Thrombophlebitis	343
4.1.56	Tuberculosis	343
4.1.57	Urology	344
4.1.58	Warts	348
4.1.59	Whiplash-associated disorders	348
4.1.60	Vitiligo	349
4.1.61	Wound healing	351
4.1.62	Zoster	372
4.2	**Indications in the pipeline**	**374**
4.2.1	Alzheimer's disease	375
4.2.2	Bisphosphonate-induced osteonecrosis	375
4.2.3	Botox failures	376
4.2.4	Cellulites	377
4.2.5	Cholesterol reduction	377
4.2.6	Eczema	377
4.2.7	Erectile dysfunction	378
4.2.8	Familial amyotrophic lateral sclerosis (FALS)	378
4.2.9	Obesity	379
4.2.10	Parkinson's disease	381
4.2.11	Post-menstrual stress	382
4.2.12	Withdrawal periods	382
4.2.13	Wrinkles	383

Chapter 5 Dental LPT 385

5.1	**The dental laser literature**	**386**
5.2	**On which patients can LPT be used?**	**386**

5.3	**Dental indications**	**387**
5.3.1	Alveolitis	388
5.3.2	Anaesthetics	388
5.3.3	Aphthae (canker sores)	389
5.3.4	Bleeding	391
5.3.5	Caries	393
5.3.6	Dentitio dificilis (pericoronitis)	396
5.3.7	Endodontics	396
5.3.8	Extraction	399
5.3.9	Gingivitis	403
5.3.10	Herpes zoster	407
5.3.11	Hypersensitive dentine	407
5.3.12	Implantology	411
5.3.13	Jaw fractures	415
5.3.14	Leukoplakia	415
5.3.15	Lingua geographica (glossitis)	415
5.3.16	Lip wounds	416
5.3.17	Mucositis	416
5.3.18	Nausea	417
5.3.19	Nerve injury	417
5.3.20	Oedema	417
5.3.21	Oral surgery	417
5.3.22	Orthodontics	419
5.3.23	Pain	426
5.3.24	Mild dental pain	426
5.3.25	Paediatric dental treatment	426
5.2.26	Periodontics	427
5.2.27	Prosthetics	437
5.2.28	Secondary dentine formation	439
5.3.29	Temporo-mandibular disorders (TMD)	440
5.4	**Other dental laser applications**	**448**
5.4.1	Dental photo dynamic therapy	448
5.4.2	Composite curing	449
5.4.3	Tooth bleaching	450
5.4.4	Caries detection	450
5.5	**Case reports**	**450**

Chapter 6 Non-coherent light sources 454

1.	**Light Emitting Diodes**	**456**
2.	**Linear polarised light**	**462**

Chapter 7 Veterinary use 465

Chapter 8 Contra indications 473

8.1	**Pacemaker**	**474**
8.2	**Pregnancy**	**474**
8.3	**Epilepsy**	**474**

8.4	Thyroid gland	475
8.5	Children	476
8.6	Cancer	477
8.7	Irradiation of the brain	477
8.8	Radiation therapy patients	479
8.9	Diabetes	480
8.10	Tatoos	481

hapter 9 Laser therapy on the internet ... 483

9.1	Laser therapy on the Internet	484
9.2	Internet discussion groups	484
9.2.1	Tinnitus	484
9.2.2	Wavelength	484
9.2.3	Coherence	486
9.2.4	Polarisation	486
9.2.5	Laser power	487
9.2.6	Light emitting diodes (LED)	490
9.2.7	Pulse frequencies	493
9.2.8	FDA approval	494
9.2.9	HeLa cells	501
9.2.10	Soliton waves	502

hapter 10 The difficult dose and intensity ... 505

10.1	Basics about energy	506
10.2	Output power	507
10.3	Power density	508
10.4	The laser beam	510
10.5	The laser probe	512
10.6	Pulsed lasers	513
10.7	Energy density	513
10.8	Treatment dose	514
10.9	The dose does not depend on the intensity	519
10.10	Dose per point	522
10.11	More about treatment technique	523

hapter 11 The Mechanisms ... 527

11.1	Are the biostimulative effects laser specific?	528
11.1.1	Is it possible to prove that laser therapy doesn't work?	528
11.1.2	Comparisons between coherent and non-coherent light	529
11.1.2.1	What is the importance of the length of coherence?	532
11.1.2.2	Hode's hamburger	534
11.1.2.3	Hode's big burger	535
11.1.3	Abrahamsson's apple	536
11.1.4	Moonlight	537
11.1.5	How deep does light penetrate into tissue?	539
11.1.6	Bright Light Phototherapy	541
11.1.7	Similarities and differences	543

11.2	**Possible primary mechanisms**	**544**
11.2.1	Polarisation effects	545
11.2.1.1	What characterises the light in a laser speckle	546
11.2.1.2	Porphyrins and polarised light	546
11.2.1.3	Cell cultures and tissue have different optical properties	547
11.2.2	The effect of heat development in the tissue	548
11.2.2.1	Macroscopic heating	549
11.2.2.2	The microscopic heat effect	549
11.2.3	Mechanical forces	549
11.2.4	Excitation effects	550
11.2.4.1	Primary reactions due to excitation	552
11.2.4.2	Secondary reactions due to cell signaling	553
11.2.5	Fluorescence – luminescence	555
11.2.6	Multi-photon effects	555
11.2.7	Lasing effects in tissue	556
11.2.8	Non linear optical effects	557
11.2.9	Opto-acoustic waves	557
11.3	**Secondary mechanisms**	**557**
11.3.1	Effects on pain	557
11.3.2	Effects on blood circulation	559
11.3.3	Stimulatory and regulatory mechanisms	560
11.3.4	Effects on the immune system	560
11.3.5	Other interesting possibilities	561
11.4	**Summary of mechanisms**	**562**
11.5	**Diagnostics with Therapy Lasers**	**564**
11.6	**Photodynamic Therapy – PDT**	**564**
11.7	**Other medical uses of lasers**	**565**

Chapter 12 A guide for scientific work 567

12.1	**Methodology of a trial…**	**570**
12.2	**Parameters**	**571**
	Technical parameters	571
	Treatment parameters	571
	Medical parameters	572
12.2.1	Closer description of the technical parameters	572
	1) Name of instrument (producer)	572
	2) Laser type and wavelength	572
	3) Laser beam characteristics	573
	4) Number of sources	573
	5) Beam delivery system	573
	6) Pulsed or continuous emission	573
	7) Output power	574
	8) Power density at probe aperture	575
	9) Calibration of the instrument	575
12.2.2	Closer description of the treatment parameters	575
	1) Treatment area	576
	2) Dose: Energy density	576
	3) Dose per treatment and total dose	576

		4) Intensity: Power density	576
		5) Treatment method	576
		6) Treatment distance (spot size), type of movement, scanning	577
		7) Sites of treatment	577
		8) Number of treatment sessions	577
		9) Frequency of treatment sessions	578
12.2.3		Closer description of the medical parameters	578
		1) Description of the problem to be treated	578
		2) Patients (number, age, sex)	578
		3) Exclusion criteria	578
		4) Inclusion criteria	578
		5) Condition of patient	578
		6) Pre-, parallel- or post-medication	579
		7) Treated with other methods before	579
		8) Drop-out rate	579
		9) Follow up	579
		10) Outcome measures	579
		11) Statistical Analysis	579
		12) Economy	579
12.2.4		Recommendations of WALT – The World Association for Laser Therapy	580
		Conclusion	580

Chapter 13 The laser phototherapy literature ... 581

13.1 Are all the negative studies really negative? ... 582

13.1.1	"I heard it through the grapevine"	583
13.1.2	Positive from negative	583
13.1.3	Negative from negative	583
13.1.4	Dose development	584
13.1.5	Pitfalls	585
	1. Low outputs	585
	2. Inclusion criteria	595
	3. Lack of proper control groups	595
	4. Therapeutic technique	596
	5. Systemic effects	597
	6. Tissue condition	597
	7. Power density	597
	8. Mixed parameters	598
	9. The influence of ambient light	598
	10. Premature conclusions	599
	11. Meta-analyses	599
	12. Confusion between groups	599
	Our comments:	601
	Conclusion	601
	Litterature:	601

	13.2	The Cochrane LPT analyses – can they be improved?	604
	13.3	An evaluation of the evaluators	610
	13.4	Poor documentation – compared to what?	614
	13.5	Can you trust your laser?	615
	13.6	English language books on LPT	616
	13.7	Books in other languages, with ISBN	618
	13.8	Laser phototherapy journals	620

Chapter 14 References – Abbreviations ... 621

	14.1	Numeric references referred to in the book.	622
		Alphabetical register of references	733
	14.2	Abbreviations	836

Chapter 1
Some basic laser physics

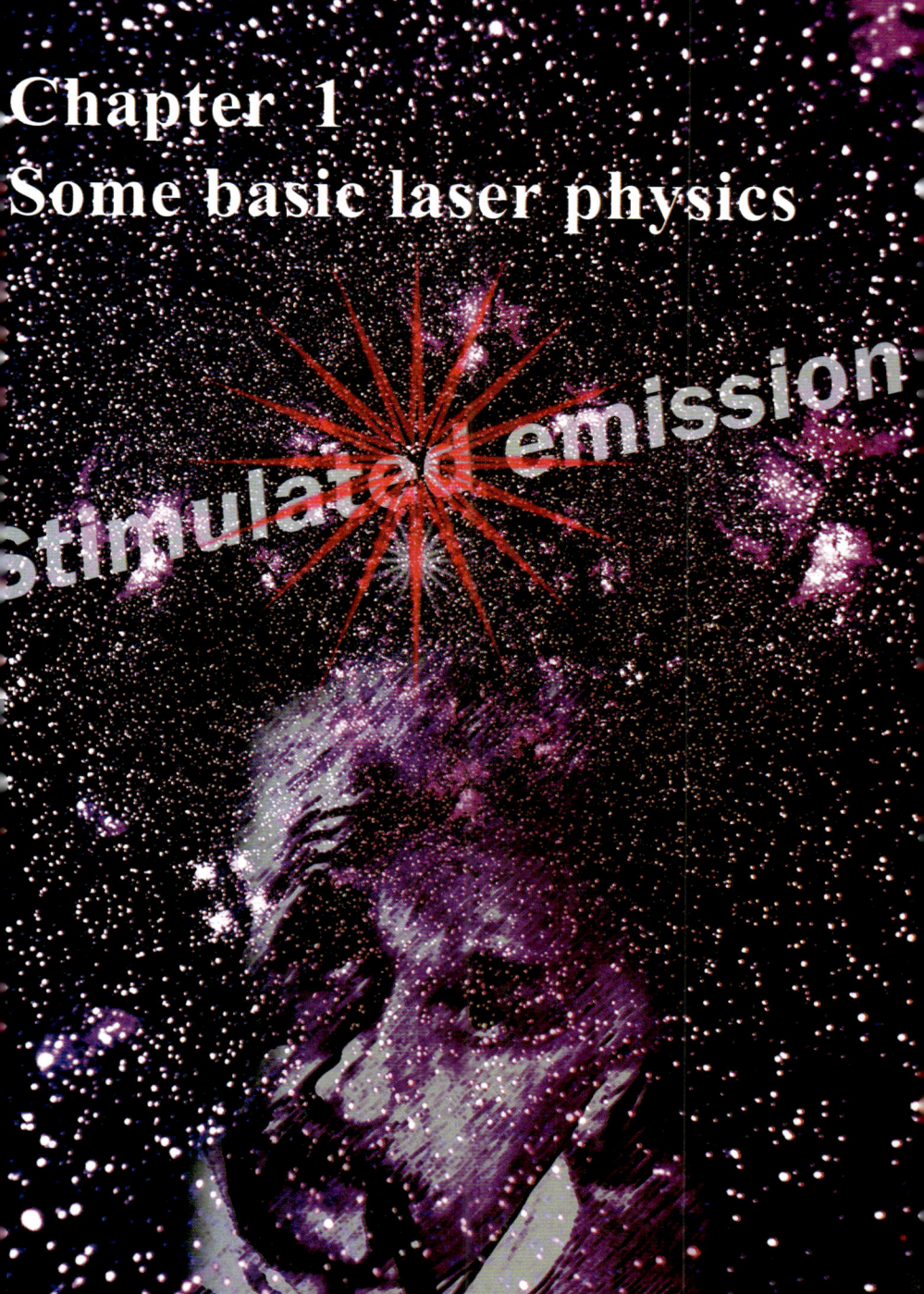

1.1 Energy

This book is not intended to be a textbook of physics. However, in order to understand some of the parts of this book, we need to know a little bit of the basic physics.

Energy is the most fundamental property of universe. Heat is energy, movement is energy, radiation is energy and even matter is a form of energy. There is a law, from which we have never found any exception; the principle of energy. It is also called "the general law of conservation of energy". This law has a simple interpretation: Energy can never be destroyed, energy can never be created, energy can only be converted from one form to another!

Amount of energy is measured in joules, named from the English physicist James Joule (1818-1889). The unit is written J. Older unit is the calorie. One calorie is 4.18 J. One calorie is the amount of energy needed to raise the temperature of one gram of water with 1 degree Celsius (Anders Celsius, Swedish physicist, 1701-1744).

1.1.1 Electromagnetic radiation

The radiation emitted by the sun, light bulbs, fires, radio transmitters, etc., is called electromagnetic radiation. This form of energy consists of photons - packets of energy - that travel at the speed of light, i.e. approximately 300.000 kilometers per second in a vacuum. Photons can be seen as wave particles or wave packets. Each photon is thus a small packet of energy in the form of a wave element, in which the wave (in the same way as water waves or sound waves) has a defined wavelength and a frequency related to that wavelength.

1.1.2 Wavelength and frequency

The relationship between wavelength (λ) and frequency (ν) is:

$$\lambda \times \nu = c$$

where c = the speed of light in the medium of interest. (In media other than a vacuum the formula will be: $\lambda \times \nu = c/n$ where n is the index of refraction.) See further Appendix.

Within the part of the electromagnetic spectrum that we call the radio frequency field, frequency is often used instead of wavelength (e.g. for FM radio stations – 87-108 MHz). In the other parts of the spectrum we would have to use unmanageably high numbers and therefore use the wavelength in all but a few cases. Another reason to use wavelength, rater than frequency, is that "frequency" often arises in discussions about pulsed radiation and is used to denote pulse frequency (number of pulses per second).

1.1.3 Photon energy

Photons of different wavelengths have different energy levels. Photon energy (E) is proportional to frequency (λ) and can be expressed as

$$E = h \times v = h \times c / \lambda$$

where h is equal to Planck's constant. If we use wavelength instead of frequency, photon energy would be inversely proportional to the photon's wavelength. Photons with a long wavelength therefore have a low energy, while photons with a short wavelength have a high energy.

1.1.4 The electromagnetic spectrum

Electromagnetic radiation spans an enormous range of wavelengths, often referred to as the wavelength spectrum, and the different parts of this spectrum have been given different names. The table on next page shows each part in terms of its name, range of wavelength, a description of its use, and an example of the source of the radiation. The electromagnetic spectrum, subranges, wavelengths, use and typical sources

Name	Wavelengths	Used for	Source
Radio waves	1000 - 1 m	Radio, TV, telecommunications, cellular telephones	Radio transmitters, electric cables
Microwaves	1000 - 1 mm	Radar, telecom, microwave ovens, speed measuring	Klystrons, magnetrons, masers
Infrared (IR)	1000 - 0.8 μm	Radiation heaters, infrared heating, remote control	Hot objects, IR lamps, fires, LEDs, lasers
Visible light	800 - 400 nm	Illumination, photography, imaging, holography	Light-bulbs, flash lamps, candles, LEDs, lasers
Ultraviolet (UV)	400 - 1 nm	Solarium, curing of plastics, sterilisation	UV lamps, lasers, accelerators
X-rays	1000 - 1 pm	X-raying, radiation treatment of tumours	X-ray tubes, accelerators
Gamma Rays	1000 - 1 fm	Radiation treatment of cancer, sterilisation of food	Radioactive isotopes, particle accelerators

Table 1.1 The electromagnetic spectrum

1.1.5 The optical field

The spectrum of electromagnetic radiation that follows the laws of optics includes wavelengths between approximately 1 nm and 1000 μm and is usually referred to as "optical radiation", even though most of it lies outside the visible spectrum (wavelengths of about 400-800 nm). Both infrared (IR) and ultraviolet (UV) radiation exhibit many similarities to visible light and are therefore regarded as part of the optical field. When using the term "light" from now on, we will be referring to infrared and ultraviolet radiation as well as visible light.

1.1.6 Radiation risks

Special considerations relating to the eyes will not be discussed in this section; See chapter 1.2.15 "Risk of eye injury" on page 20.

Because different wavelengths have different energy levels, the risks of exposure to various kinds of electromagnetic radiation are also of varying magnitude. High-energy photons (gamma rays, X-rays and ultraviolet light) can "break" (ionise) atoms and break up chemical bonds in molecules which they encounter, while low-energy photons (radio waves and microwaves, infrared and visible light) do not cause ionisation but only excitation and heating. Photons in the optical field, either as visible light, ultraviolet or infrared, can be reflected, transmitted (that is, go right through) or absorbed when they come in contact with matter. Tissue is generally more transparent to wavelengths near infrared (800-1200 nm) than to visible light. When a photon is absorbed, it sheds all of its energy into the matter and is annihilated. The energy shed is transformed into another type of energy, most often thermal. Consequently, if high-power radiation (many watts = many photons per second) encounters an object, a great deal of heat can result (for example, a stone in the sun becomes hot). By concentrating a beam on a small area, e.g. by focusing it, a high power density is achieved in that small area and the heat built up during the absorption of the radiation can be so great that the beam burns, melts or vaporises the material in the area encountered. This technique is used in surgical lasers. In this way, all radiation (if sufficiently intense) can injure an individual or an object.

However, those types of radiation involving photons in which the energy level is so high that they can ionise are dangerous even at low intensities, because ionisation is by nature damaging. This type of radiation is usually called ionising radiation.

In principle, all ionising radiation is carcinogenic, since cell damage may result from exposure to it. All electromagnetic radiation with a wavelength shorter than 320 nm (UVB radiation, UVC radiation, X-rays, and gamma radiation) is ionising, and thus in principle dangerous to us even in relatively low quantities. In the range from 320 nm to 400 nm (the UVA band), long-term exposure - to sunlight or in a solarium, for example - has been shown to cause some cell damage, though only rarely cancer.

As far as the visible band (400-800 nm) goes, there are people who are oversensitive to light (photo allergy), and who can only tolerate red light (light with wavelengths over 600 nm) and therefore cannot go out in daylight.

1.1.7 Can electromagnetic radiation cause cancer?
Electromagnetic radiation can injure living organisms if it

1) is of sufficient intensity to burn (many watts) and/or
2) contains high-energy photons (short wavelength).

N.B. Whether the photons come from a "natural" or from an artificial light source is of no significance - one photon with a certain energy is exactly the same as another one with the same energy!

There is a fairly clear wavelength limit at which photon energy becomes so high that the photons can ionise matter that they meet. This limit is 320 nm, (for physicists: this corresponds to 3.91 eV) so that photons with a shorter wavelength than this are capable of ionising molecules or atoms in tissue and hence can cause cancer (they are carcinogenic).

An example of a source of radiation which produces carcinogenic ultraviolet radiation is the quartz lamp. The casing of such a lamp is not made of glass but of quartz. This material, unlike glass, allows ultraviolet radiation to pass through it and tolerates much higher temperatures. Quartz lamps produce much of their radiation in the wavelength field around 250 nm. Ultraviolet radiation with such a short wavelength is very aggressive and is used, for example, to kill bacteria and other microorganisms. Because the radiation from quartz lamps is carcinogenic, these lamps were banned in most countries about 40 years ago. A laser with the same wavelength and the same strength is just as dangerous - no more, no less. (See chapter 3.6 "Risks and side effects" on page 131.) The risk factor depends on both the dose (input energy, measured in joules per cm^2 of skin) and the power density (intensity) of the radiation.

1.1.8 Protective mechanisms
Human beings have always been subjected to solar radiation. The sun emits all of the types of radiation shown in the table on the previous page, though only radio waves, microwaves, infrared radiation (thermal radiation), visible light, and the longwave part of ultraviolet radiation are not absorbed by the atmosphere and therefore reach the surface of the earth. Of those types of radiation that reach the ground, only a small part of the ultraviolet radiation (known as UVB) is dangerous to human beings. We have as a consequence developed protective mechanisms against it. Special cells (melanocytes) in the outer skin produce melanin, which absorbs UV radiation and prevents it from reaching the deeper and more sensitive tissues.

1.2 Various sources of radiation

1.2.1 Natural sources of radiation
The sun is our main natural source of radiation and energy. Like the light used for general illumination, it has a very wide spectrum (i.e. it is composed

of photons with considerably varying wavelengths). On the earth's surface, solar radiation has its highest intensity at 440 nm, blue light, above and below which it decreases. The sun, then, is actually blue, though any self-respecting child will draw it in yellow. It looks yellow to us because our eyes are most sensitive to yellow - 550 nm. Below 440 nm, the intensity of solar radiation drops, falling to zero at 290 nm (with the ozone layer in its present state). The carcinogenic part of solar radiation lies between 290 and 320 nm, and is known as UVB radiation. There is no upper limit to the sun's long wave radiation, but at very long wavelengths - radio waves - the intensity is low. (See Figure 1.1 "Wavelength distribution of light from various sources" on page 7.)

1.2.2 Man-made sources of radiation

All conventional light sources are more or less broadband. The most narrow-banded are low-pressure gas discharge lights, such as neon lights (red) or sodium lights (yellow). These often feature a dominant wavelength, meaning that most photons have this wavelength or a wavelength close to it. These light sources have a function in some ways reminiscent of a laser's.

Of all the hundreds of types of lamps, we have chosen to study only two types in more detail: the light emitting diode and the laser. They are both used in therapeutic instruments and it is important to know the difference between them.

1.2.3 The light-emitting diode (LED)

Another light source, which is relatively narrow-banded, is the light-emitting diode. This is a small, inexpensive semiconductor lamp, which should not be confused with a laser. Typical LEDs produce red, yellow, green, blue or even white light (three LEDs in one case). There are LEDs which emit infrared radiation, generally with wavelengths around 950 nm (entirely invisible). These are often used in television remote control units.

According to the European Standard IEC 601, an LED is: "*Any semiconductor p-n junction device which can be made to produce electromagnetic radiation by radiative recombination in the semiconductor in the wavelength range from 180 nm to 1 mm, produced primarily by the process of spontaneous emission.*"

The diagram shows the wavelength distribution of light from various sources, including sunlight, filament lamps, fluorescent lamps, and several different lasers. Note that the spectrum of a laser is shown as a narrow vertical line; the laser emits light of only "one" wavelength. This line has nothing to do with the fact that laser light is sometimes collimated to a narrow beam!

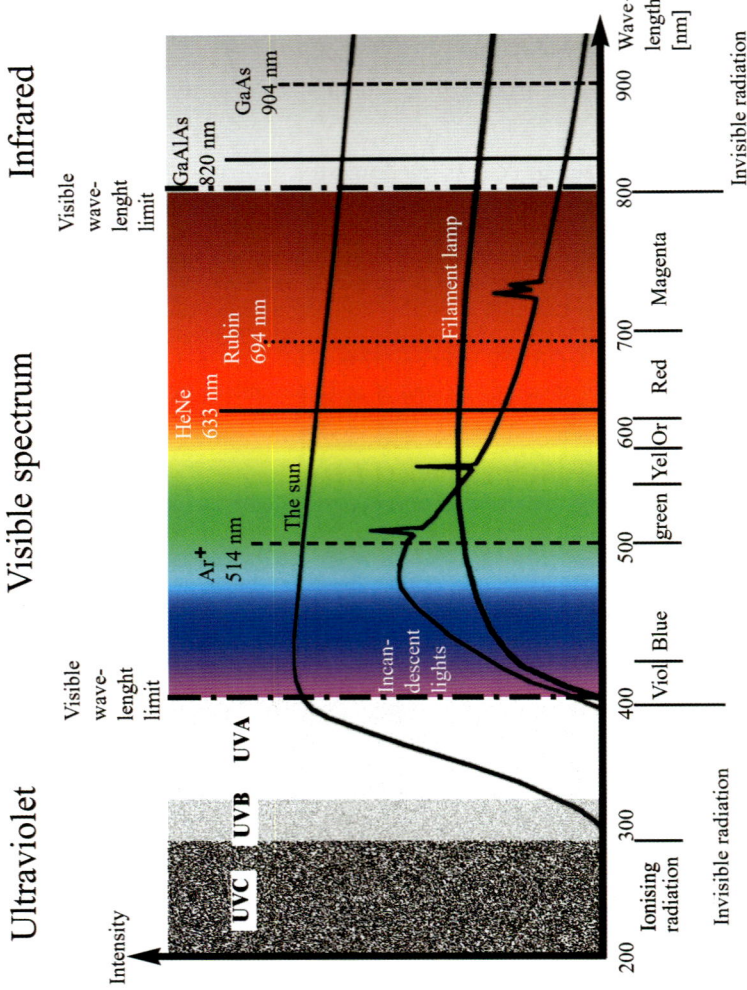

Figure 1.1   Wavelength distribution of light from various sources

1.2.4 The laser

The laser is the most advanced of our light sources. The word LASER is an acronym for **L**ight **A**mplification by **S**timulated **E**mission of **R**adiation.

As a point of interest, the first name suggested for the laser was "Light Oscillation by Stimulated Emission of Radiation" - but this resulted in the unfortunate acronym LOSER.

Credit for the development of laser theory is generally given to Albert Einstein. In his theory "Zur Quantum Theories der Strahlung", published in 1916, he first used the name stimulated emission. Other and more important steps have been taken by Arthur Shawlow, Charles Townes and Theodor Maiman. Maiman presented the first working laser, a ruby laser, at a press conference on 7th July 1960.

Strictly speaking, a laser is a light amplifier if the radiation produced is within the visible range or a radiation amplifier if the radiation produced is within the infrared or ultraviolet radiation ranges. A predecessor of the laser was the MASER (Microwave Amplification by Stimulated Emission of Radiation). It works on the same principle as the laser, but within the microwave range.

According to the European Standard IEC 601, the definition of a laser is: *"Any device which can be made to produce or amplify electromagnetic radiation in the wavelength range from 180 nm to 1 mm primarily by the process of controlled stimulated emission"*.

1.2.5 Laser design

A laser, whether large or small, always includes the following parts:

Energy source	(power supply)
Lasing (amplifying) medium	(solid, liquid or gas)
Resonating cavity[1]	(mirrors)

How energy is supplied to the lasing medium depends on the structure of the medium. The energy source may be an electrical current, optical radiation from a flash lamp or another (pumping) laser, radio waves or microwaves, or a chemical reaction.

---

1. There exist lasers without resonating cavity but we will not go into that as it would lead too far away.

"Star wars" chemical laser

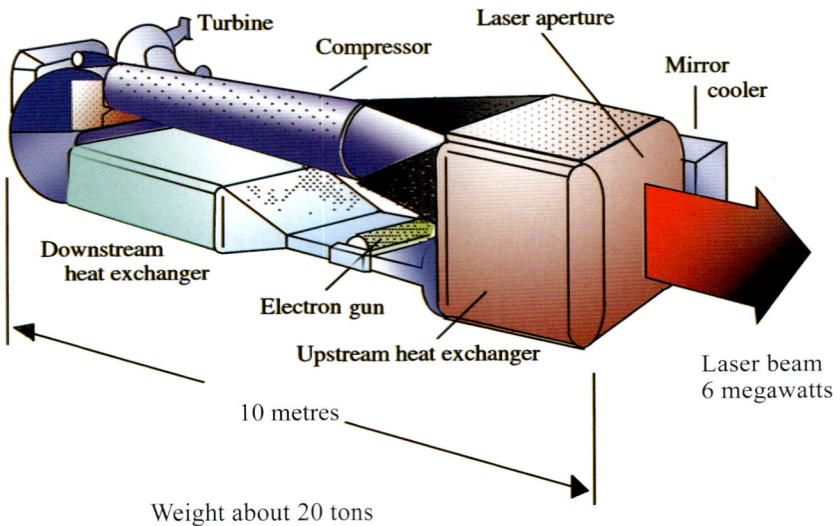

GaAs laser diode

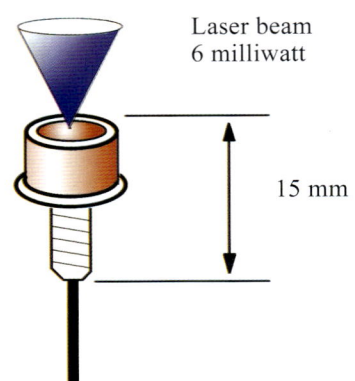

Laser beam
6 milliwatt

15 mm

A laser can be seen as a tool: Tools have different shapes and sizes and different use

Two different lasers are shown here: Weight 20 tons and 2 grams, respectively. One for destruction (but was never built) and one for healing.

Figure 1.2 Star wars

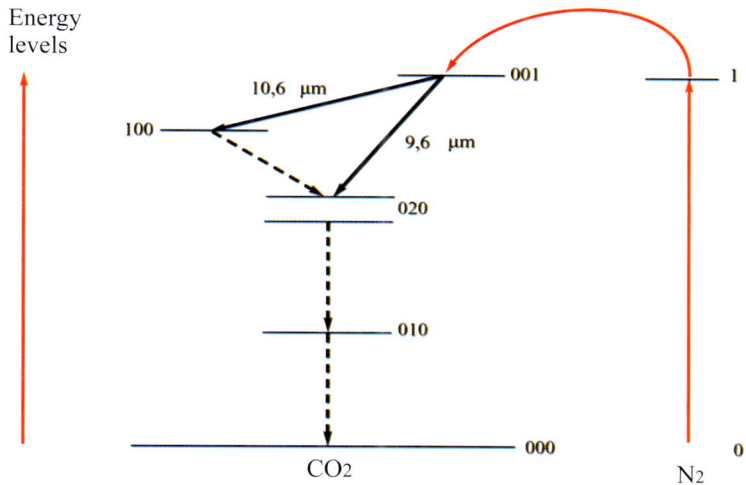

Energy diagram for CO$_2$ laser

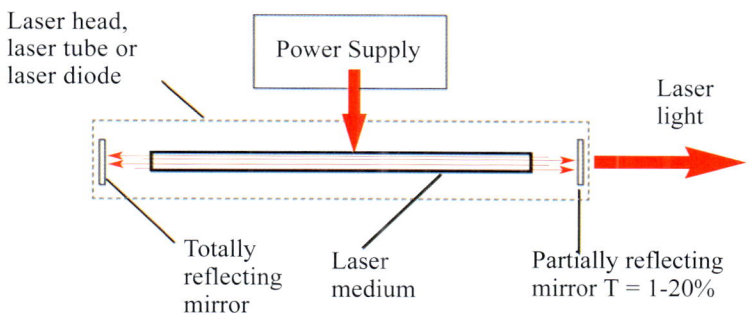

Figure 1.3 Principle design of a laser

The lasing medium must be able to store the energy supplied, which it does by a process called population inversion. This stored energy can then be emitted in an organized fashion, known as stimulated emission of radiation. When a photon with the right photon energy enters the electromagnetic field of the excited atom with energy stored in this way, some of the energy is emitted by the creation of an identical photon. The first photon is not absorbed. Hence, both the new and the old photon can then stimulate other atoms in the lasing medium to emit their stored energy. It is like a chain reaction, causing an "avalanche" of light in which all the photons have exactly the same photon energy.

Hence, the radiation from a laser always has a certain fixed wavelength, which is determined by the structure of the lasing medium and does not, like the radiation from other light sources, consist of a wide range of wavelengths. There are currently thousands of different types of laser, and these produce light, UV, or IR radiation of various wavelengths. Usually a laser has one characteristic wavelength, though it is sometimes possible to choose within a range of wavelengths. This is most common among semiconductor lasers. There are a few lasers designed in such a fashion that the wavelength can be changed, even during operation - tunable lasers.

> Summary: Stimulated emission only occurs when the incident photon has exactly the same energy as the released photon; the first photon causes release of the second photon simultaneously, i.e. the second photon must follow the oscillations of the first photon, so that the two photons oscillate in phase. This phase-locked, wavelength specific, photon chain reaction results in the monochromatic (one wavelength), coherent (fixed phase relation) characteristics of laser light.

Further, the lasing medium is generally elongated in shape, often in the form of a channel (gas lasers) or a narrow rod (solid state lasers) or doped channel (semiconductor lasers), and is fitted with mirrors at its ends. These mirrors form the resonating cavity. The light produced in the lasing medium is reflected back into the lasing medium several times and stimulates new light production. The resonating cavity is of two-fold importance: it increases the lasing medium's amplification and makes the light more coherent. (See chapter 1.2.7 "Coherence" on page 12.) The elongation and mirror arrangement also make it possible for the light to emerge as a relatively parallel beam (that may be focused to a very small point). To extract the light from the laser, one mirror is made somewhat transparent - most often 1-20% transparency, so that between 99% and 80% of the light is reflected back. Hence, the light intensity inside a laser is always higher than the output power.

Other optical components may be arranged between the mirrors, permitting wavelength selection, polarisation of the laser light, or Q-switching (a pulsing method making it possible to achieve very intense and very short pulses). By inserting a non linear crystal, optical overtones (e.g. double frequency) can be generated - one example of this is the KTP laser. (See chapter 1.4.7 "KTP/532-laser (frequency doubled Nd:YAG laser)" on page 40.)

1.2.6 The properties of laser light

Laser light has two essential characteristics which differentiate it from "normal" light:

(1) its very narrow bandwidth
(2) its high level of coherence

Coherence means that the photons are well ordered - they are connected and build light waves that remain synchronised with one another over long distances, (See Figure 1.6 "Coherent and non-coherent light" on page 15.) A narrow bandwidth is necessary for a high degree of coherence. These two characteristics are typical of all laser light and are important with regard to laser therapy. Neither of them, however, has any major significance in the use of lasers as surgical instruments. Two other characteristics that many people believe are typical of lasers are:

(3) parallel beams
(4) high intensity

These characteristics can often be brought about in a laser by chosing the size and geometric design of the lasing medium and resonating cavity as mentioned above, **but laser light does not need to be parallel or particularly strong**. These two characteristics are, however, most important with respect to lasers as surgical instruments. They are also the properties of laser light that make it harmful to the eye under certain circumstances. Narrow and parallel beams can allow the entire volume of light to pass through the pupil of an unprotected eye - it is thus not difficult to imagine how an intense laser light source can be dangerous to our light-sensitive eyes. (See Figure 1.9 "Laser and eye-risk" on page 24.)

1.2.7 Coherence

Coherence generally means order, or synchronicity. When a troop of soldiers is marching, it moves coherently, but if the soldiers are free to leave, they start to move incoherently. The same is true of the sound emanating from a flute (a flute is a typical "sound laser" - it has a resonance cavity, and its sound is monochromatic and coherent).

Soldiers marching (moving coherently) over a bridge will influence the mechanical structure other than they would if they were walking or running (moving incoherently) over the same bridge.

The tone of a flute may cause a crystal glass to break due to interference and resonance, but a wide-band, incoherent sound of the same intensity cannot break the glass. Interference is the effect of adding two or more waves. This addition may result in either amplification (constructive interference) or attenuation (destructive interference) of the resulting amplitude. Amplification is what makes extra high peaks when water waves meet, or what makes one pitch sound particularly strong when we sing at various pitches in the bathroom.

When a rough surface is illuminated with visible laser light, a kind of grainy quality can be observed in the light. These grainy elements, or granules, are called laser speckles, (See Figure 1.5 "Laser speckles" on page 15.) and occur as a result of interference between different light beams. This is because light with a sufficiently high coherence length can be "combined" in the same way that waves of water combine when they meet. (More about speckles and their medical importance in chapter 11.1.3.)

Waves of coherent light stay in phase in long trains of waves. The length of these trains of waves, the coherence length, vary from one light source to another. An ordinary light bulb has a low coherence length, a matter of thousandths of a millimetre. A HeNe laser, on the other hand, may have a very high coherence length - decimetres or even several metres. A semiconductor laser usually has a coherence length of no more than a millimetre or so.

N.B. In a laser beam, the different parts of the wave field can have a fixed phase relation but are usually not "in phase". (See Figure 1.6 "Coherent and non-coherent light" on page 15.)

The concept of coherence consists of both spatial and temporal coherence and it is mainly the former that is of interest here. However, the two are related to each other through the relation: $\Delta\omega \times \Delta t \geq 2\pi$ where $\Delta\omega$ represents the frequency interval within which the radiation is emitted and where Δt is close to the coherence time - higher Δt means a higher degree of temporal coherence.

> Coherency: Coherency in general is the property of wave-like states that enables them to exhibit interference. It is also the parameter that quantifies the quality of the interference, also known as the degree of coherence. The degree of coherence is equal to the interference visibility, a measure of how perfectly the waves can cancel out each other due to destructive interference.
>
> Two types of coherency are at hand, temporal coherency, where phase synchronization is valid for a certain time and, spatial coherency meaning that light waves show coherency when they are emitted from different locations of an extended light source.

Literature:

Nicola [511] developed a technique of causing highly reproducible inflammatory lesions on the skin of rats. HeNe light at 1 J/cm² produced an acceleration of the healing process. Incoherent light of the same wavelength and dose was less favourable.

In a study by Rosner [493] the effect of HeNe laser in the regeneration process of crushed optical nerves was estimated. While HeNe laser postponed the degenerative process, non-coherent infrared light was ineffective or affected the injured nerves adversely.

Read more in chapter 11.12. "Comparison between coherent and non-coherent light".

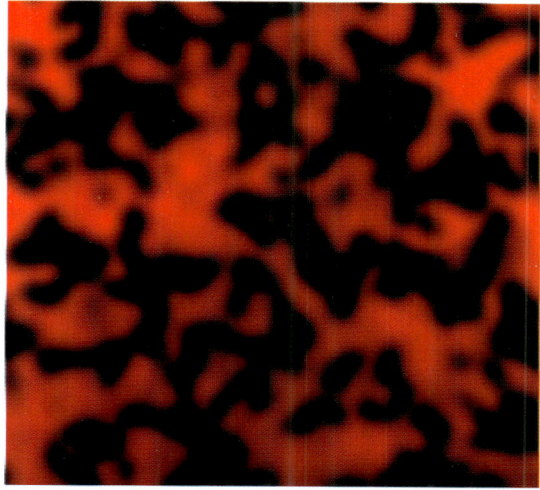

Figure 1.4   Photographed laser speckles

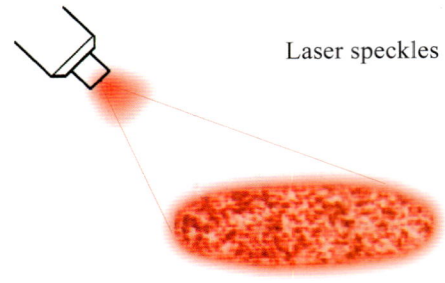

Laser speckles

If a rough surface is illuminated by visible laser light, the laser light shows a speckled structure due to interference. This phenomenon is called laser speckles and occurs in the eye of the viewer.

Figure 1.5 Laser speckles

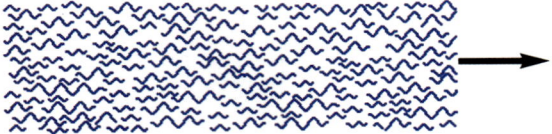

A parallel beam of light with short coherence length. This is often called "incoherent" or non-coherent light - lamp light.

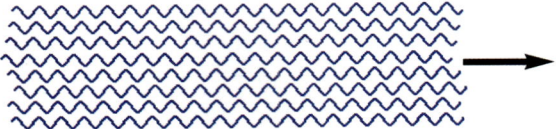

A parallel beam of light with long coherence length. This is often called "coherent" light - laser light.
N.B. Coherence has nothing to do with parallelity and the waves do not have to be in phase.

Figure 1.6 Coherent and non-coherent light

1.2.8 Polarisation

Light - whether from a laser or another source - can be non-polarised or polarised. It can also be more or less polarised (partially polarised). There are two types of polarisation: linear and circular, which can be described using the following analogy. We can take a long rope and tie one end round a tree, then stretch the rope so that it does not touch the ground. We then create wave motion by moving the rope up and down - the waves move vertically in accordance with the up and down movement. The wave is vertically linearly polarised. If we instead move the rope from side to side, the wave is horizontally linearly polarised. Finally, if we rotate the rope, a corkscrew-like wave motion results. This is circular polarisation, and we can differentiate between right and left rotational circular polarisation. (Both linear and circular polarisation are special cases of the more general elliptical polarisation, which - as well as the circular polarisation - can be left or right handed rotational).

Polarised light can be achieved by filtering with "polarisation" filters. Special prisms or other optical components (e.g. a Brewster window) can also be used. Most lasers (gas- and solid state lasers) and other light sources are not equipped with polarising means and consequently emit non-polarised light. Diode lasers, however, usually emit polarised light. (For more information about the importance of polarisation, read chapter 11.1).

1.2.9 Output power

Power is measured in watts (W). The strength or power output of a laser is thus measured in watts or milliwatts (mW = a thousandth of a watt). Higher output power is of some consequence in that at a higher power output one achieves a higher power density, which is often desirable. Also, a higher output power means that a certain desired dose (input energy, measured in joules per cm^2 of skin) is more quickly reached because energy is the same as power multiplied by time.

When you buy an ordinary lamp, it is always its power consumption, i.e. its <u>input power</u>, that is specified, and almost never its output power (radiance). Hence a 60 W lamp consumes 60 watts and yields, typically, 1 - 2 watts of visible light power. The remaining 98 – 99% of the input power is converted to heat in the glass casing and metal socket and to directly emitted, invisible infrared radiation. The power specified for a laser is always its <u>output power</u>. Hence a 60 W laser consumes more than 60 watts but yields 60 watts of (visible or invisible) radiation power.

1.2.10 Continuous and pulsed lasers

A light source usually emits light at a constant intensity. This is known as continuous wave (cw) emission. However, it is also possible to make lasers and other lamps with varying intensity, known as amplitude modulated emission. The variability of modulated light may be small (low degree of modulation) or large (high degree of modulation). In the extreme case (100%

modulation), the intensity periodically reaches zero. If the light intensity only varies between a maximum and zero, the modulation is known as square-wave amplitude modulation, and the light source is said to be pulsed – the same as switching it on and off. (See Figure 1.7 "Different types of pulsing" on page 19.)

A pulsed light source can be pulsed either electrically, by switching its electrical power on and off, or by interrupting the light, for example, by using a chopper (mechanical shutter, Kerr cell, Pockels cell, etc.). It may be pulsed at a high or a low frequency, i.e. with many or few pulses per second. If the lamp (or laser) emits visible light and is pulsed at a low frequency (up to about 30 pulses per second), we can see that the light is blinking.

If the lengths of the periods of light are equal to the lengths of the periods of zero intensity, the "duty cycle" is 50%, as light is emitted during 50% of the overall time.

Some lasers and other lamps can be pulsed like flash bulbs with extremely short and very intense light pulses and rather long intermission times (very low duty cycle). This type of rather extreme pulsing is usually called superpulsing. Examples of lasers that can be superpulsed are YAG lasers, CO_2-lasers and GaAs lasers.

Note 1. Pulse frequency has nothing to do with the frequency of the light itself - the carrier wave. (See chapter 1.1.2 "Wavelength and frequency" on page 2)

Note 2. "Frequency modulation" has nothing to do with this. It refers to the variation of the frequency of the carrier wave.

1.2.11 The pulse peak power

When a laser is pulsed, the laser light power varies between the pulse peak output power and zero. It is possible to design a laser to achieve extremely high pulse peak output power - even trillions of watts. However, the pulse duration is then correspondingly low. The peak pulse power value is of importance for the penetration of light into tissue. The power density during these very high power pulses is of course also very high, yielding an extremely high photon flux with an increased probability of multi-photon effects. (See chapter 3.4.2.3 "How deep does the light penetrate?" on page 121 and chapter 11.2.6 "Multi-photon effects" on page 555.)

1.2.12 Average power output

For pulsed lasers, the output power value to be used for dose calculation is the laser's average power. (See chapter 3.3.1.7 "Calculation of doses" on page 78.) When a laser is chopped, the pulsing can have different duty cycles. If the light is "on" for 30% of the time and "off" for 70% of the time, the duty cycle is 30%. Then the average power is 30% of the peak power (if the switching is momentary, i.e. a true square wave). The duty cycle of the

GaAs-laser is extremely low - in the order of 0.001. (See Figure 1.7 "Different types of pulsing" on page 19.)

1.2.13 Power density

Power density is another way of saying "light intensity" or "light concentration", and is the light output power per unit area of the target being illuminated by the laser light. This is usually measured in watts per square centimetre (W/cm^2). High power density is achieved, for instance, at the focal point of a magnifying glass. If the magnifying glass is moved closer to the objective point, so that the light spot grows, the light is spread over a wider area and the power density is correspondingly lower. Spreading the light over a larger area leads to a directly proportional reduction of power density.

For example, a 10 mW laser with the light focused on an area of 1 mm^2 gives a power density of 1 W/cm^2. A surgical laser with 10 W output power focused on a spot with a diameter of 0.1 mm, gives a power density of more-than 100 000 W/cm^2. Power density is of significance both in laser surgery and laser therapy.

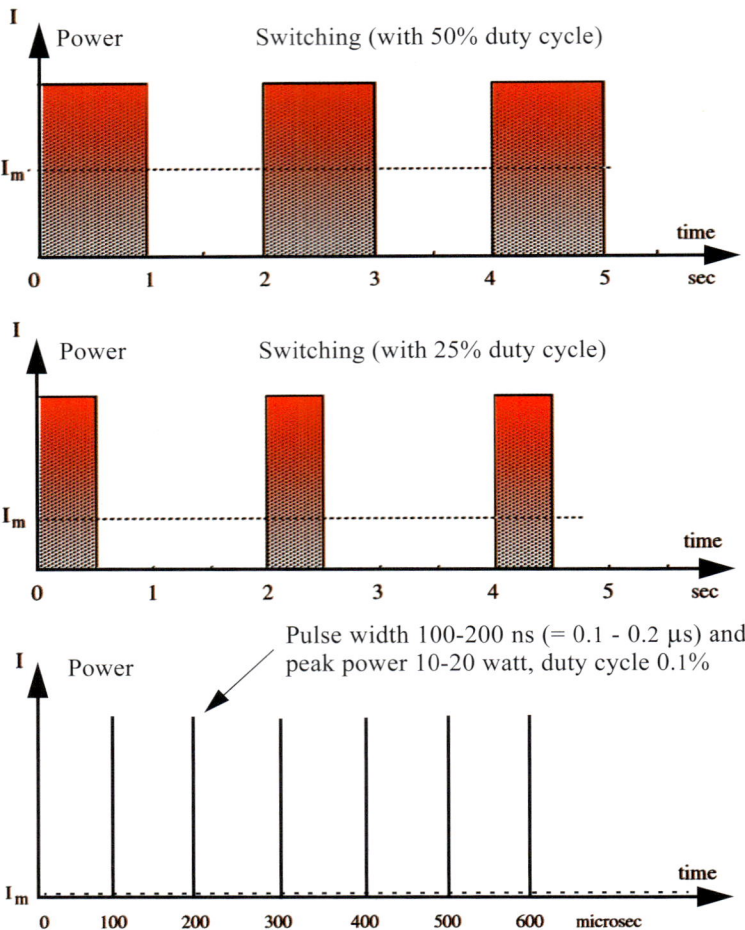

This diagram shows typical superpulsing: i.e. the ratio between the peak power and average power is very high.

Figure 1.7 Different types of pulsing

1.2.14 Collimation

It is a common misconception that light from a laser is always in the form of a parallel beam. The light from a gas laser is usually rather parallel (typically in the order of milliradian), while the light from a diode laser (without collimating optics) is ordinarily much more divergent, with an angle of "spread" of around 30-90 degrees. This is mainly due to diffraction when the light is emitted from the resonator mirror on the semiconductor crystal. If a collimating lens or lens system is placed in front of the diode, the light's parallelity can be increased. This is called collimation. A collimated beam is quite parallel, and with such a beam, we can irradiate from a distance and still achieve high power density over a small area.

1.2.15 Risk of eye injury

Even in the infancy of laser technology there was an awareness of the increased risk of eye damage compared to conventional light sources. Hence, new rules were introduced to handle this hazard. Lasers were divided into five categories (Class 1, 2, 3A, 3B and 4) according to their potential to damage the eye. Classes 1-3A are considered safe, whereas Class 3B involves a certain risk and Class 4 a definite risk. Class 4, for example, comprises strong industrial and surgical lasers capable of burning and cutting. Note that this classification has nothing to do with the medical use, efficiency or quality of lasers but refers solely to the possible risk of eye injury.

In most countries only physicians and dentists are allowed to use Class 4 lasers (and veterinarians, in the treatment of animals). The practical job can then usually be delegated to nurses or other staff members.

To date, only a handful of accidents involving lasers have been reported and the only severe accidents concern contact with high voltage power supplies. Reports on eye injuries are very rare, and, when they do occur, injuries involve either the use of very strong industrial lasers where protective measures have been ignored or laboratories where people, over time, have become careless. Furthermore, in several cases the person in question has not even been aware of an eye injury, although there has been a visible scar on the retina. In the book "Therapeutic lasers", professor David Baxter writes: "In the only reported case of eye injury during therapeutic laser treatment, a chartered physiotherapist using a treatment unit on loan from a supplier suffered 60% corneal abrasion from the protective wings on the side of the goggles provided with the apparatus".

Another aspect is that, in the treatment of diabetic retinopathy, a strong argon or diode laser beam is directed right into the eye, and often some hundreds of laser pulses are fired. Still, the patient is not aware of any injury and reports that his vision is fine. In the treatment of cataract, a strong Nd:YAG laser is directed and fired right into the eye. Vision corrections are performed with an Excimer laser, evaporating parts of the cornea. CO_2-lasers, too, are used in eye surgery. All these lasers are strong and capable of burning tissue!

So, even though there are lasers capable of causing eye damage, the risk should not be exaggerated. Too often the fear of laser light is a greater risk than the laser itself! For example: a car driver being blinded by a laser pointer can lose control of his vehicle out of fear because he realises that he has been hit by a laser (and he "knows" this is very dangerous). But if he is blinded by a sunbeam, he will not be frightened, just blinded for a spell. Usually a sunbeam blinds a person much more than a laser pointer, because the laser pointer can only hit one eye at a time and for a much shorter time due to the narrowness of the beam.

A lot has been written about the laser as a military weapon to make soldiers blind. Well, that is not possible. At close range and with large lasers, it would be possible to inflict eye injury if an invisible beam were to be used. But in reality, no laser makes a person blind. Pilots could be disturbed by visible laser light but not made blind. Also, the user of the laser weapon would reveal his position and turn himself into a target. Still, the common military use of lasers is as distance measuring devices, beam-riding missiles and target designators – a laser points at a target and a "smart" bomb or missile sees the laser spot and flies to it. Amendations have been proposed to the Geneva Convention to forbid the use of laser as a weapon, but we think it would be much more sensible to suggest that guns be forbidden, as a bullet can do much more harm than a beam of light.

There are light sources which are more hazardous to the eyes than the corresponding lasers [1294]. One such device usually called IPL (Intense Pulsed Light) using a powerful flash lamp with a band-pass filter. It emits light pulses in the wavelength region 600 to 900 nm and with pulse energies around 50 joules per cm^2 aperture area. The aperture is usually rectangular and in the order of one by three cm. Like ruby and alexandrite lasers, this instrument is used in hair removal – the light is absorbed in dark hairs and then converted to heat, which burns the surrounding follicle to destruction or injury. This is called photo epilation. If this aperture is directed towards an unprotected eye, this can cause a much more severe injury than staring into the beam of e.g. an uncollimated ruby laser with fibre-optic transmission made for hair removal. But as these flash lamp devices are not lasers, there are no restrictions in their use!

Our recommendation is to use protective googles on the patient when performing laser phototherapy in the head and neck area. This gives the patient a feeling of safety and "high tech" and saves the therapist from any negative physchological reactions. However, irradiating a naked eye with a visible non collimated beam below 100 mW is completely harmless. We often do this on ourselves during lectures and it seems to suprise most participants who already "knew" how dangerous this is. And as can be seen later in this book, even invisible LPT in this energy range has been used to treat macular degeneration.

Laser and lightbulb

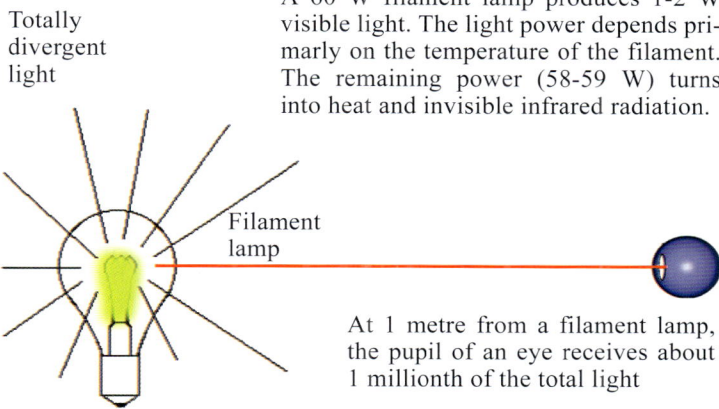

Totally divergent light

A 60 W filament lamp produces 1-2 W visible light. The light power depends primarily on the temperature of the filament. The remaining power (58-59 W) turns into heat and invisible infrared radiation.

Filament lamp

At 1 metre from a filament lamp, the pupil of an eye receives about 1 millionth of the total light

Laser with collimated beam

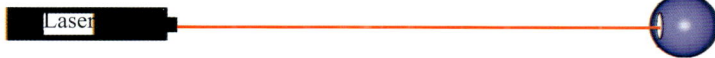

Here, the eye can receive 100% of the light from the laser, even at a fairly large distance

Laser with divergent beam. (e.g. 0.1 radian)

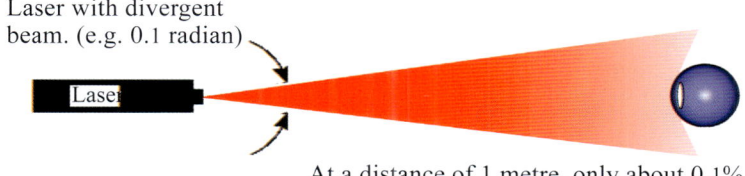

At a distance of 1 metre, only about 0.1% of the laser light passes into the eye. At 20 cm, only 25% passes into the eye.

The risk to the eye depends primarily on the parallelity and diameter of the laser beam

Figure 1.8 Laser and light-bulb

Decisive factors in the risk of eye injury

In 1998 there was an outbreak of laser hysteria in the Danish press. A train engineer was reported to have suffered a 20% loss of vision after having been irradiated by two young boys, using a laser pointer. In addition, a car driver was reported to have been injured in a similar fashion. This is, of course, pure nonsense. Laser pointers do not injure the eye! They are far too low-powered and the blink reflex will automatically reduce the exposure time.

Reidenbach [1303] has controlled the blink reflex of the human eye when hit by visible lasers of 1 mW. For 670 nm only 15.9% of the tested persons showed a blink reflex, for 635 nm 17.2% and for 532 nm 20.3%. This may seem alarming, but a 1 mW visible laser will never harm the eye and at higher power the blink reflex will increase gradually and work well long before the beam reaches a risky level.

The restrictions in the use of class 3B lasers as therapeutic instruments have been lifted in Europe since no reports of eye damages from these lasers have ever been reported.

1.2.16 Decisive factors in the risk of eye injury
The following factors are of importance in the eye risk of various lasers. (See Figure 1.9 "Laser and eye-risk" on page 24.)
- The divergence of the light beam: A parallel light beam of small diameter is by far the most dangerous. It can enter the pupil in its entirety and be focused by the eye's lens to a spot with a diameter of hundredths of a millimetre. The entire light output is concentrated on this small area. With a 10 mW beam, the power density can be up to 12 000 W/cm^2.
- The output power of the laser: It is fairly obvious that a powerful laser (many watts) is more hazardous to stare into than a weak laser.
- The exposure time: The shorter the exposure time is, the stronger the light can be without risk of injuries. For visible light, the blink reflex affords a good protection.
- The wavelength of the light: Within the visible wavelength range, we respond to strong light with a quick blink reflex. This reduces the exposure time and thereby the light energy which enters the eye. Light sources which emit invisible radiation, whether an infrared laser or an infrared diode, always entail a higher risk than the equivalent source of visible light Radiation at wavelengths over 1400 nm is absorbed by the eye's lens and thus rendered safe, provided the power of the beam is not too high. Radiation at wavelengths over 2500 nm is absorbed by the cornea and is less dangerous. (See Figure 1.9 "Laser and eye-risk" on page 24.)

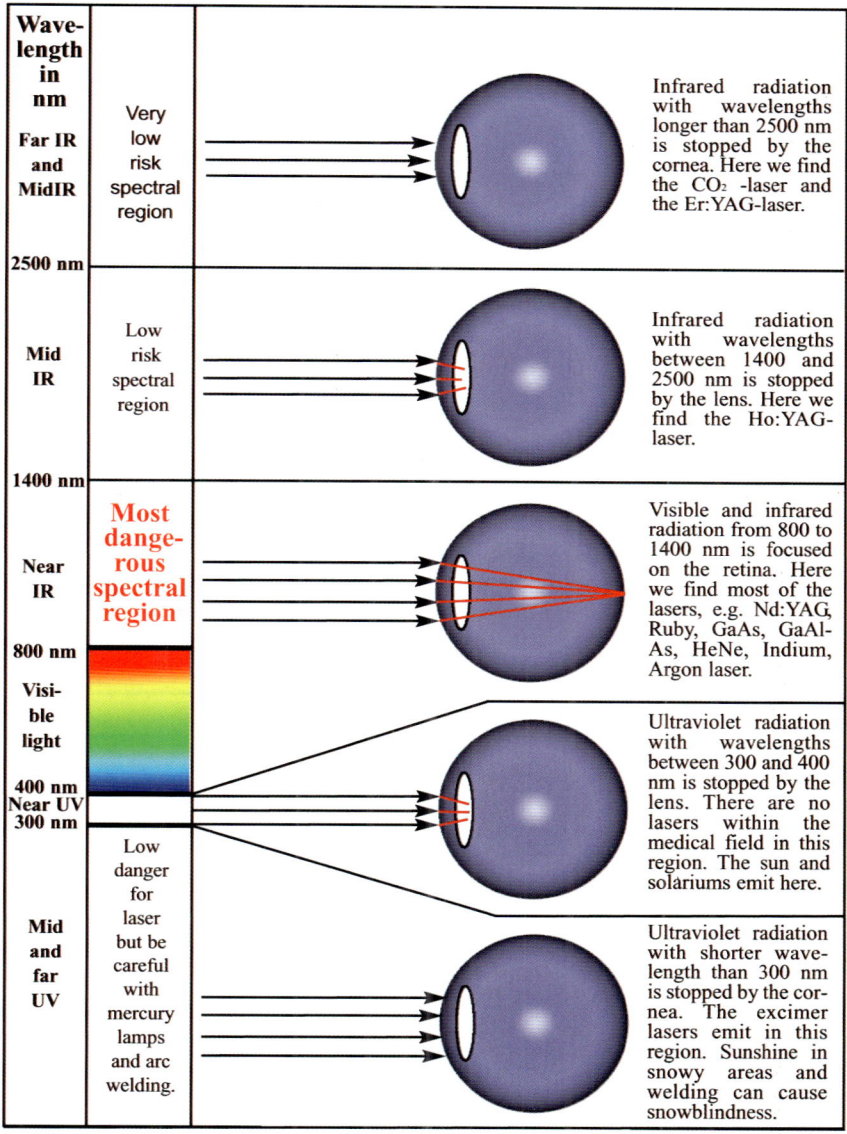

Figure 1.9   Laser and eye-risk

- <u>The distribution of the light source:</u> When looking at a light source, an image of the source is projected on the retina. If the light source is concentrated, as is often the case with lasers, the image will be projected as a point, provided it lies within our accommodation range, i.e. the area in which we can see clearly. A widely spread light source is projected onto the retina in a correspondingly wide image, with the light spread over a larger area, and with a lower power density as a consequence. For example: a clear light bulb (which is apprehended as a more concentrated light source) is worse to look at than a "pearl" light bulb. A laser system with several light sources spaced apart, such as a multiprobe with several laser diodes (the probe is the part of the laser you hold and apply to the area to be treated: a single probe means there is only one laser diode in the probe, as opposed to a multiprobe, which has several laser diodes) may be very powerful as a whole, yet constitutes a lesser hazard to the eye than it would if the entire power output was emitted by one laser diode, because the diodes' separate placement means that they are reproduced in different places on the retina.

We have often heard this kind of remark: "If it's a class 3B laser then it's fine, otherwise it is not effective!" This is, of course, entirely incorrect, and has led manufacturers to produce lasers that meet the 3B classification in order to sell higher volumes.

Let us look at two examples:
A GaAlAs laser with a wavelength of 830 nm, an output of 1 mW and a well-collimated beam (1 mrad divergence) is classified as laser class 3B as it is judged to be hazardous to the eye. The reason for this is partly the collimated beam, and partly the wavelength, which is just outside the visible range and hence provokes no blink reflex in strong light.
- A HeNe laser with a wavelength of 633 nm, an output of 10 mW (10 times stronger than the laser in the previous example) and divergent beams (1 rad divergence, which corresponds to a cone of light with a top angle of about 57°, which is often the divergence of light from a fibre-optic cable) is classified as laser class 3A because, owing to its divergence, it cannot damage the eye (only a small portion of the light will hit the pupil). The light from a laser diode is usually rather divergent unless it is fitted with a collimating lens or lens system.
- A CO_2-laser (10 600 nm wavelength) of EDL (defocused) type, with 15 watt output and with the radiation uniformly spread out over a surface with a diameter of 5 cm, will be classified as a class 4 instrument. If instead it is spread out over a surface of 10 cm diameter, it will be classified as a class 1 instrument (only class 1 and 4 have this wavelength) and is hence regarded as absolutely eye-safe in spite of its high output power.

A laser pointer uses an InGaAlP laser with a wavelength usually between 650 and 670 nm (red light). The output power is in the order of 0.5 to 3 mW, focussed in a well-collimated beam. The spot size is usually 5 to 10 mm in diameter at a distance of 1 metre. If you look straight into the beam, the light looks very strong. However, these devices are completely harmless and no eye injury has been reported. But many people are afraid of them. As a comparison, an arrow or a dart can completely destroy an eye - a laser pointer is harmless.

As for therapeutic lasers, patients often ask: "Is it enough to shut your eyes if you receive laser treatment to the face, or must you have protective glasses?" Yes, it is enough to close your eyes! It is actually sufficient to shut your eyes even if a very powerful laser is being used. It is quite possible to treat a stye on the eyelid without risk, even if it is located right in front of the pupil [129]. The reason for this is that the eyelid spreads the light so that the lens cannot focus it. The light is spread over the entire retina and, with a 10 mW laser, we get a power density over the retina of 0.001 W/cm^2, which is about ten million times lower than if the eye were open and the beam parallel.

However, the use of protective glasses can be of benefit, particularly if powerful, collimated lasers in the infrared spectral region are used. In any case, protective glasses give the patient a sense of security. Furthermore, therapists never run the risk of a claim for damages from a patient if they make sure the patient always wears protective glasses during treatment. (Patients may well convince themselves that the laser has a negative effect on their eyes.)

Bear in mind, though, that protective glasses for HeNe or InGaAlP lasers are of no use whatsoever when using other laser types.

Warning: The use of normal sunglasses increases the risk of eye injury. The filtration mechanism of sunglasses is a wide band attenuation, giving a much lower absorption of a particular laser wavelength than real protection goggles give. In addition to this, the darkness of the glasses makes the pupil dilate and let in more light. They provide a false sense of security!

Summary: Although most lasers are harmless, some lasers certainly can cause eye injury. The most dangerous types combine power (> 100 mW) with a collimated beam and have a wavelength in the interval 700 nm – 1400 nm. So called laser pointers are harmless. A divergent beam can be quite strong and still carry a low risk; the more divergent, the less risk.

Literature:
Dushin [1783] reports that 60 patients with chronic dacryocystitis with partially retained patency of the lacrimal duct were treated by HeNe laser. The patients received 3-5 min sessions twice a week, 5-8 sessions per course. Positive effect was attained in 56 patients: complete cessation of excessive lacrimal discharge in 38 patients and subjective improvement in 18. HeNe laser exposure brought about a good antiinflammatory effect; in

combination with antibiotic therapy it promoted rapid sanitization of the lacrimal duct, removed edema, and rapidly normalized lacrimal discharge.

Safe doses of LPT exposure for the structures of the eye were searched for in rabbit experiments by Prokofeva [1217], and the potentials of such lasers in ophthalmology were assessed. A 890 nm diode laser was used. The doses varied from 0.0001 to 1.0 J/cm^2, corresponding to exposure duration of 0.3 to 45 min. Experiments were carried out on 20 animals. The right eyes were exposed, and the left ones were control. An increase of intraocular pressure was recorded at a dose of 0.1 J/cm^2 (4.5 min) and higher; morphological study showed dilated, well-filled and newly formed vessels in the ciliary body and iris, as well as edema and destruction of the external layers of the retina. Exposure to a dose of 0.05 J/cm^2 and lower did not lead to destruction of ocular structures and increase of intraocular pressure. The maximal LPT dose causing no side effects for the organ of vision was established at 0.05 J/cm^2, this corresponding to 2.5 min exposure.

1.3 Laser types in medicine and surgery

In the table below, the names, wavelengths, working modes, and uses of the most common laser systems in medicine are listed. .

Laser name	Wavelength	Pulsed or cont.	Medical use
Crystalline laser medium:			
KTP/532	532 nm	p/c	leg vein treatment
Ruby	694 nm	p	tattoo and hair removal
Alexandrite	755 nm	p	bone cut, hair removal
Nd:YAG	1064 nm	p/c	coagulation of tumours
Ho:YAG	2130 nm	p	surgery, root canal, lithotripsia
Er:YAG	2940 nm	p	dental drill, laser peeling
Ti:sapphire	tuneable	p	two-photon PDT
Semiconductor lasers:			
InGaAlP	630-700 nm	c	biostimulation
GaAlAs	780-820-870 nm	c	biostimulation and surgery
GaAs	904, 905 nm	p	biostimulation
Liquid laser medium:			
Dye laser	tuneable	p/c	kidney stones
Rhodamine	560-650 nm	p/c	PDT, dermatology
Gas lasers:			
Excimer	193, 248, 308 nm	p	eye, vascular surgery
Argon	350-514 nm	c	dermatology, retinopathy
Copper	578 nm	p/c	dermatology
HeNe	633, 3390 nm	c	biostimulation
CO_2	10 600 nm	p/c	dermatology, surgery

Table 1.2 Different lasers, their wavelengths and use

There are other types, but those mentioned above are the most common. The Dye laser is expensive to buy and to run and is gradually being replaced by other laser types. The semiconductor lasers can also be tuned, (± 10 nm) simply by varying the working temperature. The Ti:sapphire laser can produce extremely short pulses, down to the femtosecond region.

1.4 The surgical lasers

The most typical surgical lasers and their wavelengths:

CO_2-laser	10 600 nm
Nd:YAG laser	1064 nm
Ho:YAG	2130 nm
Er:YAG	2940 nm
Argon laser	514 nm
Copper vapour laser	578 nm
KTP laserfrequency-doubled Nd:YAG	532 nm
Ruby laser	694 nm
Alexandrite	755 nm
Stronger types of GaAlAs laser	typically 800-870 nm
Dye laser	400-900 nm
Ti:sapphire laser	700-900 nm
Excimer laser	193, 248, 308, 351 nm

Table 1.3 Typical surgical lasers and their wavelengths

In order for a laser to be suitable for use as a surgical laser, it must be powerful enough to heat up the tissue to temperatures over 50 °C. A surgical laser can either be used in continuous wave or pulsed mode. These lasers can be broadly divided into three groups, according to their output:

1. vaporising (superficial complaints, e.g. condyloma) 1-5 W.
2. light cutting (superficial incisions, e.g. plastic surgery) 5-20 W.
3. deep cutting (conisation, major surgical operations) 20-100 W.

The main aim of this book is not to instruct colleagues in the profession who work with or are thinking of working with surgical lasers - a great deal of literature on this subject already exists. Nevertheless, in this chapter we will be describing some of the surgical lasers on the market so that the reader can appreciate the difference between surgical and therapeutic lasers and thereby answer their patients' questions.

For those who already have a surgical laser, it is worth knowing that it can usually also be used in biostimulation - even powerful, destructive lasers do have laser therapy effects. It is well known that surgery with carbon dioxide lasers means less postoperative pain compared with conventional surgical techniques, and this may partly be due to its biostimulatory effect. Laser surgery, for instance, is followed by minimal scarring. This is suggested by Calderhead [304] to be an "alpha-phenomenon", meaning that the lower laser light intensities in the periphery of the target area have biostimulative effects. Surgical laser can also be used as primary biostimulators just by irraditing from a distance and thereby reduce the power density. This takes a few minutes of calculation but it worth the trouble, since it adds a biostimulative laser into the clinic at no extra cost. Surgical and biostimulative lasers can be said to be "two sides of the same coin".

The surgical application of lasers is not within the scope of this book but in the following a brief orientation is presented.

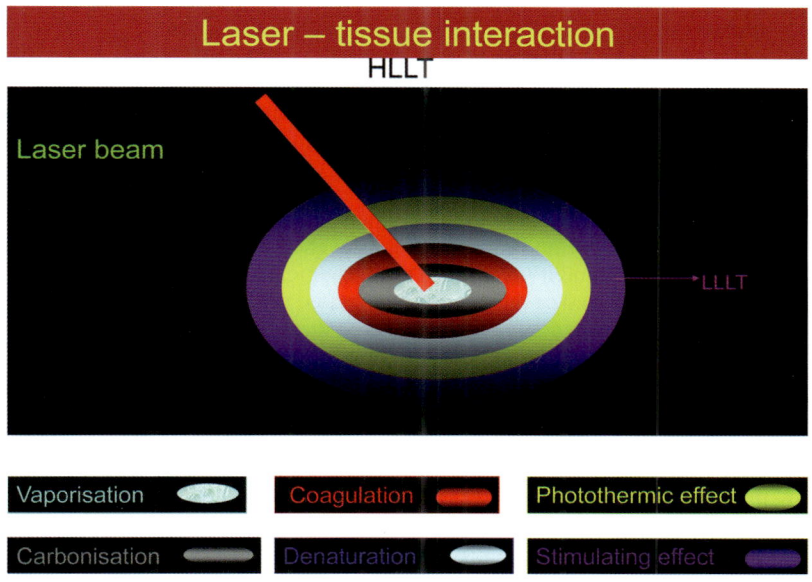

Figure 1.10 Theoretical model of laser-tissue interaction.
Courtesy: Edson Nagib

1.4.1 The Carbon dioxide laser (CO_2-laser)

As mentioned earlier, most types of laser are named after a combination of the components (or the main component) of the lasing medium. The main component of the CO_2-laser is thus carbon dioxide. This laser usually produces radiation with a wavelength of 10.6 micrometers (10 600 nanometers), which is high in the infrared band of the spectrum. The advantage of radiation with a long wavelength is that it is absorbed by water to a great extent, and by objects which contain water, such as tissue. This makes the CO_2-laser largely non-hazardous to the eye. See Figure 1.9 "Laser and eye-risk" on page 24, chapter 1.2.15 "Risk of eye injury" on page 20 and chapter 1.2.16 "Decisive factors in the risk of eye injury" on page 23. Ordinary spectacles or glass or plastic discs in a suitable frame are a sufficient protection for this wavelength.

Because of the high absorption rate in water and organic matter, the CO_2-laser beam has a shallow depth of penetration; 99% is absorbed within 0.2 mm [296]. (See chapter 1.1.6 "Radiation risks" on page 4.) This also makes it very easy to evaporate and remove tissue without causing a deeper burn. Papilloma virus warts, for example, can be vaporised with only minor damage to the underlying tissue. The colour and melanin content of the tissue are not significant in relation to the rate of absorption.

A disadvantage associated with the long wavelength is that it is difficult to produce optical fibres with satisfactory transmission properties. There are fibres made from silver halide salts, which appear to be usable. Thin, flexible wave-guides in the form of small tubes of single-crystal sapphire can also be used to conduct the CO_2-laser beam. Up until now, the best way to get the light out from the laser tube has been to use mirror optics in articulated arms. However, this is relatively expensive and sensitive to knocks and bumps. The mirror setting requires a high level of precision, and the articulated arms are consequently sensitive to mechanical shocks.

Also, small plastic tubes, internally coated with dielectric layers, have been tested as wave-guides. Internally coated metal tubes are also being used in spite of some disadvantages. The most promising wave-guide technique may be small flexible glass tubes, internally coated with dielectric layers.

A CO_2-laser can be made very powerful - with an output of millions of watts - though such a laser would be as big as a house and very nearly require its own power station! Powerful lasers of this kind are used in industry to cut and process metal. Modern CO_2-lasers with an output under 200 W are often radio-wave excited with sealed gas systems, and do not require, as their predecessors did, any gas supply, gas refilling, or high voltage. Their lifetime is usually very long.

Today's surgical CO_2-lasers can also be superpulsed. This means that the laser light is emitted in a train of short but very intense pulses. In the case of tissue evaporation, this results in less burning under and around the vaporisation zone.

1.4.1.1 Carbon dioxide lasers in surgery

One of the advantages of the carbon dioxide laser is that the energy it produces is strongly absorbed by water and all organic matter. This means that layer after layer of tissue can be removed without nearby tissue being affected to any great extent. At the same time, the CO_2-laser coagulates blood in small vessels, making it possible to work in a controlled fashion.

Imagine the removal of pre-cancer cells on the uterus or a fungal infection from the floor of a patient's mouth, when the instruments you have to choose between are a scalpel and a carbon dioxide laser. It is not difficult to see the advantages of the laser. The scalpel causes profuse bleeding, making it difficult to see where the healthy tissue starts, and the practitioner is working with a knife close to well-vascularised tissue. With the laser we can vaporise fractions of a millimetre at a time and our vision is not impeded as there is generally no bleeding, and, furthermore, sutures are unnecessary. The same applies to an operation on a haemangioma on the lip. No bleeding, no sutures. The whole operation takes a couple of minutes and can be done on an outpatient basis. Subsequent check-ups are generally unnecessary. By focusing the beam, it can also be used like a scalpel, so it is possible to take a biopsy with a CO_2-laser.

Another interesting property of the CO_2-laser is that, when cutting, evaporating or coagulating the tissue, pain persists for only a few seconds after the burning has stopped. This is in contrast to when you burn yourself on a hot iron, your oven or hot water, leaving a pain for 20 to 30 minutes unless cold water or ice is applied to the site of the burn. The reason for this difference in pain perception is not known.

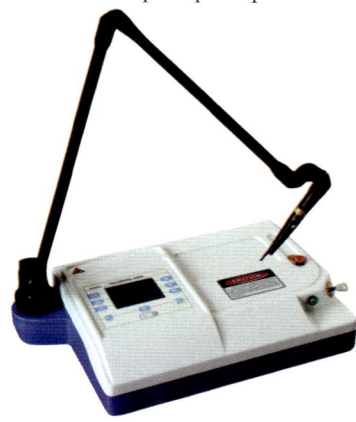

Figure 1.11 Small CO_2-laser

The mucosa consists of 80-90% water, which argues for the use of carbon dioxide lasers. In the target area of a focused laser the temperature is between 150 and 300 degrees, depending on the laser output and the cross section of the beam, while from a distance of 0.5 mm from the "laser gun" the temperature drops to around 50 degrees. The power output used should be determined from case to case. The volume of liquid covering the mucous membrane must also be taken into consideration, as it affects the energy uptake of the tissue. Mucous membrane conditions such as lichen and leucoplakia can be removed by vaporising the tissue once a biopsy has been performed.

The healing process after an operation using a carbon dioxide laser is a little slower than after conventional surgery, but, on the other hand, the postoperative discomfort is considerably milder and the final cosmetic result much more acceptable (the latter is of course more important in cases of treatment of the face). The absence of bleeding may be the cause of the slower healing. The laser beam also kills off any residual infection in the operating area, which contributes to the healing process.

It is important to remove tissue with a certain extra margin, in order to remove clinically invisible change in the transitional zone between healthy and cancerous or infected tissue.

The disadvantages of carbon dioxide lasers used to be their size and price. Around 100 kg and US $30 000 - $40 000 has been a rough guide. The latest technical advances have led to lighter (around 15 - 20 kg) and cheaper

(US$15 000 - US$25 000) lasers. They use sealed-off laser tubes without the need for gas refilling or high voltage. They may also be completely silent and may even be made battery powered and thereby mobile. Carbon dioxide lasers can be made very powerful, but for dermatological and ENT use, 1-10 W usually suffices.

In general surgery, the CO_2-laser has been used for a long time. One good indication for the laser is haemorrhoidectomy. Other good indications are fimosis and circumcision. The healing after excision of penis cancer has proved to be very good. In sleep apnea, CO_2-laser is used for uvulopalatoplasty in the treatment of snoring. The laser can also be used in laparoscopy. Typical benefits of laser surgery are less pronounced postoperative oedema and pain compared to conventional methods. Sutures are often not required.

Another use of CO_2-laser is so called transmyocardial revascularisation (TMR), in which a number of small holes are made through the heart muscle wall [572]. TMR is a modern therapeutic approach in the treatment of patients with severe chronic ischemic cardiac disease. Clinical data from 1800 worldwide TMR-treated patients show that TMR can improve cardiac status in cases without preoperative congestive heart failure. The mechanisms underlying beneficial TMR effects are not well understood, but there seems to be some evidence that biostimulation plays a role. Channels made by mechanical tools do not give the same favourable result. In a recent study the following result was presented: In a follow-up at 6 months, clinical data indicate that CO_2-laser TMR was able to improve clinical status in 50 of 61 laser-treated patients, whereas 5 did not show any benefit and 6 died. Histopathological investigations revealed tissue remodelling comparable with different stages of wound healing. The cicatricial tissue in the original laser-created channels displayed a stronger immunostaining for collagen type III than for type I. And the authors conclude: "Clinically, TMR improves cardiac function in some patients with severe ischemic cardiac disease, but pathophysiological data as well as morphological features from human myocardium could not explain this phenomenon. Therefore, TMR treatment should be used only as 'the last chance' in patients with severe angina pectoris. "

Another surgical use of CO_2-laser is as a drilling tool in laser-assisted hair transplantation [573]. These lasers deliver high bursts of energy of short duration and vaporise the hair transplantation recipient sites, which are consistent in depth and diameter.

Gynaecology was the first main field of use for the CO_2-laser. It can be used to evaporate genital condyloma, cervical neoplasia etc. In the case of conisation a rather strong CO_2-laser is needed, due to the deep incision needed in the blood rich tissue.

In dermatology, the CO_2-laser is very well suited for excision of superficial tumours, evaporation of angioma, verrucae, syringoma, tricho-epithelioma, adenoma sebaceum, steatocystoma, hidradenitis suppurativa, condyloma, neurofibromatosis, xanthelasma, rhinophyma, actinic cheilitis, venous lacuna, spider naevi, hematoma, telangiectasia, superficial basaloma, lentigo solaris, lentigo senilis etc.

A good field for the CO_2-laser is plastic surgery, such as eyelid operations (blepharoplasty). Even in tattoo treatment, this laser can be very useful. Our own experience is that the safest method is to evaporate very superficially over the tattoo and not to go down to the tattoo pigments, especially on shoulders and trunk, as the risk of keloid scarring is high in these areas. The CO_2-laser has also been used for so called laser peeling - a very superficial tissue ablation in the face - for the removal of wrinkles and acne scars. The mechanism is partly thermic by remodelling and contraction of the collagen, partly biostimulative.

An interesting application is to use a relatively low powered CO_2-laser to weld or solder tissue instead of suturing. Tissue welding gives less risk of scarring and can be done with high precision. Human albumin (HAS) can be used as a solder.

1.4.1.2 Carbon dioxide lasers in dental applications

In dentistry, the carbon dioxide laser has been used experimentally in cariotic tissue. If caries is removed with a carbon dioxide laser, a number of positive effects result. The residual infection in the dentinal tubuli is removed, the cavity bottom is almost vitrified, and a secondary dentine-stimulating effect can be achieved in the odontoblasts. Some promising experiments have been conducted relating to the treatment of pulp lesions, although the disadvantages currently outweigh the advantages. It is only possible to get at open caries, which must first be uncovered with a rotating instrument. The enamel contains only 10% water, so the temperature soon reaches destructive levels if hit by the carbon dioxide laser. Intraoral access has been improved by "wave conductors", bendable tubes, but access (and wave conductors) are still not good enough for the method to be used on a routine basis within cariology. A powerful suction system is needed to remove smoke and malodorous vapour.

Aphthae can be treated with small doses of carbon dioxide laser.

Dental necks can be successfully treated by CO_2-laser by closing the dentinal tubules [442].

Flap operation is an interesting indication for carbon dioxide lasers. All granulation on the inside of the flap can be removed, and the flap edge can be contoured. Rossman [236] and Israel [237] note in their studies that the normally unavoidable epithelium down-growth in the pocket is reduced after the flap is treated in this way.

Frenectomy is performed much more quickly with a carbon dioxide laser as compared to a scalpel. No suturing is required, and the subsequent course of healing is very positive.

Gingivectomies have been described in the literature, but are not a recommended operation for the inexperienced laser operator, in view of the damage to the dental hard tissue and prosthetic replacements which can result. However, special tools which protect the tooth substance have been developed. The CO_2-laser can, on the other hand, be used in flap operations to remove granulation and to treat the exposed root surface. Necrotic cement can be removed and dentine tubuli can be sealed. It has been reported that by changing the structure of the root surface, the regeneration of fibroblasts is improved. A special form of gingivectomy is that performed on patients on Dilantine and related medicines. The strong hyperplasia is well suited to carbon dioxide lasers as the bleeding is minimal. A gingivectomy is first performed with a focused beam, and then the gingiva is contoured with a defocused beam.

Haemangiomas are also appropriately removed with laser once the size of the tumour has been carefully determined. Bear in mind that many haemangiomas are like the tip of the iceberg. The majority of laser-treated oral soft tissues are left to heal "per secundam", that is, by secondary intention without sutures.

Hyperplasia of various kinds is appropriately removed by incision. After anaesthetics, the tissue is stabilised with a pair of tweezers, and then an incision is made using single pulses.

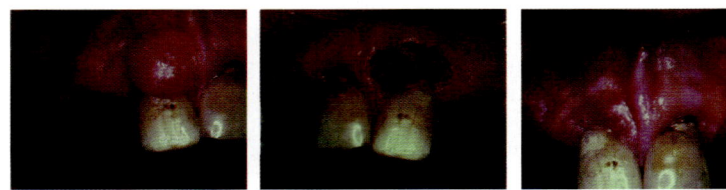

Preprosthetic surgery can be performed with a carbon dioxide laser. Hypertrophic tubera and "flabby ridges" can be peeled off layer by layer. The patient can start using dentures much more quickly than after conventional surgery because the oedema is much smaller than if a scalpel were used. In crown and bridge therapy, the uncovering of the preparation margin is a good indication if access is acceptable. There is no retraction of the tissue as with electro-surgery.

Retention cysts such as ranula and mucocele can either be removed in their entirety or fenestrated by laser. By comparison with conventional surgery, a lower recurrence frequency has been reported when lasers are used.

Root canals can be sterilised by carbon dioxide laser [441]. The laser energy helps kill off the root canal's microflora, and partially seals the side canals and apex delta. A special adapter is needed to allow the laser beam to reach the apical region of the tooth. Laser can, in certain situations, replace the retrograde root filling in apical surgery. The laser energy kills infections and seals the side canals.

1.4.2 The Nd:YAG laser

This type of laser produces light in a single crystal of Yttrium-Aluminium-Garnet doped with an additional substance. The most common such substance is elemental neodymium (Nd). The full name of this laser is thus Nd:YAG. Normally the laser is pumped by a very strong flash lamp.

Another new type of Nd:YAG-laser is the diode laser pumped YAG-laser. Here, powerful GaAlAs-lasers are used to pump optical energy to the Nd:YAG-laser rod instead of using a flash lamp. The output wavelength is then the typical 1064 nm. The advantage of this laser is its smaller size.

In spite of its high output power, the Nd:YAG laser also has biostimulating effects [152, 202, 218, 1062].

1.4.2.1 Nd:YAG lasers in surgery

The Nd:YAG laser has been used in general surgery for many years but is being replaced more and more by the CO_2-laser, which has better evaporation and cutting properties. However, the Nd:YAG laser is very good for coagulation and is a good tool for coagulating tumours. This is called hyperthermia and the effect on cancer is based on the fact that healthy tissue can be heated to a higher temperature than the tumour cells before being killed. Usually the laser beam is brought to the centre of the tumour by means of an optical fibre.

1.4.2.2 Nd:YAG lasers in dentistry

The output of the dental Nd:YAG laser is variable, and can be anything between 0 and 15 watts. Its pulsing can also be varied. Both these parameters should be adjusted to suit the type of treatment, even during the operation itself.

The Nd:YAG laser for "drilling" was a pioneer in the area but has now been replaced by the Er:YAG laser, which is much more suited for "drilling". Some of the possibilities of the dental YAG lasers are presented below.

<u>Analgesia.</u> It is possible to cut soft tissue without causing much pain. The mechanism is unclear.

<u>Anaesthesia</u> of teeth. By irradiating a tooth for a few minutes with increasing intensity, local anaesthesia of the tooth can be brought about using energy densities ranging from 2 to 40 J/cm^2, preferably starting with short pulses, slightly below the pain threshold, and gradually increasing until anaesthesia is achieved. No lasting damage to the pulp as a result of this treatment has been observed. The anaesthesia is most easily achieved on young teeth. The more sclerotic the pulp space, the poorer the effect.

<u>Caries.</u> Superficial caries in the enamel can be treated without removing tooth substance. A defect does remain, in the form of a small pit, but the surface is more resistant to caries than normal enamel.

<u>Fissure sealing.</u> Laser-treated enamel is restructured and made more acid-resistant. This restructuring is possible through laser treatment of the

fissure system. It is also thought that the bacteria in the bottom of the fissure can be killed and that it is possible to fuse the fissure. It is still possible to seal with resin, if so desired. The enamel can be etched by the laser but acid etch is considered to give better bonding.

Herpes simplex. As any other dental laser, with proper dosage, Nd:YAG will successfully treat herpes simplex lesions. When treated with a higher intensity than in conventional laser therapy, the lesions will shrink within seconds and will then fall off after a few days.

Hypersensitive dentine. The sensitive root surface is "painted" with the laser, using water-cooling. Organic matrix is coagulated and the tubuli are closed.

Periodontics. Nd:YAG laser has been tested for a number of purposes within periodontics. A typical treatment could be as follows. The probe is moved down close to the bottom of the pocket and is then moved in a sweeping motion around the tooth. By this procedure, a large part of the bacterial flora in the pocket is eliminated. The laser probe is then moved in all directions over the root cement. The calculus is loosened up, and can be more easily removed, using the conventional methods. The probe is then finally moved into the pocket epithelium. The granulation tissue is vaporised, and the result is pocket curettage. No anaesthetic is generally required. Substantial regeneration of bone has been observed after Nd:YAG treatment in deep bony pockets. Different outputs and pulsation times are used for different operations. Nd:YAG lasers can be used with and without water cooling.

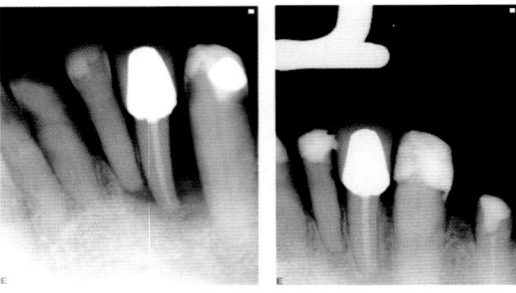

Figure 1.12 Bone regeneration after Nd:YAG laser treatment Baseline and one year control.
Courtesy: Talat Qadri

Bi- and trifurcations are a challenging indication for Nd:YAG treatment. The flexible fibre will reach areas where the curette often fails.

Soft tissue treatment. It is possible to cut soft tissue without causing bleeding and without the need for anaesthetics. The uncovering of preparation margins is also possible, as are smaller operations, such as the removal of hyperplasia and minor frenectomies. The cutting output is, however, low and the operation takes longer than with carbon dioxide lasers. The tissue tends to stick to the probe. Unlike electrocautery, there will be no tissue retraction

<u>Sterilisation of root canals.</u> The biggest problem with the treatment of non-vital teeth is the apical infection. By moving the thin laser probe down into the apical area, and slowly moving it back, one can kill off bacteria in both the apex delta and the side canals.

Further literature: [926, 927, 1582, 1583, 1584, 1585, 1792]

1.4.3 Ho:YAG lasers

The Ho:YAG-laser (short for CTH:YAG-laser, with the dopant substances chromium, thulium and holmium in the YAG host), emits a wavelength of 2130 nm in the infrared part of the spectrum. This wavelength couples well into water and body fluids and can be transmitted through a silica fibre for easy and accurate beam delivery.

The Ho:YAG-laser is used for fragmentation of gall stones, kidney stones and stones in the urinary bladder. It has also been used successfully in the treatment of endometriosis. It can cut, evaporate and coagulate tissue. Further, it is used for shrinking of cartilage in e.g. knee joints and in the spinal cord.

It is not known if biostimulative effects occur when it is used but this is probable. The Ho:YAG-laser is not dangerous to eyes unless directly focused on the eye.

1.4.4 Er:YAG lasers

The Er:YAG laser has elemental erbium as dopant. It works at a wavelength of 2940 nm and is, like the other members of the YAG family, pulsed. A great benefit of this wavelength is that it is not as harmful to the eyes (unless directly focused on the cornea) as the Nd:YAG laser. The main use of this laser type in surgery is for laser peeling. Compared with the CO_2-laser, it is less painful during treatment and the healing is somewhat faster. However, it has not quite as good an effect on wrinkles and acne scars as the CO_2-laser unless used for more than one session.

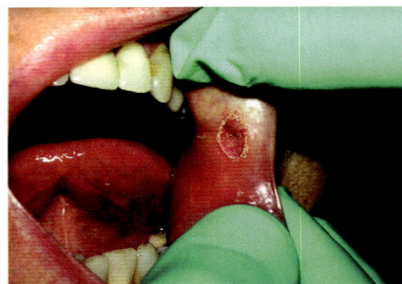

Figure 1.13 Hyperplasia removed with Er:YAG laser
Courtesy: Continuum Lasers

In dentistry, the Er:YAG family is excellent for dental hard tissue and is therefore more suited for the treatment of caries than Nd:YAG-lasers. The wavelength 2940 nm is optimally absorbed by the water in the tooth substance and by the OH-ion in the hydroxy apatite. To avoid overheating, a jet of water accompanies the laser beam, in the same way as with a conventional drill. The treatment is generally painless and the concept is obviously very interesting. Enamel, dentin and composites can be removed with this laser, but not metals such as amalgam. Apart from working as a "drill" the Er:YAG laser can be used in minor surgical procedures such as frenectomies, tongue ties and pulpectomies, frequently with just topical anaesthesia. It can also be used to treat aphthae and herpes simplex. Using thin fibres it is also possible to reduce the microbic infection in root canals and to reduce bacterial growth in periodontal pockets. The Er:YAG "drill" is a bit slower than the traditional drill but has the advantage of requiring no anaesthesia (in most cases), so several quadrants can be treated during the same session. There is no temperature rise in the pulp; on the contrary the temperature is reduced by the water spray. With the Er:YAG laser, dentistry has taken a large leap from the old "extension for prevention" to "minimal invasive dentistry".The Er:YAG laser is excellent for treating hypersensitive dentine. Several studies have confirmed this fact but have only been looking at morphological changes as possible explanations. Zeredo [1311, 1588] has, however, shown that this wavelength has a pain modulating effect in itself, just like all the other lasers used in dentistry. As always, it is not a matter of the laser used but of the dosage applied. Pourzarandian [1606, 1646] confirms the pain relieving effect of Er:YAG as well as the stimulatory effect.

A newcomer in the Er:YAG family is the ErCr:YSGG laser (Erbium-Chromium:Yttrium-Scandium-Gallium-Garnet) with a wavelength of 2870 nm. The water spray is claimed not only to serve as a coolant but also to give a "hydrokinetic" action in order to make the ablation more effective. If so, this is the same with the Er:YAG as well, since water is always needed for "drilling".

One of the difficult parts of the Erbium lasers is beam delivery. The first lasers used articulated arms with mirrors, a solution that is expensive and clumsy since the dentist has to move it at different angles. To make an optical fibre, the light conducting materials available were not transparent enough. Typically a one meter fibre reduced the output to 50% and a two meter fibre reduced it to 25%. Also, the fibres were easily burned at the input end. Today, there are flexible fibres of very pure quartz, transmitting more than 80% over a length of two meters.

Another method is to use a hollow wave guide with a dielectric surface material reflecting the beam. There are basically two problems with this solution, namely that the output power depends on the bending angles and that it easily breaks if bent too much.

Further literature: [201, 160, 1156, 1157, 1158, 1581, 1792].

1.4.5 Argon laser

Like the CO_2-laser, the argon laser (or rather, the argon ion laser) is a gas laser, usually emitting light with a wavelength of 514.5 nm (green light). It is much used in the treatment of diabetic retinopathy. However, other lasers, such as semiconductor laser types or KTP-lasers, are gradually replacing the argon laser. In the same way, the argon laser has been used in dermatology to coagulate haemangiomas but is now being replaced by the KTP/532-laser, the Dye laser or the Copper vapour laser. Argon laser at 488 nm has also been used to cure composite fillings and for tooth bleaching.

1.4.6 Copper vapour laser

This laser type is the strongest of the neutral metal vapour lasers. In its most typical form, it emits light at a wavelength of 578 nm (yellow). It is used in dermatology to coagulate haemangiomas and telangiectasis.

1.4.7 KTP/532-laser (frequency doubled Nd:YAG laser)

If a Nd:YAG laser is combined with a non-linear crystal (such as KDP, KTP, LiNbO3, etc.), light can be emitted at other wavelengths. One such combination is a Nd:YAG laser and a KTP crystal (Potassium Titanyl Phosphide), which is used for frequency doubling and hence also halves the wavelength to 532 nm (green light). Such instruments are often called KTP/532. A laser with this wavelength is a better alternative to the argon laser for treating haemangiomas, small telangiectasis, and red tattoos.

These lasers are normally pulsed (which the argon laser is not) with typical pulse lengths from microseconds to milliseconds. They can also be made to yield pulse trains.

Further, it has been observed that the KTP-laser radiation also has an effect on wrinkles, sometimes called "Non-Ablative Laser Treatment" of wrinkles. The energy density is set lower than the pain threshold, which makes the treatment painless. Practically no side effects have been noted. If the KTP-laser treatment is combined with a Ruby-laser treatment or Nd:YAG-laser treatment, even better results are obtained. The mechanism behind this is biostimulation.

The 532 nm wavelength used to be exclusive but is now available in inexpensive laser pointers The wavelength has sucessfully been used for wound healing but the literature is still scarse.

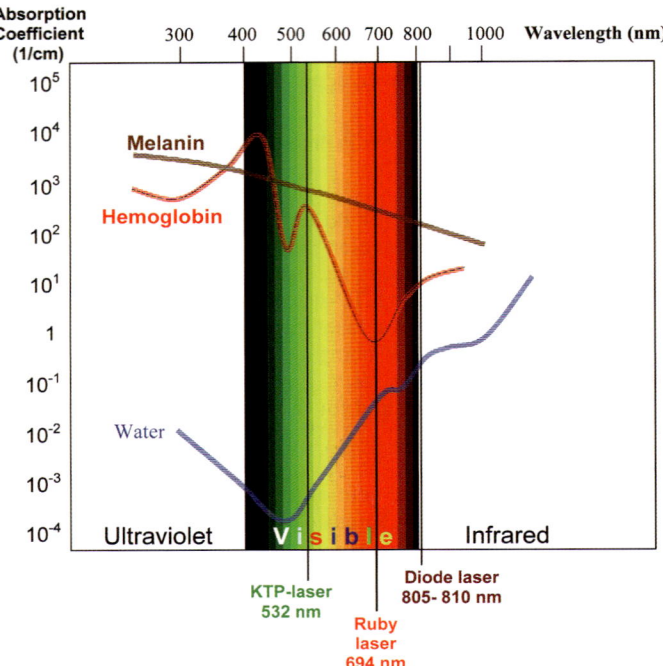

Figure 1.14   Absorption coefficient for melanin and hemoglobin

1.4.8 Ruby laser

This is the oldest of all lasers. The first working laser, presented at a press conference arranged at the Hughes Aircraft Laboratory in Los Angeles, on July 7, 1960, was a Ruby laser. This laser is a solid-state laser using a single, rod-shaped ruby crystal. It emits pulsed light at a wavelength of 694 nm (red light). This laser is currently used in dermatology to remove unwanted hair and to treat blue or green tattoos. In dentistry the ruby laser has been used to produce double-pulse holograms.

  It is worth remembering that it was a Ruby laser that Endre Mester used when he discovered what he called biostimulation. The Ruby laser is still a useful instrument in the treatment of leg ulcers, decubitus, herpes labialis, herpes zoster, scars etc.

  In the diagram above, it can be seen that the ruby laser has minimal absorption in blood and that KTP laser has hundred times higher absorbtion.

1.4.9 Alexandrite
This laser is also pulsed and can be made tuneable, usually within a range of 720-800 nm. Normally, it emits deep red visible light at a wavelength of 755 nm. It is primarily used to remove unwanted hair, as in cases of hirsutism. Q-switched, mode-locked versions are sometimes used to drill and cut bone.

1.4.10 High power semiconductor lasers
Today, semiconductor lasers of the GaAlAs type (with several stacked diode chips) can emit up to 200 W in continuous mode. Typical wavelengths range from 800-880 nm. This laser type can replace the Nd:YAG in surgery and coagulation. It has also been used with some success for hair removal. Its advantages are that it is small, relatively inexpensive, and relatively insensitive to mechanical shock and vibrations.

1.4.11 Dye laser
The active medium in a dye laser is a fluorescent organic dye dissolved in a liquid solvent, usually water. The input energy usually comes from another, external laser (such as an argon, nitrogen, or XeCl laser) or from a flash lamp. The main feature of the dye laser is its tuneable wavelength output and ability to produce ultra-short pulses. Dye lasers are used in dermatology to coagulate certain skin problems such as unwanted tattoos, haemangiomas, and telangiectasis. A version that can produce extreme pulsing can be connected to an optical fibre to blast kidney stones.

A method for detecting and destroying cancer tumours with dye lasers, is photodynamic therapy. It is often performed in two steps: detection and destruction. Detection is based on the following. HPD (hematoporphyrin derivate), a light sensitive flourescensing substance, at a dose of 10 mg/kg, or Photofrin Photosan etc, labelled with an antibody specific to the kind of tumour in question, is injected in the patient intravenously 24 hours prior to light irradiation. By irradiating the patient with green light and looking at the irradiated area through red bandpass filters, fluorescence can be seen. Fluorescence will occur at areas with higher concentrations of the dye, indicating the presence of a tumour. By irradiating the tumour area with light with a wavelength around 630 nm, the HPD will split, releasing toxic agents in the tumour area, possibly killing the tumour. The dye laser is often used as it is strong and can be tuned to the most efficient wavelength. It has been established [24], [25] that the depth of laser light penetration is sufficient to obtain a biological response (necrosis) as far down as 10 mm in the tissue

1.4.12 Excimer laser
The Excimer laser (193, 248, 308, 351 nm) is mainly used for vision correction. The most promising technique, the LASIK surgery is a procedure that corrects for near- or far-sightedness by evaporation of the surface of the cornea. The curvature of the cornea makes it work like a lens as a part of the

eye's lens system, and by changing the curvature, the focus length and refraction quality of this system can be adjusted. The short wavelength of the Excimer laser enables it to be absorbed by the surface of the cornea, and the evaporation process can be very carefully controlled by means of a computer. Both nearsighted and farsighted persons can be helped, and the technique can also be used to adjust astigmatism. This method is very safe nowadays and the whole procedure is a matter of hours.

1.5 Therapeutic lasers

The most typical therapeutic lasers and their wavelengths:

HeNe laser	633 nm	Gas laser
InGaAlP lasers	633-700 nm	Semiconductor laser
GaAlAs lasers	780-890 nm	Semiconductor laser
GaAs laser	904 nm	Semiconductor laser
Defocused CO_2-laser	10 600 nm	Gas laser
Defocused Ruby laser	694 nm	Solid state laser
Defocused Nd:YAG laser	1064 nm	Solid state laser

Table 1.4 Typical therapeutic lasers and their wavelengths

We recognise here three typical surgical laser types - the CO_2-laser, the Ruby laser and the Nd:YAG laser. The Ruby laser was actually the very first biostimulative laser, used by Endre Mester. As a matter of fact, the other surgical lasers could also be used as therapeutic instruments. When strong lasers are used for biostimulation, one only needs to make the beam wide enough not to burn. The patient will then feel only a mild heat. An alternative is to scan rapidly over the area to be treated with a narrow beam. In this case, it is important to have a safety mechanism to ensure that laser light cannot be emitted unless the scanning system is really working, to prevent the patient being burned if the scanning beam stops.

1.5.1 The Helium-Neon laser (HeNe)

This laser, the oldest in laser therapy use after ruby laser, consists of a large laser tube of glass containing a low-pressure gas mixture, which is connected to a high voltage source. It emits visible, red light with a wavelength of 633 nm. The laser generally works continuously, but can be pulsed by switching the electric power supply or by means of a beam chopper or similar unit. In that case, half the output is lost (if the duty cycle is 50%) compared to the continuous working mode. Typical output is 1-10 mW, sent directly (parallel beams) or via fibre optics to a treatment probe (usually divergent light). Instruments containing a HeNe laser are usually rather large and fragile because of the sensitive laser tube. There are laser tubes that are well protected by cushioning material, though the size problem still remains.

The HeNe laser is the most coherent of the different therapeutic types, having a coherence length of centimetres to metres. This is an important factor for the biological result. (See Table 3.3 "Dose ranges for different lasers and indications" on page 81 and Figure 11.4 "Different light sources have different spectra" on page 536.)

In a therapeutic instrument, the HeNe laser light is aimed at the area to be treated either directly, via scanning mirrors, or transferred via a fibre-optic light conductor. The light conductor can either be a mono-fibre or consist of a number of small, thin fibres (fibre bundle). Mono-fibres have much less power loss (typically 1-10%), but are more expensive. Fibre bundles often give a power loss between 20% and 50%, depending on quality. As can be seen, there are a number of practical disadvantages associated with HeNe laser equipment.

For treatment with skin contact, the depth of penetration of a useful level of light from a HeNe laser is 6-8 mm at 3.5 mW output and 8-10 mm for a laser with 7 mW output. (For a more detailed explanation, see chapter 3.4.2 "Depth of penetration, greatest active depth" on page 118.) The depth of penetration thus increases only minimally with increased output.

1.5.2 Indium-Gallium-Aluminium-Phosphide lasers (InGaAlP)

The InGaAlP is named GaAlInP laser in some of the literature. It belongs to a group of semiconductor lasers in which the crystal contains gallium, aluminium, indium, and phosphorus. They are related to the GaAlAs lasers and emit light in the wavelength range of 630-700 nm. Small lasers of this kind within the 650-700 nm wavelength range are often used as pointers in lectures. Developments in this field have taken the InGaAlP laser wavelength down towards and even below the HeNe laser's 633 nm, and the HeNe laser is gradually being replaced by the cheaper, smaller and more robust 633-700 nm InGaAlP laser. InGaAlP lasers make this wavelength available in a more practical form than the HeNe laser, with its expensive, large, and sensitive laser tube. The InGaAlP laser is still often referred to as "GaAlAs" in laser papers.

One should bear in mind, though, that diode lasers emit light with a shorter coherence length than gas lasers, and we have noticed that the biological effects of light from these types of 633 nm lasers are less obvious than using He-Ne laser light. With higher output – e.g. 25-50 mW – similar results seem obtainable through using higher power densities and higher doses.

1.5.3 Gallium-Aluminium-Arsenide lasers (GaAlAs)

This type of laser comprises an entire family of semiconductor lasers. The wavelength can be selected within the 780-890 nm range, but in therapeutic use is usually between 800 and 830 nm, which is invisible, being just inside the infrared area. (However, if one looks straight into a GaAlAs laser probe without protection goggles, one can see a small red glowing point due to the remnant eye sensitivity at that wavelength). These lasers are continuous in their method of operation, but can be pulsed, in which case they are not superpulsed like the GaAs laser, but switched, which means that around half the power output (with a 50% duty cycle) is lost compared to when not pulsed. The depth of penetration of this type of laser is around 2-3 cm.

The GaAlAs laser has grown increasingly popular during the 1990s as it is very easy to run electrically. Small rechargeable lasers have been put on the market, not much larger than an electrical toothbrush. They can run on regular or rechargeable batteries. 30-100 mW laser diodes are now relatively cheap and the GaAlAs laser provides "a lot of mW for the money". There are also GaAlAs lasers on the market with an output of more than 1000 mW. A warning should be issued about these lasers - the dangers of eye injury are very real at such high outputs, particularly if the beam is collimated. One way of avoiding these problems is to use GaAlAs lasers which can be activated only on contact with tissue.

Many GaAlAs lasers have well-designed, exchangeable, sterilisable intra-oral probes. Output meters are essential, because the light from this type of laser is largely invisible. The price tag for a GaAlAs laser of around 100 mW can be between US $2000 and $5000. Price differences depend on factors such as output, ergonomics, standard of hygiene, and dose calculating electronics, to name but a few.

In recent years GaAlAs lasers of 500-1000 mW have entered the market. Prices range from $4000 to $10 000. These lasers require proper protection for the eyes and can produce a noticeable heat sensation, especially in hairy or pigmented areas.

1.5.4 The Gallium-Arsenide laser (GaAs)

This is also a semiconductor laser, and consequently it can be quite small. It emits an infrared (invisible) beam with a wavelength of 904 nm. A laser diode emits a divergent beam (usually 10 to 20 degrees), which can be made parallel by the use of a collimating lens. The GaAs laser is always operated in a pulsed fashion, with very short pulses (100-200 ns) of high peak power (10-100 W maximum output), more or less like a flash bulb. This is often called super-pulsing.

The average output of most of the conventional GaAs treatment lasers on the market varies in direct proportion to the pulse repetition frequency. This means that at 1000 pulses per second, for example, the average output is ten times higher than at 100 pulses per second. There are, however, some lasers that use pulse trains, in which the average output can be kept constant and independent of the set pulse frequency. This simplifies dosage calculation and shortens treatment time considerably.

Because of the GaAs laser's "flash bulb" method of working, with very intense light pulses, it reaches deeper than a laser of the same wavelength that is not superpulsed but has the same average output power. Measurements have shown that the depth of penetration can be as much as 30-50 mm, depending on the type of tissue.

In the treatment of horses, the GaAs laser has been utilised as a diagnostic tool due to the fact that the horse often feels the effect of this laser's radiation and hence reacts when a probe is held over a site of injury. See chapter Chapter 7 "Veterinary use" on page 465

1.5.5 The defocused strong lasers

A more detailed description these lasers has been presented in the previous section. In therapy, they are defocused or combined with scanners so that the power density or average power is kept low enough to avoid burning. These laser types have also made it possible to investigate these wavelengths with some interesting results.

Literature:

Basford [1062] performed a double-blind, placebo-controlled, randomised clinical trial on patients with low back pain. The subjects were 63 ambulatory men and women between the ages of 18 and 70 years with symptomatic non-radiating low back pain of more than 30 days' duration and normal neurological examination results. Subjects were bloc randomized into two groups with a computer-generated schedule. All underwent irradiation for 90 seconds at eight symmetric points along the lumbosacral spine three times a week for 4 weeks by a masked therapist. The Nd:YAG laser emitted 542 mW/cm^2. Subject's perception of benefit, level of function, as assessed by the Oswestry Disability Questionnaire, and lumbar mobility were evaluated. The treated group had a time-dependent improvement in two of the three outcome measures: perception of benefit and level of function. These results were most marked at the midpoint evaluation and end of treatment but tended to lessen at the 1-month follow-up. Lumbar mobility did not differ between the groups at any time.

The aim of a study by Morrone [898] was to verify the effects of laser therapy performed with GaAlAs (780 nm, 2500 mW) on human cartilage cells in vitro. The cartilage sample used for the biostimulation treatment was taken from the right knee of a 19-year-old patient. After the chondrocytes were isolated and suspended for cultivation, the cultures were incubated for 10 days. The culture was divided into four groups. Groups I, II, III were subject to biostimulation with the following laser parameters: 300 J, 1 W, 100 Hz, 10 min. exposure, pulsating emission; 300 J, 1 W, 300 Hz, 10 min. exposure, pulsating emission; and 300 J, 1 W, 500 Hz, 10 min. exposure, pulsat-

ing emission, respectively. Group IV did not receive any treatment. The laser biostimulation was conducted for five consecutive days. The data showed good results in terms of cell viability and levels of Ca and Alkaline Phosphate in the groups treated with laser compared to the untreated group. The results obtained confirm previous positive in vitro results from the same authors, that the GaAlAs laser provides biostimulation without cell damage.

Kim [545] used 1.2 J in plastic and aesthetic surgery. The energy was delivered either by a 1000 mW or a 60 mW 830 nm laser (1000 mW × 1.2 sec or 60 mW x 200 sec). Both were effective, but the 60 mW laser was more effective in the initial period of wound healing, while the 1000 mW laser was more effective in the later stage.

1.5.6 Some "exotic lasers"

Of course laser therapy has been performed with all kinds of existing lasers, such as the argon laser. Some of them may be worth mentioning:

1.5.7 The krypton laser

The krypton laser (or krypton ion laser) is a gas laser, usually emitting light at a wavelength of 647 nm (red light). It has been used in the treatment of herpes [63]. However, it is an expensive laser and is thus not often used for laser therapy.

1.5.8 The nitrogen laser

The nitrogen laser, emitting at a wavelength of 337 nm is a gas laser in the ultraviolet region of the spectrum. It has been used in wound healing studies [1641] and in the treatment of tuberculosis [715, 1283, 1540, 1641].

Chapter 2
Therapeutic instruments

GaAs

Output

Class 3B

He

Super pulsing

Visible or infrared

Continuous

D-laser

650 - 980 nm

2.1 A customer's guide

In the following chapter we will only discuss laser instruments. Even though other light sources also produce biological effects, few articles have been published showing that light emitting diodes (LED) or other incoherent sources have as good an effect as lasers when using the same parameters, except for superficial structures.

If an instrument has both LED (e.g. used as indicators or warning lights) and laser components we regard it as a laser instrument if the power from the laser or lasers clearly dominates the output power.

2.1.1 History

The first commercial therapeutic lasers appeared in the late seventies. They featured a HeNe laser with a fibre-optic cable and were often billed as "soft lasers". The purchasers consisted primarily of cosmetologists. Output powers ranged from 0.5-2 mW for many years.

GaAs lasers came onto the scene in the early 1980's. These lasers were also quite low-powered in the beginning, 1-4 mW being typical. Pulse-train modulated GaAs lasers ("constant power pulse") entered the market in the late 1980's.

Low-powered GaAlAs lasers appeared in the late-80's. 10-30 mW were typical powers. They have grown in popularity and now dominate the market. In the late 1990's lasers of 500-1000 mW were introduced.

Carbon dioxide lasers were introduced as tools for laser therapy in the mid 1990's.

Also in the mid 1990's, the InGaAlP laser arrived, offering an alternative to HeNe lasers.

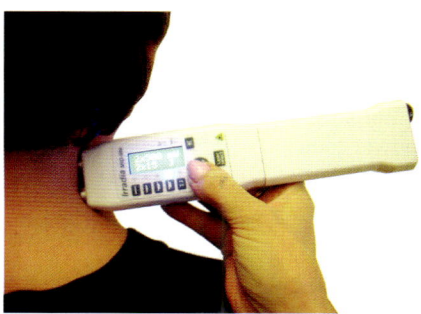

Figure 2.1 Small rechargeable 2 x 500 mW GaAlAs laser

2.1.2 What will tomorrow's lasers look like

The lasers used in many clinics today are still only producing a handful of milliwatts [2103]. Equipment produced commercially in the 1970's were very low powered and generally only of HeNe type, often equipped with a fibre-optic cable conducting the light from the laser tube to a handheld probe. This cable usually reduced the light intensity by more than 50%. The HeNe lasers of today can produce up to 60 mW. With an optical mono-fibre or a scanning system, most of the power from the laser tube can be utilised.

The first GaAs laser, had a typical output of 0.1 – 4 mW per laser diode. Today, there are pulse-train modulated GaAs-lasers with an average output of 100 mW, independent of the envelope frequency.

GaAlAs lasers had an output in the 1-5 mW range. Later on in the 1990's the output from these lasers rose to between 5 and 50 mW. In the new millennium, the power level has gone up to a thousand mW or more, providing new and interesting possibilities.

Many of these old lasers still are around. Taking into account losses in fibres and aging laser diodes (do test your laser!), a large number of today's laser therapists are using rather low outputs. If you don't have a power meter, you may very well have a true "placebo laser"!

The next generation of therapeutic lasers will not necessarily offer higher outputs but rather a radically different design. Holding a laser pen over an area for 10-15 minutes is not very productive work. Lasers in the form of attachable bracelets or shields have already appeared; whole-body approaches may come, laser pens for home care are already available for the general public, and so forth. Some new thinking is already mature in Russia, where adapters for irradiation via rectum and urethra are in use. We

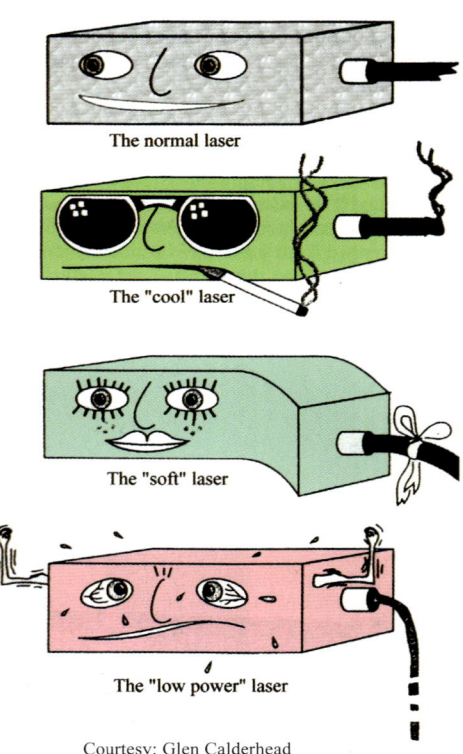

"Lasers I have known"

The normal laser

The "cool" laser

The "soft" laser

The "low power" laser

Courtesy: Glen Calderhead

may not be able to imagine what the next generation will look like, but as soon as the market is ripe, it will be here. It is not that we do not have the technology. It is rather the small market and the small players on the market which slow down development.

Within ten years, and looking back, we will no doubt think that the lasers and techniques of the 90's were rather primitive.

2.1.3 Hand held lasers and automatic devices

A laser beam can be formed into almost any geometrical form through the use of lenses and mirrors. If the light from a laser with a narrow beam (collimated light) is to illuminate a larger surface, this can be done either by expanding the laser beam with lenses or by means of moving mirrors, scanning the beam to cover the surface area. The shape of a scanned area is usually quadratic or rectangular. In the case of expanding the beam by lenses, the illuminated area is usually circular.

In the early 80's therapeutic laser "guns" or laser scanners were in fashion. These instruments - often on big metal stands - definitely look more impressive than smaller hand held devices. An impressive laser gives a higher degree of placebo, no doubt, but the actual efficiency of those instruments was usually not related to their price and size.

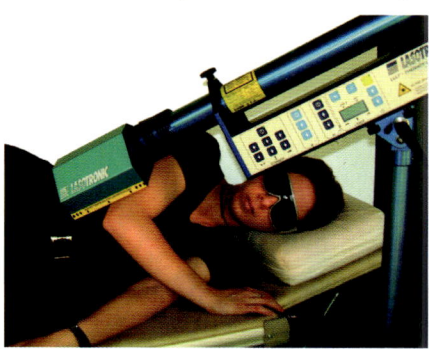

Figure 2.2   Typical scanner

The classical scanning laser was the Space Laser, using a 5-10 mW HeNe-laser mixed with light from two or more 1-5 mW GaAs-laser diodes. The value 1 mW corresponds to a 1000 Hz pulse repetition rate and 5 mW is achieved at 5000 Hz. The width and length of the area to scan could be set, as well as the scanning speed. These instruments lost a great deal of popularity when their clinical performance was not up to expectation.

The disadvantage of scanners (and laser "guns") is that they are less efficient than hand held instruments with probes that can be used for treatment with skin contact. Furthermore, they are very expensive - the price per milliwatt is especially high.

However, scanners are still useful for various conditions, such as the treatment of large wounds and other skin conditions like herpes zoster. And if used in combination with contact mode treatment, scanners have been shown to have an additional therapeutic effect. The scanners of today also have higher a output power and give a higher power density.

An advantage of a scanner is, of course, that it runs by itself so that the therapist can treat other patients in the meantime. This may, on the other hand, in turn lead to a deterioration in patient contact and information exchange between therapist and patient.

Generally, we consider the hand held devices to be more efficient than scanners in the treatment of most indications.

2.1.4 Which type of laser is best suited to which task?

There are three main types of laser on the market: HeNe (now being gradually replaced by the InGaAlP laser), GaAs, and GaAlAs. They can be installed in separate instruments or combined in the same instrument. It is not possible to give a straightforward answer to the question in the headline. There are overlapping areas of effect, and individual sensitivity. Sometimes the wavelength may not be optimal, but it may be the only possible one, due to its superior penetration to the target. The following is a brief outline of the experience of the authors and the documentation found in the literature.

2.1.4.1 HeNe laser and InGaAlP laser

The HeNe and the InGaAlP lasers are used to treat skin wounds, wounds to mucous membrane, herpes simplex, herpes zoster (shingles), gingivitis, pains in skin and mucous membrane, conjunctivitis, neuralgia, etc.

The HeNe laser has now been used for wound healing for more than 30 years and the InGaAlP laser for more than 15 years. One advantage is the documented beneficial effect on mucous membrane and skin (the types of problem it is best suited to), and another advantage is the absence of risk of injury to the eyes. Maeno [129] has treated calves with keratoconjunctivitis with excellent results, irradiating the eye through the eyelid. Schindl [350] also used HeNe lasers for experimental eye treatment. Normal HeNe output is 3-15 mW, although apparatuses with up to 60 mW are available. The optimal dosage when using a HeNe laser for wound healing is about 2.0 J/cm^2 around the edge of the wound and approximately 0.5 J/cm^2 in the open wound. The dose levels for InGaAlP lasers are higher due to the lower degree of coherence – typically twice as high.

2.1.4.2 GaAs laser

The GaAs laser is best used for the treatment of deeper situated problems and of pain and inflammations, and is less well suited to the treatment of wounds and mucous membrane. Very low dosages should be administered to mucous membranes! Most GaAs equipment are intended for extra-oral use, but there are special lasers adapted for intra-oral use. We have only found a few positive studies of GaAs lasers which demonstrate effects on wound healing. It is likely that dosage is a critical factor.

Prices are usually between US $2000 and $4000 for outputs between 10 and 100 mW. A GaAs laser must have an integral output meter that indicates that there is a beam and shows its power in milliwatts. This is necessary because the light is completely invisible. Protective glasses for the patient may be appropriate in view of the invisible nature of the light, especially if the beam is collimated (though it rarely is).

In older systems, the power output is proportional to the pulse frequency. A GaAs laser that has an average output of 10 mW when pulsed at 10 000 Hz thus produces just 1 mW when pulsed at 1000

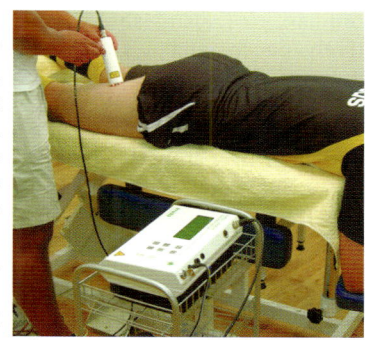

Laser treatment with superpulsed 904 nm GaAs laser.

Hz, and merely 0.1 mW at 100 Hz. If you wish to administer treatment at pulse repetition rates (PRR) with such an instrument, around, for example, 20 Hz (for the treatment of pain), the output power is, clinically speaking, unusable. However, there are GaAs lasers with "constant power pulse", meaning that the power output is held constant at all PRR:s. This might be of interest to a physiotherapist, for example, considering that the GaAs laser has the deepest penetration of the common therapeutic lasers. Good doses can be administered to deep-lying tissue over a short period of time. A GaAs multi-probe can also shorten treatment times for conditions involving larger areas (neck/shoulders).

The GaAs laser is, like the GaAlAs and the InGaAlP laser, a semiconductor laser. A purely practical advantage of this type of laser is that the laser diode is located in the hand-held probe. This means that there is no sensitive fibre-optic light conductor running from the laser apparatus to the probe, just an ordinary, cheap, robust electric cable. Optimum treatment dosages with GaAs lasers are lower than with GaAlAs lasers.

The GaAs laser is most effective in the treatment of pain, inflammations and functional disorders in muscles, tendons and joints (e.g. epicondylitis, tendinitis and myofascial pain, gonarthrosis, etc.), and for deep-lying disorders in general. As mentioned above, GaAs has not been shown to be as effective on wounds and other superficial problems as the HeNe laser (InGaAlP laser) and GaAlAs laser. GaAs can, nevertheless, be used successfully on wounds in combination with HeNe or InGaAlP, but the dosages should be very low in open wounds.

2.1.4.3 GaAlAs lasers

The GaAlAs lasers have become increasingly popular in the nineties. They are very easy to power electrically, and small rechargeable lasers, not much larger than an electric toothbrush, are on the market. (They can run on ordinary or rechargeable batteries.) 30-500 mW laser diodes are now relatively cheap, and a GaAlAs laser provides "a lot of milliwatts for the money". Recently, GaAlAs lasers have appeared on the market with an output of over 1000 mW. Wavelengths normally vary between 800 and 810 nm but 980 nm is also offered. There are indications that the clinical effect of 780 nm differs from the very frequently used 800-830 nm.

Many GaAlAs lasers also have well-designed, exchangeable, sterilisable intra-oral probes. Output meters are essential because the light from this type of laser is largely invisible. For 800 nm wavelength the sensitivity of the human eye is only about 1% of its sensitivity at 550 nm. In a dark surrounding, the 830 nm red light is faintly visible, however.

The GaAlAs laser normally works continuously, like the HeNe and the InGaAlP, and is used mainly on skin and mucous membranes, but can also be used on more deep-lying problems, especially the high powered lasers. Indications are difficult-to-heal wounds, rheumatoid arthritis, muscle attachments (preferably in small joints), pain and various oral conditions.

2.1.4.4 Combination probes

There are probes on the market that combine two different laser wavelengths. There are also probes that combine one or more laser diodes with LEDs of various wavelengths - known as "cluster probes". (Here we do not mean the LEDs that are used only as indicator lamps.) The authors themselves prefer equipment with only one wavelength in the probe, and there are several reasons for this. The combination of laser and LED is problematic. There is no doubt that LED light has a biological effect, though less pronounced. The incoherent light from LEDs may even counteract the effect of the laser or lasers in the probe. (See chapter 11.1.2 "Comparisons between coherent and non-coherent light" on page 529.) Also, how are we to know which of the wavelengths gives the best results under particular conditions? How do the different light sources affect each other? How is the dosage to be calculated if the probe's light sources have differing physical characteristics? Are there wavelengths that are unsuitable for some indications but will always be used because of the probe's design? How should the results of the laser + LED probes be evaluated, since they cannot be compared to "pure" laser therapy studies? In fact, a result obtained with a laser + LED probe can only be obtained with and compared to one performed with an identical probe. A comparison could be made with pharmacology, in which the preparation is refined as much as possible to isolate the desired effect.

2.1.4.5 Therapeutic CO_2-lasers

Therapeutic treatment with these lasers has become more and more popular. Instruments designed expressly for the purpose are not required. Practically any carbon dioxide laser can be used, as long as the beam can be spread out over an appropriate area and the power can be regulated to avoid burning. This can always be achieved with an additional lens of germanium or zinc selenide, if it is impossible with the standard accessories accompanying the apparatus. There are small, portable CO_2-lasers on the market today - even battery-operated units - producing up to 10-15 watts, which is more than enough power output. There is a general misconception about these lasers, implying that they can penetrate into deep areas due to their high power. In fact, the contrary applies. You will find more about this issue in chapter 11, section 1.6. The main advantage of therapeutic carbon dioxide lasers is their ability to give high doses over large areas.

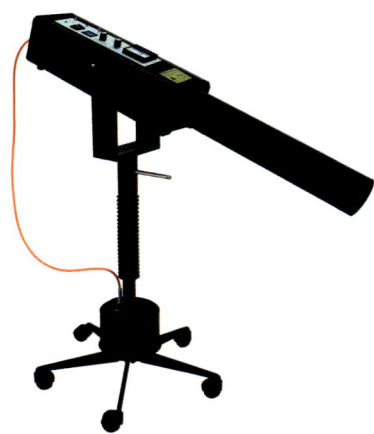

Figure 2.4   Therapeutic CO_2-laser, 10-15 W to tissue

2.1.5 Which laser should I buy?

There is no simple answer to this question. You have to ask yourself a number of questions: "What is the laser to be used for?", "How much am I prepared to pay?", "Must the probe be sterilisable?", "Should it be portable?", "Should it contain a microprocessor to aid in dose calculations?", "Should it be used for veterinary treatments?" and so on.

The small pen-like GaAlAs lasers are a popular choice. They are easy to handle because they have no electric cable, and can therefore be moved easily from one treatment room to another. Those with rechargeable batteries are the best choice but are more expensive than the models that run on ordinary batteries. The latter consume batteries at an alarming rate, and cannot always maintain a constant output. They are, on the other hand, very small and a little cheaper. The small rechargeable lasers are probably the most versatile for a dentist. Modern batteries are becoming more durable but still cause problems with the output.

If you want to treat muscle, tendon, and joint problems (whether in humans or animals), a GaAs laser with a single or multiple probe is, in our opinion, an appropriate choice. Though GaAlAs still has much to offer in these areas, the GaAs penetrates deeper and has a different biological effect. A multiprobe allows shorter treatment times.

If you want to treat ulcers, skin, pain, myoses, etc., a laser with a variety of wavelengths would be a good choice, such as an InGaAlP or GaAlAs, or at least equipment to which new wavelengths can be added at a later stage.

If you are worried about the (minimal) risk of eye injury, particularly if you plan to delegate the laser work to assisting staff, you may prefer a GaAlAs laser which can be activated only on contact with tissue, or to use non collimated light.

Are you particular about dosage and not so good at mathematics? Some laser systems can calculate the dosage, or provide only the dosage you tell them to give. However, applying the "correct" dosage is not only a matter of mathematics, as will be shown later on in this book. For practical clinical purposes a "beep" indicating each Joule may be enough.

A question that is often asked is: "Should I wait until the lasers have become more sophisticated and even cheaper?" They will probably be cheaper in five years. But they will be even cheaper in ten years, and by the time you have retired, they will be cheaper still, and better...

It is clearly not an easy choice, so read this chapter carefully before making a decision - and particularly before talking to a salesperson!

2.1.6 Stronger = better?

The power output of therapeutic lasers has increased radically during the nineties. McKibbin reports that there were about 1800 therapeutic laser units in Canada in 1990. 22% of them were HeNe lasers with an output of 1 mW or less, 35% HeNe lasers with 1-2 mW, 13% 830 nm units with an output up to 5 mW, 3% 830 nm units with an output up to 30 mW, 26% GaAs units with an output of 5 mW or less, and 1% units in the 760-780 range nm with an output up to 30 mW.

Now in 2009, the situation is quite different. HeNe units are being replaced by stronger InGaAlP lasers up to 500 mW, GaAlAs units of 7 000 mW are on the market, and GaAs units of 100 mW and more are available.

Even though it is possible to attain some effects with a 1-2 mW laser, there is no doubt that with a laser 100 times stronger, it is much easier to achieve biostimulating effects, at least if one intends to use treatment periods of the same length. Power density is also very important!

The authors used to have certain misgivings about an "inflation" with respect to the output power of therapeutic lasers. One misgiving was, and still is, the obvious risk of eye damage. The need for protective glasses has previously been exaggerated, but is now becoming more important. Another misgiving is the lack of research in the field of "high-power" therapeutic lasers. So far, insufficient data have been published on these powerful lasers. For the moment, we must rely primarily on our own clinical experience. That experience, however, is so encouraging that it cannot be ignored, even with the lack of scientific support. It would appear that "high-powered" therapeutic lasers will be able to further expand the scope of laser therapy, epsecially in pain therapy.

The doses previously recommended for laser therapy still hold true, in a way. However, much of what we know about dosage is based upon wound healing studies. This is the field in which both stimulating and inhibiting doses have generally been observed. But a wound is superficial, and the superficial tissue will absorb most of the laser energy. So treating a condition in the inner ear through the bone behind the ear is quite a different matter. The dense bone behind the ear

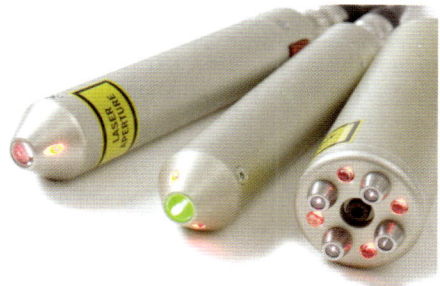

Figure 2.5 Examples of laser probes: red 650 nm, green 532 nm and superpulsed 904 nm.

absorbs some 90% of the light energy. Skin and blood absorb another 5%. Thus, 100 J in contact mode means only some 5 J or less in the inner ear. For pain and inflammation in large joints, such as the knee, quite a few joules may be required on the surface before the actual target receives the energy needed.

Using the same amount of energy but with different energy densities will not necessarily trigger the same biological response. Kim [545] used 1.2 J in plastic and aesthetic surgery. The energy was delivered either by a 1000 mW or a 60 mW 830 nm laser (1000 mW × 1.2 sec or 60 mW × 200 sec). Both were effective, but the 60 mW laser was more effective in the initial period of wound healing, while the 1000 mW laser was more effective in the late period.

Hoteya [624] previously conducted a double-blind study in the field of orthopaedics. A 150 mW GaAlAs laser was used in a group of patients suffering from chronic pain. The overall efficacy rate was 70.6%. In a later study, a 1000 mW GaAlAs laser was used. The spot size was adjusted so that the incident power density was 670 mW/cm^2, thereby avoiding any possible photo-thermal effects and any sensations of heat from the real laser as compared with the dummy laser. The overall efficacy was 75.5% with a "no change" in 24.5%. Thus, the efficacy rate was not greatly improved, but the treatment time was certainly shortened.

It is speculated that "high-powered" therapeutic lasers actually can put sufficient energy into much deeper layers of tissue, due to the high power density of the beam. Previous treatment efforts may have been somewhat less successful due to inadequate power density in deeper tissues. Increased treatment time cannot completely compensate for lower power density. For instance: 5 minutes of 30 mW = 9 J. 20 seconds × 450 mW = 9 J. The same energy is delivered, but the superior power density of the 450 mW diode will deliver energy above the response level to deep-lying areas, while the 30 mW diode will be less successful.

It is important not to over-stimulate superficial tissues with these powerful lasers. When treating wounds, the probe should be kept at a distance to reduce the power density. It should be emphasised that healthy tissues do not react adversely. Thus, the healthy tissues covering a deep target will not be damaged.

For tissue regeneration low output and long time is much more useful than high output and short time.

A GaAlAs 830 nm for wound healing was used by Ihara [925]. The 1000 mW laser was defocused to give a power density of 669 mW/cm^2. Five patients with persistent skin ulcers, which had proved resistant to past conservative treatment, were irradiated. The probe was held at 5 cm above the surface of the ulcer giving 2.1 - 6.3 J/cm^2 twice a week during the treatment period. The ulcers responded well to the laser therapy.

The important thing is not only the nominal output of the diode; the power density is also very important. If the spot size of a 30 mW laser is very small at the tissue, the beam may even cause a burn – especially if the skin is pigmented. The spot size of a 1000 mW diode can be made large enough to treat even sensitive areas such as the lip without any sensation of warmth.

The examples below illustrate the fact that high power densities may be useful for pain but not necessarily for superficial cell stimulation. Again, however, it is not a matter of milliwatts, it is a matter of power density at tissue, and dosage.

Finally, time in itself is an important parameter. Castano [1840] tested LPT on rats that had zymosan injected into their knee joints to induce inflammatory arthritis. The author compared illumination regimens consisting of a high and low fluence (3 and 30J/cm^2), delivered at high and low irradiance (5 and 50 mW/cm^2) using 810 nm laser light daily for 5 days, with the positive control of conventional corticosteroid (dexamethasone) therapy. Illumination with 810 nm laser was highly effective (almost as good as dexamethasone) at reducing swelling and a longer illumination time (10 or 100 minutes compared to 1 minute) was more important in determining effectiveness than either the total fluence delivered or the irradiance. LPT induced reduction of joint swelling correlated with reduction in the inflammatory marker serum prostaglandin E_2 (PGE_2).

The lesson here is probably that high power densities and high energies are suitable for pain conditions whereas low power densities and longer time of irradiation are more efficient for stimulation of biological processes.

Literature:

Yamada [418] reports better and faster results in treating postherpetic neuralgia with a 150 mW GaAlAs laser than with a 60 mW GaAlAs laser. The patients were treated the same number of minutes, but at different energies.

The number of patients treated was small (17), and the patients in the 60 mW group also benefited from the treatment.

Shiroto [205] compared the reaction of human neutrophils in vitro, using 830 nm 60 mW, 830 nm 100 mW, and 904 nm 3 mW lasers. The highest stimulation was achieved with the 830 nm 60 mW laser, followed by the 904 nm 3 mW laser, while the 830 nm 100 mW laser actually retarded activity.

In a double blind study by Sattayut [924] patients with TMD for more than 6 months were treated with laser therapy. 1/3 of the patients were rendered free of symptoms (assessed at 3 months) by laser therapy alone while the other 2/3 needed additional treatment. Joint and muscular trigger points were irradiated. A GaAlAs laser, with 300 mW output and a dose of 20 J per point (100 J/cm^2) was much more effective than 60 mW and 4 J per point.

Shiroto [1286] has treated tenth of thousands of pain patients and followed up the therapy through questionnaires [53]. Most of the therapy has been performed with a GaAlAs laser of 60 mW. In order to compare the possible advantages of stronger lasers, Shiroto selected 48 pain patients for treatment with either 60 mW, 150 mW or "SuperLizer", which is a high-powered polarised light source. The patients were followed weekly for 14 weeks. The results were similar but the 150 mW laser showed a faster pain relieving effect. However, at 14 weeks there was a negative tendency in this group.

2.1.7 How much should a laser cost?

Lasers are fairly expensive instruments relative to their technical complexity, primarily because they are produced in small numbers. The most important factor is not how much the laser costs, but how good it is. An instrument costing US $3000 without any noticeable treatment benefits (and there are such instruments, unfortunately) is in reality much more expensive than a US $7000 laser that effectively alleviates symptoms or cures the ailments you are treating. Many laser producers or importers have gone bankrupt or disappeared, which has left their customers in an unenviable position when their instruments break down. And remember: it is never easy to sell a second-hand laser!

2.1.8 Is a therapeutic laser really worth the money?

Are there other benefits over and above those relating to treatment? Could you, for example, successfully treat a number of conditions that are beyond your colleagues' ability, doing so without pain? Many therapists have to compete for patients and would very much like to extend their customer base. If patients can recommend their friends and acquaintances a therapist who can treat conditions that other therapists normally cannot, then that person has a much better chance of coping with the competition. However, the simple fact of using a laser does not automatically create such market advantages. Medical competence always comes first. But no matter what your degree of medical competence, a thorough knowledge of laser therapy basics is needed to achieve successful medical results with a laser. If you have both, you will be able to buy the right laser, and you will find it very profitable.

2.1.9 Do you need to update your laser?

If you already are the owner of a laser, it may be a good laser or a bad laser. To know if it is good or bad you need to find out what output power it has. And not the output power stated in the manual and not even what possibly was measured when you bought it. It is not uncommon that the output decreases by time and even that it comes close to zero. You should be able to measure the output on a regular basis with a power meter made for the actual wavelength used.

If the output is low, it can be quite money- and time saving to update your laser or even to buy a new one. How much time and money would you save in a year if you could obtain the same dose in two minutes, that you now need twenty minutes to obtain? Should you decide to buy a new laser, read the next section to get some advice.

2.1.10 Microcomputer features

Some laser units have pre-set programmes where the therapist can push a multitude of pre-programmed settings for various conditions. While this can be useful for a beginner, there are obvious drawbacks. No programme can make an individual estimation of the depth to target, tissue condition, chronic or acute, skin colouration etc. This has to be taken into consideration in all cases. Further, pushing all those knobs to find the "right" dosage takes time. So, even if such programmes can be helpful in the beginning, there should preferably be a "continuous" button to make the laser just that - a continuous beam, allowing the therapist to use his/her own estimation of the suitable dosage.

2.2 Ten points to consider when choosing an instrument

The laser market is very complicated and full of pitfalls. How do you know which instruments are good? What is expensive? Will it be expensive in the long run to buy something cheap? It is easy to make hasty decisions when faced with a skilful salesman. Before you know it, you've signed on the dotted line.

Here are a number of questions, which you should ask both the salesman and yourself. You are well advised to read these carefully, or you may regret it later on!

1. "Laser instruments" have been sold which do not even contain a laser, instead being equipped with LEDs or even ordinary light bulbs. These instruments have been sold for between US $3000 and $10 000. How can you acquire proof that the instrument really does contain a laser?

2 In a number of products, laser diodes have been combined with LEDs. This may be kept secret and the salesman only talks about a laser. Are all light sources in the apparatus (except guide lights and warning lights) really lasers? What output power has the laser or lasers compared to the other sources?

3 For oral work and wound healing, HeNe, InGaAlP and GaAlAs are the most common types, GaAlAs being the most versatile. Sterilisable probes are normally only available for the latter two. For injuries to joints, vertebrae, the back, and muscles - that is, for the treatment of more deep-lying problems - the GaAs laser is the best documented. Veterinary work requires a laser designed so that the light can pass through the coat and penetrate to the desired depth. It is very important that the light source is in skin contact in order to make the light penetrate into the tissue under the fur of a horse or dog. For superficial tendon and muscle attachments, the required depth can be reached with the GaAlAs laser. Many companies have only one type of laser, such as a GaAlAs, and the salesman will naturally tell you that it is the best model for everything, and that it is irrelevant which type of laser is used. However, research tells quite a different story.

4 Size, colour, shape, appearance, and price vary a great deal from manufacturer to manufacturer. Because a piece of equipment is large, it does not necessarily follow that its medical efficacy is high, or vice versa. The most important factor is the dosage that enters the tissue. Make sure the laser you buy is designed in such a way that most of the light really enters the tissue. Ask the salesman: how is the dosage measured? Is there a power meter available? How do you know if the power of your laser has decreased? Design is nice but doesn't do the job.

5 Some companies that import lasers have insufficient knowledge of medicine, laser physics and technology. If a piece of equipment is faulty, it may have to be sent to the country of manufacture for repair. How long would you be without your equipment in such a case, and what would it cost to repair? Can the importer document his expertise? Who can you speak to who has used the apparatus in question for a long period of time? Is there a well-known professional who uses this laser? What does it cost to change a laser diode or laser tube after the guarantee has expired? Can you get written confirmation of this? Try to get a list of references that you can call and ask. How long is your guarantee - one or two years? Two years guarantee is becoming more and more common.

6 The difference between a colourful brochure and reality is often considerable. There are examples of brochures that describe an output ten times that which the equipment actually provides. How can you find out the real performance of the equipment (e.g. its output to tissue)? For pulsed lasers (usually GaAs-lasers), some manufacturers specify only the

peak power of the pulse output in their technical specifications - 70 watt peak pulse output naturally seems more impressive than 35 milliwatts average output ("70 watt output" is a power that in continuous wave could cut deep in tissue). Are measurement results available from an independent agency? Is it possible to borrow an apparatus in order to measure its performance? Is there a power meter on the apparatus that can measure what is emitted and display it numerically? It is not enough simply to have a light indicator as it cannot tell you if the output power has decreased over time.

7 Some dealers might know that their products are sub-standard. Customers should beware of dealers who are overeager to get them to sign a contract. If a product is good, the dealer will have no qualms about selling it on sale-or-return basis and putting the agreement in writing. What happens if the medical effects are not as promised? Is it possible to get a written guarantee of sale-or-return?

8 In most countries, therapeutic lasers must be approved. Find out what the law says about lasers in your country.

9 Many companies organise courses and "training" events of markedly varying quality. Serious importers or manufacturers will take pains to ensure that their equipment is used properly and ensure that the customer receives some training in its use. What are the instructor's background and qualifications? Has he or she published anything? Is there a course description? What does the training material cost? Is a training course included in the cost of the equipment? Is the training material included? Is it possible to buy the training material only?

10 Development is proceeding rapidly. Suddenly, you have out-of-date laser equipment and a new and perhaps more efficient type of laser comes onto the market. What happens if your laser becomes outmoded? Do you have to buy a new laser, or can your equipment be updated with future components and probes?

1. "Laser instruments" should contain a laser as the primary light source.
2. If it has LEDs, they should only be guide lights or warning lights.
3. For oral work an exchangeable and sterilisable light conductor is best.
4. For veterinary work it must be designed to let the light pass through the coat.
5. Make sure the laser you buy has a power meter with a display.
6. Make sure that your laser instrument can be repaired after the guarantee has expired.
7. Make sure that the output as stated in the brochure is correct.
8. Is your laser approved by the authorities in your country?
9. Do you get proper training included in the price?
10. Can your equipment be updated with future components?

2.3 How do I maintain my laser?

We have seen many examples of laser instruments that have been badly treated – sometimes you wonder if the owner had his instrument hanging from a rope behind his car! This applies especially to instruments used for treating horses. Although for most people the following recommendations are obvious, we want to point them out anyway:

- Avoid mechanical shock and vibrations.
- Temperatures too high (> +40 °C) or too low (< 0 °C) may be harmful to your instrument.
- Dust or smoke may collect on optical components and obstruct the path of light from source to target. Oil used in physiotherapy must not come in direct contact with the probe.
- Water or high humidity may destroy electronics.
- High voltage peaks in the mains can damage electronics. Be sure to disconnect your instrument in case of a thunderstorm.
- Cables and mechanical switches usually break first.
- Never try to repair your laser yourself. Usually this voids your guarantee.
- Like most other equipment, a laser requires care and attention. If the laser has an electric cable, it should be checked regularly to prevent electrical hazards. The laser's output should also be checked on a regular basis to

ensure that dose calculations are correct. A loss of power can occur when laser diodes start to age, or when light conductors age or are subjected to mechanical stress. The laser probe aperture should be washed with alcohol and soft cotton wool, for example. When the laser is used directly on skin, small amounts of dirt and grease can enter the probe opening and gradually cause a loss of output.

- If the laser beam is invisible and collimated, the laser should (for safety reasons) not be left in a state in which it is emitting light when you are not actually working with it. This can be ensured by removing the key or by separating the laser probe and battery.
- If the probe is not sterilisable, it may be covered by ordinary cling film during treatment, after which the cling film is disposed of. In any case, the aperture can be wiped with alcohol afterwards.
- Do not use the laser in direct contact with skin oils, use protective cling film. Even moving the probe in contact with skin will finally make grease penetrate the optics.

Chapter 3
Biostimulation

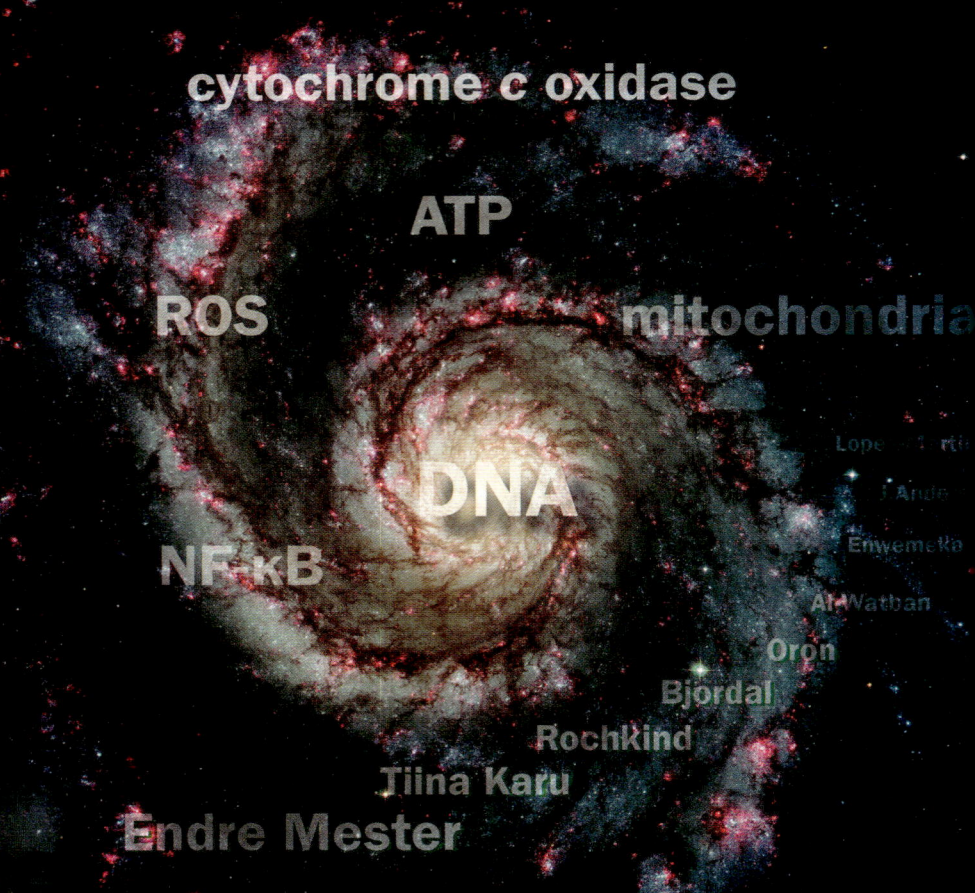

We would like your comment

If you have any comments on the contents of this book, positive or negative, we would be pleased to have an e-mail from you. Please send your opinion to info@prima-books.com.

Visit our website for other laser therapy books:
www.prima-books.com

Prima Books AB
Spjutvägen 11
772 32 Grängesberg
Sweden
Fax +46 240 23037
www.prima-books.com

About the authors

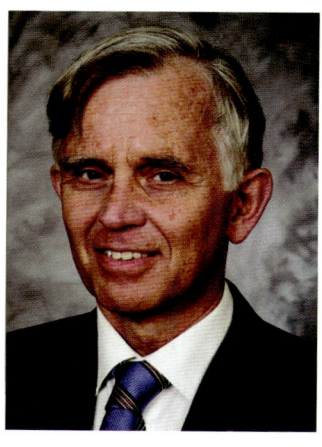 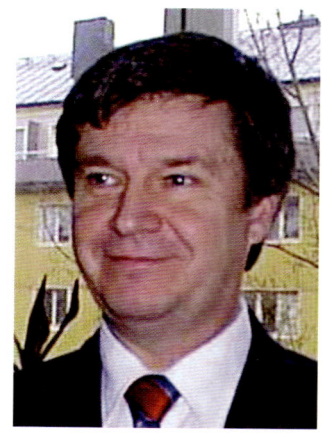

Jan Tunér is a dentist in private practise, working with lasers since 1986. He is a board member of the World Association for Laser Therapy.

Lars Hode is a physicist, specialised in medical laser applications and working with laser therapy since 1985. He is the president and founder of the Swedish Laser-Medical Society.

Find a laser therapist

The World Association for Laser Therapy is sponsoring a global search function for persons looking for a laser therapist in their area. This service can be found at www.findalasertherapist.com. WALT is not endorsing any therapist appearing on this site, only allowing therapists of all kinds to advertise their presence.

Tooth bleaching 450
Tourette's syndrome 111
Treatment dose 78, 514
Treatment interval 81, 91
Treatment technique 76, 95, 523
Trigeminal neuralgia 89, 129, 342
Trigger point 85, 97, 109
Trismus 98, 288, 418, 440
Tuberculosis 47, 72

U
Urology 344
Uveitis 290

V
Vaginitis 237
Vasoconstriction 391
Vasodilatation 99, 138, 391
Venous ulcer 214
Vertigo 330, 332, 336, 337, 339, 452
Veterinary 64, 466, 564
Virus 31, 123, 126, 131, 242, 246, 272
Vitiligo 349

W
Warts 348
Wavelength 2, 3
Withdrawal periods 382
Wound healing 351
Wrinkles 34, 38, 40, 383, 528

X
Xerostomia 202, 308
X-ray 3, 4, 94, 136, 267

Y
Yttrium 36, 39

Z
Zoster 41, 91, 109, 242, 372

S

Salivary glands	305
Scanner	46, 52, 152, 214, 573
Scattering	509, 515, 528, 536, 538, 540, 547
Schizophrenia	111
Schlatter	477
Schwann cell	272
Sciatic nerve	271, 274, 280, 296
Secondary dentine	128, 396, 397, 439
Secondary mechanisms	557
Semiconductor laser	28, 42, 43
Serotonin	300, 541, 542, 543, 556
Shingles	53, 372
Shoulder tendinitis	145, 232, 531
Sialoadenitis	308
Side effects	131
Singlet oxygen	71, 94, 555, 558
Sinuitis	309
Sjögren's syndrome	305
Sluder	265
Snake bites	311
Soft laser	50
Soliton	497, 502 503, 504
Somatosensory tinnitus	337, 338, 340
Speckle Interferometry	565
Speckles	13, 15, 486, 534, 535, 536, 546
Spectrum	3, 5, 7
Sperm	344, 345
Spinal cord	109, 274, 276, 310
Sports injuries	76, 313
Stellate ganglion	133, 283, 300, 374
Steroid	145, 232, 440, 441
Stimulatory and regulatory mechanisms	560
Stye	26, 290, 291
Superpulse	17, 31, 45, 46, 86, 118
Suppression	73, 192, 207, 271
Swimmers Ear	335
Synovia	133, 164, 165, 167, 441
synovial membrane	159
Systemic effect	72, 73, 121, 226, 352, 516, 539, 576, 582, 591, 597

T

Tattoo	28, 34, 40, 41, 42, 481
Teats	467
Temporo-mandibular disorders	338, 440
Tendinitis	143, 145, 232, 322, 323
Tennis elbow	109, 532
Tensile strength	72, 139, 427
Therapeutic window	128, 517, 531
Thermography	99, 138, 165, 228, 265, 301
Thrombophlebitis	343
Thyroid gland	195, 248, 475
Tissue condition	123
Titanium implant	411, 413, 414
TMD	338, 440, 443, 444
TNF-alpha	159
Tonsillitis	342

PDT	28, 246, 427, 531, 539, 555, 564
Peak pulse power	17, 63, 121
Penetration depth	17, 31, 42, 44, 45, 46, 76, 77, 96, 118, 120, 121
Periodontics	37, 427
Periostitis	313, 451
PGE	160, 164, 165, 171, 250, 251, 255, 256, 297, 303, 327, 354, 404, 419
PGE1	157
PGE2	154, 160, 161, 165, 404
Phantom pain	300
Pharyngitis	128
Photo Activated Disinfection	448
Photo dynamic therapy	448, 531
Photobiomodulation	73
Photon energy	3, 10, 450, 538, 555, 557, 563
Photosensitivity	274
Pituitary gland	73, 296
Plantar fasciitis	304
Plaque	406, 407
Plaque (dental)	394, 404, 405
Plaque (viral)	243
Pneumonia	111
Polarisation	16, 486, 528, 531, 546, 560
Polarisation effects	545
Porphyrin	71, 486, 546, 547, 557, 558
Possible primary mechanisms	544
Postherpetic neuralgia	59, 243, 300, 372, 374
Post-menstrual stress	382
Pregnancy	474
Prostaglandin	157, 419
Prostatitis	346, 347
Prosthetics	437
Proximal priority	313
Psoriasis	126
Psoriatic arthritis	153, 164
Pulp capping	396
Pulse frequency	2, 17, 46, 54, 89, 124, 298, 306, 344, 466, 487, 488, 493
Pulse train	40, 46, 574
Pulsed lasers	513

Q

Q-switched	11, 42

R

Radiation risks	4
Radiation therapy patients	479
RANKL	414, 419, 420, 422, 423
Ranula	35
Raynaud's disease	138, 265, 374
Recommendations of WALT	580
Retention cyst	35
Rheumatoid arthritis	129, 138, 164, 606
Risks and side effects	131
RNA	72, 164, 356, 404, 412
Root canal	28, 35, 38, 39, 396
Ruby laser	8, 29

M

Macrophage	555, 560
Macroscopic heating	549
Mastitis	197, 237, 369, 468
Ménière	238, 330, 336
Menstrual pain	236
Meta analysis	43, 168, 294, 353, 371, 607
Metalloproteinase	406, 434
Methodology of a trial	570
Microcirculation	110, 259, 260, 310
Migraine	238
Mitochondria	267, 344, 361, 430, 547, 552, 553, 554, 558, 559
MMP	157, 204, 294
Mononucleated cell	266
Moxa	97, 109
mRNA	159, 172, 177, 248, 251, 253, 254, 277, 295, 296, 299, 354, 375
MRSA	449
Mucocele	35
Mucositis	94, 190, 198
Muscle regeneration	266
Myofibroblast	72, 428
Myoses	57, 440
Myotube	191, 266

N

NADH	554
Naloxone	296, 558
Nausea	97, 417
Nd:YAG	389, 390, 408
Nd:YAG (dental)	36
Nd:YAG (surgical)	36
Nd:YAG (therapeutic)	128
Nephritis	111
Nerve conduction	271
Nerve regeneration	76

O

Oedema	98, 109, 208, 216, 217, 248, 285, 297, 310, 311, 315, 322, 348, 359, 360, 365, 379, 383, 389, 399, 403, 404, 438
OPH gestosis	111
Ophthalmic problems	289
Opioid	530
Optical field	3, 4
Opto-acoustic waves	557
Oral surgery	417
Orthodontics	419
Osteoarthritis	153, 155, 164, 166, 167, 168, 169
Osteoblast	175, 176, 177, 178, 181, 183, 185, 188, 194, 196
Osteoclast	420
Osteocyte	196

P

Pacemaker	474
Paediatric patients	200, 426
Pain	293
Pain reaction	132
Paraesthesia	129, 210, 280, 282, 417
Parkinson's disease	381

I

IL-1 .... 250, 355
IL-6 159
IL-8 159
Immune system 72, 110, 114, 131, 190, 246
Impacted wisdom teeth 399, 400
Implantology 411
Incoherent polarised light 231, 528, 532
Infected wounds 369
Infertility 236, 346
Inflammation 89, 94, 123, 142, 160, 232, 247, 287, 290, 308, 323, 347, 348, 365
Inhibition 82, 124
Inner ear 120, 256, 330
Inorganic bovine bone graft 179
Interleukin 154, 356, 419, 441
interleukin IL-1beta 159
Intraligamental anaesthesia 389, 426
Irradiation of the brain 477
Ischemia 96, 597
Ischemic heart conditions 111, 207

J

Jaw fracture 415
Joule 77, 78

K

Keloid 34, 129
Keratinocyte 123, 356, 545, 597
Keratoconjunctivitis 53, 290
Krypton laser 47, 243, 358
KTP 28, 40

L

Laryngitis 256
Laser acupuncture 89, 97, 100, 138
Laser cytofluorometry 565
Laser Doppler Velocimeter 565
Laser microscopy 565
Laser phototherapy journals 620
Laser speckle flowmetry 263
Laser spectroscopy 565
Lasing effects in tissue 556
LED 6, 50, 55, 61, 89, 429, 449, 485, 490, 492, 513, 528, 529, 530, 535, 536, 547
Length of coherence 532
Leukoplakia 415, 450
Lichen 32, 256
Lingua geographica 415
Lip fissure 416
Lip wounds 416
Liver 360
Low back pain 46, 257
Lumbago 128
Lumbar disc herniation 257
Luminescence 555
Lung abscess 111
Lymph nodes 96, 244, 252, 255, 396, 426
Lymphatic system 72, 285, 286, 288, 352
Lymphocytes 124, 132, 246, 247, 342, 346, 560
Lymphoedema 194, 285, 286, 288

E

Eczema	377
Effects on blood circulation	559
Effects on the immune system	560
Elastase	406, 434
Electromagnetic radiation	2, 3, 4, 5
Endodontics	396
Endorphin	299, 530, 557
English language books on LPT	616
Epicondylitis	127, 230, 323
Epilepsy	474, 578
Epithelium down-growth	34, 427
Er:YAG	28, 383
Er:YAG (dental)	388, 389
Er:YAG (surgical)	36, 38
ErCr:YSGG	39
Erectile dysfunction	378
Excimer laser	20, 29, 42
Excitation	550
Extraction	98, 399
Eye hazard	512

F

Familial amyotrophic lateral sclerosis (FALS)	378
Fibrin network	285, 391
Fibroblast	35, 71, 77, 82, 91, 123, 129, 157, 159, 192, 272, 355, 365, 389, 400, 403, 404, 430
Fibromyalgia	164, 235, 451
Flap operatio	34, 35, 129, 430
Fluorescence	42, 450, 547, 555, 564
Fractures	180, 186, 188, 415
Frenectomy	37, 39
Frequency	2, 17
Frequency doubled Nd:YAG	40

G

GaAlInP laser	44
GaAs laser	45
Gagging	417
GAlAs laser	45
Genital	33, 242, 348
Gingivectomy	35, 405
Gingivitis	403
Glossitis	415
Goggles (protective)	20, 26, 45, 289
Gynaecology	33, 236

H

Haemangioma	32, 35, 40, 120
Haemoglobin	121, 285, 391, 540, 561
Haemorrhoids	239
Hair laser	240
Headache	100, 238, 338
Heat sensation	43, 45, 58, 71, 114, 138
HeNe laser	43, 53
Herpes simplex	37
Hologram	41
Hyperaemia	393
Hyperplasia	35, 39
Hyperreflexic bladder	237
Hypersensitive dentine	407

Cancer	5, 36, 42, 124, 131, 389
Candida albicans	89
Canker sore	389
Carbon dioxide laser (acupuncture)	98, 109
Carbon dioxide laser (surgical)	30
Carbon dioxide laser (therapeutic)	126
Cardiac conditions	203
Caries	393, 448
Caries detection	450
Carpal tunnel	208
Cartilage	158
Case reports	374, 450
cDNA	176, 357, 554
Cellulites	377
Cerebral palsy	214
C-fibre	271, 557
Chemiluminescence	76, 123, 140
Cholesterol reduction	377
Chondrocytes	158
Chromophore	71, 285, 547, 548
Chronic pain	222, 299, 313, 530, 558
Circulatory encephalopathy	111
Cluster probe	598
Coagulation	98, 360, 399, 469
Cochrane	218, 604
Collagen	69, 71, 82, 124, 128, 129, 139
Collimation	20, 118, 535, 540
Combination probe	513
Composite curing	449
Contraindications	473
Copper vapour laser	40
Corticosteroid	232, 282
COX-2	161, 171, 250, 251, 279, 297, 327
C-reactive protein	401
Cross-over study	100, 231, 373
Crural ulcer	214, 529
Cumulative effect	91, 92, 299
Cytochrome	71, 547, 552, 554, 689
Cytochrome-c-oxidase	160, 554
Cytotoxin	389, 479

D

de Quervain's disease	231
Delayed onset muscle soreness	313
Dentitio dificilis	301, 396
Depolarisation	271, 558
Depression	110, 222, 528, 541
Diabetes	480
Diabetes foot ulcers	228
Diagnostics with Therapy Lasers	564
Divergence	23, 25, 118, 489, 512, 595
DNA	1, 125, 158, 159, 175, 192, 193, 224, 344, 356, 404, 412
Dosage	77, 78, 80, 323, 331
Double blind studies	582
Dressings	371
Dry socket	388
Duodenal ulcer	229
Duty cycle	17, 19, 43, 574
Dye laser	28, 40, 42, 197, 360, 369

Alphabetic index

A

Absorption	4, 26, 31, 41
Acetylcholine	558
Achilles	314, 323, 324
Acne	34, 38, 128, 151
Acne	151
ACTH	299, 530
Acute calculous pyelonephritis	111
Acyclovir	243
Adhesion	95, 286, 323, 324
Alexandrite	21, 28, 29, 42
Alkaline phosphatase	176, 177, 180, 193, 213, 316
Allergy	4, 150, 152
Alveolitis	98, 293, 388, 418
Alzheimer's disease	375
An evaluation of the evaluators	610
Anaesthesia	36, 98, 388
Anaesthetics	98, 388, 389
Angiogenesis	203, 597
Angular cheilitis	416
Ankle sprain	314, 600
Ankylosing spondylarthritis	167
aPDT	448
Aphthae	39, 389, 390, 417, 418
Apoptosis	266, 550, 554
Argon	20, 28, 29, 40, 42
Arndt-Schulz law	514
Arthritis	153
Artificial insemination	470
Asthma	171
ATP	125, 247, 344, 559, 562
Autologous bone graft	175, 179
Average power output	17

B

Bacteria	74, 131, 190, 246, 394
Bechterew	153, 167
Bell's paralysis	282
Biostimulation	28, 29, 33, 40, 41, 43, 46, 67, 80, 126, 127, 145
Bisphosphonate-induced osteonecrosis	375
Bleeding	98, 391, 392
Blink reflex	23, 25
Blood flow	89, 114, 138, 139, 260, 265, 285, 352, 373, 392, 429
Blood pressure	173
Bone morphogenetic protein	178, 179, 187
Bone regeneration	128, 398
Books in other languages	618
Botox failures	376
Bright Light Phototherapy	541
Burns	362
Bursitis	164, 232

C

Calcium ion balance	71
cAMP	159
Can you trust your laser?	615

ROM	Range Of Movement
SEM	Sweep Electron Microscopy
SOD	Super Oxide Dismutase
SPIE	The International Society for Optical Engineering
TBO	Tolouidine Blue
TMD	Temporo Mandibular Disorders
TMJ	Temporomandibular joint
TMR	Transmyocardial Revascularisation
VAS	Visual Analogue Scale
YAG	Yttrium Aluminium Garnet

EDL	Emitted Defocused Laser-Light
EMG	Electromyogram
ENT	Ear-Nose-Throat
Er:YAG	Erbium Yttrium-Aluminium-Garnet
FCS	Fetal Calf Serum
FDA	Food and Drug Administration
GaAlAs	Gallium Aluminium Arsenide
GaAs	Gallium Arsenide
Gy	Gray
HeNe	Helium Neon
Ho:YAG	Holmium Yttrium-Aluminium-Garnet
HSV	Herpes Simplex Virus
IL	Interleukin
InGaAlP	Indium Gallium Aluminium Phosphide
IR	Infra Red
IRB	Institutional Review Board
KTP	Potassium (Kalium) Titanyle Phosphide
LED	Light Emitting Diode
MRI	Magnetic Resonance Imaging
Nd:YAG	Neodymium Yttrium-Aluminium-Garnet
NMRI	Nuclear Magnetic Resonance Imaging
NO	Nitric Oxide
NSAID	Non-Steriodal Anti-Inflammatory Drug
OA	Osteoarthritis
PD	Power Density
PDT	Photodynamic Therapy
PGE	Prostaglandine E
PHN	Postherpetic Neuralgia
RA	Rheumatic Arthritis
RNA	Ribonucleic Acid

Zhou Y C. Effect of HeNe laser irradiation of acupoint on analgesia and met-enkephalin contents in different regions in the rat. Laser Journal. 1986; 7: 41-. (in Chinese with English abstract)

Zhou, Chuannong; Song, Xuyan; Deng, Jinsheng; Liang, Junlin; Zhang, Hua; Huang, Wenjia; Liu, Tao; Ha, Xian-Wen Photodynamic effect of copper-vapor pumped-dye laser, HeNe laser, and noncoherent red light to the liver in normal mice. Proc. SPIE. 1993; Vol 1616: 239-245. (International Conference on Photodynamic Therapy and Laser Medicine, Jun-Heng Li; Ed.)

Zhu Q, Yu W, Yang X et al. Photoirradiation improved functional preservation of the isolated rat heart. Laser Surg Med. 1997; 20: 332-339.

Zhu X, Chen Y, Sun X. [A study on expression of basic fibroblast growth factors in periodontal tissue following orthodontic tooth movement associated with low power laser irradiation]. Hua Xi Kou Qiang Yi Xue Za Zhi. 2002; 20 (3): 166-168. (in Chinese)

Zimin A A, Zhevago N A, Buiniakova A I, Samoilova K A. [Application of low-power visible and near infrared radiation in clinical oncology]. Vopr Kurortol Fizioter Lech Fiz Kult. 2009; 6: 49-52. (in Russian)

Zinman L H, Ngo M, Ng E T et al. Low-intensity laser therapy for painful symptoms of diabetic sensorimotor polyneuropathy: a controlled trial. Diabetes Care. 2004; 27 (4): 921-924.

Zivin J A, Albers G W, Bornstein N, Chippendale T, Dahlof B, Devlin T, Fisher M, Hacke W, Holt W, Ilic S, Kasner S, Lew R, Nash M, Perez J, Rymer M, Schellinger P, Schneider D, Schwab S, Veltkamp R, Walker R, Streeter J. Effectiveness and safety of transcranial laser therapy for acute ischemic stroke. Stroke. 2009; 40 (4): 1359-1364.

Zubkova S T. [The use of helium-neon laser radiation in the treatment of trophic disorders in patients with diabetes mellitus]. Klin Khir. 1992; 3: 47-49. (in Russian with English abstract)

Zyss J. Renewed perspectives in Molecular Photonics and Biophotonics at the micro- and nano-scales. Proceedings of the Symposium on Photonics Technologies for 7th Framework Program, Wroclaw, Poland, 12-14 October 2006.

14.3 Abbreviations

Abbreviations used in this book are explained but not everywhere you meet them in the text. The following is a list of some of these abbreviations.

ASA	Acetylsalicylic Acid
ATP	Adenosine Triphosphate
BMP	Bone Morphogenetic Protein
CL	Chemiluminescence
CO_2	Carbon Dioxide
CTS	Carpal Tunnel Syndrome
CW	Continuous Wave
DNA	Deoxyribonucleic Acid
ED	Energy Density

Zalesskiy V N, Belousova I A, Frolov G V. Laser-acupuncture reduces cigarette smoking: a preliminary report. Acupunct Electrother Res. 1983; 8 (3-4): 297-302.

Zalewska-Kaszubska J, Obzejta D. Use of low-energy laser as adjunct treatment of alcohol addiction. Lasers Med Sci. 2004; 19 (2): 100-104.

Zan-Bar T, Bartoov B, Segal R, Yehuda R, Lavi R, Lubart R, Avtalion R R. Influence of visible light and ultraviolet irradiation on motility and fertility of mammalian and fish sperm. Photomed Laser Surg. 2005; 23 (6): 549-555.

Zanin I C, Goncalves R B, Aldo Brugnera Junior A, Hope K C, Pratten J. Susceptibility of Streptococcus mutans biofilms to photodynamic therapy: an in vitro study. Journal of Antimicrobial Chemotherapy. 2005; 56 (2): 324-330.

Zanin T, Zanin F, Carvalhosa A, Castro P H, Brugnera Jr A. Diode laser 660 nm in the prevention and treatment of oral mucositis. Proc. 7th Internat Congr of WALT, Sun City, South Africa, October 2008, page 28.

Zarkovic J et al. Use of HeNe laser for treatment of soft tissue trauma: evaluation by Gallium-67 citrate scanning. J Orthop and Sports Physical Therapy. 1986; 8 (2): 93-96.

Zati A, Fortuna D, Valent A, Pulvirenti F, Bilotta T W. Treatment of low back pain caused by intervertebral disk displacement: comparison between high power laser, TENS and NSAIDs. Medicina Dello Sport. 2004; 57 (1): 77-82.

Zazzio M. Pain threshold improvement for chronic hyperacusis patients in a prospective clinical study. Photomed Laser Surg. Accepted for publication 2009.

Zeredo J L, Sasaki K M, Fujiyama R et al. Effects of low power Er:YAG laser on the tooth pulp-evoked jaw-opening reflex. Laser Surg Med. 2003; 33 (3): 169-172.

Zeredo J L, Sasaki K M, Takeuchi Y, Toda K. Antinociceptive effect of Er:YAG laser irradiation in the orofacial formalin test. Brain Res. 2005; 1032 (1-2): 149-153.

Zeredo J L, Sasaki K M, Toda K. High-intensity laser for acupuncture-like stimulation. Lasers Med Sci. 2007; 22 (1): 37-41. [Epub 2006 Nov 21]

Zhang D, Gao Q. Treatment of facial paralysis with laser and acupuncture: report of 76 cases. Int J Clin Acupunct 1993; 4 (3): 327-329.

Zhang D, Zhou Y, Xiao B, Li G. The effect of postoperative irradiation with low incident levels of CO2 laser irradiation on skin flap survival and the possible mechanisms. Laser Therapy. 1992; 4 (2): 75-80.

Zhang Y, Song S, Chi-Chun Fong C C et al. cDNA Microarray Analysis of Gene Expression Profiles in Human Fibroblast Cells Irradiated with Red Light. Journal of Investigative Dermatology. 2003; 120: 849-857.

Zhang L, Xing D, Zhu D, Chen Q. Low-power laser irradiation inhibiting Abeta25-35-induced PC12 cell apoptosis via PKC activation. Cell Physiol Biochem. 2008; 22 (1-4): 215-222.

Zheng H, Qin J, Xin H, Xin S: The activation action of low level Helium Neon laser radiation on macrophages in the mouse model. Laser Therapy. 1992; 4 (2): 55-58.

Zhevago N A, Samoilova K A, Obolenskaya K D. The regulatory effect of polychromatic (visible and infrared) light on human humoral immunity. Photochem Photobiol Sci. 2004; 3 (1): 102-108.

Zhong X et al. Correlation between endogenous opiate-like peptides and serotonin in laseracupuncture analgesia. Am J Acupunct. 1989; 17: 39-43.

Zhong-Quan Zhao, Paul W. Dependence of light transmission through human skin on incident beam diameter at different wavelengths. Proc.SPIE. 1998; 3254: 354-361.

Zhou Y C. An Advanced Clinical Trial with Laser Acupuncture Anaesthesia for Minor Operations in the Oro-maxillofacial Region. Laser Surg Med. 1984; 4: 297-303.

Yew DT, Li WW, Pang KM, Mok YC, Au C. Stimulation of collagen formation in the intestinal anastomosis by low dose He-Ne laser. Scanning Microsc. 1989; 3 (1): 379-385; discussion 386.

Yilmaz S, Kuru B, Kuru L et al. Effect of galium arsenide diode laser on human periodontal disease: A microbiological and clinical study. Lasers Surg Med. 2002; 30 (1): 60-66.

Yo-Chen Zhou. Practical Applications of Non-contact laser therapy in Various Fields. In: Low Level Laser Therapy. A Practical Introduction, Eds. Ohshiro & Calderhead. John Wiley & Sons. 1988: 71.

Yokoyama K, Sugiyama K. Influence of Linearly Polarized Near-Infrared Irradiation on Deformability of Human Stored Erythrocytes. J Clinical Laser Medicine & Surgery. 2003; 21 (1): 19-22.

Yokoyama K, Sugiyama K. Temporomandibular joint pain anelgesia by linearly polarized near-infrared irradiation. Clin J Pain. 2001; 17: 47-51.

Yonaga T, Kimura Y, Matsumoto K. Treatment of cervical dentin hypersensitivity by various methods using pulsed Nd:YAG laser. Journal of Clinical Laser Medicine and Surgery. 1999; 17 (5): 205-210.

Yoo C, Lee W K, Kemmotsu O. Efficacy of polarized light therapy for musculoskeletal pain. Laser Therapy. 1993; 5 (4): 153-157.

Youssef M, Ashkar S, Hamade E, Gutknecht N, Lampert F, Mir M. The effect of low-level laser therapy during orthodontic movement: a preliminary study. Lasers Med Sci. 2008; 23 (1): 27-33.

Yoshida K, Kato M, Ishida S, Arao M, Fukaya M. The management of the facial palsy patients using lower power output laser irradiation. 4th International Congress on Lasers in Dentistry, Singapore, 1994: 39.

Yoshida T et al. Pain reduction effect of soft laser in orthodontic therapy. Proc. Annual Meeting Jpn Orthodont Soc. 1992: 69.

Young JM, Altschuler BR. Laser holography in dentistry. J Prosthet Dent. 1977; 38 (2): 216-225.

Yousefi-Nooraie R, Schonstein E, Heidari K, Rashidian A, Pennick V, Akbari-Kamrani M, Irani S, Shakiba B, Mortaz Hejri S, Mortaz Hejri S, Jonaidi A. Low level laser therapy for nonspecific low-back pain. Cochrane Database Syst Rev. 2008; 16 (2): CD005107.

Yu H S et al. Low energy helium-neon laser irradiation stimulates interleukin-1 alpha and interleukin-8 release from cultured human keratinocytes. J Invest Dermatol. 1996; 107 (4): 593-596.

Yu Hsin-Su, Wu Chieh-Shan, Yu Chia-Li et al. Helium-neon laser irradiation stimulates migration and proliferation in melanocytes and induces repigmentation in segmental-type vitiligo. J Invest Dermatol. 2003; 120 (1): 56-64.

Yu W, Naim J O, Lanzafame R J Effects of photostimulation on wound healing in diabetic mice. Laser Surg Med. 1997; 20 (1): 56-63.

Yu W et al. Improvement of host response to sepsis by photobiomodulation. Lasers in Surg Med. 1997; 21: 262-268.

Yu W, Naim J O, Lanzafame R J. The effect of laser irradiation on the release of bFGF from 3T3 fibroblasts. Photochem Photobiol. 1994; 59 (2): 167-170.

Yu W, Naim JO, McGowan M, Ippolito K, Lanzafame RJ. Photomodulation of oxidative metabolism and electron chain enzymes in rat liver mitochondria. Photochem Photobiol 1997; (6): 866-871.

Yu, I. Low Power Laser Therapy for carpal tunnel syndrome.Proc X Internat Congress Int Soc Laser Surg Med, Bangkok 1993, p. 197.

Yamada H, Kameya T, Abe N, Miyahara K. Low Level Laser Therapy in Horses. Laser Therapy. 1989; 1 (2): 31-36.

Yamada H, Ogawa H. Comparative study of 60 mW diode laser therapy and 150 mW diode laser therapy in the treatment of postherpetic neutralgia. Laser Therapy. 1995; 7 (2): 71-74.

Yamada H, Yamanaka Y, Orihara H et al. Preliminary clinical study comparing the effect of low level laser therapy (laser therapy) and corticosteroid therapy in the treatment of facial palsy. Laser Therapy. 1995; 7 (4): 157-162.

Yamada K. Biological effects of low power laser irradiation on clonal osteoblastic cells (MC3T3-E1). Nippon Seikeigeka Gakkai Zasshi. 1991; 65 (9): 787-799.

Yamada K. Effect of low power laser irradiation on osteoblastic cell growth. Surgical and Medical Lasers. 1989; 2-3 (2): 67. (abstract)

Yamaguchi M et al. Clinical study on the treatment of hypersensitive dentine by GaAlAs laser diode using the double blind test. Aichi Gakuin Daigaku Shigakkai Shi - Aichi-Gakuin Journal of Dental Science 1990; 28(2): 703-707. (In Japanese)

Yamamoto H et al. Pain clinic. 1987; 8: 43-48. (In Japanese)

Yamamoto J.et al. Effect of long-term aerobic exercise on helium-neon-laser-induced thrombogenesis in rat mesenteric arterioles and platelet aggregation. Haemostasis. 1993; 23 (3): 129-134.

Yamamoto Y, Kono T, Kotani H, Kasai S, Mito M. Effect of low-power laser irradiation on procollagen synthesis in human fibroblasts. J Clin Laser Med Surg. 1996; 14 (3): 129-132.

Yamaya M, Shiroto C, Kobayashi Mechanistic approach to GaAlAs diode laser effects on production of reactive oxygen species from human neutrophils as a model for therapeutic modality at cellular level. Laser Therapy. 1993; 5 (3): 111-116.

Yamazaki M, Miura Y, Tsuboi R, Ogawa H. Linear polarized infrared irradiation using Super Lizer is an effective treatment for multiple-type alopecia areata. Int J Dermatol. 2003; 42: 738-740.

Yamaura M E, Min E, Yao M E, Yaroslavsky I V, Cohen R et al. Low level laser therapy for reduction of chronic joint pain: in vitro studies. BiOS 2008, Proceedings of SPIE; Volume 6846-8.

Yamaura M, Yao M, Yaroslavsky I, Cohen R, Smotrich M, Kochevar I E. Low level light effects on inflammatory cytokine production by rheumatoid arthritis synoviocytes. Lasers Surg Med. 2009; 41 (4): 282-290.

Yan Li, Timon Cheng-Yi Liu, Rui Duan. Effects of some anaesthetics on wound healing: laser biomodulation mechanisms. Laser Surg Med. 2001; Suppl 13: 9. Laser Surg Med. 2001; Suppl 13: 9.

Yarita T et al. Effect of low power laser on gingival microcirculation. Proc. X Internat Congress Int Soc Laser Surgery and Medicine, Bangkok 1993, p 235.

Yasuda, Kubota J, Ohshiro T. The effects of diode laser low reactive-level laser therapy (laser therapy) on musculocutaneous flaps. Laser Therapy. 1993; 5 (4): 159-163.

Yasukawa A, Hrui H, Koyama Y, Nagai M, Takakuda K. The effect of low reactive-level laser therapy (LLLT) with helium-neon laser on operative wound healing in a rat model. J Vet Med Sci. 2007; 69 (8): 799-806.

Yeager R L, Franzosa J A, Millsap D S, Angell-Yeager J L et al. Effects of 670-nm phototherapy on development. Photomed Laser Surg. 2005; 23 (3): 268-272.

Yew D T et al. Low dose laser and the developing retina. A histochemical and scanning electronmicroscopic study. Acta Morphol Neerl Scand. 1982; 20: 57-63.

Yew D T et al. Responses of astrocytes in culture after low dose laser irradiation. Scand Microscopy. 1990; 4: 151-159.

Wozniak P, Stachowiak G, Pieta-Dolinska A, Oszukowski P. Laser acupuncture and low-calorie diet during visceral obesity therapy after menopause. Acta Obstet Gynecol Scand. 2003; 82 (1): 69-73.

Wright E F, Bifano S L. The Relationship between Tinnitus and Temporomandibular Disorder (TMD) Therapy. Int Tinnitus J. 1997; 3: 55-61.

Wright E F, Syms C A 3rd, Bifano S L. Tinnitus, dizziness, and nonotologic otalgia improvement through temporomandibular disorder therapy. Mil Med. 2000; 165: 733-736.

Wu J, Sanchez de la Pena S, Hallberg F et al. Chronosynergistic effects of lighting schedule-shift and cefodizime on plasmacytoma growth and host survival time. Chronobiologia. 1988; 15 (1-2) : 105-128.

Wu XB. 100 cases of facial paralysis treated with He-Ne laser irradiation on acupoints. J Tradit Chin Med 1990; 10 (4) :300-301.

Wu C S, Hu S C, Lan C C, Chen G S, Chuo W H, Yu H S. Low-energy helium-neon laser therapy induces repigmentation and improves the abnormalities of cutaneous microcirculation in segmental-type vitiligo lesions. Kaohsiung J Med Sci. 2008; 24 (4): 180-189.

Wu Wen-hsien, Ponnudurai R, Katz J et al. Failure to confirm report of light-evoked response of peripheral nerve to low power helium-neon laser light stimulus. Brain Research. 1987; 407-408.

Xian-Qiang M I, Chen J Y, Liang Z J, Zhou L W. In vitro effects of helium-neon laser irradiation on human blood: bloodviscosity and deformability of erythrocytes. Photomed Laser Surg. 2004; 22 (6): 477-482.

Xiaoa X, Donga J, Chua X et al. A single photon emission computed tomography of the therapy of intravascular low intensity laser irradiation on blood for brain infarction. Laser Therapy. 2001; 13: 110-113.

Xijing Wu et al. Observations on the effect of HeNe laser acupoint radiation in chronic pelvic inflammation. J Trad Chin Med. 1983; 7 (4): 263-265.

Xu D, Klaus Schulten K. Coupling of Protein Motion to Electron Transfer in a Photosynthetic Reaction Center: Investigating the Low Temperature Behavior in the Framework of the Spin-Boson Model. Department of Physics and Beckman Institute, University of Illinois at Urbana-Champaign, Urbana, IL 61801, USA. August 23, 2000.

Xu Xiao-Yang, Zhao Xiu-Feng et al. Cellular research on photobiomodulation on excercise induced skeletal muscular fatigue. Laser Surg Med. 2006; Abstract issue, p. 52, abstract 174.

Xu M, Deng T, Mo F, Deng B, Lam W, Deng P, Zhang X, Liu S. Low-intensity pulsed laser irradiation affects RANKL and OPG mRNA expression in rat calvarial cells. Photomed Laser Surg. 2009; 27 (2): 309-315.

Xu Yong-Qing et al. Experimental study of the effects of helium-neon laser radiation on repair of injured ten-don. Proc. SPIE. 1993; Vol 1616: 598-604. (International Conference on Photodynamic Therapy and Laser Medicine)

Yaakobi T et al. Promotion of bone repair in the cortical bone of the tibia in rats by low energy laser (He-Ne) irradiation. Calcif Tissue Int. 1996; 59 (4): 297-300.

Yaakobi T, Oron U. Enhancement of bone repair in the rat tibia by low energy laser irradiation. Laser Therapy. 1996; 8 (1):19. (abstract)

Yaakov N, Ben-Haim S, Oron U. Low level laser irradiation reduces interstitial scarring in the isoproternol-induced hypertrohpic rat heart. Laser Therapy. 1999; 11 (4): 190-197.

Yaakov N, Bdolah A, Wollberg Z et al. Recovery from Sarafotoxin-b induced cardiopathological effects in mice following low energy laser irradiation. Basic Research Cardiology. 2000; 95: 385-389.

Yagci I, Elmas O, Akcan E, Ustun I, Gunduz O H, Guven Z. Comparison of splinting and splinting plus low-level laser therapy in idiopathic carpal tunnel syndrome. Clin Rheumatol. 2009 Jun 21. [Epub ahead of print]

Williams R, Havoonjian H, Isagholian K, Menaker G, Moy R. A clinical study of hair removal using the long-pulsed ruby laser. Dermatol Surg. 1998; 24 (8): 837-42.

Wilson M et al. Bacteria in supragingival plaque samples can be killed by low-power laser light in the presence of a photosensitizer. J Appl Bacteriol 1995; 78 (5): 569-74.

Wilson M, Pratten A. Lethal photosensitisation of Staphylococcus aureus in vitro: effect of growth phase, serum, and pre-irradiation time. Lasers Surg Med. 1995; 16 (3): 272-276.

Vinck E, Coorevits P, Cagnie B, De Muynck M et al. Evidence of changes in sural nerve conduction mediated by light emitting diode irradiation. Lasers in Medical Science. 2005; 20 (1): 35-40.

Vinck E M, Cagnie B J, Cornelissen M J et al. Increased fibroblast proliferation induced by light emitting diode and low power laser irradiation. Lasers in Medical Science. 2003; 18 (2): 95-99.

Vinck E M, Cagnie B J, Cornelissen M J, Declercq H A, Cambier D C. Green light emitting diode irradiation enhances fibroblast growth impaired by high glucose level. Photomed Laser Surg. 2005; 23 (2): 167-171.

Vinck E, Cagnie B, Coorevits P, Vanderstraeten G, Cambier D. Pain reduction by infrared light-emitting diode irradiation: a pilot study on experimentally induced delayed-onset muscle soreness in humans. Lasers Med Sci. 2006; 21 (1): 11-18.

Winther A, Laserklinikken, Copenhagen, Denmark. 1997. Personal communication.

Winterle J S, Einarsdóttir O. Photoreactions of cytochrome C oxidase. Photochem Photobiol. 2006; 82 (3): 711-719.

Wirz-Justice A. Beginning to see the light. Arch Gen Psychiatry. 1998; 55 (10): 861-862. Review.

Witt U, Felix C. Selektive photo-Biochemotherapie in der Kombination Laser und Ginkgo-Pflanzenextrakt nach der Methode Witt. Neue Möglichkeiten bei Innerohrstörungen. (1989). Unpublished material.

Wollman Y et al. Low power laser irradiation enhances migration and neurite sprouting of cultured rat embryonal brain cells. Neurol Res. 1996; 18 (5); 467-470.

Wong E et al. Successful management of female office workers with "repetitive stress injury" or "carpal tunnel syndrome" by a new treatment modality - application of low level laser. Int J Clin Pharmacol Ther. 1995; 33 (4): 208-211.

Wong E et al. Efficacy of Low Power Laser Therapy in the Pain Relief of Migraine Headaches. Proc Ninth Congress Soc Laser Surgery and Medicine, Anaheim, California, USA: 2-6 November 1991.

Wong E, Lee G, Mason D T. Temporal headaches and associated symptoms related to the styloid process and its attachments. Annn Acad Med Singapore. 1995; 24: 124-128.

Wong F. Laser treatment for headaches of neurogenic and neuromuscular origin. Laser Surg Med. Suppl 12, 2000: 13.

Wong S F, Wilder-Smith P. Pilot study on laser effects on oral mucositis in patients receiving chemotherapy. Cancer J. 2002; 8 (3): 247-254.

Wong-Riley M T, Liang H L, Eells JT, Chance B et al. Photobiomodulation directly benefits primary neurons functionally inactivated by toxins: role of cytochrome c oxidase. J Biol Chem. 2005; 11; 280 (6): 4761-4771.

Voskanian KSh, Simonian N V, Avakian TsM, Arutiunian A G. [Effect of helium-neon laser radiation on the radiosensitivity of Escherichia coli K-12 cells]. Radiobiologiia. 1985; 25 (4): 557-560. [in Russian]

Voskanian KSh, Arzumanian G M. [Radiation protective effects of laser irradiation with wavelength 532 nm]. Radiats Biol Radioecol. 1996; 36 (5): 731-733. [in Russian]

Wetterberg L. Light and biological rhythms. J Intern Med. 1994; 235 (1): 5-19.

Wetterberg L. Light therapy of depression; basal and clinical aspects. Pharmacol Toxicol 1992; 71, Suppl 1: 96-106.

Wetterberg L. Lighting. Nonvisual effects. Scand J Work Environ Health. 1990; 16 Suppl 1: 26-28.

Wetterberg L. Melatonin and affective disorders. Ciba Found Symp. 1985; 117: 253-65.

Wetterberg L. The importance of light for health and well-being. Läkartidningen. 1991; 30; 88 (5): 295-296. (in Swedish)

Wetterberg L. The significance of lighting for health and wellbeing. Nord Med. 1991; 106 (3): 90-91. (in Swedish)

Wetterberg L. Light and biological rhythms. Läkartidningen. 1992; 89 (37): 2915-2918. (in Swedish)

Whelan H T, Smits R L Jr, Buchman E V, Whelan N T et al. Effect of NASA light-emitting diode irradiation on wound healing. J Clin Laser Med Surg. 2001; 19 (6): 305-314.

Whelan H T, Buchmann E V, Dhokalia A, Kane M P et al. Effect of NASA light-emitting diode irradiation on molecular changes for wound healing in diabetic mice. J Clin Laser Med Surg. 2003; 21(2): 67-74.

Whelan H T, Connelly J F, Hodgson B D, Barbeau L, Post AC et al. NASA light-emitting diodes for the prevention of oral mucositis in pediatric bone marrow transplant patients. J Clin Laser Med Surg. 2002; 20 (6): 319-324.

White AR, Rampes H, Ernst E. Acupuncture for smoking cessation. Cochrane Database Syst Rev. 2002; (2): CD000009.

Whittaker P. Laser acupuncture: past, present, and future. Lasers in Medical Science. 2005; 19 (2): 69-80.

Vidal L, Pérez de Vargas I, Ruiz C, Parrado C, Peláez A. Effect of IR laser radiation in thyroid follicular cells: fine structural and stereological study. Proc. SPIE 1992; 1981: 273-277.

Vidal L, Ortíz M, Pérez de Vargas I. Ultrastructural Changes in Thyroid PerifollicularCapillaries During Normal Postnatal Development and After Infrared Laser Radiation. Lasers Med Sci. 2002; 17: 187-197.

Wiederrecht G P, Seibert M, Govindjee,Wasielewski M R. Femtosecond photodichroism studies of isolated photosystem II reaction centers. Proc Natl Acad Sci USA. 1994; 91 (19): 8999-9003.

Viegas V N, Marcelo Abreu E R, Viezzer C, Cantarelli Machado D, Sant'Anna Filho M et al. Effect of Low-Level Laser Therapy on Inflammatory Reactions during Wound Healing: Comparison with Meloxicam. Photomed Laser Surg. 2007; 25 (6): 467-473.

Wikner J, Andersson D E, Wetterberg L, Röjdmark S. Impaired melatonin secretion in patients with Wernicke-Korsakoff syndrome. J Intern Med. 1995; 237 (6): 571-575.

Wilden L, Dindinger D. Treatment of chronic diseases in the inner ear with low level laser therapy (laser therapy): pilot project. Laser Therapy. 1996; 8 (2): 209-212.

Wilden L, Ellerbrock D. Verbesserung der Hörkapazität durch Low-Level-Laser-Licht (LLLL). [Amelioration of the hearing capacity by low-level-laser-light (LLL)]. Lasermedizin. 1999; 14: 129-138.

Wilden L. The effect of low level laser light on innear ear diseases. In: Low Level Laser Therapy, Clinical Practice and Scientific Background. Eds. Jan Tunér and Lars Hode. Prima Books in Sweden AB (1999). ISBN 91-630-7616-0.

Wilden L, Karthein R. Import of radiation phenomena of electrons and therapeutic low-level laser in regard to the mitochondrial energy transfer. J Clin Med Surg. 1998; 16 (3): 159-165.

Wang Ya Zhu Jing et al. Vascular low level laser irradiation therapy in treatment of brain injury. Acta Laser Biol Sinica. 1999; 8 (2).

Vasheghani M M, Bayat M, Rezaei F, Bayat A, Karimipour M. Effect of low-level laser therapy on mast cells in second-degree burns in rats. Photomed Laser Surg. 2008; 26 (1): 1-5.

Wasserman I, Rabau M Y, Shoshan S. Collagen metabolism in lowpower CO_2 laser welded intesitinal anastomosis in rats. Proc Ninth Congress of the International Society for Laser Surgery and Medicine, Anaheim, Cal., 2-6 November 1991.

Watanabe H, Ishikawa I, Susuki M et al. Clinical assessment of the Erbium:YAG laser for soft tissue surgery and scaling. J Clin Laser Med Surg. 1996; 14 (2): 67-75.

Waylonis G W, Wilke S, O'Toole D et al. Chronic myofascial pain: management by low-output helium-neon laser therapy. Arch Phys Med Rehab. 1988; 69 (12): 1017-1020.

Webb C et al. Stimulatory effect of 660 nm low level laser energy on hypertrophic scar-derived fibroblasts. Possible mechanisms for increase in cell count. Laser Surg Med. 1998; 22: 294.

Webb C, Dyson M, Lewis W H. Stimulatory effect of 660 nm low level laser energy on hypertrophic scar-derived fibroblasts: possible mechanisms for increase in cell counts. .Laser Surg Med. 1998; 22 (5): 294-301.

Weber J B, Pinheiro A L, de Oliveira M G et al. Laser therapy improves healing of bone defects submitted to autologous bone graft. Photomed Laser Surg. 2006; 24 (1): 38-44.

Weber J B, Pinheiro A L, de Oliveira M G et al. Laser therapy improves healing of bone defects submitted to autologus bone graft. PhD dissertation. 2005; School of Dentistry, Pontificia Universidade Católica do Rio Grande do Sul, Porto Alegre, Brazil.

Wee JS, Jung JC, Han JY, Lee SG, Rowe SM. Effects of Stellate Ganglion Irradiation by the Low-level Laser Therapy on Reflex Sympathetic Dystrophy of the Hemiplegic Arm. Chonnam Med J. 2001; 37 (1): 49-54.

Wedel H, Calero L, Walger M et al. Soft-laser/Ginkgo therapy in chronic tinnitus. A placebo-controlled study. Adv Otorhinolaryngol. 1995; 49: 105-108.

Wedlock P, Shephard R A, Little C, McBurney F. Analgesic effects of cranial laser treatment in two rat nociception models. Physiol Behav. 1999; 59 (3): 445-448.

Weintraub M I. Noninvasie laser neurolysis in carpal tunnel syndrome. Muscle Nerve. 1997; 20 (8): 1029-1031.

Weiss N, Oron U. Enhancement of muscle regeneration in the rat gastrocnemius muscle by low energy laser irradiation. Anat Embryol. 1992; 186: 497-503.

Weiss R A, McDaniel D H, Geronemus R G, Munavalli G M, Bellew S G. Clinical Experience with Light-Emitting Diode (LED) Photomodulation. Dermatol Surg. 2005; 31(Pt 2): 1199-1205.

Wenzel G I, Pikkula B, Choi C H, Anvari B, Oghalai J S. Laser irradiation of the guinea pig basilar membrane. Lasers Surg Med. 2004;35 (3): 174-180.

Wenzel G I, Anvari B, Mazhar A, Pikkula B, Oghalai JS. Laser-induced collagen remodeling and deposition within the basilar membrane of the mouse cochlea. J Biomed Opt. 2007; 12 (2): 021007.

Wenzel G I, Balster S, Zhang K, Lim H H, Reich U, Massow O, Lubatschowski H, Ertmer W, Lenarz T, Reuter G. Green laser light activates the inner ear. J Biomed Opt. 2009; 14 (4): 044007.

Vescovi P, Merigo E, Manfredi M, Meleti M, Fornaini C, Bonanini M, Rocca J P, Nammour S. Nd:YAG laser biostimulation in the treatment of bisphosphonate-associated osteonecrosis of the jaw: clinical experience in 28 cases. Photomed Laser Surg. 2008; 26 (1): 37-46.

Wetterberg L et al. Light therapy of depression. Läkartidningen. 1991; Jan 30; 88 (5): 310-312. (in Swedish)

von Ahlften U et al. Erfahrungen bei der Behandlung aphtöser und herpetiformer Mundschleimhauterkrankungen mit einem neuen Infrarotlaser. Die Quintessenz. 1987; 5: 927-933.

Voronin I T et al. [The use of laser therapy for restoring the fertilizing capacity of the ejaculate in men with chronic genital inflammation.] Vopr Kurortol Fizioter Lech Fiz Kult. 1994; 2: 24-26.

Vulliez C et al. Éffet du Laser Infra Rouge a Diode sur le Tissue Conjuctif. Innov. Tech Biol. Med. 1990; 11(1): 143-.

Wafa F et al. A clinical study of laser therapy in fixed posthodontic pain control after tooth preparation to receive a crown.. 1990; 2 (2): 83-88.

Wahl G, Bastianer S. Soft laser in postoperative care in dentoalveolar treatment. ZWR. 1991; 100 (8): 512-515.

Waiz M, Saleh A Z, Hayani R, Jubory S O. Use of the pulsed infrared diode laser (904 nm) in the treatment of alopecia areata. J Cosmet Laser Ther. 2006; 8 (1): 27-30.

Wakabayashi H et al. Effect of Irradiation by Semiconductor Laser on Responses Evoked in Trigeminal Caudal Neurons by Tooth Pulp Stimulation. Laser Surg Med. 1993; 13: 605-.

Wakabayashi H et al. Treatment of dentine hypersensitivity by GaAlAs soft laser irradiation. J Dent Research. 1988; 67: 182.

Walker J B, Swartzwelder H S, Bondy S C. Suppression of Hippocampal Epileptiform Activity In Vitro After Laser Exposure. Laser Therapy. 1989; 1 (1): 19-22.

Walker J B et al. Laser therapy for pain of rheumatoid arthritis. Laser Surg Med. 1986; 6: 171-.

Walker J B et al. Laser Therapy for pain of trigeminal neuralgia. Pain 1987; 29: 585-.

Walker J B et al. Laser Therapy for pain of Rheumatoid Arthritis. The Clinical Journal of Pain. 1987; 3 (53): 54-59.

Walker J B. Relief from Chronic Pain by Low Power Laser Irradiation. Neuroscience Letters. 1983; 43: 339-344.

Walker J B. Temporary suppression of clonus in humans by brief photo-stimulation. Brain Research. 1985; 340: 109-113.

Walker J. Treatment of human neurological problems by laser photostimulation. U.S. patent 4,671,285, 1987.

Walker M D, Rumpf S, Baxter G D, Hirst D G, Lowe A S. Effect of low-intensity laser irradiation (660 nm) on a radiation-impaired wound-healing model in murine skin. Lasers Surg Med. 2000; 26 (1): 41-47.

Walsh D et al. The effect of low intensity laser irradiation upon conduction and skin temperature in the superficial radial nerve. Double blind placebo controlled investigation using experimental ischaemic pain. Proc. Second Meeting of the International Laser Therapy Association, London Sept 1992.

Walsh D, Baxter D, Allen J. Lack of effect of pulsed low-intensity infrared (820) nm laser irradiation on nerve conduction in the human superficial radial nerve. Lasers in Surg Med. 2000; 26: 485-490.

Walsh L J. The use of lasers in implantology: an overview. J Oral Implantol. 1992; 18: 335-340.

Walter Wintsch, Switzerland, personal communication

Wang F, Wang Z. Observation on clinical effect of 70 cases of acute otitis media treated by He-Ne laser radiation on acupoints. Chin J Acupunct Moxibustion. 1991; 4 (1): 30-33.

Wang L-S, Kameya T, Yamada H. A Review of Clinical Applications of Low Level Laser Therapy in Veterinary Medicine. Laser Therapy. 1989; 1 (4): 183-190.

Vecchio P et al. A double-blind study of the effectiveness of low level laser treatment of rotator cuff tendinitis. Br J Rheum. 1993; 32: 740-742.

Vekshin N A. Light-dependent ATP synthesis in mitochondria. Mol. Biol. (Moscow). 1991; 25: 54.

Vélez-González M et al. Activation of the subcutanus absorbtion of drugs previous laser irradiation. Proc. Ninth Congress of the International Society for Laser Surgery and Medicine, Anaheim, California, USA: 2-6 November 1991.

Vélez-Gonzáles M A. Absorción subcutaneo del salicilato de dietilamina tras la irradiación laser. Boletín CDL. 1987; 4 (12): 4-8.

Vélez-González M et al. Treatment of relapse in Herpes Simplex on labial & facial areas and of primary herpes simplex on genital areas and "area pudenda" with low power laser (HeNe) or Acyclovir administred orally. Proc SPIE. 1995; Vol 2630: 43-50.

Velizhanina I A et al. [The laser therapy of hypertension patients in the initial stages.] Voprosy Kuror Fizioter Lecheb Fiziches Kult. 1998; 1: 9-11.

Venancio R A, Camparis CM, Lizarelli R F. Low intensity laser therapy in the treatment of temporomandibular disorders: a double-blind study. J Oral Rehabil. 2005; 32 (11): 800-807.

Verbruggen L A et al. Low-power laser therapy in chronic rheumatic diseases: Western and Soviet experiences. Phys Med Rehab. 1991; 1: 101.

Verdote-Robertson R, Munchua M M, Reddon J R. The use of low intensity laser therapy (LILT) for the treatment of open wounds in psychogeriatric patients: A pilot study. Physical and Occupational Therapy in Geriatrics. 2000, 18 (2): 1-19.

Verhoeven M A. Electronic and Spatial Characteristics of the Retinylidene Chromophore of Rhodopsin. Dissertation, University of Leiden, The Netherlands, November 2005.

Verplanken M. Stimulation of wound healing after tooth extraction using low intensity laser therapy. Revue Belge de Medecine Dentaire. 1987; 42: 134-138.

Vieira A H, Passos V F, de Assis J S, Mendonça J S, Santiago S L. Clinical Evaluation of a 3% Potassium Oxalate Gel and a GaAlAs Laser for the Treatment of Dentinal Hypersensitivity. Photomed Laser Surg. 2009 Aug 28. [Epub ahead of print]

Villa G E P, Catirse A B, Lia R C, Lizarelli R F Z. Analysis in vivo on the effects of low power laser irradiation at stimulation of reactional dentin. Proc. 3rd Congress of ESOLA, Barcelona, Spain, May 2005, p. 52.

Villaplana L A, Sarti M A, Trelles M A et al. Changes in albino rat testicle interstitial cells after pituitary stimulation in vivo with HeNe laser. Laser Therapy. 1995; 7 (1): 19-22.

Villaplana-Torres L A, Sarti-Martinez M A, Montesinos M, Smith-Agreda V, Trelles M A. Morphofunctional aspects of the follicular cells of the thyroid of albino rats after pituitary activation with low power laser. Laser in Medicine and Surgery. 1985; 1 (3): 124-129.

Vizi E, Mester E, Tisza S, Mester A. Acetylcholine releasing effect of laser irradiation on Auerbach's plexus in guinea-pig ileum. J. Neural Transmission. 1977; 40: 305.

Vitreshchak T V, Mikhailov V V, Piradov M A, Poleshchuk V V et al. Laser modification of the blood in vitro and in vivo in patients with Parkinson's disease. Bull Exp Biol Med. 2003; 135 (5): 430-432.

Vladimirov Y, Borisenko G, Boriskina N et al. NO-hemoglobin may be a light-sensitive source of nitric oxide both in solution and in red blood cells. J Photochem. Photobiol. B Biol. 2000; 59: 115.

Vlassov V V, Pechatnikov L M, MacLehose H G. Low level laser therapy for treating tuberculosis. Cochrane Database Syst Rev. 2002; (3):CD003490.

Volkov V, Svirko Y P, Kamalov V F, Song L, El-Sayed M A. Optical rotation of the second harmonic radiation from retinal in bacteriorhodopsin monomers in Langmuir-Blodgett film: evidence for nonplanar retinal structure. Biophys J. 1997; 73 (6): 3164-3170.

Uchida K et al. Treatment of chronic prostatitis and prostatodynia with low reactive laser. Laser Therapy. (ILTA Okinawa Congr Abstr Issue) 1990; 2 (1): 36.

Ueda Y, Shimizu N. Pulse irradiation of low-power laser stimulates bone nodule formation. Journal of Oral Science. 2001; 43 (1): 55-56.

Ulrich M et al. Influence of laser light (830 nm) on the growth kinetics of rat rhabdomyosarcomas. University of Hamburg, Department of Accident Surgery. Part of M.D. thesis

Umeda Y et al. Blood pressure controlled by low reactive level diode laser therapy (laser therapy). Laser Therapy. 1990; 2 (2): 59-64.

Umetov M A. Effects of laser therapy on psychophysiological parameters and arterial blood pressure in drivers with hypertension. Med Tr Prom Ekol. 1996; 8: 10-12. (in Russian)

Urazalin Zh B et al. Laser therapy in the combined treatment of mandibular fractures. Stomatologiia. 1983; 62: 34-.

Utsunomiya T A histopathological study of the effects of low-power laser irradiation on wound healing of exposed dental pulp tissues in dogs, with special reference to lectins and collagens. J Endod. 1998; 24 (3): 187-193.

Vacca R A et al. Activation of mitochondrial DNA replication by He-He laser irradiation. Biochem Biophys Res Commun. 1993; 195 (2): 704-709.

Valiente-Zaldivar C et al. Laserterapía en la neuralgía trigeminal. Informa preliminar. Rev Cubana de Estomat. 1990; 2 (22): 166-171.

Valiente-Zaldivar C et al. Lasers en estomatología. Rev Cubana de Estomat. 1989: 26: 336-343.

Velizhanina I A, Gapon L I, Shabalina M S et al. [Efficiency of low-intensity laser radiation in essential hypertension]. Klinicheskaia Meditsina (Mosk). 2001; 79 (1): 41-44.

van Breugel H et al. Low energy HeNe laser irradiation effects proliferation and laminin production of rat Schwann cells in vitro. Laser Surg Med. 1991;Suppl 3:10.

van Breugel HH, Bär PR. Power Density and Exposure Time of HeNe Laser Irradiation Are More Important Than Total Energy Dose in Photo-Biomodulation of Human Fibroblasts in Vitro. Laser Surg Med. 1992; 12 (5): 528-537.

van den Brande P. Effect of HeNe - IR laser on cutaneous microcirculation in vascular patients. Proc. Lasertherapy III, Vrije Universiteit Brussel, October 1987.

van der Veen P, Lievens P. Low level laser therapy (laser therapy): The influence on the proliferation of fibroblasts and the influence of the regeneration process of lymphatic, muscular and cartilage tissue. In: Simunovic, Z (ed), Lasers in Medicine and Dentistry. Basic science and an up-to-date clinical application of low energy laser therapy. 2000: 187-217.

van der Ven P et al. The influence of IR-laser on the proliferation of fibroblasts: an in-vitro study. Proc. 2nd Congress World Assn for Laser Therapy, Kansas City, Sept 1998; p. 120-122.

van Dieten H E et al. Systematic review of the cost effectiveness of prophylactic treatments in the prevention of gastropathy in patients with rheumatoid arthritis or osteoarthritis taking nonsteroidal anti-inflammatory drugs. Ann Rheum Dis. 2000; 59 (10): 753-759.

van Rensburg S D, Wiltshire W A. The effect of soft laser irradiation on fluoride release of two fluoride-containing orthodontic bonding materials. J Dent Assoc S Afr. 1994; 49 (3): 127-131.

van Thor J J, Mackeen M, Kuprov I et al. Chromophore structure in the photocycle of the cyanobacterial phytochrome CPH1. Biophys J BioFAST, published on June 2, 2006.

Vasilotta A. I.R. laser: a new therapy in rhino-sino-nasal bronchial syndrome with asthmatic component. Proc X. Internat Congr Soc Laser Surg Med, Bangkok 1993, p. 161.

Vasseljen O et al. Low Level Laser versus placebo in the treatment of tennis elbow. Scand J Rehab Med. 1992; 24: 37-42. Also in Physiotherapy. 1992; 5: 329-334.

Tsai J-C, Kao M-C. The Biological Effects of Incident Low Power Density Laser Irradiation on Cultivated Rat Glial and Glioma Cells. Laser Therapy. 1989; 1 (4): 191-202.

Tsang D, Yew D T, Hui BS. Further studies on the effect of low-dose laser irradiation on cultured retinal pigment cells of the chick. Acta Anat (Basel) 1986; 125 (1):10-13.

Tsuchiya K et al. Diode laser irradiation selectively diminishes slow component of axonal volleys to dorsal roots from the saphenous nerve in the rat. Neuroscience Letters. 1993; 161: 65-68. Also: Tsuchiya K, Kawatani M, Takeshige C, et al.Laser irradiation abates neuronal responses to nociceptive stimulation of rat-paw skin.Brain Res Bull. 1994; 34 (4): 369-374

Tsurko V V, Muldiyarov PY, Sigidin YA. Laser therapy of rheumatoid arthritis. A clinical and morphological study. Terap Arkh. 1983; 55: 97-102. (in Russian)

Tsushima T et al. Effects of two-point linear polarised near-infrared irradiation in difficult temporomandibular joint disorders. Proc. 2nd Congress World Assn for Laser Therapy, Kansas City, September 1998; p. 29-30.

Tuby H, Maltz L, Oron U. Modulations of VEGF and iNOS in the rat heart by low level laser therapy are associated with cardioprotection and enhanced angiogenesis. Lasers Surg Med. 2006; 38 (7): 682-688.

Tuby H, Maltz L, Oron U. Low-level laser irradiation (LLLI) promotes proliferation of mesenchymal and cardiac stem cells in culture. Lasers Surg Med. 2007; 39 (4): 373-378.

Tuby H, Maltz L, Oron U. Implantation of low-level laser irradiated mesenchymal stem cells into the infarcted rat heart is associated with reduction in infarct size and enhanced angiogenesis. Photomed Laser Surg. 2009; 27 (2): 227-233.

Tulebaev R K et al. Indicators of the activity of the immune system during laser therapy of vasomotor rhinitis. Vestn. Otorinolaringol. 19989; 1: 46-49. (in Russian)

Tullberg M, Alstergren P J, Ernberg M M. Effects of low-power laser exposure on masseter muscle pain and microcirculation. Pain. 2003; 105 (1-2): 89-96.

Tullberg M, Ernberg M. Long-term effect on tinnitus by treatment of temporomandibular disorders: a two-year follow-up by questionnaire. Acta Odontol Scand. 2006; 64 (2): 89-96.

Tumilty S, Munn J, Abbott J H, McDonough S, Hurley D A, Baxter G D. Laser therapy in the treatment of achilles tendinopathy: a pilot study. Photomed Laser Surg. 2008; 26 (1): 25-30.

Tumilty S, Munn J, McDonough S, Hurley D A, Basford J R, Baxter G D. Low Level Laser Treatment of Tendinopathy: A Systematic Review with Meta-analysis. Photomed Laser Surg. 2009 Aug 26. [Epub ahead of print]

Tuncel A, Görgü M, Ayhan M et al. Treatment of anogenital warts by pulsed dye laser. Dermatol Surg. 2002; 28 (4): 350-352.

Tunér J, Hode L. It's all in the parameters: a critical analysis of some well-known negative studies on low-level laser therapy. J Clin Laser Med Surg. 1998; 16 (5): 245-248.

Tunér J, Hode L. Are all the negative studies really negative? Laser Therapy. 1998; 10 (4): 165-174.

Tunér J. 100 positive double-blind studies: enough or too little? Proc. SPIE. 1999; Vol. 4166: 226-232.

Tunér J. The Cochrane analyses - can they be improved? Laser Therapy. 1999; 11 (3): 138-143.

Tunér J. Is low-power pulsed laser ineffective in neural growth? Microsurgery. 2009; 29 (3): 251.

Turhani D, Scheriaub M, Kapralb D, Beneschc T et al. Pain relief by single low-level laser irradiation in orthodontic patients undergoing fixed appliance therapy. Am J Orthodont Dentofac Orthoped. 2006; 130 (3): 371-377.

Tuz H H, Onder E M, Kisnisci R S. Prevalence of otologic complaints in patients with temporomandibular disorder. Am J Orthod Dentofacial Orthop. 2003; 123: 620-623.

Timirgalef M J et al. [Laser therapy of the inflammatory diseases of the accessory nasal sinuses]. Vestn Otorin. 1985; 3: 56-60.

Tiphlova O, Karu T I. Action of low-intensity laser radiation on *Escherichia coli*. CRC Critical Rev. Biomed. Eng. 1991; 18: 387.

Tiphlova O, Karu T I. Dependence of *Escherichia coli* growth rate on irradiation with He-Ne laser and growth substrates. Lasers Life Sci. 1991; 4: 161.

Tiukhin N S et al. Laser therapy in patients with inflammatory pleural exudates. Problemy Tuberkuleza. 1997; 4: 38-40. (in Russian)

Toida M, Watanabe F, Kazumi Goto K, Shibata T. Usefulness of Low-Level Laser for Control of Painful Stomatitis in Patients with Hand-Foot-and-Mouth Disease. Journal of Clinical Laser Medicine & Surgery. 2003; 21 (6): 363-367.

Tolle R. Psychotherapy of depressive disorders: on the theoretical background and its clinical relevance. Ner-venarzt. 1997; 68 (7): 602-605.

Torres C S, dos Santos J N, Monteiro J S, Amorim P G, Pinheiro A L. Does the use of laser photobiomodulation, bone morphogenetic proteins, and guided bone regeneration improve the outcome of autologous bone grafts? An in vivo study in a rodent model. Photomed Laser Surg. 2008; 26 (4): 371-377.

Torriceilli P, Giavaresi G, Fini G A, Guzzardella G et al. Laser biostimulation of cartilage: in vitro evaluation. Biomed Pharmacother. 2001; 55: 117-120.

Tortamano A, Lenzi D C, Haddad A C, Bottino M C, Dominguez G C, Vigorito J W. Low-level laser therapy for pain caused by placement of the first orthodontic archwire: a randomized clinical trial. Am J Orthod Dentofacial Orthop 2009; 136 (5) 662-667.

Toscani A, Bombelli G. [Laser therapy in post-extraction alveolitis]. Dent Cadmos. 1987; 55 (9): 73-74. (In Italian)

Toya S, Motegi M, Inomata K, Ohshiro T. Report on a computer-randomized double blind clinical trial to determine the effectiveness of the GaAlAs (830 nm) diode laser for pain attenuation in selected pain. Laser Therapy 1994; 6 (3): 143-148.

Trelles M et al. Bone Fracture Consolidates Faster With Low-Power Laser. Laser Surg Med. 1987; 7: 36-45.

Trelles M A, Rigau J, Soto P et al. Infrared Diode Laser in Low Reactive-Level Laser Therapy (laser therapy) for Knee Osteoarthroses. Laser Therapy. 1991; 3 (4): 149-154.

Trelles M, Mayayo E, Miro L, Rigau J, Baudin G, Calderhead G. The action of low reactive level laser therapy (laser therapy) on mast cells. Laser Therapy. 1989; 1: 27-30.

Trelles M, Mayayo E. Mast cells are implicated in low power laser effect on tissue. A preliminary study. Lasers in Medical Science. 1992; 7: 73-.

Trelles M A, Rotinen S. He/Ne laser treatment of hemorrhoids. Acupuncture & Electro-Therapeutics Research. 1983; 8 (3-4): 289-95.

Treutlein H, Schulten K, Brünger A T, Karplus M, Deisenhofer J, Michel H. Chromophore-protein interactions and the function of the photosynthetic reaction center: a molecular dynamics study. Proc Natl Acad Sci USA. 1992; 89 (1): 75-79.

Trimmer P A, Schwartz K M, Borland M K, De Taboada L, Streeter J, Oron U. Reduced axonal transport in Parkinson's disease cybrid neurites is restored by light therapy. Mol Neurodegener. 2009; 17; 4 (1): 26.

Trümpler F, Oez S, Stähli P, Brenner H D, Jüni P. Acupuncture for alcohol withdrawal: a randomized controlled trial. Alcohol Alcohol. 2003; 38 (4): 369-375.

Tsai CL et al. Effect of CO2 laser on healing of cultured meniscus. Laser Surg Med. 1997; 20 (2): 172-178.

Taradaj J, Franek A, Cierpka L et al. Failure of low-level laser therapy to boost healing of venous leg ulcers in surgically and conservatively treated patients. Phlebologie 2008; 37 (5): 241-246.

Tardivo J P et al. Effect of low power laser over cells infected by herpes s mplex virus (HSV). Laser Surg Med. 1989; Suppl 1: 31.

Tasaki E et al. Application of low power laser therapy for relief of of low back pain. Proc Ninth congress of the International Society for Laser Surgery and Medicine, Anaheim, California, USA: 2-6 November 1991.

Tasaki et al. Application of low power laser therapy in closed lock temporomandibular joint dysfunction. Laser Surg Med. 1992; suppl 4: 84.

Tascioglu F, Armargan O, Tabak Y, Corapci I, Oner C. Low power laser treatment in patients with knee osteoarthritis. Swiss Med Wkly. 2004; 134 (17-18): 254-258.

Taube S, Piironen J, Ylipaavalniemi P. Helium-neon laser therapy in the prevention of postoperative swelling and pain after wisdom tooth extraction. Proc Finn Dent Soc 1990; 86: 23-27.

Tauber S, Baumgartner R, Schorn K, Beyer W. Lightdosimetric quantitative analysis of the human petrosus bone: experimental study for laser irradiation of the cochlea. Laser Surg Med. 2001; 28: 18-26. Also: Transmeatal cochlear laser (TCL) treatment of cochlear dysfunction: A feasibility study for chronic tinnitus. Lasers Med Sci. 2003;18 (3): 154-161.

Tay E J, Lee L I, Yee S, Loh H S. Laser-induced reduction of post-operative pain following third molar surgery. Laser Surg Med. 2001; Suppl 13: 17.

Teggi R T, Bellini C, Fabiano B, Bussi M. Efficacy of Low-Level Laser Therapy in Ménière's Disease: A Pilot Study of 10 Patients. Photomed Laser Surg. 2008; 26 (4): 249-253.

Tekeyoshi S, Takiyama R, Tsuno S et al. Low reactive-level infrared diode laser therapy (laser therapy) of the area over the stellate ganglion, and conventional anaestethic stellate ganglion block in treatment of allergic rhinitis: a preliminary comparative study. Laser Therapy. 1996; 8 (2): 159-164.

Telfer J, Filonenko N, Salansky N M. Leg ulcer plastic surgery descent by laser therapy. Proc. SPIE. 1994; Vol 2086: 258-263. (Medical Applications of Lasers)

Tenenbaum J. The epidemiology of nonsteroidal anti-inflammatory drugs. Can J Gastroenterol. 1999; 13: 119-122.

Tengroth B. [Ban the laser weapons! Invisible rays may cause permanent blindness in thousands of war victims!] [Article in Swedish]. Läkartidningen. 1995; 92 (9): 837.

Terashima H et al. Low Energy Laser Irradiation for Lateral Humeral Epycondylitis and de Quervains Disease. Laser Therapy. (ILTA Okinawa Congr Abstr Issue) 1990; 2 (1): 27.

Thalén B E, Kjellman B F, Mörkrid L, Wetterberg L. Melatonin in light treatment of patients with seasonal and nonseasonal depression. Acta Psychiatr Scand 1995; (4): 274-284.

Thalén B E, Kjellman B F, Mörkrid L, Wibom R, Wetterberg L. Light treatment in seasonal and nonseasonal depression. Acta Psychiatr Scand 1995; 91 (5): 352-360.

Thaweboon B, Sa-Nguansin S, Thaweboon S, Buajeeb W. In vitro enhanced neutrophils phagocytosis by Ga-Al-As diode laser. J Dent Res. 1995; 74 (Spec Issue): 570, Abstract 1354.

Thomasson T L.(Facial Pain/TMJ Centre, Denver, CO). Effects of Skin-Contact Monochromatic Infrared Irradiation on Tendonitis, Capsulitis and Myofascial Pain. 1995. 19th Annual Scientific Meeting, American Academy of Neurological & Orthopaedic Surgeons.

Thorsen H. [Low energy laser treatment-effect in localized fibromyalgia in the neck and shoulder regions.] Ugeskrift for Laeger. 1991; 17; 153 (25):1801-1804. (in Danish)

Thwee T, Kato J , Hashimoto M et al. Pulp reaction after pulpotomy with He-Ne laser irradiation. In: Abstract handbook. Vol 4. Internat Soc Laser in Dentistry. 1994. Denics Pacific Ltd, Hong Kong. HeNe laser in combination with calcium hydroxide created dentin-like calcified layer after pulpotomy in Wistar rats.

Taha M F, Valojerdi M R. Quantitative and qualitative changes of the seminiferous epithelium induced by Ga. Al. As. (830 nm) laser radiation. Lasers Surg Med. 2004; 34 (4): 352-359.

Tajali S B, Bayat M, Ebrahimi E et al. Effects of low power He-Ne laser on bone regeneration in rabbits from biomechanical point of view. Proc. 3rd Congr World Assn for Laser Therapy, Athens, Greece, May 2000, p. 86-87.

Taly A B, Sivaraman Nair K P, Thyloth Murali T, Archana J. Efficacy of multiwavelength light therapy in the treatment of pressure ulcers in subjects with disorders of the spinal cord: A randomized double-blind controlled trial. Archives of Physical Medicine and Rehabilitation. 2004; 85 (10): 1657-1661.

Takac S. Treatment of menstrual pain with GaAs-laser therapy. Novi Sad, Yugoslavia. 1992 (personal communication).

Takamoto M, Magalhães Da Cruz F, Ladalardo T C; Tarso Mugnai Marraccini; Brugnera Júnior A, De Carvalho Campos R A. Evaluation of the effect of Laser Therapy in the treatment of trigeminal neuralgia. Photomed Laser Surg. 2005; 23 (1). Abstracts from the 5th Congress of the World Association for Laser Therapy, São Paulo, Brazil, November 2004. Poster no 28, page 121.

Takashi K. Clinical evaluation of a GaAlAs semiconductor unilaser irradiation on solitary aphta erosion and hypersensitive dentine. Shikwa Gauko. 1987; 87 (2): 295-.

Takahashi Y, Hitomi S, Hirata T, Fukuse T, Yamazaki F, Cho K, Wada H. Neovascularization effect with HeNe laser in the rat trachea. Thoracic & Cardiovascular Surgeon. 1992; 40 (5): 288-291.

Takahashi T, Fukuda M, Ohnuki T et al. Nd:YAG LLLT in the treatment of temporomandibular disorders: a treatment protocol and preliminary report. Laser Therapy. 1998; 10 (1): 7-15.

Takeda Y. Irradiation effect of low-energy laser on alveolar bone after tooth extraction. Experimental study in rats. Int J Oral Maxillofac Surg. 1988; 17: 388-391.

Takeda Y. Irradiation effect of low-energy laser on rat submandibular salivary gland. J Oral Pathol. 1988; 17: 91-94.

Takema T, Yamaguchi M, Abiko Y. Reduction of plasminogen activator activity stimulated by lipopolysaccharide from periodontal pathogen in human gingival fibroblasts by low-energy irradiation. Lasers Med Sci. 200; 15 (1): 35-42.

Taly A B, Sivaraman Nair K P, Murali T, John A. Efficacy of multiwavelength light therapy in the treatment of pressure ulcers in subjects with disorders of the spinal cord: A randomized double-blind controlled trial. Archives of Physical Medicine and Rehabilitation. 2004; 85 (10): 1657-1661.

Tam G. Low power laser therapy and analgesic action. J Clin Laser Med Surg. 1999; 17 (1): 29-33.

Tamachi Y. Enhancement of antitumor chemotherapy effect by low level laser irradiation. Tokyo Medical College Newsletter 1991: 888-893.

Tamagawa S, Otsuka H, Kemmotsu O. Severe intractable facial pain attenuated by a combination of infrared diode low reactive-level laser therapy and stellate ganglion block. Laser Therapy. 1996; 8 (2): 155-158.

Tan C H, Sin Y M. The use of laser acupuncture point for smoking cesssation. American J Acupuncture. 1987; 15: 137-141.

Tang X M, Chai B P. Effect of CO2 laser irradiation on experimental fracture healing: a transmission electron microscopy study. Laser Surg Med. 1986; 6: 346-352.

Tang J, Godlewski G, Rovy S et al. Morphologic changes in collagen fibers after 830 nm diode welding. Laser Surg Med. 1997; 21: 438-443.

Taniguchi D, Dai P, Hojo T, Yamaoka Y, Kubo T, Takamatsu T. Low-energy laser irradiation promotes synovial fibroblast proliferation by modulating p15 subcellular localization. Lasers Surg Med. 2009; 41 (3): 232-239.

Stadler I, Lanzafame R J, Oskoui P, Zhang R Y, Coleman J, Whittaker M. Alteration of skin temperature during low-level laser irradiation at 830 nm in a mouse model. Photomed Laser Surg. 2004; 22 (3): 227-231.

Stergioulas A. Low-level laser treatment can reduce edema in second degree ankle sprains. J Clin Laser Med Surg. 2004; 22 (2): 125-128.

Stergioulas A, Stergioula M, Aarskog R, Lopes-Martins R A, Bjordal J M. Effects of Low-Level Laser Therapy and Eccentric Exercises in the Treatment of Recreational Athletes With Chronic Achilles Tendinopathy. Am J Sports Med. 2008; 36 (5): 881-887.

Stergioulas A. Effects of Low-Level Laser and Plyometric Exercises in the Treatment of Lateral Epicondylitis. Photomed Laser Surg. 2007; 25 (3): 205-213.

Stergioulas A. Low-Power Laser Treatment in Patients with Frozen Shoulder: Preliminary Results. Photomed Laser Surg. 2008; 26 (2): 99-105

Streeter J, De Taboada L, Oron U. Mechanisms of action of light therapy for stroke and acute myocardial infarction. Mitochondrion. 2004; 4 (5-6): 569-576.

Strupinska E. Low-power-laser therapy used in tendon damage. Proc. SPIE. 1996; Vol 2781: 177-183. (Lasers in Medicine)

Sudoh A et al. Effect of low power laser irradiation on experimental tooth movement. J Dent Res 74 (IADR Abstracts). 1995; p. 457. abstr. 453.

Sugrue M E et al. The use of infrared laser therapy in the treatment of venous ulceration. Ann Vasc Surg. 1990; 4 (2): 179-181.

Sun X H, Zhu X, Xu C, Ye N, Zhu H. [Effects of low energy laser on tooth movement and remodeling of alveolar bone in rabbits]. Hua Xi Kou Qiang Yi Xue Za Zhi. 2001; 19 (5): 290-293. (in Chinese)

Sun X H, Wang R, Zhang X Y. [Effects of He-Ne laser irradiation on the expression of transforming growth factor beta1 during experimental tooth movement in rabbits]. Shanghai Kou Qiang Yi Xue. 2006; 15 (1): 52-57. (in Chinese)

Sun Y, Oberley L W. Redox regulation of transcriptional activators. Free Rad Biol Med. 1996; 21: 335-338.

Supiev T K. Action of laser radiation on the course of an inflammatory process in the maxillofacial area. Stomatologiia (Mosk). 1984; 5: 17-19.

Svaasand L. O. Biostimulering med lav-intensitetslasere. Fysikk eller metafysikk? ["Biostimulation with low intensity laser: Physics o or metaphysics?"] Nordisk Medicin. 1990; 103 (3): 72-.(in Norwegian)

Swoboda R, Schott A. Behandlung neurotologischer Erkrankungen mit Gingko biloba Hevert, Hyperforat und Low-Power-Laser-Therapie. Medizinische Akademie Erfurt. (1992)

T-W Marín V. Experimental wound healing with coherent and non-coherent radiation. Laser & Technology. 1992; 2 (3): 121-134.

Tabau C. Contributions from Midlaser in the treatment of lateral ankle sprain. Medical Laser Report. 1984; 1: 29-32.

Takaduma K. Possible application of the laser in immunobiology. Keio J Med. 1993; 42 (4): 180-182.

Taghawinejag M Fricke R. Laser Therapie in der Behandlung kleiner Gelenke bei chronischer Polyarthritis. Z Phys Med Baln Med Klin. 1985; 14: 402-408.

Taguchi T et al. Thermographic Changes Following Laser Irradiation for Pain Relief. J Clin Laser Med Surg. l99l; 9 (2): 143-.

Taguchi Y. Clinical experiences of laser applications in physical therapy. Proc. 2nd Congress World Assn for Laser Therapy, Kansas City, September 1998; p. 106.

Soroor N. Comparison between the effects of low level laser therapy (LLT) and Magnetic low level laser therapy (MLLLT) in treatment of knee osteoarthritis. Abstract. WALT2006, Lemesos, Cyprus, October 2006.

Soudry M et al. Action d' un laser hélium-néon sur la croissance cellulaire: étude in vitro sur fibroblastes gingivaux humains. J Biol Buccale. 1988; 16: 129-.

Soukos N S, Som S, Abernethy A D et al. Phototargeting oral black-pigmented bacteria. Antimicrob Agents Chemother. 2005; 49 (4): 1391-1396.

Sussai D A, Carvalho P D, Dourado D M, Belchior A C, Dos Reis F A, Pereira D M. Low-level laser therapy attenuates creatine kinase levels and apoptosis during forced swimming in rats. Lasers Med Sci. 2009 Jun 25. [Epub ahead of print]

Souza S C, Munin E, Alves L P, Salgado M A, Pacheco M T. Low power laser radiation at 685 nm stimulates stem-cell proliferation rate in Dugesia tigrina during regeneration. J Photochem Photobiol B. 2005; 80 (3): 203-207.

Sousa L R, Cavalcanti B N, Marques M M. Effect of Laser Phototherapy on the Release of TNF-alpha and MMP-1 by Endodontic Sealer-Stimulated Macrophages. Photomed Laser Surg. 2009 Jan 30. [Epub ahead of print]

Spanner D C. The active transport of water under temperature gradient. Symp. Soc. Exp. Biol. 1954; 8: 76.

Spivak J M, Grande D A et al. The effect of low-level Nd:YAG laser energy on adult articular cartilage in vitro. Arthroscopy. 1992; 8 (1): 36-43.

Stadler I, Oskoui P, Ellie C et al. Alteration of skin temperature in a mouse model during low energy level laser irradiation at 830 nm. Laser Surg Med. Abstract issue, 2002: 11.

Stadler I, Evans R, Kolb B et al. In vitro effects of low-level laser irradiation at 660 nm on peripheral blood lymphocytes. Laser Surg Med. 2000; 27: 255-261.

Stadler I, Lanzafame R J, Evans R et al. 830 nm irradiation increases the wound tensile strength in a diabetic murine model. Lasers in Surg Med. 2001; 28 (3): 220-226.

Stadler I, Lanzafame R J, Oskoui P, Zhang R Y, Coleman J, Whittaker M. Alteration of skin temperature during low-level laser irradiation at 830 nm in a mouse model. Photomed Laser Surg. 2004; 22 (3): 227-231

Stein A, Kraicer P, Oron U. Effect of low energy (He-Ne) irradiation on embryo implantation rate in the rat. In: Proc. Low Power Light Effects in Biological Systems. Proc. SPIE. 1997; Vol. 3198: 24-30.

Stein A, Benayahu D, Maltz L, Oron U. Low-level laser irradiation promotes proliferation and differentiation of human osteoblasts in vitro. Photomed Laser Surg. 2005; 232: 161-166.

Stein E, Koehn J, Sutter W, Wendtlandt G, Wanschitz F, Thurnher D, Baghestanian M, Turhani D. Initial effects of low-level laser therapy on growth and differentiation of human osteoblast-like cells. Wien Klin Wochenschr. 2008; 120 (3-4): 112-117.

Steinlechner C, Dyson M. The effect of low level laser therapy on the proliferation of keratinocytes. Laser Therapy; 1993; 5 (2): 65-74.

Stelian J, Gil I, Habot B et al. Improvement of Pain and Disability in Elderly Patients with Degenerative Osteoarthritis of the Knee Treated with Narrow-Band Light Therapy. 1992. J Am Geriatr Soc; 40: 23-26.

Stoffel M et al. Low-energy He-Ne-laser irradiation of the bovine mammary gland. Zentralbl Veterinarmed A. 1989; 36 (8): 596-602.

Strada G et al. Semi-conductor laser ray therapy for the treatment of abacterial chronic prostatitis, induratio penis plastica and urethral stenosis. In: Lasers in Medicine and Dentistry. Ed. Simunovic Z. 2000. European Medical Laser Assn. ISBN 953-6059-30-4.

Smithdeal C D et al. Carbon dioxide laser-assisted hair transplantation. The effect of laser parameters on scalp tissue - a histological study. Dermatol. Surg. 1997; 23 (9): 835-840.

Smolyaninova N K, Karu T I, Fedoseyeva G E, Zelenin A V. Effect of He-Ne laser irradiation on chromatin properties and nucleic acids synthesis of human blood lymphocytes, Biomed. Sci. 1991; 2: 121.

Snyder S K, Byrnes K R, Borke R C, Sanchez A, Anders J J. Quantitation of calcitonin gene-related peptide mRNA and neuronal cell death in, facial motor nuclei following axotomy and 633 nm low power laser treatment. Lasers Surg Med. 2002; 31 (3): 216-222.

Snyder-Mackler L, Bork C, Bourbon B et al. Effect of Helium-Neon Laser on Musculoskeletal Trigger points. Physical Therapy. 1986; 66 (7): 1087-1090.

Snyder-Mackler L et al. Effect of helium-neon laser irradiation on peripheral sensory nerve latency. Physical Therapy. 1988; 68: 223-227.

Snyder-Mackler L et al. Effect of helium-neon laser irradiation on skin resistance and pain in patients with trigger points in the neck or back. Physical Therapy. 1989; 69: 336-341.

Sobanko J F, Alster T S. Efficacy of Low-Level Laser Therapy for Chronic Cutaneous Ulceration in Humans: A Review and Discussion. Dermatol Surg. 2008; 34 (8): 991-1000.

Sokolova I et al. Low-intensity laser radiation in complex treatment of inflammatory diseases of parodontium. Proc SPIE. 1995; Vol 1984: 234-237.

Soldo I et al. Effects of GaAs laser combined with radiotherapy on murine sarcoma depends on tumor size. Laser Surg Med. 1989; Suppl 1: 40.

Sommer, A.P. Components for NOA of Biosystems and Nanoscale Resolution, in: Proc. 1st International Workshop on Nearfield Optical Analysis, Reisensburg, Germany, November 2000, (ed. A.P. Sommer). J Clin Laser Med & Surg. 2001., 19: 112.

Sommer, A P, Franke, R P. Hydrophobic optical elements for near-field optical analysis (NOA) in liquid environment - a preliminary study. Micron. 2002; 33: 227-231.

Sommer, A P, Franke R P. Near-Field Optical Analysis of Living Cells in Vitro. Journal of Proteome Research; 2001 1: 111-114.

Sommer, A P. Novel Low Intensity Light Activated Biostimulation Paradigm, in: Abstracts of the Second Congress of the North American Association for Laser Therapy & First Consensus Conference on Laser Medicine, Photobiology and Bioengineering of Tissue Repair, Atlanta, GA, March 2002.

Soriano F et al. Low level laser therapy response in patients with chronic low back pain. A double blind study. Laser Surg Med. 1998. Suppl 10, p. 6.

Soriano F. GaAs laser treatment of venous ulcers. Proc. 2nd Congress World Assn for Laser Therapy, Kansas City, September 1998; p. 128-130.

Soriano F. Venous leg ulcers healed with GaAs laser. Argentine experience. Proc Congr Int Soc Laser Surg Med, Bangkok 1993, p. 35.

Soriano F et al. The analgesic effect of 904 nm gallium arsenide semiconductor low level laser therapy (laser therapy) on osteoarticular pain: a report on 938 irradiated patients. Laser Therapy. 1995; 7 (2): 75-80.

Soriano F, Campaña V, Soriano M, Soriano R.Vasculitis Ulcers Irradiated with Ga. As. Laser: Ten years of experience. Soriano F, Campana V, Soriano M, Soriano R. Photomed Laser Surg. 2005; 23 (1). Abstracts from the 5th Congress of the World Association for Laser Therapy, São Paulo, Brazil, November 2004. Abstract no 050, p.102.

Soriano F, Campaña V, Moya M, Gavotto A et al. Photobiomodulation of pain and inflammation on microcrystalline arthropathies: experimental and clinical results. Photomed Laser Surg. 2006; 24 (2): 140-150.

Simunovic-Soskic M, Pezelj-Ribaric S, Brumini G, Glazar I, Grzic R, Miletic I. Salivary Levels of TNF-alpha and IL-6 in Patients with Denture Stomatitis Before and After Laser Phototherapy. Photomed Laser Surg 2009 Oct 1 [Epub ahead of print].

Sinev I V et al. [The local treatment of chemical burns of the esophagus via an endoscope by means of laser therapy and adhesive application.] Vestnik Khirurgii Imeni i - i - Grekova 1990; 145 (11): 62-64.

Singer R, Sagiv M, Barnet M et al. Low energy narrow band non-coherent infrared illumination of human semen and isolated sperm. Androl.1991; 23: 181-184.

Siposan D, Lukacs A. Effect of low-level laser radiation (lllr) in some rheological factors in human blood: an in vitro study. Clin J Laser Med Surg. 2000; 18 (4): 185-195.

Siposan D, Lukacs A. Relative variation to received dose of some erythrocytic and leukocytic indices of human blood as a result of low.level laser radiation: An in vitro study. J Clin Laser Med Surg. 2001; 19 (2): 89-103.

Siposan D. An in vitro study of the effects of low-level laser radiation on human blood.Laser in Medical Science. 2002; 17 (4). Proc. 14th Annual Meeting of Deutsche Gesellschaft für Lasermedizin, Munich, Germany, June 2003.

Sirenko I N et al. Changes in the parameters of central and regional hemodynamics in the patiens with unstable stenocardia treated by the methods of quantum hemotherapy. Lik Sprava. 1992; (6): 70-73.

Sitnikov V P et al. [Use of helium-neon lasers in the treatment of postoperative wounds of the pharynx]. Vestnik Otorinolaringologii. 1989; (5): 46-49.

Skinner S M, Gage J P, Wilce P A, Shaw R M. A preliminary study of the effects of laser radiation on collagen metabolism in cell culture. Aust Dent J 1996; 41 (3):188-192.

Skobelkin O K et al. [Use of lasers in the treatment of acute suppurative lactation mastitis]. Vestn Khir Im I I Grek. 1988; 141 (9): 46-49.

Skobelkin O K, Michailov V A, Zakharov S D. Preoperative activation of the immune system by low reactive level laser therapy (laser therapy) in oncologic patients: A preliminary report. Laser Therapy. 1991; 3 (4): 169-176.

Skopin M D, Molitor S C. Effects of near-infrared laser exposure in a cellular model of wound healing. Photodermatol Photoimmunol Photomed. 2009; 25 (2): 75-80.

Skoric T et al. Laser biostimulation: application of the gallium-arsenide laser in the therapy of ulcus cruris. Laser Surg Med. 1998; Suppl. 10: 7.

Slattery K, Amy R, Pinto J et al. Treatment of chronic neck and shoulder pain with 635 nm low level laser therapy. A randomized, multi-center, double blind, clinical study on 100 patients. Proc. Of the North American Association for Laser Therapy, Atlanta, GA, USA, March 2002, p. 23.

Sliney D, Aron-Rosa D, DeLori F, Fankhauser F, Landry R, Mainster M, Marshall J, Rassow B, Stuck B, Trokel S, West T M, Wolffe M. Adjustment of guidelines for exposure of the eye to optical radiation from ocular instruments: statement from a task group of the International Commission on Non-Ionizing Radiation Protection (ICNIRP). Appl Opt. 2005; 44 (11): 2162-2176.

Sliney D H. Risks of occupational exposure to optical radiation. Med Lav. 2006; 97 (2): 215-220.

Smesny D B. Acupuncture laser in treating headache pain. 1989. Proc. SPIE.Vol 1353: 234-237.

Smith C F, Vangsness C T, Anderson T & Good W. Treatment of repetitive use carpal tunnel syndrome. Proc. SPIE. 1995; Vol 2395: 658-661. Lasers in Surgery: Advanced Characterization, Therapeutics, and Systems V, R. Rox Anderson; Ed.

Smith R J et al. The effect of low-energy laser on skin-flap survival in the rate and porcine animal models. Plastic and Reconstruct Surg. 1992; 89 (2): 306-310.

Silveira P C L, Streck E L, Pinho R A. Evaluation of mitochondrial respiratory chain activity in wound healing by low-level laser therapy. J Photochem and Photobiol B: Biology. 2007; 86 (3): 279-282.

Simões A, Nicolau J, de Souza D N, Ferreira L S, de Paula Eduardo C, Apel C, Gutknecht N. Effect of defocused infrared diode laser on salivary flow rate and some salivary parameters of rats. Clin Oral Investig. 2008; 12 (1): 25-30.

Simões A, Siqueira W L, Lamers M L, Santos M F, Eduardo C D, Nicolau J. Laser phototherapy effect on protein metabolism parameters of rat salivary glands. Lasers Med Sci. 2009; 24 (2): 202-208.

Simões A, de Freitas P M, Tunér J, de Paula Eduardo C. Laser as a new auxiliary therapy for Stevens Johnson Syndrome: a case report. Accpted for publication 2010. Photomed Laser Surg.

Simões A, Platero M D, Campos L, Aranha A C, Eduardo Cde P, Nicolau J. Laser as a therapy for dry mouth symptoms in a patient with Sjögren's syndrome: a case report. Spec Care Dentist. 2009; 29 (3): 134-137.

Simões A, de Campos L, de Souza D N, de Matos J A, Freitas P M, Nicolau J. Laser Phototherapy as Topical Prophylaxis Against Radiation-Induced Xerostomia. Photomed Laser Surg. 2009 Oct 9. [Epub ahead of print]

Simões A, Nogueira FN, Eduardo CD, Nicolau J. Diode Laser Decreases the Activity of Catalase on Submandibular Glands of Diabetic Rats. Photomed Laser Surg. 2009 Oct 5. [Epub ahead of print]

Simões A, de Oliveira E, Campos L, Nicolau J. Ionic and histological studies of salivary glands in rats with diabetes and their glycemic state after laser irradiation. Photomed Laser Surg. 2009; 27(6): 877-883.

Simunovic Z, Simunovic K. Status after multiple teeth extractions treatment with low level laser therapy: A randomised clinical study with control group. Laser Surg Med. 2001; Suppl 13: 11.

Simunovic Z, Trobonjaca T, Trobonjaca Z. Treatment of medial and lateral epicondylitis - tennis and golfer's elbow with low level laser therapy: a multicenter double blind, placebo-controlled clinical study on 324 patients. J Clin Laser Med & Surg. 1998; 16 (3): 145-151.

Simunovic Z, Trobonjaca T. Comparison between low level laser therapy and visible incoherent polarised light in the treatment of lateral epicondylitis - tennis elbow. A pilot clinical study on 20 patients. Laser Surg Med. 2001; Suppl 13: 9.

Simunovic Z, Trobonjaca T. Low level laser therapy in the treatment of osteoarthrosis of joints of the upper extremity: a multicenter, double blind, placebo controlled clinical study of 154 patients. Lasers in Surg Med. Suppl 12, 2000: 7

Simunovic Z, Trobonjaca T. Low level laser therapy in the treatment of cervical syndrome: a multi center, double blind placebo controlled clinical study on 128 patients. Laser Surg Med. Suppl 12. 2000: 8.

Simunovic Z, Trobonjaca T. Low level laser therapy of acne and scars applied as monotherapy and complimentary treatment modality to tetracycline: a multi centre clinical study on 80 patients with control group. Lasers in Surg Med. Suppl 12, 2000: 7

Simunovic Z, Trobonjaca T. Soft tissue injury during sport activities and traffic accidents - treatment with low level laser therapy. A multicenter double blind, placebo controlled clinical study on 132 patients. Laser Surg Med. 1999; Suppl 11:5

Simunovic Z. Curing stomatological and maxillo-facial diseases with MID laser therapy. QLT. 1984: 1-.

Simunovic Z. Low level laser therapy with trigger points technique: a clinical study on 243 patients. J Clin Laser Med Surg. 1996; 14 (4): 163-167.

Shiomi Y et al. Efficacy of transmeatal low power laser irradiation on tinnitus: a preliminary report. Auris Nasus Larynx. 1997; 24: 39-42.

Shiomi Y et al. [Effect of low power laser irradiation on innear ear.] Pract Otol (Kyoto). 1994; 87: 1135-1140. (in Japanese)

Shiroto C et al. Effects of diode laser radiation in vitro on activity of human neutrofils. Laser Therapy. 1989; 1 (3): 135-.

Shiroto C et al: Retrospective study of diode laser therapy for pain attenuation in 3635 patients: Detailed analysis by questionnaire. Laser Therapy. 1989; 1 (1): 41-44.

Shiroto C. Clinical results of pain relief with low lever laser therapy. Laser Bologna '92, p. 25. Monduzzi Editore S.p.A., Bologna, Italy.

Shiroto C, Nakaji S, Umeda T. Current state-of-the-art of the clinical laser in Japan. Proc. 4th Congress of the World Ass. for Laser Therapy, Tokyo, Japan 2002. Pages 59-69. Monduzzi Editore, Bologna, Italy.

Shishkin S A. Use of low intensity laser irradiation in the treatment of thrombophlebitic complications during subclavian vein catheterization. Anesteziol Reanimatol. 1993; (6): 66-68.

Schuhfried O, Korpan M, Fialka-Moser V. Helium-Neon Laser Irradiation: Effect on the Experimental Pain Threshold. Lasers Med Sci. 2000; 15: 169-173.

Shoji N, de Oliveira C, Magacho T A, Chavantes M C. Low Potency Laser treatment for acute dehiscence saphenactomy process. Photomed Laser Surg. 2005; 23 (1). Abstracts from the 5th Congress of the World Association for Laser Therapy, São Paulo, Brazil, November 2004. Abstract no 082, p.110.

Shore S E, Vass Z, Wyss N L,Altschuler R A. Trigeminal ganglion innervates the auditory brainstem. J Comparative Neurology. 2000; 419: 271-285.

Shliakhova L N, Itkes A V, Manteifel V M, Karu T I. Expression of c-myc gene in irradiated at 670 nm human lymphocytes: a preliminary report. Lasers Life Sci. 1996; 7: 107.

Shu B, Wu Z, Hao L, Zeng D, Feng G, Lin Y. Experimental study on He-Ne laser irradiation to inhibit scar fibroblast growth in culture. Chin J Traumatol. 2002;5 (4): 246-249.

Shuvalova I N, Klimenko I T, Zhukova L P et al. [The effect of low-intensity laser radiation in the infrared and red ranges on arterial pressure regulation in patients with borderline hypertension]. Lik Sprava. 1998; (7): 141-143.

Shuvalova I N et al. [The effect of low-intensity laser radiation in the infrared and red ranges on arterial pres-sure regulation in patients with borderline hypertension]. Likarska Sprava. 1998; (7): 141-143.

Siedentopf C M, Golaszewski S M, Mottaghy F M, Ruff C C, Felber S, Schlager A. Functional magnetic resonance imaging detects activation of the visual association cortex during laser acupuncture of the foot in humans. Neurosci Lett. 2002; 327 (1): 53-56.

Siedentopf C M, , Koppelstaetter F, Haala I A et al. Laser acupuncture induced specific cerebral cortical and subcortical activations in humans. Lasers Med Sci. 2005; 20 (2): 68-73.

Siebert W et al. What is the efficacy of "soft" and "mid" lasers in therapy of tendinopathies? A double blind studie. Arch Ortop and Traum Surg. 1987; 106: 358-363.

Silva Junior A N, Pinheiro A L B, Oliveira M G et al. Computerized morphometric assessment of the effect of low-level laser therapy on bone repair: an experimental animal study. J Clin Laser Med Surg. 2002; 20 (2): 83-87.

Silveira L B, Ribeiro M S, Garrocho A A et al. In vivo study on mast cells behaviour following low-intensity visible and near infrared laser radiation. Laser Surg Med. Supplement 14, 2002, abstract 304.

Silveira L B, Prates R A, Novelli M D, Marigo H A, Garrocho A A, Amorim J C, Sousa G R, Pinotti M, Ribeiro M S. Investigation of mast cells in human gingiva following low-intensity laser irradiation. Photomed Laser Surg. 2008; 26 (4): 315-321.

Senda A, Gomi A et al. A clinical study of Soft Laser 632, a Helium-Neon low energy medical laser. 1st report. The effect in releiving pain just after irradiation. Aichi-Gakuin J Dent Sci. 1985; 23 (4): 773-780.

Senda N, Ito K, Sugano N et al. Inhibitory effect of yellow He-Ne laser irradiation mediated by crystal violet solution on early plaque formation in human mouth. Lasers Med Sci. 2000; 15 (3): 174-180.

Senhorino H C, Bichinho G L, Nohama P, Gariba M A. Morphometric effects of different energy densities of diode laser on adipose tissue in rats. BiOS 2008. Proceedings of SPIE; Volume 6846-59.

Sepp W, Haina D et al. Laserstrahlen in der Dermatologie- Der Deutsche Dermatologe. 1978; 11 (26): 557-575.

Severtsev A N et al. The preliminary results of the immunomodulatory effects of HeNe-laser irradiation in human mixed lymphocytes culture. Laser Surg Med, Suppl 5. 1993; 10.

Shamir M H, Rochkind S, Sandbank J, Alon M. Double-blind randomized study evaluating regeneration of the rat transected sciatic nerve after suturing and postoperative low-power laser treatment. Journal of Reconstructive Microsurgery. 2001; 17 (2): 133-137.

Shand M L, Chance R R. Raman photoselection and conjugation-length dispersion in conjugated polymer solutions. Physical Review B. 1982; 25 (7): 4431-4436.

Sharp RE, Chapman S K. Mechanisms for regulating electron transfer in multi-centre redox proteins. Biochem Biophys Acta. 1999; 1432: 143.

Shchepetkin I A The effect of He-Ne laser radiation on the chemiluminescence of human neutrophils. Radio-biologiia. 1993; 33 (3): 377-382.

Shear J B, Xu C, Webb W W. Multiphoton-excited visible emission by serotonin solutions. Photochem Photobiol 1997; 65 (6): 931-936.

Shefer G, Oron U, Irintchev A. Low energy laser irradiation activates specific signal transduction pathways in skeletal muscle cells. J Cell Physiol. 2001; 187: 73-80.

Shefer G, Partridge T A, Heslop L et al. Low-energy laser irradiation promotes the survival and cell death entry of skeletal muscle satellite cells. J Cell Sci. 2002; 115: 1461-1469.

Shefer G, Ben-Dov N, Halevy O, Oron U. Primary myogenic cells see the light: improved survival of transplanted myogenic cells following low energy laser irradiation. Lasers Surg Med. 2008; 40 (1): 38-45.

Shen-Zheng, Xiao-Jian, Lin S Z, Wang L H. Effects of laser guided by optic fiber into rat brain on conditioned avoidance response and brain chemistry. Lasers Surg Med. 1983; 2 (3): 231-239.

Shesterina M V. [Effects of laser therapy on immunity in patients with bronchial asthma and pulmonary tuberculosis.] Probl Tuberk. 1994; 5: 23-26.

Shi K, Lu R, Xu X. Influence of low energy HeNe laser on the regeneration of peripheral nerves. Chung Kuo Hsiu Fu Chung Chien Wai Ko Tsa Chih. 1997; 11 (1): 14-8. (in Chinese)

Shibli J A, Martins M C, Nociti F H Jr, Garcia V G, Marcantonio E Jr. Treatment of ligature-induced peri-implantitis by lethal photosensitization and guided bone regeneration: a preliminary histologic study in dogs. J Periodontol. 2003; 74 (3): 338-345.

Shimizu N et al. Prospect of relieving pain due to tooth movement during orthodontic treatment utilizing a GaAlAs diode laser. Proc. SPIE. 1995; Vol 1984: 275-280.

Shimizu N, Yamaguchi M, Goseki T et al. Inhibition of prostaglandin E2 and interleukin 1-ß production by low-power laser irradiation in stretched human periodontal ligament cells. J Dent Res. 1995; 74 (7): 1382-1388.

Shin D H, Lee E, Hyun J K, Lee S J et al. Growth-associated protein-43 is elevated in the injured rat sciatic nerve after low power laser irradiation. Neurosci Lett. 2003; 344 (2): 71-74.

Schindl L, Kainz A, Kern H. Effect of Low Level Laser Irradiation on Indolent Ulcers Caused by Bürgers Disease. Laser Therapy. 1992; 4 (1): 25-32.

Schindl A, Schindl M, Pernerstorfer-Schön H et al. Low-intensity laser therapy: a review. J Invest Med. 2000; 48 (5): 312-326.

Schindl A, Schindl M, Pernerstorfer-Schoen H, Schindl L. Low intensity laser therapy in wound healing - A review with special respect to diabetic angiopathies. Acta Chirurgica Austriaca. 2001; 33: 3.

Schindl M, Schindl A, Polzleitner D et al. Healing of bone affections and gangrene with low-intensity laser irradiation in diabetic patients suffering from foot infections. Forch Komplementarmed. 1998; 5: 244-247.

Scoletta M, Arduino P G, Reggio L, Dalmasso P, Mozzati M. Effect of Low-Level Laser Irradiation on Bisphosphonate-Induced Osteonecrosis of the Jaws: Preliminary Results of a Prospective Study. Photomed Laser Surg. 2009 Oct 1. [Epub ahead of print]

Shirani A M, Gutknecht N, Taghizadeh M, Mir M. Low-level laser therapy and myofacial pain dysfunction syndrome: a randomized controlled clinical trial. Lasers Med Sci. 2008; Nov 12. [Epub ahead of print]

Schlager A et al. Laser stimulation of acupuncture point P6 reduces postoperative vomiting in children undergoing strabismus surgery. Br J Anaesth. 1998; 81 (4): 529-532

Schlager A, Kronberger P, Petschke F et al. Low-power laser light in the healing of burns: a comparison between two different wavelengths (635 nm and 690 nm) and a placebo group. Lasers in Surg Med. 2000; 27: 39-42.

Schoop U, Moritz A, Kluger W, Patruta S et al. The Er:YAG laser in endodontics: results of an in vitro study. Lasers Surg Med. 2002; 30 (5): 360-364.

Shooshtari S M, Badiee V, Taghizadeh S H, Nematollahi A H, Amanollahi A H, Grami M T. The effects of low level laser therapy in clinical outcome and neurophysiological results of carpal tunnel syndrome. Electromyogr Clin Neurophysiol. 2008; 48 (5): 229-231.

Schubert V. Effects Of Phototherapy (LLLT) On Pressure Ulcer Healing In Elderly Patients After A Falling Trauma. A Prospective, Randomized, Controlled Study. Photodermatol Photoimmunol Photomed. 2001; 17 (1): 32-38.

Schubert M M, Eduardo F P, Guthrie K A, Franquin J C, Bensadoun RJ, Migliorati CA et al. A phase III randomized double-blind placebo-controlled clinical trial to determine the efficacy of low level laser therapy for the prevention of oral mucositis in patients undergoing hematopoietic cell transplantation. Support Care Cancer. 2007 Mar; [Epub ahead of print].

Schultz R J, Krishnamurthy S, Thelmo W et al. Effects of varying intensities of laser energy on articular cartilage: A preliminary study. Laser Surg Med. 1985; 5: 557-588.

Schuster M A et al. [Treatment of vasomotor rhinitis, trigeminal neuralgia and Sluder's syndrome by helium-neon laser irradiation of the pterygopalatine ganglion]. Vest. Otorinolar. 1988; 4: 35-40.

Schwartz F et al. Effect of low energy laser irradiation on cytokines secretion from skeletal muscle cells - involvement of calcium in the process. Proc SPIE. 1997. Vol 3198: 48-54.

Schwartz M et al. Effect of low-energy HeNe laser irradiation on posttraumatic degeneration of adult rabbit optic nerve. Lasers Sur Med. 1987; 7: 51-55.

Scudds R A et al. A double-blind crossover study of the effectiveness of low-power gallium arsenide laser on the symptoms of fibrositis. Physiotherapy Canada. 1989; 41: (suppl 3):2.

Seaton E D, Charakida A, Mouser P E et al. Pulsed-dye laser treatment for inflammatory acne vulgaris: randomised controlled trial. The Lancet. 2003; 362: 1347-1352.

Seifi M, Shafeei HA, Daneshdoost S, Mir M. Effects of two types of low-level laser wave lengths (850 and 630 nm) on the orthodontic tooth movements in rabbits. Lasers Med Sci. 2007; 22 (4): 261-264.

Saygun I, Karacay S, Serdar M, Ural AU, Sencimen M, Kurtis B. Effects of laser irradiation on the release of basic fibroblast growth factor (bFGF), insulin like growth factor-1 (IGF-1), and receptor of IGF-1 (IGFBP3) from gingival fibroblasts. Lasers Med Sci. 2008; 23 (2): 211-215.

Sazonov A M, Romanov G A, Portnoy L M et al. Low-intensity noncoherent red light in complex healing of peptic and duodenal ulcers. Sov Med. 1985; 42 (12). (in Russian)

Sbarra A J, Strauss R R. Eds. The Respiratory Burst and Its Photobiological Significance. Plenum Press, New York, 1988.

Schaffer M et al. Biomodulative effects induced by 805 nm laser light irradiation of normal and tumor cells. J Photochem Photobiol B:Biol. 1997; 40: 253-257.

Schaffer M et al. Magnetic resonance imaging (MRI) controlled outcome of side effects caused by ionizing radiation, treated with with 780-nm diode laser - preliminary results. J Photochemistry and Photobiology B: Biology. 2000; 59: 1-8.

Schaffer M et al. Mitotic rate of normal mouse fibroblast cells and human tumor cells after diode laser irradiation. Laser Therapy. 1996; 8 (1) 23. (abstract)

Schaffer M, Bonel H, Sroka-R et al. Effects of 780 nm diode laser irradiation on blood microcirculation: Preliminary findings on time-dependent T1-weighted contrast-enhanced magnetic resonance imaging (MRI). J Photochemistry and Photobiology B: Biology 2000; 54 (1): 55-60.

Shao XH, Yang YP, Dai J, Wu JF, Bo AH. Effects of He-Ne laser irradiation on chronic atrophic gastritis in rats. World J Gastroenterol. 2005; 7; 11 (25): 3958-3961.

Schenk P et al. Elektronenmikroskopische Untersuchungen von oralen Schleimhautepithelien nach bestrahlung mit dem Helium-Neon-laser. Dtsch Z Mun Kiefer Gesischts Chir. 1985; 9: 278-.

Shibata Y, Ogura N, Yamashiro K et al. Anti-inflammatory effect of linear polarized infrared irradiation on interleukin-1-induced chemokine production in MH7A rheumatoid synovial cells. Lasers in Medical Science. 2005; July 27.

Schindl A et al. Increased dermal neovascularization after low dose laser therapy of chronic radiation ulcer determined by a video measuring system. Proc. 2nd Congress World Assn for Laser Therapy, Kansas City, September 1998; p. 34.

Schindl A et al. Low intensity laser irradiation improves skin circulation in patients with diabetic microangiopathy. Diabetes Care. 1998; 21 (4): 580-584.

Schindl A et al. Low intensity laser irradiation in the treatment of recalcitrant radiation ulcers in patients with breast cancer - long term results of 3 cases. Photodermatol-Photoimmunol-Photomed. 2000; 16 (1): 34-37.

Schindl A, Merwald H, Schindl L. Low intensity laser irradiation stimulates endothelial cell proliferation in an vitro model of diabetic microangiopathy. Laser Surg Med. 2001; Suppl 13: 7.

Schindl A, Neuman R. Low-intensity laser therapy is an effective treatment for recurrent herpes simplex infection. Results from a randomized double-blind placebo controlled study. J Investigative Dermatology. 1999; 113 (2): 221-223.

Schindl A, Schindl L. Systemic increase in blood flow in conditions of disturbed microcirculation after low-power laser irradiation. Proc. SPIE. 1996, Vol 2929: 63-69.

Schindl L et al. Effects of low power laser-irradiation on differential blood count and body temperature in endotoxin-preimmunized rabbits. Life Sci. 1997; 60 (19): 1669-1677.

Schindl L et al. Topical low power laser irradiation shows a systemic increase in blood flow in conditions of disturbed microcirculation. Laser Therapy. 1996; 8 (1): 58. (abstract)

Schindl L et al. Influence of low-power laser irradiation on "arthus phenomenon" induced in rabbit cornea. Laser Therapy. 1994; 6 (1); 23. (abstract)

Sandoval M C, Mattiello-Rosa S M, Soares E G, Parizotto N A. Effects of Laser on the Synovial Fluid in the Inflammatory Process of the Knee Joint of the Rabbit. Photomed Laser Surg. 2009 Feb 2. [Epub ahead of print]

Sanseverino N T M, Sanseverino C A M, Ribeiro M S et al. Clinical evaluation of the low intensity laser antialgic action of GaAlAs (wavelength=785 nm) in the treatment of the temporomandibular disorders. Laser Surg Med. Abstract issue, 2002: 18.

Sant'Anna G R et al. Photodynamic therapy using low level laser as a disinfecting approach to carious dentine: in vivo microbiological study. Proc. 7th Int Congr Lasers in Dentistry, ISLD, Brussels, Belgium, July 2000, abstr. 43.

Sant'Anna G R, Duarte D A, Brugnera Jr A et al. Dye-assisted laser therapy as a disinfecting approach to caries dentine. In vivo microbiology study. Proc. 3rd Congr World Assn for Laser Therapy, Athens, Greece, May 2000, p. 62.

Santoianni P et al. Inadequate effect of helium-neon laser on venous leg ulcers. Photodermatology. 1984; 1: 245-249.

Saperia D, Glassberg E, Lyons R F et al. Demonstration of elevated type I and type III laser. Biochem and Biophys Res Communic. 1986; 138 (3): 1123-1128.

Sapiera D et al. Demonstration of elevated type I and type III procollagen mRNA levels in cutaneous wounds treated with helium-neon laser. Biochem Biophys Res Com. 1986; 3 (138): 1123-1128.

Sasaki K, Ohshiro T, Hoshino T. A preliminary double blind controlled study on free amino acid analysis in burn wounds in the mouse following 830 nm diode laser therapy. Laser Therapy. 1997; 9 (2): 59-66.

Sasaki K et al. Low level laser therapy (laser therapy) for thromboangitis obliterans. Proc. 2nd Congress World Association for Laser Therapy, Kansas City, USA, September 2-5 1998; p 95-96.

Sasaki K, Calderhead R G, Chin I, Inomata K. To examine the adverse photothermal effects of extended dosage laser therapy in vivo on the skin and subcutaneous tissue in the rat model. Laser Therapy. 1992; 2: 69-74.

Sasaki K, Ohshiro T. Role of Low Reactive-Level Laser Therapy (laser therapy) in the Treatment of Aquired and Cicatricial Vitiligo. Laser Therapy. 1989; 1 (3): 141-146.

Satino J, Markou M. Hair Regrowth and Increased Hair Tensile Strength Using the HairMax LaserComb for Low-Level Laser Therapy. Int J Cosmetic Surg Aest Derm. 2003; 5 (2): 113-117.

Sato H. The effects of laser light on sperm motility and velocity in vitro. Andrologia. 1984; 16 (1): 23-25.

Sato K, Kaseno S, Takigawa C et al. A double blind assessment of low power laser therapy in the treatment of postherpetic neuralgia. Surgical and Medical Lasers. 1990; 3 (3): 134. (abstract)

Sato T, Kawatani M, Takeshige C, Matsumoto I. Ga-Al-As laser irradiation inhibits neuronal activity associated with inflammation. Acupunct Electrother Res. 1994; 19 (2-3): 141-151.

Sattayut S, Bradley P F. Low intensity laser therapy (LILT) for TMD myofascial pain: results from a pilot study. 1998. Proc. 6th Int Congr Lasers in Dentistry. University of Utah Press. Ed: J Frame. ISBN 0-87480-606-2, p. 152-156.

Sattayut S, Hughes F, Bradley P. 820 nm gallium aluminium arsenide laser modulation of prostaglandin E2 production in interleukin-1 stimulated myoblasts. Laser Therapy. 1999; 11 (2): 88-95.

Sattayut S A study on the influence of low intensity laser therapy on painful temporomandibular disorders 1999;. University of London PhD thesis (prof. P Bradley).

Saunders L. The efficacy of low-level laser therapy in supraspinatus tendinitis. Clin Rehab. 1995; 9: 126-134.

Ryabykh T, Karu T. Action of pulsed visible and near IR laser radiation on oxidative metabolism of cells evaluated by chemiluminescence measurement. Proc SPIE. 1995; Vol 2630: 12-21.

Rydén H, Persson L, Preber H, Bergström J. Effect of low-energy laser on gingival inflammation. Swedish Dent J. 1994; 18: 35-41.

Safavi S M, Kazemi B, Esmaeili M, Fallah A, Modarresi A, Mir M. Effects of low-level He-Ne laser irradiation on the gene expression of IL-1beta, TNF-alpha, IFN-gamma, TGF-beta, bFGF, and PDGF in rat's gingiva. Lasers Med Sci. 2008; 23 (3): 331-335.

Sagalovich E E. Secretory immunity changes in patients with acute and chronic herpetic stomatitis by laser therapy. Clin Immunol Immunopathol. 1995. 1 (7): 385-.

Saito K. Effects of 830 nm diode laser irradiation on superficial blood circulation in college sumo wrestlers. Meeting report from the 1st Congr of the IALSM 1997. Laser Therapy. 1997; 9 (4): 187.

Saito S, Shimizu N. Stimulatory effects of low-power laser irradiation on bone regeneration in midpalatal suture during expansion in the rat. Am J Ortod Dentofac Orthop. 1997; 11 (5): 525.

Sakihama I. Effect of a helium-neon laser on cutaneous inflammation. Karume Medical J. 1995; 52 (4): 299-305.

Sakurai Y; Yamaguchi M; Abiko Y. Inhibitory effect of low-level laser irradiation on LPS-stimulated prostaglandin E2 production and cyclooxygenase-2 in human gingival fibroblasts. Eur J Oral Sci. 2000; 108 (1): 29-34.

Salate A C, Barbosa G, Gaspar P et al. Effect of Ga-Al-As Diode Laser Irradiation on Angiogenesis in Partial Ruptures of Achilles Tendon in Rats. Photomed Laser Surg. 2005; 23 (5): 470-475.

Saldo I et al. Effects of GaAs-laser combined with radiotherapy on murine sarcoma depends on tumor size. Laser Surg Med. 1989; Suppl 1: 40.

Salinas E O, Hakim-Kreis C M, Piketty M L et al. Hypersecretion of melatonin following diurnal exposure to bright light in seasonal affective disorder: preliminary results. Biol Psychiatry. 1992; Sep 1; 32 (5) : 387-398.

Salet C, Moreno G, Vinzens F. A study of beating frequency of a single myocardial cell. III. Laser microirradiation of mitochondria in the presence of KCN or ATP. Exp. Cell Res. 1979; 120: 25.

Salet C. A study of beating frequency of a single myocardial cell. I. Q-switched laser microirradiation of mitochondria. Exp Cell Res. 1972; 73: 360.

Salet C. Acceleration par micro-irradiation laser du rhythme de contraction de cellular cardiaques en culture. C.R. Acad Sci. Paris. 191; 272: 2584.

Samoilova K, Snopov S. A key role on whole circulating blood modification in therapeutic effects of ultraviolet and visible light. Proc. 2nd Congress World Assn for Laser Therapy, Kansas City, September 1998; p. 92-94.

Samoilova K A, Kukui L M. Photochemotherapy in clinical and veterinary medicine: therapeutic effects and mechanisms. Laser Therapy. 1996; 8 (1): 62. (abstract)

Samoilova K A, Bogacheva O N, Obolenskaya K D, Blinova M I, Kalmykova NV, Kuzminikh E V. Enhancement of the blood growth promoting activity after exposure of volunteers to visible and infrared polarized light. Part I: stimulation of human keratinocyte proliferation in vitro. Photochem Photobiol Sci. 2004; 3 (1): 96-101.

Samoilova K A, Zhevago N A, Menshutina M A, Grigorieva N B. Role of nitric oxide in the visible light-induced rapid increase of human skin microcirculation at the local and systemic level: I. diabetic patients. Photomed Laser Surg. 2008; 26 (5): 433-442.

Sandford M A, Walsh L J. Thermal effects during desensitisation of teeth with gallium-aluminum-arsenide lasers. Periodontol 1994; 15 (1): 25-30.

Rochkind S, Drory V, Alon M, Nissan M, Ouaknine G E. Laser Phototherapy (780 nm), a New Modality in Treatment of Long-Term Incomplete Peripheral Nerve Injury: A Randomized Double-Blind Placebo-Controlled Study. Photomed Laser Surg. 2007; 25 (5): 436-442.

Rodrigues M T J, Ribeiro M S, Groth E B et al. Evaluation of effects of laser therapy (wavelength=830 nm) on oral ulcertation induced by fixed orthodontic appliances. Laser Med Surg Abstract issue, 2002: 15.

Rodrigues de Sant'anna G. Development anomalies as Amelogenesis.Laser. Photomed Laser Surg. 2005; 23 (1). Abstracts from the 5th Congress of the World Association for Laser Therapy, Sao Paulo, Brazil, November 2004. Abstract no 029, p. 96.

Rogowski M, Menich S, Gindzienska E, Lazarczyk B. [Low-power laser in the treatment of tinnitus - a placebo-controlled study]. Laser niskoenergetyczny w leczeniu szumow usznychóbadania porownawcze z placebo. Otolaryngologia polska. Otolaryngol-Pol. 1999; 53 (3): 315-320.

Rogvi Hansen B et al. Low level laser treatment of chondromalacia patellae. Int Orthopaedics. 1991; 15: 359-361.

Roig J, Fleites A, Bécquer R. Tratamiento del síndrome del túnel carpiano con láser HeNe e infrarojo. Evaluación clínica y electrofisiológica de los resultados.[Treatment of the carpal tunnel syndrome with HeNe and infrared laser. Clinical and electrophysical evaluation of the results]. Rev Cubana Ortop Traumatol. 1992; 6 (2): 139-143.

Romanos, G E. Treatment of periimplant lesions using different laser systems. J Oral Laser Applications. 2002; 2: 75-81.

Romanos G E, Nentwig G H. Diode laser (980 nm) in oral and maxillofacial surgical procedures: Clinical observations based on clinical applications. J Clin Laser Med Surg. 1999; 17: 193–197.

Rosen H S., Klebanoff S J. Federal Proceedings, 1976; 35: 1391.

Roshal L. Application of Low-Level Laser in Pediatry and Pediatric Surgery in the USSR. In: Progress in Laser Therapy. Editors: Ohshiro & Calderhead. John Wiley & Sons. 1991, p. 112.

Rosner M, Caplan M, Cohen S et al. Dose and temporal parameters in delaying injured optic nerve degeneration by low-energy laser irradiation. Laser Surg Med. 1993; 13 (6): 611-617.

Rossetti V et al. Experimental studies on the in vivo effects of HeNe laser irradiation in rat brain. Lasermedizin - Laser in Med Surg. 1995; 11 (2): 24 .

Rossman J A. Current research using the CO2 laser in guided tissue regeneration: animal studies. Proc Second Annual Advanced Application Seminar. Luxar Corp, USA., 1993.

Rotola A, Cassai E, Farina R, Caselli E, Gentili V, Lazzarotto T, Trombelli L. Human herpesvirus 7, Epstein-Barr virus and human cytomegalovirus in periodontal tissues of periodontally diseased and healthy subjects. J Clin Periodontol. 2008; 35 (10): 831-837.

Roumeliotis D, Emmanouilidis O, Diamantopoulos C. C.W. 820nm 15mW 4J/cm^2, laser diode application in sports injunes. A double blind study. Proc. Fifth Annual Congress, 28-30 January 1987. British Medical Laser Association.

Røynesdal A et al. The effect of soft-laser application on postoperative pain and swelling. A double-blind, cross-over study. J Oral Maxillofac Surg. 1993; 22: 242-245.

Rubinov A N. Physiological grounds for biological effect of laser radiation. J Phys D: Appl Phys, 2003; 36: 2317-2330.

Ruffolo P et al. Impiego della Laser-terapia nelle leucoplachie del cavo orale. Int Congress on Laser Med and Surg, Bologna June 1985, p. 279 Monduzzi Editore S.p.A., Bologna, Italy.

Ruiz I et al.. Histological and clinical responses of articular cartilage to low level laser therapy: Experimental study. Lasers in Medical Science. 1997; 12 (2): 117-121.

Ribeiro I W, Sbrana M C, Esper L A, Almeida A L. Evaluation of the effect of the GaAlAs laser on subgingival scaling and root planing. Photomed Laser Surg. 2008; 26 (4): 387-391.

Ribeiro M A, Albuquerque R L, Ramalho L M, Pinheiro A L, Bonjardim L R, Da Cunha S S. Immunohistochemical Assessment of Myofibroblasts and Lymphoid Cells During Wound Healing in Rats Subjected to Laser Photobiomodulation at 660 nm. Photomed Laser Surg. 2009; 27 (1): 49-55.

Rice J, Mayor J, Tucker HA, Bielski RJ. Effect of light therapy on salivary melatonin in seasonal affective disorder. Psychiatry Res. 1995; 56 (3): 221-228.

Riendeau F. An in vivo study of the effects of Helium-Neon laser on the breaking force and histological characteristics of wound. Proc Int Congr of Lasers in Dentistry, Tokyo, August 5-6. 1988: 20.

Rigau J, Trelles M A. Effects of the 633 nm laser on the behaviour and morphology of primary fibroblast culture. Proc SPIE. 1995; Vol 2630: 38-42.

Rizzi C F, Mauriz J L, Freitas Correa D S, Moreira A J et al. Effects of low-level laser therapy (LPT) on the nuclear factor (NF)-kappaB signaling pathway in traumatized muscle. Lasers Surg Med. 2006; 38 (7): 704-713.

Robinson J F et al. Wound healing in porcine skin following low output carbon dioxide laser irradiation of the lesion. Annals Plastic Surgery. 1987; 18 (6): 449-505.

Rocha Júnior A M, Vieira B J, de Andrade L C, Aarestrup F M. Low-level laser therapy increases transforming growth factor-beta2 expression and induces apoptosis of epithelial cells during the tissue repair process. Photomed Laser Surg. 2009; 27 (2): 303-307.

Rochkind S, Barr-Nea L, Bartal A et al. New method of treatment of severely injured sciatic nerve and spinal cord. An experimental study. Acta Neurochirurgica. 1988; Suppl 43: 91-93.

Rochkind S, Nissan M, Lubart A. A single Transcutaneous Light Irradiation to Injured Peripheral Nerve: Comparative Study with Five Different Wavelengths. Lasers in Medical Sciences. 1989; 4: 259-263.

Rochkind S, Ouaknine G E. New trand in neuroscience: Low-power laser effect on peripheral and central nerve system (basic science, preclinical and clinical studies). Neurol Res. 1992; 14: 2-11.

Rochkind S, Alon M, Drory V et al. Laser therapy as a new modality in the treatment of incomplete peripheral nerve and brachial plexus injuries: prospective clinical double blind placebo-controlled randomized study. In: Abstract book of the Annual Meeting 2001, American Society for Peripheral Nerve, San Diego, California, USA, January 2001, p. 21.

Rochkind S, Nissan M, Alon M et al. Effects of laser irradiation on the spinal cord for the regeneration of crushed peripheral nerve in rats. Laser Surg Med. 2001; 28 (3): 216-219.

Rochkind S, Rousso M, Nissan M et al. Systemic effects of low-power laser irradiation on the peripheral and central nervous system, cutaneous wounds and burns. Laser Surg Med. 1989; 9: 174-182.

Rochkind S, Nissan M, Razon N et al. Electrophysiological Effect of HeNe Laser on Normal and Injured Sciatic Nerve in the Rat. Acta Neurochir. (Vienna). 1986; 83: 125-130.

Rochkind S et al. Double-blind Randomized Study Using Neurotube and Laser Therapy in the Treatment of Complete Sciatic Nerve Injury of Rats. Proc. 2nd Congr World Assoc. for Laser Therapy, Kansas City, 1998.

Rochkind S, Shahar A, Alon M, Nevo Z. Transplantation of embryonal spinal cord nerve cells cultured in biodegradable microcarriers followed by low power laser irradiation for the treatment of traumatic paraplegia in rats. Neur Res. 2002; 24 (4): 355-360.

Rochkind S, Kogan G, Luger E G et al. Molecular structure of the bony tissue after experimental trauma to the mandibular region followed by laser therapy. Photomed Laser Surg. 2004; 22 (3): 249-253.

Reddy G K et al. The effects of laser stimulation on wound healing in diabetic rats. Proc. 2nd Congress World Assn for Laser Therapy, Kansas City, September 1998; p. 124-125.

Reddy K, Stehno-Bittel L, Enwemeka C. Laser photostimulation accelerates wound healing in diabetic rats. Wound Repair and Regeneration. 2001, 9 (3): 248-255.

Reidenbach H D, Dollinger K, Hoffman J. Field trials with low power lasers concerning the blink reflex. Biomed Tech (Berl.). 2002; 47 Suppl 1 Pt 2: 600-6001.

Reis S R, Medrado A P, Marchionni A M, Figueira C, Fracassi L D, Knop L A. Effect of 670-nm laser therapy and dexamethasone on tissue repair: a histological and ultrastructural study. Photomed Laser Surg. 2008; 26 (4): 307-313.

Renno A C, de Moura F M, dos Santos N S et al. Effects of 830-nm laser, used in two doses, on biomechanical properties of osteopenic rat femora. Photomed Laser Surg. 2006; 24 (2): 202-206.

Renno A C, de Moura F M, dos Santos N S, Tirico R P, Bossini P S, Parizotto N A. Effects of 830-nm laser light on preventing bone loss after ovariectomy. Photomed Laser Surg. 2006; 24 (5): 642-645.

Renno A C, McDonnell P A, Parizotto N A, Laakso E L. The Effects of Laser Irradiation on Osteoblast and Osteosarcoma Cell Proliferation and Differentiation in Vitro. Photomed Laser Surg. 2007; 25 (4): 275-280.

Reznikov L L et al. Urol Nefrol. 1991; 2: 45-49.

Reznikov L L et al. Biomechanism of low-energy laser irradiation is similar to a general adaptive reaction. Proc. SPIE. 1994; Vol 2086: 380-449.

Reznikov L L et al. Similarity between the mechanisms of soft-laser radiation and chemical adaptogen action. Proc. SPIE. 1993; Vol 1883: 91-98.

Reznikov, Leonid; Personal communication, Dec 1998.

Rezvani M et al. Prevention of x-radiation induced dermal necrosis in pig skin by monochromatic light. Laser Surg Med. 1991; suppl 3: 11

Ribari O et al. [Closure of tympanic perforations with low-energy HeNe laser irradiation]. Acta Chir Academ Scient Hungaricae. 1980; 21 (3): 229-238. (in Hungarian with English abstract)

Ribeiro D A, Matsumoto M A. Low-level laser therapy improves bone repair in rats treated with anti-inflammatory drugs. J Oral Rehabil. 2008; 35 (12): 925-933.

Ribeiro M S, Zezell D M, Fontenele J D, Pellegrini C M R, Zorn T M T. Incorporation of [3H]-Proline in the Dermis of Mice Following He-He Polarized Laser Radiation in the Wound Healing Process. A preliminary Study. Proc. 2nd Congress World Assn for Laser Therapy, Kansas City, Sept 1998; p. 13-15.

Ribeiro M S, Freitas A Z, Silva D F et al. Comparison of polarization degree in healthy and wounded rat skin. Proc. SPIE. Vol. 4433.

Ribeiro M S, Zezell D M, Maldonado E P et al. Histological study of wound healing in rats following He-Ne and GaAlAs laser radiation. Proc. SPIE. Vol. 3569: 50-55.

Ribeiro M S, Zezell D M, Carbone K et al. Effects of He-Ne polarized laser radiation on skin wound repair: a morphological study. Proc. SPIE. Vol. 3198.

Ribeiro M S, Da Silva D de F, De Araujo C E, De Oliveira S F et al. Effects of low-intensity polarized visible laser radiation on skin burns: a light microscopy study. J Clin Laser Med Surg. 2004; 22 (1): 59-66.

Ribeiro M S, Silva D F, Maldonado E P, de Rossi W, Zezell D M. Effects of 1047-nm neodymium laser radiation on skin wound healing. J Clin Laser Med Surg. 2002; 20 (1): 37-40.

Ribeiro M, Sugayama S T, Nogueira G, Franca C A et al. Angiogenesis induced by low-intensity laser therapy: comparative study between single and fractionated dose on burn healing. BiOS 2008. Proceedings of SPIE; Volume 6846-12.

Qadri T, Bohdanecka P, Miranda L, Tunér J, Altamash M, Gustafsson A. The importance of coherence length in laser phototherapy of gingival inflammation - a pilot study. Lasers in Med Sci. 2007; 22 (4): 245-251.

Quah-Smith J I, Tang WM, Russell J. Laser acupuncture for mild to moderate depression in a primary care setting - a randomised controlled trial. Acupunct Med. 2005; 23 (3): 103-111.

Quickenden T R, Daniels L L, Byrne L T. Does low-intensity He-Ne radiation affect the intracellular pH of intact E. coli? Proc. SPIE. Vol 2391. 1995: 535.

Radelli J, Cieslar G, Sieron A, Grzybek H. Influence of low-power laser radiation on carbohydrate metabolism and insulin-glycemic balance in experimental animals. Proc. SPIE. 1996, Vol 2929: 94-102.

Radelli, J et al. Metabolism and insulin-glycemic balance in rats. Laser Therapy. 1996; 8 (1): 26. (abstract)

Radmayr C, Schlager A, Studen M, Bartsch G. Prospective randomized trial using laser acupuncture versus desmopressin in the treatment of nocturnal enuresis. Eur Urol. 2001; 40 (2): 201-205.

Radwan N M, El Hay Ahmed N A, Ibrahim K M, Khedr M E, Aziz M A, Khadrawy Y A. Effect of infrared laser irradiation on amino acid neurotransmitters in an epileptic animal model induced by pilocarpine. Photomed Laser Surg. 2009; 27 (3): 401-409.

Ragnarsson S-I. Vision Research. 1972; 12: 411

Rajab A A. A study on the effect of low intensity laser therapy on the osseointegration of hydroxylapatite implants. 1999. University of London PhD thesis.

Rajaratuan S, Bolton P, Dyson M. Macrophage responsiveness to laser therapy with varying pulsing frequencies. Laser Therapy. 1994; 6: 107-102.

Rakcheev A P et al. Experimental and clinical substantiation of laser therapy of wounds and throphic ulcers. Ortop Travmatol Protez. 1989; 10: 66-70. (in Russian with English abstract)

Rallis T R. Low-intensity laser therapy for recurrent herpes labialis. J Invest Dermatol. 2000; 115 (1): 131-132.

Ramos L, Penna S, Marcos R L et al. Low level infrared laser therapy (810 nm) in experimental skeletal muscle strain: functional and biochemical evaluation. Proc. 7th Internat Congr of WALT, Sun City, South Africa, October 2008, page 132.

Rao M L, Muller-Oerlinghausen B, Mackert A et al. The influence of phototherapy on serotonin and melatonin in non-seasonal depression. Pharmacopsychiatry. 1990; 23 (3): 155-158.

Rao M L, Muller-Oerlinghausen B, Mackert A, Strebel B, Stieglitz RD Volz HP. Blood serotonin, serum melatonin and light therapy in healthy subjects and in patients with nonseasonal depression. Acta Psychiatr Scand. 1992; 86 (2): 127-132.

Rappl T, Laback C, Quasthoff S et al. Low-level-laser therapy in mild and moderate CTS - a double blind, randomised study. Proc. Laser Florence 2003.

Rattanayatikul C, Limpanichkul W, Godfrey K, Srisuk N. Effects of low-level laser therapy on the rate of orthodontic tooth movement. Orthod Craniofacial Res. 2006. 9: 38-43.

Raulin C, Gündogan C, Greve B, Gebert S. [Excimer laser therapy of alopecia areata - side-by-side evaluation of a representative area]. JDDG - J Ger Soc of Dermatol. 2005; 3: 524-526. (in German with English abstract)

Read A, Beaty P, Corner J, Sommerville Ville C. Reducing naltrexone-resistant hyperphagia using laser acupuncture to increase endogenous opiates. Brain Inj. 1996; 10 (12): 911-919.

Reddy G K et al. Biochemistry and biomechanics of healing tendon: Part II. Effects of combined laser therapy and electrical stimulation. Med Sci Sports Exerc. 1998; 30 (6): 794-800.

Reddy G K et al. Laser photostimulation of collagen production in healing rabbit achilles tendons. Lasers in Medicine and Surgery. 1998; 22: 281-287.

Pourreau-Schnedier N et al. Soft-Laser Therapy for Iatrogenic Mucositis in Cancer Patients Receiving High-Dose Fluorouacil: A preliminary report. J Nat Cancer Inst. 1992; 5 (84): 358-.

Pourreau-Schneider N et al. Helium-Neon Laser Treatment Transforms Fibroblasts into Myofibroblasts. Am J Pathol. 1990; 137: 171-178.

Pourzarandian A, Watanabe H, Ruwanpura SM, Aoki A, Ishikawa Effect of low-level Er:YAG laser irradiation on cultured human gingival fibroblasts. J Periodontol. 2005; 76 (2): 187-193.

Pourzarandian A, Watanabe H, Ruwanpura SM, Aoki A, Noguchi K, Ishikawa I. Er:YAG laser irradiation increases prostaglandin E_2 production via the induction of cyclooxygenase-2 mRNA in human gingival fibroblasts. J Periodontal Res. 2005; 40 (2): 182-186.

Powell K, Laakso L, Low P, Ralph S. The in vitro effects of laser irradiation on human breast carcinoma and immortalised human mammary epithelial cell lines. Proc. 7th Internat Congr of WALT, Sun City, South Africa, October 2008, page 104.

Pozza D H, Fregapani P W, Weber J B, de Oliveira M G, de Oliveira M A, Ribeiro Neto N, de Macedo Sobrinho J B. Analgesic action of laser therapy (LLLT) in an animal model. Med Oral Patol Oral Cir Bucal. 2008; 13 (10): 648-652.

Prado R P, Liebano R E, Hochman B, Pinfildi C E, Ferreira L M. Experimental model for low level laser therapy on ischemic random skin flap in rats. Acta Cir Bras. 2006; 21 (4):258-262.

Prezotto Villa G E, Catirse A B, Lizarelli R F. Evaluation of secondary dentin formation applying two fluences of Low Level Laser.Photomed Laser Surg. 2005; 23 (1). Abstracts from the 5th Congress of the World Association for Laser Therapy, Sao Paulo, Brazil, November 2004. Abstract no 024, p. 95.

Prochazka, Koci K. Non-invasive laser therapy of morbus perronie - induratio penis placstica. Abstracts of 7th Int Congr European Medical Laser Assn, Dubrovnik, Croatia 2000, p. 39.

Prochazka M, Tejnska R. Noninvasive laser in therapy of tinnitus. In: A window on the laser medicine world. Proc. SPIE. 1999, Vol 4166: 222-223. Also: Prochazka M, Hahn A. Comprehensive laser rehabilitation therapy of tinnitus: long-term double blind study in a group of 200 patients in 3 years. Laser Partner. 2002; 51. www.laserpartner.org/lasp/web/en/2002/0051.htm.

Prokofeva G L, Kravchenko E V, Mozherenkov V P. [Effects of low-intensity infrared laser irradiation on the eye. An experimental study]. Vestn-Oftalmol. 1996; 112 (1): 31-32

Prokopova L V et al. Effect of intravascular laser therapy on rheologic properties of blood in children with bilateral destructive pneumonia. Klin Khir. 1992; (6): 7-9.

Prokopowisch I, Kleine B M, Youssef M N, Lage-Marques L J. The low power GaAlAs action in the postoperative pain control in human teeth after root canal preparation. Proc. 3rd Congress of ESOLA, Barcelona, Spain, May 2005, p. 33.

Pugliese LS, Medrado AP, Reis SR, Andrade Zde A. The influence of low-level laser therapy on biomodulation of collagen and elastic fibers. Pesqui Odontol Bras. 2003; (4): 307-313.

Puri M M, Arora K. Role of Gallium Arsenide Laser Irradiation at 890 nm as an Adjunctive to Anti-tuberculosis Drugs in the Treatment of Pulmonary Tuberculosis. Indian J Chest Dis Allied Sci. 2003; 45: 13-19.

Pyczek M, Sopala M, Dabrowski Z. Effect of low-energy laser power on the bone marrow of the rat. Folia Biol (Krakow) 1994; 42 (3-4): 151-156

Pöntinen P. LEPT for preoperative care and early rehabilitation. Proc. 4th Congress of the World Ass. for Laser Therapy, Tokyo, Japan 2002. Pages 75-79. Monduzzi Editore, Bologna, Italy.

Qadri T, Miranda L, Tunér J, Gustavsson A. The short-term effects of low-level lasers as adjunct therapy in the treatment of periodontal inflammation. J Clin Periodontol. 2005; 32 (7): 714-719.

Pinheiro A L, Limeira Júnior F, Gerbi M M et al. Effect of Low Level Laser Therapy on the Repair of Bone Defects Grafted with Inorganic Bovine Bone. Braz Dent J. 2003; 14 (3): 177-181.

Pinheiro A L B, Gerbi M E M, Ponzi E A C, Ramalho L M P, Marques A M C et al. Infrared Laser Light Further Improves Bone Healing When Associated with Bone Morphogenetic Proteins and Guided Bone Regeneration: An in Vivo Study in a Rodent Model. Photomed Laser Surg. 2008; 26 (2): 167-174.

Pires Oliveira D A, de Oliveira R F, Zangaro R A, Soares C P. Evaluation of low-level laser therapy of osteoblastic cells. Photomed Laser Surg. 2008; 26 (4): 401-404

Plavnik L, Crosa M, Malberti A. Effect of low power laser radiation on guinea pig submandibular glands: a structural and biomechanical study. J Dent Res. 2000; 79 (5): 1010-.

Plavnik L, de Crosa M, Malberti A. Effect of low-power radiation (helium/neon) upon submandibular glands. J Clin Laser Med Surg. 2003; 21 (4): 219-225.

Plog F. Biophysical application of the laser beam. 1980. In Koebner H.K: Lasers in Medicine. John Wiley, New York.

Pluzhnikov S M et al. Use of intracavitary low-energy laser therapy in the complex treatment of inflammatory diseases in the sphenoid sinus. Vest Otoringolaringol. 1986; 4: 72-73. (in Russian with English abstr)

Podelinskaia L V et al. Effects of low-intensity laser irradiation on several parameters of microcirculation in the bulbar conjunctiva of patients with scleroderma. Vestn Oftalmol. 1995; 111 (2): 10-12.

Podolskaya E et al. Radiation damage of lips and its treatment by low-intensity laser irradiation. Proc SPIE. 1995; Vol 1984: 245-246.

Polonskii A K, Kharlampovich S I, Maschanova D D et al. [Effect of laser irradiation on a dystrophic process in the liver due to x-ray irradiation]. Med Radiol. 1983; 28: 59-61.

Polosukhin V V. Ultrastructure of the blood and lymphatic capillaries of the respiratory tissue during inflammation and endobronchial laser therapy. Ultrastructural Pathology. 2000; 24 (3): 183-189.

Ponnudurai R N et al. Hypoalgesic effect of laser photobiostimulation shown by rat tail flick test. Intern J Acup and Electrother Res. 1987; 12: 93-100.

Pöntinen P et al. Comparative effects of exposure to different light sources (He-Ne laser, InGaAl diode laser, a specific type of noncoherent LED) on skin blood flow for the head. Acupunct Electrother Res. 1996; 21 (2): 105-118.

Poon V K, Huang L, Burd A. Biostimulation of dermal fibroblasts by sublethal Q-switched Nd:YAG 532 nm laser: collagen remodeling and pigmentation. J Photochem Photobiol B. 2005: 1-8.

Popov B. Trigeminal neuralgia with local laser irradiation and laserpuncture. Stomatologiia Bulgaria. 1986; 68: 25-29.

Popova M et al. Effect of Helium-Neon laser beam in regeneration of irradiated transplanted skeletal muscle. Biull Exp Biol Med. 1978; 80: 333. (Russian with English abstract)

Porras M D, Bermudez D, Parrado C. Effects biologicos de la radiation laser IR sobre el epitelio seminifero. Invest Clin Laser. 1986; 3: 57-60.

Porteder H. Einsatz des Helium-Neon-Lasers zur Förderung der Wundheilung. Z Stomat. 1983; 80: 333-339.

Posso I P, Goncalves S A, Posso M B, Filipini R. Control of nipple pain during breastfeeding using low level laser therapy. Reg Anesth Pain Med. 2007; 32 (2) (Supplement): 185-185.

Pothman R, Yeh H L. The effects of treatment with antibiotics, laser and acupuncture upon chronic maxillary sinusitis in children. Am J Chin Med. 1982; 10 (1-4): 555-558.

Pereira A N, Eduardo C P, Matson E et al. Effect of low-power laser irradiation on cell growth and procollagen synthesis of cultured fibroblasts. Lasers Surg Med. 2002; 31: 263-267.

Pereira C L, Sallum E A, Nociti F H Jr, Moreira R W. The effect of low-intensity laser therapy on bone healing around titanium implants: a histometric study in rabbits. Int J Oral Maxillofac Implants. 2009; 24 (1): 47-51.

Pérez de Vargas I, Parrado C, González V, Vidal L, Rius F. Histological study of the thyroid gland following IR laser radiation. Proc. SPIE. 1992; 1981: 267-272.

Perrin D, Jolivald J R, Triki H et al. Effect of laser irradiation on latency of herpes simplex virus in a mouse model. Pathol Biol. 1997; 45 (1) : 24-27.

Pesevska S, Nakova M, Ivanovski K, Angelov N, Kesic L, Obradovic R, Mindova S, Nares S. Dentinal hypersensitivity following scaling and root planing: comparison of low-level laser and topical fluoride treatment. Lasers Med Sci. 2009 Jun 1. [Epub ahead of print]

Peters A. Blinding laser weapons. Med Confl Surviv. 1996; 12 (2): 107-113.

Petersen S L, Botes C, Olivier A, Guthrie A J. The effect of LLLT on wound healing in horses. Equine Vet J. 1999; 31 (3): 228-231.Petrek M et al. Immunomodulatory effects of laser therapy in the treatment of chronic tonsillitis. Acta Univ Palacki Olomuc Fac Med. 1991; 129: 119-126.

Pfander D, Jorgensen B, Rohde E, Bindig U, Muller G, Eric Scheller E. [The influence of laser irradiation of low-power density on an experimental cartilage damage in rabbit knee-joints: an in vivo investigation considering macroscopic, histological and immunohistochemical changes] Biomed Tech (Berlin). 2006; 51 (3):131-138. [in German]

Petrischev N N, Leontjeva N V, Leontjeva T A. Influence of irradiation of helium-neon laser on microcirculation blood vessels. Proc. SPIE. 1996; Vol 2929: 198-.

Petterborg L J, Kjellman B F, Thalén B E, Wetterberg L. Effect of a 15 minute light pulse on nocturnal serum melatonin levels in human volunteers. J Pineal Res. 1991; 10 (1): 9-13.

Pesevska S, Nakova M, Ivanovski K, Angelov N, Kesic L, Obradovic R, Mindova S, Nares S Dentinal hypersensitivity following scaling and root planing: comparison of low-level laser and topical fluoride treatment. Lasers Med Sci. 2009 Jun 1. [Epub ahead of print]

Pessoa E S, Melhado R M, Theodoro L H, Garcia V G. A histologic assessment of the influence of low-intensity laser therapy on wound healing in steroid-treated animals. Photomed Laser Surg. 2004; 22 (3): 199-204.

Piller N B, Thelander A, Esterman A. The objective assessment of the effect of low level laser therapy on chronic secondary arm and leg lymphoedemas. Proc. 3rd Cong World Ass for Laser Therapy, Athens, Greece, May 2000, p. 78.

Piller N B, Thelander A. Treatment of chronic postmastectomy lymphoedema with low level laser therapy: A 2.5 year follow-up. Lymphology. 1998; 31: 74-86.

Pinfildi C E, Liebano R E, Hochman B S, Ferreira L M. Helium-neon laser in viability of random skin flap in rats. Lasers Surg Med. 2005; 37 (1): 74-77.

Pinheiro A L, Carneiro Nascimento S, De Barros Vieira A L et al. Effects of low-level laser therapy on malignant cells: In vitro study. J Clin Med Surg. 2002; 20 (1): 23-26.

Pinheiro A L et al. Low-level laser therapy in the management of disorders of the maxillofacial region. J Clin Laser Med Surg. 1997; 15 (4): 181-183.

Pinheiro A, Oliveira M G, Martins P P M et al. Biomodulatory effects of LLLT bone regeneration. Laser Therapy. 2001; 13: 73-79.

Pinheiro A. Biomodulatory effects of LLLT on bone regeneration. Proc. 2nd ENSOMA Congress, Houston, Texas, USA. 2001, p. 14-22.

Pinheiro A L, Limeira Jr F de A, Gerbi M E et al. Effect of 830-nm laser light on the repair of bone defects grafted with inorganic bovine bone and decalcified cortical osseous membrane. J Clin Laser Med Surg. 2003; 21 (5): 301-306.

Parizotto N A, Baranauskas V. Structural analysis of collagen fibrils after HeNe laser photostimulated regenerating rat tendon. Proc. 2nd Congress World Assn for Laser Therapy, Kansas City, September 1998; p. 66.

Park S, Kim E Y, Yoon S H, Chung K S, Lim JH. Enhanced hatching rate of bovine IVM/IVF/IVC blastocysts using a 1.48-micron diode laser beam. J Assist Reprod Genet. 1999; 16: 97-101.

Parker J, Dowdy D, Harkness E et al. The effects of laser therapy on tissue repair and pain control. A meta analysis of the literature. Proc. 3rd Congress of the World Ass for Laser Therapy, Athens, Greece, 2000, page 77. Submitted Laser Surg Med 2001.

Parman E M. [Low-intensity laser radiation in combined treatment of urinary system tuberculosis]. Probl Tuberk. 1999; 6: 34-37.

Parrado C et al. Quantitative study of the Morphlogical Changes in the Thyroid Gland Following IR Laser Radiation. Lasers in Med Sciences. 1990; 5: 77-.

Parrado C, Carrillo de Albornoz F, Vidal L et al. A quantitative investigation of microvascular changes in the thyroid gland after infrared (IR) laser radiation. Histol H stopathol. 1999; 14 (4): 1067-1071.

Parshad R, Sanford K. Proliferative response of human diploid fibroblasts to intermittent light exposure. J Cell Physiol. 1977; 92: 481-.

Partheniadis-Stumpf M, Maurer J, Mann W. Soflasertherapie in Kombination mit Tebonin i.v. bei Tinnitus. Laryngorhinoootologie 1993; 72 (1): 28-31

Partonen T, Vakkuri O, Lönnqvist J. Suppression of melatonin secretion by bright light in seasonal affective disorder. Biol Psychiatry. 1997; Sep 15;42 (6): 509-513.

Paschaud Y et al. Effet du soft-laser sur la néofromation d'un pont dentinaire après coiffage pulpaire direct de dents humaines à l' hydroxyde de calcium. Rev Mens Suisse Odont-Stomatol. 1988; 98 (4): 345-349.

Passarella S et al. Increase in the ADP/ATP exchange in rat liver mitochondria irradiated in vitro by helium-neon laser. Biochem Biophys Res Commun. 1988; 156 (2): 978-986.

Passarella S et al. Increase of proton electrochemical potential and ATP synthesis in rat liver mitochondria irradiated in vitro by helium-neon laser. FEBS Letters. 1984; 175 (1): 95-99.

Passeniouk A M, Mikhailov V A. Application of low-level laser therapy for the treatment of vaginitis. In: A window on the laser medical world. Longo L ed. Proc. SPIE. 1999; Vol 4166: 316-318.

Pastore D et al. Stimulation of ATP synthesis via oxidative phosphorylation in weak mitochondria irradiated with helium-neon laser. Biochem Mol Biol Int. 1996; 39 (1): 149-157.

Pavlova R N. et al. Soft-laser radiation bioeffect: is laser a physical adaptogen? Proc. SPIE. 1993; Vol 1922: 225-229.

Pavlova, R N.; Gomberg, V. G.; Boiko, V. N.; Pupkova, L. S.; Reznikov, Leonid L.; Dadali, V. A. Effects of low-energy laser isolation upon the development of postradiation syndrome. Proc. SPIE. 1996; Vol 2769: 78-81. (Laser Optics '95: Biomedical Applications of Lasers)

Payer M, Jakse N, Pertl C, Truschnegg A et al. The clinical effect of LLLT in endodontic surgery: a prospective study on 72 cases. Oral Surg Oral Med Oral Pathol Oral Radiol Endod. 2005; 100 (3): 375-379.

Pedrola M et al. Acute cervical pain relieved with gallium arsenurio (GaAs) laser irradiation. A double blind study. Laser Surg Med. 1995, suppl 7, p 10.

Pekli F F, Kruchinina I L. [Physiological functions of the nose before and after laser treatment of acute and chronic maxillary sinusitis in children]. Vestn Otorinolaringol. 1988; (3): 53-55.

Peláez A et al. Growing cartilage after IR laser radiation - utlrastructural study. Proc SPIE. 1993;. Vol 2086: 356-364.

Ozen T, Orhan K, Gorur I, Ozturk A. Efficacy of low level laser therapy on neurosensory recovery after injury to the inferior alveolar nerve. Head Face Med. 2006; 15; (2): 3.

Ozcelik O, Cenk Haytac M, Kunin A, Seydaoglu G. Improved wound healing by low-level laser irradiation after gingivectomy operations: a controlled clinical pilot study. J Clin Periodontol. 2008; 35 (3): 250-254.

Ozcelik O, Cenk Haytac M, Seydaoglu G. Enamel matrix derivative and low-level laser therapy in the treatment of intra-bony defects: a randomized placebo-controlled clinical trial. Clin Periodontol. 2008; 35 (2): 147-156.

Ozkan N, Altan L, Bingol U et al. Investigation of the supplementary effect of GaAs laser therapy on the rehabilitation of human digital flexor tendons. J Clin Laser Med Surg. 2004; 22 (2): 105-110.

Padua L et al. Clinical outcome and neurophysiological results of low power laser irradiation in carpal tunnel syndrome. Lasers Med Sci. 1999; 14 (3); 196-202.

Padulles J et al. [Laser treatment of spinal pinching due to discal hernias in dogs]. Boletín CDL. 1986; 2: 11-14. (in Spanish)

Palchun V T et al. [Low-energy laser irradiation in the combined treatment of sensorineural hearing loss and Ménière's disease]. Vestnik Otorinolaring. 1996; (1): 23-25. (in Russian)

Paleev NR, Slinchenko O, Ilchenko VA et al. Influence of He-Ne laser blood irradiation on morphofunctional state of monocytes in asthmatic patients. In: Effects of low-power light on biological systems. Proce. SPIE. 1999; Vol 2630: 142-146.

Palma J et al. Blockade of inflammatory signals by laser radiation. Lasers in Surgery and Medcine. 1991; suppl 3: 11

Palmgren N et a. Low Level Laser Therapy of infected abdominal wounds after surgery. Laser Surg Med. 1991; Suppl 3:11.

Palmgren N, Jensen G F, Kaae K et al. Low-Power Laser Therapy in Rheumatoid Arthritis. Lasers in Medical Science. 1989; 4: 193-196.

Palmieri B A double blind stratified cross over study of amateur tennis players suffering from tennis elbow using infrared laser therapy. Medical Laser Report. 1984; 1: 3-14.

Palto S P, Durand G. Friction Model of Photo-induced Reorientation of Optical Axis in Photo-oriented Langmuir-Blodgett Films. J. Phys. II France. 1995; 5: 963-978.

Pankov O P. Low-level therapy in ophthalmology. In: Novel Laser Methods in Medicine and Biology. Eds. Prokhorov A M, Pustovoy V I, Kuzmin G P. Proc. SPIE. 1998; Vol 3829:13-17.

Paolini D, Paolini-Pisani L. Tratamiento de la lesion del tendón manguito de los rotadores con láser de baja potencia. Estúdio prospectivo. Proc. II Congr Internat Assn for Laser and Sports Medicine. Rosario, Argentina. March 2000.

Paolini L E et al. Tratamiento de la lesion Osgood-Schlatter con láser de baja potencia - estúdio prospectívo.Proc. II Congr Internat Assn for Laser and Sports Medicine. Rosario, Argentina. March 2000.

Paolini L E, Paolini D. Tratamiento de la parálisis de Bell con láser de baja potencia. Estúdio prospectivo. Proc. II Congr Internat Assn for Laser and Sports Medicine. Rosario, Argentina. March 2000.

Papadopoulos E S, Smith R W, Cawley M I D. Low-level laser therapy does not aid the management of tennis elbow. Clinical Rehabilitation. 1996; 10: 9-11.

Parascandalo S et al. Azione della Laser-terapia nella sindrome di Sluder: considerazioni clinico-etiopatogenetiche. Int Congress on Laser in Med and Surg, Bologna June 1985, p 325.

Parascandolo S et al. Azione della Laser-terapia nella nevralgia essenziale del trigemino. Int Congress on Laser in Med and Surg, Bologna June 1985, p 317. Monduzzi Editore S.p.A., Bologna, Italy.

Onizawa K, Muramatsu T, Matsuki M, Ohta K, Matsuzaka K, Oda Y, Shimono M. Low-level (gallium-aluminum-arsenide) laser irradiation of Par-C10 cells and acinar cells of rat parotid gland. Lasers Med Sci. 2009; 24 (2): 155-161.

Orchardson R, Whitters C J. Effect of HeNe and pulsed Nd:YAG laser irradiation on intradental nerve responses to mechanical stimulation of dentine. Laser Surg Med 2000; 26: 241-249.

O'Reilly B A, Dwyer P L, Hawthorne G et al. Transdermal posterior tibial nerve laser therapy is not effective in women with interstitial cystitis. J Urol. 2004; 172 (5 Pt 1): 1880-1883.

Oron U, Yaakobi T, Oron A et al. Attenuation of the formation of scar tissue in rats and dogs post myocardial infarction by low energy laser irradiation. Laser Surg Med. 2001; 28: 1-7.

Oron U, Yaakobi T, Oron A et al. Attenuation of infarct size in rats and dogs after myocardial infarction by low-energy laser irradiation. Laser Surg Med. 2001; 28 (3): 204-211.

Oron U. Photoengineering of tissue repair in skeletal and cardiac muscles. Photomed Laser Surg. 2006; 24 (2): 111-120.

Oron A, Oron U, Chen J, Eilam A et al. Low-level laser therapy applied transcranially to rats after induction of stroke significantly reduces long-term neurological deficits. Stroke. 2006; 37 (10): 2620-2624.

Oron A, Oron U, Streeter J, de Taboada L, Alexandrovich A, Trembovler V, Shohami. E. low-level laser therapy applied transcranially to mice following traumatic brain injury significantly reduces long-term neurological deficits. J Neurotrauma. 2007; 24 (4): 651-656.

Oron U, Ilic S, De Taboada L, Streeter J. Ga-As (808 nm) Laser Irradiation Enhances ATP Production in Human Neuronal Cells in Culture. Photomed Laser Surg. 2007; 25 (3): 180-182.

Ortutay J, Koo E, Mester A. Psoriatic arthritis treatment with low power laser irradiation. A double blind clinical study. Lasermedizin - Laser in Med Surg. 1998; 13 (3-4): 140-.

Ortutay J, Mester A. Laserstimulation therapy in the rehabilitation medicine. Proc. Laser Florence '97, 5th Congr , p. 22.

Otsuka H, Numasawa R, Okubo K et al. Effects of helium-neon laser therapy on herpes zoster pain. Laser Therapy. 1995; 7 (1): 27-32.

Otsuka K et al. Low reactive level laser therapy near the stellate ganglion for postherpetic facial pain. Jpn J Anaesthes. 1991; 41: 1809-1813. [In Japanese with abstract in English]

Otsuka H, Okubo K, Imai M, Kaseno S, Kemmotsu O. [Polarized light irradiation near the stellate ganglion in a patient with Raynaud's sign]. Masui. 1992; 41 (11): 1814-1817. [Article in Japanese]

Oudoff HAF; van der Kuiji P. Inquiry about the application of low reactive level laser therapy in dental clinics in The Netherlands. Laser Therapy. 1996; 8 (1): 42. (abstract)

Oulamara A. et al. Biological activity measurement on botanical specimen surfaces using a temporal decorrelation effect of laser speckle. Journal of Modern Optics. 1989; 36 (2): 165-.

Oyamada Y et al. Trials in treatment of RA-related diseases by HeNe-laser. Surg Med Lasers. 1989; 2: 18. Also in: Oyamada Y, Satodate R, Nishida J et al. Estudio en double ciego del efecto del laser de baja potencia HeNe en la artritis reumatoidea. Bol. CDL. 1988; 17: 8-12.

Oyamada Y et al. A double blind study of low power HeNe laser therapy in rheumatoid arthritis. In: Optoelectronics in Medicine. 1987; p 747-750. Springer Verlag, Berlin. (abstract) Complete study in Boletín de CDL. 1988; 17: 8-12.

Ozawa Y, Shimizu N, Abiko Y. Low-energy diode laser irradiation reduced plasminogen activator activity in human periodontal ligament cells. Laser Surg Med. 1997; 21: 456-463.

Ozawa Y et al. Stimulatory effects of low-power laser irradiation on bone formation in vitro. Proc SPIE. 1995; Vol 1984: 281-288.

Ozawa Y, Shimizu N, Kariya G et al. Low-energy laser irradiation stimulates bone nodule formation at early stages of cell culture in rat calvarial cells . Bone. 1998; 22 (4): 347-354.

Ohbayashi E, Matsushima K, Hosoya S et al. Stimulatory effect of laser irradiation on calcified nodule formation in human dental fibroblasts. J Endod. 1999. 25; 1: 30-33.

Ohno T. Pain suppressive effect of low power laser irradiation. A quantitative analysis of substance P in the rat spinal dorsal root ganglion. Nippon Ika Daigaku Zasshi (J Nippon Med School). 1997; 64 (5): 395-400. (in Japanese with English abstract)

Ohshiro T etr al. The Japanese experience in sumo wrestling. Proc. II Congr Internat Assn for Laser and Sports Medicine. Rosario, Argentina. March 2000.

Ohshiro T. Fujii S, Sasaki K et al. Laser therapy as an adjunct treatment for severe female infertility - a preliminary report. Laser Therapy. 1999; 11 (2): 96-102.

Ohshiro T. To publish, or not to publish.Editorial. Laser Therapy. 1989; 1 (2): 61-62.

Ohshiro T. Treatment techniques to achieve superficial and intermediate laser therapy irradiation. Laser Therapy. 1989; 3 (1): 153-155.

Ohshiro T. Alleviating Sport-relating pain with the diode laser. J Jap Soc Laser Med Surg. 1985; 5 (3): 221-.

Ohta A, Abergel P, Uitto J. Laser modulation of human immune system: Inhibition of lymphocyte proliferation by a gallium-arsenide laser at low energy. Laser Surg Med. 1987; 7: 199-.

Ohtsuka H et al. Low recative-level laser therapy near the stellate ganglion for postherpetic facial neuralgia. Masui. 1992; 41 (11): 1809-1813. (in Japanese)

Okamoto H, Iwase T, Morioka T. Dye-mediated bactericidal effffect of HeNe laser irradiation on oral microorganisms. Laser Surg Med. 1992; 12 (4): 450-458.

Oken O, Kahraman Y, Ayhan F, Canpolat S, Yorgancioglu Z R, Oken O F. The short-term efficacy of laser, brace, and ultrasound treatment in lateral epicondylitis: a prospective, randomized, controlled trial. J Hand Ther. 2008; 21 (1): 63-67.

Olban M, Wachowicz B, Koter M, et al. The biostimulatory effect of red laser irradiation on pig blood platelet function. Cell Biol Int. 1998: 22 (3): 245-248.

Oliveira N M, Parizzotto N A, Salvini T F. GaAs (904-nm) laser radiation does not affect muscle regeneration in mouse skeletal muscle. Laser Surg Med. 1999; 25: 13-21.

Oliveira Lopes C, Zangaro R A, Rigau J. Prevention of xerostomia induced by radiotherapy using low level laser. Photomed Laser Surg. 2005 (1). Abstracts from the 5th Congress of the World Association for Laser Therapy, November 25-27, 2004, São Paulo, Brazil. Abstr 001, p.90.

Oliveira F S, Pinfildi C E, Parizoto N A, Liebano R E, Bossini P S, Garcia E B, Ferreira L M. Effect of low level laser therapy (830 nm) with different therapy regimes on the process of tissue repair in partial lesion calcaneous tendon. Lasers Surg Med. 2009; 41 (4): 271-276.

Olivier J, Plath P. Combined low power laser therapy and extracts of Gingo Biloba in a blind trial of treatment for tinnitus. Laser Therapy. 1993; 5 (3): 137-140.

Olofsson M. Studying linear polarization of laser light when propagating through tissue. University of Linkoping, Sweden. Thesis, 2006. Prima Books AB, 2007.

Omura Y, Losco B M, Omura A K et al. Common factors contributing to intractable pain and medical problems with sufficient drug uptake in areas to be treated, and their pathologies and treatment. Acupunct Electrother Res. 1992; 17 (2): 107-

Onac I et al. Histological study regarding the effects of HeNe (632.8 nm) laser biostimu-lation upon the tegument of Cavia Cobaia as compared with that of monochromatic red light (618 nm). Proc. 2nd Congress World Assn for Laser Therapy, Kansas City, September 1998; p. 52-53.

Önal B et al. Preliminary report on the application of pulsed CO_2 laser radiation on root canals with AgCl fibers: a scanning and transmission electron microscopic study. J Endodontics. 1993; 19 (6): 272-276.

Novogrodski A. Lymphocyte activation induced by modifications of surface. In: Immune Recognition. Rosenthal S. Ed, Academic Press, New York, 1975, p. 43.

Novoselova E G, Glushkova O V, Cherenkov D A, Chudnovsky V M, Fesenko E E. Effects of low-power laser radiation on mice immunity. Photodermatol Photoimmurol Photomed. 2006; 22 (1): 33-38.

Numazawa R, Kemmotsu O, Otsuka H et al. The role of laser therapy in intensive pain management of postherpetic neuralgia. Laser Therapy. 1996; 8 (2): 143-148.

Núñez S C, Nogueira G E, Ribeiro M S, Garcez AS, Lage-Marques J L. He-Ne laser effects on blood microcirculation during wound healing: a method of in vivo study through laser Doppler flowmetry. Lasers Surg Med. 2004; 35 (5): 363-368.

Nuñez SC, Garcez AS, Suzuki SS, Ribeiro MS. Management of mouth opening in patients with temporomandibular disorders through low-level laser therapy and transcutaneous electrical neural stimulation. Photomed Laser Surg. 2006; 24 (1): 45-49.

Nussbaum E et al. Comparison of ultrasound/ultraviolet-C and laser for treatment of pressure ulcers in patients with spinal cord injury. Phys Ther. 1994; 74: 812-823.

Nussbaum E L. Low-intensity laser therapy for benign fibrotic lumps in the breast following reduction mammaplasty. Physical Therapy. 1999; 79 (7): 691-698.

Nussbaum E L, Lilge L, Mazzulli T. Effects of low-level laser therapy (LLLT) of 810 nm upon in vitro growth of bacteria: relevance of irradiance and radiant exposure. J Clin Laser Med Surg. 2003; 21 (5): 283-290.

Oasevich I A, Shargorodskii A G. [Low-intensity infrared laser radiation in the diagnosis and combined treatment of acute nonspecific lymphadenitis of the face and neck in children] Infrakrasnoe nizkointensivnoe lazer-noe izluchenie v diagnostike i kompleksnom lechenii ostrogo nespetsificheskogo limfadenita litsa i shei u detei. Stomatologiia (Mosk). 1999; 78 (2): 28-30.

Obata J et al. Clinical effects of total laser irradiation for the control of disease activity of chronic rheumatoid arthritis. Surgical and Medical Lasers. 1990; 3 (3): 140. (abstract)

Obata J et al. Evaluation of acute pain-relief effects of low power laser therapy on rheumatoid arthritis by thermography. Laser Therapy. 1990; 2: 28-

Obata J et al. The pain relief of low energy laser irradiation on rheumatoid arthritis. Pain Clin. 1987; 8: 18-.

Obata J, Yanse M. Evaluation of the effects of low power laser therapy on rheumatoid arthritis joints by roentgenographic survey. Laser Bologna '92, p. 41. Monduzzi Editore S.p.A., Bologna, Italy.

Obradovic R R, Kesic L G, Peševska S. Influence of low-level laser therapy on biomaterial osseointegration: a mini-review. Lasers Med Sci. 2009; 24 (3): 447-451.

Ocaña-Quero J M et al. Biological effects of helium-neon (He-Ne) laser irradiation on acrosome reaction in bull sperm cells. J Photochem Photobiol. B - Biol. 1997; 40 (3): 294-298.

Ocaña-Quero J M, Gomez-Villamandos R, Moreno-Millan M, Santisteban-Valenzuela J M. Helium-Neon (He-Ne) Laser Irradiation Increases the Incidence of Unreduced Bovine Oocytes During the First Meiotic Division In Vitro. Lasers Med Sci. 1998. 13 (4): 260-264.

Odud A M, Potapenko P I. [The effectiveness of laser puncture in hypertension patients]. Vrach Delo. 1990; (6): 19-21. (in Russian)

Odud A M, Potapenko P I. [The use of laser puncture for managing hypertensive crises]. Vrach Delo. 1991; (7): 34-36. (in Russian)

Özdemir F, Birtane M, Kokino S. The clinical efficacy of low-power laser therapy on pain and function in cervical osteoarthritis. Clinical Rheumatology. 2001; 20 (3): 181-184.

Ng G Y, Fung D T, Leung M C, Guo X. Comparison of single and multiple applications of GaAlAs laser on rat medial collateral ligament repair. Laser Surg Med. 2004; 34 (3): 285-289.

Ng G Y F, Fung D T C. The Combined Treatment Effects of Therapeutic Laser and Exercise on Tendon Repair. Photomed Laser Surg. 2008; 26 (2): 137-141.

Ng G Y, Fung D T. Combining therapeutic laser and herbal remedy for treating ligament injury: an ultrastructural morphological study. Photomed Laser Surg. 2008; 26 (5): 425-432.

Nicola J H et al. The role of coherence in wound healing stimulation by non-thermal laser radiation. Surgical and Medical Lasers. 1989; 2-3 (2): 70 (abstract)

Nicola J H, Nicola E M D, Simões M, Paschoal J R. Role of polarization and Coherence of Laser Light on Wound Healing. Laser Tissue Interaction. V S.L. Jacques, ed. Proc SPIE. 1994; Vol 2134A: 448-450.

Nicola E M, Nicola J H. Low-power CO_2 laser in the treatment of chronic pharyngitis: a five-year experience. Proc. SPIE. 1994; Vol 2128: 85-87. (Laser Surgery: Advanced Characterization, Therapeutics, and Systems IV).

Nicolau R A, Jorgetti V, Rigau J et al. Effect of low power laser Ga-Al-As (660 nm) in the bone tissue remodelation in mice. Proc. 4th Congress of the World Association for Laser Therapy, Tokyo, Japan, June 27-30. 2002; p. 127.

Nicolau R A, Jorgetti V, Rigau J, Marcos T T. Effect of low-power GaAlAs laser (660 nm) on bone structure and cell activity: an experimental animal study. Lasers in Medical Science. 2003; 18 (2): 89-94.

Nicolopoulos C et al. Clinical application of helium neon (632 nm) plus infrared diode laser GaAlAs (830 nm) and CO_2 laser in the treatment of onychomycotic nails. Foot. 1999; 9 (4): 181-184.

Nicolopoulos N, Dyson M et al. The use of laser surgery in the subtotal meniscectomy and the effect of low-level laser therapy on the healing potential of rabbit meniscus: an experimental study. Lasers Med Sci. 1996; 11 (2): 109-115.

Nikitin A V, Karpukhina E P. The effect of endovascular laser therapy on the clinical course and on the mechanisms of antioxidant protection in brochical asthma patients. Ter Arkh. 1992; 64 (1): 62-64. (in Russian)

Nikitin A V, Kashin A V, Karpukhina EP. Correction of the antioxidant defence in patients with bronichial asthma by the method of intravascular laser irradiation. Probl Tuberk. 1993; 3: 46-47.

Nishida J, Satoh T, Satodate R et al. Histological evaluation of the effect of HeNe laser irradiation on the synovial membrane in rheumatoid arthritis. Jap J Rheumatol. 1990; 2: 251-260.

Nissan J, Binderman I. Effect of soft laser on bone healing of surgical defect in rat mandible. J Dent Res. 1993; 72 (4) :776, Abstract 53.

Nissen L R et al. [Low-energy laser therapy in medial tibial stress syndrome]. Ugeskrift Læger. 1994; 156 (49): 7329-7331. (in Danish)

Nivbrant B, Friberg S. Knee - Therapeutic Laser Treatment in Gonarthroses. Acta Orthop Scand. 1989; 60 (suppl 231): 33.

Nomura K, Yamaguchi M, Abiko Y. Inhibition of Interleukin-1-beta production and gene expression in human gingival fibroblasts by low-energy laser irradiation. Lasers Med Sci. 2001; 16 (3): 218-223.

Noro S. Semi-conductor laser application for pain attenuation in the temporo-mandibular joint following facial contusion and facial fracture. Meeting report from the 1st Congr of the IALSM 1997. Laser Therapy. 1997; 9 (4): 184.

Novak C, Spelman L. Low energy fluence CO_2 laser treatment of lymphangiectasia. Australas J Dermatol. 1998; (4): 277-278.

Naim JO, Yu W, Ippolito K M L et al. The effect of low level laser irradiation on nitric oxide production by mouse macrophages. Lasers Surg. Med. 1996; Suppl. 8, 7 (abstr. 28).

Naeser M A. Treatment of carpal tunnel syndrome: research and clinical studies with laser acupuncture and microamps TENS. Proc. 2nd Congress World Assn for Laser Therapy, Kansas City, September 1998; p. 145-146.

Naeser M A, Hahn K, Lieberman B E. Carpal tunnel syndrome pain treated with low-level laser and microamps TENS, a controlled study. Arch Phys Med Rehabil. 2002; 83: 978-988.

Nagao M, Yamaguchi S, Okuda Y. [Effects of low reactive level laser, linear polarized light and Xenon-ray irradiation on the stellate ganglion in dogs]. Masui. 2001; 50 (9): 958-963. [Article in Japanese]

Nagasawa A et al. Fundamental studies in reactive histological changes in pulp tissue of lased teeth. J Jap Soc Laser Med Surg.

Nagasawa A, Negishi A, Kato K. Clinical Applications of laser therapy in Dental and oral Surgery in the Urawa Clinic. Laser Therapy. 1991; 3 (3): 119-122.

Nagasawa A. Application of laser therapy in Dentistry.In: Low-Reactive Laser Therapy - Practical Application. T. Ohshiro. John Wiley & Sons. 1991: 76-.

Nakashima T, Ueda H, Misawa H et al. Transmeatal low-power laser irradiation Nakashima T, Ueda H, Misawa H et al. Transmeatal low-power laser irradiation for tinnitus. Otology & Neurotology. 2002; 23 (3): 296-300.

Nakamura H, Nakamura K, Yodoi J. Redox regulation of cellular activation, Annu Rev Immunol. 1997; 15: 351-369.

Nara Y et al. Stimulative effect of HeNe laser irradiation on cultured fibroblasts derived from human dental pulp. Lasers in the Life Sciences. 1992; 4 (4): 249-.

Nascimento P M, Pinheiro A L, Salgado M A, Ramalho L M. A preliminary report on the effect of laser therapy on the healing of cutaneous surgical wounds as a consequence of an inversely proportional relationship between wavelength and intensity: histological study in rats. Photomed Laser Surg. 2004; 22 (6): 513-518.

Nascimento R X, Callera F. Low-level laser therapy at different energy densities (0.1-2.0 J/cm^2) and its effects on the capacity of human long-term cryopreserved peripheral blood progenitor cells for the growth of colony-forming units. Photomed Laser Surg. 2006; 24 (5): 601-604.

Nasu F, Tomiyasu K, Inomata K, Calderhead R G. Cytochemical Effects of GaAlAs Diode Laser Radiation on Rat Saphenous Artery Calcium Ion Dependent Adenosine Triphosphatase Activity. Laser Therapy. 1989; 1 (2): 89-92.

Naveh N et al. Low-energy laser. a new measure for suppression of arachidonic acid metabolism in the optic nerve. J Neurosci Res. 1990; 26: 386-389.

Neckel C. The effect of low level laser therapy with a GaAlAs diode laser on the bony regeneration of extraction sockets. ESOLA congress Abu Dhabi, October 7-8, 2004. Clinical Experiences in Laser Dentistry.

Neira R, Arroyave J, Ramirez H, Ortiz C L, Solarte E, Sequeda F, Gutierrez M I. Fat liquefaction: effect of low-level laser energy on adipose tissue. Plast Reconstr Surg. 2002; 110 (3): 912-22; discussion 923-925.

Nelson A J, Friedman M H. Somatosensory trigeminal evoked potential amplitudes following low level laser and sham irradiation over time. Laser Therapy. 2001; 13: 60-64.

Nelson R.D,. Mills E.L,. Simmons R.L. et al. Infect. Immun., 1976; 14: 29-33.

Nes A G, Posso M B. Patients with moderate chemotherapy-induced mucositis: pain therapy using low intensity lasers. Int Nurs Rev. 2005; 52 (1): 68-72.

Neuman I, Finklestein Y, Lubart R. Low energy phototherapy in allergic rhinitis and nasal polyposis. Laser Therapy. 1996. 1: 37. (abstract)

Morrone G et al. Muscular trauma treated with GaAlas diode laser: in vivo experimental study. Lasers in Medical Science. 1998; 13 (4): 293-298.

Morrone G, Guzzardella G A, Tigani D et al. Biostimulation of human chondrocytes with Ga-Al-As diode laser: 'In vitro' research. Artificial Cells, Blood Substitutes, and Immobilization Biotechnology. 2000; 28 (2): 193-201.

Morrone G, Guzzardella G A, Torricelli P et al. Osteochondral lesion repair of the knee in the rabbit after low-power diode Ga-Al-As laser biostimulation: an experimental study. Artificial Cells, Blood Substitutes, and Immobilization Biotechnology. 2000; 28 (4): 321-336.

Morselli M et al. Effects of very low energy-density treatment of joint pain by CO2 laser. Laser Surg Med. 1985; 5:150-.

Morton A R, Fazio S M, Miller D. Efficacy of laser-acupuncture in the prevention of exercise-induced asthma. Ann Allergy 1993; 70 (4): 295-298.

Motomura K et al. Effects of various laser irradiation on callus formation after osteotomy. J Jpn Soc Laser Med. 1984; 4: 195-196.

Mousques T. Étude en double aveugle des effets du traitment unilateral au laser hélium-néon lors de chirurgies parodontales bilàterales simultanés. [Double blind study on the effects of helium-neon laser in simultaneous bilateral periodontical surgery] Quest Odontostomatol. 1986; 11: 245-254

Mousques T: Étude en double aveugle des effets du hélium-néon en chirurgie parodontale [Double blind study on the effects of helium-neon laser in periodontal surgery]. Quest Odonto-Stomatol 1986; 11: 233-244.

Moustsen P et al. Laserbehandling af bihulebetændelse i almen lægepraxis vurderet ved en dobbeltblind kontrolleret undersøgelse. [Laser Treatment of Sinuitis in General Medical Praxis Evaluated in a Double Blind Study]. Ugeskrift Læger. 1991; 153 (32): 2232-2234. (in Danish)

Mozgunov V N et al. [Method of treatment of common warts with low-energy laser irradiation.] Vestnik Dermatologii i Venerologii. 1985; (2): 55-56.

Mrowiec J et al. Analgesic effect of low-power infrared laser radiation in rats. Proc SPIE. 1997; Vol 3198: 83-89.

Mrowiec J et al. The antinociceptive effect of infrared laser radiation in experimental animals. Laser Therapy. 1996; 8 (1): 25. (abstract)

Muldiyarov P et al. Effect of Monochromatic Helium-Neon Laser Red Light on the Morphology of Zymosan Arthritis in Rats. Biull Eksp Biol Med. 1983; 1: 55-.

Müller K P, Rodrigues C R, Núnez S C et al. Effects of low power red laser on induced-dental caries in rats. Archives of Oral Biology. 2007; 52 (7): 648-654.

Mulligan S et al. The effect of low energy HeNe laser irradiation on the neurite elongation in vitro. Laser Surg Med. 1991; Suppl 3: 10.

Murakami F, Kemmotsu O, Kawano Y et al.. Diode low reactive level laser therapy and stellate ganglion block compared in the treatment of facial paralysis. Laser Therapy. 1993; 5 (3):131-135.

Murphy PJ, Campbell SS. Enhanced performance in elderly subjects following bright light treatment of sleep maintenance insomnia. J Sleep Res. 1996 ; (3): 165-72.

Mvula B, Mathope T, Moore T, Abrahamse H. The effect of low level laser irradiation on adult human adipose derived stem cells. Lasers Med Sci. 2008; 23 (3): 277-282.

Mvula B, Moore T J, Abrahamse H. Effect of low-level laser irradiation and epidermal growth factor on adult human adipose-derived stem cells. Lasers Med Sci. 2010; 25 (1): 33-39.

Myrhaug H. The theory of otosclerosis and Morbus Ménière (Labyrintine vertigo) being caused by the same mechanism: physical irritants, an otognathic syndrome. Bergmanns Boktrykkeri A/S, Bergen, Norway. 1981.

Molina Soto J J, Moller I. La laserterapía como coadyuvante en el tratamiento de la A.R. (Artritis Reumatoidea). Bol. C.D.L. 1987; 14: 4-8.

Moller K I, Kongshoj B, Philipsen P A et al. How Finsen's light cured lupus vulgaris. Photodermatol Photoimmunol Photomed. 2005 Jun;21(3):118-124.

Monich V A, Malinovskaja S, Lockhmachova E et al. Effect of low-power luminescent irradiation on surgical and burn wounds of soft tissues. Proc. SPIE. 1996; Vol 2929: 58-62.

Monstrey S, Hoeksema H, Depuydt K et al. The effect of polarized light on wound healing. Eur J Plast Surg. 2002; 24: 377-382.

Montag M, Rink K, Delacretaz G, van der Ven H. Laserinduced immobilization and plasma membrane permeabilization in human spermatozoa. Hum Reprod. 2000; 15: 846-852.

Monteforte P, Baratto L, Molfetta L, Rovetta G. Low-power laser in osteoarthritis of the cervical spine. Int J Tissue React. 2003; 25 (4): 131-136.

Monteiro Martins P P et al. P.P.M.M. implant system has osseointegration improved by laser therapy. Proc. 3rd Congr World Assn for Laser Therapy, Athens, Greece, May 2000, p. 124.

Montes-Molina R, Madroñero-Agreda M A, Romojaro-Rodríguez A B, Gallego-Mendez V, Prados-Cabiedas C, Marques-Lucas C, Pérez-Ferreiro M, Martinez-Ruiz F. Efficacy of Interferential Low-Level Laser Therapy Using Two Independent Sources in the Treatment of Knee Pain. Photomed Laser Surg. 2009 Apr 30. [Epub ahead of print]

Montesinos M. et al. Experimental Effects of Low Power Laser in Encephalin and Endorphin Synthesis. LASER. Journ Eur Med Laser Ass. 1988; 1 (3): 2-6.

Moore K C. Postherpetic neuralgia as a complication of malignant disease and its treatment using a GaAlAs diode laser. Laser Therapy. 1996; 8 (1): 49. (abstract)

Moore K, Hira N, Kumar. Ohshiro T. Double blind crossover trial of low level laser therapy in the treatment of post herpetic neuralgia. Laser Therapy. 1988; (pilot issue): 7-10.

Moore K, Hira N, Broome I J, Cruikshank J A. The effect of infra-red diode laser irradiation on the duration and severity of postoperative pain. A double-blind trial. Laser Therapy. 1992; 4 (4): 145-150.

Moore K. Laser therapy in post herpetic neuralgia. Laser Therapy. 1996; 8 (1): 48 (abstract)

Moreira L A, Santos M T, Campos V F, Genovese W J. Efficiency of laser therapy applied in labial traumatism of patients with spastic cerebral palsy. Braz Dent J. 2004;15 Spec No: 29-33.

Moritz A et al. Advantage of a pulsed CO_2 laser in direct pulp capping. A long-term in vivo study.Laser Surg Med. 1998; 22: 288-293.

Moritz A et al. Irradiation of infected root canals with a diode laser in vivo: results of microbiological examinations. Laser Surg Med. 1997; 21: 221-226.

Moritz M D et al. The advantage of CO_2 treated dental necks, in comparison with a standard method: Results from an in vitro study. J Clin Laser Med Surg. 1996; 14 (1): 27.

Moritz A, Schoop U, Goharkhay K, Jakolitsch S et al. The bactericidal effect of Nd:YAG, Ho:YAG, and Er:YAG laser irradiation in the root canal: an in vitro comparison. J Clin Laser Med Surg. 1999; 17 (4): 161-164.

Moriyama Y, Moriyama EH, Blackmore K, Akens MK, Lilge L. In vivo study of the inflammatory modulating effects on low-level laser therapy on iNOS expression using bioluminescence imaging. Photochem Photobiol. 2005; 81 (6): 1351-135.

Moriyama Y, Nguyen J, Akens M, Moriyama E H, Lilge L. In vivo effects of low level laser therapy on inducible nitric oxide synthase. Lasers Surg Med. 2009; 41 (3): 227-231.

Morozova S V et al. [Possibilities of helium-neon lasers in olfactory disorders]. Vestn Otorinolaringol. 1995; 5: 35-36.

Mirz F, Zachariae R, Andersen S E et al. The low-power laser in the treatment of tinnitus. Clin Otolaryngol 1999; 24: 346-354.

Mirzaei M, Bayat M, Mosafa N, Mohsenifar Z et al. Effect of Low-Level Laser Therapy on Skin Fibroblasts of Streptozotocin-Diabetic Rats. Photomed Laser Surg. 2007; 25 (6): 519-525.

Mirzaii-Dizgah I, Ojaghi R, Sadeghipour-Roodsari H R, Karimian S M, Sohanaki H. Attenuation of morphine withdrawal signs by low level laser therapy in rats. Behav Brain Res. 2009; 196 (2): 268-270.

Mischenkin N V et al. [Effects of helium-neon laser energy on the tissues of the middle ear in the presence of biological fluids and drug solutions]. Vestn Otorinolaringol. 1990; 5: 18-21.

Mizutani K, Musya Y, Wakae K, Kobayashi T et al. A clinical study on serum prostaglandin E_2 with low-level laser therapy. Photomed Laser Surg. 2004; 22 (6): 537-539.

Miyagi K. Double-blind comparative study of the effect of low-energy laser irradiation to rheumatoid arthritis. In: Current awareness of Excerpts Medica. Amsterdam. Elsevier Science Publishers BV. 1989; 25: 315. Also: J Jap Assoc Physical Med Balneol & Climatol. 1989; 52 (3): 117-126.

Miyajima K, Yoshida K, Iwata T, et al. Effects of HeNe laser irradiation on gingival fibroblasts. Aichi-Gakuin Dent Sci. 1994; 7: 1-5.

Mizokami T et al. Effect of diode laser for pain: A clinical study on different pain types. Laser Therapy. 1990; 2 (4): 171-174.

Mizokami T, Aoki K, Iwabuchi S et al. Laser therapy (Low Reactive Level Laser Therapy) - a clinical study: relationship between pain attenuation and the serotonergic mechanism. Laser Therapy. 1993; 5 (4): 165-168.

Mochizuki O N, Kataoka Y, Cui Y et al. Effects of near-infra-red laser irradiation on adenosine triphosphate and adenosine diphosphate contents of rat brain tissue. Neuroscience letters. 2002; 323 (3): 207-210.

Mochizuki-Oda N, Kataoka Y, Cui Y, Yamada H, Heya M, Awazu K. Effects of near-infra-red laser irradiation on adenosine triphosphate and adenosine diphosphate contents of rat brain tissue. Neurosci Lett. 2002; 323 (3): 207-210.

Moges H, Vasconcelos O M, Campbell W W, Borke R C, McCoy J A, Kaczmarczyk L, Feng J, Anders J J. Light therapy and supplementary Riboflavin in the SOD1 transgenic mouse model of familial amyotrophic lateral sclerosis (FALS). Lasers Surg Med. 2009; 41 (1): 52-59.

Mognato M, Squizzato F, Facchin F, Zaghetto L, Corti L. Cell growth modulation of human cells irradiated in vitro with low-level laser therapy. Photomed Laser Surg. 2004; 22 (6): 523-526.

Mok YC, Pang KM, Au CY, Yew DT. Preliminary observations on the effects in vivo and in vitro of low dose laser on the epithelia of the bladder, trachea and tongue of the mouse. Scanning Microsc. 1988; 2 (1): 493-502.

Mokhtar B et al. A double blind placebo controlled investigation of the hypoalgesic effects of low intensity laser irradiation of the cervical roots using experimental ischaemic pain. ILTA Congress, London l992, abstracts p 61.

Mokhtar B et al. The possible significance of pulse repetition rate in laser-mediated analgesia: a double blind placebo controlled investigation using experimental ischaemic pain. ILTA Congress, London l992, abstracts p 62.

Mokmeli S, Bishe Sh, Kahe Kh, Shakhes M. Intravascular laser therapy (IVL) in pre-hypertension and hypertension conditions. Proc. 7th Internat Congr of WALT, Sun City, South Africa, October 2008, page 140.

Mokmeli S, Khazemikho N, Niromanesh S, Vatankhah Z. The Application of Low-Level Laser Therapy after Cesarean Section Does Not Compromise Blood Prolactin Levels and Lactation Status. Photomed Laser Surg. 2009 Apr 30. [Epub ahead of print]

Migliorati C, Massumoto C, Eduardo C P et al. Low-energy laser therapy in oral mucositis. J Oral Laser Applications. 2001; 1 (2): 97.101-.

Mijailovic B, Karadaglic D, Mladenovic T et al. Painful piezogenic pedal papules - successful low level laser therapy. Acta Dermatovenerologica, Pannonica, Alpina et Adriatica. 2001; 10 (3).

Mika T et al. [Infrared laser radiation in the treatment of low back pain syndrome]. Wiad Lek. 1990; 43 (11): 511-516. (in Polish)

Mikhailov V A et al. Results of treatment of the patients with IInd - IIIrd st. breast cancer by combination of low level laser therapy (laser therapy) and surgery -10-years experience. In: A window on the laser medicine world. Longo L ed. Proc. SPIE. 1999; Vol 4166: 40-42.

Mikhailov V A et al. Results of treatments of patients with stomach cancer advanced form treated by combination of low level laser therapy (laser therapy) and other methods (10-years experience). In: A window on the laser medicine world. Longo L ed. Proc. SPIE. 1999; Vol 4166: 43-47.

Mikhailov V A et al. The immunomodulating action of low-energy laser radiation in the treatment of bronchial asthma. Vopr Kurortol Fizioter Lech Fiz Kult. 1998; (4): 23-25.

Mikhailov V A et al. Use of immunomodulative influence of low-level laser radiation in the treatment of an autoimmune thyroiditis. In: A window on the laser medicine world. Longo L ed. Proc. SPIE. 1999, Vol 4166: 319-322.

Mikhailov V A , Skobelkin O K, Denisov I N, Frank G A, Voltchenko N N. Investigations on the influence of Low Level Diode Laser irradiation of the growth of experimental tumors. Laser Therapy. 1993; 5 (1): 33-38.

Mikhailov V A, Denisov I N. Activation of the immune system by low level laser therapy (laser therapy) for treating patients with stomach cancer in advanced form. Laser & Technology. 1997; 7 (1): 31-44.

Mikhailova R I et al. The laser therapy and laser acupuncture of patients with chronic recurrent aphtous stomatitis. Stomatologiia (Moscow). 1992; 3-6: 27-28.

Miles V, Klein. Optics. John Wiley & Sons inc. New York. Chapter 10.3, page 507-520

Millson C E, Wilson M et al. The killing of Helicobacter pylori by low-power laser light in the presence of a photosensitiser. J Med Microbiol. 1996; 44 (4): 245-52.

Milojevic M, Kuruc V. [Low power laser biostimulation in the treatment of bronchial asthma]. Biostimulacija laserom niske snage u lecenju bronhijalne astme. Medicinski pregled. 2003; 56 (9-10): 413-418.

Miloro M, Repasky M. Low-level laser effect on neurosensory recovery after sagittal ramus osteotomy. Oral surgery, oral medicine, oral pathology, oral radiology,and endodontics. 2000; 89 (1): 12-18.

Miloro M, Miller J J, Stoner J A. Low-Level Laser Effect on Mandibular Distraction Osteogenesis . J Oral Maxillofac Surg. 2007; 65 (2): 168-176.

Minatel D G, Frade M A, França S C, Enwemeka C S. Phototherapy promotes healing of chronic diabetic leg ulcers that failed to respond to other therapies.Lasers Surg Med. 2009; 41 (6): 433-441.

Miro L et al. Estudio capilaroscópico de la acción de un laser AsGa sobre la microcirculación. Investig Clínica Láser. 1984; 1/2: 9-14.

Miroshnikov B I, Reznikov L L, Ogurtsov R P, Khachatrian S A. [Immunological characteristics of the course of acute nonspecific epididymitis in relation to the treatment performed]. Vestn Khir Im I I Grek. 1992; 148: 156-161.

Mirsky N, Krispel Y, Shoshany Y, Maltz L, Oron U. Promotion of angiogenesis by low energy laser irradiation. Antioxid Redox Signal. 2002; 4 (5): 785-790.

Melnichenko E M et al. [The clinico-experimental validation of the use of low-intensity laser radiation for the treatment of exacerbated recurrent herpetic stomatitis in children]. Stomatologiia. 1992; (2): 76-78.

Melo C A, Lima A L, Brasil I et al. Characterization of light penetration in rat tissues. J Clin Laser Med Surg. 201;19 (4): 175-179.

Meneguzzo D T, Pallotta R, Ramos L, Penna S, Marcos R L, Teixeira S, Muscará M N, Bjordal J M, Lopes-Martins R A, Ribeiro M S. Near infrared laser therapy (810 nm) on lymph nodes: Effects on acute inflammatory process. Proc. 7th Internat Congr of WALT, Sun City, South Africa, October 2008, page 11.

Merli L A, Santos M T, Genovese W J, Faloppa F. Effect of low-intensity laser irradiation on the process of bone repair. Photomed Laser Surg. 2005; 23 (2): 212-215.

Mester A et al. Irradiation of arthritis with 820 and 830 nm diode lasers. Laser Therapy. 1996; 8 (1): 33. (abstract)

Mester A, Ortutay J, Barabás K. Laser therapy in rheumatology. Abstracts of 7th Int Congr European Medical Laser Assn, Dubrovnik, Croatia 2000, p. 36.

Mester A. Biostimulative effect in wound healing by continous wave 820 nm laser diode double-blind randomized cross-over study. Lasers in Med Science, abstract issue July 1988.

Mester Andrew, Mester Adam. Scientific background of laser biostimulation. LASER. Journ Eur Med Laser Ass. 1988; 1 (1): 23-.

Mester E et al. Effect of laser-rays on wound healing. Am J Surg. 1971; 122: 532-.

Mester E, Mester A F, Mester A. The biomedical effects of laser application. Laser Surg Med. 1985; 5: 31-39.

Mester E, Szende B, Tota J. Die Wirkung der Laser-Strahlen auf den Haarwuchs der Maus. Radiobiol. Radiother. 9: 621-626. Original paper: Mester E, Szende B, Tota JG. Effect of laser on hair growth of mice. Kiserl Orvostud. 1967; 19: 628-631.

Mester E. et al. Auswirkungen direkter Laserbestrahlung auf menschliche Lymphozyten. Arch Dermatol Res. 1978; 5: 31-

Mester E. et al. The Biostimulating Effect of Laser Beam. Proc from Laser - 81, Opto-Elektronik, Munich 1981.

Mester E. et al. Untersuchungen über die hemmende bzw. fördernde Wirkung der Laserstrahlen. Arch Klin Chir. 1968; 322: 1022-.

Mester A F, Snow J B Jr, Shaman P. Photochemical effects of laser irradiation on neuritic outgrowth of olfactory neuroepithelial explants. Otolaryngol Head Neck Surg. 1991; 105 (3): 449-456.

Meyers A, Joyce J, Cohen J. Effects of low-watt Helium Neon laser radiation on human lymphocyte cultures. Laser Surg Med. 1987; 6: 540-.

Mezawa S et al. The possible analgesic effect of soft-laser irradiation on heat nociceptors in the cat tounge. Ach Oral Biol. l988; 33 (9): 693-694.

Mi X Q, Chen J Y, Zhou L W. Effect of low power laser irradiation on disconnecting the membrane-attached hemoglobin from erythrocyte membrane. J Photochem Photobiol B. 2006; 1: 832: 146-150.

Michels H. Erfahrungen mit dem HeNe Laser bei Herpes Erkrankungen. Proc. 7th Int Congr Laser 1985. Edit. W Waidelinch. 1986; 116-119. Springer-Verlag (Berlin).

Midamba E D, Haanaes H R. Low reactive-level 830 nm GaAlAs diode laser therapy (laser therapy) successfully accelerates regeneration of peripheral nerves in human. Laser Therapy, 1993; 5 (3): 125-130.

Midamba E D, Haanaes H. Effect of low level laser therapy (laser therapy) on inferior alveolar, mental and lingual nerves after traumatic injury in 15 patients. A pilot study. Laser Therapy. 1993; 5 (2): 89-94.

McCaughan J S Jr, Bethel B H, Johnston T, Janssen W. Effect of low-dose argon irradiation on rate of wound closure. Lasers Surg Med. 1985; 5 (6): 607-614.

McGuff P E, Deterling R A Jr, Gottlieb L S. Tumoricidal effect of laser energy on experimental and human malignant tumors. N Engl J Med. 1965; 273 (9): 490-492.

McGuff P E, Deterling R A Jr, Gottlieb L S, Fahimi H D, Bushnell D, Roeber F. Effects Of Laser Radiation On Tumor Transplants. Fed Proc. 1965; 24: Suppl 14: 150-154.

McGuff P E, Bell E J. The effect of laser energy radiation on bacteria. Med Biol Illus. 1966; 16 (3): 191-193.

McGuff P E, Gottlieb L S, Katayama I, Levy C K. Comparative study of effects of laser and/or ionizing radiation therapy on experimental or human malignant tumors. Am J Roentgenol Radium Ther Nucl Med. 1966; 96 (3): 744-748.

McGuff P E, Deterling R A Jr, Gottlieb L S. Laser radiation for metastatic malignant melanoma. JAMA. 1966; 31; 195 (5): 393-394.

McGuff P E. Laser radiation for basal cell carcinoma. Dermatologica. 1966; 133 (5): 379-383.

McGuff P E. Tumoricidal effect of laser radiation on malignant tumors. Int Ophthalmol Clin. 1966; 6 (2): 379-386.

McKibbin L. Low Level Laser Therapy in Veterinary Practice on Standardbred Horses. In: Low Level Laser Therapy. A Practical Introduction, Eds Ohshiro & Calderhead. John Wiley & Sons. 1988: 77-80.

McKibbin L et al. Treatment of post herpetic neuralgia using a 904 nm (infrared) low energy laser: A clinical study. Laser Therapy. 1991; 3 (1): 35-40.

McKibbin L, Paraschak D A. Study of the Effects of Lasering on Chronic Bowed Tendons at Whitney Hall Farm Limited, Canada. Laser Surg Med. 1983; 3 (1): 55-59.

McMeeken J, Stillman B. Perceptions of the clinical efficacy of laser therapy. Australian J Physiotherapy. 1993; 39 (2): 101-105.

McNamara D C, Rosenberg I, Jackson P A et al. Efficacy of arthroscopic surgery and midlaser treatment for chronic temporomandibular joint articular disc derangement following motor vehicle accident. Austr Den J. 1996; 41 (6): 377-387.

Medenica L, Lens M. The use of polarised polychromatic non-coherent light alone as a therapy for venous leg ulceration. J Wound Care. 2003; 12: 37-40.

Medrado R A P, Pugliese L S, Reis S R A, Andreade Z A A. The influence of low level laser therapy on wound healing and its biological action upon myofibroblasts. Lasers Surg Med. 2003; 32 (3): 239-244.

Medrado AP, Trindade E, Reis SR, Andrade ZA. Action of low-level laser therapy on living fatty tissue of rats. Lasers Med Sci. 2006; 21 (1): 19-23.

Meersman P. Laser pharmacology and achilles tendinopathy. Laser Therapy. 1999; 11 (3): 144-150.

Meguro D, Yamaguchi M, Kasai K. Laser irradiation inhibition of open gingival embrasure space after orthodontic treatment. Aust Orthod J. 2002; 18 (1): 53-63.

Meirelles G C S, Santos J N, Chagas P O, Moura A P, Pinheiro A L B. A Comparative Study of the Effects of Laser Photobiomodulation on the Healing of Third-Degree Burns: A Histological Study in Rats. Photomed Laser Surg. 2008; 26 (2): 159-166.

Mehdi M S, al Magsosy R. Design and Construction of a System to Study the Effect of Laser Radiation on the Absorption of the Antibiotics in Blood. Thesis for PhD. 2005. Department of Laser and Optoelectronics Engineering, Al-Nahrain University, Al-Jaderia, Baghdad, Iraq.

Meier J-L, Kerkour K. Traitement laser de la tendinite. Méd et Hyg. 1988; 46: 907-911.

Melges F T. Efficacy of therapies for depression. Am J Psychiatry. 1981; 138 (11): 1513.

Maricic B et al. Analgetic effect of laser in dental therapy. Acta Stomat Croat. 1987; 21 (4): 291-295.

Marino A, Giavelli S, Galanti A et al. Low level laser therapy of chronic wounds of geriatric patients: preliminary report. Laser & Technology. 1996; 6 (1/2): 41-47.

Markovic A B, Kokovic V, Todorovic L. The influence of low-power laser on healing of bone defects: an experimental study. J Oral Laser Applications. 2005; 5: 169-172.

Markovic A B, Todorovic L. Postoperative analgesia after lower third molar surgery: contribution of the use of long-acting local anesthetics, low-power laser, and diclofenac. Oral Surg Oral Med Oral Pathol Oral Radiol Endod. 2006; 102 (5): 4-8.

Marks, R, de Palma F. Clinical efficacy of low power laser therapy in osteoarthritis. Physiother Res Int. 1999; 4 (2): 141-157.

Marques M M, Fujihara N A. Effect of dexamethasone and LILT on adhesion, proliferation and protein synthesis of cultured osteoblast cells. Proc. 3rd Congress of ESOLA, Barcelona, Spain, May 2005, p. 11.

Márquez de Martínez Gerbi M E, Limeira Jr F, Pinheiro A et al. Efeito de laserterapia de 830 nm sobre o reparo de defeitos ósseos com implantes de osso bovino e mineral. Proc. Laser Dental Show, São Paulo, Brazil, November 2003, p 11.

Márquez Martínez M E, Pinheiro A L, Ramalho L M. Effect of IR laser photobiomodulation on the repair of bone defects grafted with organic bovine bone. Lasers Med Sci. 2008; 23 (3): 313-317.

Marshall J. The safety of laser pointers: myths and realities. Br J Ophthalmol. 1998; 82 (11): 1335-1338.

Marsilio A L, Rodrigues J R, Borges A B. Effect of the clinical application of the GaAlAs laser in the treatment of dentine hypersensitivity. J Clin Laser Med Surg. 2003; 21 (5): 291-296.

Martelli M R A. A clinico statistical investigation of laser effect in the treatment of pain and dysfunction of temporo-mandibular joint (T.M.J.). J Dental Proth. 1990; (18): 31-36.

Martin D et al. Effect of laser pulse repetition rate upon peripheral blood flow in human volunteers. Laser Surg Med. 1991; Suppl 3: 83.

Martin J L, Migus A, Poyart C et al. Ultra-fast events in biological systems. Laboratoire d'Optique Appliquee INSERM U275. Ecole Polytechnique-ENSTA, Palaiseau. p. 218.

Masse J-F et al. Effectiveness of soft laser treatment in periodontal surgery. Int Dent J. 1993; 43: 121-127.

Matouskova I. [Reaction of the palatal tonsils after the application of a HeNe laser]. Acta Universitatis Palackianae Olomucensis Facultatis Medicae. 1984;107: 315-320.

Matsushita H, Kakami K, Ito A et al. Effect on the action potential of the low power Nd:YAG laser as irradiated directly to the nerve. Aichi Gakuin Dent Sci. 1989; 2: 19-28.

Matulis A A, Vasilenkaitis V V, Raistensky I L et al. Laser therapy and laseracupuncture in rheumatoid arthritis, osteoarthritis deformans and psoriatic arthropathy. Ther Arkh. 1983; 55 (7): 92-97.

Mayayo E, Trelles M, Calderhead R, Santafe M, Tomas J, Rigau J. Short term ultrastructural changes in soft tissue (Endomysium) after laser therapy Helium-Neon laser treatment. Laser Therapy. 1989; 1 (3): 119-126.

Mayordomo M M et al. Laser in painful process of locomotor system: our experience. 1985. Proc. of Laser Bologna 1985. Monduzzi Editore, Bologna.

Mazo V. Transrectal laser therapy in prostatic problems' management.Proc. X Internat Congr Soc Laser Surgery and Medicine, Bangkok. 1993, p. 153.

McAuley R et al. Soft laser: A treatment for osteoarthritis of the knee. Arch Phys Med Rehab. 1985; 66: 553-554. (abstract)

Manteifel V M, Andreichuk T N, Karu T I. Influence of He-Ne laser radiation and phytohemagglutinin on the ultrastructure of chromatin of human lymphocytes. Lasers Life Sci. 1994; 6: 1.

Manteifel V M, Karu T I. Activation of chromatin in T-lymphocytes nuclei under the He-Ne laser radiation. Lasers Life Sci. 1998; 8: 117.

Manteifel V M, Karu T I. Ultrastructural changes in human lymphocytes under He-Ne laser radiation. Lasers Life Sci. 1992; 4: 235.

Manteifel V, Bakeeva L, Karu T I. Ultrastructural changes in chondriome of human lympocytes after irradiation with He-Ne laser: appearance of giant mitochondria. J Photochem Photobiol B Biol. 1997; 38: 25.

Manukhin I B, Matafonov V A, Mamedov F M. [The efficacy of the transcutaneous magnetic-laser irradiation of the blood in acute salpingo-oophoritis] Voprosy kurortologii, fizioterapii, i lechebnoi fizicheskoi kultury. 2000; (1): 32-35.

Maiti S, Shear JB, Williams RM, Zipfel WR, Webb WW Measuring serotonin distribution in live cells with three-photon excitation. Science. 1997; 275 (5299): 530-532.

Maiya GA, Kumar P, Rao L. Effect of low intensity helium-neon (He-Ne) laser irradiation on diabetic wound healing dynamics. Photomed Laser Surg. 2005; 23 (2): 187-190.

Makihara E, Makihara M, Masumi S, Sakamoto E. Evaluation of facial thermographic changes before and after low-level laser irradiation. Photomed Laser Surg. 2005; 232: 191-195.

Makk A, Pollera M. Multicenter study related to laser treatment of TMJ syndrom. Proc. Internat Congress LASERMED, Munich, 1995, p. 104.

Malm M, Lundeberg T. Effect of low power gallium arsenide laser on healing of venous ulcers. Scand J Plast Reconstr Hand Surg. 1991; 25: 249-251.

Maloney R. Presentation at 29th Annual Conference of the American Society for Laser Medicine and Surgery (ASLMS) in National Harbor, Maryland, USA, 2009.

Malta J et al. The influences of Low Level Laser Therapy on Wound Healing after Palatinal Surgery in Beagle Dogs. EOS. 1990; 122: 82-.

Mamedova F M et al. Microbiological estimate of parodontitis laser therapy efficiency. Proc SPIE. 1995; Vol 1984: 247-249.

Mandel A Sh, Dunaeva L P. Effect of laser therapy on blood levels of serotonin and dopamine scleroderma patients. Vestn Dermatol Venerol. 1982; (8):13-17. (in Russian)

Manne J. Le laser arséniure de gallium 6 watts, étude clinique en odonto-stomatologie. Le Chirurgien Dent de France 1985; 284: 15-.

Manteifel V, Andreichuk T, Karu T, Chelidze P, Zelenin A. Activation of transcription in lymphocytes after exposure to a HeNe laser. Mol.Biol. 1990; 24: 860-867.

Manteifel V, Andreichuk T, Karu T. Reaction of the mitocondrial apparatus of the lymphocytes to irradiation by a HeNe laser and to the mitogen phytohema-glutinin. Mol.Biol. 1991; 25: 229-235.

Marchesini R, Dasdia T, Melloni E, Rocca E. Effect of low-energy laser irradiation on colony formation capability in different human tumor cells in vitro. Laser Surg Med. 1989; 9 (1): 59-62.

Marcos R L, Bjordal J M, Pallota R C et al. The effect of low level laser therapy (infrared, 810 nm) on collagenase induced rat achilles tendinitis: COX-1 and COX-2 expression and prostaglandin E2 production. Proc. 7th Internat Congr of WALT, Sun City, South Africa, October 2008, page 128.

Marei M K. Effect of low-energy laser application in the treatment of denture-induced mucosal lesions. J Prosthet Dent. 1997; 77 (3): 256-264.

Lubart R, Eichler M, Lavi R, Friedman H, Shainberg A. Low-energy laser irradiation promotes cellular redox activity. Photomed Laser Surg. 2005; 23 (1): 3-9.

Lucas C, Coenen C, De Haan R. The effect of low level laser therapy (laser therapy) on stage III decubitus ulcers (pressure sores); a prospective randomised single blind, multicentre pilot study. Lasers in Medical Science. 2000; 15 (2): 94-100.

Lucas C, Stanborough RW, Freeman CL, de Haan RJ. Efficacy of low-level laser therapy on wound healing in human subjects: a systematic review. Lasers Med Sci. 2000; 15: 84-93.

Lucas C. Efficacy of low level laser treatment in the management of chronic wounds. Thesis. Hogeschool van Amsterdam, The Netherlands. 2001. ISBN 90-9015244-X.

Luger E J, Rochkind S et al. Effect of low-power laser irradiation on the mechanical properties of bone fracture healing in rats. Laser Surg Med. 1998; 22 (2): 97-102.

Lukashevich I G. HeNe laser in facial pain. Stomatologiia. 1985; 64: 29-31.

Lundeberg T, Haker E, Thomas M. Effect of laser versus placebo in tennis elbow. Scand J of Rehab Med. 1987; 19: 135-138.

Lundeberg T, Hode L, Zhou J. A comparative study of the pain-relieving effect of laser treatment and acupuncture. Acta Physiol Scand. 1987; 131 (1): 161-162.

Lundeberg T, Hode L, Zhou J. Effect of low power laser irradiation on nociceptive cells in Hirudo medicinalis. Acupunct Electrother Res. 1988; 13 (2-3): 99-104.

Lundeberg T, Malm M. Low power HeNe laser treatment of venous leg ulcers. Ann Plast Surg. 1991; 27: 537-539.

Luomanen M. A comparative study of healing of laser and scalpel incision wounds in rat oral mucosa. Scand J Dent Res. 1987; 95 (1): 65-73.

Lupton J R, Alster T S. Nonablative laser skin resurfacing using a 1540 nm erbium glass laser: a clinical and histologic analysis. Dermatol Surg. 2002; 28 (9): 833-835.

Lutsyk L et al. [Use of a helium-neon laser in the combined treatment of oral mucosa diseases in children]. Stomatologiia (Mosk). 1981; 60 (6): 15-16.

Lyons R et al. Biostimulation of wound healing in vivo by a helium neon laser. Annals Plastic Surg. 1987; 18: 47-.

Mach E S et al. Helium-Neon (Red Light) Therapy of Arthritis. Rhevmatologia. 1983; 3: 36.

Machnikowski I et al. [Application of therapeutic laser in treatment of the selected chronic illnesses of the oral cavity]. Protet Stomatol. 1989; 39 (3): 147-150.

Maeda T et al. Histological, thermographic and thermometric study in vivo and excised 830 nm diode laser irradiated rat skin. Laser Therapy. 1990; 2 (1): 32. (abstract)

Maegawa Y, Itoh T, Hosokawa T et al. Effects of near-infrared low-level laser on microcirculation. Lasers Surg Med. 2000; 27: 427-437.

Maeno N, Kameya T,Yamada H, Abe N. Effects of laser therapy, Using Helium-Neon Laser on Infectious Bovine Keratoconjunctivitis. Laser Therapy. 1989; 1 (2): 79-82.

Mahdavi Z, Jalalian D M, Fekrazad R. Evaluation of low level laser therapy on desensitivity of vital abutment teeth in fix prosthesis.10th. International Congress of the International Society for Lasers in Dentistry, Berlin, 18.5.-20.5.2006.

Maier M, Haina D, Landthaler M. Effect of Low Energy Laser on the Growth and Regeneration of Capillaries. Lasers in Medical Sciences. 1990; 5: 381-385.

Majlesi G. GaAs laser treatment of bilateral eyelid ptosis due to complication of botulinum toxin type A injection. Photomed Laser Surg. 2008; 26 (5): 507-509.

Makihara E, Makihara M, Masumi S, Sakamoto E. Evaluation of facial thermographic changes before and after low-level laser irradiation. Photomed Laser Surg. 2005; 23 (2): 191-195.

Longo L, Tamburini A, Monti A et al. Treatment with 904 nm and 10 600 nm laser of acute lumbago - double blind control. LASER. Journ Eur Med Laser Ass. 1988; 1 (3): 16-20.

Lopes C B, Pinheiro A L, Sathaiah S, Duarte J, Martins C M. Infrared laser light reduces loading time of dental implants: a Raman spectroscopic study. Photomed Laser Surg. 2005; 23 (1): 27-31.

Lopez V J. El láser en el tratiamento de las disfunciones de ATM. Revista de Actualidad de Odontoestomatologica Española. 1986; (Jun): 35-.

Lopes-Martins R A, Albertini R, Lopes-Martins P S et al. Steroids receptor antagonist Mifepristone inhibits the anti-inflammatory effects of photoradiation. Photomed Laser Surg. 2006; 24 (2): 197-201.

Lopes-Martins R A, Albertini R, Martins P S, Bjordal J M, Faria Neto H C. Spontaneous effects of low-level laser therapy (650 nm) in acute inflammatory mouse pleurisy induced by carrageenan. Photomed Laser Surg. 2005; 23 (4): 377-381.

Lopes-Martins R A, Marcos R L, Leonardo P S, Prianti A C, Muscara M, Aimbire F N, Frigo L, Iversen V V, Bjordal J M. The Effect of Low Level Laser Irradiation (Ga-Al-As - 655nm) On Skeletal Muscle Fatigue induced by Electrical Stimulation in Rats. J Appl Physiol. 2006 Apr 20; [Epub ahead of print]

Lowe A et al. Effect of low intensity monochromatic light therapy (890 nm) on a radiation-impaired, wound healing model in murine skin. Lasers in Surg Med. 1998; 23: 291-298.

Lowe A S, Baxter G D, Walsh D M et al. Low-intensity laser irradiation of the human median nerve: effect of energy density upon conduction and skin temperature. Abstracts 'London Laser 1992', Second Meeting of the International Laser Therapy Association: 56.

Lowe A, Baxter D, Walsh D, Allen J. Effect of low intensity laser (830 nm) irradiation on skin temperature and antidromic conduction latencies in the human median nerve: Relevance of radiant exposure. Laser Surg Med. 1994; 14: 40-46.

Lubart R et al. Changes in calcium transport in mammalian sperm mitochondria and plasma membrane due to 630 nm and 780 nm laser irradiation. Proc. LASERMED Munich 1995, p. 104.

Lubart R, Friedmann H, Levinshal T, Lavie R, Breitbart H. Effect of light in calcium transport in bull sperm cells. J Photochem Photobiol B Biol. 1992; 15: 337-341.

Lubart R et al. Changes in calcium transport in mammalian sperm mitochondria and plasma membranes caused by 780 nm irradiation. Lasers in Surg Med. 1997; 21: 493-499.

Lubart R et al. Photosensitized biostimulation of fibroblasts by low energy visible light. Laser Therapy. 1996; 8 (1): 16. (abstract)

Lubart R, Friedmann H, Peled I, Grossman N. Light effect on fibroblast proliferation. Laser Therapy. 1993; 5 (2): 55-58.

Lubart R, Rochkind S, Sharon U, Nissan M.. A light source for phototherapy. Laser Therapy. 1991; 3 (1): 15-18.

Lubart R, Wollman Y, Friedman H, Rochkind S, Laulicht I. Effects of visible and near-infrared lasers on cell cultures. J. Photochem. Photobiol. B. 1992; 12: 305-310.

Lubart R. et al. A possible Mechanism of Low Level Laser - Living Cell Interaction. Laser Therapy. 1990; 2 (2): 65-68.

Lubart R, Breitbart H, Sofer Y, Lavie R. He-Ne irradiation of human spermatozoa: enhancement in hamster egg penetration. Laser Therapy. 1999; 11 (4): 171-176.

Lubart R, Breitbart H. Biostimulative effects of low energy lasers. 3rd Congress of the North American Association for Laser Therapy, Bethesda, Md, USA, March 2003.

Lubart R, Friedman H, Lavie R. Photostimulation as a function of different wavelengths. Laser Therapy. 2000; 12: 38-41.

Lizarelli R F, Lamano-Carvalho T, Brentegani G. Histometrical evaluation of the healing of the dental alveolus in rats after irradiation with a low-powered GaAlAs laser. In Lasers in Dentistry V. Proceedings SPIE. 1999; Vol 3593: 49-56.

Lizarelli R F, Ciconelli K P, Braga C A, Berro R J. Low-powered laser therapy associated with oral implantology. Proc SPIE. 1999; Vol 3593: 69-73, Lasers in Dentistry V, John D. Featherstone; Peter Rechmann; Daniel Fried; Eds.

Lizarelli R F, Marcello O Mazzetto M O, Bagnato V S. Low-intensity laser therapy to treat dentin hypersensitivity: comparative clinical study using different light doses. Proc. SPIE. 2000; Vol. 4422.

Lizarelli R F Z, Pizzo R CA, Mazzetto M O. The antialgetic effect of the low intensity laser in the internal disorders of the temporo-mandibular joint. Proc. 3rd Congress of ESOLA, Barcelona, Spain, May 2005, p. 52.

Loevscall H. The Application of Low Level Laser in Dentistry - A Critical Review. Dept of Oral Pathology, Royal Dental College, Aarhus University, Vennelyst Boulevard, DK-8000 Aarhus C, Denmark. 1992.

Loevschall H et al. Effect of Low Level Diode Laser Effect in Cultures of Human Oral Mucosa. Proc. Second Meeting of the Intern Laser Therapy Association, London, Sept 1992, p 55.

Loevschall H et al. Low Level Laser Irradiation of Human Oral Mucosa Fibroblast in Vitro in Cultures of Human Oral Fibroblasts. Laser Surg Med. 1994; 14: 347-354.

Lögdberg-Andersson M, Mützell S, Hazel Å. Low Level Laser Treatment of Tendonitis and Myofascial Pains - a Randomized, Double-Blind Study. Laser Therapy. 1997; 9 (3): 79-86.

Loginov A S, Sokolova G N, Sokolova S V et al. [The content of biologically active substances in the margin of a stomach ulcer being treated with a copper-vapor laser]. Ter Arkh. 1991; 63 (8): 75-78. (in Russian)

Loginov A S, Sokolova G N, Trubitsyna I E et al. [Biogenic amines and cyclic nucleotides in the laser therapy of long-term nonhealing stomach ulcers]. Vrach Delo 1991; (1): 24-27. (in Russian)

Lomelí-Rivas A, Krötzsch E, Michtchenko A. Effect of 650 nm laser stimulation with clinical doses on cultivated human fibroblasts proliferation. [Efecto de la estimulación láser de 650 nm, utilizando dosis de uso clínico, sobre la proliferación de fibroblastos humanos cultivados]. Rev Mex Med Fis Rehab. 2003; 15 (3-4): 69-71.

Lomnitski I, Bibiashevski E V. Substantiation of the optimal exposure to monochromatic red light for stimulating osteogenesis. Stomatologiia. 1982; 2 (61):14-.

Lomnitski I. The mechanism of stimulation of reparative osteogenesis with laser radiation. Stomatologiia (Mosk). 1983; 5: 18-20.

Lomnitski I. Clinical X-ray characteristics of the healing of mandibular fractures following the use of HeNe laser radiation. Stomatologiia (Mosk). 1985; 3: 38-40.

Lonauer G. Controlled double blind study on the efficacy of HeNe-laser beams versus HeNe-plus Infrared-laser beams in the therapy of activated osteoarthritis of finger joints. Clin Experim Rheuma. 1987; 5 (suppl 2): 39. Also in Laser Surg Med. 1986; 7: 172.

Longo L, Evangelista S, Tinacci G, Sesti A G. Effects of diodes-laser silver Arsenide-Aluminium (Ga-Al-As) 904 nm on healing of experimental wounds. Laser Surg Med. 1987; 7 (5): 444-447.

Longo L, Simunovic Z, Postiglione M, Postiglione M.. Laser therapy for fibromyositic rheumatism. J Clin Laser Med Surg. 1997; 15 (5): 217-220.

Longo L et al. Laser therapy of La Peyronie's syndrome: a review. Abstr. Laser Florence '97. European Medical Laser Assn. p. 18.

Longo L et al. Laser treatment of induratio penis plastic: advantages and limitations. Proc. 2nd Congress World Assn for Laser Therapy, Kansas City, September 1998; p. 104-105.

Lievens P, van der Veen P. The influence of low level infrared laser therapy on the regereration of cartilage tissue. Laser in Medical Science. 2002; 17 (4). Proc. 14th Annual Meeting of Deutsche Gesellschaft für Lasermedizin, Munich, Germany, June 2003.

Light therapy for winter depression. Health News. 1998; 4 (14): 6-.

Light therapy. Health News. 1998; Mar 10;4 (3): 5.

Lihong S. He-Ne laser auricular irradiation plus body acupuncture for treatment of acne vulgaris in 36 cases. J Tradit Chin Med. 2006; 26 (3): 193-194.

Lilge L, Tierney K, Nussbaum E. Low-level laser for wound healing: feasibility of wound dressing transillumination. J Clin Laser Med Surg. 2000; 18 (5): 235-240.

Lilveria P, Syeck E L, Pinhoa R A. Evaluation of mitochondrial respiratory chain activity in wound healing by low-level laser therapy. Journal of Photochemistry and Photobiology B: Biology. 2007; 86 (3): 279-282.

Lim, Hong Meng et al. A clinical investigation of the efficacy of low level laser therapy in reducing orthodontic postadjustment pain. Am J Orthod Dentofac Orthop. 1995; 108: 614-22.

Lin S W, Mathies R A. Orientation of the protonated retinal Schiff base group in bacteriorhodopsin from absorption linear dichroism. Biophys. J. 1989; 56: 653-660.

Lin Y S, Huang M H, Chai C Y, Yang R C. Effects of helium-neon laser on levels of stress protein and arthritic histopathology in experimental osteoarthritis. Am J Phys Med Rehabil. 2004; 83 (10): 758-765.

Lin YS, Huang MH, Chai CY. Effects of helium-neon laser on the mucopolysaccharide induction in experimental osteoarthritic cartilage. Osteoarthritis Cartilage. 2006; 14 (4): 377-383.

Lindén L-Å. Enhanced curing of dental lasers. Swedish Dental J. 1997; 6: 242.

Lindholm A, de Mitri N, Swensson U. Clinical effect of non-fucuses CO2 laser on traumatic arthritis in horses. Lasers Med Surg. Supplement 12, 2000: 51.

Lindholm A C, Swensson U, de Mitri N,Collinder E. Clinical Effects of Betamethasone and Hyaluronan, and of Defocalized Carbon Dioxide Laser Treatment on Traumatic Arthritis in the Fetlock Joints of Horses. J Vet Med. 2002: 189-194.

Lipson E D. Action spectroscopy: methodology, in CRC Handbook of Organic Chemistry and Photobiology. Horspool W H. and Song P.-S, Eds. CRC Press, Boca Raton, FL, 1995, p. 1257.

Litscher G et al. Specific effects of laserpuncture on the cerebral circulation. Lasers in Medical Science. 2000; 15 (1): 57-62.

Litscher G. Cerebral and peripheral effects of laser needle-stimulation. Neurol Res. 2003; 25 (7): 722-728.

Litscher G, Rachbauer D, Ropele S, Wang L, Schikora D, Fazekas F, Ebner F. Acupuncture using laser needles modulates brain function: first evidence from functional transcranial Doppler sonography and functional magnetic resonance imaging. Lasers Med Sci. 2004; 19 (1): 6-11.

Litscher G, Nemetz W, Smolle J, Schwarz G et al. [Histological investigation of the micromorphological effects of the application of a laser needle - results of an animal experiment]. Biomed Tech (Berl). 2004; 49 (1-2): 2-5. (in German)

Liu et al. The effectiveness of semiconductor laser in the treatment of post-endodontic filling pain. Proc. 7th Int Congr Lasers in Dentistry, ISLD, Brussels, Belgium, July 2000, abstr. 28.

Liu H-C, Lan W-H. The combined effectiveness of the semiconductor laser with Duraphat in the treatment of dentin hypersensitivity. J Clin Laser Med Surg. 1994; 12 (6): 315-319.

Liu X, Lyon R, Meier H T, Thometz J, Haworth S T. Effect of Lower-Level Laser Therapy on Rabbit Tibial Fracture. Photomed Laser Surg. 2007; 25 (6): 487-494.

Lee, Chang Woo and Kim, Ki Suk. Study on the Effect of Low Denisty Power Laser Radiation in Treating Gingival Inflammation. Clinical, Microbiological, Histological Study. J Korean Acad Oral Med 1987; 1 (12).

Lee K-H., Kim K-S. Effects of low level laser irradiation on the ALP activity and calcified nodule formation of rat osteoblastic cell. J of Korean Academy of Oral Medicine. 1996; 21: 279-292.

Lenzi A, Claroni F, Gandini L, Lombardo F, Barbieri C, Lino A, Dondero F. Laser radiation and motility patterns of human sperm. Arch Androl. 1989; 23: 229-234.

Lerner LA. Effectiveness of laser therapy in Bechterew's disease. Terapevticheskii Arkhiv. 1988, 60(4): 134-136. (in Russian)

Leung M C, Lo S C, Siu F K, So K F. Treatment of experimentally induced transient cerebral ischemia with low energy laser inhibits nitric oxide synthase activity and up-regulates the expression of transforming growth factor-beta 1. Lasers Surg Med. 2002; 31 (4): 283-288.

Levine RA, Abel M, Cheng H. CNS somatosensory-auditory interactions elicit or modulate tinnitus. Exp Brain Res. 2003; 153 (4): 643-648.

Lewith G T, Machin D. A randomized trial to evaluate the effect of infrared stimulation of local trigger points, versus placebo, on the pain caused by cervical osteoarthrosis. Acupunct Electro-Ther Res, 1981; 6: 277-284.

Lewy AJ, Bauer VK, Cutler NL, Sack RL, Ahmed S, Thomas KH, Blood ML, Jackson JM. Morning vs evening light treatment of patients with winter depression. Arch Gen Psychiatry. 1998; 55 (10): 890-896.

Li J, Yao G, Wang L V. Degree of polarization in laser speckles from turbid media: implications in tissue optics. J Biomed Opt. 2002; 7 (3):307-312.

Li X H. Laser in the Department of Traumatology. With a report of 60 cases of soft tissue injury. Laser Therapy. 1990; 2 (3): 119-122.

Lichtenstein D, Morag B. Low level laser therapy in ambulatory patients with venous stasis ulcers. Laser Therapy. 1999; 11 (2): 71-78.

Lichtenstein D, Morga B. Laser therapy in ambulatory patients with venous stasis ulcers. Proc. 2nd Congress World Assn for Laser Therapy, Kansas City, September 1998; p. 31-32.

Leichliter S G, Williams K, Whitehorse T et al. Low level laser therapy in the treatment of cervical strain in active duty military. Proc. 3rd Congr World Assn for Laser Therapy, Athens, Greece, May 2000.

Lievens P C. The effect of a combined HeNe and I.R. laser treatment on the regeneration of the lymphatic system during the process of wound healing. Lasers in Medical Science. 1991; 6: 193-199.

Lievens P C. The effect of I.R. laser irradiation on the vosomotricity of the lymphatic system. Lasers in Medical Science. 1991; 6: 189-191

Lievens P, Lippens E. The influence of low level infra red lasertherapy on the regeneration of cartilage tissue. Laser Surg Med. 1998; Suppl 10: 5.

Lievens P, Mohebbian M. The effect of IR-laser irradiation on the regeneration of muscle fibres. In: Laser Therapy in Dentistry and Medicine. Prima Books in Sweden AB. Eds Jan Tunér and Lars Hode. 1996, p. 164-179.

Lievens P. Effects of Laser Treatment on the Lymphatic System and Wound Healing. LASER. Journ Eur Med Laser Ass. 1988; 1 (2): 12-15.

Lievens P. Infrared lasertherapy and bedsores. Laser Surg Med. 1992; Suppl 4:11.

Lievens P. The Influence of Laser Irradiation on the Motricity of Lymphatical System and on the Wound Healing Process. Proc Int Congr on Laser in Med and Surg. Bologna, June 26-28, 1985; p. 171.

Lam R W, Terman M, Wirz-Justice A. Light therapy for depressive disorders: indications and efficacy. Mod Probl Pharmacopsychiatry. 1997; 25: 215-234.

Lam L K, Cheing G L. Effects of 904-nm low-level laser therapy in the management of lateral epicondylitis: a randomized controlled trial. Photomed Laser Surg. 2007; 25 (2): 65-67.

Lampl Y, Zivin J A, Fisher M, Lew R, Welin L, Dahlof B, Borenstein P, Andersson B, Perez J, Caparo C, Ilic S, Oron U. Infrared laser therapy for ischemic stroke: a new treatment strategy: results of the NeuroThera Effectiveness and Safety Trial-1 (NEST-1). Stroke. 2007; 38 (6): 1843-1849.

Lan C C, Wu C S, Chiou M H, Hsieh P C, Yu H S. Low-energy helium-neon laser induces locomotion of the immature melanoblasts and promotes melanogenesis of the more differentiated melanoblasts: recapitulation of vitiligo repigmentation in vitro. J Invest Dermatol. 2006; 126 (9): 2119-2126.

Lancaster C R, Michel H. The coupling of light-induced electron transfer and proton uptake as derived from crystal structures of reaction centres from Rhodopseudomonas viridis modified at the binding site of the secondary quinone, QB. Structure. 1997; 5 (10): 1339-1359.

Landau Z. Topical hyperbaric oxygen and low energy laser for the treatment of diabetic foot ulcer. Archives of Orthopaedic & Trauma surgery. 1998; 117 (3): 156-158.

Landthaler M et al. Behandlung von Zoster, postzosterischen Schmerzen und Herpes simplex recidivans in loco mit Laser-Licht. Fortschr. Med. 1983; 101 (22): 1039-1042.

Landyshev I, Avdeeva N V, Goborov N D et al. [Efficacy of low intensity laser irradiation and sodium nedocromil in the complex treatment of patients with bronchial asthma]. Ter Arkh. 2002; 74: 25-28.

Lanyi J K, Luecke H. Bacteriorhodopsin. Current Opinion in Structural Biology 2001, 11: 415-419.

Lanzafame R J, Stadler I, Coleman J, Haerum B, Oskoui P, Whittaker M, Zhang R Y. Temperature-controlled 830-nm low-level laser therapy of experimental pressure ulcers. Photomed Laser Surg. 2004; 22 (6): 483-488.

Laor Y et al. The pathology of laser irradiation of the skin and body wall of the mouse. 1965; 47 (4): 643-662.

Lapchak P A, Wei J, Zivin J A. Transcranial infrared laser therapy improves clinical rating scores after embolic strokes in rabbits. Stroke. 2004; 35 (8): 1985-1988.

Lapchak P A, Han M K, Salgado K F, Streeter J, Zivin J A. Safety profile of transcranial near-infrared laser therapy administered in combination with thrombolytic therapy to embolized rabbits. Stroke. 2008; 39 (11): 3073-3078.

Lapina V A, Veremei E T, Pancovets E. Effects of laser irradiation for healing of the skin-muscle wounds in animals. Proc. SPIE. Vol. 3907.

Lavor Z V, Bortkevich A S, Pozdniakova et al. Quantum therapy in the treatment of patients suffering from allergic rhinitis and bronchial asthma. Laser in Medical Science. 2002; 17 (4). Proc. 14th Annual Meeting of Deutsche Gesellschaft für Lasermedizin, Munich, Germany, June 2003, p. 157.

Leal Junior E C, Lopes-Martins R A, Dalan F, Ferrari M, Sbabo F M, Generosi R A, Baroni B M, Penna S C, Iversen V V, Bjordal J M. Effect of 655-nm low-level laser therapy on exercise-induced skeletal muscle fatigue in humans. Photomed Laser Surg. 2008; 26 (5): 419-24.

Lederer H et al. Influence of light on human immunocompetent cells in vitro. Proc. Laser Opto-Elektronik, Munich 1981.

Lee G et al. New concepts in pain management in the application of low-power laser for relief of cervicothoracic pain syndromes. Am Heart J. 1996; 132 (6): 1329-1334.

Lee P, Kim Kibeom and Kim Ki-Suk. Effects of low incident energy levels of infrared laser irradiation on helaing of infected open skin wounds in rats. Laser Therapy 1993; 5 (2): 59-64.

Kurumada F A study on the application of Ga-As semiconductor laser to endodontics. The effects of laser irradiation on the activation of inflammatory cells and the vital pulpotomy. Ohu Daigaku Shigakushi. 1990; 17 (3) :233-244.

Kurumada F. The effect of laser irradiation on the activation of inflammatory cells and the vital pulpotomy. A study of the application of Ga-As semiconductor laser to endodontics. J Clinical Pediatric Dentistry. 1995; 19: 232.

Kusakari H, Orikasa N, Tani H. Effects of low power laser on wound healing of gingiva and bone. Laser Bologna '92, p. 49-55. Monduzzi Editore S.p.A., Bologna, Italy.

Kusakari H. The use of lasers to dental implant. Proc X Internat Congr Soc Laser Surg Med, Bangkok, 1993, p 332.

Kujawa J, Zavodnik I B, Lapshina A, Labieniec M, Bryszewska M. Cell survival, DNA, and protein damage in B14 cells under low-intensity near-infrared (810 nm) laser irradiation. Photomed Laser Surg. 2004; 22 (6): 504-508.

Kuznetsova M Iu, Zueva S M, Gunenkova I V et al. [The use of the Optodan laser physiotherapeutic apparatus for the prevention of complications and the acceleration of the time in treating anomalies in the position of individual teeth with fixed orthodontic appliances]. Stomatologiia (Mosk). 1998; 77 (3): 56-60. (in Russian)

Kwon K, Son T, Lee KJ, Jung B. Enhancement of light propagation depth in skin: cross-validation of mathematical modeling methods. Lasers Med Sci. 2009. 24 (4): 605-615.

Laakso E L, Cramond T, Richardson C, Galligan J P. Plasma ACTH and ß-endorphin levels in response to low level laser therapy for myofascial trigger points. Laser Therapy. 1994; (3) 6: 133-142.

Laakso L. Richardson. C. Cramond T. Quality of light - is laser necessary for effective photo-biostimulation? Australian Journal of Physiotherapy. 1993; 39 (2): 87-92.

Laakso EL, Cabot PJ. Nociceptive scores and endorphin-containing cells reduced by low-level laser therapy (LLLT) in inflamed paws of Wistar rat. Photomed Laser Surg. 2005; 23 (1): 32-35.

Labajos M et al. ß-endorphine levels modification after GaAs and HeNe laser irradiation on the rabbit. Comparative study. Investigación clínica láser. 1988; 1-2: 6-8.

Labajos M et al. Effect of the irradiation of GaAs diode laser on intestinal absorption: in vitro and in vivo studies. Lasers in Medical Science. 1986; 1: 21-25.

Labbe R et al. Laser photobioactivation mechanisms: in vitro studies using ascorbic acid uptake and hydroxyproline formation as biochemical markers of irradiation response. Lasers in Surgery and Medicin. 1990; 10: 201-207.

Labbe R, Skogerboe K, Davis H, Rettmer R: Laser photobioactivation mechanisms: In vitro studies using ascorbic acid uptake and hydroxyproline formation as bio-chemical markers of irradiation response. Laser Surg Med. 1990; 10: 201.

Ladalardo T, Brugnera A, Pinheiro A et al. Comparative clinical study of the effects of LLLT in the immediate and late treatment of hypoesthesia due to surgical procedures. Proc. SPIE Vol 4610, 2002; p. 183-186. Lasers in Dentistry VIII.

Ladalardo T, Mangabeira A, Pedro L et al. Comparative clinical evaluation of the immediate and late analgesic effect of GaAlAs diode lasers of 830 and 660 nm in the treatment of dentine pain: a preliminary report. 2002; Proc. SPIE. Vol. 4610. p. 178-182. Lasers in Dentistry III.

Ladalardo T C, Tirapelli B, Marraccini T M et al. The effects of phototherapy on oral mucositis in bone marrow transplant patients—Preliminary results. Photomed Laser Surg. 2005; 23 (1). Abstracts from the 5th Congress of the World Association for Laser Therapy, São Paulo, Brazil, November 2004. Poster no 81, page 134.

Lagan K M, McDonough S M, Clements B A, Baxter G D. A case report of low intensity laser therapy (LILT) in the management of venous ulceration: potential effects of wound debridement upon efficacy. Journal of Clinical Laser Medicine & Surgery. 2000; 18 (1): 15-22.

Kruchinina I et al. Effect of laser therapy on the local synthesis of class A immunoglubulin in children with acute and chronic maxillary sinuitis. Vestn Otorinolaringol. 1988; 2: 19-21. (in Russian with English abstr)

Kruchinina I et al. Therapeutic effect of helium-neon laser on microcirculation of nasal mucosa in children with acute and chronic maxillary sinuitis as measured by conjunctival biomocroscopy. Vestn Otorinolaringol. 1991; 3: 26-30. (in Russian with English abstr)

Kubasova T, Kovács L, Somosy Z, Unk P, Kókai A. Biological effect of HeNe laser: Investigations on functional and micromorphological alterations of cell membranes, in vitro. Lasers in Surgery and Medicin. 1984; 4: 381.

Kubasova T, Horwvath M, Kocsis K et al. Effect of visible light on some cellular and immune parameters. Immunol Cell Biol. 1995; 73: 239-244.

Kubota J, Ohshiro T. The effect of diode laser laser therapy on flap survival: measurement of flap microcirculation with the laser specle method. Laser Therapy. 1996; 8 (4): 241-246.

Kubota J, Ohshiro T. The effects of diode laser low reactive-level laser therapy (laser therapy) on flap survival in a rat model. Laser Therapy. 1989; 1 (3): 127-134.

Kubota J. Defocused diode laser therapy (830 nm) in the treatment of unresponsive skin ulcers: a preliminary trial. J Cosmet Laser Ther. 2004; 6 (2): 96-102.

Kucerová H J. et al. Effect of laser modulatory frequency on the secretion of IgA and albumin levels after the extraction of human molars in the lower jaw. In: Progress in Biomedical Optics, Proc. of Low-power Light on Biological Systems. Proc SPIE. 1997; Vol 3198: 98-101.

Kucerová H et al. Modulatory frequency of lasers in connection to laser beam therapeutic effect Proc. SPIE. 1998; Vol: 191-195 (Lasers in Dentistry IV)

Kucerová H, Dostálová T, Himmlová L et al. Low-level laser therapy after molar extraction. J Clin Laser Med Surg. 2000; 18 (6): 309-315.

Kudoh Ch et al. Effects of 830 nm Gallium Aluminium Arsenide Dioce Laser Radiation on Rat Saphenous Nerve Sodium-Potassium-Adenosine Triphosphatase Activity: A Possible Pain Attenuation Mechanism Exam-ined. Laser Therapy. 1989; 1 (2): 63-67.

Kuhn A, Porto F A, Miragliaz P, Brunetto A L. Low-level infrared laser therapy in chemotherapy-induced oral mucositis: a randomized placebo-controlled trial in children. J Pediatr Hematol Oncol. 2009; 31 (1) :33-37.

Kulikova N G. The effect of low-intensity infrared laser therapy on the endocrine function of patients with climacteric disorders. Vopr Kurortol Fizioter Lech Fiz Kult. 1996; 5: 25-26.

Kulekcioglu S, Sivrioglu K, Ozan O, Parlak M. Effectiveness of low-level laser therapy in temporomandibular disorder. Scan J Rheumatol. 2003; 32: 114-118.

Kumæ T, Arakawa H. In vitro effects of therapeutic laser on superoxice generation from rat alveolar macrophage. Laser Therapy. 1999; 11 (3): 119-129.

Kunin A A, Bykov E I, Podolskaya E E et al. Clinical and morphological indications for laser treatment of patients with precancerous diseases of the oral cavity. Proc. SPIE. 1996; Vol 2929: 185-197.

Kunin A A. et al. Biological effects caused by low power laser light in the treatment of the dentition, parodontium and mucosa of the oral cavity and lip diseases. Proc. SPIE. 1997. Vol 3198: 37-47.

Kunin S, Pankova Y, Oleinik T et al. The influence of low level lasers together with modern filling materials and bonding systems on mineral metabolism of hard tissues. Proc. European Conf Biomed Optics, Munich, Germany, June 2001, p. 18.

Kurland H D. Releif of low back pain with low-reactive laser acupuncture techniques. Aku. 1999; 27 (4). (abstract)

Koukoui L M et al. The differential approach to the application of laser, ultraviolet and roentgenological auto-blood irradiation for the correction of homeostatis. Laser Therapy. 1996; 8 (1): 60. (abstract)

Kourmanov B. Light torque induced by polarized laser beam in an optical trap. Thesis for the Degree of Master in Science. Wake Forest Univiersity. N.C., USA. 2002.

Kovács I, Mester E, Görög P. Stimulation of wound healing with laser beam in the rat. Experientia. 1974; 30 (11): 1275-1276.

Kovács I et al. Laser-Induced Stimulation of the Vascularization of the Healing Wound. Separatum Experientia. 1974; 30: 341-.

Kovács L. The stimulatory effect of laser on the physiological healing process of portio surface. Lasers in Surgery & Medicine 1981; 1 (3): 241-52

Kovalev E V. [The effect of low-intensity laser irradiation on spermatogenesis in men]. Voprosy Kurortol, Fizioter Lechebnoi Fizicheskoi Kultury. 1990; (5): 33-36.

Kovalev E V. The effect of low-intensity laser radiation on spermatogenesis in men. Vopr Kurortol Fizioter Lech Fiz Kult. 1990; (5): 33-36.

Kovalev M I. et al. [Prevention of lactation mastitis by the use of low-intensity laser irradiation]. Akush Ginekol (Mosk.). 1990; (2): 57-61.

Kozanoglu E, Basaran S, Paydas S, Sarpel T. Efficacy of pneumatic compression and low-level laser therapy in the treatment of postmastectomy lymphoedema: a randomized controlled trial. Clin Rehabil. 2009; 23 (2):117-124.

Kozlov V et al. Lasers in diagnostics and treatment of microcirculation disorders under parodontitis. Proc SPIE. 1995; Vol 1984: 253-264.

Krasheninnikoff M, Ellitsgaard B, Rogvi-Hansen B et al. No effect of low power laser in lateral epicondylitis. Scand J Rheum. 1994; 23: 260-263.

Kramer J F, Sandrin M. Effects of Low-Power Laser and white light on sensory conduction rate of the superficial radial nerve. Physiotherapy Canada. 1993; 45 (3): 165-170.

Krechina E K, Shidova A V, Maslova V V. [Comparative evaluation of influence of low-intensity laser radiation of different spectrum components and regimen of laser work upon microcirculation in comprehensive treatment of chronic parodontitis]. [Article in Russian] Stomatologiia (Mosk). 2008; 87 (3): 24-27.

Kreisler M, Christoffers A B, Willershausen B et al. Effect of low-level GaAlAs laser irradiation on the proliferation rate of human periodontal ligament fibroblasts: an in vitro study. J Clin Periodontol. 2003; 30 (4): 353-358.

Kreisler M, Christoffers A B, Al-Haj H et al. Low level 809-nm diode laser-induced in vitro stimulation of the proliferation of human gingival fibroblasts. Laser Surg Med. 2002; 30: 365-369.

Kreisler M B, Haj H A, Noroozi N, Willershausen B. Efficacy of low level laser therapy in reducing postoperative pain after endodontic surgery - a randomized double blind clinical study. Int J Oral Maxillofac Surg. 2004; 33 (1): 38-41.

Kreisler M, Christoffers A B, Willershausen B, d'Hoedt B et al. Low-level 809 nm GaAlAs laser irradiation increases the proliferation rate of human laryngeal carcinoma cells in vitro. Lasers in Medical Science. 2003; 18 (2): 100-103.

Kreisler M, Al-Haj H, d'Hoedt B. Clinical efficacy of semiconductor laser application as an adjunct to conventional scaling and root planning. Lasers Surg Med. 2005; 37 (5): 350–355.

Kreczi T, Klinger D A. A comparison of laser acupuncture versus placebo in radicular and pseudoradicular pain syndromes as recorded by subjective responses of patients. Acupunct Electrotherap Res. 1986; 11: 207-216.

Kripke DF. Light treatment for nonseasonal depression: speed, efficacy, and combined treatment. J Affect Disord. 1998; May;49 (2): 109-117.

Komerik N, Nakanishi H, MacRobert A J, Henderson B, Speight P, Wilson M. In vivo killing of Porphyromonas gingivalis by toluidine blue mediated photosensitization in an animal model. Antimicrob Agents Chemother. 2003; 47 (3): 932-940.

Konchugova T V et al. The enhancement of immune supression by local laser irradiation in rats exposed to cyclophosphane. Eksp Klin Farm. 1993; 56 (2): 42-43.

Kono A, Fujumasa I. The evaluation of pain therapy with low power laser: comparative study on thermography and double blind test. Thermologie Österreich. 1995: 5 (3): 112

Konstantinovic L et al. [Combined low-power laser therapy and local infiltration of corticosteroids in the treatment of radial-humeral epicondylitis.] Vojnosanit Pregl. 1997; 54 (5): 459-463. (in Croatian)

Konstantinovic L M, Kanjuh Z M, Milovanovic A N, Cutovic M R, Djurovic A G, Savic V G, Dragin A S, Milovanovic N D. Acute Low Back Pain with Radiculopathy: A Double-Blind, Randomized, Placebo-Controlled Study. Photomed Laser Surg. 2009 [Epub ahead of print]

Kopera D, Kokol R, Berger C, Haas J. Does the use of low-level laser influence wound healing in chronic venous ulcers? J Wound Care. 2005; 14 (8): 391-394.

Kopf K et al: Endothelregeneration nach Laserbestrahlung - tierexperimentelle Untersuchungen an Kaninchen. Fortschr Kiefer u Gesichtschir. 1983; 28: 140-142.

Korchemskaya E Y, Stepanchikov D A, Druzhko A B Dyukova T V. Mechanism of Nonlinear Photoinduced Anisotropy in Bacteriorhodopsin and its Derivatives. J Biol Phys. 1999; 24: 201-215.

Korochkin I M et al. [Clinico-biochemical parallels against background of traditional treatment and laser therapy of patients with ischemic heart disease]. Ter Arkh. 1988; 60 (12): 40-44.

Korochkin I M et al. [Helium-neon laser therapy in multimodal treatment of acute pneumonia]. Sov Med. 1990; (3): 12-5.

Korochkin I M et al. [Helium-neon laser therapy in patients with ischemic heart disease]. Kardiologiia 1990; 30 (3): 24-28.

Korochkin I M et al. [Intravenous laser therapy in multimodal treatment of acute pneumonia]. Sov Med. 1989; (7): 22-26.

Korolev Iu N, Panova L N, Geniatulina M S. [The correction of the subcellular postradiation changes in the hypothalamus and parathyroid gland by using low-intensity laser radiation. An experimental study]. Vopr Kurortol Fizioter Lech Fiz Kult. 2000; (3): 3-4.

Korytny D L. [Use of Helium-Neon laser in therapeutic stomatology]. Stomatologiia (Mosk). 1978; 57 (5): 21-.

Kosilov K V. [The treatment of neurogenic hyperreflexic bladder dysfunctions in girls with low-intensity laser radiation.] Urol Nefrologiia. 1995; (2): 16-19. (in Russian)

Koslov V I et al. The microcirculation of patients with arterial ischemia of the lower extremities during laser therapy. Fiziol Zh SSSR Im I M Sechenova. 1991; 77 (6): 55-67. (in Russian)

Kotani H. Effects of low power laser stimulation on wound healing in rats. Lasermedizin - Laser in Med Surg. 1995; 11 (2): 25-29 .

Kotlyar A, Borovok N, Hazani M, Szundi I, Einarsdóttir O. Photoinduced intracomplex electron transfer between cytochrome c oxidase and TUPS-modified cytochrome c. Eur J Biochem. 2000; 267 (18): 5805-5809.

Koultchavenia E V. Low-Level Laser as device for increase of drug concentration in the kidney. Proc. SPIE Vol. 4156. 2001: 218-221.

Koutna M, Janisch R, Unucka M, Svobodnik A, Mornstein V. Effects of low-power laser irradiation on cell locomotion in protozoa. Photochem Photobiol. 2004; 80 (3): 531-534.

Klebanov G I et al. Effects of endogenous photosensitizers on the laser.induced priming of leucocytes. Membr. Call Biol. 1998; 12 (3): 339-354.

Klebanov G I et al. Low-power laser irradiation induces leukocyte priming. Gen Physiol Biophys. 1998; 17: 365-375.

Klein E, Fine S, Laor Y et al. Interaction of laser radiation with biologic systems. II. Experimental tumors. Fed Proc. 1965; 24: Suppl 14: 147.

Klein R et al: Low-energy laser treatment and exercise for chronic low back pain: a double-blind controlled trial. Arch Phys Med Rehabil. 1990; 71: 34-37.

Kleinman , Simmer S, Braksma Y et al. Low power laser therapy in pateints with diabetic foot ulcers: early and long term outcome. Laser Therapy. 1996; 8 (2): 205-208.

Kleinman Y et al. Low level laser therapy in patients with venous ulcers: early and long-term outcome. Laser Therapy. 1996; 8 (3): 205-208.

Klima H, Haas O, Roschger P. In Photoemission from Biological Systems (Ed J. Slavinski, B. Kochel) World Publishing House, Singapore, 1987.

Klima H, Haas O, Roschger P. In Photon emission from Biological Systems (Ed. J. Slawinsky, B. Kochel), World Publishing House, Singapore, 1987.

Klima H. Effect of Weak Laser Light and Oxygen Activation in Open Biological Systems. LASER - Journ Eur Med Laser Ass. 1988; 1 (2): 16-.

Klimenko I T, Shuvalova I N. [Low intensity laser radiation in complex therapy of patients with vascular obliterating atherosclerosis of low extremities]. Lik Sprava. 2002; (8): 98-102. (in Polish)

Klinke T, Klimm W, Gutknecht N. Antibacterial effects of Nd:YAG laser irradiation within root canal dentin. J Clin Laser Med Surg. 1997; 15 (1): 29-31.

Ko et al . Clinical evaluation of low level laser therapy on the trigger points. Proc. 7th Int Congr Lasers in Dentistry, ISLD, Brussels, Belgium, July 2000, abstr. 25.

Kobayashi M et al. Studies of the diode laser therapy on blood supply in the rat model. Proc. 2nd Congress World Assn for Laser Therapy, Kansas City, September 1998; p. 70-71.

Kohli R, Gupta P K. Irradiance dependence of the He-Ne laser-induced protection against UVC radiation in E. coli strains. J Photochem Photobiol B. 2003; 69 (3): 161-167.

Kohli R, Gupta PK, Dube A. Helium-neon laser preirradiation induces protection against UVC radiation in wild-type E. coli strain K12AB1157. Radiat Res. 2000; 153 (2): 181-185.

Kólarová H et al. Effect of HeNe laser irradiation on phagocytic activity of leukocytes in vitro. Acta Universitatis Palackianae Olomucensis Facultatis Medicae. 1991; 129: 127-132.

Kolárová H, Ditrichová D, Wagner J. Penetration of the laser light into the skin in vitro. Laser Surg Med. 1999; 24: 231-235.

Kolomiyets L A et al. Mechanism of treatment effect of low-energy laser irradiation. Proc SPIE. 1996; Vol 2728: 63-67.

Kolyakov S F, Pyatibrat L V, Mikhailov E L et al. Changes in the spectra of circular dichroism of suspension of living cells after low intensity laser radiation at 820 nm, Dokl Akad Nauk (Moscow). 2001; 377: 824.

Komatsu M, Kubo T, Kogure S, Matsuda Y, Watanabe K. Effects of 808 nm low-power laser irradiation on the muscle contraction of frog gastrocnemius. Lasers Surg Med. 2008; 40 (8): 576-583.

Komelkova L V, Vitreshchak T V, Zhirnova I G, Poleshchuk V V et al. [Biochemical and immunological induces of the blood in Parkinson's disease and their correction with the help of laser therapy]. Patol Fiziol Eksp Ter. 2004; (1): 15-18.

Kim Y G. Laser mediated production of reactive oxygen and nitrogen species; implications for therapy. Free Radic Res. 2002; 36 (12): 1243-1250.

Kim S S, Min M W, Lee C J. Phototherapy of androgenetic alopecia with low level narrow band 655-nm red light and 780-nm infrared light. J Am Acad Dermatol. 2007; 56 (2), Suppl 2, P. AB112.

Kim Y D, Kim S S, Hwang D S, Kim S G, Kwon Y H et al. Effect of low-level laser treatment after installation of dental titanium implant-immunohistochemical study of RANKL, RANK, OPG: an experimental study in rats. Lasers Surg Med. 2007; 39 (5): 441-450.

Kim S J, Moon SU, Kang S G, Park Y G.Effects of low-level laser therapy after Corticision on tooth movement and paradental remodeling. Lasers Surg Med. 2009 Jul 28. [Epub ahead of print]

Kim H, Zarif N. MID-laser therapy - a potential approach to reduce pain in dysmenorrhea. Presented at NAALT2009, San Francisco, USA, June 2009.

Kimura Y, Wilder-Smith P, Yonaga K, Matsumoto K. Treatment of dentine hypersensitivity by laser: a review. J Clin Periodontol. 2000; 27: 715-721.

Kimura Y, Fujiwara M, Ikegami A. Anisotropic electric properties of purple membrane and their change during the photoreaction cycle. Biophys J. 1984; 45: 615-625.

King D L, Steinhauer W, Garcia-Godoy F, Elkins C J. Herpetic gingivostomatitis and teething difficulty in infants. Pediatr Dent. 1992; 14 (2): 82-85.

King C E et al. Effect of helium-neon laser auriculotherapy on experimental pain threshold. Phys Ther. 1990; 70 (1): 24-30.

King P. Low Level Laser Therapy: A Review. Lasers in Medical Science. 1989; 4: 141-.

Kipshidze N et al. Photoremodeling of arterial wall reduces restenosis after balloon angioplasty in an athero-sclerotic rabbit model. J Am Coll Cardiol. 1998; 31 (5): 1152-1157.

Kipshidze N N et al.[Lecitin-induced chemiluminiscence of peripheral blood neutrophils in patients with ischemic heart disease before and after blood irradiation with helium-neon laser]. Kardiologiia. 1992; 32 (1): 53-56.

Kipshidze N N et al. Treatment of acute myocardial infarction with a low-intensity Helium-Neon laser. Proc X Internat Congr Soc Laser Surg Med, Bangkok 1993, p. 309.

Kipshidze N N. [Changes in lecitin-induced chemiluminiscence of neutrophilic granulocytes after irradiation of blood with Helium-Neon lasers]. Biull Eksp Biol Med. 1992; 113 (1): 24-26.

Kipshidze N N. Our experience in the use of a low intensity HeNe laser in the treatment of acute myocardial infarction. Laser Therapy. 1996; 8 (1): 28. (abstract)

Kipshidze N N, Nikolaychik V, Keelan M et al. Low-power helium:neon laser irradiation enhances production of vascular endothelial growth factor and promotes growth of endothelian cells in vitro. Laser Surg Med. 2001; 28: 355-364.

Kipshidze N N, Petersen J, Vassoughi J et al. Low-power laser irradiation increases cyclic GMP synthesis in penile smooth muscle cells in vitro. J Clin Laser Med Surg. 2000; 18 (6): 291-294.

Kirichuk V F et al. Influence of low power laser radiation on platlet aggregation in pathological stress. Laser Therapy. 1996; 8 (1): 63. (abstract)

Kiritsi O, Tsitas K, Malliaropoulos N, Mikroulis G. Ultrasonographic evaluation of plantar fasciitis after low-level laser therapy: results of a double-blind, randomized, placebo-controlled trial.

Kitzes M, Twigg G, Berns M W. Alteration of membrane electrical activity in rat myocardial cells following selective laser microbeam irradiation. J Cell Physiology. 1977; 93: 99-104

Kiyoizumi T. Low Level Diode Laser Treatment for Hematomas under Grafted Skin and its Photobiological Mechanisms. Keio J Med. 1988; 37: 415-428.

Khullar S M et al. Enhanced sensory reinnervation of dental target tissues in rats following low level laser (LLL) irradiation. Lasers Med Sci. 1999; 14 (3): 177-184.

Khullar S M, Brodin P, Barkvoll P et al. Preliminary study of low-level laser for treatment of long-standing sensory aberrations in the inferior alveolar nerve. J Oral Maxillofac Surg. 1996; 54 (2): 2-7.

Khullar S M et al. The effects of low level laser treatment on recovery of nerve conduction and motor function after compression injury in the rat sciatic nerve. Europ J Oral Sci. 1995; 103: 299-305.

Khullar S M et al. Upregulation of growth associated protein (GAP) 43 expression and neural co-expression with neuropeptide Y (NPY) following inferior alveolar nerve (IAN) axotomy in the rat. J Periph Nerv Syst. 1998, 3 (2): 79-90.

Khullar S M. Reinnervation after nerve injury: the effects of low level laser treatment. In: Low Level Laser Therapy, clinical practice and scientific background. Eds Tunér-Hode. 1999; p. 280-302. Prima Books in Sweden. ISBN 91-630-7616-0.

Kiernicka M, Owczarek B, Galkowska E, Wysokinska-Miszczuk J. Comparison of the effectiveness of the conservative treatment of the periodontal pockets with or without the use of laser biostimulation. Ann Univ Mariae Curie Sklodowska [Med]. 2004; 59 (1): 488-494.

Kim Jin Wang, Lee Joung Ok. Double blind cross-over clinical study of 830 nm diode laser and 5 years clini-cal experience of biostimulation in plastic surgery & aesthetic surgery in Asians. Laser Surg Med. 1998; Suppl 10: 59.

Kim K et al. An experimental study on the effects of low power density laser (GaAs) on the wound healing of rat tongue and skin. J Korean Acad Oral Med. 1985; 10: 91-104.

Kim K et al. Study on the effect of low power laser irradiation in treating gingival inflammation. Clinical, microbiological, histoloical study. J Korean Acad Oral Med. 1987; 12: 5-16.

Kim K S, Hun L D, Kun K S. Effects of Low Incident Energy Levels of Infrared Laser Irradiation on the Proliferation of Streptococcus Mutans. Laser Therapy. 1992; 4 (2): 81-86.

Kim K S; Kim, Saeng Kon. An experimental study of the effects of low power density laser on the human gingival fibroblast. J Korean Acad. Oral Med 1987; 12 (1): 17-.

Kim K-S, Kim J-K, Kim S-W et al Effects of low level laser irradiation (LLLI) with 904 nm pulsed diode laser on osteoblasts: a controlled trial with the rat osteoblast model. Laser Therapy. 1996; 8 (4): 223-232.

Kim K-S, Kim S-K, Lee P-Y et al. Effects of low incident energy levels of infrared laser irradiation on the proliferation of candida albicans. Part 1: A long term study on the pulse types. Laser Therapy. 1994; 6 (3): 161-166.

Kim K-S et al. Effects of low level laser irradiation with 904 nm pulsed diode laser on the extraction wound. J of Korean Academy of Oral Medicine. 1998; 23: 301-307.

Kim, Ki-Suk and Kim, Saeng Kon. An experimental study on the effect of low power density laser on the human gingival fibroblasts. J Korean Acad Oral Med. 1987; 1 (12): 17-.

Kim, Ki-Suk and Kim, Young-Ku. Comparative study of the clinical effects of splint, laser acupuncture and laser therapy for temporomandibular disorders. J Dental College, Seoul Nat Univ. 1988: 1 (12): 195-.

Kim S-Y, Park J-S. The effect of low level laser therapy at the trigger points in masseter and other muscles. J Korean Acad Med. 1996; 21 (1): 3.

Kim S-Y, Park J-S. The effect of low level laser therapy at the trigger points in masseter and other muscles. J Korean Acad Oral Med. 1996; 21 (1): 1-3.

Kim, Dong-Won. The healing effects of low power density laser to the experimental periodontitis; histopathologic study. Thesis for M.S., Dept. of Dentistry, Dankook University, Korea. Advisor: Prof. Chung, Chin-Hyung. 1993.

Kazemi-Khoo N. Successful treatment of diabetic foot ulcers with low-level laser therapy. The Foot. 2006; 16 (4): 184-187.

Kazemi-kho N, Babazadeh K, Lajevardi M, Noudeh Y J. Application of low-level laser therapy after coronary artery bypass grafting (CABG) surgery. Proc. 7th Internat Congr of WALT, Sun City, South Africa, October 2008, page 135.

Kazemi-Kho N, Dabaghian F. Effect of blue light intravenous laser on blood sugar in diabetic type 2 patients. Proc. 7th Internat Congr of WALT, Sun City, South Africa, October 2008, page 94.

Kazmina S et al. Laser prophylaxis and treatment of primary caries. Proc. SPIE. Vol 984; 1994: 231-233.

Kemmotsu M D at al. Laser therapy for pain attenuation - the current experience in the pain clinic. In: Progress in Laser Therapy. 1991: 197-200. John Wiley & Sons, Chichester, Engl. ISBN 0-471-93154-3.

Kemmotsu O et al. Laser therapy for pain attenuation. Proc. 2nd Congress World Assn for Laser Therapy, Kansas City, September 1998; p. 7-8.

Kerns T. HeNe Lasers Show Promise in Treating Equine Injuries. Lasers & Applications. 1986; Dec: 39.

Khadra M, Kassem N, Haanaes H R, Ellingsen J E, Lyngstadaas S P. Enhancement of bone formation in rat calvarial bone defects using low-level laser therapy. Oral Surg Oral Med Oral Pathol Oral Endod. 2004; 97: 693-700.

Khadra M, Ronold H J, Lyngstadaas S P, Ellingsen J E, Haanaes H R. Low-level laser therapy stimulates bone-implant interaction: an experimental study in rabbits. Clin Oral Implants Res. 2004; 15 (3): 325-332.

Khadra M, Kasem N, Lyngstadaas S P, Haanæs H, Mustafa K. Laser therapy accelerates initial attachment and subsequent behaviour of human oral fibroblasts cultured on titanium implant material. A scanning electron microscopic and histomorphometric analysis. Clinical Oral Implants Research. 2005; 16 (2): 168-175.

Khadra M, Lyngstadaas S P, Haanaes H R, Mustafa K. Effect of laser therapy on attachment, proliferation and differentiation of human osteoblastic-like cells cultured on titanium implant material. Biomaterials.2005; 26: 3503-3509.

Khadra M, Lyngstadaas S P, Haanaes H R, Mustafa K. Determining optimal dose of laser therapy for attachment and proliferation of human fibroblasts cultured on titanium implant material. J Biomed Mater Res. 2005; 73A: 55-62.

Khan A, Syed A, Shah A M, Ahmad F, Qadri T. Early experience on the effect of 820 nm LLLT on musculoskeletal pain. Proc. 4th Congress of the World Association for Laser Therapy, Tokyo, Japan, June 27-30. 2002; page 133.

Khanna A, Shankar LR, Keelan MH et al. Augumentation of the expression of proangiogenic genes in cardiomyocytes with low dose laser irradiation in vitro. Cardiovasc Radiat Med. 1999; 265-269.

Khomeriki S G, Kubatiev A A, Shliapnikov V N.[Lecitin-induced aggregation of neutrophilic granulocytes before and after irradiation of the blood with a helium-neon laser]. Gematol Transfuziol. 1993; 38 (7): 26-28.

Khorsand T N, Mokmeli S, Daneshvar L, Soror N, Hosseini H. Comparison between the effect of low level laser therapy and injection of Botox in treatment of anal fissure (clinical trial, case control). Proc. 7th Internat Congr of WALT, Sun City, South Africa, October 2008, page 138.

Khullar S M, Emami B, Westermark A et al. Effect of low-level laser treatment on neurosensory deficits subsequent to sagittal split ramus osteotomy. Oral Surg Oral Med Oral Pathol Oral Radiol Endod. 1996; 82 (2): 132-138.

Karu T I. Ryabykh T P., Fedoseyeva G E, Puchkova N I. Induced by He-Ne laser radiation respiratory burst on phagocytic cells. Lasers Surg. Med. 1989; 9: 585.

Karu T I. Effects of visible radiation on cultured cells. Photochem Photobiol. 52:1089- 1090.

Karu T I, Pyatibrat L V, Kalendo G S. Donors of NO and pulsed radiation at lambda = 820 nm exert effects on cell attachment to extracellular matrices. Toxicol Lett. 2001; 121 (1): 57-61.

Karu T I, Pyatibrat L V, Afanasyeva N I. Cellular effects of low power laser therapy can be mediated by nitric oxide. Lasers Surg Med. 2005; 36 (4):307-314.

Karu T, Pyatibrat L, Kalendo G. Irradiation with He-Ne laser increases ATP level in cells cultivated in vitro. J Photochem Photobiol B. 1995; 27 (3): 219-223.

Kasai S et al. Effects of low-power laser irradiation on impulse conductions in anaesthetized rabbits. J Clin Laser Med Surg. 1996; 14 (3): 107-109.

Kato M et al. Clinical studies of low power density HeNe laser irradiation on stellate ganglion. Jpn J Oral Maxillofac Surg. 1987; 33 (12): 1-11.

Kats A .et al. [Use of laser in nonspecific inflammatory processes of the temporomnadibular joint]. Stomatologiia (Mosk). 1983; 62: 42-45

Kats A et al. [Laser therapy in fracture of the mandible]. Vestn Kir. 1986; 136: 93 (in Russian with English abstract)

Kats A G et al. [Remote results of the complex treatment of chronic sialadenitis with the use of helium-neon lasers]. Vestnik Khirurgii Imeni i-i- Grekova. 1985; 135: 39-42.

Kats A. [Treatment of erosive-ulcerative forms of lichen planus with low-energy laser irradiation]. Vestnik Khirurgii Imeni i - i - Grekova 1990 144 (4): 121-123.

Kato I T, Pellegrini V, Prates R A, Wetter N U, Ribeiro M S, Sugaya N N. Infrared laser irradiation applied to the treatment of burning mouth syndrome. Proc. 7th Internat Congr of WALT, Sun City, South Africa, October 2008, page 140.

Katsuyama I et al. Suppressive effect of diode laser irradiation on picryl contact sensitivity. Laser Therapy 1998, 10 (3): 117-122.

Kaul U, Singh B, Sudan D et al. Red light laser therapy after coronary stenting: angiographic and clinical follow up study in humans. J Invas Cardiol. 1998; 10: 269-273.

Kaviani A, Fateh M, Nooraie R Y, Alinagi-Zadeh M R, Ataie-Fashtami L. Low-level laser therapy in management of postmastectomy lymphedema. Lasers Med Sci. 2006; 21 (2): 90-94.

Kawalec J S, Hetherington J, Pfennigwerth C et al Effect of a diode laser on wound healing by using diabetic and nondiabetic mice. Journal of Foot and Ankle Surgery. 2004; 43 (4): 214-220.

Kawalec J S, Pfennigwerth C, Hetherington J et al. A review of lasers in healing diabetic ulcers.The Foot. 2004; 14: 68-71.

Kawamura M et al. Effect of Nd:YAG and diode laser irradiation on periodontal wound healing. Innov. Techn. Biol. Med. 1990; 11 (1) :113.

Kawasaki K, Shimizo N. Effects of low-energy laser irradiation on bone remodelling during experimental tooth movement in rats. Laser Surg Med. 2000; 26: 282-291.

Kawato S, Sigel E, Carafoli E, Cherry R J. Cytochrome oxidase rotates in the inner membrane of intact mitochondria and submitochondrial particles. J Biol Chem. 1980; 255 (12): 5508-5510.

Kawato S, Kinoshita K. Time-dependent absorption anisotropy and rotational diffusion of proteins in membranes. Biophys J. 1981; 36: 277-296.

Kayano T. Effect of Er:YAG laser irradiation on human extracted teeth. J Clinical Laser Med Surg 1991; 9 (2): 147-.

Karu T I, Pyatibrat L V, Kalendo G S. Cell attachment modulation by radiation from a pulsed semiconductor light diode (820 nm) and various chemicals. Lasers Surg Med. 2001; 28: 227-236.

Karu T I, Pyatibrat L V, Kalendo G S. Cell attachment to extracellular matrices is modulated by pulsed radiation at 820 nm and chemical that modify the activity of enzymes in the plasma membrane. Lasers Surg Med. 2001; 29: 274-281.

Karu T I, Pyatibrat L V, Kalendo G S. Donors of NO and pulsed radiation at (820 nm) exert effects on cells attachment to extracellular matrices. Toxicol Lett. 2001; 121:57.

Karu T I, Pyatibrat L V, Kalendo G S. Thiol reactive agents and semiconductor light diode radiation (820 nm) exert effects on cell attachment to extracellular matrix. Laser Therapy. 2001; 11: 177.

Karu T I, Pyatibrat L V, Ryabykh T P. Nonmonotonic behaviour of the dose dependence of the radiation effect on cells *in vitro* exposed to pulsed laser radiation at 820 nm. Lasers Surg Med. 1997; 21: 485.

Karu T I, Pyatibrat L V, Kalendo G S, Esenaliev R O. Effects of monochromatic low intensity light and laser irradiation on adhesion of HeLa cells *in vitro*. Lasers Surg Med. 1996; 18: 171.

Karu T I, Pyatibrat L V, Kalendo G S. Biostimulation of HeLa cells by low-intensity visible light. V. Stimulation of cell proliferation *in vitro* by He-Ne laser radiation. Il Nuovo Cimento D. 1987; 9: 1485-1494.

Karu T I, Pyatibrat L V, Kalendo G S. Studies into the action specifics of a pulsed GaAlAs laser (820 nm) on a cell culture. I. Reduction of the intracellular ATP concentration: dependence on initial ATP amount. Lasers Life Sci. 2001; 9: 203.

Karu T I, Ryabykh T P, Letokhov V S. Different sensitivity of cells from tumor-bearing organisms to continuous-wave and pulsed laser radiation (632.8 nm) evaluated by chemiluminescence test. III. Effect of dark period between pulses. Lasers Life Sci. 1997; 7: 141.

Karu T I, Ryabykh T P, Sidorova T A, Dobrynin Ya V. The use of a chemiluminescence test to evaluate the sensitivity of blast cells in patients with hemoblastoses to antitumor agents and low-intensity laser radiation. Lasers Life Sci. 1996; 7: 1.

Karu T I, Smolyaninova N K, Zelenin A V. Long-term and short-term responses of human lymphocytes to He-Ne laser radiation. Lasers Life Sci. 1991; 4: 167.

Karu T I, Tiphlova O A, Fedoseyeva G E et al. Biostimulating action of low-intensity monochromatic visible light: is it possible? Laser Chem. 1984; 5: 19.

Karu T I, Tiphlova O A, Matveyets Yu A et al Comparison of the effects of visible femtosecond laser pulses and continuous wave laser radiation of low average intensity on the clonogenicity of *Escherichia coli*. J Photochem Photobiol B Biol. 1991; 10: 339.

Karu T I, Tiphlova O, Esenaliev R, Letokhov V. Two different mechanisms of low-intensity laser photobiological effects on *Escherichia coli*. J Photochem Photobiol B Biol. 1994; 24: 155.

Karu T I. Local pulsed heating of absorbing chromophores as a possible primary mechanism of low-power laser effects. In: *Laser Applications in Medicine and Surgery.* Galletti, G, Bolognani L, Ussia G, Eds. Monduzzi Editore, Bologna, 1992, p. 253.

Karu T I. Low-power laser effects, in *Lasers in Medicine*. Waynant R, Ed. CRC Press, Boca Raton, FL. 2002, p. 169.

Karu T I. Mechanisms of low-power laser light action on cellular level. In: *Lasers in Medicine and Dentistry.* Simunovic Z, Ed., Vitgraf, Rijeka (Croatia), 2000, p. 97.

Karu T I. Molecular mechanism of the therapeutic effect of low-intensity laser radiation. Lasers Life Sci. 1988; 2: 53.

Karu T I. Primary and secondary mechanisms of action of visible-to-near IR radiation on cells. J Photochem Photobiol B Biol. 1999; 49: 1.

Karu T I et al. Biostimulation of HeLa-cells by low-Intensity Visible Light. Nuovo Cimento. 1982; 1D (6): 828-.

Karu T I. Low Intensity Laser Light Action upon Fibroblast and Lymphocytes. Progress in Laser Therapy, Eds. T. Ohshiro and R.G. Calderhead, John Wiley & Sons, England. 1991 p. 175.

Karu T I. Photobiological Fundamentals of Low Power Laser Therapy. IEEE Journal of Quantum Electronics. 1987; 23 (10): 1703-.

Karu T I. Photobiology of low-power laser effects. Health Physics. 1989; 56 (5): 691-704.

Karu T I, Kolyakov S, Pyatibrat V et al. Irradiation with a diode at 820 nm induces changes in circular dichroism spectra (270-780 nm) of living cells. IEEE J Selected Topics in quantum Electronics. 2001; 7 (6): 976-981.

Karu T I, Afanasyeva N, Kolyakov S et al. Changes in absorbance of momolayer of living cells induced by laser radiation at 633, 670, and 820 nm. IEEE J Selected Topics in quantum Electronics. 2001; 7 (6): 982-988.

Karu T I, Afanasyeva N I, Kolyakov S F et al. Changes in absorbance of monolayer of living cells induced by laser radiation at 633, 670, and 820 nm. IEEE J Sel Top Quantum Electron. 2001; 7: 982.

Karu T I, Afanasyeva N I, Kolyakov S F, Pyatibrat L V. Changes in absorption spectra of monolayer of living cells after irradiation with low intensity laser light. Dokl Akad Nauk (Moscow). 1998; 360: 267.

Karu T I, Afanasyeva N I. Cytochrome oxidase as primary photoacceptor for cultured cells in visible and near IR regions. Dokl Akad Nauk (Moscow). 1995; 342: 693.

Karu T I, Andreichuk T N, Ryabykh T P. On the action of semiconductor laser radiation (Ξ?= 820 nm) on the chemiluminescence of blood of clinically healthy humans. Lasers Life Sci. 1995; 6: 277.

Karu T I, Andreichuk T, Ryabykh T. Changes in oxidative metabolism of murine spleen following diode laser (660–950 nm) irradiation: effect of cellular composition and radiation parameters. Lasers Surg Med. 1993; 13: 453.

Karu T I, Andreichuk T, Ryabykh T. Suppression of human blood chemiluminescence by diode laser radiation at wavelengths 660, 820, 880 or 950 nm. Laser Therapy. 1993; 5: 103.

Karu T I, Kalendo G S, Letokhov V S, Lobko V V. Biological action of low-intensity visible light on HeLa cells as a function of the coherence, dose, wavelength, and irradiation dose, Sov J Quantum Electron. 1982; 12: 1134.

Karu T I, Kalendo G S, Letokhov V S, Lobko V V. Biological action of low-intensity visible light on HeLa cells as a function of the coherence, dose, wavelength, and irradiation regime. II. Sov J Quantum Electron. 1983; 13: 1169.

Karu T I, Kalendo G S, Letokhov V S, Lobko V V. Biostimulation of HeLa cells by low intensity visible light. II. Stimulation of DNA and RNA synthesis in a wide spectral range. Nuov Cim. 1984; D, 3: 309.

Karu T I, Kalendo G S, Letokhov V S, Lobko V V. Biostimulation of HeLa cells by low intensity visible light. III. Stimulation of nucleic acid synthesis in plateau phase cells. 1984; Nuov Cim. 1984; D, 3: 319.

Karu T I, Kalendo G S, Letokhov V S. Control of RNA synthesis rate in tumor cells HeLa by action of low-intensity visible light of copper laser. Lett. Nuov. Cim. 1981; 32: 55.

Karu T I, Piatibrat L V, Kalendo G S. [The effect of He-Ne laser radiation on the survival of HeLa cells subjected to ionizing radiation]. Radiobiologiia. 1992; 32 (2): 202-206. [in Russian]

Kami T, Yoshimura Y, Nakajima T et al. Effect of low-powered diode lasers on flap survival. Ann Plast Surgery. 1985; 14 (3): 278-283.

Kamikawa K, Kyoto J. Double blind experiences with mid-Lasers in Japan. 1985. Int Congr on Lasers in Med and Surg, Bologna June 1985, 165-169. Moduzzi Editore S.p.A., Bologna

Kamikawa K et al. Essential mechanisms of low power laser effects. Laser Bologna '92, p. 11. Monduzzi Editore S.p.A., Bologna, Italy.

Kamikawa K Studies on low power laser therapy of pain. Lasers in Dentistry. 1989; page 29-38. Elsevier Science Publisher B.V. Amsterdam

Kana J, Hutschenreiter G, Haina D, Waidelich W. Effect of low-power density laser radiation on healing of open skin wounds in rats. Arch surg. 1981; 116: 293-296.

Kaneko M et al. The application of Nd:YAG laser for low energy laser therapy in the intraoral region. Laser in Dentistry. Proceedings of the Intern Congr of Lasers in Dentistry, Tokyo, August 1988, p. 131-136. Excerpta Medica, Elsevier Science Publishers, Amsterdam.

Kaneps A, Hultgren B, Riebold T, Shires G. Laser therapy in the horse: Histopathologic response. Am J Vet Res. 1984; 45 (3): 581-.

Kapinosov I K et al. Reaction of lymphoid organs to laser radiation with different pulsation rates. Proc. SPIE. 1996; Vol 2678: 530-533. (Optical Diagnostics of Living Cells and Biofluids)

Karabegovic A, Kapidzic-Durakovic S, Ljuca F. Laser therapy of painful shoulder and shoulder-hand syndrome in treatment of patients after the stroke. Bosn J Basic Med Sci. 2009; 9 (1): 59-65.

Karpen M. Low-level laser therapy in trials for urologiclal applications. J Clin Laser Med Surg. 1995; 13 (4): 293-294.

Karu T I, Letokhov V S, Lobko V V, Novikov V F, Paramonov L V. [Phototherapy of gastric and duodenal peptic ulcer patients based on cellstimulation with low-intensity red light]. Vopr Kurortol Fizioter Lech Fiz Kult. 1984; (1): 36-39. (in Russian)

Karu T I, Pyatibrat L, Kalendo G. Irradiation with HeNe laser can influence the cytotoxic response of HeLa cells to ionizing radiation. Int. J Radiation Biology. 1994; 65 (6): 691-697.

Karu T I, Ryabykh T P, Antonov S N. Different sensitivity of cells from tumor-bearing organisms to countinuous-wave and pulsed laser radiation (=632.8 nm) evaluated by chemiluminescence test. II. Comparison of responses of human blood: healthy persons and patients with colon cancer. Lasers in the Life Sciences. 1996; 7 (2): 99-106.

Karu T I, Ryabykh T P, Antonov S N. Different sensitivity of cells from tumor-bearing organisms to countinuous-wave and pulsed laser radiation (=632.8 nm) evaluated by chemiluminescence test. I. Comparison of responses of murine splenocytes: intact mice and mice with transplanted leukemia EL-4. Lasers in the Life Sciences. 1996; 7 (2): 91-98.

Karu T I, Andreichuck T, Ryabykh T. Supression of human blood chemi-luminescence by diode laser irradiation at wavelengths 660, 820, 880 or 950 nm. Laser Therapy. 1993; 5 (3): 103-110.

Karu T I , Tiphlova O. Stimulation of E. Coli growth by laser and incoherent red light. Nuovo Cimento. 1983; 2 (4): 1138-.

Karu T I. Depression of the genome after irradiation of human lymphocytes with HeNe laser. Laser Therapy. 1992. 4 (1): 5-24

Karu T I. Mechanism of interaction of monochromatic visible light with cells. Proc. SPIE. 1995; Vol 2630: 10-.

Karu T I. Mechanisms of interaction of monochromatic visible light with cells. Proc. SPIE. 1995; Vol 2630: 2-9

Karu T I. Low power laser therapy. In: Biomedical Photonics Handbook, Chapter 48. CRC Press LLC. 2003.

Jensen I, Harms-Ringdahl K. Strategies for prevention and management of musculoskeletal conditions. Neck pain. Best Pract Res Clin Rheumatol. 2007; 21 (1): 93-108.

Jia Y K, Luo H C, Zhan L, Jia T Z, Yan M. A study on the treatment of schizophrenia with He-Ne laser irradiation of acupoint. J Tradit Chin Med 1987; 7 (4): 269-272.

Jia Y L, Guo Z Y. Effect of low-power He-Ne laser irradiation on rabbit articular chondrocytes in vitro. Lasers Surg Med. 2004; 34 (4): 323-328.

Jih Ming H, Friedman P M, Kimyai A A, Goldberg L H. Successful treatment of a chronic atrophic dog-bite scar with the 1450-nm diode laser. Dermatologic Surgery 2004; 30 (8): 1161-11633.

Jimbo K, Noda K, Suzuki K, Yoda K. Suppressive effects of low-power laser irradiation on bradykinin evoked action potentials in cultured murine dorsal root ganglion cells. Neurosci Lett. 1998; 9; 240 (2): 93-96.

Jin-zhi He. Clinical analysis of 100 cases of scald injury cured by HeNe laser acupuncture in combination with scanning laser therapy. Laser Therapy. 1990; 2 (4): 179-180.

Johannsen F et al. Low energy laser therapy in rheumatiod arthritis. Scand J Rheumatol. 1994; 23 (3): 145-147.

Johnson D et al. Low-level laser therapy for Peyronie's disease. Proc. SPIE. 1995; Vol 2395: 108-110.

Joyce K M, Downes C S, Hannigan B M. Radioadaptation in Indian muntjac fibroblast cells induced by low intensity laser irradiation. Mutat Res. 1999; 435 (1): 35-42.

Junior E C, Lopes-Martins R A, Baroni B M, De Marchi T, Rossi R P, Grosselli D, Generosi R A, de Godoi V, Basso M, Mancalossi J L, Bjordal J M. Comparison Between Single-Diode Low-Level Laser Therapy (LPT) and LED Multi-Diode (Cluster) Therapy (LEDT) Applications Before High-Intensity Exercise. Photomed Laser Surg. 2009 Mar 20. [Epub ahead of print]

Juri H et al. Efectos del láser HeNe sobre las concentraciones de fibrinogeno en el plasma de ratas en lesiones tistulares. Boletín CDL. 1986; 10: 5-6.

Juri H et al. Effects of Nd:YAG laser radiation on PGE2 level in experimental arthtitis. Proc X Internat Congr Soc Laser Surg Med, Bangkok 1993, p. 314.

Jöbsis-van der Vliet F F, Jöbsis P D. Biochemical and physiological basis of medical near-infrared spectroscopy. Biomed. Opt. 1999; 4: 397.

Jöbsis-van der Vliet F F. Dicovery of the near-infrared window in the body and the early development of near-infrared spectroscopy. J Biomed. Opt. 1999; 4: 392.

Kaihøj P. Low Level Lasers Effekt på Følsomme Tandhalse - en klinisk pilottest. [The Effect of Low Level Lasers on Sensitive Toothnecks - a Clinical Pilot Study] . Odont Pract. 1991; 6 (2): 229-. (in Danish)

Kaiser C, Manso F, Zaragoza J R.. Estúdio en doble ciego randomizado sobre la eficacia del HeNe en el tratamiento de la sinuitis maxilar aguda: en pacientes con exacerbación de una infección sinusal crónica. (Double blind randomized study on the effect of HeNe in the treatment of acute maxillary sinuitis: in patients with exacerbation of a chronic maxillary sinuitis). Boletín CDL. 1986; 9: 15-19.

Kalivradzhiyan E et al. Usage of low-intensity laser radiation for the treatment of the inflammatory processes of the oral cavity mucosa after applying removable plate dentures. Proc SPIE. 1995; Vol 1984: 225-230.

Kamali F, Bayat M, Torkaman G, Ebrahimi E, Salavati M. The therapeutic effect of low-level laser on repair of osteochondral defects in rabbit knee. J Photochem Photobiol B. 2007; 88 (1): 11-15.

Kamata H, Hirata H. Redox regulation of cellular signaling. Cell Signal. 1999; 11: [1]: 1-14.

Irvine J, Chong S L, Amirjani N, Chan K M. Double-blind randomized controlled trial of low-level laser therapy in carpal tunnel syndrome. Muscle Nerve. 2004; 30 (2): 182-187.

Ishikawa I, Aoki A, Takasaki A A. Potential applications of Erbium:YAG laser in periodontics. J Periodontal Res 69. 2004; (4): 275–285.

Israel M. Current research using the CO_2 laser in guided tissue regeneration. Clinical studies. Proc Second Annual Advanced Application Seminar. Luxar Corp, USA. 1993.

Israel N, Gougerot-Pocidalo M-A, Aillet F, Verelizier J-L. Redox status of cells influences constitutive or induced NF-B translocation and HIV long terminal repeat activity in human T-lymphocytes and monocytic cell lines. J Immunol. 1992; 149: 3386.

Ito A et al. Studies of Nd:YAG low power laser irradiation on stellate ganglion. In: Lasers in dentistry. Ed. H Yamamoto. 1989; p. 271. Elsevier Science Publishers B.V.

Ito A, Kakami K, Matsushita H, Fukaya M. Effects of Nd:YAG low power laser irradiation on the ulnar nerve. Aichi Gakuin Dent Sci. 1989; 2: 1-8.

Itoh T et al. The protective effect of low power HeNe laser against erythrocytic damage caused by artificial heart-lung machines. Horoshima J Med Sci. 1996; 45 (1): 15-22.

Itoh T, Murakami H, Orihashi K et al. Low power laser protects human erythrocytes in an in vitro model of artificial heart-lung machines. Artificial Organs. 2000; 24 (11): 870-873.

Iusim M et al. Evaluation of the degree of effectiveness of Biobeam low level narrow band light on the treatment of skin ulcers and delayed postoperative wound healing. Orthopedics. 1992; 15: 1023-1026.

Ivandic B T, Ivandic T. Low-Level Laser Therapy Improves Vision in Patients with Age-Related Macular Degeneration. Photomed Laser Surg. 2008; 2 (3): 241-245.

Ivandic B T, Hoque N N, Ivandic T. Early diagnosis of ocular hypertension using a low-intensity laser irradiation test. Photomed Laser Surg. 2009; 27 (4): 571-575.

Ivanov A S et al. [Effect of Helium-Neon laser radiation on the course of temporomandibular joint arthritis and arthrosis.] Stomatologiia (Mosk). 1985; 64: 81-82.

Ivanov A S et al. [The morphofunctional status of the synovial membrane of the temporomandibular joint under exposure to helium-neon laser]. Morfologia. 1996; 109 (3): 59-63.

Iwase T, Saito T, Nara Y, Morioka T. Inhibitory effect of HeNe laser on dental plaque deposition in hamsters. J Periodont Research. 1989; 24: 282-283.

Iwase T, Hori N, Morioka T et al. Low power laser irradiation reduces ischemic damage in hippocampal slices in vitro. Laser Surg Med. 1996; 19 (4): 465-470.

Izzo A D, Richter C P, Jansen E D, Walsh J T Jr. Laser stimulation of the auditory nerve. Lasers Surg Med. 2006; 38 (8): 745-753.

Jackeviciute I. Low power laser treatment for bronchial asthma and chronic bronchitis. Proc. Scand Soc for Laser Therapy. 3rd Congress, Örebro, Sweden. Oct 2-4, 1991.

Jackson Z et al. Killing of the yeast and hyphal forms of candida albicans using a light-activated antimicrobial agent. Lasers in Medical Science. 1999; 14 (2): 150-157.

Jaguar G C, Prado J D, Nishimoto I N, Pinheiro M C, de Castro D O Jr, da Cruz Perez D E, Alves F A. Low-energy laser therapy for prevention of oral mucositis in hematopoietic stem cell transplantation. Oral Dis. 2007; 13 (6): 538-543.

Jankiewicz, Zdzislaw; Zajac, A. Detection of laser radiation in biological experiments. Proc. SPIE. 1995; Vol 2203: 148-161. (Laser Technology IV: Applications in Medicine, Wieslaw Wolinski; Tadeusz Kecik; Eds.)

Jarry G, Debray S, Perez J, Lefebvre J P et al. In vivo transillumination of the hand using near infrared laser pulses and differential spectroscopy. J Biomed Eng 1989; 11 (4): 293-299.

Jensen H et al. [Is infra-red laser effective in painful arthrosis of the knee?] (In Danish) Ugeskr Laeger 1987; 149: 3104-3106.

Idrisova L T, Enikeev D A, Vasileva T V. [The effect of intravenous laser irradiation of the blood on the brain bioelectrical activity in patients in the postcomatose period]. Vopr Kurortol-Fizioter-Lech-Fiz-Kult. 2000; (2): 28-31.

Igarashi H, Inomata K. Effects of low-power gallium aluminium arsenide diode laser irradiation on the development of synapses in the neonatal rat hippocampus. Acta Anat (Basel). 1991; 140 (2): 150-155.

Igic M, Kesic L, Apostolovic M, Kostadinovic L. [Low-level laser efficiency in the therapy of chronic gingivitis in children] [in Serbian]. Vojnosanit Pregl. 2008; 65 (10): 755-757.

Ihara N, Kubota J, Ban I. Defocused diode laser therapy for wound management. Proc. 3rd Cong World Ass for Laser Therapy, Athens, Greece, May 2000, p. 78.

Ihsan F R. Low-level laser therapy accelerates collateral circulation and enhances microcirculation. Photomed Laser Surg. 2005; 23 (3): 289-294.

Ihsan F R, Al-Mustawfi N, Kaka L N. Promotion of Regenerative Processes in Injured Peripheral Nerve Induced by Low-Level Laser Therapy. Photomed Laser Surg, 2007, 25 (2): 107-111.

Iijima K, Shimoyama N, Shimoyama M, Mizuguchi T. Evaluation of Analgesic Effect of Low Power HeNe laser on Postherpetic Neuralgia Using VAS and Modified McGill Pain Questionaire. J Clin Laser Med Surg . 1991; 9 (2): 121-126.

Iijima K et al. Evaluation of analgesic effect of low-power laser for outpatients in pain clinic. J Jpn Soc Med Lasers. l988; 9: 3-10. (in Japanese)

Iijima K, Shimoyama N, Shimoyama M et al. Effect of repeated irradiation of low-power Ne-He laser in pain relief from postherpectic neuralgia. Clin J Pain. 1989; 5 (3): 271-274.

Iilima K, Shimoyama N, Shimoyama M, Mizuguchi T. Red and green low-powered HeNe lasers protect human erythrocytes from hypotonic hemolysis. J Clin Laser Med Surg. 1991; 9: 385-.

Ilbuldu E, Cakmak A, Disci R, Aydin R. Comparison of laser, dry needling, and placebo laser treatments in myofascial pain syndrome. Photomed Laser Surg. 2004; 22 (4): 306-311.

Ilic S, Leichliter S, Streeter J, DeTaboada L, Oron U. Effects of Dose, Mode and Frequency of Low Level Laser Therapy on the Rat Brain. Photomed Laser Surg. 2006; 24 (4): 458-66.

Ilich-Stoianovich O, Nasonov E L, Balabanova R M. [Effects of low-intensity infrared impulse laser therapy on inflammation activity markers in patients with rheumatoid arthritis]. Terapevticheskii Arkhiv. 2000; 72 (5): 32-34.

Illnerova H, Vanecek J, Krecek J, Wetterberg L, Sääf J. Effect of one minute exposure to light at night on rat pineal serotonin N-acetyltransferase and melatonin. J Neurochem. 1979; 32 (2): 673-675.

Imbronito A V, Okuda O S, Maria de Freitas N, Moreira Lotufo R F, Nunes F D. Detection of Herpesviruses and Periodontal Pathogens in Subgingival Plaque of Patients With Chronic Periodontitis, Generalized Aggressive Periodontitis, or Gingivitis. J Periodontol. 2008; 79(12): 2313-2321.

Inkova G A, Ionin A P, Ionina G I. [The treatment of posttraumatic uveitis with low-intensity laser Radiation]. Vestnik oftalmologii. 1999; 115 (5): 20-21.

Inoue K et al. Altered lymphocyte proliferation by low dosage laser irradiation. Clin Exp Rheumatol. 1989; 7 (5): 521-523.

Inoue K et al. Suppressed tuberculine reaction in guinea pigs following laser irradiation. Laser Surg Med, 1989; 9: 271-275.

Iordanou P, Baltopoulos G, Giannakopoulou M et al. Effect of polarized light in the healing process of pressure ulcers. Int. J Nurs Pract. 2002; 8: 49-55.

Iruzubieta J N. Effects of soft laser (HeNe) irradiation on corneal wound healing. An experimental study in the rabbit. Chibret Int J Ophthalm. 1991; 8: 25-33.

Hothersall J S, Cunha F Q, Neild G H, Norohna-Dutra A. Induction of nitric oxide synthesis in J774 cell lowers intracellular glutathione: effect of oxide modulated glutathione redox status on nitric oxide synthase induction. Biochem J. 1997; 322: 477.

Hou J F, Zhang H, Yuan X, Li J, Wei Y J, Hu S S. In vitro effects of low-level laser irradiation for bone marrow mesenchymal stem cells: proliferation, growth factors secretion and myogenic differentiation. Lasers Surg Med. 2008; 40 (10):726-733.

Rallis T R. Low-intensity laser therapy for recurrent herpes labialis. J Invest Dermatol. 2000; 115 (1): 131-132.

Houghton P E, Brown J L. Effects of low level laser on healing of wounded fetal mouse limbs. Laser Therapy. 1999; 11 (2): 54-70.

Houreld N, Abrahamse H. Effectiveness of Helium-Neon Laser Irradiation on Viability and Cytotoxicity of Diabetic-Wounded Fibroblast Cells. Photomed Laser Surg. 2007; 25 (6): 474-481.

Houreld N, Abrahamse H. In Vitro Exposure of Wounded Diabetic Fibroblast Cells to a Helium-Neon Laser at 5 and 16 J/cm^2. Photomed Laser Surg. 2007; 25 (2): 78-84.

Houreld N, Abrahamse H. Irradiation with a 632.8 nm helium-neon laser with 5 J/cm^2 stimulates proliferation and expression of interleukin-6 in diabetic wounded fibroblast cells. Diabetes Technol Ther. 2007; 9 (5): 451-459.

Houreld N, Abrahamse H. Laser light influences cellular viability and proliferation in diabetic-wounded fibroblast cells in a dose- and wavelength-dependent manner. Lasers Med Sci. 2008; 23 (1): 11-18.

Howell R M et al. The use of low energy laser therapy to treat aphtous ulcers. Ann Dent. 1988; 47 (2): 16-18.

Hrnjak M et al. Stimulatory effect of low-power density HeNe laser radiation on human fibroblasts in vitro. Vojnosanitetski Pregled. 1995; 52 (6): 539-546.

Hronková H, Navrátil L, Krymplová J, Knizek J. Possibilities of the analgesic therapy of ultrasound and-non-invasive laser on plantar fasciitis. Laser Partner Clinixperience. No 21. May 2001. www.laserpartner.org.

Hsu J et al. Combined effects of laser irradiation/solution fluoride ion on enamel demineralization. J Clin Laser Med Surg. 1998; 16 (2): 93-105.

Hubacek J et al. Lymphocyte reaction in the palatine tonsils after use of the HeNe laser. Ceskoslov Gastroen-terol a Vyziva. 1983; 37 (8): 467-471.

Hubacek J, Olomouc CZ. Experience with the use of laser therapy in ENT medicine. Laser Partner No 22. December 19, 2001.

Hübler R, Blando E, Gaião L, Kreisner P E, Post L K, Xavier C B, de Oliveira M G. Effects of low-level laser therapy on bone formed after distraction osteogenesis. Lasers Med Sci. 2009 Jun 23. [Epub ahead of print]

Hudson S J. Eye injuries from laser exposure: a review. Aviat Space Environ Med. 1998; 69 (5): 519-524.

Humzah M D, Diamantopoulos C, Dyson M. Multi-wavelength low reactive-level laser therapy (laser therapy) as an adjunct in malignant ulcers; case reports. Laser Therapy. 1993; 5 (4): 149-152.

Iakovleva NE, Liapina LA, Novoderzhkina IS et al. [The effect of low-intensity laser radiation on the parameters of the blood anticoagulation system in the early postresuscitation period]. Anesteziol Reanimatol. 1997 ; (4): 36-8

Ibanez J C, Medico R O. [Laser therapy in temporomandibular dysfunction]. Rev Fac Odont Univ Nac (Córdoba). 1989; 17 (1-2): 21-30. (in Spanish)

Hietanen M. Health risks of exposure to non-ionizing radiation - myths or science-based evidence. Med Lav. 2006; 97 (2): 184-188.

Hirsch D, Leupold W. [Placebo-controlled study on the effect of laser acupuncture in childhood asthma]. Atemwegs Lungenkr. 1994; 20 (12): 701-705.

Hirschl M, Katzenschlager R, Ammer K et al. Double-blind, randomised, placebo controlled low level laser therapy study in patients with primary Raynaud's phenomenon. Vasa - Journal of Vascular Diseases. 2002; 31 (2): 91-94.

Hode L, Biedermann K. Observation of surface deformation in real time using laser speckles. Proc Conference in Physics, Lund, Sweden, June 12-14. 1972.

Hode L. Elektronisk bildbehandling för speckelinterferometri i reell tid. Proj 1006. Institutet för Optisk Forskning, Kungl. Tekniska Högskolan. Oktober 1973. (in Swedish)

Hode L, Tunér J. Dose distribution in living tissue at different wavelengths, power densities and incident target areas. Proc. SPIE. 1999; Vol. 4166: 294-302.

Hode L, Tunér J. Low-level laser therapy (LLLT) versus light-emitting diode therapy (LEDT: What is the difference? Proc. SPIE. 1999; Vol. 4166: 90-97.

Hode L, Tunér J. Wrong parameters can give just any result. Laser Surg Med. 2006; 38: 343 (Letter to the editor).

Hoens-Alison M. Low intensity Nd:YAG laser irradiation for lateral epicondylitis. Clin J Sport Medicine. 2002; 12 (1): 55-.

Hoffman B, Bär Th. Reaktionen der Hautoberflächentemperatur - ein Vergleich zwischen Verum- und Placebo-Laserstimulation am Akupunkturpunkt Di 4. Dtsch. Zschr. Akup. 1994; 37 (2): 28-.

Hoffmann B, Bar T. The reactions of the skin surface temperature - a comparison between real and placebo laser acupuncture stimulation of LI 4.]. Dtsch Z Akupunkt 1994; 37 (2): 28-32.

Hong J N, Kim T H, Lim S D: Clinical trial of low reactive-level laser therapy in 20 patients with postherpetic neuralgia. Laser Therapy. 1990; 2 (4): 167-170.

Honmura A et al. Analgesic Effect of Ga-Al-As Diode Laser Irradiation on Hyperalgesia in Carrageenin-Induced Inflammation. Laser Surg Med. 1993; 13: 463-469.

Honmura A et al. Therapeutic effects of GaAlAs diode laser irradiation on experimentally inducedinflammation in rats. Laser Surg Med 1992; 12: 441-449.

Hopkins G O et al. Double blind cross over study of laser versus placebo in the treatment of tennis elbow. Proc Internat Congr in laser, "Laser Bologna". 1985; p 210. Monduzzi Editore S.p.A., Bologna.

Hopkins J T, McLoda T A, Seegmiller J G, Baxter G D. Low-Level Laser Therapy Facilitates Superficial Wound Healing in Humans: A Triple-Blind, Sham-Controlled Study. J Athl Train. 2004; 39 (3): 223-229.

Horch H et al. Erfahrungen mit der Laserbehandlung oberflächlicher Mundschleimhauterkrankungen. Dtsch Z Mund-, Kiefer- u Gesichtschir. 1983; 7:31-35

Horowitz I et al. Infrared spectroscopy analysis of the effect of low power laser irradiation on calvarial bone defect healing in the rat. Laser Therapy. 1996; 8: 29. (abstract)

Hort O, Vanpel T. Die verteilung von Na+ und K+ unter dem Einfluss von Temperaturgradienten. Pflügers Arch. 1971; 323: 158-.

Horvath I, Tanos E. The situation of low level laser therapy in Hungary. Proc. 3rd Congress of the World Ass for Laser Therapy, Athens, Greece 2000. Poster, p. 118.

Hoteya K et al. Effects of a 1 W GaAlAs diode laser in the field of orthopedics. In: Meeting Report: The first Congress of the International Association for Laser and Sports Medicine. Tokyo, 1997. Laser Therapy 1997; 9 (4): 185.

Hashimoto T, Kemmutso O, Otsuka H et al. Efficacy of laser irradiation on the area near the stellate ganglion is dose-dependent: a double-blind crossover placebo-controlled study. Laser Therapy. 1997; 9 (1): 7-12.

Hatano Y. Lasers in the diagnosis of the TMJ problems. In: Lasers in dentistry. Eds. Yamamoto Y et al. 1989; p. 169-172. Elsevier Science Publishing B.V, Amsterdam.

Havlik I. Use of low level laser therapy (laser therapy) in gynaecology and obstetrics. Laser-Partner. 2000, No 14.

Hawkins D, Abrahamse H. The role of laser fluence in cell viability, proliferation, and membrane integrity of wounded human skin fibroblasts following helium-neon laser irradiation. Lasers Surg Med. 2006; 38 (1): 74-83.

Hawkins D, Abrahamse H. Biological effects of helium-neon laser irradiation on normal and wounded human skin fibroblasts. Photomed Laser Surg. 2005; 23 (3): 251-259.

Hawkins D, Abrahamse H. Effect of multiple exposures of low-level laser therapy on the cellular responses of wounded human skin fibroblasts. Photomed Laser Surg. 2006; 24 (6): 705-714.

Hawkins D, Abrahamse H. Influence of broad-spectrum and infrared light in combination with laser irradiation on the proliferation of wounded skin fibroblasts. Photomed Laser Surg. 2007; 25 (3): 159-169.

Hedner E. [Herpes simplex virus type 1 and intraoral wound healing]. J of the S D A, 1994, 1: 8-10. (in Swedish)

Hegedus B, Viharos L, Gervain M, Gálfi M. The Effect of Low-Level Laser in Knee Osteoarthritis: A Double-Blind, Randomized, Placebo-Controlled Trial. Photomed Laser Surg. 2009 Jun 16. [Epub ahead of print]

Hemvani N, Chitnis D S, Bhagwanani N S. Helium-neon and nitrogen laser irradiation accelerates the phagocytic activity of human monocytes. Photomed Laser Surg. 2005;23 (6): 571-574.

Hemvani N, Chitnis DS, George M, Chammania S. In vitro effect of nitrogen and He-Ne laser on the apoptosis of human polymorphonuclear cells from burn cases and healthy volunteers. Photomed Laser Surg. 2005; 23 (5): 476-479.

Henderson A R. Laser radiation hazards. Optics and Laser Technology, 1984; 2: 75.

Herbert K E et al. Effect of laser light at 820 nm on adeonsine nucleotide levels in human lymphocytes. Lasers Life Sci. 1989; 3: 37-.

Herman J et al. In vitro Effects of Nd:YAG Laser Radiation on Cartilage Metabolism. J Rheum. 1988; 15: 181-8.

Herman J, Khosla R. Nd:YAG laser modulation of synovial tissue metabolism. Clinic Exp Rheumatol. 1989; 7: 505-512.

Hernández L C, Santisteban P, del Valle-Soto M E et al: Changes in mRNA of thyryglobulin, cytoskeleton of thyroid cells and thyroid hormone levels induced by IR-laser radiation. Laser Therapy. 1989; 1 (4): 203-208.

Herzog C, Luzern, Switzerland. Low level lasertherapie un der Stillzeit. Reagieren Läsionen der Mammillen auf die Low Level Lasertherapie? On file, Swedish Laser-Medical Society. www.laser.nu.

Heussler J K et al. A double blind randomized trial of low power laser treatment in rheumatoid arthritis. Annals Rheum Diseases. 1993; 52: 703-706.

Heyn M P, Borucki B, Otto H. Chromophore reorientation during the photocycle of bacteriorhodopsin: experimental methods and functional significance. Biochim Biophys Acta. 2000; 1460 (1): 60-74.

Hicks M J et al. Root caries in vitro after low fluence argon laser and fluoride treatment. Compend Contin Educ Dent. 1997; 18 (6): 543-548.

Hagiwara S, Iwasaka H, Hasegawa A, Noguchi T. Pre-Irradiation of blood by gallium aluminum arsenide (830 nm) low-level laser enhances peripheral endogenous opioid analgesia in rats. Anesth Analg. 2008; 107 (3): 1058-1063.

Hagiwara S, Iwasaka H, Okuda K, Noguchi T. GaAlAs (830 nm) low-level laser enhances peripheral endogenous opioid analgesia in rats. Lasers Surg Med. 2007; 39 (10): 797-802.

Haimovici N et al. Clinical use of antiinflammatory action of the laser in activated osteoarthritis of small peripheral joints. LASER. Journ Eur Med Laser Ass. 1988; 1 (2): 4-11.

Haina D et al. Temperature of the skin during application of softlaser. Laser in Medicine and Surgery. 1988; 4 (1): 26-29.

Haina D, Brunner R, Landthaler M, Waidelich W. Stimulierung der Wundheilung mit Laserlicht - Klinische und tierexperimentelle Untersuchungen. Verhandlungen der Deutschen Dermatologischen Gesellschaft XXXII Tagung. Der Hausartz. Supplementum V 32. 1981: 429-431.

Haina D, Brunner R, Landthaler O et al. Animal Experiments on Light-Induced Woundhealing. Biophysica Berlin. 1973; 35 (3): 227-230.

Haker E, Lundeberg T. Is Low-Energy Laser Treatment Effective in Lateral Epicondylalgia? J Pain Symptom Managment. 1991; 6 (4): 241-246.

Haker E, Lundeberg T. Laser treatment applied to acupuncture points in lateral humeral epicondylalgia. A double-blind study. Pain. 1990; 43: 243-.

Halevy S et al. 780 nm low power laser therapy for wound healing - in vivo and in vitro studies. Laser Therapy. 1996; 8 (1): 20. (abstract)

Hall G et al. Effect of low level energy laser irradiation on wound healing. An experimental study in rats. Sw Dental J. 1994; 18 (1-2): 29-34.

Hall G et al. Effect of low level energy laser irradiation on wound healing. An experimental study in rats. Swed Dent J. 1994; 18: 29-34.

Hall J et al. Low level laser therapy is ineffective in the management of rheumatoid arthritic finger joints. British J Rheumat. 1994; 33: 142-147.

Hamajima S, Hiratsuka K, Kiyama-Kishikawa M, Tagawa T et al. Effect of low-level laser irradiation on osteoglycin gene expression in osteoblasts. Lasers in Medical Science. 2003; 18 (2): 78-82.

Hamblin M R. The role of nitric oxide in LLLT. BiOS 2008. Proceedings of SPIE. Volume 6846-1.

Hansen H, Thorøe U. Low power laser biostimulation of chronic orofacial pain. A doubleblind placebo controlled cross-over study in 40 patients. Pain. 1990; 43: 169-179.

Hansson T. Infrared laser in the treatment of craniomandibular disorders, arthrogenous pain. Journ of Prosthetic Dentistry. 1989; 61: 614-617.

Harada G et al. A clinical application of the 1 W Ga-Al-As diode laser - double blind study. J Phys Med. 1998; 9 : 99-103.

Harazaki M, Isshiki Y. Soft laser irradiation effects on pain reduction in orthodontic treatment. Bull Tokyo Dent Coll. 1997; 38 (4): 291-5.

Harris M D, Lincoln A E, Amoroso P J, Stuck B, Sliney D. Laser eye injuries in military occupations. Aviat Space Environ Med. 2003; 74 (9): 947-952.

Hartman K M. Action spectroscopy, in Biophysics, Hoppe W, Lohmann W, Marke H and Ziegler H, Eds. Springer-Verlag, Heidelberg, 1983, p. 115.

Hasan P, Rijadi S A, Purnomo S, Kainama H.. The possible application of low reactive laser therapy (laser therapy) in the treatment of male infertility. Laser Therapy. 1989; 1 (1): 49-50.

Hashieh I A et al. Helium-neon laser irradiation is not a stressful treatment: a study on heatshock protein (HSP70) level. Laser Surg Med. 1997; 20 (4): 451-460.

Gür A, Karakoc M, Nas Ket al. Effects of low power laser and low dose amitriptyline therapy on clinical symptoms and quality of life in fibromyalgia: a single-blind, placebo-controlled trial. Rheumatol Int. 2002; 22 (5): 188-193.

Gür A, Cosut A, Sarac A J et al. Effect of different therapy regimes of low power laser in painful osteoarthritis of the knee: A double-blind and placebo-controlled trial. Laser Surg Med. 2003; 33: 330-338.

Gür A, Karakoc M, Cevik R et al. Efficacy of low power laser therapy and exercise on pain and functions in chronic low back pain. Laser Surg Med. 2003; 32 (3): 233-238.

Gür A, Sarac A J, Cevik R, Altindag O, Sarac S. Efficacy of 904 nm gallium arsenide low level laser therapy in the management of chronic myofascial pain in the neck: a double-blind and randomize-controlled trial. Laser Surg Med. 2004; 35 (3): 229-235.

Gürsoy B, Bradley P F. Penetration studies of low intensity laser therapy (laser therapy) wavelengths. Laser Therapy, 1996; 8 (1): 18. (abstract)

Guzzardella G A, Torricelli P, Nicolo-Aldini N et al. Osseointegration of endosseous ceramic implants after postoperative low-power laser stimulation: an in vivo comparative study. Clin Oral Implants Res. 2003; 14 (2): 226-232.

Guzzardella G A, Fini M, Torricelli P et al. Laser stimulation on bone defect healing: an in vitro study. Lasers Med Sci. 2002; 17 (3): 216-220.

Guzzardella G A, Torricelli P, Nicoli Aldini N et al. Laser technology in orthopedics: preliminary study on low power laser therapy to improve the bone-biomaterial interface. Int J Artif Organs. 2001; 24 (12): 898-902.

Gutknecht N, Moritz A, Dercks H W et al. Treatment of hypersensitivity teeth using neodymium: ytrium-aluminum-garnet lasers: a comparison of the use of various settings in an in vivo study. J Clinical Laser Medicine and Surgery. 1997; 15 (4): 171-174

Gutknecht N, Moritz A, Conrads G, Sievert T, Lampert F. Bactericidal effect of the Nd:YAG laser in in vitro root canals. J Clin Laser Med Surg. 1996; 14 (2): 77-80.

Gutknecht N, Kaiser F, Hassan A, Lampert F. Long-term clinical evaluation of endodontically treated teeth by Nd:YAG lasers. J Clin Laser Med Surg. 1996; 14 (1): 7-11.

Gutknech N, ed: Proceedings of the 1st International Workshop of Evidence Based Dentistry on Lasers in Dentistry. 2007. Quintessenz Verlags-GmbH.

Guzzardella G A, Morrone G, Torricelli P et al. Assessment of low-power laser biostimulation on chondral lesions: an "in vivo" experimental study. Artificial Cells, Blood Substitutes, and Immobilization Biotechnology. 2000; 28 (5): 441-449.

Haas R, Dortbudak O, Mensdorff-Pouilly N, Mailath G. Elimination of bacteria on different implant surfaces through photosensitization and soft laser. An in vitro study. Clin Oral Implants Res. 1997; 8 (4): 249-254.

Haberland U, Blazek V, Schmitt H. Chirp Optical Coherence Tomography of Layered Scattering Media. Journ. Biomedical Optics, July 1988, Vol 3, No 3, p. 259-266.

Hachenberger I. Laserstrahlen bei Herpeserkrankungen. Ärztliche Kosmetologie. 1981; 11: 142-.

Hahn A, Sejna I, Stolbova K et al. Combined laser-EGb 761 tinnitus therapy. Acta Otolaryngol Suppl. 2001; 545: 92-93.

Haffmans J et al. Suicide after bright light treatment in seasonal affective disorder: a case report. J Clin Psychiatry. 1998; (9): 478-.

Hage R, Duarte J, Silva C M et al. The Low Level Laser Therapy (LLLT) in the prevention and repair of the muscle injury induced by bothrops jararaca poison injected in rats. Photomed Laser Surg. 2005; 23 (1). Abstracts from the 5th Congress of the World Association for Laser Therapy, São Paulo, Brazil, November 2004. Poster no 100, page 139.

Grossman N, Schneid N, Reuveni H, Halevy S, Lubart R. 780 nm low power diode laser irradiation stimulates proliferation of keratinocyte cultures: involvement of reactive oxygen species. Lasers Surg Med. 1998; 22 (4): 212-218.

Groth E B. Treatment of dentine hypersensitivity with low power laser of Ga-Al-As. J Dent Res. 1995; 74 (3): 794, Abstract 163.

Gruber W, Eber E, Malle-Scheid D, Pfleger A et al. Laser acupuncture in children and adolescents with exercise induced asthma. Thorax. 2002; 57 (3): 222-225.

Grubnik V V et al. [Combined laser therapy of diabetic gangrene of the lower limbs]. Klin Khir. 1994; 7: 20-22. (in Russian with English abstract)

Gruszka M et al. Effects of low energy laser therapy on herniated lumbar discs. Laser Surg Med. 1998. Suppl 10, p. 6

Grzesiak-Janas, Grazyna A A. Low-power-laser therapy in Costen's syndrome. Proc. SPIE. 1996; Vol 2781: 126-128. (Lasers in Medicine)

Grzesiak-Janas G, Janas A. Conservative closure of antro-oral communication stimulated with laser light. Journal of Clinical Laser Medicine and Surgery. 2001; 19 (4): 181-184.

Grzesiak-Janas G, Kobos J. Influence of laser radiation on acceleration of postextraction wound healing. Proc. SPIE. Vol. 3188.

Grzesiak Janas G, Janas A. Laser biostimulation in treatment of actinomycosis. Proc SPIE ; Vol. 5229: 135-139.

Guang Hua Wang et al. A study on the analgesic effect of low power HeNe-laser and its mechanism by electrophysiological means. In: Lasers in Dentistry. Excerpta Medica. Elsevier Science Publishers, Amsterdam. 1989: p. 277.

Gudmundsen J, Vikne J. Laserbehandling av epicondylitis humeri og rotatorcuffsyndrom. Dobbelt blindstudie - 200 pasienter. Telemark Sentralsjukehus, Norge. ["Laser Treatment of Epicondylitis Humeri and Rotator Cuff Syndrome. A Double-Blind Study - 200 Patients."] (In Norwegian.) Norsk Tidskrift for Idrettsmedisin 1987; 2: 6-11.

Guerino M R, Baranauskas V, Guerino A C, Parizotto N. Laser treatment of experimentally induced chronic arthritis. Applied Surface Science. 2000; 154-155: 561-564.

Gundogan C, Greve B, Raulin C. Treatment of alopecia areata with the 308-nm xenon chloride excimer laser: case report of two successful treatments with the excimer laser. Lasers Surg Med. 2004; 34 (2): 86-90.

Guerra A, Munoz P, Esquivel T, Boullón F, Tunér J. The effect of 670 nm Laser Therapy on herpes simplex and aphtae. Photomed Laser Surg. 2005 (1). Abstracts from the 5th Congress of the World Association for Laser Therapy, November 25-27, 2004, São Paulo, Brazil. Abstr. 003, p. 90.

Gum S L et al. Combined ultrasound, electrical stimulation, and laser promote collagen synthesis with moderate changes in tendon biomechanics. Am J Phys Med Rehabil. 1997; 76 (4): 288-296.

Guirro R R, Weis L C. Radiant power determination of low-level laser therapy equipment and characterization of its clinical use procedures. Photomed Laser Surg. 2009; 27 (4): 633-639.

Gungor A, Dogru S, Cincik H, Erkul E, Poyrazoglu E. Effectiveness of transmeatal low power laser irradiation for chronic tinnitus. Laryngol Otol. 2008; 122 (5): 447-451.

Gupta A , Filolenko N, Salansky N. Low energy photon therapy of leg ulcers. J Dermatol Treat. 1997; 8: 103-108.

Gupta A K. The use of low-energy photon therapy in the treatment of leg ulcers - a preliminary report. J Dermatol Treat. 1997; 8 (2): 103-108.

Gür A, Karakoc M, Nas K et al. Efficacy of low power laser therapy in fibromyalgia. A single-blind, placebo-controlled trial. Lasers in Medical Science. 2002; 17: 57-61.

Gomberg V G et al. Endolymphatic laser therapy in management of acute nonspecific epididymitis. Proc. 2nd Congress World Assn for Laser Therapy, Kansas City, Sept 1998; p. 27

Gomez-Villamandos R J. HeNe laser therapy by fibroendoscopy in the mucosa of the equine upper airway. Laser Surg Med. 1995; 16: 184-188.

Gomi A et al. A clinical study of soft Laser 632 Helium Neon low energy medical laser. 2nd report. The effects in the relieving the pain of hypersensitive dentine and the pain during seating inlay. Aichi Gukuin J Dent Sci. 1986; 24 (3): 390-399.

González V, Chiquini J. Low level laser therapy in ortognathic surgery. Proc. 3rd Congress of ESOLA, Barcelona, Spain, May 2005, p. 12.

Gordjestani M, Dermaut L, Thierens H. Infrared laser and bone metabolism: a pilot study. Int J Oral Maxillofac Surg. 1994; 23: 54-56.

Gottlieb T, Jörgensen B, Rohde E, Müller G, Schellera E E. The influence of irradiation with low-level diode laser on the proteoglycan content in arthrotically changed cartilage in rabbits. Medical Laser Application. 2006; 21 (1): 53-59.

Gottschling S, Meyer S, Gribova I, Distler L, Berrang J, Gortner L, Graf N, Shamdeen MG. Laser acupuncture in children with headache: A double-blind, randomized, bicenter, placebo-controlled trial. Pain. 2007 Nov 15. [Epub ahead of print]

Goulart C S, Nouer P R, Mouramartins L, Garbin I U, Lizarelli R. Photoradiation and orthodontic movement: experimental study with canines. Photomed Laser Surg. 2006; 24 (2): 192-196.

Götte S, Keyl W, Wirzback E. Doppelblindstudie zur überprüfung der Wirksamkeit und Verträglichkeit einer niederenergetischen Lasertherapie bei Patienten mit aktiver Gonarthrose. Jaros Orthopädie. 1995; 10: 30-34.

Gou, Jing-Zhen. Effects of HeNe regional irradiation on 53 cases in the field of pediatric surgery. In: Lasers in Dermatology and Tissue Welding. Proc. SPIE. 1991; Vol 1442: 9.

Grande S R, Imbronito A V, Okuda O S, Lotufo R F, Magalhães M H, Nunes F D. Herpes viruses in periodontal compromised sites: comparison between HIV-positive and - negative patients. J Clin Periodontol. 2008; 35 (10): 838-845.

Grbavac R A, Veeck E B, Bernard J P, Ramalho L M, Pinheiro A L. Effects of laser therapy in CO_2 laser wounds in rats. Photomed Laser Surg. 2006; 24 (3): 389-396.

Gray R J M, Quale A A, Hall C A et al. Physiotherapy in the treatment of temporomandibular joint disorders: a comparative study of four treatment methods. Br J Dent. 1994; 176: 257-261.

Greguss P. Biostimulation of tissue by laser radiation. Lasers and Medicine. 1989; 1353: 79-.

Greguss P. Interaction of optical radiation with living matter. Optics and Laser Technology. 1985; 3: 151-.

Greguss P. Letter to the editor. Biological effects of low power laser radiation. Optics and Laser Technology. 1985; 3: 161-.

Gretzinger H et al. An in vivo study of the effect of helium-neon laser on human fibroblast migration. Proc Int Congr of Lasers in Dentistry, Tokyo, August 5-6. 1988: p 23.

Greulich K O. Low level laser therapy (laser therapy) - does it damage DNA? LaserWorld Editorial; 2, 2000. www.laser/nu/lllt/lllt_editorial5.htm (May 2001).

Gross A J, Jelkmann W. Helium-neon laser irradiation inhibits the growth of kidney epithelial cells in culture. Laser Surg Med. 1990;10 (1): 40-44.

Grossman N, Schneid N, Reuveni H, et al. 780 nm low power diode laser irradiation stimulates proliferation of keratinocyte cultures: involvement of reactive oxygen species. Laser Surg Med. 1998; 22 (4): 212-218.

Georgadze A K et al. [Treatment of non-healing wounds and trophic ulcers by low-intensity laser irradiation in an outpatient clinic]. Khirurgiia (Mosk). 1990; 12: 93-96. (in Russian)

Gerbi M E, Pinheiro A L, Marzola C, Limeira Junior Fde A et al. Assessment of bone repair associated with the use of organic bovine bone and membrane irradiated at 830 nm. Photomed Laser Surg. 2005; 23 (4): 382-388.

Gerschman J A, Ruben J, Gebart-Eaglemont J. Low Level Laser for dentinal tooth hypersensitivity. Australian Dent J. 1994; 39 (6): 353-357.

Ghamsari S M, Acorda J A, Taguchi K et al. Evaluation of wound healing of the teat with and without low level laser therapy in diary cattle by laser Doppler flowmetry in comparison with histopathology, tensiometry and hydroxyproline analysis. Br Vet J. 1996; 152 (5): 583-592.

Ghamsari S M, Taguchi K, Abe N et al. Histopathological effect of low-level laser therapy on sutured wounds of the teat in diary cattle. Vet Q. 1996; 18 (1): 17-21.

Ghamsari S M, Taguchi K et al. Evaluation of low level laser therapy on primary healing of experimentally induced full thickness wounds in diary cattle. Vet Surg. 1997; 26 (2): 114-120.

Ghoreyshian M, Fazilat F, Fekrazad R, Deyhimi P. Cellular and molecular effect of low level laser on velocity and quality of bone formation in craniofacial distraction osteogenesis. 10th. International Congress of the International Society for Lasers in Dentistry, Berlin, 18.5.-20.5.2006.

Giavelli F et al. [Low-level laser therapy in osteoarticular diseases in geriatric patients]. Radiol Med (Torino). 1998; 5 (4): 303-309. (in Italian)

Giavelli S, Fava G, Castronuovo G et al. Low power laser in the treatment of knee osteoarthritis in geriatric patients. Laser & Technology. 1994; 4 (1/2): 39-48.

Gigo-Benato D, Geuna S, de Castro Rodrigues A, Tos P et al. Low-power laser biostimulation enhances nerve repair after end-to-side neurorrhaphy: a double-blind randomized study in the rat median nerve model. Lasers in Medical Science, 2004; 19 (1): 57-65.

Gilioli G et al. Studio ultrastrutturale di colture cellulari "vero" infettate con virus Herpes Simplex e sot-toposte all'azione Laser. Int Congress on Laser Med and Surg, Bologna June 1985, p 207. Monduzzi Editore S.p.A, Bologna, Italy.Also in: Medical Laser Report 1985; 3: 28-31.

Giuliani A, Fernandez M, Farinelli M, Baratto L et al. Very low level laser therapy attenuates edema and pain in experimental models. Int J Tissue React. 2004; 26 (1-2): 29-37.

Gius D, Boreto A, Shah S, Curry H A., Intracellular oxidation reduction status in the regulation of transcription factors NF-kappaB and AP-1. Toxicol Lett. 1999; 106: 93-106.

Gladkova N D, Karachistov A B, Komarova L G et al. Clinical effectiveness of low-power laser radiation of hemosalivary barrier in patients with rheumatic disease. Proc. SPIE. 1996; Vol 2929: 124-131.

Glazewski J B. Application of low-intensity lasers in rheumatology. The results of four-year observation in 224 patients. Proc. SPIE. 1996; Vol 2929: 80-91.

Glinkowski W et al. Sprained ankles treatment with use of laser therapy. Lasermedizin -Laser in Med Surg. 1995; 11 (2): 42.

Glinkowski W, Rowinski J. Effect of low incident levels of infrared laser energy on the healing of experimental bone fractures. Laser Therapy. 1995; 7 (2): 67-70.

Godfrey R. Photoselection and circular dichroism in the purple membrane. Biophys J. 1982; 38:1-6.

Godoy B M, Arana-Chavez V E, Nunez S C, Ribeiro M S. Effects of low-power red laser on dentine-pulp interface after cavity preparation. An ultrastructural study. Arch Oral Biol. 2007; 52 (9): 899-903.

Goldman J, Chiapella J, Bass N et al. Laser Therapy for Rheumatoid Arthritis.Lasers Surg Med. 1980; 1 (1): 93-101.

Garcez A S, Ribeiro M S, Tegos G P, Nunez S C, Jorge A O, Hamblin M R. Antimicrobial photodynamic therapy combined with conventional endodontic treatment to eliminate root canal biofilm infection. Lasers Surg Med. 2007; 39 (1): 59-66.

Garcia V G, Fernandes L A, de Almeida J M, Bosco A F, Nagata M J, Martins T M, Okamoto T, Theodoro L H. Comparison between laser therapy and non-surgical therapy for periodontitis in rats treated with dexamethasone. Lasers Med Sci. 2009 May 14. [Epub ahead of print]

Garkavoy D V et al. Use of the Helium-Neon laser in the treatment of ulcer disease. Proc X. Internat Congr Soc Laser Surgery and Medicine, Bangkok 1993; p. 160.

Gasparyan L, Brill G, Makela A. Activation of vascuilar endothelial (VEGF) and fibroblast growth factor (FGF) induced angiogenesis under influence of low level laser radiation in vitro. In: Progesss in Biomedical Optics and imaging. Proc. SPIE.Volume 6140; 614009: 1-7.

Gasparyan L, Brill G, Makela A. Influence of laser radiation on migration of stem cells. In: Progesss in Biomedical Optics and imaging. Proc. SPIE.Volume 6140; 61400P 1-6.

Gärtner C. Low reactive-level laser therapy (laser therapy) in rheumatology: a review of the clinical experience in the author's laboratory. Laser Therapy. 1992; 4 (3): 107-115.

Gärtner C. Analgesy by low power laser (LPL): a controlled double blind study in ankylosing spondarthritis (SPA). Laser Surg Med. 1989; Suppl 1: 30.

Gáspar L et al. Oral lesions induced by scalpel, electrocautery and CO2 laser compared with light scanning and electron microscopy. J Clin Laser Med Surg October 1991; 9: 34-9.

Gasparyan L. Investigations of sensations, associated with laser blood irradiation. Proc. 2nd Congress World Assn for Laser Therapy, Kansas City, September 1998; p. 87-88.

Gasparyan L. Low level laser therapy of male genital tract chronic inflammations. Proc. 2nd Congress World Association for Laser Therapy, Kansas City, USA, September 2-5 1998; p. 82-83.

Gassler N et al. Clinical data and histological features of trans-myocardial revascularuzation with CO2 laser. Eur J Cardiothorac Surg. 1997; 12 (1): 25-30.

Gaudel Y et al. Pico second study of free radical reactions in organized assemblies: Kinetics of univalent reduction of b-NAD+. Laboratoire d'Optique Appliquee INSERM U275. École Polytechnique-ENSTA, Palaiseau. p 219.

Gavish L, Asher Y, Becker Y, Kleinman Y. Low level laser irradiation stimulates mitochondrial membrane potential and disperses subnuclear promyelocytic leukemia protein. Lasers Surg Med. 2004; 35 (5): 369-376.

Gavish L, Perez L S, Reissman P, Gertz S D. Irradiation with 780 nm diode laser attenuates inflammatory cytokines but upregulates nitric oxide in lipopolysaccharide-stimulated macrophages: implications for the prevention of aneurysm progression. Lasers Surg Med. 2008; 40 (5): 371-378.

Gavish L, Perez L S, Gertz S D. Low-level laser irradiation modulates matrix metalloproteinase activity and gene expression in porcine aortic smooth muscle cells. Lasers Surg Med. 2006; 38 (8): 779-786.

Gaydess E et al. The effects of laser stimulation on cell and bacterial growth in a cell culture wound model. Proc. 2nd Congress World Assn for Laser Therapy, Kansas City, Sept 1998; p. 72-73.

Gelskey S C, White J M, Pruthi V K. The effectiveness of the Nd:YAG laser in the treatment of dentinal hypersensitivity. J Can Dent Assoc. 1993; 59 (4): 337-386.

Genkin V M. [Effects of low-intensity laser irradiation on the state of blood proteins]. Biull Eksp Biol Med 1989. 108 (8): 188-190.

Genot M T, Klasterksy J. Low-level laser for prevention and therapy of oral mucositis induced by chemotherapy or radiotherapy. Curr Opin Oncol. 2005;17 (3): 236-240.

Fujimaki Y, Shimoyama T, Liu Q et al. Low-Level Laser Irradiation Attenuates Production of Reactive Oxygen Species by Human Neutrophils. J Clinical Laser Medicine & Surgery. 2003; 21 (3): 165-170.

Fukuuchi A, Suzuki H, Inoue K. A double-blind trial of low reactive level laser therapy in the treatment of chronic pain. Laser Therapy. 1998; 10 (2): 59-64.

Fulga C, Fulga IG, Predescu M. Clincal study on the effect of laser therapy in rheumatic degenerative diseases. Rev Roum Med Int. 1994; 32 (3): 227-233.

Fung D T, Ng G Y, Leung M C et al. Therapeutic low energy laser improves the mechanical strength of repairing medial collateral ligament. Lasers Surg Med. 2002; 31 (2): 91-96.

Funk J O et al. Helium-Neon laser irradiation induces effects on cytokine production at the protein and the mRNA level. Experimental Dermatology. 1993; 2: 75-83.

Funk J O, Kruse A, Kirchner H. Cytokine production after helium-neon laser irradiation in cultures of human peripheral blood mononuclear cells. J Photochem Photobiol B. 1992; 16 (3-4): 347-355.

Fursinn G et al. Effects of Nd:YAG laser irradiation on human cartilage cell metabolism. Proc of Laser-81, Opto-Elektronik. München 1981. Abstr 200.

Gabel P. A pilot study on Low Level Laser Therapy (LLLT) for otitis externa - swimmer's ear. Implications for competitive swimmers. Proc. WALT2002, Tokyo, Japan, June 2002.

Gabel, C. P. (1995). Does Laser enhance bruising in acute sporting injuries? Aust. J. Physio. 1995; 41 (4): 267-269.

Gabor D. LaseLow-Energy Density CO2 Laser as Deep Tissue Stimulator: A Comparative Study. J. Clin. Laser Medicine & Surg. 1991; 9: 179-

Gaida K, Koller R, Isler C et al. Low Level Laser Therapy-a conservative approach to the burn scar? Burns. 2004; 30 (4): 362-367.

Gál P, Vidinsky B, Toporcer T, Mokry M et al. Histological assessment of the effect of laser irradiation on skin wound healing in rats. Photomed Laser Surg. 2006; 24 (4): 480-488.

Gál P, Mokrý M, Vidinský B, Kilík R, Depta F, Harakacová M, Longauer F, Mozeš S, Sabo J. Effect of equal daily doses achieved by different power densities of low-level laser therapy at 635 nm on open skin wound healing in normal and corticosteroid-treated rats. Lasers Med Sci. 2008 Aug 21. [Epub ahead of print]

Gamaleja N F, Polischuuk E I. The experience of skin tumours treatment with laser radiation. Panminerva Med. 1975; 17: 238-240. In Enwemeka, C.S. 1988, 'Laser Biostimulation of healing wounds: Specific effects and mechanisms of action'. The Journal of Orthopaedic and Sports Physical Therapy, 9 (10): 333-338.

Gamaleya N F, Shishko E D, Yanish G B. New data about mammalian cells photosensitivity and laser biostimulation. Dokl Akad Nauk S.S.S.R. (Moscow). 1983; 273:224.

Gan L, Tse C, Pilliar R M, Kandel R A. Low-power laser stimulation of tissue engineered cartilage tissue formed on a porous calcium polyphosphate scaffold. Lasers Surg Med. 2007; 39 (3): 286-293.

Gao, Yun-Qing; Liu, Song-Hao; Zhang, You; Liu, T. C. 367 cases of CO2 laser therapy on facial acne. Proc. SPIE. 1996; Vol 2887: 60-62. (Lasers in Medicine and Dentistry: Diagnostics and Treatment)

Garavello-Freitas I, Baranauskas V, Joazeiro P P et al. Low-power laser irradiation improves histomorphometrical parameters and bone matrix organization during tibia wound healing in rats. J Photochem Photobiol B. 2003; 70 (2): 81-89.

Garavello I, Baranauskas V, Cruz-Hoefling MA. The effects of low laser irradiation on angiogenesis in injured rat tibiae. Histology and Histopathology. 2004; 19 (1): 43-48.

Fontana C R, Kurachi C, Mendonca C R, Bagnato V S. Temperature variation at soft periodontal and rat bone tissues during a medium-power diode laser exposure. Photomed Laser Surg. 2004; 22 (6): 519-522.

Forman N J, Boveris A. Superoxide radical and hydrogen peroxide in mitochondria. In Free Radicals in Biology. Vol. 5. Pryor A, Ed, Academic Press, New York, 1982, p. 65.

Forney R, Mauro T. Using lasers in diabetic wound healing. Diabetes Technology & Therapeutics. 1999; 1 (2): 189-192.

Fortuna D, Rossi G, Zati A et al. Pilot study of the Nd:YAG laser in experimentally induced chronic degenerative osteoarthritis in an animal model. Atti della Fondazione Giorgio Ronchi. 2002; 62 (2)179-193.

Foyaca-Sibat H, Ibañez-Valdés L. Laser therapy in zoster neuropathy - HIV related. Proc. 7th Internat Congr of WALT, Sun City, South Africa, October 2008, page 100.

Fracher Abramoff M M, Petrilli A S; Monteiro Caran E, Almeida Lopes L, Fontana Lopes N N. Preliminary study of prevention and treatment of oral mucositis due to chemotherapy in children, adolescents and young adults through the use of Laser Therapy. Photomed Laser Surg. 2005; 23 (1). Abstracts from the 5th Congress of the World Association for Laser Therapy, São Paulo, Brazil, November 2004. Abstract no 048, p.101.

França C M, Núñez S C, Prates R A, Noborikawa E, Faria M R, Ribeiro M S. Low-intensity red laser on the prevention and treatment of induced-oral mucositis in hamsters. J Photochem Photobiol B. 2009; 94 (1): 25-31.

Frauenfelder H. The Conformational Energy Surface. Princeton University. http://wwwphy.princeton.edu/~austin/hf_book/chapter23.pdf.

Freitas A C, Pinheiro A, Miranda P et al. Assessment of anti-inflammatory effect of 830 nm laser light using C-reactive protein levels. Braz Dent J. 2001; 12 (3): 187-190.

Fridberger A, Ren T. Local mechanical stimulation of the hearing organ by laser irradiation. Neuroreport. 2006;17(1): 33-37.

Friedman et al. Somatosensory trigeminal evoked potential amplitudes following low level laser irradiation over time. Proc. 7th Int Congr Lasers in Dentistry, ISLD, Brussels, Belgium, July 2000, abstr. 14.

Friedman H et al. A possible explanation of laser-induced stimulation and damage of cell cultures. J Photochem Photobiol B Biol. 1991; 11: 87-95.

Friedman H, Lubart R. Nonlinear photobiostimulation: the mechanisms of visible and infrared laser-induced stimulation and reduction of neural excitability and growth. Laser Therapy. 1993; 5 (1): 39-42.

Friedman H, Lubart R. Towards an explanation of visible and infrared laser induced stimulation and damage of cell cultures. Laser Therapy. 1992; 4 (1): 39-42.

Friedman S, Liu M, Dörscher-Kim J, Kim S. In situ testing of CO2 laser on dental pulp function: Effects on microcirculation. Laser Surg Med. 1991; 11: 325-330.

Friedmann H, Lubart R. Competition between activayting and inhibitory processes in photobiology. Proc. SPIE. 1995; Vol 2630: 60-64.

Fructuoso F J G, Moset J M. Randomized double blind study on the biostimulatory effect of laser irradiation of the parotid gland in patients suffering of Sjögren syndrome. Invest y Clinica Laser. 1987; 1: 18-25. In Sp with E abstr. Also published in Centro Documentación Láser. 1987: 4 (13): 4.

Frugoni P. Shoulder calcified periarthritis recovery with low power laser therapy. Proc X Internat Congr Soc Laser Surg Med, Bangkok 1993, p. 200.

Fujihara NA, Hiraki KR, Marques MM. Irradiation at 780 nm increases proliferation rate of osteoblasts independently of dexamethasone presence. Lasers Surg Med. 2006; 38 (4): 332-336.

Fagnoni V, Fontolan D. Importanza della laser-terapia di bassa potenza per la riduzione dei tempi di guarigione dopo interventi di chirurgia parodontale. Laser Abstracts. 3 (2): 25-33.

Farina C G, Duarte M, Mori M et al. Effects of Low Intensity Laser Therapy (780 nm) in temporomandibular disorders: electromiographic, pain and bite force analysis. Photomed Laser Surg. 2005; 23 (1). Abstracts from the 5th Congress of the World Association for Laser Therapy, Sao Paulo, Brazil, November 2004. Abstract no 035, p.98.

Faxén K, Gilderson G, Ädelroth P, Brzezinski P. A mechanistic principle for proton pumping by cytochrome c oxidase. Nature. 2005; 437: 286-289.

Fedoseyeva G E, Smolyaninova N K, Karu T I, Zelenin A V. Human lymphocyte chromatin changes following irradiation with a He-Ne laser. Lasers Life Sci. 1998; 2: 197.

Fekrazad R, Jafari Sh, Kalhori K. The effects of Pulsed Nd:YAG Laser Therapy on Recurrent Aphtous Ulcers. Internat Congress of. ESOLA, Vienna, Austria, May 2001, p. 40-

Fekrazad R, Atabaki M, Eslami B, Kalhori K. A study on the effects of low level laser therapy. Proc. 3rd Congress of ESOLA, Barcelona, Spain, May 2005, p. 12.

Fenyö M et al. Theoretical and experimental basis of biostimulation by laser irradiation. Optics and Laser Technology. 1984: No 4: 209.

Fernando S et al. A randomised double blind comparative study of low level laser therapy following surgical extraction of lower third molar. Br J Oral Maxillofac Surg 1993; 31 (3): 170-172.

Ferreira D M, Zangaro R A, Villaverde A B, Cury Y, Frigo L et al. Analgesic effect of He-Ne (632.8 nm) low-level laser therapy on acute inflammatory pain. Photomed Laser Surg. 2005; 23 (2):177-181.

Ferreira A N S, Silveira L, Genovese W J, Cavalcante de Araujo V, Frigo L et al. Effect of GaAlAs Laser on Reactional Dentinogenesis Induction in Human Teeth. Photomed Laser Surg. 2006; 24 (3): 358-365.

Ferreira Dde C, Martins F O, Romanos M T. [Impact of low-intensity laser on the suppression of infections caused by Herpes simplex viruses 1 and 2: in vitro study] Rev Soc Bras Med Trop. 2009; 42 (1): 82-85.

Fikackova H, Dostalova T, Navratil L, Klaschka J. Effectiveness of Low-Level Laser Therapy in Temporomandibular Joint Disorders: A Placebo-Controlled Study. Photomed Laser Surg. 2007; 25 (4): 297-303.

Filho W, Nogueira T et al. Effects of irradiation with a HeNe laser on the healing of the hard tissue. Surgical and Medical Lasers. 1989; 2-3 (2): 71-

Fillipin L I, Mauriz J L, Vedovelli K, Moreira A J, Zettler C G, Lech O, Marroni N P, González-Gallego J. Low-level laser therapy (LLLT) prevents oxidative stress and reduces fibrosis in rat traumatized Achilles tendon. Lasers Surg Med. 2005; 37 (4): 293-300.

Fine S, Klein E, Nowak W, Scott R E, Laor Y et al.. Interaction of laser irradiation with biological systems. I. Studies on interaction with tissues. Fed Proc 1965; 24, Supplement 14: 40.

Fitz-Ritson D. Low energy laser therapy efficacy in the extension neck muscle recovery after whiplash injury. Lasers Surgery and Medicine. 1993; 13: 9.

Flöter T, Rehfisch H P. Pain treatment with laser: a double blind study. Proc. of the 4th Internat Symposium. Acup & Electroteher Res. 1988; 13 (4): 236-237.

Fong K. Bronchial asthma treated by He-Ne laser radiation on ear points. Chin J Acupunct Moxibustion 1990 ; 3 (4): 272-273.

Fontana C R, Kurachi C, Mendonca C R, Bagnato V S. Microbial reduction in periodontal pockets under exposition of a medium power diode laser: an experimental study in rats. Lasers Surg Med. 2004; 35 (4): 263-268.

Enwemeka C, Reddy G K. The biological effects on laser therapy and other physical modalities on connective tissue repair processes. Laser Therapy. 2000; 12: 22-30.

Enwemeka C. Depth of low intensity helium-neon and gallium-arsenide lasers through rabbit dermal and subderml tissues. Laser Therapy. 2001; 13: 95-101.

Enwemeka C. Attenuation and penetration of visible 632.8 nm and invisible infra-red 904 nm light in soft tissues. Laser Therapy. 2001; (13): 95-101.

Enwemeka C S. Standard Parameters in Laser Phototherapy. Editorial. Photomed Laser Surg. 2008; 26 (5): 411.

Enwemeka C S, Williams D, Enwemeka S K, Hollosi S, Yens D. Blue 470-nm light kills methicillin-resistant Staphylococcus aureus (MRSA) in vitro. Photomed Laser Surg. 2009; 27(2): 221-226.

Escola R et al. Beitrag zur ultrastrukturellen Untersuchung von Zahnfleischbeweben mit dem Soft-Laser. Zahnarztpraxis. 83: 110-115.

Esnouf A, Wright P A, Moore J C, Ahmed S. Depth of penetration of an 850 nm wavelength low level laser in human skin. Acupunct Electrother Res. 2007; 32 (1-2): 81-86.

Estep T N E, Thompson T E. Energy transfer in lipid bilayers. Biophys J. 1979: 26: 195-208.

Estola-Partanen M. Muscular tension and tinnitus (thesis). ISBN 951-44-4972-X.

Esquerra R M, Che D, Shapiro D B, Lewis J W, Bogomolni R A, Fukushima J, Kliger D S. Chromophore reorientations in the early photolysis intermediates of bacteriorhodopsin. Biophys J. 1996; 70 (2): 962-970.

Exner K. Sitzber. Akad. Wiss., Wien 76II, 522 (1877).

Fagnoni V et al. Considerazioni clinico terapeutiche sull'ieffetto della luce laser di bassa potenza nell Herpes Simple Labiale. Laser Abstracts. 1984; 1: 28-33.

Fagnoni V et al. Il laser di bassa potenza come coadiuvante nella terapia della sindrome algico-dizfunzionale dell'iarticolazione temporo-mandibulare. Laser Abstracts. 1985; 3: 16-26.

Fagnoni V et al. Laser therapy in dentistry and stomatology. Observations on 200 cases treated, Medical Laser Report 1984; 1: 36-40.

Fagnoni V et al. Studio sulla guarigione di ferite chirurgiche eseguite sulla mucosa orale di coniglio trattata con soft-Laser. Int Congress on Laser in Med and Surg, Bologna June 1985, p 269.

Fagnoni V et al. Studio sulla guarigione di ferite chirurgiche della mucosa di coniglio precedentemente irradiate con laser I.R. a dosaggi diversi. Laser Abstracts. 1985; 3: 32-37.

Fagnoni V et al. Study of behaviour of dental enamel in acid solution after treatment with fluorine combined with low power laser. Laser Abstracts. 2 (1): 30-34.

Fagnoni V et al. Su di un caso di emangioma della mucosa orale trattato mediante irraggiamento con laser di bassa potenza. Minerva Stomatologica. 1983; 32 (5): 701-703.

Fagnoni V et al. Trattamento delle nevralgie trigeminali con laser di bassa potenza. Laser Abstracts. 1985; 2: 23-36.

Fagnoni V et al. Use of HeNe soft-laser in 32 cases of mouth aphta. Laser Abstracts (Rivista Europea di Laser Terapia Medica e Chirurgia). 2 (2): 25-29.

Fagnoni V et al. Verifica sperimentale delle variazioni degli oppioidi endogeni plasmatici in pazienti affetti da nevralgie trigeminali e trattati con laser di bassa potenza. Laser Abstracts. 1985: 3 (2): 35-42.

Fagnoni V et al. Verifica sperimentale sulle variazioni termiche nella cavità pulpare di denti humani estratti, durante irraggiamento con laser di bassa potenza. Laser Abstracts, 1985; 3: 27-31.

Eckerdal A. Kliniske erfaringer fra et 5-års icke-kontroleret studie af low power laserbehandling af periorale neuropatier. (Clinical experiences from a 5 year non-controlled study of low power laser treatment of perioral neuropatias. In Danish). Tandlægebladet. 1994; 98 (11): 526-529.

Eduardo C de P et al. Benefits of low-power lasers on oral soft tissue. Proc. SPIE. 1996; Vol 2672: 27-33. (Lasers in Dentistry II)

Eduardo C d P, Freitas P M, Esteves-Oliveira M, Correa Aranha A C, Müller Ramalho K, Simões A, Bello-Silva M S, Tunér J. Laser Phototherapy in the Treatment of Periodontal Disease: A literature review. Submitted for publication 2009.

Eduardo F de P, Bueno D F, de Freitas P M, Marques M M, Passos-Bueno M R, Eduardo C de P, Zatz M. Stem cell proliferation under low intensity laser irradiation: a preliminary study. Lasers Surg Med. 2008; 40 (6): 433-438.

Efanov O I. Laser therapy for periodontitis. Proceedings of SPIE Vol. 4422 (2001). Low-Level Laser Therapy, Tatiana I. Solovieva, Ed.

Efendiev AI et al. [Increasing the scar strength after preventive skin irradiation with low-intensity laser]. Klin Khir 1992; (1): 23-25.

Ekim A, Armagan O, Tascioglu F, Oner C, Colak M. Effect of low level laser therapy in rheumatoid arthritis patients with carpal tunnel syndrome. Swiss Med Wkly. 2007; 137 (23-24): 347-352.

el Sayed S O, Dyson M. Effect of laser pulse repetition rate and pulse duration on mast cell number and degranulation. Laser Surg Med. 1996; 19 (4): 433-437.

el Sayed S. et al. The Effect of Low Level Laser Irradiation on Mast Cell Degranulation. Proc 7th Ann Meeting of Am Soc Laser Med Surg 1987.

Eliseeva E V, Shusterov I A, Vakhrushev B N. [Intravasal laser irradiation of autologous blood in the treatment of eye diseases]. Vestn Oftamol. 1994; 110 (2): 23-24.

Elman M, Lebzelter J. Light therapy in the treatment of acne vulgaris Dermatol Surg. 2004; 30 (2): 139-146.

Elwakil T F. An in-vivo experimental evaluation of He-Ne laser photostimulation in healing Achilles tendons. Lasers Med Sci. 2007; 22 (1): 53-59.

Elwakil T F, Elazzazi A, Shokeir H. Treatment of carpal tunnel syndrome by low-level laser versus open carpal tunnel release. Lasers Med Sci. 2007; 22 (4) :265-270.

Emmanoulidis O et al. CW IR low-power laser application significantly accelerates chronic pain relief rehabilitation of professional athletes. A double blind study. Laser Surg Med. 1986; 6: 173.

Emshoff R, Bösch R, Pümpel E, Schöning H, Strobl H. Low-level laser therapy for treatment of temporomandibular joint pain: a double-blind and placebo-controlled trial. Oral Surg Oral Med Oral Pathol Oral Radiol Endod. 2008; 105 (4): 452-456.

England S, Farrell A J, Coppock J S. Low power laser therapy of shoulder tendonitis. Scand J Rheumatology. 1989; 18 (6): 427-431.

Enwemeka C et al. Corrective ultrastructural and biomechanical changes induced in regenerated tendons exposed to laser photostimulation. Laser Surg Med. 1990; (Suppl 2): 12-19.

Enwemeka C et al. Effect of HeNe photostimulation on tendon fibroblast protein synthesis: preliminary report. Proc Ninth Congress of the International Society for Laser Surgery and Medicine, Anaheim, Calif, USA: 2-6 Nov 1991.

Enwemeka C. Laser biostimulation of healing wounds: specific effects and mechanisms of action. J Orthop Sports Physical Therapy. 1988; 9: 333-.

Enwemeka C, Rodriguez O, Gall N et al. Morphometries of collagen fibril populations in HeNe photostimulated tendons. J Clin Laser Med Surg. 1990; 47-52.

Dotsenko A P et al. [[Use of carbon dioxide laser in the treatment of acute lactation mastitis]. Sov Med. 1989; 9: 39-42.

Dougherty T J. Photodynamic therapy. Innovations in Radiation Oncology. Withers H, Peters L, eds. Berlin/ Heidelberg, Springer-Verlag, 1988, p. 175.

Dougherty T J. Photosensitizers: Therapy and detection of malignant tumors. Photochem Photobio. 1987; 45 (6): 879-889.

Dourado D M, Cruz-Höfling M A. LLLT on damaged muscle caused by bothrops moojeni snake venom. Laser Surg Med. 2003; 33: 352-357.

Douris P, Southard V, Ferrigi R, Grauer J et al. Effect of phototherapy on delayed onset muscle soreness. Photomed Laser Surg. 2006; 24 (3): 377-382.

Drugova O V, Monich V A, Zhitnikova O V. [Effects of red light on postischemic myocardium during reperfusion]. Bull Exp Biol Med. 2001;131 (4): 325-326. Translation in: Bulletin of Experimental Biology and Medicine, No. 4, 2001. Biophysics and biochemistry.

Duan R, Liu C-Y, Li Y et al. Signal transduction pathways involved in low intensity He-Ne laser-induced respi-ratory burst in bovine neutrophils: a potential mechanism of low intensity laser biostimulation. Laser Surg Med. 2001; 29: 174-178.

Dube A, Gupta P K, Bharti S. Redox absorbance changes of the respiratory chain components of E. coli following He-Ne laser irradiation. Lasers Life Sci. 1997; 7: 173.

Dube A, Bock C, Bauer E, Kohli R, Gupta P K, Greulich K O. HeNe laser irradiation protects B-lymphoblasts from UVA-induced DNA damage. Radiat Environ Biophys. 2001; 40 (1): 77-82.

Dube A , Jayasankar K, Prabakaran L et al. Nitrogen laser irradiation (337 nm) causes temporary inactivation of clinical isolates of Mycobacterium tuberculosis. Lasers in Medical Science. 2004; 19 (1): 52-56.

Dudenko G I et al. [Treatment of acute trombophlebitis of the lower limbs with laser irrradiation]. Khirurgiia (Mosk). 1989; 9; 97-99. (in Russian)

Durnov L A, Gusev L I, Balakirev S A et al [Low-intensity lasers in pediatric oncology].Vestn Ross Akad Med Nauk. 2000; (6): 24-27.

Dyson M, Young S. Effect of Laser Therapy on Wound Contraction and Cellularity in Mice. Lasers in Medical Science. 1986; (1): 125-130.

Dyson M. Laser therapy in wound management. Proc. 7th Congr European Medical Laser Ass., Dubrovnik, Croatia, June 2000, p. 22.

Dyson M: Cellular and subcellular aspects of low level laser therapy. In: Progress in Laser Therapy. Eds. T. Ohshiro and R.G. Calderhead, John Wiley & Sons, England. 1991, p. 221-.

Dyson S. Primary, secondary and tertiary effects of phototherapy: a review. In: Progesss in Biomedical Optics and imaging. Proc. SPIE.Volume 6140; 614005 1-12.

Dörtbudak O, Haas R, Mailath-Pokorny G. Effect of low-power laser irradiation on bony implant sites. Clin Oral Implants Res. 2002; 13 (3): 288-292.

Eells J T, Henry M M, Summerfelt P, Wong-Riley M T, Buchmann E V et al. Therapeutic photobiomodulation for methanol-induced retinal toxicity. Proc Natl Acac Sci U S A. 2003; 18; 100 (6): 3439-3444.

Ebert D W, Bertone A L. Effect of irradiation with low intensity diode laser on the metabolism of equine articular cartilage in vitro. Am J Vet Res. 1998; 59 (12): 1615-1618.

Ebneshahidi N S, Heshmatipour M, Moghaddami A, Eghtesadi A P. The effects of laser acupuncture on chronic tension headache - a randomised controlled trial. Acupuncture in Medicine. 2005; 23 (1): 13-18.

Eckerdal A, Lehmann Bastian H. Can low reactive-level laser therapy be used in the treatment of neurogenic facial pain? A double-blind, placebo controlled investigation of patients with trigeminal neuralgia. Laser Therapy. 1996; 8 (4): 247-252.

Desmettre T, Maurage C A, Mordon S. Transpupillary thermotherapy (TTT) with short duration laser exposures induce heat shock protein (HSP) hyperexpression on choroidoretinal layers. Lasers Surg Med. 2003; 33 (2): 102-107.

Delibasi E, Turan B, Yucel E. The quantitative investigation of infrared laser effects on the levels of copper and zinc in various tissues. Clin Phys Physiol Meas. 1988; 9: 375-377.

Deltito J A, Moline M, Pollak C et al. Effects of phototherapy on non-seasonal unipolar and bipolar depressive spectrum disorders. J Affect Disord. 1991; 23 (4): 231-237.

Demir H, Yaray S, Kirnap M, Yaray K. Comparison of the effects of laser and ultrasound treatments on experimental wound healing in rats. J Rehabil Res Dev. 2004; 41 (5): 721-728.

Demir H, Menku P, Kirnap M, Calis M, Ikizceli I. Comparison of the effects of laser, ultrasound, and combined laser + ultrasound treatments in experimental tendon healing. Lasers Surg Med. 2004; 35 (1): 84-89.

Deng Q Z, Han Z Y. Therapy of female infertility under defocused CO_2 and HeNe laser acupoint irradiation. Laser Therapy. 1990; 2 (3): 117-118.

Derr V E, Klein E, Fine S. Free radical occurrence in some laser-irradiated biologic materials. Federal Proc. 1965; 24 (No 1, Suppl 14): 99-103.

Dillon K. Healing photons. Scientia Press, Washington D.C. 1998. ISBN 0-9642976-5-5.

Dima F V et al. Doserelated immunological and morphological changes observed in rats with Walker-256 carcinosarcoma after photodynamic therapy: a controlled study. Laser Therapy. 1991; 3 (3): 159-168.

Dima F V, Vasiliu V, Ionescu M D, Dima S V. Studies on some biological functions of macrophages activated by HeNe laser photodynamic treatment as compared to coryne-bacterium parvum and interferon activation. Laser Therapy. 1993; 5 (3): 117-124.

Dimitriadis V et al. Effect of HeNe Laser on the Midgut Cells of Drosophila Auraria Larvae and its Correlation with Acupuncture. Acup & Electro-Therap Res. Int J. 1985; 10: 67-.

Ditrichova D. Application of biostimulative effects of HeNe laser in the therapy of crural ulcers. Ultrastructural findings in irradiated tissue. Acta Universitatis Palackianae Olomucensis Facultatis Medicae. 1988; 119: 337-346.

Djavid GE, Mehrdad R, Ghasemi M, Hasan-Zadeh H et al. In chronic low back pain, low level laser therapy combined with exercise is more beneficial than exercise alone in the long term: a randomised trial. Aust J Physiother. 2007; 53 (3): 155-160.

Dong-Sheng Zhan et al. The effect of postoperative irradiation of Low Level CO_2 laser on the skin flap survival and its mechanism. Laser Therapy, (ILTA Okinawa Congr Abstr Issue). 1990; 2 (1): 36.

Doin-Silva R, Baranauskas V, Rodrigues-Simioni L, da Cruz-Höfling M A. The Ability of Low Level Laser Therapy to Prevent Muscle Tissue Damage Induced by Snake Venom. Photochem Photobiol. 2008 Jul 17. [Epub ahead of print]

Donko Z. Possible ab-initio explanation of laser "biostimulation" effects. Laser Applications in Medicine and Surgery. G. Galletti et al, Eds.: Proc 3rd World Congr - Int Soc Low Power Laser Appl in Medicine.: 1992: 57. Monduzzi Editore S.p.A., Bologna.

Dortbudak O, Haas R, Mallath-Pokorny G. Biostimulation of bone marrow cells with a diode soft laser. Clin Oral Implants Res. 2000; 11 (6): 540-545.

Dortbudak O, Haas R, Bernhart T, Mailath-Pokorny G. Lethal photosensitization for decontamination of implant surfaces in the treatment of peri-implantitis.Clin Oral Implants Res. 2001; 12 (2): 104-108.

Dos Reis F A, Belchior A C, de Carvalho P D, da Silva B A, Pereira D M, Silva I S, Nicolau R A. Effect of laser therapy (660 nm) on recovery of the sciatic nerve in rats after injury through neurotmesis followed by epineural anastomosis. Lasers Med Sci. 2008 Dec 23. [Epub ahead of print]

Damjanova J, Manolov V. [Therapeutic influence on patients with epiconoylitis and myotendinitis of upper extremity by the means of low-intensity laser]. Fizikalna Kurortna i Rekhabilitatsiona Meditsina. 2000; 39 (1): 15. (in Russian)

Danhof S. Laser treatment and smoking cessation. Dissertation. Dutch Medical Acupuncture Assn. 2000.

Darrre E M et al. [Laser treatment of achilles tendonitis]. Ugeskr Læger. 1994; 156 (45): 6680-6683. (in Danish)

da Silva R V, Camilli J A. Repair of bone defects treated with autogenous bone graft and low-power laser. J Craniofac Surg. 2006; 172: 297-301.

David L, Abergel P. Laser for cosmetic surgery. Laser Surg Med. 1989; Suppl 1: 32.

David R, Nissan M, Cohen I et al. Effects of low-power He-Ne laser on fracture healing in rats. Laser Surg Med. 1996; 19: 458-464.

Dcabrowska E et al. [Intravital treatment of the pulp with simultaneous laser biostimulation] Rocz Akad Med Bialymst. 1997; 42 (1): 168-176. (in Polish)

de Assis Limeira F. Assessment of bone repair following the use of anorganic bone graft and membrane, associated or not to 830 nm laser light. In: Proc. 3rd NOA Congress, Sao Paulo, Brazil, June 25-26 2002.

de Braekt M M H et al: Effect of low level laser therapy of wound healing after palatal surgery in beagle dogs. Laser Surg Med. 1991; 11: 462-.

de Castro e Silva Júnior O, Zucoloto S, Menegazzo L A G et al. Laser enhancement in hepatic regeneration for partially hepatectomized rats. Laser Surg Med. 2001; 29: 73-77.

de Jesus Guirro R R, de Oliveira Guirro E. Analysis of the transmissivity of Low Power Laser radiation in different occlusive dressings. Photomed Laser Surg. 2005; 23 (1). Abstracts from the 5th Congress of the World Association for Laser Therapy, São Paulo, Brazil, November 2004. Abstract no 055, p.103.

Delbari A, Bayat M, Bayat M. Effect of Low-Level Laser Therapy on Healing of Medial Collateral Ligament Injuries in Rats: An Ultrastructural Study. Photomed Laser Surg. 2007; 25 (3): 191-196.

de Lima F, Costa M S, Albertini R, Silva J A Jr, Aimbire F. Low level laser therapy (LLLT): Attenuation of cholinergic hyperreactivity, beta2-adrenergic hyporesponsiveness and TNF-alpha mRNA expression in rat bronchi segments in E. coli lipopolysaccharide-induced airway inflammation by a NF-kappaB dependent mechanism. Lasers Surg Med. 2009; 41 (1): 68-74.

de Medeiros JS, Vieira GF, Nishimura PY. Laser application effects on the bite strength of the masseter muscle, as an orofacial pain treatment. Photomed Laser Surg. 2005; 23 (4): 373-376.

Demura S, Yamaji S, Ikemoto Y. Effect of linear polarized near-infrared light irradiation on flexibility of shoulder and ankle joint. J Sport Med Phys Fitness. 2002; 42: 438-445.

Derkacz A, Bialy D, Protasiewicz M et al. Photostimulation of coronary arteries with low power laser radiation: preliminary results for a new method in invasive cardiology therapy. Medical Science Monitor. 2003; 9 (7): 335-339.

Derkacz A, Protasiewicz M, Kipshidze N, Bialy D et al. Endoluminal phototherapy for prevention of restenosis: preliminary results at 6-month follow-up. Photomed Laser Surg. 2005; 23 (6): 536-542.

de Scheerder I K et al. Intravascular low-power red laser light as an adjunct to coronary stent implantation. Initial clinical experience. Catheter Cardiovasc Intervent. 2000; 49 (4): 468-471.

de Scheerder I, Wang K, Zhou X R et al. Intravascular low power red laser light as an adjunct to coronary stent implantation evaluated in a porcine coronary model. J Invas Cardiol. 1998; 10: 534-538.

De Scheerder I, Wang K, Nikolaychik V, Kaul U et al. Long-term follow-up after coronary stenting and intravascular red laser therapy. Am J Cardiol. 2000; 86 (9): 927-930.

Corrral-Baqués M I, Riveira M M, Rodríguez-Gil J E, Rigau J. The effect of low-level laser irradiation on dog spermatozoa motility is dependent on laser output power. Lasers in Medical Science. September 12, 2008. [Epub ahead of print]

Corazza V A, Jorge J, Kurachi C, Bagnato V S. Photobiomodulation on the Angiogenesis of Skin Wounds in Rats Using Different Light Sources. Photomed Laser Surg. 2007; 25 (2): 102-106.

Correa F, Lopes Martins R A, Correa J C, Iversen V V, Joenson J, Bjordal J M. Low-Level Laser Therapy (GaAs=904 nm) Reduces Inflammatory Cell Migration in Mice with Lipopolysaccharide-Induced Peritonitis. Photomed Laser Surg. 2007; (4): 245-249.

Cowen D et al. Low energy helium neon laser in the prevention of oral mucositis in patients undergoing bone marrow transplant: results of a double blind randomized trial. Int J Radiat Oncol Biol Phys. 1997; 38 (4): 697-707.

CRA Newsletter. 1997; 21(4). Clinical Research Associates, Provo, Utah, USA.

Craig J A, Barlas P, Baxter G D, Walsh D M, Allen J M. Delayed-onset muscle soreness: lack of effect of combined phototherapy/low-intensity laser therapy at low pulse repetition rates. J Clin Laser Med Surg. 1996; 14 (6): 375-380.

Craig J A, Barron J, Walsh D M, Baxter G D. Lack of effect of combined low intensity laser therapy/phototherapy (CLILT) on delayed onset muscle soreness in humans. Lasers Surg Med. 1999; 24 (3): 223-230. Erratum in: Lasers Surg Med 1999; 25 (1): 88.

Crespi R et al. Periodontal tissue regeneration in beagle dogs after laser therapy. Lasers Surg Med. 1997. 21: 395-402.

Cressoni M D, Dib Giusti H H, Casarotto R A, Anaruma C A. The Effects of a 785-nm AlGaInP Laser on the Regeneration of Rat Anterior Tibialis Muscle After Surgically-Induced Injury. Photomed Laser Surg. 2008 Sep 18. [Epub ahead of print]

Croley T. Laser treatment of fibroconnective tissue scarring. Proc. 2nd Congress World Assn for Laser Therapy, Kansas City, September 1998; p. 35-39.

Cruz-Höfling A, Garavello Freitas Z, Baranauskas I B. SEM and AFM studies of rat injured tibiae after HeNe radiation. Medical Science. 2002; 17 (4). Proc. 14th Annual Meeting of Deutsche Gesellschaft für Lasermedizin, Munich, Germany, June 2003.

Cruz D R, Kohara E K, Ribeiro M S, Wetter N U. Effects of low-intensity laser therapy on the orthodontic movement velocity of human teeth: a preliminary study. Laser Surg Med. 2004; 35 (2): 117-120.

Cruz L B, Ribeiro A S, Rech A, Rosa L G, Castro C G Jr, Brunetto A L. Influence of low-energy laser in the prevention of oral mucositis in children with cancer receiving chemotherapy. Pediatr Blood Cancer. 2007; 48 (4): 435-440.

Cuda D, De Caria A. Combined counselling and low level laser stimulation effectiveness in the treatment of disturbing chronic tinnitus. The International Tinnitus Journal. 2008; 14 (2): 175-80.

da Cunha S S, Sarmento V, Ramalho L M, De Almeida D, Veeck E B, Da Costa N P, Mattos A, Marques A M, Gerbi M, Freitas A C. Effect of laser therapy on bone tissue submitted to radiotherapy: experimental study in rats. Photomed Laser Surg. 2007; 25 (3): 197-204.

da Cunha L A, Firoozmand L M, da Silva A P, Esteves S A, Oliveira W. Efficacy of low-level laser therapy in the treatment of temporomandibular disorder. Int Dent J. 2008; 58 (4): 213-217.

Dadras S, Mohajerani E, Eftekhar F, Hosseini M. Different photoresponses of Staphylococcus aureus and Pseudomonas aeruginosa to 514, 532, and 633 nm low level lasers in vitro. Curr Microbiol. 2006; 53 (4): 282-286.

Damante C A, Greghi S L, Sant'Ana A C, Passanezi E, Taga R. Histomorphometric study of the healing of human oral mucosa after gingivoplasty and low-level laser therapy. Lasers Surg Med. 2004; 35 (5): 377-384.

Chor A, Sotero Caio A B, de Azevedo A M. Amelioration of oral mucosal lesions of acute graft-versus-host disease by low-level laser therapy. Haematologica. 2001; 86 (12): 1321-.

Chow R. Dose dilemmas in low level laser therapy - the effects on different paradigms and historical perspectives. Laser Therapy. 2001: 13: 102-109.

Chow R T, Barnsley L. Systematic review of the literature of low-level laser therapy (LLLT) in the management of neck pain. Lasers Surg Med. 2005; 37 (1): 46-52.

Chow R T, Heller G Z, Barnsley L. The effect of 300mW, 830 nm laser on chronic neck pain: A double-blind, randomized, placebo-controlled study. Pain. 2006; 124 (1-2): 201-210.

Chow R. Laser acupuncture studies should not be included in systematic reviews of phototherapy. Photomed Laser Surg. 2006; 24 (1): 69. Comment on: Photomed Laser Surg. 2005; 23 (4): 425-30.

Chow R T, David M A, Armati P J. 830 nm laser irradiation induces varicosity formation, reduces mitochondrial membrane potential and blocks fast axonal flow in small and medium diameter rat dorsal root ganglion neurons: implications for the analgesic effects of 830 nm laser. J Peripher Nerv Syst. 2007; 12 (1): 28-39.

Cojocariu C, Rochon P. Synthesis and optical storage properties of a novel polymethacrylate with benzothiazole azo chromophore in the side chain. J Mater Chem. 2004; 14: 2909-2916.

Ciais G et al. La laserthérapie dans la prévention et le traitement des mucities liées à la chimothérapie antican-céreuse. Bull Cancer. 1992; 79: 183.

Cieslar G, Sieron A, Adamek M et al. Effect of low-power laser radiation in the treatment of the motional system overloading syndromes. Proc SPIE. 1997; Vol 3198: 76-82.

Corona S A, Nascimento T N, Catirse A B et al. Clinical evaluation of low-level laser therapy and fluoride varnish for treating cervical dentinal hypersensitivity. J Oral Rehabil. 2003; 30 (12): 1183-1189.

Ciuchita T et al. Low energy laser treatment in lichen planus and finger pulpitis infections. Lasers in Surg Med. 1999; Suppl 11: 6.

Ciuchita T. Low-energy laser in the treatment of alopecia of the scalp. Proc. SPIE. 1997; Vol 3198: 116-126.

Clokie C et al. The effects of helium-neon laser on postsurgical discomfort: A pilot study. Canadian Dent Assn Journal. 1991; 7 (57): 584-586.

Cohen N, Lubart R, Rubenstein S et al. Laser irradiation of mouse spermatozoa enhances in vitro fertilization and Ca2+ uptake via reactive oxygen species. Proc. SPIE. 1996; Vol 2929 :27-37.

Colvard M, Kuo P. Managing aphtous ulcers: laser treatment applied. J Am Dent Assoc. 1991; 122 (7): 51-53.

Conlan M J et al. Biostimulation of wound healing low-energy laser irradiation. A review. J Clin Periodontol. 1996; 23 (5): 492-496.

Conti P C. Low level laser therapy in the treatment of temporomandibular disorders (TMD): a double-blind pilot study. Cranio. 1997; 15 (2): 144-149.

Corona S A, Nascimento T N, Catirse A B, Lizarelli R F, Dinelli W, Palma-Dibb R G. Clinical evaluation of low-level laser therapy and fluoride varnish for treating cervical dentinal hypersensitivity. J Oral Rehabil. 2003; 30 (12): 1183-1189.

Corral-Baques M-I, Rigau J. About time to get to speak the same language. Proc. 4th Congress of the World Association for Laser Therapy, Tokyo, Japan, June 27-30. 2002; page 123. Also on http://www.laser.nu/lllt/lllt_editorial10.htm

Corral-Baques M I, Rigau T, Rivera M, Rodriguez J E, Rigau J. Effect of 655-nm diode laser on dog sperm motility. Lasers Med Sci. 2005; 20 (1): 28-34.

Abstracts from the 5th Congress of the World Association for Laser Therapy, São Paulo, Brazil, November 2004. Abstract no 096, p.113.

Chaves de Vasconcelos Catão M H, Gerbi M E, Cavalcanti Gonçalves R. A laserterapia no tratamento da radiomucosite em paciente com carcinoma espino celular no palato mole - relato de caso. Proc. Laser Dental Show, São Paulo, Brazil, November 2003, p. 8.

Chavrier C et al. Immunohistochemical localization of type I, ,III and IV collagen in healthy human gingiva. J de Biologie Buccale. 1981; 9: 271-277.

Checkley S A, Murphy D G, Abbas M J et al.Melatonin rhythms in seasonal affective disorder. Br J Psychiatry. 1993; 163: 332-337.

Cheetham M J, Young R S, Dyson M. Histological effects of 820 nm laser irradiation on the healthy growth plate of the rat. Laser Therapy 1992; 4 (2): 59-64.

Chen M et al. Application of a pain alleviating effect of low power laser irradiation to patients in orthodontic treatment. J Jpn Soc Laser Med. 1933; 14: 5-11. (in Japanese)

Chen, Ji-wei, Zhou, Yo-cheng. Effect of low level carbon dioxide laser radiation on biochemical metabolism of rabbit mandibular bone callus. Laser Therapy. 1989; 1 (2): 83-88.

Chen Y S, Hsu S F, Chiu C W, Lin J G, Chen C T, Yao C H. Effect of low-power pulsed laser on peripheral nerve regeneration in rats. Microsurgery. 2005; 25 (1): 83-89.

Chen CH, Hung HS, Hsu SH. Low-energy laser irradiation increases endothelial cell proliferation, migration, and eNOS gene expression possibly via PI3K signal pathway. Lasers Surg Med. 2008; 40 (1): 46-54.

Chen K H, Hong C Z, Kuo F C, Hsu H C, Hsieh Y L. Electrophysiologic effects of a therapeutic laser on myofascial trigger spots of rabbit skeletal muscles. Am J Phys Med Rehabil. 2008; 87 (12): 1006-1014.

Cheng ZY, Zhao CX, Zhang YH, et al. Superficial acupuncture combined with He-Ne laser radiation in the treatment of facial spasm. Int J Clin Acupunct 1991; 2 (1): 95-97.

Chernoff W G et al. Cutaneous Laser Surfacing. Operative Techniques in Otolaryngology - Head & Neck Surgery. 1994; 5: 281-284.

Chernoff W G. Cutaneous Laser Resurfacing. Clinical Laser Monthly. December 1994.

Cherry R J. Measurement of protein rotation diffusion in membranes by flash photolysis. Methods in Enzymology. 1978; 54: 47-61.

Chio C-C, Lin S-J, Kao M-C. Cytogenic effects of low level laser irradiation of human leukocytes. Laser Therapy. 1990; 2 (3): 111-116.

Chistov V B. [The effect of low-intensity radiation from a helium-neon laser on the alkaline phosphatase activity in an uncomplicated mandibular fracture and in traumatic osteomyelitis]. Stomatologiia 1989; 68 (6): 13-15.

Cho H J, Lim S C, Kim S G et al. Effect of low-level laser therapy on osteoarthropathy in rabbit. In Vivo. 2004; 18 (5): 585-591.

Choi J et al. A comparison of electroacupuncture, transcutaneous electrical nerve stimulation and laser photo-biostimulation on pain relief and glucocorticoid excretion. Int J Acupunct Electrotherp Res. 1986; 11: 45-51.

Chomette G, Auriol M, Zeitoun R et al. Effet du soft-laser sur le tissu conjunctif gingival. I - Effet sur les fibroblastes. Étude d'histoenzymologie et de microscopie eléctronique. J Biol Buccale. 1987; 15: 45-50.

Chomette G, Auriol M, Zeitoun R et al. Effet du soft-laser sur le tissu conjunctif gingival. II - Effet sur la cicatrisation. Étude en microscopie optique, histoenzymologie et de microscopie électronique. J Biol Buccale. 1987; 15: 51-57.

Chopp H, Chen Q, Dereski M O, Hetzel F W. Chronic metabolic measurement of normal brain tissue response to photodynamic therapy. Photochem. Photobiol. 1990; 52: 1033-1036.

Cassone MC, Lombard A, Rossetti V, Urciuoli R, Rolfo PM. Effect of in vivo HeNe laser irradiation on biogenic amine levels in rat brain. J Photochem Photobiol B 1993; 18 (2-3): 291-294.

Castano A P, Dai T, Yaroslavsky I, Cohen R, Apruzzese W A, Smotrich M H, Hamblin M R. Low-level laser therapy for zymosan-induced arthritis in rats: Importance of illumination time. Lasers Surg Med. 2007; 39 (6): 543-550.

Castro D J, Abergel R P, Johnston K et al. Wound healing: biological effects of Nd:YAG laser on collagen metabolism in pig skin in comparison to thermal burn. Ann Plast Surg 1983; 11: 131-.

Castro D J, Abergel R P, Meweker C et al. Effects of the Nd:YAG laser on DNA synthesis and collagen production in human skin fibroblast cultures. Ann Plast Surg. 1983; 1 (3): 214-222.

Castronuovo G. et al. The skin role during a low level laser therapy. Laser Bologna '92, p. 19. Monduzzi Editore S.p.A., Bologna, Italy.

Castro-e-Silva O Jr, Zucoloto S, Marcassa L G, Marcassa J et al.Spectral response for laser enhancement in hepatic regeneration for hepatectomized rats. Lasers Surg Med. 2003; 32 (1): 50-53.

Catão M H, Pinheiro A L, Costa J L et al. Low energy AsGaAl Laser (830nm) for the prevention of chemo-induced mucositis in oral cavity cancer patients. Photomed Laser Surg. 2005; 23 (1). Abstracts from the 5th Congress of the World Association for Laser Therapy, São Paulo, Brazil, November 2004. Poster no 111, page 142.

Ceccherelli F et al. Diode laser in cervical myofascial pain: A double blind study versus placebo. The Clinical J Pain. 1989; 5: 301-304.

Cedillo Valle B. An evaluation of the enantiomeric recognition of amino acid based polymeric surfactants and cyclodextrins using spectroscopic and chromatographic methods. Dissertation Faculty of the Louisiana State University and Agricultural and Mechanical College December 2005.

Celani M F, Gilioli G, Fano AR, Montanini V, Morrama P. The effect of laser radiation on Leydig cells: Functional and morphological studies. IRCS Med Sci. 1984; 12: 883-884.

Celani M F, Gilioli G, Montanini V, Morrama P. Further evidence that mid laser radiations may stimulate Leydig cell steroidogenesis. IRCS Med Sci. 1985; 13: 336-337.

Celani M F, Grandi M, Gilioli G. Changes in mouse Leydig cell streoidogenesis following infrared and helium-neon laser irradiation. Exp Clin Endocrinol. 1987; 80: 16-22.

Chagas-Oliveira P, Meireles G C S, dos Santos N R, de Carvalho C M et al. The Use of Light Photobiomodulation on the Treatment of Second-Degree Burns: A Histological Study of a Rodent Model. Photomed Laser Surg. 2008; 26 (4): 289-299.

Cetiner S, Kahraman SA, Yucetas S. Evaluation of low-level laser therapy in the treatment of temporomandibular disorders. Photomed Laser Surg. 2006; 24 (5): 637-641.

Chance B. Cellular oxygen requirements, Fed. Proc. Fed. Am. Soc. Exp. Biol. 1957; 16: 671.

Chang W D, Wu J H, Jiang J A, Yeh C Y, Tsai C T. Carpal tunnel syndrome treated with a diode laser: a controlled treatment of the transverse carpal ligament. Photomed Laser Surg. 2008; 26 (6): 551-557.

Changjun C et al. The Preoperative Period of the Veterinary Anaesthesia by Laser. Sichuan Agricultural College, Sichuan. Acupuncture Res. 1984; 9 (1): 16.

Chavantes M C. Pilot study : new treatment applying LLLT in tracheal stenosis. Using biomodulated effect. Photomed Laser Surg. 2005; 23 (1). Abstracts from the 5th Congress of the World Association for Laser Therapy, São Paulo, Brazil, November 2004. Abstract no 095, p.113.

Chavantes M C, Baptista I M, Kajita G, Shoji N. Prevention or acute treatment right after a risky surgery: does LLLT decrease complications? Photomed Laser Surg. 2005; 23 (1).

Calderhead G. Watt's A Joule?: On the Importance of Accurate and Correct Reporting of Laser Parameters in Low Reactive-Laser Therapy and Photobioactivation Research: Laser Therapy 1991; 3 (4): 177-182.

Calderhead R G, Inomata K. A study of the possible haemorrhagic effects of extended infrared diode laser irradiation on encapsulated and exposed synovial membrane articular tissue in the rat. Laser Therapy. 1992; 4 (2): 65-74.

Calderhead R G. Simultaneous low reactive-level laser therapy in laser surgery: the "alpha-phenomenon" explained. In: Progesss in Laser Therapy. 1991. John Wiley & Sons. P. 209-213.

Calkhoven C F, Geert A B. Multiple steps in regulation of transcription-factor level and activity. Biochemistry. 1996; 317: 329-342.

Cambier D C et al. Low-level laser therapy: the experience in Flanders. Eur J Phys Med Rehab. 1997; 7: 102-105.

Cameron R, Tabisz G C. Observation of two-photon optical rotation by molecules. Molecular Phys. 1997; 90 (2): 159-164.

Campaña V, Moya M, Gavotto A et al. Effects of helium-neon laser on microcrystalline arthropaties. Laser Surg Med. 2001; Suppl 13: 11.

Campaña V, Moya M, Gavotto A et al. He-Ne laser on microcrystalline arthropathies. J Clin Laser Med Surg. 2003; 21 (2): 99-103.

Campaña V R, Moya M, Gavotto A, Spitale L, Soriano F, Palma J A. Laser therapy on arthritis induced by urate crystals. Photomed Laser Surg. 2004; 22 (6): 499-503.

Campbell S S, Murphy P J. Extraocular circadian phototransduction in humans. Science 1998; 279 (5349): 396-399.

Carati C J, Anderson S N, Gannon B J, Piller N B. Treatment of postmastectomy lymphedema with low-level laser therapy. A double blind, placebo-controlled trial. Cancer. 2003; 98 (6): 1114-1122.

Carney S A et al. The effect of light from a ruby laser on the metabolism of skin in tissue culture. Biochem Biophys Acta. 1967; 148: 525-530.

Carniel R. The 780 laser and the CO2-laser in chronic achilles tendinitis: Different methods compared. Proc. 2nd Congress World Assn for Laser Therapy, Kansas City, Sept 1998; p. 40-42.

Carrasco T G, Mazzetto M O, Mazzetto R G, Mestriner W Jr. Low intensity laser therapy in temporomandibular disorder: a phase II double-blind study. Cranio. 2008; 26 (4): 274-281.

Carrillo J, Calatayud J, Manso F J et al. A randomized double-blind clinical trial on the effectiveness of helium-neon laser in the prevention of pain, swelling and trismus after removal of impacted third molars. Int Dent Journal. 1990; 40: 31-36.

Carrinho P M, Renno A C, Koeke P, Salate A C, Parizotto N A, Vidal B C. Comparative study using 685-nm and 830-nm lasers in the tissue repair of tenotomized tendons in the mouse. Photomed Laser Surg. 2006; 24 (6): 754-758.

Carvalho Baptista I, Chavantes M C, Soji N. A new application of Low Level Laser Therapy for treatment pain in patients submitted to a cardiac surgery. Photomed Laser Surg. 2005; 23 (1). Abstracts from the 5th Congress of the World Association for Laser Therapy, Sao Paulo, Brazil, November 2004. Abstract no 038, p.99.

Carvalho C, Nascimento F, Cangussu M, Gerbi M M, Marques A M, Pinheiro A L. The association of wavelengths is effective on the reduction of TMJ pain. A clinical study in a Brazilian population. Proc. 7th Internat Congr of WALT, Sun City, South Africa, October 2008, page 33.

Cassese M et al. Laser-terapia nelle sindromi algico-disfunzionali delle articolazioni temoporo-mandibolari. Int Congress on Laser in Med and Surg, Bologna June 1985, p 337. Monduzzi Editore S.p.A, Bologna, Italy.

Brown S A, Rohrich R J, Kenkel J et al. Effect of low-level laser therapy on abdominal adipocytes before lipoplasty procedures. Plast Reconstr Surg. 2004; 113 (6): 1796-1804; discussion 1805-1806.

Brugnera A et al. Clinical results evaluation of dentinary hypersensitivity patients treated with laser therapy. Proc. SPIE. 1999; Vol 3593: 66-68.

Brugnera A et al. Low-reactive level laser treatment in facial paralysis. In: Lasers in Dentistry VI. Ed Featherstone J D et al. Proc. SPIE. 2000; Vol 3910: 68-74.

Brugnera A. LLLT in treating dentinary hypersensibility: A histological study and clinical application. Proc. 2nd ENSOMA Congress, Houston, Texas, USA. 2001, p. 23-31.

Brugnera Jr A et al. Low level laser therapy in treatment of lesions in the inferior alveolar and mental nerves. Proc. 3rd Congr World Assn for Laser Therapy, Athens, Greece, May 2000, p.126.

Brugnera Junior A, Garrini A E, Pinheiro A et al. Laser therapy in the treatment of dental hypersensitivity - a histologic study and clinical application. Laser Therapy. 2000; 12: 16-21

Bucek M et al. Morphology of epithelizing varicose ulcers following HeNe laser therapy. Acta Universitatis Palackianae Olomucensis Facultatis Medicae. 1991; 131: 303-316.

Buliakova N V et al. Effects of helium-neon laser on regeneration capacity of skeletal muscles of adult guinea pigs. Biull Eksp Biol Med. 1992; 113 (4): 411-414.

Buliakova N V. Regereration of the x-ray irradiated gastrocnemius muscle in old rats after stimulation. Biull Eksp Biol Med. 1989; 108 (7): 123-126. (in Russian with English abstract)

Bülow P M, Jensen H, Danneskiold-Samsoe B. Low power Ga-Al-As laser treatment of painful osteoarthritis of the knee. Scan J Rehan Med. 1994; 26: 155-159.

Burch J M. Interferometry with Scattered Light. Optical Instruments and Techniques. J. Home, Dickson ed. (Reading Conf. 1969) p. 213. Oriel Press, New Castle upon Tyne 1970.

Burns T, Wilson M, Pearson G J Killing of cariogenic bacteria by light from a gallium aluminium arsenide diode laser. J Dent. 1994; (5) :273-278.

Bykov V L et al. [Low-energy laser irradiation in the complex treatment of patients with ear diseases]. Voprosy Kurortologii, Fizioterapii i Lechebnoi Fizicheskoi Kultury. 1985; (2): 60-62. (in Russian)

Bylesjö EI, Boman K, Wetterberg L. Obesity treated with phototherapy: four case studies. Int J Eat Disord. 1996; (4): 443-46.

Byrnes K R, Waynant R W, Ilev I K et al. Cellular invasion following spinal cord lesion and low power laser irradiation. Laser Surg Med. Abstract issue, 2002: 11.

Byrnes K R et al. Low power laser treatment of cutaneous wounds in psammomys obesus. Laser Surg Med. 2000; Supplement 12: 4.

Byrnes K R, Barna L, Chenault V M et al. Photobiomodulation improves cutaneous wound healing in an animal model of type II diabetes. Photomed Laser Surg. 2004; 22 (4): 281-290.

Byrnes KR, Waynant RW, Ilev IK Wu X et al. Light promotes regeneration and functional recovery and alters the immune response after spinal cord injury. Lasers Surg Med. 2005; 36 (3): 171-185.

Byrnes K R, Wu X, Waynant R W, Ilev I K, Anders J J. Low power laser irradiation alters gene expression of olfactory ensheathing cells in vitro. Lasers Surg Med. 2005; 37 (2): 161-117.

Calderhead G. Meeting report: International low power laser symposium, Vienna, Austria, October 7th-8th, 1994. Laser Therapy. 1995; 7 (1): 39.

Calderhead G. Meeting report: Proc Ninth Congress of the International Society for Laser Surgery and Medicine, Anaheim, California, USA: 2-6 November 1991. Laser Therapy. 1992; 4: 43.

Bossy J et al. In Vitro Survey of Low Energy Laser Beam Penetration in Compact Bone. Faculté de Médecine et CHRU de Nimes, BP 26, 3000 Nimes, France. (1985).

Boulton M et al. HeNe-Laser Stimulation of Human Fibroblasts and Attachment in vitro. Lasers in Life Sciences. 1986; 1 (2): 125-.

Bounkeo J M, Brannon W M, Dawes Jr K S et al. The efficacy of laser therapy in the treatment of wounds: a meta analysis of the literature. Proc. 3rd Congress of the World Ass for Laser Therapy, Athens, Greece, 2000, page 79. Submitted 2001.

Boussignac G et al. Thermal effects of semiconductor lasers in men. Proc 6th Congress of The Internat Soc for Laser Surg Med. 1985; 77.

Boxer S G, Roelofs M G. Chromophore organization in photosynthetic reaction centers: High-resolution magnetophotoselection. Proc Natl Acad Sci USA. 1979; 76 (11): 5636-5640.

Bradley F G, Reynolds P A. Low reactive level laser therapy in Oral and Maxillofacial Surgery. Review of 100 cases. Laser Therapy. 1994; 6 (1): 67. (abstract)

Bradley P F, Rebliini Z. Low intensity laser therapy (LILT) for temporomandibular joint pain: a clinical electromyographic and thermographic study. Laser Therapy. 1996; 8 (1): 47 (abstract)

Bradley P. Thermographic Evaluation of Response to Low Level Laser Acupuncture. Proc. Second Meeting of the International Laser Therapy Association, London Sept 1992. p 32.

Branco K, Naeser M A. Carpal tunnel syndrome: clinical outcome after low-level laser acupuncture, microamps transcutaneous electrical nerve stimulation, and other alternative therapies - an open protocol study. J Alternat Complem Med. 1999; 5: 5-26.

Braverman B, McCarthy R, Ivankovich A D et al. Effect of Helium-Neon and Infrared Laser Irrradiation on Wound Healing in Rabbits. Laser Surg Med. 1989; 9: 50-58.

Brill A G, Brill G E, Shenkman B et al. Low power laser irradiation of blood inhibits platlet function: role of cyclic GMP. Proc. SPIE. 1998; Vol 3569: 4-11.

Brill G et al. Influence of HeNe laser irradiation on giant chromosomes. Proc.SPIE. 1995; Vol 2630: 51-59.

Brill G, Brill A. [Guanilate cyclase and nitric oxide synthetsase as possible primary acceptors of low level laser radiation energy]. J Laser Medicine. 1997; 39-42. (in Russian)

Brill G E, Budnik I A, Gasparyan L V. Influence of helium-neon laser radiation on platelet function. BiOS 2008. Proceedings of SPIE; Volume 6846-20.

Bringman W. Lasertherapie beim chronischen Schultertrauma. DZA. 1998; 4: 109-120.

Brondon P, Stadler I, Lanzafame R J. Pulsing influences photoradiation outcomes in cell culture. Lasers Surg Med. 2009; 41 (3): 222-336.

Brosseau L et al. Low level laser therapy for osteoarthritis and rheumatoid arthritis: a metaanalysis. J Rheumatol. 2000; 27 (8): 1961-1969.

Brosseau L, Welch V, Wells G et al. Low level laser therapy (classes I, II and III) for treating rheumatoid arthritis. In: The Cochrane Library. Issue 4, 2000. Oxford: Update Software.

Brosseau L, Welch V, Wells G et al. Low level laser therapy (classes I, II and III) for treating oesteoarthritis. In: The Cochrane Library. Issue 4, 2000. Oxford: Update Software. Withdrawn 2007.

Brosseau L, Wells G, Marchand S, Gaboury I et al. Randomized controlled trial on low level laser therapy (LLLT) in the treatment of osteoarthritis (OA) of the hand. Lasers Surg Med. 2005; 36 (3): 210-219.

Brown G C. Control of respiration and ATP synthesis in mammalian mitochondria and cells. Biochem. J. 1992; 284: 171.

Brown G C. Nitric oxide and mitochondrial respiration. Biochem Biophys Acta. 1999; 1411: 351.

Bjorne A, Agerberg G. Symptom relief after treatment of temporomandibular and cervical spine disorders in patients with Ménière´s disease: A 3-year follow-up. J Crandomandib Pract. 2003; 21 (1): 50-60.

Bjorne A, Agerberg G. Reduction in sick leave and costs to society of patients with Ménière´s disease after treatment of temporomandibular and cervical spine disorders: A controlled 6-year cost-benefit study. Cranio. 2003; 21 (2): 136-143.

Blay A, Blay C C, Groth E B et al. Effects of visible NIR low intensity laser on implant osseointegration in vivo. Laser Surg Med, Supplement 14, 2002: 11.

Blaya D S, Guimarães M B, Pozza D H, Weber J B, de Oliveira M G. Histologic study of the effect of laser therapy on bone repair. J Contemp Dent Pract. 2008; 9 (6): 41-48.

Bliddal H et al. Soft laser therapy of rheumatoid arthritis. Scand J Rheuma. 1987; 16: 225-228.

Boboreko B A. [Helium-neon laser irradaition in the therapy of urinary bladder and uretral tubercolosis]. Probl Tuberk. 1999; 6: 38-40.

Boerner E, Podbielska H, Nesterowicz M et al. Double-blind study on the efficacy of the lasertherapy. Proc. SPIE; Vol. 2929: 75

Bogomilskii M R et al. [Effects of low-energy laser irradiation on the functional state of the acoustic analyzer.] Vestn Otorinolaringol. 1989; 2: 29-34.

Bolton P A, Dyson M, Young S R. The effect of polarised light on the release of growth factors from the U-937 macrophage-like cell line. Laser Therapy. 1992; 4 (1): 33-42.

Bolton P A, Young S R, Dyson M.. Macrophage responsiveness to light therapy. A dose response study. Laser Therapy. 1990; 2 (3): 101-106.

Bolton P, Young S, Dyson M. The direct effect of 860 nm light on cell proliferation and on succinic dehydrogenase activity of human fibroblasts in vitro. Laser Therapy. 1995; 7 (2): 55-60.

Bolton P, Young S, Dyson M. Macrophage responsiveness to light therapy with varying power and energy densities. Laser Therapy. 1991; 3 (3): 105-112.

Bolton P, Dyson M, Young S. The effect of polarized light on the release of growth factors from the U-937 magraophage cell line. Laser Therapy. 1992; 4 (1): 33-37.

Bonin K D, Kourmanov B, Walker T G. Light torque nanocontrol, nanomotors and nanorockers. Optic Express. 2002; 10 (19): 984-989.

Bonome Salate A C, Barbosa G, Gaspar P, Nivaldo Antonio Parizotto N A et al. Effects of 660 nm GaAsAl with 10 mW and 40 mW on neoangiogenesis after partial ruptures of Achilles tendon (Tendocalcaneus). Photomed Laser Surg. 2005; 23 (1). Abstracts from the 5th Congress of the World Association for Laser Therapy, São Paulo, Brazil, November 2004. Poster no 60, page 129.

Bortone F, Santos H A, Albertini R, Pesquero J B, Costa M S, Silva J A Jr. Low level laser therapy modulates kinin receptors mRNA expression in the subplantar muscle of rat paw subjected to carrageenan-induced inflammation. Int Immunopharmacol. 2008; 8 (2): 206-210.

Bosatra M, Lucci A, Olliaro P et al. In vitro fibroblast activation by laser irradiation at low energy. Dermatologica. 1984; 168: 157-162.

Boschi E S, Leite C E, Saciura V C, Caberlon E, Lunardelli A, Bitencourt S, Melo D A, Oliveira J R. Anti-Inflammatory effects of low-level laser therapy (660 nm) in the early phase in carrageenan-induced pleurisy in rat. Lasers Surg Med. 2008; 40 (7): 500-508.

Boss W K Jrc, Usal H, Thompson R C, Fiorillo M A. A comparison of the long-pulse and short-pulse Alexan-drite laser hair removal systems. Ann Plast Surg 1999; 42 (4): 381-384.

Bossini P S, Fangel R, Habenschus R M, Renno A C, Benze B, Zuanon J A, Neto C B, Parizotto N A. Low-level laser therapy (670 nm) on viability of random skin flap in rats. Lasers Med Sci. 2009; 24 (2): 209-213.

Bjordal J M. Low level laser therapy in shoulder tendinitis/bursitis, epicondylalgia and ankle sprain. A critical review on clinical effects. Master thesis in Physiotherapy Science, Div Physiotherapy Science, University of Bergen, Norway. 1997.

Bjordal J M, Greve G. What may alter the conclusions of reviews? Physical Therapy Reviews. 1998; 3: 121-132.

Bjordal J M, Couppe C, Ljunggren A. Low level laser therapy for tendinopathies. Evidence of a dose-response pattern. Physical Therapy Reviews. 2001; 6 (2): 91-100.

Bjordal J M, Couppè C, Chow R T, Tunér J, Ljunggren A E. A systematic review of low level laser therapy with location-specific doses for pain from chronic joint disorders. Australian J Physiotherapy. 2003; 49: 107-116.

Bjordal JM, Ljunggren AE, Klovning A, Slordal L. Non-steroidal anti-inflammatory drugs, including cyclo-oxygenase-2 inhibitors, in osteoarthritic knee pain: meta-analysis of randomised placebo controlled trials. Br Med J. 2004; 329 (7478): 1317-. '

Bjordal J M, Ljunggren A E, Klovning A, Slordal L. NSAIDs, including coxibs, probably do more harm than good, and paracetamol is ineffective for hip OA. Ann Rheum Dis. 2005; 64 (4):655-656; author reply 656. Comment on: Ann Rheum Dis. 2005; 64 (5): 669-681.

Bjordal J M, Lopes-Martins R A, Iversen V V. A randomised, placebo controlled trial of low level laser therapy for activated Achilles tendinitis with microdialysis measurement of peritendinous prostaglandin E2 concentrations. Br J Sports Med. 2006; 40 (1): 76-80.

Bjordal J M. Can a Cochrane review in controversial areas be biased? A sensitivity analysis based on the protocol of a systematic Cochrane review Low Level Laser Therapy in Osteoarthritis. Photomed Laser Surg. 2005; 23 (5): 453-458.

Bjordal J M, Johnson M I, Iversen V, Aimbire F, Lopes-Martins R A. Photoradiation in acute pain: a systematic review of possible mechanisms of action and clinical effects in randomized placebo-controlled trials. Photomed Laser Surg. 2006; 24 (2): 158-168.

Bjordal J M, Baxter G D. Ineffective dose and lack of laser output testing in laser shoulder and neck studies. Photomed Laser Surg. 2006; 24 (4):533-534; author reply 534.

Bjordal J M, Klovning A, Ljunggren A E, Slordal. L. Short-term efficacy of pharmacotherapeutic interventions in osteoarthritic knee pain: A meta-analysis of randomised placebo-controlled trials. Eur J Pain. 2007; 11 (2): 125-138.

Bjordal J M, Tunér J, Iversen V V, Frigo L, Gjerde, K, Lopes-Martins A B. A systematic review of post-operative pain relief by Low Level Laser Therapy (LLLT) after third molar extraction. Abstract Congr. Of the European Division of the World Federation for Laser Dentistry, Nice, May 2007.

Bjordal J M, Lopes-Martins R A, Joensen J, Couppe C, Ljunggren A E, Stergioulas A, Johnson M I. A systematic review with procedural assessments and meta-analysis of low level laser therapy in lateral elbow tendinopathy (tennis elbow). BMC Musculoskelet Disord. 2008; 9: 75.

Bjordal J M, Johnson M I, Lopes-Martins R A, Bogen B, Chow R, Ljunggren A E. Short-term efficacy of physical interventions in osteoarthritic knee pain. A systematic review and meta-analysis of randomised placebo-controlled trials. BMC Musculoskelet Disord. 2007; 8:51.

Bjordal J M. A systematic review of Low Level Laser Therapy (LLLT) in chemotherapy-induced oral mucositis. Annual Congress of the Federation Dentaire International, Singapore, August 2009.

Bjordal J M, Bensadoun R J, Lopes–Martins R A, Tunér J, Pinheiro A, Ljunggren A E. A systematic review of low level laser therapy (LLLT) in cancer therapy-induced oral mucositis. Submitted for publication 2010.

Bjorne A, Berven A, Agerberg G. Cervical signs and symptoms in patients with Ménière's disease: a controlled study. J Cranomandib Practice. 1998; 16 (3): 194-202.

Bermudez D, Carrasco F, Diaz F, Vargas I P. Germ cell DNA quantification shortly after IR laser radiation. Andrologia. 1991; 23: 303-307.

Barkana Y, Belkin M. Laser eye injuries. Surv Ophthalmol. 2000; 44 (6): 459-478.

Bernal G. Helium Neon and Diode Laser Therapy is an effective adjunctive therapy for facial paralysis. Laser Therapy. 1993; 5 (2): 79-87

Bernardini U D, Longo L. Terapia laser nella nevralgia del trigemino. Proc. Atti dell'í VIII Congresso Nazionale A.I.S.D., Verona. 1985: 80-81.

Bernhardt O, Gesch D, Schwahn C, Bitter K et al. Signs of temporomandibular disorders in tinnitus patients and in a population-based group of volunteers: results of the Study of Health in Pomerania. J Oral Rehabil. 2004; 31 (4): 311-319.

Bernhardt J H. [Electrosmog, cellular phones, sunbeds etc. - adverse health effects from radiation? Health aspects of non-ionizing radiation] Bundesgesundheitsblatt Gesundheitsforschung Gesundheitsschutz. 2005; 48 (1): 63-75. [Article in German]

Berns M W, Gross D C L, Cheng W K, Woodring D. Argon laser microirradiation of mitochondria in rat myocardial cell in tissue culture. II. Correlation of morphology and function in single irradiated cells. J Mol Cell Cardiol. 1972; 4: 71.

Bertoloni G, Sacchetto R, Baro E et al. Biochemical and morphological changes in Escherichia coli irradiated by coherent and non-coherent 632.8 nm light, J Photochem Photobiol B Biol. 1993; 18: 191-.

Bertolucci L E, Grey T. Clinical analysis of Mid-laser versus placebo treatment of arthralgic TMJ degenerative joints. J Craniomandib Practice. 1995; 13 (1): 26-29.

Beyer W et al. Light dosimetry and preliminary clinical results for low level laser therapy in cochlear dysfunction. Proc. Laser Florence '99.

Bezuur N J, Hansson T L. The effect of therapeutic laser treatment in patient with cranomandibular disorders. J Cranomandib Disorders. 1988; 2: 83-86.

Bhagwanani N S et al. Low level nitrogen laser therapy in pulmonary tuberculosis. J Clin Laser Med Surg. 1996; 14 (1): 23-25.

Bibikova A et al. Enhancement of angiogenesis in regenerating gastrocnemius muscle of the toad (Bufo viridis) by low-energy laser irradiation. Anatomy & Embryology. 1994; 190 (6): 597-602.

Bibikova A, Oron U. Attenuation of the process of skeletal muscle regeneration by low energy laser irradiation. Laser Therapy. 1996; 8 (1): 19. (abstract)

Bibokova A, Oron U. Attenuation of the process of muscle regeneration in the toad gastrocnemius muscle by low energy laser irradiation. Laser Surg Med. 1994; 14: 355-361.

Bibikova A, Oron U. Regeneration in denervated toad (Bufo viridis) gastrocnemius muscle and the promotion of the process by low energy laser irradiation. The Anatomical Record. 1995; 241: 123-128

Bihari I, Mester A. The biostimulative effect of low level laser therapy of long-standing crural ulcer using Helium Neon laser, Helium Neon plus infrared lasers and noncoherent light: Preliminary report of a randomized double blind comparative study. Laser Therapy. 1989; 1 (2): 97-102.

Bingöl Ü, Altan L, Yurtkuran M. Low-Energy Laser Treatment for Shoulder Pain. Photomed Laser Surg. 2005; 23 (5): 459-464.

Bisht D et al. Effect of low intensity laser radiation on healing of open skin wounds in rats. Indian J Medical Research. 1994; 100: 43-46.

Bisht D, Mehrotra R, Singh P A et al. Effect of helium-neon laser on wound healing. Indian Journal of Experimental Biology. 1999; 37(2): 187-189.

Bisland S K. Priming cells for photodynamic therapy using low intensity light therapy. Proc. NAALT2006, Toronto, Canada, June 3-4 2006.

Baumler W, Neff S, Landthaler M et al. Laser Assisted Hair Removal: Comparison of a Normal Mode Ruby Laser and a High Power Laser Diode. Abstract volume, Laser Florence. 14:th International Congress of Laser Medicine, pp 11, Florence 1999.

Baxter G D et al. Low level laser therapy: Current clinical practice in Northern Ireland. Physiotherapy 1991; 3:171-178.

Baxter G D. Therapeutic Lasers. 1994; p 148. Churchill Livingstone.

Bayat M, Vasheghani M M, Razavi N et al. Effect of low-level laser therapy on the healing of second-degree burns in rats: a histological and microbiological study. J Photochem Photobiol B. 2005; 78 (2): 171-177

Bayat M, Delbari A, Almaseyeh M A et al. Low-level laser therapy improves early healing of medial collateral ligament injuries in rats. Photomed Laser Surg. 2005; 23 (6): 556-560.

Bayat M, Vasheghani M M, Razavie N, Jalili M R. Effects of low-level laser therapy on mast cell number and degranulation in third-degree burns of rats. J Rehabil Res Dev. 2008; 45 (6): 931-938.

Beckerman H et al. Efficacy of physiotherapy for musculoskeletal disorders: what can we learn from research? Br J Gen Pract. 1993; 43 (367): 73-77.

Beck-Friis J, Borg G, Wetterberg L: Rebound increase of nocturnal melatonin levels following evening suppression by bright light exposure in healthy men: relationship to cortisol levels and morning exposure. In: The Medical and Biological Effects of Light. Wurtman RJ, ed. Ann. NY Acad Sci. 1985; 453: 371-375.

Behling A A. Low Level Laser Therapy and Women's Health. Swedish Laser Medical Society Symposium, Stockholm, Sweden, May 2008.

Belchior A C, Dos Reis F A, Nicolau R A, Silva I S, Perreira D M, de Carvalho P D. Influence of laser (660 nm) on functional recovery of the sciatic nerve in rats following crushing lesion. Lasers Med Sci. 2009 Feb 6. [Epub ahead of print]

Ben-Dov N, Shefer G, Irinitchev A et al. Low energy laser irradiation affects satellite cell proliferation and differentiation in vitro. Biochem Biophys Acta. 1999; 1448: 372-380.

Belkin M, Schwartz M. Evidence for the existence of low-energy laser bioeffects on the nervous system. Neurosurg Rev 1994;17 (1): 7-17.

Belkin M, Schwartz M. Ophthalmic effects of low-energy laser irradiation. Survey of Ophthalmology. 1994; 39 (2): 113-122.

Bellina J H. Laser in gynecology. Excerpts from Leventhal, J.M. et al (eds.): Current Problems in Obstetrics and Gynecology. Year Book Medical Publishers, Inc., Chicago. 1981.

Ben Hatit Y. The Nd:YAG Laser in Dentistry. LASER. Journ Eur Med Laser Ass. 1991; 4 (1-2): 17.

Ben Hatit B Y, Lammens J P. Laser therapy with 10 600 nm defocused CO2 laser. Laser Therapy. 1992; 4 (4): 175-178.

Benedicenti B. Valoración radioimunológica del nivel de ß-endorfina en el líquido encefaloraquídeo antes y después de irradiar con laser 904 nm, en neuralgia del trigemino. Inv. Clin Láser. 1984; 1 (3): 7-12.

Bensadoun R-J, Franqiun J C, Ciais C et al. Low energy He/Ne laser in the prevention of radiation-induced mucositis: A multicenter phase III randomized study in patients with head and neck cancer. Support Care Cancer. 1999; 7 (4): 244-252.

Bensadoun R-J, Ciais G. Radioation- and chemotherapy-induced mucositis in oncology: results of multicenter phase III studies. J Oral Laser Applications. 2000; 2: 115-120.

Berki T, Németh, Hegedüs J. Effect of low-power continous-wave HeNe laser irradiation on in vitro cultured lymphatic cell lines and macrophages. Stud Biophys. 1985; 105: 141-

Berki T et al. Biological Effect of Low-power Helium-Neon (HeNe) Laser Irradiation. Lasers in Medical Science. 1988; 3: 35-.

ovial membranes performed with neodym phosphate glass laser irradiation. Proc. 7th Congr Internat Soc for Laser Surg and Med, Munich June 1987. Abstract no 216a.

Barabash A G et al. [Experience in treating patients with lichen ruber planus by using a helium-neon laser.] Stomatologiia; 1995; 74 (1): 20-21.

Barasch A, Peterson D, Tanzer J M et al. Helium-neon laser effects on conditioning-induced oral mucositis in bone marrow transplan-tation patients. Cancer. 1995; 76 (12): 2550-2556.

Baratto L, Capra R, Farinelli M et al. A new type of very low-power modulated laser: soft-tissue changes induced in osteoarthritic patients revealed by sonography. International Journal of Clinical Pharmacology Research. 2000; 20 (1-2): 13-6.

Barber A, Luger J E, Karpf A et al. Advances in laser therapy for bone repair. Laser Therapy. 2001: 13: 80-85.

Barberis G et al. In vitro synthesis of prostaglandin E2 by synovial tissue after helium-neon laser radiation in rheumatoid arthritis. J Clin Laser Med Surg. 1996; 14 (4): 175-177.

Barbarosa Lopes C. Laser biostimulation in bone implants. A Raman spectral study. In: Proc. 3rd NOA Con-gress, Sao Paulo, Brazil, June 25-26 2002.

Barbosa A M, Villaverde A B, Guimarães-Souza L, Ribeiro W, Cogo J C, Zamuner S R. Effect of low-level laser therapy in the inflammatory response induced by Bothrops jararacussu snake venom. Toxicon. 2008; 51 (7): 1236-1244.

Barbosa A M, Villaverde A B, Sousa L G, Munin E, Fernandez C M, Cogo J C, Zamuner S R. Effect of Low-Level Laser Therapy in the Myonecrosis Induced by Bothrops jararacussu Snake Venom. Photomed Laser Surg. 2009 Jun 16. [Epub ahead of print]

Barnes J et al. Electronic Acupuncture and Cold Laser Therapy as Adjuncts to Pain Treatment. J Cranomandibular Pract. 1977; 2 (2): 614-.

Barushka O, Yaakobi T, Oron U. Effect of low-energy laser (He-Ne) irradiation on the process of bone repair in rat tibia. Bone. 1995; 16 (1): 147-155.

Basford J R et al. Low-energy Helium Neon laser treatment of thumb osteoarthritis. Arch Phys Med Rehab. 1987; 68: 794-797.

Basford J R, Malanga G A, Krause D A, Harmsen W S. A randomized controlled evaluation of low-intensity laser therapy: plantar fasciitis. Arch Phys Med Rehab. 1998; 79 (3): 249-254.

Basford J R, Sheffield C G, Harmsen W S. Laser therapy: a randomized, controlled trial of the effects of low-intensity Nd:YAG laser irradiation on musculoskeletal back pain. Arch Phys Med Rehabil. 1999; 80 (6): 647-652.

Basford, J R, Sheffield C G , Cieslak K R. Laser therapy: a randomized, controlled trial of the effects of low intensity Nd:YAG laser irradiation on lateral epicondylitis. Arch Phys Med Rehabil. 2000; 81 (11): 1504-1510.

Basford J R, Sandroni P, Low P A, Hines S M et al. Effects of linearly polarized 0.6-1.6 microM irradiation on stellate ganglion function in normal subjects and people with complex regional pain (CRPS I). Lasers Surg Med. 2003; 32 (5): 417-423.

Bashardoust Tajali S, Macdermid J C, Houghton P, Grewal R. Effects of low power laser irradiation on bone healing in animals: a meta-analysis. Lasers Med Sci. 2010 Feb 6. [Epub ahead of print]

Basirnia A, Sadeghipoor G, Djavid E G et al. The effect of low power laser therapy on osteoarthritis of the knee.Laser in Medical Science. 2002; 17 (4). Proc. 14th Annual Meeting of Deutsche Gesellschaft für Lasermedizin, Munich, Germany, June 2003.

Basko I:. A New Frontier: Laser Therapy. California Veter. 1983; 10: 17.

Baumann M, Jörgensen B, Rohde E et al. Influence of wavelength, power density and exposure time of laser radiation on chondrocyte cultures - An in-vitro investigation. Medical Laser Application. 2006; 21 (3): 191-198.

Ataie L. Djavid G E. Efficacy of low power laser GaAlAs (630 nm) in the treatment of vitiligo patients. Laser in Medical Science. 2002; 17 (4). Proc. 14th Annual Meeting of Deutsche Gesellschaft für Lasermedizin, Munich, Germany, June 2003.

Atsumi K et al. Biostimulation effect of low-power energy diode laser for pain relief. Laser Surg Med. 1987; 7: 77-.

Attia M A, El-Kashef H. Low level laser therapy in the treatment of arteriosclerosis of the lower limbs. Laser Therapy. 1999; 11 (1): 26-29.

Avery D H. A turning point for seasonal affective disorder and light therapy research? Arch Gen Psychiatry. 1998; Oct;55 (10): 863-864. Review.

Avila R et al. Histological effects of HeNe laser on chick embryo. Proc X Internat Congress Int Soc Laser Surg Med, Bangkok 1993, p. 164.

Avni D, Levkovitz S, Maltz L, Oron U. Protection of skeletal muscles from ischemic injury: low-level laser therapy increases antioxidant activity. Photomed Laser Surg. 2005 23 (3): 273-277.

Avram M R, Rogers N E. The use of low-level light for hair growth: part I. J Cosmet Laser Ther. 2009; 11 (2): 110-117.

Axelsen S M, Bjerno T. [Laser therapy of ankle sprain]. Ugeskr Læger. 1993; 155 (48): 3908-3911. (in Danish)

Axelsson R, Tullberg M, Ernberg M, Hedenberg-Magnusson B. Temporomandibular conditions in patients with sudden sensorineural hearing loss. Swed Dental J 2005; 29 (4): 175-176. (abstract)

Azevedo L H, Correa Aranha A C, Stolf S F, Eduardo C P, Vieira M M. Evaluation of Low-Level Laser Therapy for the Thyroid Gland of Male Mice. Photomed Laser Surg. 2005; 23 (6): 567-570.

Babcock G, Vickery L E, Palmer G. Electronic state of Heme in cytochrome-c oxidase. J Biol Chem. 1976; 251 (24): 790-791.

Bach G, Neckel C, Mall, Krekeler G. Conventional versus laser-assisted therapy of periimplantitis: a five-year comparative study. Implant Dent. 2000; 9: 247–251.

Bae C S, Lim S C, Kim K Y, Song C H et al. Effect of Ga-as laser on the regeneration of injured sciatic nerves in the rat. In Vivo. 2004; 18 (4): 489-495.

Bagis S, Comelekoglu U, Coskun B, Milcan A et al. No effect of GA-AS (904 nm) laser irradiation on the intact skin of the injured rat sciatic nerve. Lasers in Medical Science. 2003; 18 (2): 83-88.

Bahn J. Biostimulation laser: reality and perspectives. LASER. Journ Eur Med Laser Ass. 1988; 1 (1): 17-22.

Bakhtiary A H, Rashidy-Pour A. Ultrasound and laser therapy in the treatment of carpal tunnel syndrome. Aust J Physiother. 2004; 50: 147-151.

Balaban P et al. HeNe laser irradiation of single neurons. Laser Surg Med. 1992; 12 (3): 329-337.

Balakirev S A, Gusev L I, Kazanova M B et al. [Nizkointensivnaia lazernaia terapiia v detskoi onkologii] Voprosy onkologii. 2000; 46 (4): 459-461.

Balakirev S A, Gusev L I, Kazanova M et al. [Low-intensity laser therapy in pediatric oncology]. Voprosy Onkologii. 2000; 46 (4): 459-61.

Barabas K, Balint G, Gaspardy G et al. Kontrollierte klinische und experimentelle Untersuchungen mit Nd-Phosphat-Glas-Laser bei Patienten mit rheomatoid Athritis bzw. ihre Wirkung auf due Synovilamembrane [Controlled clinical and experimental studies with Nd-Phosphate-Glass laser in patients with rheumatoid arthri-tis and its effect on the synovial membrane]. Zeitschrif für Physiotherapie. 1989; 41 (5): 293-296. Also in: Barabás K et al. Controlled clinical and experimental examinations on rheumatoid arthritis patients and syn-

Arao M et al. The clinical study of low power laser treatment for temporomandibular arthrosis. Proc. 4th Int Congr Lasers in Dentistry. Ed. Hong-Sai L. 1995, p. 245-250. Munduzzi Editore, Italy.

Aras M H, Güngörmüs M. Placebo-controlled randomized clinical trial of the effect two different low-level laser therapies (LLLT) - intraoral and extraoral - on trismus and facial swelling following surgical extraction of the lower third molar. Lasers Med Sci. 2009 May 31. [Epub ahead of print]

Arbuliev MG, Mikhailov SK, Alibekova SA. [Choice of the treatment method in patients with acute inflammatory diseases of the scrotal organs]. Urol Nefrol (Mosk) 1989; 3: 17-20.

Armino L, Fornari B, Longo L, Losito A. Laser therapy in post-episiotomic nevralgie. LASER. Journ Eur Med Laser Ass. 1988; 1 (1): 7-.

Armino L, Longo L. Effects of laser treatment on vulvar dystrophy. LASER. Journ Eur Med Laser Ass.; 1991:4 (1-2): 10-13.

Arora H, Pai KM, Maiya A, Vidyasagar M S, Rajeev A. Efficacy of He-Ne Laser in the prevention and treatment of radiotherapy-induced oral mucositis in oral cancer patients. Oral Surg Oral Med Oral Pathol Oral Radiol Endod. 2008; 105 (2): 180-186.

Arun Maiya A, Sagar M S, Fernandes D. Effect of low level helium-neon (He-Ne) laser therapy in the prevention & treatment of radiation induced mucositis in head & neck cancer patients. Indian J Med Res. 2006; 124 (4): 399-402.

Arvanitaki A, Chalazonitis N. Reactiones bioeléctriques à la photoactivation des cytochromes. Arch. Sci. Physiol. 1947; 1: 385.

Asada K, Yutani Y, Shimazu A. Diode Laser Therapy for Rheumatoid Arthritis: A Clinical Evaluation of 102 Joints Treated with Low Reactive-level Laser Therapy (laser therapy). Laser Therapy. 1989; 1 (3): 147-152.

Asagai Y et al. Application of low reactive-level laser therapy (laser therapy) in the functional training of cerebral palsy patients. Proc. 2nd Congress World Assn for Laser Therapy, Kansas City, September 1998; p. 99-100.

Asagai Y, Imakiire A, Ohshiro T. Thermographic effects of laser therapy in patients with cerebral palsy. Laser Therapy. 2000; 12: 12-15.

Asagai Y, Imakiire A, Ohshiro T. Thermographic study of low level laser therapy for acutephase injury. Laser Therapy. 2000; 12: 31-33.

Asanami S, Shiba H, Ohtaishi M et al. The Activatory Effect of HeNe laser therapy Irradiation of Hydroxy-apatite Implants in the Rabbit Mandibular Bone. Laser Therapy. 1993; 5 (1): 29-32.

Asencio-Arana F et al. Endoscopic Enhancement of the Healing of High-Risk Colon Anastomoses by Low-Power Helium-Neon Laser. Dis Colon Rectum. 1992; 35: 568-573.

Ash JB, Piazza E, Anderson JL. Light therapy in the clinical management of an eating-disordered adolescent with winter exacerbation. Int J Eat Disord. 1998; (1): 93-97.

Ashkin A. Optical trapping and manipulation of neutral particles using lasers. Proc. Natl. Acad. Sci. USA. 1997; 94: 4853-4860.

Ashman R F. Lymphocyte activation. In: Fundamental Immunology. Paul W P, Ed, Raven Press, New York, 1984, p. 267.

Assia E, Rosner M, Belkin M et al. Temporal parameters of low energy laser irradiation for optimal delay of post-traumatic degeneration of rat optic nerve. Brain Research. 1989; 476: 205-212.

Ataka I et al. Studies of Nd:YAG Low Power Laser Irradiation on Stellate Ganglion. Lasers in Dentistry. 1989; page 271. Elsevier Science Publisher B.V. Amsterdam.

Amir A et al. The influence of low energy Helium-Neon laser irradiation on the viability of skin flaps of the rat. Laser Therapy. 1996; 8 (1): 59. (abstract)

Amorim J C F, Ribeiro M S, Groth E B. Gingival healing after gingivectomy procedure and low intensity laser irradiation. A clinical and biometrical study in anima nobile. Laser Surg Med. Supplement 14, 2002: 20.

Anders J J et al. Low power laser irradiation alters the rate of regeneration of the rat facial nerve. Laser Surg Med. 1993; 13: 72-82.

Anders J J, Geuna S, Rochkind S. Phototherapy promotes regeneration and functional recovery of injured peripheral nerve. Neurol Res. 2004; 26 (2): 233-239.

Anders J, Wu X, Anton Dmitriev A, Mario T. Cardoso M T et al. Light promotes axonal regeneration and functional recovery in two spinal cord injury models BiOS 2008. Proceedings of SPIE; Volume 6846-11.

Anders J J, Ilev I. Light interaction with human central nervous system progenitor cells. Proc. 7th Internat Congr of WALT, Sun City, South Africa, October 2008, page 106.

Andersen B.R., Brendzdel A.M,. Lint T.F. Infect. Immun. 1977; 17: 62-.

Ando Y, Watanabe H, Ishikawa I. Bactericidal effect of Erbium YAG laser on periodontal bacteria. Laser Surg Med. 1996; 19: 190-200.

Angiolillo P J, Vanderkooi. J M. The Photoexcited Triplet State as a Probe of Chromophore-Protein Interaction in Myoglobin. Biophysical Journal. 1998; 75 1491-1502.

Anneroth G, Hall G, Rydén H, Zetterqvist L. The effect of Low-energy infrared laser radiation on woundhealing in rats. Brit J Oral & Max Surg. 1988; 26: 12-17.

Antikas T. Low Power Laser Treatment of Musculoskeletal Disorders and Body Measurements of the Equine Athlete. Proc. SPIE (Lasers in Medicine). 1989; Vol 1353: 92-.

Antikatzides T. G. Soft Laser Treatment of Muskuloskeletal and Other Disorders in the Equine Athlete. Equine Practice. 1986; 8 (2): 24-.

Antipa C et al. Laser biostimulation (Ne-He and Ga-As) effects as compared to the conventional therapy in several pelvic inflammatory diseases. Proc. SPIE. 1993; Vol 1879: 15-22 (Lasers in Urology, Gynecology, and General Surgery).

Antipa C et al. Low-energy laser treatment of rheumatic diseases: a long-term study Proc. SPIE. 1995; Vol 2391: 658-662. (Laser-Tissue Interaction VI)

Antipa C et al. Pulsed-laser therapy (GA-As) in combined treatment of post-traumatic swellings and some dermatological disorders. In: Medical Applications of Lasers. Proc. SPIE. 1994; Vol 2086: 371-377.

Antipa C et al. Use of pulsed laser therapy (Ga-As) in combined treatment of posttraumatic swellings and some dermatological disorders. Proc SPIE. 1993; Vol. 2086.: 371-377.

Antipa C, Pascu M, Stanciulescu V et al. Low power coherent and noncoherent light in clinical practice. Proc. SPIE. 1996; Vol 2929: 119-123.

Antipa C, Pascu M, Stanciulescu V et al. Coherent and noncoherent low-power diodes in clinical practice. Proc. SPIE Vol. 2981, p. 236-241, Coherence Domain Optical Methods in Biomedical Science and Clinical Applications; Valery V. Tuchin, Halina Podbielska M.D., Ben Ovryn; Eds.

Antipa C, Nacu M, Bunila D et al. Clinical results of the low energy laser stimulation on distal forearm posttraumatic nerve lesion.Proc. 2nd Congr World Assoc. for Laser Therapy, Jerusalem, 1996, p. 36.

Aoki A, Ishikawa I, Yamada T et al. Comparison between Er:YAG laser and conventional technique for root caries treatment in vitro. J Dent Res. 1998; 77 (6): 1404-1414.

Arao et al. The low power laser treatment for patients of xerostomia: a preliminary report. Proc. 7th Int Con Lasers in Dentistry, ISLD, Brussels, Belgium, July 2000, abstr. 2.

Almeida-Lopes L, Rigau J, Zángaro R et al. Comparison of the low level laser therapy effects on cultured human gingival fibroblast proliferation using different irradiance and same fluency. Laser Surg Med. 2001; 29: 179-184.

Almeida-Lopes L. PhD dissertation. Universidade do Vale do Paraíba, SP, Brazil, 2003.

Almeida-Lopes L, Pretel H, Moraes V et al. Effects of continuous and pulsed infrared laser application on bone repair using different energy doses. Study in rats. Proc. 7th Internat Congr of WALT, Sun City, South Africa, October 2008, page 86.

Al-Shenqiti A, Oldham J. The use of low intensity laser therapy (LILT) in the treatment of trigger points that are associated with rotator cuff tendonitis. Laser in Medical Science. 2002; 17 (4). Proc. 14th Annual Meeting of Deutsche Gesellschaft für Lasermedizin, Munich, Germany, June 2003, p. 157.

Alstergren P et al. Interleukin 1ß in the arthritic temporomandibular joint fluid and its relation to pain, mobility and anterior open bite. Swedish Dent J. 1998; 2: 247.

Alves da Cuhna M, Munin E, Castro de Abreu W. [O uso do laser terapeutico em mucosite oral e xerostomia em pacientes submetida à radioterapia]. Proc. Laser Dental Show, São Paulo, Brazil, November 2003, p.8.

Al-Watban F. Stimulation and inhibtion effects of Kr laser for wound management. Laser Surg Med. 1998; Suppl 10: 5.

Al-Watban F, Zhang X Y. Comparison of the effects of laser therapy on wound healing using different laser wavelengths. Laser Therapy. 1996; 8 (2): 127-136.

Al-Watban F, Zhang X Y. Comparison of wound healing process using argon and krypton lasers. J Clin Laser Med Surg. 1997; 15 (5): 209-215.

Al-Watban F. Laser therapy am the healthy rat model for wound healing research - is it a feasible idea? LaserWorld Guest editorial, No 10, 2000. www.laser.nu/lllt/lllt_editorial.htm.

Al-Watban F. Laser acceleration of open skin wound closure in rats and its dosimetric dependence. Laser Therapy. 1996; 8 (1): 27. (abstract)

Al-Watban F, Andres B L. Laser photons and pharmacological treatment in wound healing. Laser Therapy. 2000; 12: 3-11.

Al-Watban F A, Zhang X Y. The comparison of effects between pulsed and CW lasers on wound healing. J Clin Laser Med Surg. 2004; 22 (1): 15-18.

Al-Watban F A H, Andres B L. Polychromatic LED Therapy in Burn Healing of Non-diabetic and Diabetic Rats. J Clinical Laser Medicine & Surgery. 2003; 21 (5): 249-258.

Al-Watban F, Zhang X Y, Andres B L. Low-Level Laser Therapy Enhances Wound Healing in Diabetic Rats: A Comparison of Different Lasers. Photomed Laser Surg. 2007, 25 (2): 72-77.

Al-Watban F A. Laser Therapy Converts Diabetic Wound Healing to Normal Healing. Photomed Laser Surg. 2009 Feb 4. [Epub ahead of print]

Al-Watban F A, Zhang X Y, Andres B L, Al-Anize A.Visible lasers were better than invisible lasers in accelerating burn healing on diabetic rats. Photomed Laser Surg. 2009; 27 (2): 269-272.

Amano A et al. Histological studies on the rheumatoid synovial membrane irradiated with a low energy laser. Laser Surg Med. 1994; 15 (3): 290-294.

Amano A. Histological Studies on the Rheumatoid Synovial Membrane Irradiated with a Low Energy Laser. Laser Surg Med. 1994; 15: 290-294.

Amaral A C et al. HeNe laser action in the regeneration of the tibialis anterior muscle of mice. Proc. 2nd Con-gress World Assn for Laser Therapy, Kansas City, September 1998; pp 18-19.

Amat A, Rigau J, Nicolau R, Aalders M et al. Effect of red and near-infrared laser light on adenosine triphosphate (ATP) in the luciferine-luciferase reaction. Journal of Photochemistry and Photobiology A: Chemistry. 2004; 168 (1-2): 59-65.

Ailioaie L, Ailioaie C. Self-organizing phenomena at membrane level and low level laser therapy of rhinitis. In: A window on the laser medicine world. Longo L ed. Proc. SPIE. 1999, Vol 4166: 309-315.

Ailioaie C, Ailioaie L. The treatment of bronchial asthma with low level laser in attack-free period of children. Proc. SPIE. 2000; Vol. 4166: 303-308.

Aimbire F, Albertini R, de Magalhães R G, Lopes-Martins R A et al. Effect of LLLT Ga-Al-As (685 nm) on LPS-induced inflammation of the airway and lung in the rat. Lasers in Medical Science. 2005; 20 (1): 11-20.

Aimbire F, Albertini R, Leonardo P, Castro Faria Neto HC, Iversen V V, Lopes-Martins R A B, Bjordal J M. Low level laser therapy induces dose-dependent reduction of TNF-alpha levels in acute inflammation. Photomed Laser Surg. 2006; 24 (1): 33-37.

Aimbire F, Bjordal J M, Iversen V V, Albertini R et al. Low Level Laser Therapy restores the impaired relaxation induced by TNF-alpha of rat trachea smooth muscle via increases of cAMP. Photomed Laser Surg. 2006.

Aimbire F, Lopes-Martins RA, Albertini R, Pacheco M T et al. Effect of low-level laser therapy on hemorrhagic lesions induced by immune complex in rat lungs. Photomed Laser Surg. 2007; 25 (2): 112-117.

Aimbire F, Ligeiro de Oliveira A P, Albertini R, Corrêa J C, Ladeira de Campos C B, Lyon J P, Silva J A Jr, Costa M S. Low Level Laser Therapy (LLLT) Decreases Pulmonary Microvascular Leakage, Neutrophil Influx and IL-1beta Levels in Airway and Lung from Rat Subjected to LPS-Induced Inflammation. Inflammation. 2008; 31 (3): 189-197.

Aimbire F, de Lima F M, Costa M S, Albertini R, Correa J C, Iversen V V, Bjordal J M. Effect of low level laser therapy on bronchial hyper-responsiveness. Laser Med Sci; 20009; 24 (4): 567-576.

Albertini R, Aimbire F S, Correa F I, Ribeiro W et al. Effects of different protocol doses of low power gallium-aluminum-arsenate (Ga-Al-As) laser radiation (650 nm) on carrageenan induced rat paw ooedema. J Photochem Photobiol B. 2004; 27;74 (2-3): 101-107.

Airaksinen O et al. Effects of HeNe-laser irradiation on the trigger points of patients with chronic muscle ten-sion in the neck. Scand J of Acup & Electrotherapy. 1989; 4: 63-65.

Airaksinen O, et al. Effects of infra-red laser irradiation at the trigger points. Scand J of Acup & Electrotherapy. 1988; 3: 56-61.

Akai M et al. Laser's effect on bone and cartilage change induced by joint immobilization: an experiment with animal model. Laser Surg Med. 1997; 21 (5): 480-484.

Al-Anazi A, Al Watban F A H, Zhang X Y, Andres B L. The effects of low power laser therapy with different wavelengths in accelerating wound healing on diabetic rats. Proc. 7th Internat Congr of WALT, Sun City, South Africa, October 2008, page 96.

al Awami M, Schillinger M, Maca T, Pollanz S, Minar E. Low level laser therapy for treatment of primary and secondary Raynaud's phenomenon. Vasa. 2004;33 (1): 25-29.

Albertini R, Aimbire F S, Correa F I, Ribeiro W et al. Effects of different protocol doses of low power gallium-aluminum-arsenate (Ga-Al-As) laser radiation (650 nm) on carrageenan induced rat paw oedema. J Photochem Photobiol B. 2004; 27;74 (2-3): 101-107.

Albrecht-Büchler G. Surface extensions of 3T3 cells towards distant infrared light sources. J Cell Biol. 1991; 114: 494.

Allais G, De Lorenzo C, Quirico P E, Lupi G et al. Non-pharmacological approaches to chronic headaches: transcutaneous electrical nerve stimulation, laser therapy and acupuncture in transformed migraine treatment. Neurol Sci. 2003; 24 Suppl 2: S138-142.

Allan R C, Stjernholm R L, Steele R H. Biochem. Biophys. Res. Commun. 1972; 47: 679-

Almeida-Lopes L et al. The use of low level laser therapy for wound healing: comparative study. Proc. 3rd Congr World Assn for Laser Therapy, Athens, Greece, May 2000, p. 118.

[2126] Chow RT, Johnson MI, Lopes-Martins RA, Bjordal JM. Efficacy of low-level laser therapy in the management of neck pain: a systematic review and meta-analysis of randomised placebo or active-treatment controlled trials. Lancet. 2009; 374 (9705): 1897-1908.

14.2 Alphabetical register of references

Abe M et al. Role of 830 nm low reactive level laser on the growth of an implanted glioma in mice. Keio J Med 1993; 42 (4): 177-179.

Abeles M, Marlowe S, Ingentio F. Treatment of osteoarthritis of the hand with low power laser. Arthritis Rheum. 1988; 28: 294. (abstract)

Abergel P et al. Non Thermal Effects of Nd:YAG Laser on the Biological Functions of the Human Skin Fibro-blasts in Culture. Laser Surg Med. 1984; 3 (4): 379-384.

Abergel P, Lyons R, Castel J, Dwyer R, Uitto J. Biostimulation of wound healing by laser: Experimental approaches in animal models and in fibroblast cultures. J Dermatol Surg Oncol. 1987; 13: 127-133.

Abergel P, Meeker C A, Lam T et al. Control of connective tissue metabolism by lasers: Recent developments and future prospects. J Am Acad Dermatol. 1984; 11: 1142-1150.

Abergel P. Laser treatment of acne scars. Laser Surg Med. 1992; Suppl 4: 70.

Abiko Y. Functional genomic study on anti-inflammatory effects by low level laser irradiation. Abstract at the 8th Congress of the World Federation for Laser Dentistry, Hong Kong, July 2008.

Abramovitch-Gottlib L, Gross T, Naveh D, Geresh S, Rosenwaks S, Bar I, Vago R. Low level laser irradiation stimulates osteogenic phenotype of mesenchymal stem cells seeded on a three-dimensional biomatrix. Lasers Med Sci. 2005; 20 (3-4): 138-146.

Abramovici A, Roisman P, Hirsch et al. HeNe laser irradiation accelerate healing process of open gingival wounds in cats. In:Anderson RR, ed. Laser surgery: Advanced characterization, therapeutics, and systems. IV. Proc. SPIE Vol. 2128: 248-256.

Ad N, Oron U. Impact of low level laser irradiation on infarct size in the rat following myocardial infarction. Int J Cardiol. 2001; 80 (2-3): 109-116.

Agaev F F. [Endobronchial laser therapy in the surgery of tuberculosis]. Probl Tuberk. 1998; 1: 33-36.

Agaiby A D, Ghali L R, Wilson R, Dyson M. Laser modulation of angiogenic factor production by T-lymphocytes. Lasers Surg Med. 2000; 26 (4): 357-363.

Agambar L, Herbert K E. Scott D L. Low powered laser therapy for rheumatoid arthritis. Br J Rheum. 1992; 31 (suppl 2): 81.

Ahl P L, Cone R A. Light activates rotations of bacteriorhodopsin in the purple membrane. Biophysical Journal. 1984; 45: 1039-1049.

Ahmed N A, Radwan N M, Ibrahim K M, Khedr M E, El Aziz M A, Khadrawy Y A. Effect of three different intensities of infrared laser energy on the levels of amino acid neurotransmitters in the cortex and hippocampus of rat brain. Photomed Laser Surg. 2008; 26 (5): 479-488.

Aihara N, Yamaguchi M, Kasai K. Low-energy irradiation stimulates formation of osteoclast-like cells via RANK expression in vitro. Lasers Med Sci. 2006; 21 (1): 24-33.

Aigner N, Fialka C, Radda C, Vecsei V. Adjuvant laser acupuncture in the treatment of whiplash injuries: a prospective, randomized placebo-controlled trial. Wien Klin Wochenschr. 2006; 118 (3-4): 95-99.

Ailioaie C, Ailioaie L, Topoliceanu F. Self-organizing phenomena at membrane levels and LLLT of rhinitis. Proc. SPIE. 2000; Vol. 416: 309-315.

Ailioaie C, Lupusoru-Ailioaie L M. Beneficial effects of laser therapy in the early stagers of rheumatoid arthritis onset. Laser Therapy. 1999; 11 (2): 79-87.

[2109] Ivandic B T, Hoque N N, Ivandic T. Early diagnosis of ocular hypertension using a low-intensity laser irradiation test. Photomed Laser Surg. 2009; 27 (4): 571-575.

[2110] Tumilty S, Munn J, McDonough S, Hurley D A, Basford J R, Baxter G D. Low Level Laser Treatment of Tendinopathy: A Systematic Review with Meta-analysis. Photomed Laser Surg. 2009 Aug 26. [Epub ahead of print]

[2111] Mvula B, Moore T J, Abrahamse H. Effect of low-level laser irradiation and epidermal growth factor on adult human adipose-derived stem cells. Lasers Med Sci. 2010; 25 (1): 33-39.

[2112] Mvula B, Mathope T, Moore T, Abrahamse H. The effect of low level laser irradiation on adult human adipose derived stem cells. Lasers Med Sci. 2008; 23 (3): 277-282.

[2113] Al-Watban F A. Laser Therapy Converts Diabetic Wound Healing to Normal Healing. Photomed Laser Surg. 2009 Feb 4. [Epub ahead of print]

[2114] Al-Watban F A, Zhang X Y, Andres B L, Al-Anize A.Visible lasers were better than invisible lasers in accelerating burn healing on diabetic rats. Photomed Laser Surg. 2009; 27 (2): 269-272.

[2115] Bjordal J M, Bensadoun R J, Lopes–Martins R A, Tunér J, Pinheiro A, Ljunggren A E. A systematic review of low level laser therapy (LLLT) in cancer therapy-induced oral mucositis. Submitted for publication 2010.

[2116] Simunovic-Soskic M, Pezelj-Ribaric S, Brumini G, Glazar I, Grzic R, Miletic I. Salivary Levels of TNF-alpha and IL-6 in Patients with Denture Stomatitis Before and After Laser Phototherapy. Photomed Laser Surg 2009 Oct 1 [Epub ahead of print].

[2117] Tortamano A, Lenzi D C, Haddad A C, Bottino M C, Dominguez G C, Vigorito J W. Low-level laser therapy for pain caused by placement of the first orthodontic archwire: a randomized clinical trial. Am J Orthod Dentofacial Orthop 2009; 136 (5) 662-667.

[2118] Kiritsi O, Tsitas K, Malliaropoulos N, Mikroulis G. Ultrasonographic evaluation of plantar fasciitis after low-level laser therapy: results of a double-blind, randomized, placebo-controlled trial. Lasers Med Sci. 2009 Oct 20. [Epub ahead of print]

[2119] Simões A, Platero M D, Campos L, Aranha A C, Eduardo Cde P, Nicolau J. Laser as a therapy for dry mouth symptoms in a patient with Sjögren's syndrome: a case report. Spec Care Dentist. 2009; 29 (3): 134-137.

[2120] Simões A, de Campos L, de Souza D N, de Matos J A, Freitas P M, Nicolau J. Laser Phototherapy as Topical Prophylaxis Against Radiation-Induced Xerostomia. Photomed Laser Surg. 2009 Oct 9. [Epub ahead of print]

[2121] Simões A, Nogueira FN, Eduardo CD, Nicolau J. Diode Laser Decreases the Activity of Catalase on Submandibular Glands of Diabetic Rats. Photomed Laser Surg. 2009 Oct 5. [Epub ahead of print]

[2122] Simões A, de Oliveira E, Campos L, Nicolau J. Ionic and histological studies of salivary glands in rats with diabetes and their glycemic state after laser irradiation. Photomed Laser Surg. 2009; 27(6): 877-883.

[2123] Minatel D G, Frade M A, França S C, Enwemeka C S. Phototherapy promotes healing of chronic diabetic leg ulcers that failed to respond to other therapies. Lasers Surg Med. 2009; 41 (6): 433-441.

[2124] Konstantinovic L M, Kanjuh Z M, Milovanovic A N, Cutovic M R, Djurovic A G, Savic V G, Dragin A S, Milovanovic N D. Acute Low Back Pain with Radiculopathy: A Double-Blind, Randomized, Placebo-Controlled Study. Photomed Laser Surg. 2009 [Epub ahead of print]

[2125] Zimin A A, Zhevago N A, Buiniakova A I, Samoilova K A. [Application of low-power visible and near infrared radiation in clinical oncology]. Vopr Kurortol Fizioter Lech Fiz Kult. 2009; 6: 49-52. (in Russian)

[2091] Simões A, de Freitas P M, Tunér J, de Paula Eduardo C. Laser as a new auxiliary therapy for Stevens Johnson Syndrome: a case report.Accepted for publication 2010. Photomed Laser Surg.

[2092] Zan-Bar T, Bartoov B, Segal R, Yehuda R, Lavi R, Lubart R, Avtalion R R. Influence of visible light and ultraviolet irradiation on motility and fertility of mammalian and fish sperm. Photomed Laser Surg. 2005; 23 (6): 549-555.

[2093] Esnouf A, Wright P A, Moore J C, Ahmed S. Depth of penetration of an 850 nm wavelength low level laser in human skin. Acupunct Electrother Res. 2007; 32 (1-2): 81-86.

[2094] Kwon K, Son T, Lee KJ, Jung B. Enhancement of light propagation depth in skin: cross-validation of mathematical modeling methods. Lasers Med Sci. 2009. 24 (4): 605-615.

[2095] Bjordal J M. A systematic review of Low Level Laser Therapy (LLLT) in chemotherapy-induced oral mucositis. Annual Congress of the Federation Dentaire International, Singapore, August 2009.

[2096] Maloney R. Presentation at 29th Annual Conference of the American Society for Laser Medicine and Surgery (ASLMS) in National Harbor, Maryland, USA, 2009.

[2097] Scoletta M, Arduino P G, Reggio L, Dalmasso P, Mozzati M. Effect of Low-Level Laser Irradiation on Bisphosphonate-Induced Osteonecrosis of the Jaws: Preliminary Results of a Prospective Study. Photomed Laser Surg. 2009 Oct 1. [Epub ahead of print]

[2098] Wenzel G I, Balster S, Zhang K, Lim H H, Reich U, Massow O, Lubatschowski H, Ertmer W, Lenarz T, Reuter G. Green laser light activates the inner ear. J Biomed Opt. 2009; 14 (4): 044007.

[2099] Kim S J, Moon SU, Kang S G, Park Y G.Effects of low-level laser therapy after Corticision on tooth movement and paradental remodeling. Lasers Surg Med. 2009 Jul 28. [Epub ahead of print]

[2100] Jensen I, Harms-Ringdahl K Strategies for prevention and management of musculoskeletal conditions. Neck pain. Best Pract Res Clin Rheumatol. 2007; 21 (1): 93-108.

[2101] Kuhn A, Porto F A, Miragliaz P, Brunetto A L. Low-level infrared laser therapy in chemotherapy-induced oral mucositis: a randomized placebo-controlled trial in children. J Pediatr Hematol Oncol. 2009; 31 (1): 33-37.

[2102] de Lima F, Costa M S, Albertini R, Silva J A Jr, Aimbire F. Low level laser therapy (LLLT): Attenuation of cholinergic hyperreactivity, beta2-adrenergic hyporesponsiveness and TNF-alpha mRNA expression in rat bronchi segments in E. coli lipopolysaccharide-induced airway inflammation by a NF-kappaB dependent mechanism. Lasers Surg Med. 2009; 41 (1): 68-74.

[2103] Guirro R R, Weis L C. Radiant power determination of low-level laser therapy equipment and characterization of its clinical use procedures. Photomed Laser Surg. 2009; 27 (4): 633-639.

[2104] Olofsson M. Studying linear polarization of laser light when propagating through tissue. University of Linkoping, Sweden. Thesis, 2006. Prima Books AB, 2007.

[2105] Kim H, Zarif N. MID-laser therapy - a potential approach to reduce pain in dysmenorrhea. Presented at NAALT2009, San Francisco, USA, June 2009.

[2106] Pesevska S, Nakova M, Ivanovski K, Angelov N, Kesic L, Obradovic R, Mindova S, Nares S Dentinal hypersensitivity following scaling and root planing: comparison of low-level laser and topical fluoride treatment. Lasers Med Sci. 2009 Jun 1. [Epub ahead of print]

[2107] Vieira A H, Passos V F, de Assis J S, Mendonça J S, Santiago S L. Clinical Evaluation of a 3% Potassium Oxalate Gel and a GaAlAs Laser for the Treatment of Dentinal Hypersensitivity. Photomed Laser Surg. 2009 Aug 28. [Epub ahead of print]

[2108] Enwemeka C S, Williams D, Enwemeka S K, Hollosi S, Yens D. Blue 470-nm light kills methicillin-resistant Staphylococcus aureus (MRSA) in vitro. Photomed Laser Surg. 2009; 27(2): 221-226.

[2074] Pereira C L, Sallum E A, Nociti F H Jr, Moreira R W. The effect of low-intensity laser therapy on bone healing around titanium implants: a histometric study in rabbits. Int J Oral Maxillofac Implants. 2009; 24 (1): 47-51.

[2075] Oliveira F S, Pinfildi C E, Parizoto N A, Liebano R E, Bossini P S, Garcia E B, Ferreira L M. Effect of low level laser therapy (830 nm) with different therapy regimes on the process of tissue repair in partial lesion calcaneous tendon. Lasers Surg Med. 2009; 41 (4): 271-276.

[2076] Tuby H, Maltz L, Oron U. Implantation of low-level laser irradiated mesenchymal stem cells into the infarcted rat heart is associated with reduction in infarct size and enhanced angiogenesis. Photomed Laser Surg. 2009; 27 (2): 227-233.

[2077] Rocha Júnior A M, Vieira B J, de Andrade L C, Aarestrup F M. Low-level laser therapy increases transforming growth factor-beta2 expression and induces apoptosis of epithelial cells during the tissue repair process. Photomed Laser Surg. 2009; 27 (2): 303-307.

[2078] Ribeiro M A, Albuquerque R L, Ramalho L M, Pinheiro A L, Bonjardim L R, Da Cunha S S. Immunohistochemical Assessment of Myofibroblasts and Lymphoid Cells During Wound Healing in Rats Subjected to Laser Photobiomodulation at 660 nm. Photomed Laser Surg. 2009; 27 (1): 49-55.

[2079] Garcia V G, Fernandes L A, de Almeida J M, Bosco A F, Nagata M J, Martins T M, Okamoto T, Theodoro L H. Comparison between laser therapy and non-surgical therapy for periodontitis in rats treated with dexamethasone. Lasers Med Sci. 2009 May 14. [Epub ahead of print]

[2080] Sousa L R, Cavalcanti B N, Marques M M. Effect of Laser Phototherapy on the Release of TNF-alpha and MMP-1 by Endodontic Sealer-Stimulated Macrophages. Photomed Laser Surg. 2009 Jan 30. [Epub ahead of print]

[2081] Skopin M D, Molitor S C. Effects of near-infrared laser exposure in a cellular model of wound healing. Photodermatol Photoimmunol Photomed. 2009; 25 (2): 75-80.

[2082] Moriyama Y, Nguyen J, Akens M, Moriyama E H, Lilge L. In vivo effects of low level laser therapy on inducible nitric oxide synthase. Lasers Surg Med. 2009; 41 (3): 227-231.

[2083] Zazzio M. Pain threshold improvement for chronic hyperacusis patients in a prospective clinical study. Photomed Laser Surg. Accepted for publication 2009.

[2084] Aimbire F, de Lima F M, Costa M S, Albertini R, Correa J C, Iversen V V, Bjordal J M. Effect of low level laser therapy on bronchial hyper-responsiveness. Laser Med Sci; 2009; 24 (4): 567-576.

[2085] Moges H, Vasconcelos O M, Campbell W W, Borke R C, McCoy J A, Kaczmarczyk L, Feng J, Anders J J. Light therapy and supplementary Riboflavin in the SOD1 transgenic mouse model of familial amyotrophic lateral sclerosis (FALS). Lasers Surg Med. 2009; 41 (1): 52-59.

[2086] Radwan N M, El Hay Ahmed N A, Ibrahim K M, Khedr M E, Aziz M A, Khadrawy Y A. Effect of infrared laser irradiation on amino acid neurotransmitters in an epileptic animal model induced by pilocarpine. Photomed Laser Surg. 2009; 27 (3): 401-409.

[2087] Hawkins D, Abrahamse H. Influence of broad-spectrum and infrared light in combination with laser irradiation on the proliferation of wounded skin fibroblasts. Photomed Laser Surg. 2007; 25 (3): 159-169.

[2088] Brondon P, Stadler I, Lanzafame R J. Pulsing influences photoradiation outcomes in cell culture. Lasers Surg Med. 2009; 41 (3): 222-336.

[2089] Lanzafame R J, Stadler I, Coleman J, Haerum B, Oskoui P, Whittaker M, Zhang R Y. Temperature-controlled 830-nm low-level laser therapy of experimental pressure ulcers. Photomed Laser Surg. 2004; 22 (6): 483-488.

[2090] Stadler I, Lanzafame R J, Oskoui P, Zhang R Y, Coleman J, Whittaker M. Alteration of skin temperature during low-level laser irradiation at 830 nm in a mouse model. Photomed Laser Surg. 2004; 22 (3): 227-231.

[2058] Karabegovic A, Kapidzic-Durakovic S, Ljuca F. Laser therapy of painful shoulder and shoulder-hand syndrome in treatment of patients after the stroke. Bosn J Basic Med Sci. 2009; 9 (1): 59-65.

[2059] Ferreira Dde C, Martins F O, Romanos M T. [Impact of low-intensity laser on the suppression of infections caused by Herpes simplex viruses 1 and 2: in vitro study] Rev Soc Bras Med Trop. 2009; 42 (1): 82-85.

[2060] Yagci I, Elmas O, Akcan E, Ustun I, Gunduz O H, Guven Z. Comparison of splinting and splinting plus low-level laser therapy in idiopathic carpal tunnel syndrome. Clin Rheumatol. 2009 Jun 21. [Epub ahead of print]

[2061] Barbosa A M, Villaverde A B, Sousa L G, Munin E, Fernandez C M, Cogo J C, Zamuner S R. Effect of Low-Level Laser Therapy in the Myonecrosis Induced by Bothrops jararacussu Snake Venom. Photomed Laser Surg. 2009 Jun 16. [Epub ahead of print]

[2062] Aras M H, Güngörmüs M. Placebo-controlled randomized clinical trial of the effect two different low-level laser therapies (LLLT) - intraoral and extraoral - on trismus and facial swelling following surgical extraction of the lower third molar. Lasers Med Sci. 2009 May 31. [Epub ahead of print]

[2063] Avram M R, Rogers N E. The use of low-level light for hair growth: part I. J Cosmet Laser Ther. 2009; 11 (2): 110-117.

[2064] Montes-Molina R, Madroñero-Agreda M A, Romojaro-Rodríguez A B, Gallego-Mendez V, Prados-Cabiedas C, Marques-Lucas C, Pérez-Ferreiro M, Martinez-Ruiz F. Efficacy of Interferential Low-Level Laser Therapy Using Two Independent Sources in the Treatment of Knee Pain. Photomed Laser Surg. 2009 Apr 30. [Epub ahead of print]

[2065] Hegedus B, Viharos L, Gervain M, Gálfi M. The Effect of Low-Level Laser in Knee Osteoarthritis: A Double-Blind, Randomized, Placebo-Controlled Trial. Photomed Laser Surg. 2009 Jun 16. [Epub ahead of print]

[2066] Yamaura M, Yao M, Yaroslavsky I, Cohen R, Smotrich M, Kochevar I E. Low level light effects on inflammatory cytokine production by rheumatoid arthritis synoviocytes. Lasers Surg Med. 2009; 41 (4): 282-290.

[2067] Sandoval M C, Mattiello-Rosa S M, Soares E G, Parizotto N A. Effects of Laser on the Synovial Fluid in the Inflammatory Process of the Knee Joint of the Rabbit. Photomed Laser Surg. 2009 Feb 2. [Epub ahead of print]

[2068] Taniguchi D, Dai P, Hojo T, Yamaoka Y, Kubo T, Takamatsu T. Low-energy laser irradiation promotes synovial fibroblast proliferation by modulating p15 subcellular localization. Lasers Surg Med. 2009; 41 (3): 232-239.

[2069] Mokmeli S, Khazemikho N, Niromanesh S, Vatankhah Z. The Application of Low-Level Laser Therapy after Cesarean Section Does Not Compromise Blood Prolactin Levels and Lactation Status. Photomed Laser Surg. 2009 Apr 30. [Epub ahead of print]

[2070] Pesevska S, Nakova M, Ivanovski K, Angelov N, Kesic L, Obradovic R, Mindova S, Nares S. Dentinal hypersensitivity following scaling and root planing: comparison of low-level laser and topical fluoride treatment. Lasers Med Sci. 2009 Jun 1. [Epub ahead of print]

[2071] Taradaj J, Franek A, Cierpka L et al. Failure of low-level laser therapy to boost healing of venous leg ulcers in surgically and conservatively treated patients. Phlebologie 2008; 37 (5): 241-246.

[2072] Belchior A C, Dos Reis F A, Nicolau R A, Silva I S, Perreira D M, de Carvalho P D. Influence of laser (660 nm) on functional recovery of the sciatic nerve in rats following crushing lesion. Lasers Med Sci. 2009 Feb 6. [Epub ahead of print]

[2073] Kozanoglu E, Basaran S, Paydas S, Sarpel T. Efficacy of pneumatic compression and low-level laser therapy in the treatment of postmastectomy lymphoedema: a randomized controlled trial. Clin Rehabil. 2009; 23 (2):117-124.

[2043] Ramos L, Penna S, Marcos R L et al. Low level infrared laser therapy (810 nm) in experimental skeletal muscle strain: functional and biochemical evaluation. Proc. 7th Internat Congr of WALT, Sun City, South Africa, October 2008, page 132.

[2044] Kazemi-kho N, Babazadeh K, Lajevardi M, Noudeh Y J. Application of low-level laser therapy after coronary artery bypass grafting (CABG) surgery. Proc. 7th Internat Congr of WALT, Sun City, South Africa, October 2008, page 135.

[2045] Khorsand T N, Mokmeli S, Daneshvar L, Soror N, Hosseini H. Comparison between the effect of low level laser therapy and injection of Botox in treatment of anal fissure (clinical trial, case control). Proc. 7th Internat Congr of WALT, Sun City, South Africa, October 2008, page 138.

[2046] Mokmeli S, Bishe Sh, Kahe Kh, Shakhes M. Intravascular laser therapy (IVL) in prehypertension and hypertension conditions. Proc. 7th Internat Congr of WALT, Sun City, South Africa, October 2008, page 140.

[2047] Kato I T, Pellegrini V, Prates R A, Wetter N U, Ribeiro M S, Sugaya N N. Infrared laser irradiation applied to the treatment of burning mouth syndrome. Proc. 7th Internat Congr of WALT, Sun City, South Africa, October 2008, page 140.

[2048] Kazemi-Kho N, Dabaghian F. Effect of blue light intravenous laser on blood sugar in diabetic type 2 patients. Proc. 7th Internat Congr of WALT, Sun City, South Africa, October 2008, page 94.

[2049] Eduardo C d P, Freitas P M, Esteves-Oliveira M, Correa Aranha A C, Müller Ramalho K, Simões A, Bello-Silva M S, Tunér J. Laser Phototherapy in the Treatment of Periodontal Disease: A literature review. Submitted for publication 2009.

[2050] Trimmer P A, Schwartz K M, Borland M K, De Taboada L, Streeter J, Oron U. Reduced axonal transport in Parkinson's disease cybrid neurites is restored by light therapy. Mol Neurodegen. 2009 Jun 17; 4 (1): 26. [Epub ahead of print]

[2051] Sussai D A, Carvalho P D, Dourado D M, Belchior A C, Dos Reis F A, Pereira D M. Low-level laser therapy attenuates creatine kinase levels and apoptosis during forced swimming in rats. Lasers Med Sci. 2009 Jun 25. [Epub ahead of print]

[2052] Junior E C, Lopes-Martins R A, Baroni B M, De Marchi T, Rossi R P, Grosselli D, Generosi R A, de Godoi V, Basso M, Mancalossi J L, Bjordal J M. Comparison Between Single-Diode Low-Level Laser Therapy (LPT) and LED Multi-Diode (Cluster) Therapy (LEDT) Applications Before High-Intensity Exercise. Photomed Laser Surg. 2009 Mar 20. [Epub ahead of print]

[2053] Hübler R, Blando E, Gaião L, Kreisner P E, Post L K, Xavier C B, de Oliveira M G. Effects of low-level laser therapy on bone formed after distraction osteogenesis. Lasers Med Sci. 2009 Jun 23. [Epub ahead of print]

[2054] Kazem Shakouri S, Soleimanpour J, Salekzamani Y, Oskuie M R. Effect of low-level laser therapy on the fracture healing process. Lasers Med Sci. 2009 Apr 28. [Epub ahead of print]

[2055] Bouvet-Gerbettaz S, Merigo E, Rocca J P, Carle G F, Rochet N. Effects of low-level laser therapy on proliferation and differentiation of murine bone marrow cells into osteoblasts and osteoclasts. Lasers Surg Med. 2009; 41 (4): 291-297.

[2056] Hou J F, Zhang H, Yuan X, Li J, Wei Y J, Hu S S. In vitro effects of low-level laser irradiation for bone marrow mesenchymal stem cells: proliferation, growth factors secretion and myogenic differentiation. Lasers Surg Med. 2008; 40 (10): 726-733.

[2057] Zivin J A, Albers G W, Bornstein N, Chippendale T, Dahlof B, Devlin T, Fisher M, Hacke W, Holt W, Ilic S, Kasner S, Lew R, Nash M, Perez J, Rymer M, Schellinger P, Schneider D, Schwab S, Veltkamp R, Walker M, Streeter J. Effectiveness and safety of transcranial laser therapy for acute ischemic stroke. Stroke. 2009; 40 (4): 1359-1364.

[2027] Imbronito A V, Okuda O S, Maria de Freitas N, Moreira Lotufo R F, Nunes F D. Detection of Herpesviruses and Periodontal Pathogens in Subgingival Plaque of Patients With Chronic Periodontitis, Generalized Aggressive Periodontitis, or Gingivitis. J Periodontol. 2008; 79(12): 2313-2321.

[2028] Obradovic R R, Kesic L G, Peševska S. Influence of low-level laser therapy on biomaterial osseointegration: a mini-review. Lasers Med Sci. 2009; 24 (3): 447-451.

[2029] Vasheghani M M, Bayat M, Rezaei F, Bayat A, Karimipour M. Effect of low-level laser therapy on mast cells in second-degree burns in rats. Photomed Laser Surg. 2008; 26 (1): 1-5.

[2030] Zhevago N A, Samoilova K A, Obolenskaya K D. The regulatory effect of polychromatic (visible and infrared) light on human humoral immunity. Photochem Photobiol Sci. 2004; 3 (1): 102-108.

[2031] Samoilova K A, Bogacheva O N, Obolenskaya K D, Blinova M I, Kalmykova NV, Kuzminikh E V. Enhancement of the blood growth promoting activity after exposure of volunteers to visible and infrared polarized light. Part I: stimulation of human keratinocyte proliferation in vitro. Photochem Photobiol Sci. 2004; 3 (1): 96-101.

[2032] Samoilova K A, Zhevago N A, Menshutina M A, Grigorieva N B. Role of nitric oxide in the visible light-induced rapid increase of human skin microcirculation at the local and systemic level: I. diabetic patients. Photomed Laser Surg. 2008; 26 (5): 433-442.

[2033] Foyaca-Sibat H, Ibañez-Valdés L. Laser therapy in zoster neuropathy - HIV related. Proc. 7th Internat Congr of WALT, Sun City, South Africa, October 2008, page 100.

[2034] Meneguzzo D T, Pallotta R, Ramos L, Penna S, Marcos R L, Teixeira S, Muscará M N, Bjordal J M, Lopes-Martins R A, Ribeiro M S. Near infrared laser therapy (810 nm) on lymph nodes: Effects on acute inflammatory process. Proc. 7th Internat Congr of WALT, Sun City, South Africa, October 2008, page 11.

[2035] Carvalho C, Nascimento F, Cangussu M, Gerbi M M, Marques A M, Pinheiro A L. The association of wavelengths is effective on the reduction of TMJ pain. A clinical study in a Brazilian population. Proc. 7th Internat Congr of WALT, Sun City, South Africa, October 2008, page 33.

[2036] Almeida-Lopes L, Pretel H, Moraes V et al. Effects of continuous and pulsed infrared laser application on bone repair using different energy doses. Study in rats. Proc. 7th Internat Congr of WALT, Sun City, South Africa, October 2008, page 86.

[2037] Zanin T, Zanin F, Carvalhosa A, Castro P H, Brugnera Jr A. Diode laser 660 nm in the prevention and treatment of oral mucositis. Proc. 7th Internat Congr of WALT, Sun City, South Africa, October 2008, page 28.

[2038] Al-Anazi A, Al Watban F A H, Zhang X Y, Andres B L. The effects of low power laser therapy with different wavelengths in accelerating wound healing on diabetic rats. Proc. 7th Internat Congr of WALT, Sun City, South Africa, October 2008, page 96.

[2039] Powell K, Laakso L, Low P, Ralph S. The in vitro effects of laser irradiation on human breast carcinoma and immortalised human mammary epithelial cell lines. Proc. 7th Internat Congr of WALT, Sun City, South Africa, October 2008, page 104.

[2040] Anders J J, Ilev I. Light interaction with human central nervous system progenitor cells. Proc. 7th Internat Congr of WALT, Sun City, South Africa, October 2008, page 106.

[2041] Hou Y-H, Hou Y-Q, Fang X. Effective therapy of low level laser in 810 nm wavelength on severe acne. Proc. 7th Internat Congr of WALT, Sun City, South Africa, October 2008, page 117.

[2042] Marcos R L, Bjordal J M, Pallota R C et al. The effect of low level laser therapy (infrared, 810 nm) on collagenase induced rat achilles tendinitis: COX-1 and COX-2 expression and prostaglandin E2 production. Proc. 7th Internat Congr of WALT, Sun City, South Africa, October 2008, page 128.

[2010] Igic M, Kesic L, Apostolovic M, Kostadinovic L. [Low-level laser efficiency in the therapy of chronic gingivitis in children] [in Serbian]. Vojnosanit Pregl. 2008; 65 (10): 755-757.

[2011] Krechina E K, Shidova A V, Maslova V V. [Comparative evaluation of influence of low-intensity laser radiation of different spectrum components and regimen of laser work upon microcirculation in comprehensive treatment of chronic parodontitis]. [Article in Russian] Stomatologiia (Mosk). 2008; 87 (3): 24-27.

[2012] Cressoni M D, Dib Giusti H H, Casarotto R A, Anaruma C A. The Effects of a 785-nm AlGaInP Laser on the Regeneration of Rat Anterior Tibialis Muscle After Surgically-Induced Injury. Photomed Laser Surg. 2008 Sep 18. [Epub ahead of print]

[2013] Wu C S, Hu S C, Lan C C, Chen G S, Chuo W H, Yu H S. Low-energy helium-neon laser therapy induces repigmentation and improves the abnormalities of cutaneous microcirculation in segmental-type vitiligo lesions. Kaohsiung J Med Sci. 2008; 24 (4): 180-189.

[2014] Vescovi P, Merigo E, Manfredi M, Meleti M, Fornaini C, Bonanini M, Rocca J P, Nammour S. Nd:YAG laser biostimulation in the treatment of bisphosphonate-associated osteonecrosis of the jaw: clinical experience in 28 cases. Photomed Laser Surg. 2008; 26 (1): 37-46.

[2015] Grönqvist J, Häggman-Eriksson B, Eriksson P-O. Impaired jaw function and eating difficulties in Whiplash-associated disorders. Swed Dent J. 2008; 32 (4): 171-177.

[2016] Márquez Martínez M E, Pinheiro A L, Ramalho L M. Effect of IR laser photobiomodulation on the repair of bone defects grafted with organic bovine bone. Lasers Med Sci. 2008; 23 (3): 313-317.

[2017] Yasukawa A, Hrui H, Koyama Y, Nagai M, Takakuda K. The effect of low reactive-level laser therapy (LLLT) with helium-neon laser on operative wound healing in a rat model. J Vet Med Sci. 2007; 69 (8): 799-806.

[2018] Ng G Y, Fung D T. Combining therapeutic laser and herbal remedy for treating ligament injury: an ultrastructural morphological study. Photomed Laser Surg. 2008; 26 (5): 425-432.

[2019] Karu T, Pyatibrat L, Kalendo G. Irradiation with He-Ne laser increases ATP level in cells cultivated in vitro. J Photochem Photobiol B. 1995; 27 (3): 219-223.

[2020] Chang W D, Wu J H, Jiang J A, Yeh C Y, Tsai C T. Carpal tunnel syndrome treated with a diode laser: a controlled treatment of the transverse carpal ligament. Photomed Laser Surg. 2008; 26 (6): 551-557.

[2021] Ahmed N A, Radwan N M, Ibrahim K M, Khedr M E, El Aziz M A, Khadrawy Y A. Effect of three different intensities of infrared laser energy on the levels of amino acid neurotransmitters in the cortex and hippocampus of rat brain. Photomed Laser Surg. 2008; 26 (5): 479-488.

[2022] Shen-Zheng, Xiao-Jian, Lin S Z, Wang L H. Effects of laser guided by optic fiber into rat brain on conditioned avoidance response and brain chemistry. Lasers Surg Med. 1983; 2 (3): 231-239.

[2023] Igarashi H, Inomata K. Effects of low-power gallium aluminium arsenide diode laser irradiation on the development of synapses in the neonatal rat hippocampus. Acta Anat (Basel). 1991; 140 (2): 150-155.

[2024] Majlesi G. GaAs laser treatment of bilateral eyelid ptosis due to complication of botulinum toxin type A injection. Photomed Laser Surg. 2008; 26 (5): 507-509.

[2025] Neira R, Arroyave J, Ramirez H, Ortiz C L, Solarte E, Sequeda F, Gutierrez M I. Fat liquefaction: effect of low-level laser energy on adipose tissue. Plast Reconstr Surg. 2002; 110 (3): 912-22; discussion 923-925.

[2026] Enwemeka C S. Standard Parameters in Laser Phototherapy. Editorial. Photomed Laser Surg. 2008; 26 (5): 411.

[1993] Pozza D H, Fregapani P W, Weber J B, de Oliveira M G, de Oliveira M A, Ribeiro Neto N, de Macedo Sobrinho J B. Analgesic action of laser therapy (LLLT) in an animal model. Med Oral Patol Oral Cir Bucal. 2008; 13 (10): 648-652.

[1994] Blaya D S, Guimarães M B, Pozza D H, Weber J B, de Oliveira M G. Histologic study of the effect of laser therapy on bone repair. J Contemp Dent Pract. 2008; 9 (6): 41-48.

[1995] Shirani A M, Gutknecht N, Taghizadeh M, Mir M. Low-level laser therapy and myofacial pain dysfunction syndrome: a randomized controlled clinical trial. Lasers Med Sci. 2008; Nov 12. [Epub ahead of print]

[1996] Shooshtari S M, Badiee V, Taghizadeh S H, Nematollahi A H, Amanollahi A H, Grami M T. The effects of low level laser in clinical outcome and neurophysiological results of carpal tunnel syndrome. Electromyogr Clin Neurophysiol. 2008; 48 (5): 229-231.

[1997] Chen K H, Hong C Z, Kuo F C, Hsu H C, Hsieh Y L. Electrophysiologic effects of a therapeutic laser on myofascial trigger spots of rabbit skeletal muscles. Am J Phys Med Rehabil. 2008; 87 (12): 1006-1014.

[1998] Doin-Silva R, Baranauskas V, Rodrigues-Simioni L, da Cruz-Höfling M A. The Ability of Low Level Laser Therapy to Prevent Muscle Tissue Damage Induced by Snake Venom. Photochem Photobiol. 2008 Jul 17. [Epub ahead of print]

[1999] Hagiwara S, Iwasaka H, Hasegawa A, Noguchi T. Pre-Irradiation of blood by gallium aluminum arsenide (830 nm) low-level laser enhances peripheral endogenous opioid analgesia in rats. Anesth Analg. 2008; 107 (3): 1058-1063.

[2000] Hagiwara S, Iwasaka H, Okuda K, Noguchi T. GaAlAs (830 nm) low-level laser enhances peripheral endogenous opioid analgesia in rats. Lasers Surg Med. 2007; 39 (10): 797-802.

[2001] Gál P, Mokrý M, Vidinský B, Kilík R, Depta F, Haraka?ová M, Longauer F, Mozeš S, Sabo J. Effect of equal daily doses achieved by different power densities of low-level laser therapy at 635 nm on open skin wound healing in normal and corticosteroid-treated rats. Lasers Med Sci. 2008 Aug 21. [Epub ahead of print]

[2002] Lapchak P A, Han M K, Salgado K F, Streeter J, Zivin J A. Safety profile of transcranial near-infrared laser therapy administered in combination with thrombolytic therapy to embolized rabbits. Stroke. 2008; 39 (11): 3073-3078.

[2003] Chen Y S, Hsu S F, Chiu C W, Lin J G, Chen C T, Yao C H. Effect of low-power pulsed laser on peripheral nerve regeneration in rats. Microsurgery. 2005; 25 (1): 83-89.

[2004] Tunér J. Is low-power pulsed laser ineffective in neural growth? Microsurgery. 2009; 29 (3): 251.

[2005] Rochkind S, Ouaknine G E. New trand in neuroscience: Low-power laser effect on peripheral and central nerve system (basic science, preclinical and clinical studies). Neurol Res. 1992; 14: 2-11.

[2006] Leal Junior E C, Lopes-Martins R A, Dalan F, Ferrari M, Sbabo F M, Generosi R A, Baroni B M, Penna S C, Iversen V V, Bjordal J M. Effect of 655-nm low-level laser therapy on exercise-induced skeletal muscle fatigue in humans. Photomed Laser Surg. 2008; 26 (5): 419-24.

[2007] Ribeiro D A, Matsumoto M A. Low-level laser therapy improves bone repair in rats treated with anti-inflammatory drugs. J Oral Rehabil. 2008; 35 (12): 925-933.

[2008] Dos Reis F A, Belchior A C, de Carvalho P D, da Silva B A, Pereira D M, Silva I S, Nicolau R A. Effect of laser therapy (660 nm) on recovery of the sciatic nerve in rats after injury through neurotmesis followed by epineural anastomosis. Lasers Med Sci. 2008 Dec 23. [Epub ahead of print]

[2009] Hou J F, Zhang H, Yuan X, Li J, Wei Y J, Hu S S. In vitro effects of low-level laser irradiation for bone marrow mesenchymal stem cells: proliferation, growth factors secretion and myogenic differentiation. Lasers Surg Med. 2008; 40 (10):726-733.

[1975] Treutlein H, Schulten K, Brünger A T, Karplus M, Deisenhofer J, Michel H. Chromophore-protein interactions and the function of the photosynthetic reaction center: a molecular dynamics study. Proc Natl Acad Sci USA. 1992; 89 (1): 75-79.

[1976] Cedillo Valle B. An evaluation of the enantiomeric recognition of amino acid based polymeric surfactants and cyclodextrins using spectroscopic and chromatographic methods. Dissertation Faculty of the Louisiana State University and Agricultural and Mechanical College December 2005.

[1978] van Thor J J, Mackeen M, Kuprov I et al. Chromophore structure in the photocycle of the cyanobacterial phytochrome CPH1. Biophys J BioFAST, published on June 2, 2006.

[1979] Verhoeven M A. Electronic and Spatial Characteristics of the Retinylidene Chromophore of Rhodopsin. Dissertation, University of Leiden, The Netherlands, November 2005.

[1980] Wiederrecht G P, Seibert M, Govindjee, Wasielewski M R. Femtosecond photodichroism studies of isolated photosystem II reaction centers. Proc Natl Acad Sci USA. 1994; 91 (19): 8999-9003.

[1981] Winterle J S, Einarsdóttir O. Photoreactions of cytochrome C oxidase. Photochem Photobiol. 2006; 82 (3): 711-719.

[1982] Volkov V, Svirko Y P, Kamalov V F, Song L, El-Sayed M A. Optical rotation of the second harmonic radiation from retinal in bacteriorhodopsin monomers in Langmuir-Blodgett film: evidence for nonplanar retinal structure. Biophys J. 1997; 73 (6): 3164-3170.

[1983] Xu D, Klaus Schulten K. Coupling of Protein Motion to Electron Transfer in a Photosynthetic Reaction Center: Investigating the Low Temperature Behavior in the Framework of the Spin-Boson Model. Department of Physics and Beckman Institute, University of Illinois at Urbana-Champaign, Urbana, IL 61801, USA. August 23, 2000.

[1984] Zyss J. Renewed perspectives in Molecular Photonics and Biophotonics at the micro- and nano-scales. Proceedings of the Symposium on Photonics Technologies for 7th Framework Program, Wroclaw, Poland, 12-14 October 2006.

[1985] Nes A G, Posso M B. Patients with moderate chemotherapy-induced mucositis: pain therapy using low intensity lasers. Int Nurs Rev. 2005; 52 (1): 68-72.

[1986] Jaguar G C, Prado J D, Nishimoto I N, Pinheiro M C, de Castro D O Jr, da Cruz Perez D E, Alves F A. Low-energy laser therapy for prevention of oral mucositis in hematopoietic stem cell transplantation. Oral Dis. 2007; 13 (6): 538-543.

[1987] Tumilty S, Munn J, Abbott J H, McDonough S, Hurley D A, Baxter G D. Laser therapy in the treatment of achilles tendinopathy: a pilot study. Photomed Laser Surg. 2008; 26 (1): 25-30.

[1988] Carrasco T G, Mazzetto M O, Mazzetto R G, Mestriner W Jr. Low intensity laser therapy in temporomandibular disorder: a phase II double-blind study. Cranio. 2008; 26 (4): 274-281.

[1989] da Cunha L A, Firoozmand L M, da Silva A P, Esteves S A, Oliveira W. Efficacy of low-level laser therapy in the treatment of temporomandibular disorder. Int Dent J. 2008; 58 (4): 213-217.

[1990] França C M, Núñez S C, Prates R A, Noborikawa E, Faria M R, Ribeiro M S. Low-intensity red laser on the prevention and treatment of induced-oral mucositis in hamsters. J Photochem Photobiol B. 2009; 94 (1): 25-31.

[1991] Mirzaii-Dizgah I, Ojaghi R, Sadeghipour-Roodsari H R, Karimian S M, Sohanaki H. Attenuation of morphine withdrawal signs by low level laser therapy in rats. Behav Brain Res. 2009; 196 (2): 268-270.

[1992] Zhang L, Xing D, Zhu D, Chen Q. Low-power laser irradiation inhibiting Abeta25-35-induced PC12 cell apoptosis via PKC activation. Cell Physiol Biochem. 2008; 22 (1-4): 215-222.

[1955] Benedicenti S, Pepe I M, Angiero F, Benedicenti A. Intracellular ATP level increases in lymphocytes irradiated with infrared laser light of wavelength 904 nm. Photomed Laser Surg. 2008; 26 (5): 451-453.

[1956] Cojocariu C, Rochon P. Synthesis and optical storage properties of a novel polymethacrylate with benzothiazole azo chromophore in the side chain. J Mater Chem. 2004; 14: 2909-2916.

[1957] Esquerra R M, Che D, Shapiro D B, Lewis J W, Bogomolni R A, Fukushima J, Kliger D S. Chromophore reorientations in the early photolysis intermediates of bacteriorhodopsin. Biophys J. 1996; 70 (2): 962-970.

[1958] Estep T N E, Thompson T E. Energy transfer in lipid bilayers. Biophys J. 1979: 26: 195-208.

[1959] Faxén K, Gilderson G, Ädelroth P, Brzezinski P. A mechanistic principle for proton pumping by cytochrome c oxidase. Nature. 2005; 437: 286-289.

[1960] Frauenfelder H. The Conformational Energy Surface. Princeton University. http://wwwphy.princeton.edu/~austin/hf_book/chapter23.pdf.

[1961] Godfrey R. Photoselection and circular dichroism in the purple membrane. Biophys J. 1982; 38:1-6.

[1962] Heyn M P, Borucki B, Otto H. Chromophore reorientation during the photocycle of bacteriorhodopsin: experimental methods and functional significance. Biochim Biophys Acta. 2000; 1460 (1): 60-74.

[1963] Kawato S, Sigel E, Carafoli E, Cherry R J. Cytochrome oxidase rotates in the inner membrane of intact mitochondria and submitochondrial particles. J Biol Chem. 1980; 255 (12): 5508-5510.

[1964] Kawato S, Kinoshita K. Time-dependent absorption anisotropy and rotational diffusion of proteins in membranes. Biophys J. 1981; 36: 277-296.

[1965] Kimura Y, Fujiwara M, Ikegami A. Anisotropic electric properties of purple membrane and their change during the photoreaction cycle. Biophys J. 1984; 45: 615-625.

[1966] Korchemskaya E Y, Stepanchikov D A, Druzhko A B Dyukova T V. Mechanism of Nonlinear Photoinduced Anisotropy in Bacteriorhodopsin and its Derivatives. J Biol Phys. 1999; 24: 201-215.

[1967] Kotlyar A, Borovok N, Hazani M, Szundi I, Einarsdóttir O. Photoinduced intracomplex electron transfer between cytochrome c oxidase and TUPS-modified cytochrome c. Eur J Biochem. 2000; 267 (18): 5805-5809.

[1968] Kourmanov B. Light torque induced by polarized laser beam in an optical trap. Thesis for the Degree of Master in Science. Wake Forest Univiersity. N.C., USA. 2002.

[1969] Lanyi J K, Luecke H. Bacteriorhodopsin. Current Opinion in Structural Biology 2001; 11: 415-419.

[1970] Li J, Yao G, Wang L V. Degree of polarization in laser speckles from turbid media: implications in tissue optics. J Biomed Opt. 2002; 7 (3):307-312.

[1971] Lin S W, Mathies R A. Orientation of the protonated retinal Schiff base group in bacteriorhodopsin from absorption linear dichroism. Biophys. J. 1989; 56: 653-660.

[1972] Palto S P, Durand G. Friction Model of Photo-induced Reorientation of Optical Axis in Photo-oriented Langmuir-Blodgett Films. J. Phys. II France. 1995; 5: 963-978.

[1973] Lancaster C R, Michel H. The coupling of light-induced electron transfer and proton uptake as derived from crystal structures of reaction centres from Rhodopseudomonas viridis modified at the binding site of the secondary quinone, QB. Structure. 1997; 5 (10): 1339-1359.

[1974] Shand M L, Chance R R. Raman photoselection and conjugation-length dispersion in conjugated polymer solutions. Physical Review B. 1982; 25 (7): 4431-4436.

[1935] Sliney D H. Risks of occupational exposure to optical radiation. Med Lav. 2006; 97 (2): 215-220.

[1936] Hietanen M. Health risks of exposure to non-ionizing radiation - myths or science-based evidence. Med Lav. 2006; 97 (2): 184-188.

[1937] Bernhardt J H. [Electrosmog, cellular phones, sunbeds etc. - adverse health effects from radiation? Health aspects of non-ionizing radiation] Bundesgesundheitsblatt Gesundheitsforschung Gesundheitsschutz. 2005; 48 (1): 63-75. [Article in German]

[1938] Marshall J. The safety of laser pointers: myths and realities. Br J Ophthalmol. 1998; 82 (11): 1335-1338.

[1939] Behling A A. Low Level Laser Therapy and Women's Health. Swedish Laser Medical Society Symposium, Stockholm, Sweden, May 2008.

[1940] Boschi E S, Leite C E, Saciura V C, Caberlon E, Lunardelli A, Bitencourt S, Melo D A, Oliveira J R. Anti-Inflammatory effects of low-level laser therapy (660 nm) in the early phase in carrageenan-induced pleurisy in rat. Lasers Surg Med. 2008; 40 (7): 500-508.

[1941] Komatsu M, Kubo T, Kogure S, Matsuda Y, Watanabe K. Effects of 808 nm low-power laser irradiation on the muscle contraction of frog gastrocnemius. Lasers Surg Med. 2008; 40 (8): 576-583.

[1942] Grande S R, Imbronito A V, Okuda O S, Lotufo R F, Magalhães M H, Nunes F D. Herpes viruses in periodontal compromised sites: comparison between HIV-positive and- negative patients. J Clin Periodontol. 2008; 35 (10): 838-845.

[1943] Rotola A, Cassai E, Farina R, Caselli E, Gentili V, Lazzarotto T, Trombelli L. Human herpesvirus 7, Epstein-Barr virus and human cytomegalovirus in periodontal tissues of periodontally diseased and healthy subjects. J Clin Periodontol. 2008; 35 (10): 831-837.

[1944] Gavish L, Perez L S, Reissman P, Gertz S D. Irradiation with 780 nm diode laser attenuates inflammatory cytokines but upregulates nitric oxide in lipopolysaccharide-stimulated macrophages: implications for the prevention of aneurysm progression. Lasers Surg Med. 2008; 40 (5): 371-378.

[1945] Gavish L, Perez L S, Gertz S D. Low-level laser irradiation modulates matrix metalloproteinase activity and gene expression in porcine aortic smooth muscle cells. Lasers Surg Med. 2008; 38 (8): 779-786.

[1946] Ahl P L, Cone R A. Light activates rotations of bacteriorhodopsin in the purple membrane. Biophysical Journal. 1984; 45: 1039-1049.

[1947] Angiolillo P J, Vanderkooi. J M. The Photoexcited Triplet State as a Probe of Chromophore-Protein Interaction in Myoglobin. Biophysical Journal. 1998; 75 1491-1502.

[1948] Ashkin A. Optical trapping and manipulation of neutral particles using lasers. Proc. Natl. Acad. Sci. USA. 1997; 94: 4853-4860.

[1949] Babcock G, Vickery L E, Palmer G. Electronic state of Heme in cytochrome-c oxidase. J Biol Chem. 1976; 251 (24): 790-791.

[1950] Belevich I, Verkhovsky M I, Wikström M. Proton-coupled electron transfer drives the protonpump of cytochrome c oxidase. Nature, 2006; 440: 829-832.

[1951] Bell T D M, Habutchi S, Österling I et al. Single photon emission from dendrimer containing eight perylene diimides chromophores. Aust J Chem. 2004; 57: 1169-1173.

[1952] Bonin K D, Kourmanov B, Walker T G. Light torque nanocontrol, nanomotors and nanorockers. Optic Express. 2002; 10 (19): 984-989.

[1953] Boxer S G, Roelofs M G. Chromophore organization in photosynthetic reaction centers: High-resolution magnetophotoselection. Proc Natl Acad Sci USA. 1979; 76 (11): 5636-5640.

[1954] Cameron R, Tabisz G C. Observation of two-photon optical rotation by molecules. Molecular Phys. 1997; 90 (2): 159-164.

[1917] Fujita S, Yamaguchi M, Utsunomiya T, Yamamoto H, Kasai K. Low-energy laser stimulates tooth movement velocity via expression of RANK and RANKL. Orthod Craniofac Res. 2008; 11 (3): 143-155.

[1918] Diniz J S, Nicolau R A, de Melo Ocarino N, do Carmo Magalhães F, de Oliveira Pereira R D, Serakides R. Effect of low-power gallium-aluminum-arsenium laser therapy (830 nm) in combination with bisphosphonate treatment on osteopenic bone structure: an experimental animal study. Lasers Med Sci. 2008 Jul 22. [Epub ahead of print]

[1919] Rhee C-K, Lim E-S, Kim Y-S, Cung Y-W et al. Effect of low level laser (LLL) on cochlear and vestibular inner ear including tinnitus. Proc. SPIE. Progress in Biomedical Optics and Imaging. 2006; 7 (1). ISSN 1605-7422.

[1920] Pinheiro A L, Gerbi M E. Photoengineering of bone repair processes. Photomed Laser Surg. 2006; 24 (2): 169-178.

[1921] Ozcelik O, Cenk Haytac M, Seydaoglu G. Enamel matrix derivative and low-level laser therapy in the treatment of intra-bony defects: a randomized placebo-controlled clinical trial. Clin Periodontol. 2008; 35 (2): 147-156.

[1922] Matsumoto M A, Ferino R V, Monteleone G F, Ribeiro D A. Low-level laser therapy modulates cyclo-oxygenase-2 expression during bone repair in rats. Lasers Med Sci. 2008 Feb 29 [Epub ahead of print]

[1923] Cuda D, De Caria A. [Efficacia della terapia laser a bassa potenza (© Tinnitool) nel trattamento degli acufeni cronici associati a patologia cocleare: risultati definitivi.] Centro per lo studio e la Cura degli Acufeni Unità operativa di Otorinolaringoiatria Ospedale "G. da Saliceto" Piacenza, Italy. Unpublished material.

[1924] Desmons S O, Delfosse C J, Rochon P, Buys B, Penel G, Mordon S. Laser preconditioning of calvarial bone prior to an X-ray radiation injury: a preliminary in vivo study of the vascular response. Lasers Surg Med. 2008; 40 (1): 28-37.

[1925] Bjordal J M, Lopes-Martins R A, Joensen J, Couppe C, Ljunggren A E, Stergioulas A, Johnson M I. A systematic review with procedural assessments and meta-analysis of low level laser therapy in lateral elbow tendinopathy (tennis elbow). BMC Musculoskelet Disord. 2008; 29 (9): 75.

[1926] Houreld N, Abrahamse H. Laser light influences cellular viability and proliferation in diabetic-wounded fibroblast cells in a dose- and wavelength-dependent manner. Lasers Med Sci. 2008; 23 (1): 11-18.

[1927] Houreld N, Abrahamse H. Irradiation with a 632.8 nm helium-neon laser with 5 J/cm^2 stimulates proliferation and expression of interleukin-6 in diabetic wounded fibroblast cells. Diabetes Technol Ther. 2007; 9 (5): 451-459.

[1928] Yip S, Zivin J. Laser therapy in acute stroke treatment. Int J Stroke. 2008; 3 (2): 88-91.

[1929] Sliney D, Aron-Rosa D, DeLori F, Fankhauser F, Landry R, Mainster M, Marshall J, Rassow B, Stuck B, Trokel S, West T M, Wolffe M. Adjustment of guidelines for exposure of the eye to optical radiation from ocular instruments: statement from a task group of the International Commission on Non-Ionizing Radiation Protection (ICNIRP) Appl Opt. 2005; 44 (11): 2162-2176.

[1930] Harris M D, Lincoln A E, Amoroso P J, Stuck B, Sliney D. Laser eye injuries in military occupations. Aviat Space Environ Med. 2003; 74 (9): 947-952.

[1931] Tengroth B. [Ban the laser weapons! Invisible rays may cause permanent blindness in thousands of war victims] [Article in Swedish]. Lakartidningen. 1995; 92 (9): 837.

[1932] Peters A. Blinding laser weapons. Med Confl Surviv. 1996; 12 (2): 107-113.

[1933] Hudson S J. Eye injuries from laser exposure: a review. Aviat Space Environ Med. 1998; 69 (5): 519-524.

[1934] Barkana Y, Belkin M. Laser eye injuries. Surv Ophthalmol. 2000; 44 (6): 459-478.

[1899] Ribeiro M, Sugayama S T, Nogueira G, Franca C A et al. Angiogenesis induced by low-intensity laser therapy: comparative study between single and fractionated dose on burn healing. BiOS 2008. Proceedings of SPIE; Volume 6846-12.

[1900] Brill G E, Budnik I A, Gasparyan L V. Influence of helium-neon laser radiation on platelet function. BiOS 2008. Proceedings of SPIE; Volume 6846-20.

[1901] Senhorino H C, Bichinho G L, Nohama P, Gariba M A. Morphometric effects of different energy densities of diode laser on adipose tissue in rats. BiOS 2008. Proceedings of SPIE; Volume 6846-59.

[1902] Corrral-Baqués M I, Riveira M M, Rodríguez-Gil J E, Rigau J. The effect of low-level laser irradiation on dog spermatozoa motility is dependent on laser output power. Lasers in Medical Science. September 12, 2008. [Epub ahead of print]

[1903] Chagas-Oliveira P, Meireles G C S, dos Santos N R, de Carvalho C M et al. The Use of Light Photobiomodulation on the Treatment of Second-Degree Burns: A Histological Study of a Rodent Model. Photomed Laser Surg. 2008; 26 (4): 289-299.

[1904] Reis S R, Medrado A P, Marchionni A M, Figueira C, Fracassi L D, Knop L A. Effect of 670-nm laser therapy and dexamethasone on tissue repair: a histological and ultrastructural study. Photomed Laser Surg. 2008; 26 (4): 307-313.

[1905] Torres C S, dos Santos J N, Monteiro J S, Amorim P G, Pinheiro A L. Does the use of laser photobiomodulation, bone morphogenetic proteins, and guided bone regeneration improve the outcome of autologous bone grafts? An in vivo study in a rodent model. Photomed Laser Surg. 2008; 26 (4): 371-377.

[1906] Ribeiro I W, Sbrana M C, Esper L A, Almeida A L. Evaluation of the effect of the GaAlAs laser on subgingival scaling and root planing. Photomed Laser Surg. 2008; 26 (4): 387-391.

[1907] Silveira L B, Prates R A, Novelli M D, Marigo H A, Garrocho A A, Amorim J C, Sousa G R, Pinotti M, Ribeiro M S. Investigation of mast cells in human gingiva following low-intensity laser irradiation. Photomed Laser Surg. 2008; 26 (4): 315-321.

[1908] Pires Oliveira D A, de Oliveira R F, Zangaro R A, Soares C P. Evaluation of low-level laser therapy of osteoblastic cells. Photomed Laser Surg. 2008; 26 (4): 401-404.

[1909] Grzesiak Janas G, Janas A. Laser biostimulation in treatment of actinomycosis. Proc SPIE ; Vol. 5229: 135-139.

[1910] Bortolleto R, Silva N S, Zangaro R A, Pacheco M T T et al. Mitochondrial membrane potential after low-power laser irradiation. Laser Med Sci. 2004; 18: 204-206.

[1911] Markovic A, Todorovic L J. Effectiveness of dexemethasone and low-power laser in minimizing oedema after thrid molar surgery: a clinical trial. J Oral Maxillofac Surg. 2007; 36: 226-229.

[1912] Whittaker P, Patterson M J. Ventricular remodeling after acute myocardial infarction: effect of low-intensity laser irradiation. Laser Surg Med. 2000; 27: 29-38.

[1913] Aboelsaad N S, Soory M, Gadalla L M, Ragab L I, Dunne S, Zalata K R, Louca C. Effect of soft laser and bioactive glass on bone regeneration in the treatment of infra-bony defects (a clinical study). Lasers Med Sci. 2009; 24 (4): 527-533.

[1914] Aboelsaad N S, Soory M, Gadalla L M, Ragab L I, Dunne S, Zalata K R, Louca C. Effect of soft laser and bioactive glass on bone regeneration in the treatment of infra-bony defects (a clinical study). Lasers Med Sci. 2009; 24 (4): 527-533.

[1915] Xu M, Tietao D, Feizhi M, Bin D, Wingho L, Pingxiang D, Xiaohui Z, Songhao L. Low-Intensity Pulsed Laser Irradiation Affects RANKL and OPG mRNA Expression in Rat Calvarial Cells. Photomed Laser Surg. 2009; 27 (2): 309-315.

[1916] Lai S M, Zee K Y, Lai M K, Corbet E F. Clinical and Radiographic Investigation of the Adjunctive Effects of a Low-Power He-Ne Laser in the Treatment of Moderate to Advanced Periodontal Disease: A Pilot Study. Photomed Laser Surg. 2008 Sep 11. [Epub ahead of print]

[1882] Ferreira A N S, Silveira L B, Genovese W J, Cavalcante de Araujo V, Frigo L et al. Effect of GaAlAs Laser on Reactional Dentinogenesis Induction in Human Teeth. Photomed Laser Surg. 2006; 24 (3): 358-365.

[1883] Cuda D, De Caria A. Combined counselling and low level laser stimulation effectiveness in the treatment of disturbing chronic tinnitus. The International Tinnitus Journal. 2008; 14 (2): 175-80.

[1884] Fridberger A, Ren T. Local mechanical stimulation of the hearing organ by laser irradiation. Neuroreport. 2006;17(1): 33-37.

[1885] Gungor A, Dogru S, Cincik H, Erkul E, Poyrazoglu E. Effectiveness of transmeatal low power laser irradiation for chronic tinnitus. Laryngol Otol. 2008; 122 (5): 447-451.

[1886] Hawkins D, Abrahamse H. Effect of Multiple Exposures of Low-Level Laser Therapy on the Cellular Responses of Wounded Human Skin Fibroblasts. Photomed Laser Surg. 2006; 24 (6): 705-714.

[1886] Fikackova H, Dostalova T, Vosicka R, Peterova V, Navratil L, Lesak J. Arthralgia of the Temporomandibular Joint and Low-Level Laser Therapy. Photomec Laser Surg. 2006; 24 (4): 522-527.

[1887] Bicalho Rabelo S, Balbin Villaverde A , Amadei Nicolau R, Castillo Salgado M A et al. Comparison between Wound Healing in Induced Diabetic and Nondiabetic Rats after Low-Level Laser Therapy. Photomed Laser Surg. 2006; 24 (4): 474-479.

[1888] Douris P, Southard V, Ferrigi R, Joshua Grauer J et al. Effect of Phototherapy on Delayed Onset Muscle Soreness. Photomed Laser Surg. 2006; 24 (3): 377-382.

[1889] Bashardoust Tajali S, Macdermid J C, Houghton P, Grewal R. Effects of low power laser irradiation on bone healing in animals: a meta-analysis. Lasers Med Sci. 2010 Feb 6. [Epub ahead of print]

[1890] Tullberg M, Ernberg M. Long-term effect on tinnitus by treatment of temporomandibular disorders: a two-year follow-up by questionnaire. Acta Odontol Scand. 2006; 64 (2): 89-96.

[1891] Safavi S M, Kazemi B, Esmaeili M, Fallah A, Modarresi A, Mir M. Effects of low-level He-Ne laser irradiation on the gene expression of IL-1beta, TNF-alpha, IFN-gamma, TGF-beta, bFGF, and PDGF in rat's gingiva. Lasers Med Sci. 2008; 23 (3): 331-335.

[1892] Rallis T R. Low-intensity laser therapy for recurrent herpes labialis. J Invest Dermatol. 2000; 115 (1): 131-132.

[1893] Eduardo Fde P,, Mehnert D U, Monezi A M, Zezell D M, Schubert M M, Eduardo Fde C, Marques M M. In vitro effect of phototherapy with low intensity laser on HSV-1 and epithelial cells. Proc. SPIE.Mechanisms for Low-Light Therapy II. 2007; Vol. 6428, 642805.

[1894] Lilveria P, Syeck E L, Pinhoa R A. Evaluation of mitochondrial respiratory chain activity in wound healing by low-level laser therapy. Journal of Photochemistry and Photobiology B: Biology. 2007; 86 (3): 279-282.

[1895] Eduardo F de P, Bueno D F, de Freitas P M, Marques M M, Passos-Bueno M R, Eduardo C de P, Zatz M. Stem cell proliferation under low intensity laser irradiation: a preliminary study. Lasers Surg Med. 2008; 40 (6): 433-438.

[1896] Yamaura M E, Min E, Yao M E, Yaroslavsky I V, Cohen R et al. Low level laser therapy for reduction of chronic joint pain: in vitro studies. BiOS 2008, Proceedings of SPIE; Volume 6846-8.

[1897] Hamblin M R. The role of nitric oxide in LLLT. BiOS 2008. Proceedings of SPIE. Volume 6846-1.

[1898] Anders J, Wu X, Anton Dmitriev A, Mario T. Cardoso M T et al. Light promotes axonal regeneration and functional recovery in two spinal cord injury models BiOS 2008. Proceedings of SPIE; Volume 6846-11.

[1864] Houreld N, Abrahamse H. In Vitro Exposure of Wounded Diabetic Fibroblast Cells to a Helium-Neon Laser at 5 and 16 J/cm^2. Photomed Laser Surg. 2007; 25 (2): 78-84.

[1865] Corazza V A, Jorge J, Kurachi C, Bagnato V S. Photobiomodulation on the Angiogenesis of Skin Wounds in Rats Using Different Light Sources. Photomed Laser Surg. 2007; 25 (2): 102-106.

[1866] Ihsan F R, Al-Mustawfi N, Kaka L N. Promotion of Regenerative Processes in Injured Peripheral Nerve Induced by Low-Level Laser Therapy. Photomed Laser Surg, 2007, 25 (2): 107-111.

[1867] Rochkind S, Drory V, Alon M, Nissan M, Ouaknine G E. Laser Phototherapy (780 nm), a New Modality in Treatment of Long-Term Incomplete Peripheral Nerve Injury: A Randomized Double-Blind Placebo-Controlled Study. Photomed Laser Surg. 2007; 25 (5): 436-442.

[1868] Viegas V N, Marcelo Abreu E R, Viezzer C, Cantarelli Machado D, Sant'Anna Filho M et al. Effect of Low-Level Laser Therapy on Inflammatory Reactions during Wound Healing: Comparison with Meloxicam. Photomed Laser Surg. 2007; 25 (6): 467-473.

[1869] Renno A C, McDonnell P A, Parizotto N A, Laakso E L. The Effects of Laser Irradiation on Osteoblast and Osteosarcoma Cell Proliferation and Differentiation in Vitro. Photomed Laser Surg. 2007; 25 (4): 275-280.

[1870] Fikackova H, Dostalova T, Navratil L, Klaschka J. Effectiveness of Low-Level Laser Therapy in Temporomandibular Joint Disorders: A Placebo-Controlled Study. Photomed Laser Surg. 2007; 25 (4): 297-303.

[1871] Houreld N, Abrahamse H. Effectiveness of Helium-Neon Laser Irradiation on Viability and Cytotoxicity of Diabetic-Wounded Fibroblast Cells. Photomed Laser Surg. 2007; 25 (6): 474-481.

[1872] Oron U, Ilic S, De Taboada L, Streeter J. Ga-As (808 nm) Laser Irradiation Enhances ATP Production in Human Neuronal Cells in Culture. Photomed Laser Surg. 2007; 25 (3): 180-182.

[1873] Delbari A, Bayat M, Bayat M. Effect of Low-Level Laser Therapy on Healing of Medial Collateral Ligament Injuries in Rats: An Ultrastructural Study. Photomed Laser Surg. 2007; 25 (3): 191-196.

[1874] Stergioulas A. Effects of Low-Level Laser and Plyometric Exercises in the Treatment of Lateral Epicondylitis. Photomed Laser Surg. 2007; 25 (3): 205-213.

[1875] Correa F, Lopes Martins R A, Correa J C, Iversen V V, Joenson J, Bjordal J M. Low-Level Laser Therapy (GaAs=904 nm) Reduces Inflammatory Cell Migration in Mice with Lipopolysaccharide-Induced Peritonitis. Photomed Laser Surg. 2007; (4): 245-249.

[1876] Liu X, Lyon R, Meier H T, Thometz J, Haworth S T. Effect of Lower-Level Laser Therapy on Rabbit Tibial Fracture. Photomed Laser Surg. 2007; 25 (6): 487-494.

[1877] Maiya G A, Kumar P, Rao L. Effect of low intensity helium-neon (He-Ne) laser irradiation on diabetic wound healing dynamics. Photomed Laser Surg. 2005; 23 (2): 187-190.

[1878] Stergioulas A. Low-Power Laser Treatment in Patients with Frozen Shoulder: Preliminary Results. Photomed Laser Surg. 2008; 26 (2): 99-105.

[1879] Ng G Y F, Fung D T C. The Combined Treatment Effects of Therapeutic Laser and Exercise on Tendon Repair. Photomed Laser Surg. 2008; 26 (2): 137-141.

[1880] Meirelles G C S, Santos J N, Chagas P O, Moura A P, Pinheiro A L B. A Comparative Study of the Effects of Laser Photobiomodulation on the Healing of Third-Degree Burns: A Histological Study in Rats. Photomed Laser Surg. 2008; 26 (2): 159-166.

[1881] Pinheiro A L B, Gerbi M E M, Ponzi E A C, Ramalho L M P, Marques A M C et al. Infrared Laser Light Further Improves Bone Healing When Associated with Bone Morphogenetic Proteins and Guided Bone Regeneration: An in Vivo Study in a Rodent Model. Photomed Laser Surg. 2008; 26 (2): 167-174.

RANKL, RANK, OPG: an experimental study in rats. Lasers Surg Med. 2007; 39 (5): 441-450.

[1845] Chen C H, Hung H S, Hsu S H. Low-energy laser irradiation increases endothelial cell proliferation, migration, and eNOS gene expression possibly via PI3K signal pathway. Lasers Surg Med. 2008; 40 (1): 46-54.

[1846] Baumann M, Jörgensen B, Rohde E et al. Influence of wavelength, power density and exposure time of laser radiation on chondrocyte cultures - An in-vitro nvestigation. Medical Laser Application. 2006; 21 (3): 191-198.

[1847] Müller K P, Rodrigues C R, Núnez S C et al. Effects of low power red laser on induced-dental caries in rats. Archives of Oral Biology. 2007; 52 (7): 648-654.

[1848] Ferreira M C, Brito V N, Gameiro J, Costa M R, Vasconcellos E C, Cruz-Hofling M A, Verinaud L. Effects of HeNe laser irradiation on experimental paracoccidioidomycotic lesions. J Photochem Photobiol B. 2006; 84 (2): 141-149.

[1849] Djavid G E, Mehrdad R, Ghasemi M, Hasan-Zadeh H et al. In chronic low back pain, low level laser therapy combined with exercise is more beneficial than exercise alone in the long term: a randomised trial. Aust J Physiother. 2007; 53 (3): 155-160

[1850] Ivandic B T, Ivandic T. Low-Level Laser Therapy Improves Vision in Patients with Age-Related Macular Degeneration. Photomed Laser Surg. 2008; 2 (3): 241-245.

[1851] Komelkova L V, Vitreshchak T V, Zhirnova I G, Poleshchuk V V et al. [Biochemical and immunological induces of the blood in Parkinson's disease and their correction with the help of laser therapy]. Patol Fiziol Eksp Ter. 2004; (1): 15-18.

[1852] Vitreshchak T V, Mikhailov V V, Piradov M A, Poleshchuk V V et al. [Laser modification of the blood in vitro and in vivo in patients with Parkinson's disease]. Bull Exp Biol Med. 2003; 135 (5): 430-432.

[1853] McGuff P E, Deterling R A Jr, Gottlieb L S. Tumoricidal effect of laser energy on experimental and human malignant tumors. N Engl J Med. 1965; 273 (9): 490-492.

[1854] McGuff P E, Deterling R A Jr, Gottlieb L S, Fahimi H D, Bushnell D, Roeber F. Effects Of Laser Radiation On Tumor Transplants. Fed Proc. 1965; 24: Suppl 14: 150-154.

[1855] McGuff P E, Bell E J. The effect of laser energy radiation on bacteria. Med Biol Illus. 1966; 16 (3): 191-193.

[1856] McGuff P E, Gottlieb L S, Katayama I, Levy C K. Comparative study of effects of laser and/or ionizing radiation therapy on experimental or human malignant tumors. Am J Roentgenol Radium Ther Nucl Med. 1966; 96 (3): 744-748.

[1857] McGuff P E, Deterling R A Jr, Gottlieb L S. Laser radiation for metastatic malignant melanoma. JAMA. 1966; 31; 195 (5): 393-394.

[1858] McGuff P E. Laser radiation for basal cell carcinoma. Dermatologica. 1966; 133 (5): 379-383.

[1859] McGuff P E. Tumoricidal effect of laser radiation on malignant tumors. Int Ophthalmol Clin. 1966; 6 (2): 379-386.

[1860] Abiko Y. Functional genomic study on anti-inflammatory effects by low level laser irradiation. Abstract at the 8th Congress of the World Federation for Laser Dentistry, Hong Kong, July 2008.

[1861] Teggi R T, Bellini C, Fabiano B, Bussi M. Efficacy of Low-Level Laser Therapy in Ménière's Disease: A Pilot Study of 10 Patients. Photomed Laser Surg. 2008; 26 (4): 249-253.

[1862] Lam L K, Cheing G L. Effects of 904-nm low-level laser therapy in the management of lateral epicondylitis: a randomized controlled trial. Photomed Laser Surg. 2007; 25 (2): 65-67.

[1863] Al-Watban F, Zhang X Y, Andres B L. Low-Level Laser Therapy Enhances Wound Healing in Diabetic Rats: A Comparison of Different Lasers. Photomed Laser Surg. 2007, 25 (2): 72-77.

[1827] Gottschling S, Meyer S, Gribova I, Distler L, Berrang J, Gortner L, Graf N, Shamdeen MG. Laser acupuncture in children with headache: A double-blind, randomized, bicenter, placebo-controlled trial. Pain. 2007; 137(2): 405-412

[1828] Zeredo J L, Sasaki K M, Toda K. High-intensity laser for acupuncture-like stimulation. Lasers Med Sci. 2007; 22 (1): 37-41. [Epub 2006 Nov 21]

[1829] Lihong S. He-Ne laser auricular irradiation plus body acupuncture for treatment of acne vulgaris in 36 cases. J Tradit Chin Med. 2006; 26 (3): 193-194.

[1830] Quah-Smith J I, Tang W M, Russell J. Laser acupuncture for mild to moderate depression in a primary care setting - a randomised controlled trial. Acupunct Med. 2005; 23 (3): 103-111.

[1831] Siedentopf C M, Koppelstaetter F, Haala I A, Haid V, Rhomberg P, Ischebeck A, Buchberger W, Felber S, Schlager A, Golaszewski S M. Laser acupuncture induced specific cerebral cortical and subcortical activations in humans. Lasers Med Sci. 2005; 20 (2): 68-73.

[1832] Litscher G. Cerebral and peripheral effects of laser needle-stimulation. Neurol Res. 2003; 25 (7): 722-728.

[1833] Litscher G, Rachbauer D, Ropele S, Wang L, Schikora D, Fazekas F, Ebner F. Acupuncture using laser needles modulates brain function: first evidence from functional transcranial Doppler sonography and functional magnetic resonance imaging. Lasers Med Sci. 2004; 19 (1): 6-11.

[1834] Trümpler F, Oez S, Stähli P, Brenner H D, Jüni P. Acupuncture for alcohol withdrawal: a randomized controlled trial. Alcohol Alcohol. 2003; 38 (4): 369-375.

[1835] Siedentopf C M, Golaszewski S M, Mottaghy F M, Ruff C C, Felber S, Schlager A. Functional magnetic resonance imaging detects activation of the visual association cortex during laser acupuncture of the foot in humans. Neurosci Lett. 2002; 327 (1): 53-56.

[1836] Radmayr C, Schlager A, Studen M, Bartsch G. Prospective randomized trial using laser acupuncture versus desmopressin in the treatment of nocturnal enuresis. Eur Urol. 2001; 40 (2): 201-205.

[1837] Read A, Beaty P, Corner J, Sommerville Ville C. Reducing naltrexone-resistant hyperphagia using laser acupuncture to increase endogenous opiates. Brain Inj. 1996; 10 (12): 911-919.

[1838] Simões A, Nicolau J, de Souza D N, Ferreira L S, de Paula Eduardo C, Apel C, Gutknecht N. Effect of defocused infrared diode laser on salivary flow rate and some salivary parameters of rats. Clin Oral Investig. 2008; 12 (1): 25-30.

[1839] Sobanko J F, Alster T S. Efficacy of Low-Level Laser Therapy for Chronic Cutaneous Ulceration in Humans: A Review and Discussion. Dermatol Surg. 2008; 34 (8): 991-1000.

[1840] Castano A P, Dai T, Yaroslavsky I, Cohen R, Apruzzese W A, Smotrich M H, Hamblin M R. Low-level laser therapy for zymosan-induced arthritis in rats: Importance of illumination time. Lasers Surg Med. 2007; 39 (6): 543-550.

[1841] Ekim A, Armagan O, Tascioglu F, Oner C, Colak M. Effect of low level laser therapy in rheumatoid arthritis patients with carpal tunnel syndrome. Swiss Med Wkly. 2007; 137 (23-24): 347-352.

[1842] Saygun I, Karacay S, Serdar M, Ural A U, Sencimen M, Kurtis B. Effects of laser irradiation on the release of basic fibroblast growth factor (bFGF), insulin like growth factor-1 (IGF-1), and receptor of IGF-1 (IGFBP3) from gingival fibroblasts. Lasers Med Sci. 2008; 23 (2): 211-215.

[1843] Kamali F, Bayat M, Torkaman G, Ebrahimi E, Salavati M. The therapeutic effect of low-level laser on repair of osteochondral defects in rabbit knee. J Photochem Photobiol B. 2007; 88 (1): 11-15.

[1844] Kim Y D, Kim S S, Hwang D S, Kim S G, Kwon Y H et al. Effect of low-level laser treatment after installation of dental titanium implant-immunohistochemical study of

[1811] Voskanian K Sh, Mitsyn G V, Gaevski V N. [Radioprotective effect of helium-neon laser radiation for fibroblast cells] Aviakosm Ekolog Med. 2007; 41 (3): 32-35. [Article in Russian]

[1812] Da Cunha S S, Sarmento V, Ramalho L M, De Almeida D, Veeck E B, Da Costa N P, Mattos A, Marques A M, Gerbi M, Freitas A C. Effect of laser therapy on bone tissue submitted to radiotherapy: experimental study in rats. Photomed Laser Surg. 2007; 25 (3): 197-204.

[1813] Shefer G, Ben-Dov N, Halevy O, Oron U. Primary myogenic cells see the light: improved survival of transplanted myogenic cells following low energy laser irradiation. Lasers Surg Med. 2008; 40 (1): 38-45.

[1814] Barbosa A M, Villaverde A B, Guimarães-Souza L, Ribeiro W, Cogo J C, Zamuner S R. Effect of low-level laser therapy in the inflammatory response induced by Bothrops jararacussu snake venom. Toxicon. 2008; 51 (7): 1236-1244.

[1815] Aimbire F, Ligeiro de Oliveira A P, Albertini R, Corrêa J C, Laceira de Campos C B, Lyon J P, Silva J A Jr, Costa M S. Low Level Laser Therapy (LLLT) Decreases Pulmonary Microvascular Leakage, Neutrophil Influx and IL-1beta Levels in Airway and Lung from Rat Subjected to LPS-Induced Inflammation. Inflammation. 2008; 31 (3): 189-197.

[1816] Yousefi-Nooraie R, Schonstein E, Heidari K, Rashidian A, Pennick V, Akbari-Kamrani M, Irani S, Shakiba B, Mortaz Hejri S, Mortaz Hejri S, Jonaidi A. Low level laser therapy for nonspecific low-back pain. Cochrane Database Syst Rev. 2008; 16 (2): CD005107.

[1817] Bossini P S, Fangel R, Habenschus R M, Renno A C, Benze B, Zuanon J A, Neto C B, Parizotto N A. Low-level laser therapy (670 nm) on viability of random skin flap in rats. Lasers Med Sci. 2009; 24 (2): 209-213.

[1818] Emshoff R, Bösch R, Pümpel E, Schöning H, Strobl H. Low-level laser therapy for treatment of temporomandibular joint pain: a double-blind and placebo-controlled trial. Oral Surg Oral Med Oral Pathol Oral Radiol Endod. 2008; 105 (4): 452-456.

[1819] Desmettre T, Maurage C A, Mordon S. Transpupillary thermotherapy (TTT) with short duration laser exposures induce heat shock protein (HSP) hyperexpression on choroidoretinal layers. Lasers Surg Med. 2003; 33 (2): 102-107.

[1820] Stein E, Koehn J, Sutter W, Wendtlandt G, Wanschitz F, Thurnher D, Baghestanian M, Turhani D. Initial effects of low-level laser therapy on growth and differentiation of human osteoblast-like cells. Wien Klin Wochenschr. 2008; 120 (3-4): 112-117.

[1821] Stergioulas A, Stergioula M, Aarskog R, Lopes-Martins R A, Bjordal J M. Effects of Low-Level Laser Therapy and Eccentric Exercises in the Treatment of Recreational Athletes With Chronic Achilles Tendinopathy. Am J Sports Med. 2008; 36 (5): 881-887.

[1822] Ozcelik O, Cenk Haytac M, Kunin A, Seydaoglu G. Improved wound healing by low-level laser irradiation after gingivectomy operations: a controlled clinical pilot study. J Clin Periodontol. 2008; 35 (3): 250-254.

[1823] Arora H, Pai K M, Maiya A, Vidyasagar M S, Rajeev A. Efficacy of He-Ne Laser in the prevention and treatment of radiotherapy-induced oral mucositis in oral cancer patients. Oral Surg Oral Med Oral Pathol Oral Radiol Endod. 2008; 105 (2): 180-186.

[1824] Onizawa K, Muramatsu T, Matsuki M, Ohta K, Matsuzaka K, Oda Y, Shimono M. Low-level (gallium-aluminum-arsenide) laser irradiation of Par-C10 cells and acinar cells of rat parotid gland. Lasers Med Sci. 2009; 24 (2): 155-161.

[1825] Oken O, Kahraman Y, Ayhan F, Canpolat S, Yorgancioglu Z R, Oken O F. The short-term efficacy of laser, brace, and ultrasound treatment in lateral epicondylitis: a prospective, randomized, controlled trial. J Hand Ther. 2008; 21 (1): 63-67.

[1826] Bortone F, Santos H A, Albertini R, Pesquero J B, Costa M S, Silva J A Jr. Low level laser therapy modulates kinin receptors mRNA expression in the subplantar muscle of rat paw subjected to carrageenan-induced inflammation. Int Immunopharmacol. 2008; 8 (2): 206-210.

[1794] Elwakil T F, Elazzazi A, Shokeir H. Treatment of carpal tunnel syndrome by low-level laser versus open carpal tunnel release. Lasers Med Sci. 2007; 22 (4) :265-270.

[1795] Karu T I, Letokhov V S, Lobko V V, Novikov V F, Paramonov L V. [Phototherapy of gastric and duodenal peptic ulcer patients based on cellstimulation with low-intensity red light]. Vopr Kurortol Fizioter Lech Fiz Kult. 1984; (1): 36-39. (in Russian)

[1796] Simões A, Siqueira W L, Lamers M L, Santos M F, Eduardo C D, Nicolau J. Laser phototherapy effect on protein metabolism parameters of rat salivary glands. Lasers Med Sci. 2009; 24 (2): 202-208.

[1797] Wenzel G I, Anvari B, Mazhar A, Pikkula B, Oghalai J S. Laser-induced collagen remodeling and deposition within the basilar membrane of the mouse cochlea. J Biomed Opt. 2007; 12 (2): 021007.

[1798] Bjordal J M, Klovning A, Ljunggren A E, Slordal L. Short-term efficacy of pharmacotherapeutic interventions in osteoarthritic knee pain: A meta-analysis of randomised placebo-controlled trials. Eur J Pain. 2007; 11 (2): 125-138.

[1799] Bjordal J M, Ljunggren A E, Klovning A, Slordal L. NSAIDs, including coxibs, probably do more harm than good, and paracetamol is ineffective for hip OA. Ann Rheum Dis. 2005; 64 (4):655-656; author reply 656. Comment on: Ann Rheum Dis. 2005; 64 (5): 669-681.

[1800] Aimbire F, Lopes-Martins R A, Albertini R, Pacheco M T et al. Effect of low-level laser therapy on hemorrhagic lesions induced by immune complex in rat lungs. Photomed Laser Surg. 2007; 25 (2):112-117.

[1801] Carrinho P M, Renno A C, Koeke P, Salate A C, Parizotto N A, Vidal B C. Comparative study using 685-nm and 830-nm lasers in the tissue repair of tenotomized tendons in the mouse. Photomed Laser Surg. 2006; 24 (6): 754-758.

[1802] Chow R. Laser acupuncture studies should not be included in systematic reviews of phototherapy. Photomed Laser Surg. 2006; 24 (1): 69. Comment on: Photomed Laser Surg. 2005; 23 (4): 425-30.

[1803] Whelan H T, Connelly J F, Hodgson B D, Barbeau L, Post AC et al. NASA light-emitting diodes for the prevention of oral mucositis in pediatric bone marrow transplant patients. J Clin Laser Med Surg. 2002; 20 (6): 319-324.

[1804] Oron A, Oron U, Streeter J, de Taboada L, Alexandrovich A, Trembovler V, Shohami. E. Low-level laser therapy applied transcranially to mice following traumatic brain injury significantly reduces long-term neurological deficits. J Neurotrauma. 2007; 24 (4): 651-656.

[1805] Schubert M M, Eduardo F P, Guthrie K A, Franquin J C, Bensadoun R J, Migliorati C A et al. A phase III randomized double-blind placebo-controlled clinical trial to determine the efficacy of low level laser therapy for the prevention of oral mucositis in patients undergoing hematopoietic cell transplantation. Support Care Cancer. 2007; 15 (10): 1145-1154.

[1806] Youssef M, Ashkar S, Hamade E, Gutknecht N, Lampert F, Mir M. The effect of low-level laser therapy during orthodontic movement: a preliminary study. Lasers Med Sci. 2008; 23 (1): 27-33.

[1807] Lampl Y, Zivin J A, Fisher M, Lew R, Welin L, Dahlof B, Borenstein P, Andersson B, Perez J, Caparo C, Ilic S, Oron U. Infrared laser therapy for ischemic stroke: a new treatment strategy: results of the NeuroThera Effectiveness and Safety Trial-1 (NEST-1). Stroke. 2007; 38 (6): 1843-1849.

[1808] Mvula B, Mathope T, Moore T, Abrahamse H. The effect of low level laser irradiation on adult human adipose derived stem cells. Lasers Med Sci. 2008; 23 (3): 277-282

[1809] Tuby H, Maltz L, Oron U. Low-level laser irradiation (LLLI) promotes proliferation of mesenchymal and cardiac stem cells in culture. Lasers Surg Med. 2007; 39 (4): 373-378.

[1810] Abramovitch-Gottlib L, Gross T, Naveh D, Geresh S, Rosenwaks S, Bar I, Vago R. Low level laser irradiation stimulates osteogenic phenotype of mesenchymal stem cells seeded on a three-dimensional biomatrix. Lasers Med Sci. 2005; 20 (3-4): 138-146.

[1776] Voskanian K Sh, Simonian N V, Avakian Ts M, Arutiunian A G. [Effect of helium-neon laser radiation on the radiosensitivity of Escherichia coli K-12 cells]. Radiobiologiia. 1985; 25 (4): 557-560. (in Russian)

[1777] Voskanian K Sh, Arzumanian G M. [Radiation protective effects of laser irradiation with wavelength 532 nm]. Radiats Biol Radioecol. 1996; 36 (5): 731-733. (in Russian)

[1778] Karu T I, Piatibrat L V, Kalendo G S. [The effect of He-Ne laser radiation on the survival of HeLa cells subjected to ionizing radiation]. Radiobiologiia. 1992; 32 (2): 202-206. (in Russian)

[1779] Sun X H, Zhu X, Xu C, Ye N, Zhu H. [Effects of low energy laser on tooth movement and remodeling of alveolar bone in rabbits]. Hua Xi Kou Qiang Yi Xue Za Zhi. 2001; 19 (5): 290-293. (in Chinese)

[1780] Sun X H, Wang R, Zhang X Y. [Effects of He-Ne laser irradiation on the expression of transforming growth factor beta1 during experimental tooth movement in rabbits]. Shanghai Kou Qiang Yi Xue. 2006; 15 (1): 52-57. (in Chinese)

[1781] Godoy B M, Arana-Chavez V E, Nunez S C, Ribeiro M S. Effects of low-power red laser on dentine-pulp interface after cavity preparation. An ultrastructural study. Arch Oral Biol. 2007 Sep; 52 (9): 899-903.

[1782] Bjordal J M, Tunér J, Iversen V V, Frigo L, Gjerde K, Lopes-Martins A B. A systematic review of post-operative pain relief by Low Level Laser Therapy (LLLT) after third molar extraction. Abstract Congr. Of the European Division of the World Federation for Laser Dentistry, Nice, May 2007.

[1783] Jensen I, Harms-Ringdahl K. Strategies for prevention and management of musculoskeletal conditions. Neck pain. Best Pract Res Clin Rheumatol. 2007; 21 (1): 93-108.

[1784] Chow R T, David M A, Armati P J. 830 nm laser irradiation induces varicosity formation, reduces mitochondrial membrane potential and blocks fast axonal flow in small and medium diameter rat dorsal root ganglion neurons: implications for the analgesic effects of 830 nm laser. J Peripher Nerv Syst. 2007; 12 (1): 28-39.

[1785] Garcez A S, Ribeiro M S, Tegos G P, Nunez S C, Jorge A O, Hamblin M R. Antimicrobial photodynamic therapy combined with conventional endodontic treatment to eliminate root canal biofilm infection. Lasers Surg Med. 2007; 39 (1): 59-66.

[1786] Gan L, Tse C, Pilliar R M, Kandel R A. Low-power laser stimulation of tissue engineered cartilage tissue formed on a porous calcium polyphosphate scaffold. Lasers Surg Med. 2007; 39 (3): 286-293.

[1787] Yousefi-Nooraie R, Schonstein E, Heidari K, Rashidian A, Akbari-Kamrani M, Irani S, Shakiba B, Mortaz Hejri Sa, Mortaz Hejri So, Jonaidi A. Low level laser therapy for nonspecific low-back pain. Cochrane Database Syst Rev. 2008 Apr 16; (2): CD005107.

[1788] Bach G, Neckel C, Mall, Krekeler G. Conventional versus laser-assisted therapy of periimplantitis: a five-year comparative study. Implant Dent. 2000; 9: 247–251.

[1789] Romanos, G E. Treatment of periimplant lesions using different laser systems. J Oral Laser Applications. 2002; 2: 75–81.

[1790] Romanos G E, Nentwig G H. Diode laser (980 nm) in oral and maxillofacial surgical procedures: Clinical observations based on clinical applications. J Clin Laser Med Surg. 1999; 17: 193–197.

[1791] Kreisler M, Al-Haj H, d'Hoedt B. Clinical efficacy of semiconductor laser application as an adjunct to conventional scaling and root planning. Lasers Surg Med. 2005; 37 (5): 350–355.

[1792] Gutknecht N, ed: Proceedings of the 1st International Workshop of Evidence Based Dentistry on Lasers in Dentistry. 2007. Quintessenz Verlags-GmbH.

[1793] Ishikawa I, Aoki A, Takasaki A A. Potential applications of Erbium:YAG laser in periodontics. J Periodontal Res 69. 2004; (4): 275-285.

[1758] Cetiner S, Kahraman S A, Yucetas S. Evaluation of low-level laser therapy in the treatment of temporomandibular disorders. Photomed Laser Surg. 2006; 24 (5): 637-641.

[1759] Nuñez S C, Garcez A S, Suzuki S S, Ribeiro M S. Management of mouth opening in patients with temporomandibular disorders through low-level laser therapy and transcutaneous electrical neural stimulation. Photomed Laser Surg. 2006; 24 (1): 45-49.

[1760] Renno A C, de Moura F M, dos Santos N S et al. Effects of 830-nm laser, used in two doses, on biomechanical properties of osteopenic rat femora. Photomed Laser Surg. 2006; 24 (2): 202-206.

[1761] Renno A C, de Moura F M, dos Santos N S, Tirico R P, Bossini P S, Parizotto N A. Effects of 830-nm laser light on preventing bone loss after ovariectomy. Photomed Laser Surg. 2006; 24 (5): 642-645.

[1762] da Silva R V, Camilli J A. Repair of bone defects treated with autogenous bone graft and low-power laser. J Craniofac Surg. 2006; 172: 297-301.

[1763] Stein A, Benayahu D, Maltz L, Oron U. Low-level laser irradiation promotes proliferation and differentiation of human osteoblasts in vitro. Photomed Laser Surg. 2005; 232: 161-166.

[1764] Merli L A, Santos M T, Genovese W J, Faloppa F. Effect of low-intensity laser irradiation on the process of bone repair. Photomed Laser Surg. 2005; 23 (2): 212-215.

[1765] Soroor N. Comparison between the effects of low level laser therapy (LLT) and Magnetic low level laser therapy (MLLLT) in treatment of knee osteoarthritis. Abstract. WALT2006, Lemesos, Cyprus, October 2006.

[1766] A B, Todorovic L. Postoperative analgesia after lower third molar surgery: contribution of the use of long-acting local anesthetics, low-power laser, and diclofenac. Oral Surg Oral Med Oral Pathol Oral Radiol Endod. 2006;102 (5): e4-8.

[1767] Mi X Q, Chen J Y, Zhou L W. Effect of low power laser irradiation on disconnecting the membrane-attached hemoglobin from erythrocyte membrane. J Photochem Photobiol B. 2006; 1: 832: 146-150.

[1768] Novoselova E G, Glushkova O V, Cherenkov D A, Chudnovsky V M, Fesenko E E. Effects of low-power laser radiation on mice immunity. Photodermatol Photoimmunol Photomed. 2006; 22 (1): 33-38.

[1769] Makihara E, Makihara M, Masumi S, Sakamoto E. Evaluation of facial thermographic changes before and after low-level laser irradiation. Photomed Laser Surg. 2005; 232: 191-195.

[1770] Enwemeka C S E. Attenuation and penetration of visible 632.8 nm and invisible infrared 904 nm light in soft tissues. Laser Therapy. 2001; (13): 95-101.

[1771] Lan C C, Wu C S, Chiou M H, Hsieh P C, Yu H S. Low-energy helium-neon laser induces locomotion of the immature melanoblasts and promotes melanogenesis of the more differentiated melanoblasts: recapitulation of vitiligo repigmentation in vitro. J Invest Dermatol. 2006; 126 (9): 2119-2126.

[1772] Novak C, Spelman L. Low energy fluence CO_2 laser treatment of lymphangiectasia. Australas J Dermatol. 1998; (4): 277-278.

[1773] Dube A, Bock C, Bauer E, Kohli R, Gupta P K, Greulich K O. HeNe laser irradiation protects B-lymphoblasts from UVA-induced DNA damage. Radiat Environ Biophys. 2001; 40 (1): 77-82.

[1774] Kohli R, Gupta P K. Irradiance dependence of the He-Ne laser-induced protection against UVC radiation in E. coli strains. J Photochem Photobiol B. 2003; 69 (3): 161-167.

[1775] Kohli R, Gupta P K, Dube A. Helium-neon laser preirradiation induces protection against UVC radiation in wild-type E. coli strain K12AB1157. Radiat Res. 2000; 153 (2): 181-185.

[1739] Kim S S, Min M W, Lee C J. Phototherapy of androgenetic alopecia with low level narrow band 655-nm red light and 780-nm infrared light. J Am Acad Dermatol. 2007; 56 (2), Suppl 2, P. AB112.

[1740] Bjordal J M, Baxter G D. Ineffective dose and lack of laser output testing in laser shoulder and neck studies. Photomed Laser Surg. 2006; 24 (4): 533-534; author reply 534.

[1741] Pfander D, Jorgensen B, Rohde E, Bindig U, Muller G, Eric Scheller E. [The influence of laser irradiation of low-power density on an experimental cartilage damage in rabbit kneejoints: an in vivo investigation considering macroscopic, histological and immunohistochemical changes] Biomed Tech (Berlin). 2006; 51 (3): 131-138. (in German)

[1742] Lin Y S, Huang M H, Chai C Y. Effects of helium-neon laser on the mucopolysaccharide induction in experimental osteoarthritic cartilage. Osteoarthritis Cartilage. 2006; 14 (4): 377-383.

[1743] King D L, Steinhauer W, Garcia-Godoy F, Elkins C J. Herpetic gingivostomatitis and teething difficulty in infants. Pediatr Dent. 1992; 14 (2): 82-85.

[1744] Hawkins D, Abrahamse H. Effect of multiple exposures of low-level laser therapy on the cellular responses of wounded human skin fibroblasts. Photomed Laser Surg. 2006; 24 (6): 705-714.

[1745] Douris P, Southard V, Ferrigi R, Grauer J et al. Effect of phototherapy on delayed onset muscle soreness. Photomed Laser Surg. 2006; 24 (3): 377-382.

[1746] Cruz L B, Ribeiro A S, Rech A, Rosa L G, Castro C G Jr, Brunetto A L. Influence of low-energy laser in the prevention of oral mucositis in children with cancer receiving chemotherapy. Pediatr Blood Cancer. 2007; 48 (4): 435-440.

[1747] Elwakil T F. An in-vivo experimental evaluation of He-Ne laser photostimulation in healing Achilles tendons. Lasers Med Sci. 2007; 22 (1): 53-59.

[1748] Zhong-Quan Zhao, Paul W. Dependence of light transmission through human skin on incident beam diameter at different wavelengths. Proc.SPIE. 1998; 3254: 354-361.

[1749] Izzo A D, Richter C P, Jansen E D, Walsh J T Jr. Laser stimulation of the auditory nerve. Lasers Surg Med. 2006; 38 (8): 745-753.

[1750] Grbavac R A, Veeck E B, Bernard J P, Ramalho L M, Pinheiro A L. Effects of laser therapy in CO_2 laser wounds in rats. Photomed Laser Surg. 2006; 24 (3): 389-396.

[1751] Baptista I M C, Zangaro R A, Rigau J, Shoji N. O Laser de Baixa Potência pode Prevenir Deiscência Incisional em Esternotomia Pós-cirurgia Cardíaca [Low level laser can prevent incisional dishecence after sternotomy surgery]. Revista da Sociedade Brasileira de Laser. 2005; 3 (3): 10-16.

[1752] Gal P, Vidinsky B, Toporcer T, Mokry M et al. Histological assessment of the effect of laser irradiation on skin wound healing in rats. Photomed Laser Surg. 2006; 24 (4): 480-488.

[1753] Baptista I M C, Zangaro R A, Rigau J, Shoji N. O Laser de Baixa Potência pode Prevenir Deiscência Incisional em Esternotomia Pós-cirurgia Cardíaca [Low level laser can prevent incisional dishecence after sternotomy surgery]. Revista da Sociedade Brasileira de Laser. 2005; 3 (3): 10-16.

[1754] Shao X H, Yang Y P, Dai J, Wu J F, Bo A H. Effects of He-Ne laser irradiation on chronic atrophic gastritis in rats. World J Gastroenterol. 2005; 7; 11 (25): 3958-3961.

[1755] Maiya G A, Kumar P, Rao L. Effect of low intensity helium-neon (He-Ne) laser irradiation on diabetic wound healing dynamics. Photomed Laser Surg. 2005; 23 (2): 187-190.

[1756] Oron A, Oron U, Chen J, Eilam A et al. Low-level laser therapy applied transcranially to rats after induction of stroke significantly reduces long-term neurological deficits. Stroke. 2006; 37 (10): 2620-2624.

[1757] Dadras S, Mohajerani E, Eftekhar F, Hosseini M. Different photoresponses of Staphylococcus aureus and Pseudomonas aeruginosa to 514, 532, and 633 nm low level lasers in vitro. Curr Microbiol. 2006; 53 (4): 282-286.

[1721] Efanov O I. Laser therapy for periodontitis. Proceedings of SPIE Vol. 4422 (2001). Low-Level Laser Therapy, Tatiana I. Solovieva, Ed.

[1722] Tuz H H, Onder E M, Kisnisci R S. Prevalence of otologic complaints in patients with temporomandibular disorder. Am J Orthod Dentofacial Orthop. 2003; 123: 620-623.

[1723] Wright E F, Bifano S L. The Relationship between Tinnitus and Temporomandibular Disorder (TMD) Therapy. Int Tinnitus J. 1997; 3: 55-61.

[1724] Wright E F, Syms C A 3rd, Bifano S L. Tinnitus, dizziness, and nonotologic otalgia improvement through temporomandibular disorder therapy. Mil Med. 2000; 165: 733-736.

[1725] Silveira P C L, Streck E L, Pinho R A. Evaluation of mitochondrial respiratory chain activity in wound healing by low-level laser therapy. J Photochem and Photobiol B: Biology. 2007; 86 (3): 279-282.

[1726] Kazemi-Khoo N. Successful treatment of diabetic foot ulcers with low-level laser therapy. The Foot. 2006; 16 (4): 184-187.

[1727] Arun Maiya A, Sagar M S, Fernandes D. Effect of low level helium-neon (He-Ne) laser therapy in the prevention & treatment of radiation induced mucositis in head & neck cancer patients. Indian J Med Res. 2006; 124 (4): 399-402.

[1728] Genot M T, Klastersky J. Low-level laser for prevention and therapy of oral mucositis induced by chemotherapy or radiotherapy. Curr Opin Oncol. 2005;17 (3): 236-240.

[1729] Turhani D, Scheriaub M, Kapralb D, Beneschc T et al. Pain relief by single low-level laser irradiation in orthodontic patients undergoing fixed appliance therapy. Am J Orthodont Dentofac Orthoped. 2006; 130 (3): 371-377.

[1730] Tuby H, Maltz L, Oron U. Modulations of VEGF and iNOS in the rat heart by low level laser therapy are associated with cardioprotection and enhanced angiogenesis. Lasers Surg Med. 2006; 38 (7): 682-688.

[1731] Rizzi C F, Mauriz J L, Freitas Correa D S, Moreira A J et al. Effects of low-level laser therapy (LPT) on the nuclear factor (NF)-kappaB signaling pathway in traumatized muscle. Lasers Surg Med. 2006; 38 (7): 704-713.

[1732] Prado R P, Liebano R E, Hochman B, Pinfildi C E, Ferreira L M. Experimental model for low level laser therapy on ischemic random skin flap in rats. Acta Cir Bras. 2006; 21 (4): 258-262.

[1733] Ferreira D M, Zangaro R A, Villaverde A B, Cury Y, Frigo L et al. Analgesic effect of He-Ne (632.8 nm) low-level laser therapy on acute inflammatory pain. Photomed Laser Surg. 2005; 23 (2): 177-181.

[1734] Cho H J, Lim S C, Kim S G, Kim Y S et al Effect of low-level laser therapy on osteoarthropathy in rabbit. In Vivo. 2004; 18 (5): 585-591.

[1735] Bayat M, Vasheghani M M, Razavie N, Jalili M R. Effects of low-level laser therapy on mast cell number and degranulation in third-degree burns of rats. J Rehabil Res Dev. 2008; 45 (6): 931-938.

[1736] Miloro M, Miller J J, Stoner J A. Low-Level Laser Effect on Mandibular Distraction Osteogenesis . J Oral Maxillofac Surg. 2007; 65 (2): 168-176.

[1737] Venancio R A, Camparis CM, Lizarelli R F. Low intensity laser therapy in the treatment of temporomandibular disorders: a double-blind study. J Oral Rehabil. 2005; 32 (11): 800-807.

[1738] Nascimento R X, Callera F. Low-level laser therapy at different energy densities (0.1-2.0 J/cm^2) and its effects on the capacity of human long-term cryopreserved peripheral blood progenitor cells for the growth of colony-forming units. Photomed Laser Surg. 2006; 24 (5): 601-604.

[1703] Butkovic D, Toljan S, Matolic M, Kralik S, Radesic L. Comparison of laser acupuncture and metoclopramide in PONV prevention in children. Paediatr Anaesth. 2005; 15 (1), 37-40.

[1704] Villaplana-Torres L A, Sarti-Martinez M A, Montesinos M, Smith-Agreda V, Trelles M A. Morphofunctional aspects of the follicular cells of the thyroid of albino rats after pituitary activation with low power laser. Laser in Medicine and Surgery. 1985; 1 (3): 124-129.

[1705] Shu B, Wu Z, Hao L, Zeng D, Feng G, Lin Y. Experimental study on He-Ne laser irradiation to inhibit scar fibroblast growth in culture. Chin J Traumatol. 2002;5 (4): 246-249.

[1706] Waiz M, Saleh A Z, Hayani R, Jubory S O. Use of the pulsed infrared diode laser (904 nm) in the treatment of alopecia areata. J Cosmet Laser Ther. 2006; 8 (1): 27-30.

[1707] Leung M C, Lo S C, Siu F K, So K F. Treatment of experimentally induced transient cerebral ischemia with low energy laser inhibits nitric oxide synthase activity and up-regulates the expression of transforming growth factor-beta 1. Lasers Surg Med. 2002; 31 (4): 283-288.

[1708] Fillipin L I, Mauriz J L, Vedovelli K, Moreira A J, Zettler C G, Lech O, Marroni N P, González-Gallego J. Low-level laser therapy (LLLT) prevents oxidative stress and reduces fibrosis in rat traumatized Achilles tendon. Lasers Surg Med. 2005; 37 (4): 293-300.

[1709] Dortbudak O, Haas R, Bernhart T, Mailath-Pokorny G. Lethal photosensitization for decontamination of implant surfaces in the treatment of peri-implantitis.Clin Oral Implants Res. 2001; 12 (2): 104-108.

[1710] Haas R, Dortbudak O, Mensdorff-Pouilly N, Mailath G. Elimination of bacteria on different implant surfaces through photosensitization and soft laser. An in vitro study. Clin Oral Implants Res. 1997; 8 (4): 249-254.

[1711] Shibli J A, Martins M C, Nociti F H Jr, Garcia V G, Marcantonio E Jr. Treatment of ligature-induced peri-implantitis by lethal photosensitization and guided bone regeneration: a preliminary histologic study in dogs. J Periodontol. 2003; 74 (3): 338-345.

[1712] Anderson T E, Good W T, Shumaker B et al. Low level laser therapy in the treatment of carpal tunnel syndrome. 1995. www-ml830laser.com/gmstudy.

[1713] Kuznetsova M Iu, Zueva S M, Gunenkova I V et al. [The use of the Optodan laser physiotherapeutic apparatus for the prevention of complications and the acceleration of the time in treating anomalies in the position of individual teeth with fixed orthodontic appliances]. Stomatologiia (Mosk). 1998; 77 (3): 56-60. (in Russian)

[1714] Drugova O V, Monich V A, Zhitnikova O V. [Effects of red light on postischemic myocardium during reperfusion]. Bull Exp Biol Med. 2001;131 (4): 325-326. Translation in: Bulletin of Experimental Biology and Medicine, No. 4, 2001. Biophysics and Biochemistry.

[1715] Fontana C R, Kurachi C, Mendonca C R, Bagnato V S. Microbial reduction in periodontal pockets under exposition of a medium power diode laser: an experimental study in rats. Lasers Surg Med. 2004; 35 (4): 263-268.

[1716] Fontana C R, Kurachi C, Mendonca C R, Bagnato V S. Temperature variation at soft periodontal and rat bone tissues during a medium-power diode laser exposure. Photomed Laser Surg. 2004; 22 (6): 519-522.

[1717] Schuhfried O, Korpan M, Fialka-Moser V. Helium-Neon Laser Irradiation: Effect on the Experimental Pain Threshold. Lasers Med Sci. 2000; 15: 169-173.

[1718] Souza S C, Munin E, Alves L P, Salgado M A, Pacheco M T. Low power laser radiation at 685 nm stimulates stem-cell proliferation rate in Dugesia tigrina during regeneration. J Photochem Photobiol B. 2005; 80 (3): 203-207.

[1719] Snyder S K, Byrnes K R, Borke R C, Sanchez A, Anders J J. Quantitation of calcitonin gene-related peptide mRNA and neuronal cell death in, facial motor nuclei following axotomy and 633 nm low power laser treatment. Lasers Surg Med. 2002; 31 (3): 216-222.

[1720] Ihsan F R. Low-level laser therapy accelerates collateral circulation and enhances microcirculation. Photomed Laser Surg. 2005; 23 (3): 289-294.

[1684] Komerik N, Nakanishi H, MacRobert A J, Henderson B, Speight P, Wilson M. In vivo killing of Porphyromonas gingivalis by toluidine blue mediated photosensitization in an animal model. Antimicrob Agents Chemother. 2003; 47 (3): 932-940.

[1685] Bisland S K. Priming cells for photodynamic therapy using low intensity light therapy. Proc. NAALT2006, Toronto, Canada, June 3-4 2006.

[1686] Yamazaki M, Miura Y, Tsuboi R, Ogawa H. Linear polarized infrared irradiation using Super Lizer is an effective treatment for multiple-type alopecia areata. Int J Dermatol. 2003; 42: 738-740.

[1687] Demura S, Yamaji S, Ikemoto Y. Effect of linear polarized near-infrared light irradiation on flexibility of shoulder and ankle joint. J Sport Med Phys Fitness. 2002; 42: 438-445.

[1688] Yokoyama K, Sugiyama K. Temporomandibular joint pain anelgesia by linearly polarized near-infrared irradiation. Clin J Pain. 2001; 17: 47-51.

[1689] Goulart C S, Nouer P R, Mouramartins L, Garbin I U, Lizarelli R. Photoradiation and orthodontic movement: experimental study with canines. Photomed Laser Surg. 2006; 24 (2): 192-196.

[1690] Hawkins D, Abrahamse H. The role of laser fluence in cell viability, proliferation, and membrane integrity of wounded human skin fibroblasts following helium-neon laser irradiation. Lasers Surg Med. 2006; 38 (1): 74-83.

[1691] Hawkins D, Abrahamse H. Biological effects of helium-neon laser irradiation on normal and wounded human skin fibroblasts. Photomed Laser Surg. 2005; 23 (3): 251-259.

[1692] Yacobi Y, Sidi A. Laser light - a new, non invasive treatment for Erectile Dysfunction: a placebo-controlled, single blinded pilot study. http://www.laser.nu/lllt/lllt_editorial11.htm.

[1693] Yamaguchi M, Kasai K. Inflammation in periodontal tissue in response to mechanical forces. Arch Immunol Ther Exper. 2005; 53 (5): 388-398.

[1694] Moriyama Y, Moriyama E H, Blackmore K, Akens MK, Lilge L. In vivo study of the inflammatory modulating effects of low-level laser therapy on iNOS expression using bioluminescence imaging. Photochem Photobiol. 2005; 81 (6): 1351-135.

[1695] Aihara N, Yamaguchi M, Kasai K. Low-energy irradiation stimulates formation of osteoclast-like cells via RANK expression in vitro. Lasers Med Sci. 2006; 21 (1): 24-33.

[1696] Kaviani A, Fateh M, Nooraie R Y, Alinagi-Zadeh M R, Ataie-Fashtami L. Low-level laser therapy in management of postmastectomy lymphedema. Lasers Med Sci. 2006; 21 (2): 90-94.

[1697] Medrado A P, Trindade E, Reis S R, Andrade Z A. Action of low-level laser therapy on living fatty tissue of rats. Lasers Med Sci. 2006; 21 (1): 19-23.

[1698] Vinck E, Cagnie B, Coorevits P, Vanderstraeten G, Cambier D. Pain reduction by infrared light-emitting diode irradiation: a pilot study on experimentally induced delayed-onset muscle soreness in humans. Lasers Med Sci. 2006; 21 (1): 11-18.

[1699] Xu Xiao-Yang, Zhao Xiu-Feng et al. Cellular research on photobiomodulation on excercise induced skeletal muscular fatigue. Laser Med Surg. 2006; Abstract issue, p. 52, abstract 174.

[1700] Aigner N, Fialka C, Radda C, Vecsei V. Adjuvant laser acupuncture in the treatment of whiplash injuries: a prospective, randomized placebo-controlled trial. Wien Klin Wochenschr. 2006; 118 (3-4): 95-99.

[1701] Gottlieb T, Jörgensen B, Rohde E, Müller G, Schellera E E. The influence of irradiation with low-level diode laser on the proteoglycan content in arthrotically changed cartilage in rabbits. Medical Laser Application. 2006; 21 (1): 53-59.

[1702] Chow R T, Heller G Z, Barnsley L. The effect of 300mW, 830nm laser on chronic neck pain: A double-blind, randomized, placebo-controlled study. Pain. 2006; 124 (1-2): 201-210.

[1666] Guerino M R, Baranauskas V, Guerino A C, Parizotto N. Laser treatment of experimentally induced chronic arthritis. Applied Surface Science. 2000; 154-155: 561-564.

[1667] Aimbire F, Albertini R, Leonardo P, Castro Faria Neto H C, Iversen V V, Lopes-Martins R A B, Bjordal J M. Low level laser therapy induces dose-dependent reduction of TNF-alpha levels in rat diaphragm muscle. Lasers Surg Med. 2006; 38 (8): 773-778.

[1668] Aimbire F, Bjordal J M, Iversen V V, Albertini R, Frigo L et al. Low level laser therapy partially restores trachea muscle relaxation response in rats with tumor necrosis factor alpha-mediated smooth airway muscle dysfunction. Lasers Surg Med. 2006; 38 (8): 773-778.

[1669] Mester A F, Snow J B Jr, Shaman P. Photochemical effects of laser irradiation on neuritic outgrowth of olfactory neuroepithelial explants. Otolaryngol Head Neck Surg. 1991; 105 (3): 449-456.

[1670] Mester A F, Snow J B Jr. Effects of laser irradiation on immature olfactory neuroepithelial explants from the rat. Laryngoscope. 1988; 98 (7): 743-745.

[1671] Seifi M, Shafeei H A, Daneshdoost S, Mir M. Effects of two types of low-level laser wave lengths (850 and 630 nm) on the orthodontic tooth movements in rabbits. Lasers Med Sci. 2007; 22 (4): 261-264.

[1672] Khanna A, Shankar L R, Keelan M H et al. Augumentation of the expression of proangiogenic genes in cardiomyocytes with low dose laser irradiation in vitro. Cardiovasc Radiat Med. 1999; 265-269.

[1673] Poon V K, Huang L, Burd A. Biostimulation of dermal fibroblasts by sublethal Q-switched Nd:YAG 532 nm laser: collagen remodeling and pigmentation. J Photochem Photobiol B. 2005: 1-8.

[1674] Craig J A, Barlas P, Baxter G D, Walsh D M, Allen J M. Delayed-onset muscle soreness: lack of effect of combined phototherapy/low-intensity laser therapy at low pulse repetition rates. J Clin Laser Med Surg. 1996; 14 (6): 375-380.

[1675] Craig J A, Barron J, Walsh D M, Baxter G D. Lack of effect of combined low intensity laser therapy/phototherapy (CLILT) on delayed onset muscle soreness in humans. Lasers Surg Med. 1999; 24 (3): 223-230. Erratum in: Lasers Surg Med 1999; 25 (1): 88.

[1676] Lopes-Martins R A, Marcos R L, Leonardo P S, Prianti A C, Muscara M, Aimbire F N, Frigo L, Iversen V V, Bjordal J M. The Effect of Low Level Laser Irradiation(Ga-Al-As - 655 nm) On Skeletal Muscle Fatigue induced by Electrical Stimulation in Rats. J Appl Physiol. 2006; 101 (1): 283-288.

[1677] Branco K, Naeser M A. Carpal tunnel syndrome: clinical outcome after low-level laser acupuncture, microamps transcutaneous electrical nerve stimulation, and other alternative therapies - an open protocol study. J Alternat Complem Med. 1999; 5: 5-26.

[1678] Naeser M A, Hahn K, Lieberman B E. Carpal tunnel syndrome pain treated with low-level laser and microamps TENS, a controlled study. Arch Phys Med Rehabil. 2002; 83: 978-988.

[1679] Bakhtiary A H, Rashidy-Pour A. Ultrasound and laser therapy in the treatment of carpal tunnel syndrome. Aust J Physiother. 2004; 50: 147-151.

[1680] Soriano F, Campaña V, Moya M, Gavotto A et al. Photobiomodulation of pain and inflammation on microcrystalline arthropathies: experimental and clinical results. Photomed Laser Surg. 2006; 24 (2): 140-150.

[1681] Bjordal J M, Johnson M I, Iversen V, Aimbire F, Lopes-Martins R A. Photoradiation in acute pain: a systematic review of possible mechanisms of action and clinical effects in randomized placebo-controlled trials. Photomed Laser Surg. 2006; 24 (2): 158-168.

[1682] Oron U. of tissue repair in skeletal and cardiac muscles. Photomed Laser Surg. 2006; 24 (2): 111-120.

[1683] Hode L, Tunér J. Wrong parameters can give just any result. Laser Surg Med. 2006; 38: 343 (Letter to the editor).

[1646] Pourzarandian A, Watanabe H, Ruwanpura S M, Aoki A, Noguchi K, Ishikawa I. Er:YAG laser irradiation increases prostaglandin E2 production via the induction of cyclooxygenase-2 mRNA in human gingival fibroblasts. J Periodontal Res. 2005; 40 (2): 182-186.

[1647] Bermudez D, Carrasco F, Diaz F, Vargas I P. Germ cell DNA quantification shortly after IR laser radiation. Andrologia. 1991; 23: 303-307.

[1648] Montag M, Rink K, Delacretaz G, van der Ven H. Laserinduced immobilization and plasma membrane permeabilization in human spermatozoa. Hum Reprod. 2000; 15: 846-852.

[1649] Park S, Kim E Y, Yoon S H, Chung K S, Lim J H. Enhanced hatching rate of bovine IVM/IVF/IVC blastocysts using a 1.48-micron diode laser beam. J Assist Reprod Genet. 1999; 16: 97-101.

[1650] Miroshnikov B I, Reznikov L L, Ogurtsov R P, Khachatrian S A. [Immunological characteristics of the course of acute nonspecific epididymitis in relation to the treatment performed]. Vestn Khir Im I I Grek. 1992; 148: 156-161.

[1651] Arbuliev M G, Mikhailov S K, Alibekova S A. [Choice of the treatment method in patients with acute inflammatory diseases of the scrotal organs]. Urol Nefrol (Mosk) 1989; 3: 17-20.

[1652] Singer R, Sagiv M, Barnet M et al. Low energy narrow band non-coherent infrared illumination of human semen and isolated sperm. Androl. 1991; 23: 181-184.

[1653] Lenzi A, Claroni F, Gandini L, Lombardo F, Barbieri C, Lino A, Dondero F. Laser radiation and motility patterns of human sperm. Arch Androl. 1989; 23: 229-234.

[1654] Lubart R, Friedmann H, Levinshal T, Lavie R, Breitbart H. Effect of light in calcium transport in bull sperm cells. J Photochem Photobiol B Biol. 1992; 15: 337-341.

[1655] Porras M D, Bermudez D, Parrado C. Effects biologicos de la radiation laser IR sobre el epitelio seminifero. Invest Clin Laser. 1986; 3: 57-60.

[1656] Celani M F, Gilioli G, Fano AR, Montanini V, Morrama P. The effect of laser radiation on Leydig cells: Functional and morphological studies. IRCS Med Sci. 1984; 12: 883-884.

[1657] Celani M F, Gilioli G, Montanini V, Morrama P. Further evidence that mid laser radiations may stimulate Leydig cell steroidogenesis. IRCS Med Sci. 1985; 13: 336-337.

[1658] Celani M F, Grandi M, Gilioli G. Changes in mouse Leydig cell streoidogenesis following infrared and helium-neon laser irradiation. Exp Clin Endocrinol. 1987; 80: 16-22.

[1659] Makihara E, Makihara M, Masumi S, Sakamoto E. Evaluation of facial thermographic changes before and after low-level laser irradiation. Photomed Laser Surg. 2005; 23 (2): 191-195.

[1660] Meguro D, Yamaguchi M, Kasai K. Laser irradiation inhibition of open gingival embrasure space after orthodontic treatment. Aust Orthod J. 2002; 18 (1): 53-63.

[1661] Zhu X, Chen Y, Sun X. [A study on expression of basic fibroblast growth factors in periodontal tissue following orthodontic tooth movement associated with low power laser irradiation]. Hua Xi Kou Qiang Yi Xue Za Zhi. 2002; 20 (3): 166-168. (in Chinese)

[1662] Rattanayatikul C, Limpanichkul W, Godfrey K, Srisuk N. Effects of low-level laser therapy on the rate of orthodontic tooth movement. Orthod Craniofacial Res. 2006; 9: 38-43.

[1663] Pérez de Vargas I, Parrado C, González V, Vidal L, Rius F. Histological study of the thyroid gland following IR laser radiation. Proc. SPIE. 1992; 1981: 267-272.

[1664] Vidal L, Pérez de Vargas I, Ruiz C, Parrado C, Peláez A. Effect of IR laser radiation in thyroid follicular cells: fine structural and stereological study. Proc. SPIE 1992; 1981: 273-277.

[1665] Vidal L, Ortíz M, Pérez de Vargas I. Ultrastructural Changes in Thyroid Perifollicular-Capillaries During Normal Postnatal Development and After Infrared Laser Radiation. Lasers Med Sci. 2002; 17: 187-197.

[1629] Kiernicka M, Owczarek B, Galkowska E, Wysokinska-Miszczuk J. Comparison of the effectiveness of the conservative treatment of the periodontal pockets with or without the use of laser biostimulation. Ann Univ Mariae Curie Sklodowska [Med]. 2004; 59 (1): 488-494.

[1630] Mijailovic B, Karadaglic D, Mladenovic T et al. Painful piezogenic pedal papules - successful low level laser therapy. Acta Dermatovenerologica, Pannonica, Alpina et Adriatica. 2001; 10 (3).

[1631] Ghoreyshian M, Fazilat F, Fekrazad R, Deyhimi P. Cellular and molecular effect of low level laser on velocity and quality of bone formation in craniofacial distraction osteogenesis. 10th. International Congress of the International Society for Lasers in Dentistry, Berlin, 18.5-20.5 2006.

[1632] Mahdavi Z, Jalalian D M, Fekrazad R. Evaluation of low level laser therapy on desensitivity of vital abutment teeth in fix prosthesis.10th. International Congress of the International Society for Lasers in Dentistry, Berlin, 18.5-20.5 2006.

[1633] Axelsson R, Tullberg M, Ernberg M, Hedenberg-Magnusson B. Temporomandibular conditions in patients with sudden sensorineural hearing loss. Swed Dental J 2005; 29 (4): 175-176. (abstract)

[1634] Qadri T, Bohdanecka P, Miranda L, Tunér J, Altamash M, Gustafsson A. The importance of coherence length in laser phototherapy of gingival inflammation - a pilot study. Lasers Med Sci. 2007; 22 (4): 245-251.

[1635] Ozen T, Orhan K, Gorur I, Ozturk A. Efficacy of low level laser therapy on neurosensory recovery after injury to the inferior alveolar nerve. Head Face Med. 2006; 15; (2): 3.

[1636] De Scheerder I, Wang K, Nikolaychik V, Kaul U et al. Long-term follow-up after coronary stenting and intravascular red laser therapy. Am J Cardiol. 2000; 86 (9): 927-930.

[1637] Derkacz A, Protasiewicz M, Kipshidze N, Bialy D et al. Endoluminal phototherapy for prevention of restenosis: preliminary results at 6-month follow-up. Photomed Laser Surg. 2005; 23 (6): 536-542.

[1638] Bayat M, Delbari A, Almaseyeh M A et al. Low-level laser therapy improves early healing of medial collateral ligament injuries in rats. Photomed Laser Surg. 2005; 23 (6): 556-560.

[1639] Bayat M, Vasheghani M M, Razavi N et al. Effect of low-level laser therapy on the healing of second-degree burns in rats: a histological and microbiological study. J Photochem Photobiol B. 2005; 78 (2): 171-177.

[1640] Bayat M, Ansari A, Hekmat H. Effect of low-power helium-neon laser irradiation on 13-week immobilized articular cartilage of rabbits. Indian J Exp Biol. 2004; 42 (9): 866-870.

[1641] Hemvani N, Chitnis DS, George M, Chammania S. In vitro effect of nitrogen and He-Ne laser on the apoptosis of human polymorphonuclear cells from burn cases and healthy volunteers. Photomed Laser Surg. 2005; 23 (5): 476-479.

[1642] Hemvani N, Chitnis D S, Bhagwanani N S. Helium-neon and nitrogen laser irradiation accelerates the phagocytic activity of human monocytes. Photomed Laser Surg. 2005;23 (6): 571-574.

[1643] Gundogan C, Greve B, Raulin C. Treatment of alopecia areata with the 308-nm xenon chloride excimer laser: case report of two successful treatments with the excimer laser. Lasers Surg Med. 2004; 34 (2): 86-90. Also in: Raulin C, Gündogan C, Greve B, Gebert S. [Excimer laser therapy of alopecia areata - side-by-side evaluation of a representative area]. JDDG - J Ger Soc of Dermatol. 2005; 3: 524-526. (in German with English abstract)

[1644] Satino J, Markou M. Hair Regrowth and Increased Hair Tensile Strength Using the HairMax LaserComb for Low-Level Laser Therapy. Int J Cosmetic Surg Aest Derm. 2003; 5 (2): 113-117.

[1645] Lirani-Galvao A P, Jorgetti V, Lopes Da Silva O. Comparative Study of How Low-Level Laser Therapy and Low-Intensity Pulsed Ultrasound Affect Bone Repair in Rats. Photomed Laser Surg. 2006; 24 (6): 735-740.

[1610] Khadra M, Kassem N, Haanaes H R, Ellingsen J E, Lyngstadaas S P. Enhancement of bone formation in rat calvarial bone defects using low-level laser therapy. Oral Surg Oral Med Oral Pathol Oral Endod. 2004; 97: 693-700.

[1611] Iordanou P, Baltopoulos G, Giannakopoulou M et al. Effect of polarized light in the healing process of pressure ulcers. Int. J Nurs Pract. 2002; 8: 49-55.

[1612] Kubasova T, Horwvath M, Kocsis K et al. Effect of visible light on some cellular and immune parameters. Immunol Cell Biol. 1995; 73: 239-244.

[1613] Medenica L, Lens M. The use of polarised polychromatic non-coherent light alone as a therapy for venous leg ulceration. J Wound Care. 2003; 12: 37-40.

[1614] Monstrey S, Hoeksema H, Depuydt K et al. The effect of polarized light on wound healing. Eur J Plast Surg. 2002; 24: 377-382.

[1615] Weber J B B, Pinheiro A L B, de Oliveira M G, Oliveira A M, Ramalho L M P. Laser Therapy Improves Healing of Bone Defects Submitted to Autologus Bone Graft. Photomed Laser Surg. 2006; 24 (1): 38-44.

[1616] Payer M, Jakse N, Pertl C, Truschnegg A et al. The clinical effect of LLLT in endodontic surgery: a prospective study on 72 cases. Oral Surg Oral Med Oral Pathol Oral Radiol Endod. 2005; 100 (3): 375-379.

[1617] Markovic A B, Kokovic V, Todorovic L. The influence of low-power laser on healing of bone defects: an experimental study. J Oral Laser Applications. 2005; 5: 169-172.

[1618] de Medeiros JS, Vieira GF, Nishimura PY. Laser application effects on the bite strength of the masseter muscle, as an orofacial pain treatment. Photomed Laser Surg. 2005; 23 (4): 373-376.

[1619] Lopes-Martins R A, Albertini R, Martins P S, Bjordal J M, Faria Neto H C. Spontaneous effects of low-level laser therapy (650 nm) in acute inflammatory mouse pleurisy induced by carrageenan. Photomed Laser Surg. 2005; 23 (4): 377-381.

[1620] Gerbi M E, Marques A M, Ramalho L M, Ponzi E A, Carvalho C M, Santos Rde C, Oliveira P C, Nóia M, Pinheiro A L. Infrared laser light further improves bone healing when associated with bone morphogenic proteins: an in vivo study in a rodent model. Photomed Laser Surg. 2008; 26 (1): 55-60.

[1621] Elman M, Lebzelter J. Light therapy in the treatment of acne vulgaris Dermatol Surg. 2004; 30 (2): 139-146.

[1622] Zazzio M. Pain threshold improvement for chronic hyperacusis patients in a prospective clinical study. Improvement on hyperacusis pain thresholds. Photomedicine and Laser Surgery. 2009, ahead of publication.

[1623] Bingöl Ü, Altan L, Yurtkuran M. Low-Energy Laser Treatment for Shoulder Pain. Photomed Laser Surg. 2005; 23 (5): 459-464.

[1624] Salate A C, Barbosa G, Gaspar P et al. Effect of Ga-Al-As Diode Laser Irradiation on Angiogenesis in Partial Ruptures of Achilles Tendon in Rats. Photomed Laser Surg. 2005; 23 (5): 470-475.

[1625] Azevedo L H, Correa Aranha A C, Stolf S F, Eduardo C P, Vieira M M. Evaluation of Low-Level Laser Therapy for the Thyroid Gland of Male Mice. Photomed Laser Surg. 2005; 23 (6): 567-570.

[1626] Gasparyan L, Brill G, Makela A. Activation of vasciular endothelial (VEGF) and fibroblast growth factor (FGF) induced angiogenesis under influence of low level laser radiation in vitro. In: Progesss in Biomedical Optics and imaging. Proc. SPIE.Volume 6140; 614009: 1-7.

[1627] Gasparyan L, Brill G. Influence of laser radiation on migration of stem cells. In: Progesss in Biomedical Optics and imaging. Proc. SPIE.Volume 6140; 61400P 1-6.

[1628] Klein E, Fine S, Laor Y et al. Interaction of laser radiation with biologic systems. II. Experimental tumors. Fed Proc. 1965; 24: Suppl 14: 147.

[1592] Vinck E, Coorevits P, Cagnie B, De Muynck M et al. Evidence of changes in sural nerve conduction mediated by light emitting diode irradiation. Lasers in Medical Science. 2005; 20 (1): 35-40.

[1593] Vinck E M, Cagnie B J, Cornelissen M J et al. Increased fibroblast proliferation induced by light emitting diode and low power laser irradiation. Lasers in Medical Science. 2003; 18 (2): 95-99.

[1594] Vinck E M, Cagnie B J, Cornelissen M J, Declercq H A, Cambier D C. Green light emitting diode irradiation enhances fibroblast growth impaired by high glucose level. Photomed Laser Surg. 2005; 23 (2): 167-171.

[1595] Kopera D, Kokol R, Berger C, Haas J. Does the use of low-level laser influence wound healing in chronic venous ulcers? J Wound Care. 2005; 14 (8): 391-394.

[1596] Yew DT, Li WW, Pang KM, Mok YC, Au C. Stimulation of collagen formation in the intestinal anastomosis by low dose He-Ne laser. Scanning Microsc. 1989; 3 (1): 379-385; discussion 386.

[1597] Neckel C. The effect of low level laser therapy with a GaAlAs diode laser on the bony regeneration of extraction sockets. ESOLA congress Abu Dhabi, October 7-8, 2004. Clinical Experiences in Laser Dentistry.

[1598] Mok YC, Pang KM, Au CY, Yew DT. Preliminary observations on the effects in vivo and in vitro of low dose laser on the epithelia of the bladder, trachea and tongue of the mouse. Scanning Microsc. 1988; 2 (1): 493-502.

[1599] Levine RA, Abel M, Cheng H. CNS somatosensory-auditory interactions elicit or modulate tinnitus. Exp Brain Res. 2003; 153 (4): 643-648.

[1600] Yoshida K et al. The effect of low power semiconductor laser to the stellate ganglion. IX Congress International Society for Laser Surg Med, Anaheim, California, USA, 1991.

[1601] Avni D, Levkovitz S, Maltz L, Oron U. Protection of skeletal muscles from ischemic injury: low-level laser therapy increases antioxidant activity. Photomed Laser Surg. 2005; 23 (3): 273-277.

[1602] Yeager R L, Franzosa J A, Millsap D S, Angell-Yeager J L et al. Effects of 670-nm phototherapy on development. Photomed Laser Surg. 2005; 23 (3): 268-272.

[1603] Pinfildi C E, Liebano R E, Hochman B S, Ferreira L M. Helium-neon laser in viability of random skin flap in rats. Lasers Surg Med. 2005; 37 (1): 74-77.

[1604] Wong B J, Pandhoh N, Truong M T, Diaz S et al. Identification of chondrocyte proliferation following laser irradiation, thermal injury, and mechanical trauma. Lasers Surg Med. 2005; 37 (1): 89-96.

[1605] Weiss R A, McDaniel D H, Geronemus R G, Munavalli G M, Bellew S G. Clinical Experience with Light-Emitting Diode (LED) Photomodulation. Dermatol Surg. 2005; 31(Pt 2): 1199-1205.

[1606] Pourzarandian A, Watanabe H, Ruwanpura SM, Aoki A, Ishikawa Effect of low-level Er:YAG laser irradiation on cultured human gingival fibroblasts. J Periodontol. 2005; 76 (2): 187-193.

[1607] Khadra M, Lyngstadaas S P, Haanaes H R, Mustafa K. Effect of laser therapy on attachment, proliferation and differentiation of human osteoblastic-like cells cultured on titanium implant material. Biomaterials.2005; 26: 3503-3509.

[1608] Khadra M, Lyngstadaas S P, Haanaes H R, Mustafa K. Determining optimal dose of laser therapy for attachment and proliferation of human fibroblasts cultured on titanium implant material. J Biomed Mater Res. 2005; 73A: 55-62.

[1609] Torriceilli P, Giavaresi G, Fini G A, Guzzardella G et al. Laser biostimulation of cartilage: in vitro evaluation. Biomed Pharmacother. 2001; 55: 117-120.

[1573] Yokoyama K, Sugiyama K. Influence of Linearly Polarized Near-Infrared Irradiation on Deformability of Human Stored Erythrocytes. J Clinical Laser Medicine & Surgery. 2003; 21 (1): 19-22.

[1574] Wee JS, Jung JC, Han JY, Lee SG, Rowe SM. Effects of Stellate Ganglion Irradiation by the Low-level Laser Therapy on Reflex Sympathetic Dystrophy of the Hemiplegic Arm. Chonnam Med J. 2001; 37 (1): 49-54.

[1575] Basford J R, Sandroni P, Low P A, Hines S M et al. Effects of linearly polarized 0.6-1.6 microM irradiation on stellate ganglion function in normal subjects and people with complex regional pain (CRPS I). Lasers Surg Med. 2003; 32 (5): 417-423.

[1576] Nagao M, Yamaguchi S, Okuda Y. [Effects of low reactive level laser, linear polarized light and Xenon-ray irradiation on the stellate ganglion in dogs]. Masui. 2001; 50 (9): 958-963. (Article in Japanese)

[1577] Wajima Z, Shitara T, Inoue T, Ogawa R. [Linear polarized light irradiation around the stellate ganglion area increases skin temperature and blood flow]. Masui. 1996; 45 (4): 433-438. (Article in Japanese)

[1578] Otsuka H, Okubo K, Imai M, Kaseno S, Kemmotsu O. [Polarized light irradiation near the stellate ganglion in a patient with Raynaud's sign]. Masui. 1992; 41 (11): 1814-1817. (Article in Japanese)

[1579] Gavish L, Asher Y, Becker Y, Kleinman Y. Low level laser irradiation stimulates mitochondrial membrane potential and disperses subnuclear promyelocytic leukemia protein. Lasers Surg Med. 2004; 35 (5): 369-376.

[1580] Albertini R, Aimbire F S, Correa F I, Ribeiro W et al. Effects of different protocol doses of low power gallium-aluminum-arsenate (Ga-Al-As) laser radiation (650 nm) on carrageenan induced rat paw oedema. J Photochem Photobiol B. 2004; 27;74 (2-3): 101-107.

[1581] Schoop U, Moritz A, Kluger W, Patruta S et al. The Er:YAG laser in endodontics: results of an in vitro study. Lasers Surg Med. 2002; 30 (5): 360-364.

[1582] Moritz A, Schoop U, Goharkhay K, Jakolitsch S et al. The bactericidal effect of Nd:YAG, Ho:YAG, and Er:YAG laser irradiation in the root canal: an in vitro comparison. J Clin Laser Med Surg. 1999; 17 (4): 161-164.

[1583] Gutknecht N, Moritz A, Conrads G, Sievert T, Lampert F. Bactericidal effect of the Nd:YAG laser in in vitro root canals. J Clin Laser Med Surg. 1996; 14 (2): 77-80.

[1584] Gutknecht N, Kaiser F, Hassan A, Lampert F. Long-term clinical evaluation of endodontically treated teeth by Nd:YAG lasers. J Clin Laser Med Surg. 1996; 14 (1): 7-11.

[1585] Klinke T, Klimm W, Gutknecht N. Antibacterial effects of Nd:YAG laser irradiation within root canal dentin. J Clin Laser Med Surg. 1997; 15 (1): 29-31.

[1586] Moreira L A, Santos M T, Campos V F, Genovese W J. Efficiency of laser therapy applied in labial traumatism of patients with spastic cerebral palsy. Braz Dent J. 2004; 15 Spec No: 29-33.

[1587] Byrnes K R, Wu X, Waynant R W, Ilev I K, Anders J J. Low power laser irradiation alters gene expression of olfactory ensheathing cells in vitro. Lasers Surg Med. 2005; 37 (2): 161-117.

[1588] Zeredo J L, Sasaki K M, Takeuchi Y, Toda K. Antinociceptive effect of Er:YAG laser irradiation in the orofacial formalin test. Brain Res. 2005; 1032 (1-2): 149-153.

[1589] Streeter J, De Taboada L, Oron U. Mechanisms of action of light therapy for stroke and acute myocardial infarction. Mitochondrion. 2004; 4 (5-6): 569-576.

[1590] Ilic S, Leichliter S, Streeter J, DeTaboada L, Oron U. Effects of Dose, Mode and Frequency of Low Level Laser Therapy on the Rat Brain. Photomed Laser Surg. 2006; 24 (4): 458-66.

[1591] Mirsky N, Krispel Y, Shoshany Y, Maltz L, Oron U. Promotion of angiogenesis by low energy laser irradiation. Antioxid Redox Signal. 2002; 4 (5): 785-790.

[1555] Villa G E P, Catirse A B, Lia R C, Lizarelli R F Z. Analysis in vivo on the effects of low power laser irradiation at stimulation of reactional dentin. Proc. 3rd Congress of ESOLA, Barcelona, Spain, May 2005, p. 52.

[1556] Dortbudak O, Haas R, Bernhart T, Mailath-Pokorny G. Lethal photosensitization for decontamination of implant surfaces in the treatment of peri-implantitis. Clin Oral Implants Res. 2001; 12 (2): 104-108.

[1557] Corral-Baques M I, Rigau T, Rivera M, Rodriguez J E, Rigau J. Effect of 655-nm diode laser on dog sperm motility. Lasers Med Sci. 2005; 20 (1): 28-34.

[1558] Shibata Y, Ogura N, Yamashiro K et al. Anti-inflammatory effect of linear polarized infrared irradiation on interleukin-1-induced chemokine production in MH7A rheumatoid synovial cells. Lasers in Medical Science. 2005; July 27.

[1559] Siedentopf C M, , Koppelstaetter F, Haala I A et al. Laser acupuncture induced specific cerebral cortical and subcortical activations in humans. Lasers Med Sci. 2005; 20 (2): 68-73.

[1560] Aimbire F, Albertini R, de Magalhães R G, Lopes-Martins R A et al. Effect of LLLT Ga-Al-As (685 nm) on LPS-induced inflammation of the airway and lung in the rat. Lasers in Medical Science. 2005; 20 (1): 11-20.

[1561] Whittaker P. Laser acupuncture: past, present, and future. Lasers in Medical Science. 2005; 19 (2): 69-80.

[1562] Gigo-Benato D, Geuna S, de Castro Rodrigues A, Tos P et al. Low-power laser biostimulation enhances nerve repair after end-to-side neurorrhaphy: a double-blind randomized study in the rat median nerve model. Lasers in Medical Science, 2004; 19 (1): 57-65.

[1563] Dube A , Jayasankar K, Prabakaran L et al. Nitrogen laser irradiation (337 nm) causes temporary inactivation of clinical isolates of Mycobacterium tuberculosis. Lasers in Medical Science. 2004; 19 (1): 52-56.

[1564] Hamajima S, Hiratsuka K, Kiyama-Kishikawa M, Tagawa T et al. Effect of low-level laser irradiation on osteoglycin gene expression in osteoblasts. Lasers in Medical Science. 2003; 18 (2): 78-82.

[1565] Bagis S, Comelekoglu U, Coskun B, Milcan A et al. No effect of GA-AS (904 nm) laser irradiation on the intact skin of the injured rat sciatic nerve. Lasers in Medical Science. 2003; 18 (2): 83-88.

[1566] Nicola R A, Jorgetti V, Rigau J, Marcos T T. Effect of low-power GaAlAs laser (660 nm) on bone structure and cell activity: an experimental animal study. Lasers in Medical Science. 2003; 18 (2): 89-94.

[1567] Kreisler M, Christoffers A B, Willershausen B, d'Hoedt B et al. Low-level 809 nm GaAlAs laser irradiation increases the proliferation rate of human laryngeal carcinoma cells in vitro. Lasers in Medical Science. 2003; 18 (2): 100-103.

[1568] Fekrazad R, Jafari Sh, Kalhori K. The effects of Pulsed Nd:YAG Laser Therapy on Recurrent Aphtous Ulcers. Internat Congress of. ESOLA, Vienna, Austria, May 2001, p. 40-41.

[1569] Ebneshahidi N S, Heshmatipour M, Moghaddami A, Eghtesadi A P. The effects of laser acupuncture on chronic tension headache - a randomised controlled trial. Acupuncture in Medicine. 2005; 23 (1): 13-18.

[1570] Chow R T, Barnsley L. Systematic review of the literature of low-level laser therapy (LLLT) in the management of neck pain. Lasers Surg Med. 2005; 37 (1): 46-52.

[1571] Zanin I C, Goncalves R B, Aldo Brugnera Junior A, Hope K C, Pratten J. Susceptibility of Streptococcus mutans biofilms to photodynamic therapy: an in vitro study. Journal of Antimicrobial Chemotherapy. 2005; 56 (2): 324-330.

[1572] Whelan H T, Buchmann E V, Dhokalia A et al. Effect of NASA Light-Emitting Diode Irradiation on Molecular Changes for Wound Healing in Diabetic Mice. J Clinical Laser Medicine & Surgery. 2003; 21 (2): 67-74.

[1539] Taly A B, Sivaraman Nair K P, Murali T, John A. Efficacy of multiwavelength light therapy in the treatment of pressure ulcers in subjects with disorders of the spinal cord: A randomized double-blind controlled trial. Archives of Physical Medicine and Rehabilitation. 2004; 85 (10): 1657-1661.

[1540] Puri M M, Arora K. Role of Gallium Arsenide Laser Irradiation at 890 nm as an Adjunctive to Anti-tuberculosis Drugs in the Treatment of Pulmonary Tuberculosis. Indian J Chest Dis Allied Sci. 2003; 45: 13-19.

[1541] Toida M, Watanabe F, Kazumi Goto K, Shibata T. Usefulness of Low-Level Laser for Control of Painful Stomatitis in Patients with Hand-Foot-and-Mouth Disease. Journal of Clinical Laser Medicine & Surgery. 2003; 21 (6): 363-367.

[1542] Al-Watban F A H, Andres B L. Polychromatic LED Therapy in Burn Healing of Nondiabetic and Diabetic Rats. J Clinical Laser Medicine & Surgery. 2003; 21 (5): 249-258.

[1543] Fujimaki Y, Shimoyama T, Liu Q et al. Low-Level Laser Irradiation Attenuates Production of Reactive Oxygen Species by Human Neutrophils. J Clinical Laser Medicine & Surgery. 2003; 21 (3): 165-170.

[1544] Jih Ming H, Friedman P M, Kimyai A A, Goldberg L H. Successful treatment of a chronic atrophic dog-bite scar with the 1450-nm diode laser. Dermatologic Surgery 2004; 30 (8): 1161-11633.

[1545] Garavello I, Baranauskas V, Cruz-Hoefling MA. The effects of low laser irradiation on angiogenesis in injured rat tibiae. Histology and Histopathology. 2004; 19 (1): 43-48.

[1545] Derkacz A,Bialy D, Protasiewicz Marcin et al. Photostimulation of coronary arteries with low power laser radiation: preliminary results for a new method in invasive cardiology therapy. Medical Science Monitor. 2003; 9 (7): 335-339.

[1546] Milojevic M, Kuruc V. [Low power laser biostimulation in the treatment of bronchial asthma]. Biostimulacija laserom niske snage u lecenju bronhijalne astme. Medicinski pregled. 2003; 56 (9-10): 413-418.

[1547] Castro-e-Silva O Jr, Zucoloto S, Marcassa L G, Marcassa J et al. Spectral response for laser enhancement in hepatic regeneration for hepatectomized rats. Lasers Surg Med. 2003; 32 (1): 50-53.

[1548] Taha M F, Valojerdi M R. Quantitative and qualitative changes of the seminiferous epithelium induced by Ga. Al. As. (830 nm) laser radiation. Lasers Surg Med. 2004; 34 (4): 352-359.

[1549] Kurumada F. The effect of laser irradiation on the activation of inflammatory cells and the vital pulpotomy. A study of the application of Ga-As semiconductor laser to endodontics. J Clinical Pediatric Dentistry. 1995; 19: 232.

[1550] Fujihara N A, Hiraki K R, Marques M M. Irradiation at 780 nm increases proliferation rate of osteoblasts independently of dexamethasone presence. Lasers Surg Med. 2006; 38 (4): 332-336.

[1551] Fekrazad R, Atabaki M, Eslami B, Kalhori K. A study on the effects of low level laser therapy. Proc. 3rd Congress of ESOLA, Barcelona, Spain, May 2005, p. 12.

[1552] González V, Chiquini J. Low level laser therapy in ortognathic surgery. Proc. 3rd Congress of ESOLA, Barcelona, Spain, May 2005, p. 12.

[1553] Prokopowisch I, Kleine B M, Youssef M N, Lage-Marques L J. The low power GaAlAs action in the postoperative pain control in human teeth after root canal preparation. Proc. 3rd Congress of ESOLA, Barcelona, Spain, May 2005, p. 33.

[1554] Lizarelli R F Z, Pizzo R CA, Mazzetto M O. The antialgetic effect of the low intensity laser in the internal disorders of the temporo-mandibular joint. Proc. 3rd Congress of ESOLA, Barcelona, Spain, May 2005, p. 52.

[1521] Wozniak P, Stachowiak G, Pieta-Dolinska A, Oszukowski P. Laser acupuncture and low-calorie diet during visceral obesity therapy after menopause. Acta Obstet Gynecol Scand. 2003; 82 (1): 69-73.

[1522] Gruber W, Eber E, Malle-Scheid D, Pfleger A et al. Laser acupuncture in children and adolescents with exercise induced asthma. Thorax. 2002; 57 (3): 222-225.

[1523] Ribeiro M S, Silva D F, Maldonado E P, de Rossi W, Zezell D M. Effects of 1047-nm neodymium laser radiation on skin wound healing. J Clin Laser Med Surg. 2002; 20 (1): 37-40.

[1524] White A R, Rampes H, Ernst E. Acupuncture for smoking cessation. Cochrane Database Syst Rev. 2002; (2): CD000009.

[1525] Karu T I, Pyatibrat L V, Kalendo G S. Donors of NO and pulsed radiation at lambda = 820 nm exert effects on cell attachment to extracellular matrices. Toxicol Lett. 2001; 121 (1): 57-61.

[1526] Karu T I, Pyatibrat L V, Afanasyeva N I. Cellular effects of low power laser therapy can be mediated by nitric oxide. Lasers Surg Med. 2005; 36 (4): 307-314.

[1527] Byrnes K R, Waynant R W, Ilev I K, Wu X et al. Light promotes regeneration and functional recovery and alters the immune response after spinal cord injury. Lasers Surg Med. 2005; 36 (3): 171-185.

[1528] Brosseau L, Wells G, Marchand S, Gaboury I et al. Randomized controlled trial on low level laser therapy (LLLT) in the treatment of osteoarthritis (OA) of the hand. Lasers Surg Med. 2005; 36 (3): 210-219.

[1529] Silva J C, Lacava Z G, Kuckelhaus S, Silva L P et al. Evaluation of the use of low level laser and photosensitizer drugs in healing. Lasers Surg Med. 2004; 34 (5): 451-457.

[1530] Mehdi M S, al Magsosy R. Design and Construction of a System to Study the Effect of Laser Radiation on the Absorption of the Antibiotics in Blood. Thesis for PhD. 2005. Department of Laser and Optoelectronics Engineering, Al-Nahrain University, Al-Jaderia, Baghdad, Iraq.

[1531] Almeida Lopes L, Lopes A. Using Laser Therapy on the lymphat c drainage technique. Photomed Laser Surg. 2005; 23 (1). Abstracts from the 5th Congress of the World Association for Laser Therapy, São Paulo, Brazil, November 2004. Abstract no 042, p.100.

[1532] Monteforte P, Baratto L, Molfetta L, Rovetta G. Low-power laser in osteoarthritis of the cervical spine. Int J Tissue React. 2003; 25 (4): 131-136.

[1533] Amat A, Rigau J, Nicolau R, Aalders M et al. Effect of red and near-infrared laser light on adenosine triphosphate (ATP) in the luciferine-luciferase reaction. Journal of Photochemistry and Photobiology A: Chemistry. 2004; 168 (1-2): 59-65.

[1534] Koutna M, Janisch R, Unucka M, Svobodnik A, Mornstein V. Effects of low-power laser irradiation on cell locomotion in protozoa. Photochem Photobiol. 2004; 80 (3): 531-534.

[1535] Pugliese LS, Medrado AP, Reis SR, Andrade Zde A. The influence of low-level laser therapy on biomodulation of collagen and elastic fibers. Pesqui Odontol Bras. 2003; (4): 307-313.

[1536] Corona S A, Nascimento T N, Catirse A B, Lizarelli R F, Dinelli W, Palma-Dibb R G. Clinical evaluation of low-level laser therapy and fluoride varnish for treating cervical dentinal hypersensitivity. J Oral Rehabil. 2003; 30 (12): 1183-1189.

[1537] Zati A, Fortuna D, Valent A, Pulvirenti F, Bilotta T W. Treatment of low back pain caused by intervertebral disk displacement: comparison between high power laser, TENS and NSAIDs. Medicina Dello Sport. 2004; 57 (1): 77-82.

[1538] Lin Y S, Huang M H, Chai C Y, Yang R C. Effects of helium-neon laser on levels of stress protein and arthritic histopathology in experimental osteoarthritis. Am J Phys Med Rehabil. 2004; 83 (10): 758-765.

[1504] Eells J T, Henry M M, Summerfelt P, Wong-Riley M T, Buchmann E V et al. Therapeutic photobiomodulation for methanol-induced retinal toxicity. Proc Natl Acad Sci U S A. 2003; 18, 100 (6): 3439-3444.

[1505] Tascioglu F, Armagan O, Tabak Y, Corapci I, Oner C. Low power laser treatment in patients with knee osteoarthritis. Swiss Med Wkly. 2004; 134 (17-18): 254-258.

[1506] Lubart R, Eichler M, Lavi R, Friedman H, Shainberg A. Low-energy laser irradiation promotes cellular redox activity. Photomed Laser Surg. 2005; 23 (1): 3-9.

[1507] Bjordal J M. Can a Cochrane review in controversial areas be biased? A sensitivity analysis based on the protocol of a systematic Cochrane review Low Level Laser Therapy in Osteoarthritis. Photomed Laser Surg. 2005; 23 (5): 453-458.

[1508] Ng G Y, Fung D T, Leung M C, Guo X. Comparison of single and multiple applications of GaAlAs laser on rat medial collateral ligament repair. Laser Surg Med. 2004; 34 (3): 285-289.

[1509] Marsilio A L, Rodrigues J R, Borges A B. Effect of the clinical application of the GaAlAs laser in the treatment of dentine hypersensitivity. J Clin Laser Med Surg. 2003; 21 (5): 291-296.

[1510] Moller K I, Kongshoj B, Philipsen P A et al. How Finsen's light cured lupus vulgaris. Photodermatol Photoimmunol Photomed. 2005; 21 (3): 118-124.

[1510] Blankenau R J, Powell G, Ellis R W, Westerman G H. In vivo caries-like lesion prevention with argon laser: pilot study. J Clin Laser Med Surg. 1999; 17 (6): 241-243.

[1511] Antipa C, Pascu M, Stanciulescu V et al. Coherent and noncoherent low-power diodes in clinical practice. Proc. SPIE Vol. 2981, p. 236-241, Coherence Domain Optical Methods in Biomedical Science and Clinical Applications; Valery V. Tuchin, Halina Podbielska M.D., Ben Ovryn; Eds.

[1512] Sato T, Kawatani M, Takeshige C, Matsumoto I. Ga-Al-As laser irradiation inhibits neuronal activity associated with inflammation. Acupunct Electrother Res. 1994; 19 (2-3): 141-151.

[1513] Schubert V. Effects Of Phototherapy (LLLT) On Pressure Ulcer Healing In Elderly Patients After A Falling Trauma. A Prospective, Randomized, Controlled Study. Photodermatol Photoimmunol Photomed. 2001; 17 (1): 32-38.

[1514] Lomelí-Rivas A, Krötzsch E, Michtchenko A. Effect of 650 nm laser stimulation with clinical doses on cultivated human fibroblasts proliferation. [Efecto de la estimulación láser de 650 nm, utilizando dosis de uso clínico, sobre la proliferación de fibroblastos humanos cultivados]. Rev Mex Med Fis Rehab. 2003; 15 (3-4): 69-71.

[1515] Giuliani A, Fernandez M, Farinelli M, Baratto L et al. Very low level laser therapy attenuates edema and pain in experimental models. Int J Tissue React. 2004; 26 (1-2): 29-37.

[1516] O'Reilly B A, Dwyer P L, Hawthorne G et al. Transdermal posterior tibial nerve laser therapy is not effective in women with interstitial cystitis. J Urol. 2004; 172 (5 Pt 1): 1880-1883.

[1517] Zalewska-Kaszubska J, Obzejta D. Use of low-energy laser as adjunct treatment of alcohol addiction. Lasers Med Sci. 2004; 19 (2): 100-104.

[1518] Litscher G, Rachbauer D, Ropele S, Wang L et al. Acupuncture using laser needles modulates brain function: first evidence from functional transcranial Doppler sonography and functional magnetic resonance imaging. Lasers Med Sci. 2004; 19 (1): 6-11.

[1519] Litscher G, Nemetz W, Smolle J, Schwarz G et al. [Histological investigation of the micromorphological effects of the application of a laser needle - results of an animal experiment]. Biomed Tech (Berl). 2004; 49 (1-2): 2-5. (in German)

[1520] Allais G, De Lorenzo C, Quirico P E, Lupi G et al. Non-pharmacological approaches to chronic headaches: transcutaneous electrical nerve stimulation, laser therapy and acupuncture in transformed migraine treatment. Neurol Sci. 2003; 24 Suppl 2: S138-142.

2005; 23 (1). Abstracts from the 5th Congress of the World Association for Laser Therapy, São Paulo, Brazil, November 2004. Poster no 111, page 142.

[1486] Dourado D M, De Paula K R, De Carvalho P T et al. Gastrocnemic muscle angiogenesis relation with the irradiated Laser Ga-As and with bothropic venom injected. Photomed Laser Surg. 2005; 23 (1). Abstracts from the 5th Congress of the World Association for Laser Therapy, São Paulo, Brazil, November 2004. Poster no 108, page 142.

[1487] Hopkins J T, McLoda T A, Seegmiller J G, Baxter G D. Low-Level Laser Therapy Facilitates Superficial Wound Healing in Humans: A Triple-Blind, Sham-Controlled Study. J Athl Train. 2004; 39 (3): 223-229.

[1488] Bernhardt O, Gesch D, Schwahn C, Bitter K et al. Signs of temporomandibular disorders in tinnitus patients and in a population-based group of volunteers: results of the Study of Health in Pomerania. J Oral Rehabil. 2004; 31 (4): 311-319.

[1489] Bae C S, Lim S C, Kim K Y, Song C H et al. Effect of Ga-as laser on the regeneration of injured sciatic nerves in the rat. In Vivo. 2004; 18 (4): 489-495.

[1490] Demir H, Yaray S, Kirnap M, Yaray K. Comparison of the effects of laser and ultrasound treatments on experimental wound healing in rats. J Rehabil Res Dev. 2004; 41 (5): 721-728.

[1491] Demir H, Menku P, Kirnap M, Calis M, Ikizceli I. Comparison of the effects of laser, ultrasound, and combined laser + ultrasound treatments in experimental tendon healing. Lasers Surg Med. 2004; 35 (1): 84-89.

[1492] Stergioulas A. Low-level laser treatment can reduce edema in second degree ankle sprains. J Clin Laser Med Surg. 2004; 22 (2): 125-128.

[1493] Kawalec J S, Pfennigwerth C, Hetherington J et al. A review of lasers in healing diabetic ulcers.The Foot. 2004; 14: 68-71.

[1494] Plavnik L, de Crosa M, Malberti A. Effect of low-power radiation (helium/neon) upon submandibular glands. J Clin Laser Med Surg. 2003; 21 (4): 219-225.

[1495] Al-Watban F A, Zhang X Y. The comparison of effects between pulsed and CW lasers on wound healing. J Clin Laser Med Surg. 2004; 22 (1): 15-18.

[1496] Nussbaum E L, Lilge L, Mazzulli T. Effects of low-level laser therapy (LLLT) of 810 nm upon in vitro growth of bacteria: relevance of irradiance and radiant exposure. J Clin Laser Med Surg. 2003; 21 (5): 283-290.

[1497] Ribeiro M S, Da Silva D de F, De Araujo C E, De Oliveira S F et al. Effects of low-intensity polarized visible laser radiation on skin burns: a light microscopy study. J Clin Laser Med Surg. 2004; 22 (1): 59-66.

[1498] Mendez T M, Pinheiro A L, Pacheco M T, Nascimento P M, Ramalho L M. Dose and wavelength of laser light have influence on the repair of cutaneous wounds. J Clin Laser Med Surg. 2004; 22 (1): 19-25.

[1499] Wong-Riley M T, Liang H L, Eells JT, Chance B et al. Photobiomodulation directly benefits primary neurons functionally inactivated by toxins: role of cytochrome c oxidase. J Biol Chem. 2005; 11; 280 (6): 4761-4771.

[1500] Shin D H, Lee E, Hyun J K, Lee S J et al. Growth-associated protein-43 is elevated in the injured rat sciatic nerve after low power laser irradiation. Neurosci Lett. 2003; 344 (2): 71-74.

[1501] Kreisler M B, Haj H A, Noroozi N, Willershausen B. Efficacy of low level laser therapy in reducing postoperative pain after endodontic surgery - a randomized double blind clinical study. Int J Oral Maxillofac Surg. 2004; 33 (1): 38-41.

[1502] Soukos N S, Som S, Abernethy A D et al. Phototargeting oral black-pigmented bacteria. Antimicrob Agents Chemother. 2005; 49 (4): 1391-1396.

[1503] Whelan H T, Smits R L Jr, Buchman E V, Whelan N T et al.. Effect of NASA light-emitting diode irradiation on wound healing. J Clin Laser Med Surg. 2001; 19 (6): 305-314

Laser Surg. 2005; 23 (1). Abstracts from the 5th Congress of the World Association for Laser Therapy, São Paulo, Brazil, November 2004. Abstract no 050, p.102.

[1474] de Jesus Guirro R R, de Oliveira Guirro E. Analysis of the transmissivity of Low Power Laser radiation in different occlusive dressings. Photomed Laser Surg. 2005; 23 (1). Abstracts from the 5th Congress of the World Association for Laser Therapy, São Paulo, Brazil, November 2004. Abstract no 055, p.103.

[1475] Núñez S C, Silva Garcez A, Cardoso Jorge A O, Suzuki S S, Simões Ribeiro M. Low Intensity Laser Therapy and transcutaneous electrical neural stimulation (TENS) on the improvement of mouth opening in patients with temporomandibular disorders. Photomed Laser Surg. 2005; 23 (1). Abstracts from the 5th Congress of the World Association for Laser Therapy, São Paulo, Brazil, November 2004. Abstract no 076, p.109.

[1476] Shoji N, de Oliveira C, Magacho T A, Chavantes M C. Low Potency Laser treatment for acute dehiscence saphenactomy process. Photomed Laser Surg. 2005; 23 (1). Abstracts from the 5th Congress of the World Association for Laser Therapy, São Paulo, Brazil, November 2004. Abstract no 082, p.110.

[1477] Ramos L, Magacho T A, Magacho Da Silva A, Chavantes M A. Preliminary study of Low Potency Laser use regarding to the constrict strength of health and atrophic musculatures. Photomed Laser Surg. 2005; 23 (1). Abstracts from the 5th Congress of the World Association for Laser Therapy, São Paulo, Brazil, November 2004. Abstract no 084, p.110.

[1478] Chow R, Barnsley L, Gillian Z, Heller G Z, Siddall P J. The effect of 300mW, 830 nm laser on chronic neck pain: a prospective, double-blind, randomised, placebo-controlled study. Photomed Laser Surg. 2005; 23 (1). Abstracts from the 5th Congress of the World Association for Laser Therapy, São Paulo, Brazil, November 2004. Abstract no 088, p.112.

[1479] Chavantes M C. Pilot study : new treatment applying LLLT in tracheal stenosis. Using biomodulated effect. Photomed Laser Surg. 2005; 23 (1). Abstracts from the 5th Congress of the World Association for Laser Therapy, São Paulo, Brazil, November 2004. Abstract no 095, p.113.

[1480] Chavantes M C, Baptista I M, Kajita G, Shoji N. Prevention or acute treatment right after a risky surgery: does LLLT decrease complications? Photomed Laser Surg. 2005; 23 (1). Abstracts from the 5th Congress of the World Association for Laser Therapy, São Paulo, Brazil, November 2004. Abstract no 096, p.113. Also: Chavantes M C; Zangaro R A; Pacheco M T T, Oliveira S A. Wound Dehiscence After Sternotomy Can Be Prevented Using Low Power Laser Therapy. Lasers Surg Med. 2004; 34, supl. 1, p. 36.

[1481] Takamoto M, Magalhães Da Cruz F, Ladalardo T C; Tarso Mugnai Marraccini; Brugnera Júnior A, De Carvalho Campos R A.Evaluation of the effect of Laser Therapy in the treatment of trigeminal neuralgia. Photomed Laser Surg. 2005; 23 (1). Abstracts from the 5th Congress of the World Association for Laser Therapy, São Paulo, Brazil, November 2004. Poster no 28, page 121.

[1482] Bonome Salate A C, Barbosa G, Gaspar P, Nivaldo Antonio Parizotto N A et al. Effects of 660 nm GaAsAl with 10 mW and 40 mW on neoangiogenesis after partial ruptures of Achilles tendon (Tendocalcaneus). Photomed Laser Surg. 2005; 23 (1). Abstracts from the 5th Congress of the World Association for Laser Therapy, São Paulo, Brazil, November 2004. Poster no 60, page 129.

[1483] Ladalardo T C, Tirapelli B, Marraccini T M et al. The effects of phototherapy on oral mucositis in bone marrow transplant patients—Preliminary results. Photomed Laser Surg. 2005; 23 (1). Abstracts from the 5th Congress of the World Association for Laser Therapy, São Paulo, Brazil, November 2004. Poster no 81, page 134.

[1484] Hage R, Duarte J, Silva C M et al. The Low Level Laser Therapy (LLLT) in the prevention and repair of the muscle injury induced by bothrops jararaca poison injected in rats. Photomed Laser Surg. 2005; 23 (1). Abstracts from the 5th Congress of the World Association for Laser Therapy, São Paulo, Brazil, November 2004. Poster no 100, page 139.

[1485] Catão M H, Pinheiro A L, Costa J L et al. Low energy AsGaAl Laser (830nm) for the prevention of chemo-induced mucositis in oral cavity cancer patients. Photomed Laser Surg.

[1458] McCaughan J S Jr, Bethel B H, Johnston T, Janssen W. Effect of low-dose argon irradiation on rate of wound closure. Lasers Surg Med. 1985; 5 (6): 607-614.

[1459] Ilbuldu E, Cakmak A, Disci R, Aydin R. Comparison of laser, dry needling, and placebo laser treatments in myofascial pain syndrome. Photomed Laser Surg. 2004; 22 (4): 306-311.

[1460] Oliveira Lopes C, Zangaro R A, Rigau J. Prevention of xerostomia induced by radiotherapy using low level laser. Photomed Laser Surg. 2005; (1). Abstracts from the 5th Congress of the World Association for Laser Therapy, November 25-27, 2004, São Paulo, Brazil. Abstr 001, p. 90.

[1461] Bjordal J M, Lopes-Martins R A, Iversen V V. A randomised, placebo controlled trial of low level laser therapy for activated Achilles tendinitis with microdialysis measurement of peritendinous prostaglandin E2 concentrations. Br J Sports Med. 2006; 40 (1): 76-80.

[1462] Pessoa E S, Melhado R M, Theodoro L H, Garcia V G. A histologic assessment of the influence of low-intensity laser therapy on wound healing in steroid-treated animals. Photomed Laser Surg. 2004; 22 (3): 199-204.

[1463] Lopes-Martins R A, Albertini R, Lopes-Martins P S et al. Steroids receptor antagonist Mifepristone inhibits the anti-inflammatory effects of photoradiation. Photomed Laser Surg. 2006; 24 (2): 197-201.

[1464] Stadler I, Lanzafame R J, Oskoui P, Zhang R Y, Coleman J, Whittaker M. Alteration of skin temperature during low-level laser irradiation at 830 nm in a mouse model. Photomed Laser Surg. 2004; 22 (3): 227-231.

[1465] Rochkind S, Kogan G, Luger E G et al. Molecular structure of the bony tissue after experimental trauma to the mandibular region followed by laser therapy. Photomed Laser Surg. 2004; 22 (3): 249-253.

[1466] Prezotto Villa G E, Catirse A B, Lizarelli R F. Evaluation of secondary dentin formation applying two fluences of Low Level Laser.Photomed Laser Surg. 2005; 23 (1). Abstracts from the 5th Congress of the World Association for Laser Therapy, São Paulo, Brazil, November 2004. Abstract no 024, p. 95.

[1467] Rodrigues de Sant'anna G. Development anomalies as Amelogenesis and Laser. Photomed Laser Surg. 2005; 23 (1). Abstracts from the 5th Congress of the World Association for Laser Therapy, São Paulo, Brazil, November 2004. Abstract no 029, p. 96.

[1468] Farina C G, Duarte M, Mori M et al. Effects of Low Intensity Laser Therapy (780 nm) in temporomandibular disorders: electromiographic, pain and bite force analysis. Photomed Laser Surg. 2005; 23 (1). Abstracts from the 5th Congress of the World Association for Laser Therapy, São Paulo, Brazil, November 2004. Abstract no 035, p. 98.

[1469] Anders J J, Geuna S, Rochkind S. Phototherapy promotes regeneration and functional recovery of injured peripheral nerve. Neurol Res. 2004; 26 (2): 233-239.

[1470] Carvalho Baptista I, Chavantes M C, Soji N. A new application of Low Level Laser Therapy for treatment pain in patients submitted to a cardiac surgery. Photomed Laser Surg. 2005; 23 (1). Abstracts from the 5th Congress of the World Association for Laser Therapy, São Paulo, Brazil, November 2004. Abstract no 038, p.99.

[1471] Gerbi M E, Pinheiro A L, Marzola C, Limeira Júnior Fde A, Ramalho L M, Ponzi E A, Soares O, Carvalho LC, Lima H V, Gonçalves T O. Assessment of bone repair associated with the use of organic bovine bone and membrane irradiated at 830 nm. Photomed Laser Surg. 2005; 23 (4): 382-388.

[1472] Abramoff M M, Lopes N N, Lopes L A, Dib L L, Guilherme A, Caran E M, Barreto A D, Lee M L, Petrilli A S. Low-level laser therapy in the prevention and treatment of chemotherapy-induced oral mucositis in young patients. Photomed Laser Surg. 2008; 26 (4): 393-400.

[1473] Soriano F, Campaña V, Soriano M, Soriano R.Vasculitis Ulcers Irradiated with Ga. As. Laser: Ten years of experience. Soriano F, Campana V, Soriano M, Soriano R. Photomed

[1440] Dortbudak O, Haas R, Mallath-Pokorny G. Biostimulation of bone marrow cells with a diode soft laser. Clin Oral Implants Res. 2000; 11 (6): 540-545.

[1441] Núñez S C, Nogueira G E, Ribeiro M S, Garcez AS, Lage-Marques J L. He-Ne laser effects on blood microcirculation during wound healing: a method of in vivo study through laser Doppler flowmetry. Lasers Surg Med. 2004; 35 (5): 363-368.

[1442] Koultchavenia E V. Low-Level Laser as device for increase of drug concentration in the kidney. Proc. SPIE Vol. 4156. 2001: 218-221.

[1443] Damante C A, Greghi S L, Sant'Ana A C, Passanezi E, Taga R. Histomorphometric study of the healing of human oral mucosa after gingivoplasty and low-level laser therapy. Lasers Surg Med. 2004; 35 (5): 377-384.

[1444] Lopes C B, Pinheiro A L, Sathaiah S, Duarte J, Cristina Martins M. Infrared laser light reduces loading time of dental implants: a Raman spectroscopic study. Photomed Laser Surg. 2005; 23 (1): 27-31.

[1445] Laakso E L, Cabot P J. Nociceptive scores and endorphin-containing cells reduced by low-level laser therapy (LLLT) in inflamed paws of Wistar rat. Photomed Laser Surg. 2005; 23 (1): 32-35.

[1446] Nakaji S, Shiroto C, Yodono M, Umeda T, Liu Q. Retrospective study of adjunctive diode laser therapy for pain attenuation in 662 patients: detailed analysis by questionnaire. Photomed Laser Surg. 2005; 23 (1): 60-65.

[1447] Lanzafame R J, Stadler I, Coleman J, Haerum B, Oskoui P, Whittaker M, Zhang R Y. Temperature-controlled 830-nm low-level laser therapy of experimental pressure ulcers. Photomed Laser Surg. 2004; 22 (6): 483-488.

[1448] Xian-Qiang M I, Chen J Y, Liang Z J, Zhou L W. In vitro effects of helium-neon laser irradiation on human blood: bloodviscosity and deformability of erythrocytes. Photomed Laser Surg. 2004; 22 (6): 477-482.

[1449] Campaña V R, Moya M, Gavotto A, Spitale L, Soriano F, Palma J A. Laser therapy on arthritis induced by urate crystals. Photomed Laser Surg. 2004; 22 (6): 499-503.

[1450] Kujawa J, Zavodnik I B, Lapshina A, Labieniec M, Bryszewska M. Cell survival, DNA, and protein damage in B14 cells under low-intensity near-infrared (810 nm) laser irradiation. Photomed Laser Surg. 2004; 22 (6): 504-508.

[1451] Grossman N, Schneid N, Reuveni H, Halevy S, Lubart R. 780 nm low power diode laser irradiation stimulates proliferation of keratinocyte cultures: involvement of reactive oxygen species. Lasers Surg Med. 1998; 22 (4): 212-218.

[1452] Kim Y G. Laser mediated production of reactive oxygen and nitrogen species; implications for therapy. Free Radic Res. 2002; 36 (12): 1243-1250.

[1453] Nascimento P M, Pinheiro A L, Salgado M A, Ramalho L M. A preliminary report on the effect of laser therapy on the healing of cutaneous surgical wounds as a consequence of an inversely proportional relationship between wavelength and intensity: histological study in rats. Photomed Laser Surg. 2004; 22 (6): 513-518.

[1454] Mognato M, Squizzato F, Facchin F, Zaghetto L, Corti L. Cell growth modulation of human cells irradiated in vitro with low-level laser therapy. Photomed Laser Surg. 2004; 22 (6): 523-526.

[1455] Byrnes K R, Barna L, Chenault V M et al. Photobiomodulation improves cutaneous wound healing in an animal model of type II diabetes. Photomed Laser Surg. 2004; 22 (4): 281-290.

[1456] Agaiby A D, Ghali L R, Wilson R, Dyson M. Laser modulation of angiogenic factor production by T-lymphocytes. Lasers Surg Med. 2000; 26 (4): 357-363.

[1457] Walker M D, Rumpf S, Baxter G D, Hirst D G, Lowe A S. Effect of low-intensity laser irradiation (660 nm) on a radiation-impaired wound-healing model in murine skin. Lasers Surg Med. 2000; 26 (1): 41-47.

[1422] Lizarelli R F, Marcello O Mazzetto M O, Bagnato V S. Low-intensity laser therapy to treat dentin hypersensitivity: comparative clinical study using different light doses. Proc. SPIE. 2000; Vol. 4422.

[1423] Kawalec J S, Hetherington J, Pfennigwerth C et al. Effect of a diode laser on wound healing by using diabetic and nondiabetic mice. Journal of Foot and Ankle Surgery. 2004; 43 (4): 214-220.

[1424] Taly A B, Sivaraman Nair K P, Thyloth Murali T, Archana J. Efficacy of multiwavelength light therapy in the treatment of pressure ulcers in subjects with disorders of the spinal cord: A randomized double-blind controlled trial. Archives of Physical Medicine and Rehabilitation. 2004; 85 (10): 1657-1661.

[1425] Cho H J, Lim S C, Kim S G et al. Effect of low-level laser therapy on osteoarthropathy in rabbit. In Vivo. 2004; 18 (5): 585-591.

[1426] Irvine J, Chong S L, Amirjani N, Chan K M. Double-blind randomized controlled trial of low-level laser therapy in carpal tunnel syndrome. Muscle Nerve. 2004; 30 (2): 182-187.

[1427] Lapchak P A, Wei J, Zivin J A. Transcranial infrared laser therapy improves clinical rating scores after embolic strokes in rabbits. Stroke. 2004; 35 (8): 1985-1988.

[1428] Brown S A, Rohrich R J, Kenkel J et al. Effect of low-level laser therapy on abdominal adipocytes before lipoplasty procedures. Plast Reconstr Surg. 2004; 113 (6): 1796-1804; discussion 1805-1806.

[1429] Gaida K, Koller R, Isler C et al. Low Level Laser Therapy-a conservative approach to the burn scar? Burns. 2004; 30 (4): 362-367.

[1430] Zinman L H, Ngo M, Ng E T et al. Low-intensity laser therapy for painful symptoms of diabetic sensorimotor polyneuropathy: a controlled trial. Diabetes Care. 2004; 27 (4): 921-924.

[1431] Ozkan N, Altan L, Bingol U et al. Investigation of the supplementary effect of GaAs laser therapy on the rehabilitation of human digital flexor tendons. J Clin Laser Med Surg. 2004; 22 (2): 105-110.

[1432] Cruz D R, Kohara E K, Ribeiro M S, Wetter N U. Effects of low-intensity laser therapy on the orthodontic movement velocity of human teeth: a preliminary study. Laser Surg Med. 2004; 35 (2): 117-120.

[1433] Gür A, Sarac A J, Cevik R, Altindag O, Sarac S. Efficacy of 904 nm gallium arsenide low level laser therapy in the management of chronic myofascial pain in the neck: a double-blind and randomize-controlled trial. Laser Surg Med. 2004; 35 (3): 229-235.

[1434] Wenzel G I, Pikkula B, Choi C H, Anvari B, Oghalai J S. Laser irradiation of the guinea pig basilar membrane. Lasers Surg Med. 2004; 35 (3): 174-180.

[1435] Takahashi T, Fukuda M, Ohnuki T et al. Nd:YAG LLLT in the treatment of temporomandibular disorders: a treatment protocol and preliminary report. Laser Therapy. 1998; 10 (1): 7-15.

[1436] Gür A, Cosut A, Sarac A J et al. Effect of different therapy regimes of low power laser in painful osteoarthritis of the knee: A double-blind and placebo-controlled trial. Laser Surg Med. 2003; 33: 330-338.

[1437] Gür A, Karakoc M, Cevik R et al. Efficacy of low power laser therapy and exercise on pain and functions in chronic low back pain. Laser Surg Med. 2003; 32 (3): 233-238.

[1438] Khadra M, Ronold H J, Lyngstadaas S P, Ellingsen J E, Haanaes H R. Low-level laser therapy stimulates bone-implant interaction: an experimental study in rabbits. Clin Oral Implants Res. 2004; 15 (3): 325-332.

[1439] Khadra M, Kasem N, Lyngstadaas S P, Haanæs H, Mustafa K. Laser therapy accelerates initial attachment and subsequent behaviour of human oral fibroblasts cultured on titanium implant material. A scanning electron microscopic and histomorphometric analysis. Clinical Oral Implants Research. 2005; 16 (2): 168-175.

[1403] Karu T I, Andreichuk T, Ryabykh T. Suppression of human blood chemiluminescence by diode laser radiation at wavelengths 660, 820, 880 or 950 nm. Laser Therapy. 1993; 5: 103.

[1404] Karu T I, Pyatibrat L V, Ryabykh T P. Nonmonotonic behaviour of the dose dependence of the radiation effect on cells *in vitro* exposed to pulsed laser radiation at (820 nm). Lasers Surg Med. 1997; 21: 485.

[1405] Naim JO, Yu W, Ippolito K M L et al. The effect of low level laser irradiation on nitric oxide production by mouse macrophages. Lasers Surg. Med. 1996; Suppl. 8, 7 (abstr. 28).

[1406] Vladimirov Y, Borisenko G, Boriskina N et al. NO-hemoglobin may be a light-sensitive source of nitric oxide both in solution and in red blood cells. J Photochem Photobiol B Biol. 2000; 59: 115.

[1407] Sbarra A J, Strauss R R. Eds. The Respiratory Burst and Its Photobiological Significance. Plenum Press, New York, 1988.

[1408] Sharp R E, Chapman S K. Mechanisms for regulating electron transfer in multi-centre redox proteins. Biochem Biophys Acta. 1999; 1432: 143.

[1409] Karu T I, Andreichuk T N, Ryabykh T P. On the action of semiconductor laser radiation (820 nm) on the chemiluminescence of blood of clinically healthy humans. Lasers Life Sci. 1995; 6: 277.

[1410] Karu T I, Ryabykh T P, Sidorova T A, Dobrynin Ya V. The use of a chemiluminescence test to evaluate the sensitivity of blast cells in patients with hemoblastoses to antitumor agents and low-intensity laser radiation. Lasers Life Sci. 1996; 7: 1.

[1411] Karu T I, Andreichuk T, Ryabykh T. Changes in oxidative metabolism of murine spleen following diode laser (660–950 nm) irradiation: effect of cellular composition and radiation parameters. Lasers Surg Med. 1993; 13: 453.

[1412] Forman N J, Boveris A. Superoxide radical and hydrogen peroxide in mitochondria. In Free Radicals in Biology. Vol. 5. Pryor A. Ed, Academic Press, New York, 1982, p. 65.

[1413] Karu T I, Tiphlova O, Esenaliev R, Letokhov V. Two different mechanisms of low-intensity laser photobiological effects on *Escherichia coli*. J Photochem Photobiol B Biol. 1994; 24: 155.

[1414] Manteifel V M, Karu T I. Activation of chromatin in T-lymphocytes nuclei under the He-Ne laser radiation. Lasers Life Sci. 1998; 8: 117.

[1415] Novogrodski A. Lymphocyte activation induced by modifications of surface. In: Immune Recognition. Rosenthal S. Ed, Academic Press, New York, 1975, p. 43.

[1416] Zhang Y, Song S, Chi-Chun Fong C C et al. cDNA Microarray Analysis of Gene Expression Profiles in Human Fibroblast Cells Irradiated with Red Light. Journal of Investigative Dermatology. 2003;120: 849-857.

[1417] Rubinov A N. Physiological grounds for biological effect of laser radiation. J Phys D: Appl Phys, 2003; 36: 2317-2330.

[1418] Kulekcioglu S, Sivrioglu K, Ozan O, Parlak M. Effectiveness of low-level laser therapy in temporomandibular disorder. Scan J Rheumatol. 2003; 32: 114-118.

[1419] Gür A,Cosut A, Sarac A et al. Efficacy of different therapy regimes of low-power laser in painful osteoarthritis of the knee: a double-blind and randomized-controlled trial. Laser Surg Med. 2003; 33: 330-338.

[1420] Guerra A, Munoz P, Esquivel T, Boullón F, Tunér J. The effect of 670 nm Laser Therapy on herpes simplex and aphtae. Photomed Laser Surg. 2005 (1). Abstracts from the 5th Congress of the World Association for Laser Therapy, November 25-27, 2004, São Paulo, Brazil. Abstr. 003, p. 90.

[1421] Bjordal JM, Ljunggren AE, Klovning A, Slordal L. Non-steroidal anti-inflammatory drugs, including cyclo-oxygenase-2 inhibitors, in osteoarthritic knee pain: meta-analysis of randomised placebo controlled trials. Br Med J. 2004; 329 (7478): 1317.

[1383] Kamata H, Hirata H. Redox regulation of cellular signaling. Cell Signal. 1999; 11: (1): 1-14.

[1384] Calkhoven C F, Geert A B. Multiple steps in regulation of transcription-factor level and activity. Biochemistry. 1996; 317: 329-342.

[1385] Chopp H, Chen Q, Dereski M O, Hetzel F W. Chronic metabolic measurement of normal brain tissue response to photodynamic therapy. Photochem. Photobiol. 1990; 52: 1033-1036.

[1386] Quickenden T R, Daniels L L, Byrne L T. Does low-intensity He-Ne radiation affect the intracellular pH of intact *E. coli*? Proc. SPIE. Vol 2391. 1995: 535.

[1387] Tiphlova O, Karu T I. Dependence of *Escherichia coli* growth rate on irradiation with He-Ne laser and growth substrates. Lasers Life Sci. 1991; 4: 161.

[1388] Karu T I, Pyatibrat LV, Kalendo G S. Studies into the action specifics of a pulsed GaAlAs laser (820 nm) on a cell culture. I. Reduction of the intracellular ATP concentration: dependence on initial ATP amount. Lasers Life Sci. 2001; 9: 203.

[1389] Ashman R F. Lymphocyte activation. In: Fundamental Immunology. Paul W P, Ed, Raven Press, New York, 1984, p. 267.

[1390] Fedoseyeva G E, Smolyaninova N K, Karu T I, Zelenin A V. Human lymphocyte chromatin changes following irradiation with a He-Ne laser. Lasers Life Sci. 1998; 2: 197.

[1391] Karu T I, Smolyaninova N K, Zelenin A V. Long-term and short-term responses of human lymphocytes to He-Ne laser radiation. Lasers Life Sci. 1991; 4: 167.

[1392] Smolyaninova N K, Karu T I, Fedoseyeva G E, Zelenin A V. Effect of He-Ne laser irradiation on chromatin properties and nucleic acids synthesis of human blood lymphocytes, Biomed. Sci. 1991; 2: 121.

[1393] Shliakhova L N, Itkes A V, Manteifel V M, Karu T I. Expression of *c-myc* gene in irradiated at 670 nm human lymphocytes: a preliminary report. Lasers Life Sci. 1996; 7: 107.

[1394] Manteifel V M, Karu T I. Ultrastructural changes in human lymphocytes under He-Ne laser radiation. Lasers Life Sci. 1992; 4: 235.

[1395] Manteifel V M, Andreichuk T N, Karu T I. Influence of He-Ne laser radiation and phytohemagglutinin on the ultrastructure of chromatin of human lymphocytes. Lasers Life Sci. 1994; 6: 1.

[1396] Manteifel V, Bakeeva L, Karu T I. Ultrastructural changes in chondriome of human lympocytes after irradiation with He-Ne laser: appearance of giant mitochondria. J Photochem Photobiol B Biol. 1997; 38: 25.

[1397] Israel N, Gougerot-Pocidalo M.-A, Aillet F, Verelizier J.-L. Redox status of cells influences constitutive or induced NF-NB translocation and HIV long terminal repeat activity in human T-lymphocytes and monocytic cell lines. J Immunol. 1992; 149: 3386.

[1398] Albrecht-B,chler G. Surface extensions of 3T3 cells towards distant infrared light sources. J Cell Biol. 1991; 114: 494.

[1399] Karu T I, Pyatibrat L V, Kalendo G S. Biostimulation of HeLa cells by low-intensity visible light. V. Stimulation of cell proliferation *in vitro* by He-Ne laser radiation. Il Nuovo Cimento D. 1987; 9: 1485-1494.

[1400] Karu T I. Effects of visible radiation on cultured cells. Photochem Photobiol. 52:1089-1090.

[1401] Karu T I, Ryabykh T P., Fedoseyeva G E, Puchkova N I. Induced by He-Ne laser radiation respiratory burst on phagocytic cells. Lasers Surg. Med. 1989; 9: 585.

[1402] Karu T I, Ryabykh T P, Letokhov V S. Different sensitivity of cells from tumor-bearing organisms to continuous-wave and pulsed laser radiation (632.8 nm) evaluated by chemiluminescence test. III. Effect of dark period between pulses. Lasers Life Sci. 1997; 7: 141.

[1363] Salet C. Acceleration par micro-irradiation laser du rhythme de contraction de cellular cardiaques en culture. C.R. Acad Sci. Paris. 191; 272: 2584.

[1364] Salet C. A study of beating frequency of a single myocardial cell. I. Q-switched laser microirradiation of mitochondria. Exp Cell Res. 1972; 73: 360.

[1365] Salet C, Moreno G, Vinzens F. A study of beating frequency of a single myocardial cell. III. Laser microirradiation of mitochondria in the presence of KCN or ATP. Exp. Cell Res. 1979; 120: 25.

[1366] Walker J. Treatment of human neurological problems by laser photostimulation. U.S. patent 4,671,285, 1987.

[1367] Karu T I, Kalendo G S, Letokhov V S. Control of RNA synthesis rate in tumor cells HeLa by action of low-intensity visible light of copper laser. Lett Nuov Cim. 1981; 32: 55.

[1368] Giese A C. Photosensitization of organisms with special reference to natural photosensitizers. In: *Lasers in Biology and Medicine*. Hillenkampf F, Pratesi R, Sacchi C, Eds. Plenum Press, New York, 1980, p. 299.

[1369] Brown GC. Nitric oxide and mitochondrial respiration. Biochem Biophys Acta. 1999; 1411: 351.

[1370] Karu T I. Mechanisms of low-power laser light action on cellular level. In: Lasers in Medicine and Dentistry. Simunovic Z, Ed., Vitgraf, Rijeka (Croatia), 2000, p. 97.

[1371] Karu T I, Pyatibrat L V, Kalendo G S. Donors of NO and pulsed radiation at 820 nm exert effects on cells attachment to extracellular matrices. Toxicol Lett. 2001; 121:57.

[1372] Hothersall J S, Cunha F Q, Neild G H, Norohna-Dutra A. Induction of nitric oxide synthesis in J774 cell lowers intracellular glutathione: effect of oxide modulated glutathione redox status on nitric oxide synthase induction. Biochem J. 1997; 322: 477.

[1373] Karu T I, Tiphlova O A, Matveyets Yu A et al Comparison of the effects of visible femtosecond laser pulses and continuous wave laser radiation of low average intensity on the clonogenicity of *Escherichia coli*. J Photochem Photobiol B Biol. 1991; 10: 339.

[1374] Karu T I. Local pulsed heating of absorbing chromophores as a possible primary mechanism of low-power laser effects. In: Laser Applications in Medicine and Surgery. Galletti, G, Bolognani L, Ussia G, Eds. Monduzzi Editore, Bologna, 1992, p. 253.

[1375] Brown G C. Control of respiration and ATP synthesis in mammalian mitochondria and cells. Biochem. J. 1992; 284: 171.

[1376] Chance B. Cellular oxygen requirements, Fed. Proc. Fed. Am. Soc. Exp. Biol. 1957; 16: 671.

[1377] Karu T I, Pyatibrat L V, Kalendo G S. Cell attachment modulation by radiation from a pulsed semiconductor light diode (820 nm) and various chemicals. Lasers Surg Med. 2001; 28: 227-236.

[1378] Karu T I, Pyatibrat L V, Kalendo G S. Thiol reactive agents and semiconductor light diode radiation (820 nm) exert effects on cell attachment to extracellular matrix. Laser Therapy. 2001; 11: 177-181.

[1379] Karu T I, Pyatibrat L V, Kalendo G S. Cell attachment to extracellular matrices is modulated by pulsed radiation at 820 nm and chemical that modify the activity of enzymes in the plasma membrane. Lasers Surg Med. 2001; 29: 274-281.

[1380] Gius D, Boreto A, Shah S, Curry H A., Intracellular oxidation reduction status in the regulation of transcription factors NF-kappaB and AP-1. Toxicol Lett. 1999; 106: 93-106.

[1381] Sun Y, Oberley L W. Redox regulation of transcriptional activators. Free Rad Biol Med. 1996; 21: 335-338.

[1382] Nakamura H, Nakamura K, Yodoi J. Redox regulation of cellular activation, Annu Rev Immunol. 1997; 15: 351-369.

[1343] Karu T I, Kalendo G S, Letokhov V S, Lobko V V. Biological action of low-intensity visible light on HeLa cells as a function of the coherence, dose, wavelength, and irradiation regime. II. Sov J Quantum Electron. 1983; 13: 1169.

[1344] Karu T I, Tiphlova O A, Fedoseyeva G E et al. Biostimulating action of low-intensity monochromatic visible light: is it possible? Laser Chem. 1984; 5: 19.

[1345] Gamaleya N F, Shishko E D, Yanish G B. New data about mammalian cells photosensitivity and laser biostimulation. Dokl Akad Nauk S.S.S.R. (Moscow). 1983; 273:224.

[1346] Vekshin N A. Light-dependent ATP synthesis in mitochondria. Mol Biol. (Moscow). 1991; 25: 54.

[1347] Karu T I, Kalendo G S, Letokhov V S, Lobko V V. Biostimulation of HeLa cells by low intensity visible light. II. Stimulation of DNA and RNA synthesis in a wide spectral range. Nuov Cim. 1984; D, 3: 309.

[1348] Karu T I, Kalendo G S, Letokhov V S, Lobko V V. Biostimulation of HeLa cells by low intensity visible light. III. Stimulation of nucleic acid synthesis in plateau phase cells. 1984; Nuov Cim. 1984; D, 3: 319.

[1349] Karu T I. Molecular mechanism of the therapeutic effect of low-intensity laser radiation. Lasers Life Sci. 1988; 2: 53.

[1350] Karu T I. Primary and secondary mechanisms of action of visible-to-near IR radiation on cells. J Photochem Photobiol B Biol. 1999; 49: 1.

[1351] Karu T I, Afanasyeva N I. Cytochrome oxidase as primary photoacceptor for cultured cells in visible and near IR regions. Dokl Akad Nauk (Moscow). 1995; 342: 693.

[1352] Karu T I, Pyatibrat L V, Kalendo G S, Esenaliev R O. Effects of monochromatic low intensity light and laser irradiation on adhesion of HeLa cells *in vitro*. Lasers Surg Med. 1996; 18: 171.

[1353] Karu T I. Low-power laser effects. In: Lasers in Medicine. Waynant R, Ed. CRC Press, Boca Raton, FL. 2002, p. 169.

[1354] Tiphlova O, Karu T I. Action of low-intensity laser radiation on *Escherichia coli*. CRC Critical Rev Biomed Eng. 1991; 18: 387.

[1355] Karu T I, Afanasyeva N I, Kolyakov S F, Pyatibrat L V. Changes in absorption spectra of monolayer of living cells after irradiation with low intensity laser light. Dokl Akad Nauk (Moscow). 1998; 360: 267.

[1356] Karu T I, Afanasyeva N I, Kolyakov S F et al. Changes in absorbance of monolayer of living cells induced by laser radiation at 633, 670, and 820 nm. IEEE J Sel Top Quantum Electron. 2001; 7: 982.

[1357] Jöbsis-van der Vliet F F. Dicovery of the near-infrared window in the body and the early development of near-infrared spectroscopy. J Biomed. Opt. 1999; 4: 392.

[1358] Jöbsis-van der Vliet F F, Jöbsis P D. Biochemical and physiological basis of medical near-infrared spectroscopy. J Biomed. Opt. 1999; 4: 397.

[1359] Dube A, Gupta P K, Bharti S. Redox absorbance changes of the respiratory chain components of *E. coli* following He-Ne laser irradiation. Lasers Life Sci. 1997; 7: 173.

[1360] Kolyakov S F, Pyatibrat L V, Mikhailov E L et al. Changes in the spectra of circular dichroism of suspension of living cells after low intensity laser radiation at 820 nm, Dokl Akad Nauk (Moscow). 2001; 377: 824.

[1361] Arvanitaki A, Chalazonitis N. Reactiones bioeléctriques de la photoactivation des cytochromes. Arch Sci Physiol. 1947; 1: 385.

[1362] Berns M W, Gross D C L, Cheng W K, Woodring D. Argon laser microirradiation of mitochondria in rat myocardial cell in tissue culture. II. Correlation of morphology and function in single irradiated cells. J Mol Cell Cardiol. 1972; 4: 71.

[1325] Siposan D. An in vitro study of the effects of low-level laser radiation on human blood. Laser in Medical Science. 2002; 17 (4). Proc. 14th Annual Meeting of Deutsche Gesellschaft für Lasermedizin, Munich, Germany, June 2003.

[1326] Cruz-Höfling A, Garavello Freitas Z, Baranauskas I B. SEM and AFM studies of rat injured tibiae after HeNe radiation. Medical Science. 2002; 17 (4). Proc. 14th Annual Meeting of Deutsche Gesellschaft für Lasermedizin, Munich, Germany, June 2003.

[1327] Dourado D M, Cruz-Höfling M A. LLLT on damaged muscle caused by bothrops moojeni snake venom. Laser Surg Med. 2003; 33: 352-357.

[1328] Seaton E D, Charakida A, Mouser P E et al. Pulsed-dye laser treatment for inflammatory acne vulgaris: randomised controlled trial. The Lancet. 2003; 362: 1347-1352.

[1329] Tullberg M, Alstergren P J, Ernberg M M. Effects of low-power laser on masseter muscle pain and microcirculation. Pain. 2003; 105: 89-96.

[1330] Almeida-Lopes L. PhD dissertation. Universidade do Vale do Paraíba, SP, Brazil, 2003.

[1331] Pinheiro A L, Limeira Jr Fde A, Márquez de Martínez Gerbi M E et al. Effect of 830-nm laser light on the repair of bone defects grafted with inorganic bovine bone and decalcified cortical osseous membrane. J Clin Laser Med Surg. 2003; 21 (5): 301-306.

[1332] Cirina S A, Nascimento T N, Catirse A B et al. Clinical evaluation of low-level laser therapy and fluoride varnish for treating cervical dentinal hypersensitivity. J Oral Rehabil. 2003; 30 (12): 1183-1189.

[1333] Chaves de Vasconcelos Catão M H, Gerbi M E, Cavalcanti Gonçalves R. A laserterapia no tratamento da radiomucosite em paciente com carcinoma espino celular no palato mole - relato de caso. Proc. Laser Dental Show, São Paulo, Brazil, November 2003, p. 8.

[1334] Alves da Cuhna M, Munin E, Castro de Abreu W. O uso do laser terapeutico em mucosite oral e xerostomia em pacientes submetida à radioterapia. Proc. Laser Dental Show, São Paulo, Brazil, November 2003, p.8.

[1335] Márquez de Martínez Gerbi M E, Limeira Jr F, Pinheiro A et al. Efeito de laserterapia de 830 nm sobre o reparo de defeitos ósseos com implantes de osso bovino e mineral. Proc. Laser Dental Show, São Paulo, Brazil, November 2003, p 11.

[1336] Lubart R, Breitbart H. Biostimulative effects of low energy lasers. 3rd Congress of the North American Association for Laser Therapy, Bethesda, Md, USA, March 2003.

[1337] Carati C J, Anderson S N, Gannon B J, Piller N B. Treatment of postmastectomy lymphedema with low-level laser therapy. A double blind, placebo-controlled trial. Cancer. 2003; 98 (6): 1114-1122.

[1338] Sazonov A M, Romanov G A, Portnoy L M et al. Low-intensity noncoherent red light in complex healing of peptic and duodenal ulcers. Sov Med. 1985; 42 (12). (in Russian)

[1339] Bertoloni G, Sacchetto R, Baro E et al. Biochemical and morphological changes in *Escherichia coli* irradiated by coherent and non-coherent 632.8 nm light. J Photochem Photobiol B Biol. 1993; 18: 191-196.

[1340] Hartman K M. Action spectroscopy, in *Biophysics*. Hoppe W, Lohmann W, Marke H and Ziegler H, Eds. Springer-Verlag, Heidelberg, 1983, p. 115.

[1341] Lipson E D. Action spectroscopy: methodology, in CRC Handbook of Organic Chemistry and Photobiology. Horspool W H. and Song P.-S, Eds. CRC Press, Boca Raton, FL, 1995, p. 1257.

[1342] Karu T I, Kalendo G S, Letokhov V S, Lobko V V. Biological action of low-intensity visible light on HeLa cells as a function of the coherence, dose, wavelength, and irradiation dose, Sov J Quantum Electron. 1982; 12: 1134.

[1308] Campaña V, Moya M, Gavotto A et al. He-Ne laser on microcrystalline arthropathies. J Clin Laser Med Surg. 2003; 21 (2): 99-103.

[1309] Garavello-Freitas I, Baranauskas V, Joazeiro P P et al. Low-power laser irradiation improves histomorphometrical parameters and bone matrix organization during tibia wound healing in rats. J Photochem Photobiol B. 2003; 70 (2): 81-89.

[1310] Hahn A, Sejna I, Stolbova K et al. Combined laser-EGb 761 tinnitus therapy. Acta Otolaryngol Suppl. 2001; 545: 92-93.

[1311] Zeredo J L, Sasaki K M, Fujiyama R et al. Effects of low power Er:YAG laser on the tooth pulp-evoked jaw-opening reflex. Laser Surg Med. 2003; 33 (3): 169-172.

[1312] Karu T I. Low power laser therapy. In: Biomedical Photonics Handbook, Chapter 48. CRC Press LLC. 2003.

[1313] Fortuna D, Rossi G, Zati A et al. Pilot study of the Nd:YAG laser in experimentally induced chronic degenerative osteoarthritis in an animal model. Atti della Fondazione Giorgio Ronchi. 2002; 62 (2): 179-193.

[1314] Nomura K, Yamaguchi M, Abiko Y. Inhibition of Interleukin-1-beta production and gene expression in human gingival fibroblasts by low-energy laser irradiation. Lasers Med Sci. 2001; 16 (3): 218-223.

[1315] Landyshev I, Avdeeva N V, Goborov N D et al. [Efficacy of low intensity laser irradiation and sodium nedocromil in the complex treatment of patients with bronchial asthma]. Ter Arkh. 2002; 74: 25-28. (in Russian)

[1316] Tuncel A, Görgü M, Ayhan M et al. Treatment of anogenital warts by pulsed dye laser. Dermatol Surg. 2002; 28 (4): 350-352.

[1317] Neira R, Arroyave J, Ramirez H et al. Fat liquefaction: effect of low-level laser energy on adipose tissue. Plast Reconstruct Surg. 2002; 110 (3): 923-925.

[1318] Lavor Z V, Bortkevich A S, Pozdniakova et al. Quantum therapy in the treatment of patients suffering from allergic rhinitis and bronchial asthma. Laser in Medical Science. 2002; 17 (4). Proc. 14th Annual Meeting of Deutsche Gesellschaft für Lasermedizin, Munich, Germany, June 2003, p. 157.

[1319] Al-Shenqiti A, Oldham J. The use of low intensity laser therapy (LILT) in the treatment of trigger points that are associated with rotator cuff tendonitis. Laser in Medical Science. 2002; 17 (4). Proc. 14th Annual Meeting of Deutsche Gesellschaft für Lasermedizin, Munich, Germany, June 2003, p. 157. Also: The Use Of Low Level Laser Therapy (Lllt) In The Treatment Of Trigger Points That Are Associated With Rotator Cuff Tendonitis. Proc. SPIE 5287.2003: 91-102.

[1320] Pereira A N, Eduardo C P, Matson E et al. Effect of low-power laser irradiation on cell growth and procollagen synthesis of cultured fibroblasts. Laser Surg Med. 2002; 31: 263-267.

[1321] Yu Hsin-Su, Wu Chieh-Shan, Yu Chia-Li et al. Helium-neon laser irradiation stimulates migration and proliferation in melanocytes and induces repigmentation in segmental-type vitiligo. J Invest Dermatol. 2003; 120 (1): 56-64.

[1322] Ataie L., Djavid G E. Efficacy of low power laser GaAlAs (630 nm) in the treatment of vitiligo patients. Laser in Medical Science. 2002; 17 (4). Proc. 14th Annual Meeting of Deutsche Gesellschaft für Lasermedizin, Munich, Germany, June 2003.

[1323] Basirnia A, Sadeghipoor G, Djavid E G et al. The effect of low power laser therapy on osteoarthritis of the knee.Laser in Medical Science. 2002; 17 (4). Proc. 14th Annual Meeting of Deutsche Gesellschaft für Lasermedizin, Munich, Germany, June 2003.

[1324] Lievens P, van der Veen P. The influence of low level infrared laser therapy on the regereration of cartilage tissue. Laser in Medical Science. 2002; 17 (4). Proc. 14th Annual Meeting of Deutsche Gesellschaft für Lasermedizin, Munich, Germany, June 2003.

[1286] Shiroto C, Nakaji S, Umeda T. Current state-of-the-art of the clinical laser in Japan. Proc. 4th Congress of the World Ass. for Laser Therapy, Tokyo, Japan 2002. Pages 59-69. Monduzzi Editore, Bologna, Italy.

[1289] Ribeiro M S, Freitas A Z, Silva D F et al. Comparison of polarization degree in healthy and wounded rat skin. Proc. SPIE. Vol. 4433.

[1290] Lapina V A, Veremei E T, Pancovets E. Effects of laser irradiation for healing of the skin-muscle wounds in animals. Proc. SPIE. Vol. 3907.

[1291] Ribeiro M S, Zezell D M, Maldonado E P et al. Histological study of wound healing in rats following He-Ne and GaAlAs laser radiation. Proc. SPIE. Vol. 3569.

[1292] Ribeiro M S, Zezell D M, Carbone K et al. Effects of He-Ne polarized laser radiation on skin wound repair: a morphological study. Proc. SPIE. Vol. 3198.

[1293] Grzesiak-Janas G, Kobos J. Influence of laser radiation on acceleration of postextraction wound healing. Proc. SPIE. Vol. 3188.

[1294] Hode L. Are lasers more dangerous than IPL instruments? Lasers Surg Med. 2003; Supplement 15: 6.

[1295] Ladalardo T, Mangabeira A, Pedro L et al. Comparative clinical evaluation of the immediate and late analgesic effect of GaAlAs diode lasers of 830 and 660 nm in the treatment of dentine pain: a preliminary report. 2002; Proc. SPIE. Vol. 4610. p. 178-182. Lasers in Dentistry III.

[1296] Guzzardella G A, Torricelli P, Nicoli Aldini N et al. Laser technology in orthopedics: preliminary study on low power laser therapy to improve the bone-biomaterial interface. Int J Artif Organs. 2001; 24 (12): 898-902.

[1297] Shefer G, Partridge T A, Heslop L et al. Low-energy laser irradiation promotes the survival and cell death entry of skeletal muscle satellite cells. J Cell Sci. 2002; 115: 1461-1469.

[1298] Posso I P, Goncalves S A, Posso M B, Filipini R. Control of nipple pain during breastfeeding using low level laser therapy. Reg Anesth Pain Med. 2007; 32 (2) (Supplement): 185-185.

[1299] Dörtbudak O, Haas R, Mailath-Pokorny G. Effect of low-power laser irradiation on bony implant sites. Clin Oral Implants Res. 2002; 13 (3): 288-292.

[1300] Wong S F, Wilder-Smith P. Pilot study on laser effects on oral mucositis in patients receiving chemotherapy. Cancer J. 2002; 8 (3): 247-254.

[1301] Guzzardella G A, Fini M, Torricelli P et al. Laser stimulation on bone defect healing: an in vitro study. Lasers Med Sci. 2002; 17 (3): 216-220.

[1302] Fung D T, Ng G Y, Leung M C et al. Therapeutic low energy laser improves the mechanical strength of repairing medial collateral ligament. Laser Surg Med. 2002; 31 (2): 91-96.

[1303] Reidenbach H D, Dollinger K, Hoffman J. Field trials with low power lasers concerning the blink reflex. Biomed Tech (Berl.). 2002; 47 Suppl 1 Pt 2: 600-6001.

[1304] Gür A, Karakoc M, Cevik R et al. Efficacy of low power laser therapy and exercise on pain and functions in chronic low back pain. Lasers Surg Med. 2003; 32 (3): 233-238.

[1305] Guzzardella G A, Torricelli P, Nicolo-Aldini N et al. Osseointegration of endosseous ceramic implants after postoperative low-power laser stimulation: an in vivo comparative study. Clin Oral Implants Res. 2003; 14 (2): 226-232.

[1306] Klimenko I T, Shuvalova I N. [Low intensity laser radiation in complex therapy of patients with vascular obliterating atherosclerosis of low extremities]. Lik Sprava. 2002; (8): 98-102. (in Polish)

[1307] Kreisler M, Christoffers A B, Willershausen B et al. Effect of low-level GaAlAs laser irradiation on the proliferation rate of human periodontal ligament fibroblasts: an in vitro study. J Clin Periodontol. 2003; 30 (4): 353-358.

[1267] Estola-Partanen M. Muscular tension and tinnitus: an experimental trial of trigger point injections on tinnitus. Tampere University Press, Acta Universitatis Tamperensis, Faculty of Medicine, Otorhinolaryngology; 782, 2000-12-08, ISBN 951-44-4965-7.

[1268] Freitas A C, Pinheiro A, Miranda P et al. Assessment of anti-inflammatory effect of 830 nm laser light using C-reactive protein levels. Braz Dent J. 2001; 12 (3): 187-190.

[1269] Lundeberg T, Hode L, Zhou J. Effect of low power laser irradiation on nociceptive cells in Hirudo medicinalis. Acupunct Electrother Res. 1988; 13 (2-3): 99-104.

[1270] Medrado R A P, Pugliese L S, Reis S R A et al. The influence of low level laser therapy on wound healing and its biological action upon myofibroblasts. Lasers Surg Med. 2003; 32 (3): 239-244.

[1271] Gordjestani M, Dermaut L, Thierens H. Infrared laser and bone metabolism: a pilot study. Int J Oral Maxillofac Surg. 1994; 23: 54-56.

[1272] Skobelkin O K et al. [Use of lasers in the treatment of acute suppurative lactation mastitis]. Vestn Khir Im I I Grek. 1988; 141 (9): 46-49. (in Russian)

[1273] Kreisler M, Christoffers A B, Al-Haj H et al. Low level 809-nm diode laser-induced in vitro stimulation of the proliferation of human gingival fibroblasts. Laser Surg Med. 2002; 30: 365-369.

[1274] Bednar B, Unterberger E. Lasertherapie bei wunden Mamillen. Laktation und Stillen. 2002; 2: 57-62.

[1275] Al-Watban F A, Zhang X Y, Andres B L. Low-level laser therapy enhances wound healing in diabetic rats: a comparison of different lasers. Photomed Laser Surg. 2007; 25 (2): 72-77.

[1276] Mizutani K, Musya Y, Wakae K, Kobayashi T et al. A clinical study on serum prostaglandin E$_2$ with low-level laser therapy. Photomed Laser Surg. 2004; 22 (6): 537-539.

[1277] Schindl M, Schindl A, Polzleitner D et al. Healing of bone affections and gangrene with low-intensity laser irradiation in diabetic patiens suffering from foot infections. Forch Komplementarmed. 1998; 5: 244-247.

[1278] Meersman P. Laser pharmacology and achilles tendinopathy. Laser Therapy. 1999; 11 (3): 144-150.

[1279] Bjordal J M, Johnson M I, Lopes-Martins R A, Bogen B, Chow R, Ljunggren A E. Short-term efficacy of physical interventions in osteoarthritic knee pain. A systematic review and meta-analysis of randomised placebo-controlled trials. BMC Musculoskelet Disord. 2007; 8:51.

[1280] Lindholm A C, Swensson U, de Mitri N, Collinder E. Clinical Effects of Betamethasone and Hyaluronan, and of Defocalized Carbon Dioxide Laser Treatment on Traumatic Arthritis in the Fetlock Joints of Horses. J Vet Med. 2002: 189 -194.

[1281] Gür A, Karakoc M, Nas K et al. Effects of low power laser and low dose amitriptyline therapy on clinical symptoms and quality of life in fibromyalgia: a single-blind, placebo-controlled trial. Rheumatol Int. 2002; 22 (5): 188-193.

[1282] Rappl T, Laback C, Quasthoff S et al. Low-level-laser therapy in mild and moderate CTS - a double blind, randomised study. Proc. Laser Florence 2003.

[1283] Vlassov V V, Pechatnikov L M, MacLehose H G. Low level laser therapy for treating tuberculosis. Cochrane Database Syst Rev. 2002; (3): CD003490.

[1284] Bolton P, Dyson M, Young S. The effect of polarized light on the release of growth factors from the U-937 magraophage cell line. Laser Therapy. 1992; 4 (1) 33-37.

[1285] Pöntinen P. LEPT for preoperative care and early rehabilitation. Proc. 4th Congress of the World Ass. for Laser Therapy, Tokyo, Japan 2002. Pages 75-79. Monduzzi Editore, Bologna, Italy.

[1248] Enwemeka C, Reddy G K. The biological effects on laser therapy and other physical modalities on connective tissue repair processes. Laser Therapy. 2000; 12 (1): 22-30.

[1249] Asagai Y, Imakiire A, Ohshiro T. Thermographic study of low level laser therapy for acute-phase injury. Laser Therapy. 2000; 12: 31-33.

[1250] Lubart R, Friedman H, Lavie R. Photostimulation as a function of different wavelengths. Laser Therapy. 2000; 12: 38-41.

[1251] Nelson A J, Friedman M H. Somatosensory trigeminal evoked potential amplitudes following low level laser and sham irradiation over time. Laser Therapy. 2001; 13: 60-64.

[1252] Pinheiro A, Oliveira M G, Martins P P M et al. Biomodulatory effects of LLLT bone regeneration. Laser Therapy. 2001; 13: 73-79.

[1253] Barber A, Luger J E, Karpf A et al. Advances in laser therapy for bone repair. Laser Therapy. 2001: 13: 80-85.

[1254] Enwemeka C. Depth of low intensity helium-neon and gallium-arsenide lasers through rabbit dermal and subdermal tissues. Laser Therapy. 2001; 13: 95-101.

[1255] Chow R. Dose dilemmas in low level laser therapy - the effects on different paradigms and historical perspectives. Laser Therapy. 2001: 13: 102-109.

[1256] Xiaoa X, Donga J, Chua X et al. A single photon emission computed tomography of the therapy of intravascular low intensity laser irradiation on blood for brain infarction. Laser Therapy. 2001; 13: 110-113.

[1257] Mochizuki-Oda N, Kataoka Y, Cui Y et al. Effects of near-infra-red laser irradiation on adenosine triphosphate and adenosine diphosphate contents of rat brain tissue. Neuroscience letters. 2002; 323 (3): 207-210.

[1258] Wilden L, Karthein R. Import of radiation phenomena of electrons and therapeutic low-level laser in regard to the mitochondrial energy transfer. J Clin Med Surg. 1998; 16 (3): 159-165.

[1259] Silva Júnior A N, Pinheiro A, Oliveira M G et al. Computerized morphometric assessment of the effect of low-level laser therapy on bone repair: an experimental animal study. J Clin Laser Med Surg. 2002; 20 (2): 83-87.

[1260] Corral-Baqués M I, Rigau J. About time to get to speak the same language. Proc. 4th Congress of the World Association for Laser Therapy, Tokyo, Japan, June 27-30. 2002; page 123. Also: Corral-Baqués M, Rigau J. About time to speak the same language. Found on www.laser.nu/lllt/lllt_editorial10.htm#ABOUT.

[1261] Khan A, Syed A, Shah A M, Ahmad F, Qadri T. Early experience on the effect of 820 nm LLLT on musculoskeletal pain. Proc. 4th Congress of the World Association for Laser Therapy, Tokyo, Japan, June 27-30. 2002; page 133.

[1262] Nicolau R A, Jorgetti V, Rigau J, Pacheco M T T, dos Reis L M, Zangaro R A. Effect of low-power GaAlAs laser (660 nm) on bone structure and cell activity: an experimental animal study. Lasers Med Sci. 2003; 18: 89-94.

[1263] Prochazka M, Hahn A. Comprehensive laser rehabilitation therapy of tinnitus: long-term double blind study in a group of 200 patients in 3 years. Laser Partner. 2002; 51. www.laserpartner.org/lasp/web/en/2002/0051.htm.

[1264] Harada G et al. A clinical application of the 1 W Ga-Al-As diode laser - double blind study. J Phys Med. 1998; 9 : 99-103.

[1265] Hirschl M, Katzenschlager R, Ammer K et al. Double-blind, randomised, placebo controlled low level laser therapy study in patients with primary Raynaud's phenomenon. Vasa - Journal of Vascular Diseases. 2002; 31 (2): 91-94.

[1266] Nakashima T, Ueda H, Misawa H et al. Transmeatal low-power laser irradiation Nakashima T, Ueda H, Misawa H et al. Transmeatal low-power laser irradiation for tinnitus. Otology & Neurotology. 2002; 23 (3): 296-300.for tinnitus. Otology & Neurotology. 2002; 23 (3): 296-300.

[1229] Shore S E, Vass Z, Wyss N L, Altschuler R A. Trigeminal ganglion innervates the auditory brainstem. J Comparative Neurology. 2000; 419: 271-285.

[1230] Sommer, A P. Components for NOA of Biosystems and Nanoscale Resolution, in: Proc. 1st International Workshop on Nearfield Optical Analysis, Reisensburg, Germany, November 2000, (ed. A.P. Sommer). J. Clin. Laser Med. & Surg. 2001; 19: 112.

[1231] Sommer A P., Franke R P. Hydrophobic optical elements for near-field optical analysis (NOA) in liquid environment - a preliminary study. Micron. 2002; 33: 227-231.

[1232] Sommer A P., Franke R P. Near-Field Optical Analysis of Living Cells in Vitro. Journal of Proteome Research. 2002; 1: 111-114.

[1233] Sommer A P. Novel Low Intensity Light Activated Biostimulation Paradigm, in: Abstracts of the Second Congress of the North American Association for Laser Therapy & First Consensus Conference on Laser Medicine, Photobiology and Bioengineering of Tissue Repair, Atlanta, GA, March 2002.

[1234] Karu T I, Kolyakov S, Pyatibrat V et al. Irradiation with a diode at 820 nm induces changes in circular dichroism spectra (670-780 nm) of living cells. IEEE J Selected Topics in quantum Electronics. 2001; 7 (6): 976-981.

[1235] Karu T I, Afanasyeva N, Kolyakov S et al. Changes in absorbance of momolayer of living cells induced by laser irradiation at 633, 670, and 820 nm. IEEE J Selected Topics in quantum Electronics. 2001; 7 (6): 982-988.

[1236] Rochkind S, Shahar A, Alon M, Nevo Z. Transplantation of embryonal spinal cord nerve cells cultured in biodegradable microcarriers followed by low power laser irradiation for the treatment of traumatic paraplegia in rats. Neur Res. 2002; 24 (4): 355-360.

[1237] Fereydson E, Samieh M. The effects of adding low energy laser irradiation after skin resurfacing in lowering complication. Laser Surg Med. Supplement 14, 2002, abstract 242.

[1238] Sousa G R, Ribeiro M S, Groth E B. Bone repair of the periapical lesions treated or not with low intensity laser (904 nm). Laser Surg Med. Supplement 14, 2002, abstract 303.

[1239] Sawazaki I, Ribeiro M S, Mizuno L T et al. A comparative study of the effects of low laser radiation on mast cells in inflammatory fibrous hyperplasia coloured or not coloured by the toluidine blue. Laser Surg Med. Supplement 14, 2002, abstract 301.

[1240] Katariya P B, Ghumare S S, Jagtap H S. Low level laser therapy in treatment of psoriasis in Indian patients. Laser Surg Med. Supplement 14, 2002, abstract 257.

[1241] Silveira L B, Ribeiro M S, Garrocho A A et al. In vivo study on mast cells behaviour following low-intensity visible and near infrared laser radiation. Laser Surg Med. Supplement 14, 2002, abstract 304.

[1242] Gabel P. DOMS (Delayed Onset Muscle Soreness) Trigger Points Deactivation: Controversial Techniques - Laser and Acupuncture. Proc. WALT2002, Tokyo, Japan June 2002.

[1243] Shefer G, Partridge T A, Heslop L et al. Low-energy laser irradiation promotes the survival and cell cycle entry of skeletal muscle satellite cells. J Cell Science. 2002; 115: 1461-1469.

[1244] Gabel P. A pilot study on Low Level Laser Therapy (LLLT) for otitis externa - swimmer´s ear. Implications for competitive swimmers. Proc. WALT2002, Tokyo, Japan, June 2002.

[1245] al-Watban F, Andres B L. Laser photons and pharmacological treatment in wound healing. Laser Therapy. 2000 (1); 12: 3-11.

[1246] Asagai Y, Imakiire A, Ohshiro T. Thermographic effects of laser therapy in patients with cerebral palsy. Laser Therapy. 2000; 12 (1): 12-15.

[1247] Brugnera Junior A, Garrini A E, Pinheiro A et al. Laser therapy in the treatment of dental hypersensitivity - a histologic study and clinical application. Laser Therapy. 2000; 12 (1): 16-21. Available at www.walt.nu.

[1210] Yilmaz S, Kuru B, Kuru L et al Effect of galium arsenide diode laser on human periodontal disease: A microbiological and clinical study. Lasers Surg Med. 2002; 30 (1): 60-66.

[1211] Pinheiro A L, Carneiro N S, Vieira A L, Brugnera A Jr, Zanin F A, Barros R A, Silva P S. Effects of low-level laser therapy on malignant cells: in vitro study. J Clin Laser Med Surg. 2002; 20(1): 23-26.

[1212] Balakirev S A, Gusev L I, Kazanova M B et al. [Nizkointensivnaia lazernaia terapiia v detskoi onkologii]. Voprosy onkologii. 2000; 46 (4): 459-461. (in Russian)

[1213] Durnov L A, Gusev L I, Balakirev S A et al [Low-intensity lasers in pediatric oncology].Vestn Ross Akad Med Nauk. 2000; (6): 24-27. (in Russian)

[1214] Korolev Iu N, Panova L N, Geniatulina M S. [The correction of the subcellular postradiation changes in the hypothalamus and parathyroid gland by using low-intensity laser radiation. An experimental study]. Vopr Kurortol Fizioter Lech Fiz Kult. 2000; (3): 3-4. (in Russian)

[1215] Melo C A, Lima A L, Brasil I et al. Characterization of light penetration in rat tissues. J Clin Laser Med Surg. 2001;19 (4): 175-179.

[1216] Shuvalova I N, Klimenko I T, Zhukova L P et al, [The effect of low-intensity laser radiation in the infrared and red ranges on arterial pressure regulation in patients with borderline hypertension]. Lik Sprava. 1998; (7): 141-143. (in Polish)

[1217] Prokofeva G L, Kravchenko E V, Mozherenkov V P. [Effects of low-intensity infrared laser irradiation on the eye. An experimental study]. Vestn-Oftalmol. 1996; 112 (1): 31-32. (in Russian)

[1218] Barbarosa Lopes C. Laser biostimulation in bone implants. A Raman spectral study. In: Proc. 3rd NOA Congress, Sao Paulo, Brazil, June 25-26 2002.

[1219] de Assis Limeira F. Assessment of bone repair following the use of anorganic bone graft and membrane, associated or not to 830 nm laser light. In: Proc. 3rd NOA Congress, Sao Paulo, Brazil, June 25-26 2002.

[1220] Blay A, Blay C C, Groth E B et al. Effects of visible NIR low intensity laser on implant osseointegration in vivo. Laser Surg Med. Supplement 14, 2002: 11.

[1221] Stadler I, Oskoui P, Ellie C et al. Alteration of skin temperature in a mouse model during low energy level laser irradiation at 830 nm. Laser Surg Med. Supplement 14, 2002: 11.

[1222] Byrnes K R, Waynant R W, Ilev I K et al. Cellular invasion following spinal cord lesion and low power laser irradiation. Laser Surg Med. Supplement 14, 2002: 11.

[1223] Rodrigues M T J, Ribeiro M S, Groth E B et al. Evaluation of effects of laser therapy (830 nm) on oral ulceration induced by fixed orthodontic appliances. Laser Surg Med. Supplement 14, 2002: 15.

[1224] Sanseverino N T M, Sanseverino C A M, Ribeiro M S et al. Clinical evaluation of the low intensity laser antialgic action of GaAlAs (785 nm) in the treatment of the temporomandibular disorders. Laser Surg Med. Supplement 14, 2002: 18.

[1225] Amorim J C F, Ribeiro M S, Groth E B. Gingival healing after gingivectomy procedure and low intensity laser irradiation. A clinical and biometrical study in anima nobile. Laser Surg Med. Supplement 14, 2002: 20.

[1226] Gür A, Karakoc M, Nas K et al.Efficacy of low power laser therapy in fibromyalgia: A singleblind, placebo-controlled trial. Lasers Med Sci. 2002; 17 (1): 57-61.

[1227] Bjorne A, Agerberg G. Symptom relief after treatment of temporomandibular and cervical spine disorders in patients with Ménière´s disease: A 3-year follow-up. J Crandomandib Pract. 2003; 21 (1): 50-60.

[1228] Bjorne A, Agerberg G. Reduction in sick leave and costs to society of patients with Ménière´s disease after treatment of temporomandibular and cervical spine disorders: A controlled 6-year cost-benefit study. Cranio. 2003; 21 (2): 136-143.

[1190] Spivak J M, Grande D A et al. The effect of low-level Nd:YAG laser energy on adult articular cartilage in vitro. Arthroscopy. 1992; 8 (1): 36-43.

[1191] Ebert, D W, Bertone A L. Effect of irradiation with low intensity diode laser on the metabolism of equine articular cartilage in vitro. Am J Vet Res. 1998; 59 (12): 1613-1618.

[1192] Ghamsari S M, Taguchi K et al. Evaluation of low level laser therapy on primary healing of experimentally induced full thickness wounds in diary cattle. Vet Surg. 1997; 26 (2): 114-120.

[1193] Kim K-S et al. Effects of low level laser irradiation with 904 nm pulsed diode laser on the extraction wound. J of Korean Academy of Oral Medicine. 1998; 23: 301-307.

[1194] Lee K-H, Kim K-S. Effects of low level laser irradiation on the ALP activity and calcified nodule formation of rat osteoblastic cell. J of Korean Academy of Oral Medicine. 1996; 21: 279-292.

[1195] Migliorati C, Massumoto C, Eduardo C P et al. Low-energy laser therapy in oral mucositis. J Oral Laser Applications. 2001; 1 (2): 97-101.

[1196] Lubart R, Breitbart H, Sofer Y, Lavie R. He-Ne irradiation of human spermatozoa: enhancement in hamster egg penetration. Laser Therapy. 1999; 11 (4): 171-176.

[1197] Yaakov N, Ben-Haim S, Oron U. Low level laser irradiation reduces interstitial scarring in the isoproternol-induced hypertrohpic rat heart. Laser Therapy. 1999; 11 (4): 190-197.

[1098] Oron U, Yaakobi T, Oron A et al. Attenuation of the formation of scar tissue in rats and dogs post myocardial infarction by low energy laser irradiation. Laser Surg Med. 2001; 28: 1-7.

[1199] Yaakov N, Bdolah A, Wollberg Z et al. Recovery from Sarafotoxin-b induced cardiopathological effects in mice following low energy laser irradiation. Basic Research Cardiology. 2000; 95: 385-389.

[1200] Al Awami M, Schillinger M, Gschwandtner M E et al. Low level laser treatment of primary and secondary Raynaud's phenomenon. Vasa - Journal of Vascular Diseases. 2001; 30 (4): 281-284.

[1201] Chor A, Sotero Caio A B, de Azevedo A M. Amelioration of oral mucosal lesions of acute graft-versus-host disease by low-level laser therapy. Haematologica. 2001; 86 (12): 1321.

[1202] Johnson D E, Bertini J E, Harris J M. Low-level laser therapy for Peyronie's disease. Proc. SPIE Vol. 2395: 108-110.

[1203] Landau Z, Schattner A. Topical hyperbaric oxygen and low energy laser therapy for chronic diabetic foot ulcers resistant to conventional treatment. Yale J Biol Med. 2001; 74 (2): 95-100.

[1204] Ailioaie C, Ailioaie L. Low level laser therapy in children's allergic purpura. Laser-Partner. 2002; 1 (2). www.laserpartner.org.

[1205] Ailioaie C, Ailioaie L. The treatment of bronchial asthma with low level laser in attack-free period of children. Proc. SPIE. 2000; 4166: 303-308.

[1206] Schindl A, Schindl M, Pernerstorfer-Schön H et al. Low-intensity laser therapy: a review. J Invest Med. 2000; 48 (5): 312-326.

[1207] Slattery K, Amy R, Pinto J et al. Treatment of chronic neck and shoulder pain with 635 nm low level laser therapy. A randomized, multi-center, double blind, clinical study on 100 patients. Proc. of the North American Association for Laser Therapy, Atlanta, GA, USA, March 2002, p. 23.

[1208] Kono A, Fujumasa I. The evaluation of pain therapy with low power laser: comparative study on thermography and double blind test. Thermologie Österreich. 1995: 5 (3): 112.

[1209] Hoens-Alison M. Low intensity Nd:YAG laser irradiation for lateral epicondylitis. Clin J Sport Medicine. 2002; 12 (1) : 55.

[1171] Guzzardella G A, Morrone G, Torricelli P et al. Assessment of low-power laser biostimulation on chondral lesions: an "in vivo" experimental study. Artificial Cells, Blood Substitutes, and Immobilization Biotechnology. 2000; 28 (5): 441-449.

[1172] Morrone G, Guzzardella G A, Torricelli P et al. Osteochondral lesion repair of the knee in the rabbit after low-power diode Ga-Al-As laser biostimulation: an experimental study. Artificial Cells, Blood Substitutes, and Immobilization Biotechnology. 2000; 28 (4): 321-336.

[1173] Itoh T, Murakami H, Orihashi K et al. Low power laser protects human erythrocytes in an in vitro model of artificial heart-lung machines. Artificial Organs. 2000; 24 (11): 870-873.

[1174] Manukhin I B, Matafonov V A, Mamedov F M. [The efficacy of the transcutaneous magnetic-laser irradiation of the blood in acute salpingo-oophoritis] Voprosy kurortologii, fizioterapii, i lechebnoi fizicheskoi kultury. 2000; (1): 32-35. (in Russian)

[1175] Idrisova L T, Enikeev D A, Vasileva T V. [The effect of intravenous laser irradiation of the blood on the brain bioelectrical activity in patients in the postcomatose period]. Vopr Kurortol-Fizioter-Lech-Fiz-Kult. 2000; (2): 28-31 (in Russian)

[1176] Balakirev S A, Gusev L I, Kazanova M et al. [Low-intensity laser therapy in pediatric oncology]. Voprosy Onkologii. 2000; 46 (4): 459-461. (in Russian)

[1177] Polosukhin V V. Ultrastructure of the blood and lymphatic capillaries of the respiratory tissue during inflammation and endobronchial laser therapy. Ultrastructural Pathology. 2000; 24 (3): 183-189.

[1178] Forney R, Mauro T. Using lasers in diabetic wound healing. Diabetes Technology & Therapeutics. 1999; 1 (2): 189-192.

[1179] Schindl A, Schindl M, Pernerstorfer-Schoen H, Schindl L. Low intensity laser therapy in wound healing - A review with special respect to diabetic angiopathies. Acta Chirurgica Austriaca. 2001; 33: 3-7.

[1180] Grzesiak-Janas G, Janas A. Conservative closure of antro-oral communication stimulated with laser light. J Clin Laser Med Surg. 2001; 19 (4): 181-184.

[1181] Ueda Y, Shimizu N. Pulse irradiation of low-power laser stimulates bone nodule formation. Journal of Oral Science. 2001; 43 (1): 55-60.

[1182] Shamir M H, Rochkind S, Sandbank J, Alon M. Double-blind randomized study evaluating regeneration of the rat transected sciatic nerve after suturing and postoperative low-power laser treatment. Journal of Reconstructive Microsurgery. 2001; 17 (2): 133-137.

[1183] Cho K-A, Park J-S, Ko M-Y. The effect of low level laser therapy on pressure threshold in patients with temporomandinular disorders. A double blind study. J Korean Acad Oral Med. 1999; 24 (3): 281-300.

[1184] Lucas C. Efficacy of low level laser treatment in the management of chronic wounds. Thesis. Hogeschool van Amsterdam, The Netherlands. 2001. ISBN 90-9015244-X.

[1185] Qadri T, Miranda L, Tunér J, Gustavsson A. The short-term effects of low-level lasers as adjunct therapy in the treatment of periodontal inflammation. J Clin Periodontology. 2005; 32 (7): 714-719.

[1186] Oliveira N M, Parizzotto N A, Salvini T F. GaAs (904-nm) laser radiation does not affect muscle regeneration in mouse skeletal muscle. Laser Surg Med. 1999; 25: 13-21.

[1187] Bjordal J M, Johnson M I, Couppè C. Clinical Electrotherapy. Your guide to optimal treatment. Hoyskoleforlaget. Norwegian Academic Press. 2001. ISBN 82-7634-320-1.

[1188] Krasheninnikoff M, Ellitsgaard B, Rogvi-Hansen B et al. No effect of low power laser in lateral epicondylitis. Scand J Rheum. 1994; 23: 260-263.

[1189] Papadopoulos E S, Smith R W, Cawley M I D. Low-level laser therapy does not aid the management of tennis elbow. Clinical Rehabilitation. 1996; 10: 9-11.

[1151] Lizarelli R F, Ciconelli K P, Braga C A, Berro R J. Low-powered laser therapy associated with oral implantology. Proc SPIE. 1999; Vol 3593: 69-73, Lasers in Dentistry V, John D. Featherstone; Peter Rechmann; Daniel Fried; Eds.

[1152] Smith C F, Vangsness C T, Anderson T & Good W. Treatment of repetitive use carpal tunnel syndrome. Proc. SPIE. 1995; Vol 2395: 658-661. Lasers in Surgery: Advanced Characterization, Therapeutics, and Systems V, R. Rox Anderson; Ed.

[1153] Petersen S L, Botes C, Olivier A, Guthrie A J. The effect of LLLT on wound healing in horses. Equine Vet J. 1999; 31 (3): 228-231.

[1154] Brosseau L et al. Low level laser therapy for osteoarthritis and rheumatoid arthritis: a meta analysis. J Rheumatol. 2000; 27 (8): 1961-1969.

[1155] Timirgalef M J et al. [Laser therapy of the inflammatory diseases of the accessory nasal sinuses]. Vestn Otorin. 1985; 3: 56-60. (in Russian)

[1156] Watanabe H, Ishikawa I, Susuki M et al. Clinical assessment of the Erbium:YAG laser for soft tissue surgery and scaling. J Clin Laser Med Surg. 1996; 14 (2): 67-75.

[1157] Ando Y, Watanabe H, Ishikawa I. Bactericidal effect of Erbium YAG laser on periodontal bacteria. Laser Surg Med. 1996; 19: 190-200.

[1158] Rajaratuan S, Bolton P, Dyson M. Macrophage responsiveness to laser therapy with varying pulsing frequencies. Laser Therapy. 1994; 6 (2): 107-102.

[1159] Kumæ T, Arakawa H. In vitro effects of therapeutic laser on superoxide generation from rat alveolar macrophage. Laser Therapy. 1999; 11 (3): 119-129.

[1160] Enwemeka C. Quantum Biology of Laser Photostimulation (editorial). Laser Therapy. 1999; 11 (2): 52-53.

[1161] Enwemeka C, Rodriguez O, Gall N et al. Morphometries of collagen fibril populations in HeNe photostimulated tendons. J Clin Laser Med Surg. 1990; 47-52.

[1162] Tang J, Godlewski G, Rovy S et al. Morphologic changes in collagen fibers after 830 nm diode welding. Laser Surg Med. 1997; 21: 438-443.

[1163] Duan R, Liu C-Y, Li Y et al. Signal transduction pathways involved in low intensity He-Ne laser-induced respiratory burst in bovine neutrophils: a potential mechanism of low intensity laser biostimulation. Laser Surg Med. 2001; 29: 174-178.

[1164] Verdote-Robertson R, Munchua M M, Reddon J R. The use of low intensity laser therapy (LILT) for the treatment of open wounds in psychogeriatric patients: A pilot study. Physical and Occupational Therapy in Geriatrics. 2000, 18 (2): 1-19.

[1165] Lagan K M, McDonough S M, Clements B A, Baxter G D. A case report of low intensity laser therapy (LILT) in the management of venous ulceration: potential effects of wound debridement upon efficacy. J Clin Laser Medicine & Surgery. 2000; 18 (1): 15-22.

[1166] Velizhanina I A, Gapon L I, Shabalina M S et al. [Efficiency of low-intensity laser radiation in essential hypertension]. Klinicheskaia Meditsina (Mosk). 2001; 79 (1): 41-44. (in Russian)

[1167] Damjanova J, Manolov V. [Therapeutic influence on patients with epiconoylitis and myotendinitis of upper extremity by the means of low-intensity laser]. Fizikalna Kurortna i Rekhabilitatsiona Meditsina. 2000; 39 (1): 15. (in Russian)

[1168] Baratto L, Capra R, Farinelli M et al. A new type of very low-power modulated laser: soft-tissue changes induced in osteoarthritic patients revealed by sonography. International Journal of Clinical Pharmacology Research. 2000; 20 (1-2): 13-16.

[1169] Ilich-Stoianovich O, Nasonov E L, Balabanova R M. [Effects of low-intensity infrared impulse laser therapy on inflammation activity markers in patients with rheumatoid arthritis]. Terapevticheskii Arkhiv. 2000; 72 (5): 32-34. (in Russian)

[1170] Özdemir F, Birtane M, Kokino S. The clinical efficacy of low-power laser therapy on pain and function in cervical osteoarthritis. Clinical Rheumatology. 2001; 20 (3): 181-184.

[1131] Rochkind S, Nissan M, Alon M et al. Effects of laser irradiation on the spinal cord for the regeneration of crushed peripheral nerve in rats. Laser Surg Med. 2001; 28 (3): 216-219.

[1132] Simunovic Z, Simunovic K. Status after multiple teeth extractions treatment with low level laser therapy: A randomised clinical study with control group. Laser Surg Med. 2001; Suppl 13: 11.

[1133] Campaña V, Moya M, Gavotto A et al. Effects of helium-neon laser on microcrystalline arthropaties. Laser Surg Med. 2001; Suppl 13: 11.

[1134] Simunovic Z, Trobonjaca T. Comparison between low level laser therapy and visible incoherent polarised light in the treatment of lateral epicondylitis - tennis elbow. A pilot clinical study on 20 patients. Laser Surg Med. 2001; Suppl 13: 9.

[1135] Yan Li, Timon Cheng-Yi Liu, Rui Duan. Effects of some anaesthetics on wound healing: laser biomodulation mechanisms. Laser Surg Med. 2001; Suppl 13: 9. Laser Surg Med. 2001; Suppl 13: 9.

[1136] Schindl A, Merwald H, Schindl L. Low intensity laser irradiation stimulates endothelial cell proliferation in an vitro model of diabetic microangiopathy. Laser Surg Med. 2001; Suppl 13: 7.

[1137] Tay E J, Lee L I, Yee S, Loh H S. Laser-induced reduction of post-operative pain following third molar surgery. Laser Surg Med. 2001; Suppl 13: 17.

[1138] Rogvi Hansen B et al. Low level laser treatment of chondromalacia patellae. Int Orthopaedics. 1991; 15: 359-361.

[1139] Lewith G T, Machin D. A randomized trial to evaluate the effect of infrared stimulation of local trigger points, versus placebo, on the pain caused by cervical osteoarthrosis. Acupunct Electro-Ther Res, 1981; 6: 277-284.

[1140] Tenenbaum J. The epidemiology of nonsteroidal anti-inflammatory drugs. Can J Gastroenterol. 1999; 13: 119-122.

[1141] Zhuk N A, Levencho M V, Barinova S E. Laser therapy of chronic tuberculosis. 8th Internat Congr of the European Medical Laser Assoc, Moscow, Russia, May 23-26 2001. Book of Abstracts, p. 17.

[1142] Baumler W, Neff S, Landthaler M et al. Laser Assisted Hair Removal: Comparison of a Normal Mode Ruby Laser and a High Power Laser Diode. Abstract volume, Laser Florence. 14:th International Congress of Laser Medicine, p. 11, Florence, 1999.

[1143] Williams R, Havoonjian H, Isagholian K et al. A clinical study of hair removal using the long-pulsed ruby laser. Dermatol Surg. 1998; 24 (8): 837-842.

[1144] Boss W K Jrc, Usal H, Thompson R C, Fiorillo M A. A comparison of the long-pulse and short-pulse Alexandrite laser hair removal systems. Ann Plast Surg 1999; 42 (4): 381-384.

[1145] Bjerring R, Clement M, Heckendorff L et al. Selective non-ablative wrinkle reduction by laser. J Cutan Laser Ther. 2000; 2: 9-15.

[1146] Goldberg D, Metzler C. Skin resurfacing utilizing a low-fluence Nd:YAG laser. J Cutan Laser Ther. 1999; 1: 23-27.

[1147] Goldberg D J. Non-ablative subsurface remodeling: clinical and histological evaluation of a 1320 nm Nd:YAG laser. J Cutan Laser Ther. 1999; 1: 153-157.

[1148] Lupton J R, Alster T S. Nonablative laser skin resurfacing using a 1540 nm erbium glass laser: a clinical and histologic analysis. Dermatol Surg. 2002; 28 (9): 833-835.

[1149] Yu W, Naim J O, Lanzafame R J. The effects of photo-irradiation on the secretion of TGF-a, PDGF and bFGF from fibroblasts in vitro (abstract). Laser Surg Med. 1994; 6: 8.

[1150] Giavelli S, Fava G, Castronuovo G et al. Low power laser in the treatment of knee osteoarthritis in geriatric patients. Laser & Technology. 1994; 4 (1/2): 39-48.

[1112] Ko et al .Clinical evaluation of low level laser therapy on the trigger points. Proc. 7th Int Congr Lasers in Dentistry, ISLD, Brussels, Belgium, July 2000, abstr. 25.

[1113] Ladalardo T, Brugnera A, Pinheiro A et al. Comparative clinical study of the effects of LLLT in the immediate and late treatment of hypoesthesia due to surgical procedures. Proc. SPIE Vol 4610, 2002; p. 183-186. Lasers in Dentistry III.

[1114] Liu et al. The effectiveness of semiconductor laser in the treatment of post-endodontic filling pain. Proc. 7th Int Congr Lasers in Dentistry, ISLD, Brussels, Belgium, July 2000, abstr. 28.

[1115] Sant'Anna et al. Photodynamic therapy using low level laser as a disinfecting approach to carious dentine: in vivo microbiological study. Proc. 7th Int Congr Lasers in Dentistry, ISLD, Brussels, Belgium, July 2000, abstr. 43.

[1116] Kubota J. Defocused diode laser therapy (830 nm) in the treatment of unresponsive skin ulcers: a preliminary trial. J Cosmet Laser Ther. 2004; 6 (2): 96-102.

[1117] Barushka O, Yaakobi T, Oron U. Effect of low-energy laser (He-Ne) irradiation on the process of bone repair in rat tibia. Bone. 1995; 16 (1): 47-55.

[1118] Thwee T, Kato J , Hashimoto M et al. Pulp reaction after pulpotomy with He-Ne laser irradiation. In: Abstract handbook. Vol 4. Internat Soc Laser in Dentistry. 1994. Denics Pacific Ltd, Hong Kong.

[1119] Kim S-Y, Park J-S. The effect of low level laser therapy at the trigger points in masseter and other muscles. J Korean Acad. Oral Med. 1996; 21 (1): 1-3.

[1120] Ghamsari S M, Taguchi K, Abe N et al. Histopathological effect of low-level laser therapy on sutured wounds of the teat in diary cattle. Vet Quarterly. 1996; 18 (1): 17-21.

[1121] Ghamsari S M, Acorda J A, Taguchi K et al. Evaluation of wound healing of the teat with and without low level laser therapy in diary cattle by laser Doppler flowmetry in comparison with histopathology, tensiometry and hydroxyproline analysis. Br Vet J. 1996; 152 (5): 583-592.

[1122] Pankov O P. Low-level therapy in ophthalmology. In: Novel Laser Methods in Medicine and Biology. Eds. Prokhorov A M, Pustovoy V I, Kuzmin G P. Proc. SPIE. 1998; Vol 3829: 13-17.

[1123] Stein A, Kraicer P, Oron U. Effect of low energy (He-Ne) irradiation on embryo implantation rate in the rat. In: Proc. Low Power Light Effects in Biological Systems. Proc. SPIE. 1997; Vol. 3198: 24-30.

[1124] Kipshidze N, Nikolaychik V, Keelan M et al. Low-power helium:neon laser irradiation enhances pro-duction of vascular endothelian growth factor and promotes growth of endothelian cells in vitro. Laser Surg Med. 2001; 28: 355-364.

[1125] De Scheerder I, Wang K, Zhou X R et al. Intravascular low power red laser light as an adjunct to coronary stent implantation evaluated in a porcine coronary model. J Invas Cardiol. 1998; 10: 534-538.

[1126] Kaul U, Singh B, Sudan D et al. Red light laser therapy after coronary stenting: angiographic and clinical follow up study in humans. J Invas Cardiol. 1998; 10: 269-273.

[1127] Brugnera A. LLLT in treating dentinary hypersensibility: A histological study and clinical application. Proc. 2nd ENSOMA Congress, Houston, Texas, USA. 2001, p. 23-31.

[1128] Pinheiro A. Biomodulatory effects of LLLT on bone regeneration. Proc. 2nd ENSOMA Congress, Houston, Texas, USA. 2001, p. 14-22.

[1129] Siposan D, Lukacs A. Relative variation to received dose of some erythrocytic and leukocytic indices of human blood as a result of low.level laser radiation: An in vitro study. J Clin Laser Med Surg. 2001; 19 (2): 89-103.

[1130] Kolárová H, Ditrichová D, Wagner J. Penetration of the laser light into the skin in vitro. Laser Surg Med. 1999; 24: 231-235.

[1093] Prochazka M, Tejnska R. Noninvasive laser in therapy of tinnitus. In: A window on the laser medicine world. Proc. SPIE. 1999, Vol 4166: 222-223. Also: Laser Partner Journal 2000: 4. www.laserpartner.org.

[1094] Rogowski M, Menich S, Gindzienska E, Lazarczyk B. [Low-power laser in the treatment of tinnitus - a placebo-controlled study]. Laser niskoenergetyczny w leczeniu szumow usznychóbadania porownawcze z placebo. Otolaryngologia polska. Otolaryngol-Pol. 1999; 53 (3): 315-20.

[1095] Mishenkin N V et al. [Effects of helium-neon laser energy on the tissues of the middle ear in the presence of biological fluids and drug solutions]. Vest Otorinolaringol. 1990; 5: 18-21. (in Russian)

[1096] Bogomilskii M R et al. [Effect of low-energy laser irradiation on the functional state of the acoustic analyzer]. Vest Otorinolaryngol. 1989; 2: 29-34. (in Russian)

[1097] Oron U, Yaakobi T, Oron A et al. Attenuation of infarct size in rats and dogs after myocardial infarction by low-energy laser irradiation. Laser Surg Med. 2001; 28 (3): 204-211.

[1098] Houghton P E, Brown J L. Effects of low level laser on healing of wounded fetal mouse limbs. Laser Therapy. 1999; 11 (2): 54-70.

[1099] Lichtenstein D, Morag B. Low level laser therapy in ambulatory patients with venous stasis ulcers. Laser Therapy. 1999; 11 (2): 71-78.

[1100] Ailioaie C, Lupusoru-Ailioaie L M. Beneficial effects of laser therapy in the early stagers of rheumatoid arthritis onset. Laser Therapy. 1999; 11 (2): 79-87.

[1101] Sattayut S, Hughes F, Bradley P. 820 nm gallium aluminium arsenide laser modulation of prostaglandin E_2 production in interleukin-1 stimulated myoblasts. Laser Therapy. 1999; 11 (2): 88-95.

[1102] Ohshiro T, Fujii S, Sasaki K et al. Laser therapy as an adjunct treatment for severe female infertility - a preliminary report. Laser Therapy. 1999; 11 (2): 96-102.

[1103] Kunin S, Pankova Y, Oleinik T et al. The influence of low level lasers together with modern filling materials and bonding systems on mineral metabolism of hard tissues. Proc. European Conf Biomed Optics, Munich, Germany, June 2001, p. 18.

[1104] Liu H-C, Lan W-H. The combined effectiveness of the semiconductor laser with Duraphat in the treatment of dentin hypersensitivity. J Clin Laser Med Surg. 1994; 12 (6): 315-319.

[1105] Senda N, Ito K, Sugano N et al. Inhibitory effect of yellow He-Ne laser irradiation mediated by crystal violet solution on early plaque formation in human mouth. Lasers Med Sci. 2000; 15 (3): 174-180.

[1106] Takema T, Yamaguchi M, Abiko Y. Reduction of plasminogen activator activity stimulated by lipopolysaccharide from periodontal pathogen in human gingival fibroblasts by low-energy irradiation. Lasers Med Sci. 200; 15 (1): 35-42.

[1107] Ohbayashi E, Matsushima K, Hosoya S et al. Stimulatory effect of laser irradiation on calcified nodule formation in human dental fibroblasts. J Endod. 1999; 25: 1: 30-33.

[1108] McNamara D C, Rosenberg I, Jackson P A et al. Efficacy of arthroscopic surgery and midlaser treatment for chronic temporomandibular joint articular disc derangement following motor vehicle accident. Austr Den J. 1996; 41 (6): 377-387.

[1109] Plavnik L, Crosa M, Malberti A. Effect of low power laser radiation on guinea pig submandibular glands: a structural and biomechanical study. J Dent Res. 2000; 79 (5): 1010.

[1110] Arao M et al. The low power laser treatment for patients of xerostomia: a preliminary report. Proc. 7th Int Cong Lasers in Dentistry, ISLD, Brussels, Belgium, July 2000, abstr. 2.

[1111] Friedman et al. Somatosensory trigeminal evoked potential amplitudes following low level laser irradiation over time. Proc. 7th Int Congr Lasers in Dentistry, ISLD, Brussels, Belgium, July 2000, abstr. 14.

[1074] Rochkind S, Rousso M, Nissan M et al. Systemic effects of low-power laser irradiation on the peripheral and central nervous system, cutaneous wounds and burns. Laser Surg Med. 1989; 9: 174-182.

[1075] Petrischev N N, Leontjeva N V, Leontjeva T A. Influence of irradiation of helium-neon laser on microcirculation blood vessels. Proc. SPIE. 1996; Vol 2929: 198.

[1076] Kunin A A, Bykov E I, Podolskaya E E et al. Clinical and morphological indications for laser treatment of patients with precancerous diseases of the oral cavity. Proc. SPIE. 1996; Vol 2929: 185-197.

[1077] Antipa C, Pascu M, Stanciulescu V et al. Low power coherent and noncoherent light in clinical practice. Proc. SPIE. 1996; Vol 2929: 119-123.

[1078] Gladkova N D, Karachistov A B, Komarova L G et al. Clinical effectiveness of low-power laser radiation of hemosalivary barrier in patients with rheumatic disease. Proc. SPIE. 1996; Vol 2929: 124-131.

[1079] Glazewski J B. Application of low-intensity lasers in rheumatology. The results of four-year observation in 224 patients. Proc. SPIE. 1996; Vol 2929: 80-91.

[1080] Radelli J, Cieslar G, Sieron A, Grzybek H. Influence of low-power laser radiation on carbohydrate metabolism and insulin-glycemic balance in experimental animals. Proc. SPIE. 1996; Vol 2929: 94-102.

[1081] Karu T I, Pyatibrat L, Kalendo G. Irradiation with HeNe laser can influence the cytotoxic response of HeLa cells to ionizing radiation. Int. J Radiation Biology. 1994; 65 (6): 691-697.

[1082] Schindl A, Schindl L. Systemic increase in blood flow in conditions of disturbed microcirculation after low-power laser irradiation. Proc. SPIE. 1996, Vo. 2929: 63-69.

[1083] Brill A G, Brill G E, Shenkman B et al. Low power laser irradiation of blood inhibits platlet function: role of cyclic GMP. Proc. SPIE. 1998; Vol 3569: 4-11.

[1084] Witt U, Felix C. Selektive photo-Biochemotherapie in der Kombination Laser und Ginkgo-Pflanzen-extrakt nach der Methode Witt. Neue Möglichkeiten bei Innerohrstörungen. (1989). Unpublished material.

[1085] Swoboda R, Schott A. Behandlung neurotologischer Erkrankungen mit Gingko biloba Hevert, Hyperforat und Low-Power-Laser-Therapie. Medizinische Akademie Erfurt, Germany. (1992)

[1086] Partheniadis-Stumpf M, Maurer J, Mann W. Soflasertherapie in Kombination mit Tebonin i.v. bei Tinnitus. Laryngorhinootologie 1993; 72 (1): 28-31.

[1087] Wedel H, Calero L, Walger M et al. Soft-laser/Ginkgo therapy in chronic tinnitus. A placebo-controlled study. Adv Otorhinolaryngol. 1995; 49: 105-108.

[1088] Mirz F, Zachariae R, Andersen S E et al. The low-power laser in the treatment of tinnitus. Clin Otolaryngol 1999; 24: 346-354.

[1089] Wilden L. The effect of low level laser light on innear ear diseases. In: Low Level Laser therapy, Clinical Practice and Scientific Background. Eds Tunér J, Hode L. Prima Books in Sweden AB (1999). ISBN 91-630-7616-0.

[1090] Wilden L, Ellerbrock D. Verbesserung der Hörkapazität durch Low-Level-Laser-Licht (LLLL). [Amelioration of the hearing capacity by low-level-laser-light (LLL)]. Lasermedizin. 1999; 14: 129-138.

[1091] Tauber S, Baumgartner R, Schorn K, Beyer W. Lightdosimetric quantitative analysis of the human petrosus bone: experimental study for laser irradiation of the cochlea. Laser Surg Med. 2001; 28: 18-26. Also: Transmeatal cochlear laser (TCL) treatment of cochlear dysfunction: A feasibility study for chronic tinnitus. Lasers Med Sci. 2003;18 (3): 154-161.

[1092] Beyer W et al. Light dosimetry and preliminary clinical results for low level laser therapy in cochlear dysfunction. Proc. Laser Florence '99.

[1056] Benedicenti B. Valoración radioimunológica del nivel de ß-endorfina en el líquido encefaloraquídeo antes y después de irradiar con láser 904 nm, en neuralgia del trigémino. Inv. Clin Láser. 1984; 1 (3): 7-12.

[1057] Ruiz I, et al. Histological and clinical responses of articular cartilage to low level laser therapy: Experimental study. Lasers in Medical Science. 1997; 12 (2): 117-121.

[1058] van der Veen P, Lievens P. Low level laser therapy (laser therapy): The influence on the proliferation of fibroblasts and the influence of the regeneration process of lymphatic, muscular and cartilage tissue. In: Simunovic, Z (ed), Lasers in Medicine and Dentistry. Basic science and an up-to-date clinical application of low energy laser therapy. 2000: 187-217.

[1059] van Dieten H.E. et al.. Systematic review of the cost effectiveness of prophylactic treatments in the prevention of gastropathy in patients with rheumatoid arthritis or osteoarthritis taking non-steroidal anti-inflammatory drugs. Ann Rheum Dis. 2000. 59 (10): 753-759.

[1060] Marks, R, de Palma F. Clinical efficacy of low power laser therapy in osteoarthritis. Physiother Res Int. 1999; 4 (2): 141-157.

[1061] Bjordal J M, Couppe C, Ljunggren A. Low level laser therapy for tendinopathy. Evidence of a dose-response pattern. Physical Therapy Reviews. 2001; 6 (2): 91-100.

[1062] Basford J R, Sheffield C G, Harmsen W S. Laser therapy: A randomized, controlled trial of the effects of low-intensity Nd:YAG laser irradiation on musculoskeletal back pain. Arch Phys Med Rehabil. 1999; 80 (6): 647-52.

[1063] Iusim M et al. Evaluation of the degree of effectiveness of Biobeam low level narrow band light on the treatment of skin ulcers and delayed postoperative wound healing. Orthopedics. 1992; 15: 1023-1026.

[1064] Nussbaum E et al. Comparison of ultrasound/ultraviolet-C and laser for treatment of pressure ulcers in patients with spinal cord injury. Phys Ther. 1994; 74: 812-823.

[1065] Wang Ya Zhu Jing et al. Vascular low level laser irradiation therapy in treatment of brain injury. Acta Laser Biol Sinica. 1999; 8 (2).

[1066] Lilge L, Tierney K, Nussbaum E. Low-level laser for wound healing: feasibility of wound dressing transillumination. J Clin Laser Med Surg. 2000; 18 (5): 235-240.

[1067] Schlager A, Kronberger P, Petschke F et al. Low-power laser light in the healing of burns: a comparison between two different wavelengths (635 nm and 690 nm) and a placebo group. Laser Surg Med. 2000; 27: 39-42.

[1068] al-Watban F. Laser therapy am the healthy rat model for wound healing research - is it a feasible idea? LaserWorld Guest editorial, No 10, 2000. www.laser.nu/lllt/lllt_editorial.htm.

[1069] al-Watban F, Zhang X-Y. Comparison of wound healing process using argon and krypton lasers. J Clin Laser Med Surg. 1997; 15 (5): 209-215.

[1070] Schuster M A et al. [Treatment of vasomotor rhinitis, trigeminal neuralgia and Sluder's syndrome by helium-neon laser irradiation of the pterygopalatine ganglion]. Vest. Otorinolar. 1988; 4: 35-40. (in Russian)

[1071] Parascandalo S et al. Azione della Laser-terapia nella sindrome di Sluder: considerazioni clinico-etio-patogenetiche. Int Congress on Laser in Med and Surg, Bologna June 1985, p. 325.

[1072] Karu T I, Ryabykh T P, Antonov S N. Different sensitivity of cells from tumor-bearing organisms to countinuous-wave and pulsed laser radiation (632.8 nm) evaluated by chemiluminescence test. I. Comparison of responses of murine splenocytes: intact mice and mice with transplanted leukemia EL-4. Lasers in the Life Sciences. 1996; 7 (2): 91-98.

[1073] Karu T I, Ryabykh T P, Antonov S N. Different sensitivity of cells from tumor-bearing organisms to countinuous-wave and pulsed laser radiation (632.8 nm) evaluated by chemiluminescence test. II. Comparison of responses of human blood: healthy persons and patients with colon cancer. Lasers in the Life Sciences. 1996; 7 (2): 99-106.

[1038] Rochkind S, Alon M, Drory V et al. Laser therapy as a new modality in the treatment of incomplete peripheral nerve and brachial plexus injuries: prospective clinical double blind placebo-controlled randomized study. In: Abstract book of the Annual Meeting 2001, American Society for Peripheral Nerve, San Diego, California, USA, January 2001.

[1039] Havlik I. Use of low level laser therapy (laser therapy) in gynaecology and obstetrics. Laser Partner. 2000, No 14. www.laserpartner.org.

[1040] Gray R J M, Quale A A, Hall C A et al. Physiotherapy in the treatment of temporomandibular joint disorders: a comparative study of four treatment methods. Br J Dent. 1994; 176: 257-261.

[1041] Kipshidze N, Petersen J, Vassoughi J et al. Low-power laser irradiation increases cyclic GMP synthesis in penile smooth muscle cells in vitro. J Clin Laser Med Surg. 2000; 18 (6): 291-294.

[1042] Kucerová H, Dostálová T, Himmlová L et al. Low-level laser therapy after molar extraction. J Clin Laser Med Surg. 2000; 18 (6): 309-315.

[1043] Sagalovich E E. Secretory immunity changes in patients with acute and chronic herpes stomatitis by laser therapy. Clin Immunol Immunopathol. 1995; 1: 385-389.

[1044] Kim S-Y, Park J-S. The effect of low level laser therapy at the trigger points in masseter and other muscles. J Korean Acad Med. 1996; 21 (1): 3.

[1045] Tam G. Low power laser therapy and analgesic action. J Clin Laser Med Surg. 1999; 17 (1): 29-33.

[1046] Lucas C, Stanborough R W, Freeman C L, de Haan R J. Efficacy of low-level laser therapy on wound healing in human subjects: a systematic review. Lasers Med Sci. 2000; 15: 84-93.

[1047] Omura Y, Losco B M, Omura A K et al. Common factors contributing to intractable pain and medical problems with sufficient drug uptake in areas to be treated, and their pathologies and treatment. Acupunct Electrother Res. 1992; 17 (2): 107-.

[1048] Sasaki K, Ohshiro T, Hoshino T. A preliminary double blind controlled study on free amino acid analysis in burn wounds in the mouse following 830 nm diode laser therapy. Laser Therapy. 1997; 9 (2): 59-66.

[1049] Rochkind S, Rousso M, Nissan M et al. Systemic effects of low-power laser irradiation on the peripheral and central nervous system, cutaneous wounds and burns. Laser Surg Med. 1989; 9: 174-182.

[1050] Jin-zhi He. Clinical analysis of 100 cases of scald injury cured by HeNe laser acupuncture in combination with scanning laser therapy. Laser Therapy. 1990; 2 (4): 179-180.

[1051] Numazawa R, Kemmotsu O, Otsuka H et al. The role of laser therapy in intensive pain management of postherpetic neuralgia. Laser Therapy. 1996; 8 (2): 143-148.

[1052] Tekeyoshi S, Takiyama R, Tsuno S et al. Low reactive-level infrared diode laser therapy (laser therapy) of the area over the stellate ganglion, and conventional anaestethic stellate ganglion block in treatment of allergic rhinitis: a preliminary comparative study. Laser Therapy. 1996; 8 (2): 159-164.

[1053] Tamagawa S, Otsuka H, Kemmotsu O. Severe intractable facial pain attenuated by a combination of infrared diode low reactive-level laser therapy and stellate ganglion block. Laser Therapy. 1996; 8 (2): 155-158.

[1054] Yamada H, Yamanaka Y, Orihara H et al. Preliminary clinical study comparing the effect of low level laser therapy (laser therapy) and corticosteroid therapy in the treatment of facial palsy. Laser Therapy. 1995; 7 (4): 157-162.

[1055] Kimura Y, Wilder-Smith P, Yonaga K, Matsumoto K. Treatment of dentine hypersensitivity by laser: a review. J Clin Periodontol. 2000; 27: 715-721.

membranes performed with neodym phosphate glass laser irradiation. Proc. 7th Congr Internat Soc for Laser Surg and Med, Munich June 1987. Abstract no 216a.

[1019] Agambar L, Herbert K E. Scott D L. Low powered laser therapy for rheumatoid arthritis. Br J Rheum. 1992; 31 (suppl 2): 81.

[1020] Matulis A A, Vasilenkaitis V V, Raistensky I L et al. [Laser therapy and laseracupuncture in rheomatoid arthritis, osteoarthritis deformans and psoriatric arthropathy]. Ther Arkh. 1983; 55 (7): 92-97. (in Russian)

[1021] Schultz R J, Krishnamurthy S, Thelmo W et al. Effects of varying intensities of laser energy on articular cartilage: A preliminary study. Laser Surg Med. 1985; 5: 557-588.

[1022] Nishida J, Satoh T, Satodate R et al. Histological evaluation of the effect of HeNe laser irradiation on the synovial membrane in rheumatoid arthritis. Jap J Rheumatol. 1990; 2: 251-260.

[1023] Brosseau L, Welch V, Wells G et al. Low level laser therapy (classes I, II and III) for treating rheumatoid arthritis. In: The Cochrane Library. Issue 4, 2000. Oxford: Update Software.

[1024] Brosseau L, Welch V, Wells G et al. Low level laser therapy (classes I, II and III) for treating oesteoarthritis. In: The Cochrane Library. Issue 4, 2000. Oxford: Update Software. Withdrawn 2007.

[1025] Bülow P M, Jensen H, Danneskiold-Samsoe B. Low power Ga-Al-As laser treatment of painful osteoarthritis of the knee. Scan J Rehab Med. 1994; 26: 155-159.

[1026] Abeles M, Marlowe S, Ingentio F. Treatment of osteoarthritis of the hand with low power laser. Arthritis Rheum. 1988; 28: 294. (abstract)

[1027] Fulga C, Fulga IG, Predescu M. Clincal study on the effect of laser therapy in rheumatic degenerative diseases. Rev Roum Med Int. 1994; 32 (3): 227-233.

[1028] Basford J R, Malanga G A, Krause D A, Harmsen W S. A randomized controlled evaluation of low-intensity laser therapy: plantar fasciitis. Arch Phys Med Rehab. 1998; 79 (3): 249-254.

[1029] Dyson S. Primary, secondary and tertiary effects of phototherapy: a review. In: Progesss in Biomedical Optics and imaging. Proc. SPIE.Volume 6140; 614005 1-12.

[1030] Maegawa Y, Itoh T, Hosokawa T et al. Effects of near-infrared low- level laser on microcirculation. Lasers Med Surg. 2000; 27: 427-437.

[1031] Stadler I, Evans R, Kolb B et al. In vitro effects of low-level laser irradiation at 660 nm on peripheral blood lymphocytes. Laser Surg Med. 2000; 27: 255-261.

[1032] Nikitin A V, Karpukhina E P. [The effect of endovascular laser therapy on the clinical course and on the mechanisms of antioxidant protection in brochical asthma patients.] Ter Arkh. 1992; 64 (1): 62-64. (in Russian)

[1033] Nikitin A V, Kashin A V, Karpukhina E P. [Correction of the antioxidant defence in patients with bronichial asthma by the method of intravascular laser irradiation.] Probl Tuberk. 1993; 3: 46-47. (in Russian)

[1034] Polonskii A K, Kharlampovich S I, Maschanova D D et al. [Effect of laser irradiation on a dystrophic process in the liver due to x-ray irradiation]. Med Radiol. 1983; 28: 59-61.

[1035] Paleev N R, Slinchenko O, Ilchenko V A et al. Influence of He-Ne laser blood irradiation on morphofunctional state of monocytes in asthmatic patients. In: Effects of low-power light on biological systems. Proce. SPIE. 1999; Vol 2630: 142-146.

[1036] Hubacek J, Olomouc C Z. Experience with the use of laser therapy in ENT medicine. Laser Partner. No 22. December 19, 200. www.laserpartner.org.

[1037] Khullar S M et al. Upregulation of growth associated protein (GAP) 43 expression and neural co-expression with neuropeptide Y (NPY) following inferior alveolar nerve (IAN) axotomy in the rat. J Periph Nerv Syst. 1998, 3 (2): 79-90.

[1000] Shchepetkin I A. [The effect of He-Ne laser radiation on the chemiluminescence of human neutro-phils]. Radiobiologiia. 1993; 33 (3): 377-382. (in Russian)

[1001] Kipshidze N N. [Changes in lecitin-induced chemiluminiscence of neutrophilic granulocytes after irradiation of blood with Helium-Neon lasers.] Biull Eksp Biol Med. 1992; 113 (1): 24-26. (in Russian)

[1002] Herzog C, Luzern, Switzerland. Low level lasertherapie un der Stillzeit. Reagieren Läsionen der Mammillen auf die Low Level Lasertherapie? On file, Swedish Laser-Medical Society. www.laser.nu.

[1003] Kovalev M I. et al. [Prevention of lactation mastitis by the use of low-intensity laser irradiation]. Akush Ginekol (Mosk.) 1990; (2): 57-61. (in Russian)

[1004] Stoffel M et al. [Low-energy He-Ne-laser irradiation of the bovine mammary gland.] Zentralbl Veterinarmed A. 1989; 36 (8): 596-602. (in German)

[1005] Dotsenko A P et al. [Use of carbon dioxide laser in the treatment of acute lactation mastitis]. Sov Med. 1989; 9: 39-42. (in Russian)

[1006] Klebanov G I et al. [Effects of endogenous photosensitizers on the laser-induced priming of leucocytes.] Membr. Cell Biol. 1998; 12 (3): 339-354. (in Russian)

[1007] Klebanov G I et al. [Low-power laser irradiation induces leukocyte priming]. Gen Physiol Biophys. 1998; 17: 365-375. (in Russian)

[1008] Sakurai Y; Yamaguchi M; Abiko Y. Inhibitory effect of low-level laser irradiation on LPS-stimulated prostaglandin E2 production and cyclooxygenase-2 in human gingival fibroblasts. Eur J Oral Sci. 2000; 108 (1): 29-34.

[1009] Perrin D, Jolivald J R, Triki H et al. Effect of laser irradiation on latency of herpes simplex virus in a mouse model. Pathol Biol (Paris). 1997; 45 (1): 24-27.

[1010] Utsunomiya T. A histopathological study of the effects of low-power laser irradiation on wound healing of exposed dental pulp tissues in dogs, with special reference to lectins and collagens. J Endod. 1998; 24 (3): 187-193.

[1011] Ozawa Y, Shimizu N, Kariya G et al. Low-energy laser irradiation stimulates bone nodule formation at early stages of cell culture in rat calvarial cells . Bone. 1998; 22 (4): 347-354.

[1012] Shimizu N, Yamaguchi M, Goseki T et al. Inhibition of prostaglandin E_2 and interleukin 1-ß production by low-power laser irradiation in stretched human periodontal ligament cells. J Dent Res. 1995; 74 (7): 1382-1388.

[1013] Olban M, Wachowicz B, Koter M et al. The biostimulatory effect of red laser irradiation on pig blood platelet function. Cell Biol Int. 1998: 22 (3): 245-248.

[1014] Grossman N, Schneid N, Reuveni H et al. 780 nm low power diode laser irradiation stimulates proliferation of keratinocyte cultures: involvement of reactive oxygen species. Laser Surg Med. 1998; 22 (4): 212-218.

[1015] Iwase T, Hori N, Morioka T et al. Low power laser irradiation reduces ischemic damage in hippocampal slices in vitro. Laser Surg Med. 1996; 19 (4): 465-470.

[1016] Joyce K M, Downes C S, Hannigan B M. Radioadaptation in indian muntjac fibroblast cells induced by low intensity laser irradiation. Mutat Res. 1999; 435 (1): 35-42.

[1017] Wedlock P, Shephard R A. Little C, McBurney F. Analgesic effects of cranial laser treatment in two rat nociception models. Physiol Behav. 1999; 59 (3): 445-448.

[1018] Barabas K, Balint G, Gaspardy G et al. Kontrollierte klinische und experimentelle Untersuchungen mit Nd-Phosphat-Glas-Laser bei Patienten mit rheomatoid Athritis bzw. ihre Wirkung auf due Synovilamembrane [Controlled clinical and experimental studies with Nd-Phosphate-Glass laser in patients with rheumatoid arthritis and its effect on the synovial membrane]. Zeitschrif für Physiotherapie. 1989; 41 (5): 293-296. Also in: Barabás K et al. Controlled clinical and experimental examinations on rheumatoid arthritis patients and syn-ovial

ence. In: A window on the laser medicine world. Longo L ed. Proc. SPIE. 1999; Vol 4166: 40-42.

[981] Ailioaie L, Ailioaie C. Self-organizing phenomena at membrane level and low level laser therapy of rhinitis. In: A window on the laser medicine world. Longo L ed. Proc. SPIE. 1999, Vol 4166: 309-315.

[982] Mikhailov V A et al. Use of immunomodulative influence of low-level laser radiation in the treatment of an autoimmune thyroiditis. In: A window on the laser medicine world. Longo L ed. Proc. SPIE. 1999, Vol 4166: 319-322.

[983] Strada G et al. Semi-conductor laser ray therapy for the treatment of abacterial chronic prostatitis, induratio penis plastica and urethral stenosis. In: Lasers in Medicine and Dentistry. Ed. Simunovic Z. 2000. European Medical Laser Assn. ISBN 953-6059-30-4.

[984] Wong F. Laser treatment for headaches of neurogenic and neuromuscular origin. Laser Surg Med. Suppl 12, 2000: 13.

[985] Ailioaie C, Ailioaie L, Topoliceanu F. Self-organizing phenomena at membrane levels and LLLT of rhinitis. Proc. SPIE. 2000; 416: 309-315.

[986] Greulich K O. Low level laser therapy (laser therapy) - does it damage DNA? Laser-World Editorial; 2, 2000. www.laser/nu/lllt/lllt_editorial5.htm (May 2001).

[987] Siposan D, Lukacs A. Effect of low-level laser radiation (lllr) in some rheological factors in human blood: an in vitro study. Clin J Laser Med Surg. 2000; 18 (4): 185-195.

[988] Yamamoto J et al. Effect of long-term aerobic exercise on helium-neon-laser-induced thrombogenesis in rat mesenteric arterioles and platelet aggregation. Haemostasis. 1993; 23 (3): 129-134.

[989] Shishkin S A. [Use of low intensity laser irradiation in the treatment of thrombophlebitic complications during subclavian vein catheterization]. Anaesteziol Reanimatol. 1993; (6): 66-68. (in Russian)

[990] Khomeriki S G, Kubatiev A A, Shliapnikov V N. [Lecitin-induced aggregation of neutrophilic granulocytes before and after irradiation of the blood with a helium-neon laser]. Gematol Transfuziol. 1993; 38 (7): 26-28. (in Russian)

[991] Sirenko I N et al. [Changes in the parameters of central and regional hemodynamics in the patients with unstable stenocardia treated by the methods of quantum hemotherapy.] Lik Sprava. 1992; (6): 70-73. (in Polish)

[992] Korochkin I M et al. [Clinico-biochemical parallels against background of traditional treatment and laser therapy of patients with ischemic heart disease.] Ter Arkh. 1988; 60 (12): 40-44. (in Russian)

[993] Kipshidze N N et al. [Lecitin-induced chemiluminiscence of peripheral blood neutrophils in patients with ischemic heart disease before and after blood irradiation with helium-neon laser.] Kardiologiia. 1992; 32 (1): 53-56. (in Russian)

[994] Korochkin I M et al. [Helium-neon laser therapy in patients with ischemic heart disease]. Kardiologiia 1990; 30 (3): 24-28. (in Russian).

[995] Korochkin I M et al. [Helium-neon laser therapy in multimodal treatment of acute pneumonia]. Sov Med. 1990; (3): 12-15 (in Russian)

[996] Prokopova L V et al. Effect of intravascular laser therapy on rheologic properties of blood in children with bilateral destructive pneumonia.] Klin Khir. 1992; (6): 7-9.

[997] Korochkin I M et al. [Intravenous laser therapy in multimodal treatment of acute pneumonia.] Sov Med. 1989; (7): 22-26. (in Russian)

[998] Genkin V M. [Effects of low-intensity laser irradiation on the state of blood proteins]. Biull Eksp Biol Med 1989. 108 (8): 188-190. (in Russian)

[999] Brill G, Brill A. [Guanilate cyclase and nitric oxide synthetsase as possible primary acceptors of low level laser radiation energy]. J Laser Medicine. 1997; 39-42. (in Russian)

[963]   Passeniouk A M, Mikhailov V A. Application of low-level laser therapy for the treatment of vaginitis. In: A window on the laser medical world. Longo L ed. Proc. SPIE. 1999; Vol 4166: 316-318.

[964]   Attia M A, El-Kashef H. Low level laser therapy in the treatment of arteriosclerosis of the lower limbs. Laser Therapy. 1999; 11 (1): 26-29.

[965]   Boboreko B A. [Helium-neon laser irradaition in the therapy of urinary bladder and uretral tubercolosis]. Probl Tuberk. 1999; 6: 38-40. (in Russian)

[966]   Parman E M. [Low-intensity laser radiation in combined treatment of urinary system tuberculosis]. Probl Tuberk. 1999; 6: 34-37. (in Russian)

[967]   Schindl A et al. Low intensity laser irradiation in the treatment of recalcitrant radiation ulcers in patients with breast cancer - long term results of 3 cases. Photodermatol-Photoimmunol-Photomed. 2000; 16 (1): 34-37.

[968]   De Scheerder I K et al. Intravascular low-power red laser light as an adjunct to coronary stent implantation. Initial clinical experience. Catheter Cardiovasc Intervent. 2000; 49 (4): 468-471.

[969]   Almeida-Lopes L et al. The use of low level laser therapy for wound healing: comparative study. Proc. 3rd Congr World Assn for Laser Therapy, Athens, Greece, May 2000, p. 118.

[970]   Monteiro Martins P P et al. P.P.M.M. implant system has osseointegration improved by laser therapy. Proc. 3rd Congr World Assn for Laser Therapy, Athens, Greece, May 2000, p. 124.

[970]   Brugnera Jr A et al. Low level laser therapy in treatment of lesions in the inferior alveolar and mental nerves. Proc. 3rd Congr World Assn for Laser Therapy, Athens, Greece, May 2000, p.126.

[971]   Shuvalova I N et al. [The effect of low-intensity laser radiation in the infrared and red ranges on arterial pressure regulation in patients with borderline hypertension]. Likarska Sprava. 1998; (7): 141-143. (in Polish)

[972]   Ciuchita T et al. Low energy laser treatment in lichen planus and finger pulpitis infections. Lasers in Surg Med. 1999; Suppl 11: 6.

[973]   Morozova S V et al. [Possibilities of helium-neon lasers in olfactory disorders]. Vestn Otorinolaringol. 1995; 5: 35-36. (in Russian)

[974]   Robinson J F et al. Wound healing in porcine skin following low output carbon dioxide laser irradiation of the lesion. Annals Plastic Surgery. 1987; 18 (6): 449-505.

[975]   Haina D, Brunner R, Landthaler M, Waidelich W. Stimulierung der Wundheilung mit Laserlicht - Klinische und tierexperimentelle Untersuchungen. Verhandlungen der Deutschen Dermatologischen Gesellschaft XXXII Tagung. Der Hausartz. Supplementum V 32. 1981: 429-431.

[976]   Sepp W, Haina D et al. Laserstrahlen in der Dermatologie - Der Deutsche Dermatologe. 1978; 11 (26): 557-575.

[977]   Walsh D, Baxter D, Allen J. Lack of effect of pulsed low-intensity infrared (820) nm laser irradiation on nerve conduction in the human superficial radial nerve. Lasers in Surg Med. 2000; 26: 485-490.

[978]   In: Low Level Laser Therapy. A Practical Introduction, Eds. Ohshiro & Calderhead. John Wiley & Sons. 1988: 114-115.

[979]   Mikhailov V A et al. Results of treatment of the patients with IInd - IIIrd st. breast cancer by combination of low level laser therapy (laser therapy) and surgery -10-years experience. In: A window on the laser medicine world. Longo L ed. Proc. SPIE. 1999; Vol 4166: 40-42.

[980]   Mikhailov V A et al. Results of treatment of the patients with IInd - IIIrd st. breast cancer by combination of low level laser therapy (laser therapy) and surgery -10-years experi-

[944] Chistov V B. [The effect of low-intensity radiation from a helium-neon laser on the alkaline phosphatase activity in an uncomplicated mandibular fracture and in traumatic osteomyelitis.] Stomatologiia 1989; 68 (6): 13-15. (in Russian)

[945] Paolini L E et al. Tratamiento de la lesion Osgood-Schlatter con láser de baja potencia - estúdio prospectívo.Proc. II Congr Internat Assn for Laser and Sports Medicine. Rosario, Argentina. March 2000.

[946] Pastore D et al. Stimulation of ATP synthesis via oxidative phosphorylation in weak mitochondria irradiated with helium-neon laser. Biochem Mol Biol Int. 1996; 39 (1): 149-157.

[947] Vacca R A et al. Activation of mitochondrial DNA replication by He-He laser irradiation. Biochem Biophys Res Commun. 1993; 195 (2): 704-709.

[948] Kim K S; Kim, Saeng Kon. An experimental study of the effects of low power density laser on the human gingival fibroblast. J Korean Acad. Oral Med 1987; 12 (1): 17.

[949] Hronková H, Navrátil L, Krymplová J, Knizek J. Possibilities of the analgesic therapy of ultrasound and non-invasive laser on plantar fasciitis. Laser Partner. No 21. May 2001. www.laserpartner.org.

[950] Chavrier C et al. Immunohistochemical localization of type I, III and IV collagen in healthy human gingiva. J de Biologie Buccale. 1981; 9: 271-277.

[951] Marino A, Giavelli S, Galanti A et al. Low level laser therapy of chronic wounds of geriatric patients: preliminary report. Laser & Technology. 1996; 6 (1/2): 41-47.

[952] Ad N, Oron U. Impact of low level laser irradiation on infarct size in the rat following myocardial infarction. Int J Cardiol. 2001; 80 (2-3): 109-116.

[953] Byrnes K R et al. Low power laser treatment of cutaneous wounds in psammamys obesus. Laser Surg Med. 2000; Supplement 12: 4.

[954] Stadler I, Lanzafame R J, Evans R et al. 830 nm irradiation increases the wound tensile strength in a diabetic murine model. Lasers in Surg Med. 2001; 28 (3): 220-226.

[955] Simunovic Z, Trobonjaca T. Low level laser therapy in the treatment of osteoarthrosis of joints of the upper extremity: a multicenter, double blind, placebo controlled clinical study of 154 patients. Lasers in Surg Med. Suppl 12, 2000: 7.

[956] Simunovic Z, Trobonjaca T. Low level laser therapy in the treatment of cervical syndrome: a multi center, double blind placebo controlled clinical study on 128 patients. Laser Surg Med. Suppl 12. 2000: 8.

[957] Simunovic Z, Trobonjaca T. Soft tissue injury during sport activities and traffic accidents - treatment with low level laser therapy. A multicenter double blind, placebo controlled clinical study on 132 patients. Laser Surg Med. 1999; Suppl 11: 5.

[958] Simunovic Z, Trobonjaca T. Low level laser therapy of acne and scars applied as monotherapy and complimentary treatment modality to tetracycline: a multi centre clinical study on 80 patients with control group. Lasers in Surg Med. Suppl 12, 2000: 7.

[959] Kolárová H et al. Penetration of the laser light into the skin in vitro. Lasers in Surg Med. 1999; 24: 231-235.

[960] Paolini L E, Paolini D. Tratamiento de la parálisis de Bell con láser de baja potencia. Estúdio prospectivo. Proc. II Congr Internat Assn for Laser and Sports Medicine. Rosario, Argentina. March 2000.

[961] Ohshiro T et al. The Japanese experience in sumo wrestling. Proc. II Congr Internat Assn for Laser and Sports Medicine. Rosario, Argentina. March 2000.

[962] Tajali S B, Bayat M, Ebrahimi E et al Effects of low power He-Ne laser on bone regeneration in rabbits from biomechanical point of view. Proc. 3rd Congr World Assn for Laser Therapy, Athens, Greece, May 2000, p. 86-87.

[925] Ihara N, Kubota J, Ban I. Defocused diode laser therapy for wound management. Proc. 3rd Cong World Ass for Laser Therapy, Athens, Greece, May 2000, p. 78.

[926] Yonaga T, Kimura Y, Matsumoto K. Treatment of cervical dentin hypersensitivity by various methods using pulsed Nd:YAG laser. Journal of Clinical Laser Medicine and Surgery. 1999; 17 (5): 205-210.

[927] Gutknecht N, Moritz A, Dercks H W et al. Treatment of hypersensitivity teeth using neodymium: ytrium-aluminum-garnet lasers: a comparison of the use of various settings in an in vivo study. J Clinical Laser Medicine and Surgery. 1997; 15 (4): 171-174.

[928] Piller N B, Thelander A, Esterman A. The objective assessment of the effect of low level laser therapy on chronic secondary arm and leg lymphoedemas. Proc. 3rd Cong World Ass for Laser Therapy, Athens, Greece, May 2000, p. 78.

[929] Bensadoun R-J, Franqiun J C, Ciais C et al. Low energy He/Ne laser in the prevention of radiation-induced mucositis: A multicenter phase III randomized study in patients with head and neck cancer. Support Care Cancer. 1999; 7 (4): 244-252.

[930] Sant'Anna G R, Duarte D A, Brugnera Jr A et al. Dye-assisted laser therapy as a disinfecting approach to caries dentine. In vivo microbiology study. Proc. 3rd Congr World Assn for Laser Therapy, Athens, Greece, May 2000, p. 62.

[931] Rajab A A. A study on the effect of low intensity laser therapy on the osseointegration of hydroxylapatite implants. 1999. University of London, PhD thesis.

[932] Arao M et al. The clinical study of low power laser treatment for temporomandibular arthrosis. Proc. 4th Int Congr Lasers in Dentistry. Ed. Hong-Sai L. 1995, p. 245-250. Munduzzi Editore, Italy.

[933] Brugnera A et al. Low-reactive level laser treatment in facial paralysis. In: Lasers in Dentistry VI. Ed Featherstone J D et al. Proc. SPIE. 2000; Vol 3910: 68-74.

[934] Lagan K M, McDonough S, Clements B, Baxter D. A case report of low intensity laser therapy (LILT) in the management of venous ulceration. J Clin Lasers Med Surg. 2000; 18 (1): 15-22.

[935] Nicolopoulos C et al. Clinical application of helium neon (632 nm) plus infrared diode laser GaAlAs (830 nm) and CO2 laser in the treatment of onychomycotic nails. Foot. 1999; 9 (4): 181-184.

[936] Sandford M A, Walsh L J. Thermal effects during desensitisation of teeth with gallium-aluminum-arsenide lasers. Periodontol. 1994; 15 (1): 25-30.

[937] Padua L et al. Clinical outcome and neurophysiological results of low power laser irradiation in carpal tunnel syndrome. Lasers Med Sci. 1999; 14 (3): 196-202.

[938] Khullar S M, Brodin P, Messelt E B, Haanaes H R. Enhanced sensory reinnervation of dental target tissues in rats following low level laser (LLL) irradiation. Lasers Med Sci. 1999; 14 (3): 177-184.

[939] Kurland H D. Releif of low back pain with low-reactive laser acupuncture techniques. Aku. 1999; 27 (4). (abstract)

[940] Paolini D, Paolini-Pisani L. Tratamiento de la lesion del tendón manguito de los rotadores con láser de baja potencia. Estúdio prospectivo. Proc. II Congr Internat Assn for Laser and Sports Medicine. Rosario, Argentina. March 2000.

[941] Gupta A, Filolenko N, Salansky N. Low energy photon therapy of leg ulcers. J Dermatol Treat. 1997; 8: 103-108.

[942] David R, Nissan M, Cohen I et al. Effects of low-power He-Ne laser on fracture healing in rats. Laser Surg Med. 1996; 19: 458-464.

[943] Lucas C, Coenen C, De Haan R. The effect of low level laser therapy (laser therapy) on stage III decubitus ulcers (pressure sores); a prospective randomised single blind, multicentre pilot study. Lasers in Medical Science. 2000; 15 (2): 94-100.

[906] Almeida-Lopes L, Rigau J, Zángaro R et al. Comparison of the low level laser therapy effects on cultured human gingival fibroblast proliferation using different irradiance and same fluency. Laser Surg Med. 2001; 29: 179-184.

[907] Schaffer M et al. Magnetic resonance imaging (MRI) controlled outcome of side effects caused by ionizing radiation, treated with with 780-nm diode laser - preliminary results. J Photochemistry and Photobiology B: Biology. 2000; 59: 1-8.

[908] Schindl A, Neuman R. Low-intensity laser therapy is an effective treatment for recurrent herpes simplex infection. Results from a randomized double-blind placebo controlled study. J Investigative Dermatology. 1999; 113 (2): 221-223.

[909] Nussbaum E L. Low-intensity laser therapy for benign fibrotic lumps in the breast following reduction mammaplasty. Physical Therapy. 1999; 79 (7): 691-698.

[910] Brugnera A et al. Clinical results evaluation of dentinary hypersensitivity patients treated with laser therapy. Proc. SPIE. 1999; Vol 3593: 66-68.

[911] Webb C, Dyson M, Lewis W H. Stimulatory effect of 660 nm low level laser energy on hypertrophic scar-derived fibroblasts: possible mechanisms for increase in cell counts. Laser Surg Med. 1998; 22 (5): 294-301.

[912] Gasparyan L. Low level laser therapy of male genital tract chronic inflammations. Proc. 2nd Congress World Association for Laser Therapy, Kansas City, USA, September 2-5 1998; p. 82-83.

[913] Sasaki K et al. Low level laser therapy (laser therapy) for thromboangitis obliterans. Proc. 2nd Congress World Association for Laser Therapy, Kansas City, USA, September 2-5 1998; p 95-96.

[914] Lizarelli R, Lamano-Carvalho T, Brentegani G. Histometrical evaluation of the healing of the dental alveolus in rats after irradiation with a low-powered GaAlAs laser. In Lasers in Dentistry V. Proc SPIE. 1999; Vol 3593: 49-56.

[915] Oasevich I A. [Low-intensity infrared laser radiation in the diagnosis and combined treatment of acute nonspecific lymphadenitis of the face and neck in children] Infrakrasnoe nizkointensivnoe lazernoe izluchenie v diagnostike i kompleksnom lechenii ostrogo nespetsificheskogo limfadenita litsa i shei u detei. Stomatologiia (Mosk). 1999; 78 (2): 28-30.

[916] Shefer G, Oron U, Irintchev A. Low energy laser irradiation activates specific signal transduction pathways in skeletal muscle cells. J Cell Physiol. 2001; 187: 73-80.

[917] Kawasaki K, Shimizo N. Effects of low-energy laser irradiation on bone remodelling during experimental tooth movement in rats. Laser Surg Med. 2000; 26: 282-291.

[918] Aoki A, Ishikawa I, Yamada T et al. Comparison between Er:YAG laser and conventional technique for root caries treatment in vitro. J Dent Res. 1998; 77 (6): 1404-1414.

[919] Jackson Z et al. Killing of the yeast and hyphal forms of candida albicans using a light-activated antimicrobial agent. Lasers in Medical Science. 1999; 14 (2): 150-157.

[920] Ocaña-Quero J M, Gomez-Villamandos R, Moreno-Millan M, Santisteban-Valenzuela J M. Helium-Neon (He-Ne) Laser Irradiation Increases the Incidence of Unreduced Bovine Oocytes During the First Meiotic Division In Vitro. Lasers Med Sci. 1998, 13 (4): 260-264.

[921] Morrone G et al. Muscular trauma treated with GaAlas diode laser: in vivo experimental study. Lasers in Medical Science. 1998; 13 (4): 293-298.

[922] Reddy K, Stehno-Bittel L, Enwemeka C. Laser photostimulation accelerates wound healing in diabetic rats. Wound Repair and Regeneration. 2001, 9 (3): 248-255.

[923] Dyson M. Laser therapy in wound management. Proc. 7th Congr European Medical Laser Ass., Dubrovnik, Croatia, June 2000, p. 22.

[924] Sattayut S. A study on the influence of low intensity laser therapy on painful temporomandibular disorders. 1999; University of London, PhD thesis.

[888] Wang F, Wang Z. Observation on clinical effect of 70 cases of acute otitis media treated by He-Ne laser radiation on acupoints. Chin J Acupunct Moxibustion. 1991; 4 (1): 30-33.

[889] Wu X B. 100 cases of facial paralysis treated with He-Ne laser irradiation on acupoints. J Tradit Chin Med. 1990; 10 (4): 300-301.

[890] Zalesskiy V N, Belousova I A, Frolov G V. Laser-acupuncture reduces cigarette smoking: a preliminary report. Acupunct Electrother Res. 1983; 8 (3-4): 297-302.

[891] Zhang D, Gao Q. Treatment of facial paralysis with laser and acupuncture; report of 76 cases. Int J Clin Acupunct 1993; 4 (3): 327-329.

[892] Schlager A, Offer T, Baldissera I. Laser stimulation of acupuncture point P6 reduces postoperative vomiting in children undergoing strabismus surgery. Br J Anaesth. 1998; 81 (4): 529-532.

[893] Roig J, Fleites A, Bécquer R. Tratamiento del síndrome del túnel carpiano con láser HeNe e infrarojo. Evaluación clínica y electrofisiológica de los resultados.[Treatment of the carpal tunnel syndrome with HeNe and infrared laser. Clinical and electrophysical evaluation of the results]. Rev Cubana Ortop Traumatol. 1992; 6 (2): 139-143.

[894] Mester A, Ortutay J, Barabás K. Laser therapy in rheumatology. Abstracts of 7th Int Congr European Medical Laser Assn, Dubrovnik, Croatia 2000, p. 36.

[895] Prochazka M, Koci K. Non-invasive laser therapy of morbus peyronie - induratio penis plastica. Abstracts of 7th Int Congr European Medical Laser Assn, Dubrovnik, Croatia 2000, p. 39.

[896] Rochkind S, Alon M, Brantwien T, Nissan M, Khaigrekht M, Drory V E. Laser therapy as a new modality in the treatment of incomplete peripheral nerve injuries and brachial plexus injuries: prospective clin-ical double-blind placebo-controlled randomized study. Proc. Am Soc Peripheral Nerve. Annual Meeting, San Diego, USA, Jan. 2001, p. 21.

[897] Bisht D, Mehrotra R, Singh P A et al. Effect of helium-neon laser on wound healing. Indian Journal of Experimental Biology. 1999; 37 (2): 187-189.

[898] Morrone G, Guzzardella G A, Tigani D et al. Biostimulation of human chondrocytes with Ga-Al-As diode laser: 'In vitro' research. Artificial Cells, Blood Substitutes, and Immobilization Biotechnology. 2000; 28 (2): 193-201.

[899] Miloro M, Repasky M. Low-level laser effect on neurosensory recovery after sagittal ramus osteotomy. Oral surgery, oral medicine, oral pathology, oral radiology, and endodontics. 2000; 89 (1): 12-18.

[900] Khullar S M, Emami B, Westermark A et al. Effect of low-level laser treatment on neurosensory deficits subsequent to sagittal split ramus osteotomy. Oral Surg Oral Med Oral Pathol Oral Radiol Endod.1996; 82 (2): 132-138.

[901] Khullar S M. Reinnervation after nerve injury: the effects of low level laser treatment. In: Low Level Laser Therapy, clinical practice and scientific background. Eds Tunér J, Hode L. 1999; p. 280-302. Prima Books in Sweden. ISBN 91-630-7616-0.

[902] Khullar S M, Brodin P, Messelt E B, Haanaes H R. The effects of low level laser treatment on recovery of nerve conduction and motor function after compression injury in the rat sciatic nerve. Europ J Oral Sci. 1995; 103: 299-305.

[903] Inkova G A, Ionin A P, Ionina G I. [The treatment of posttraumatic uveitis with low-intensity laser Radiation]. Vestnik oftalmologii. 1999; 115 (5): 20-21. (in Russian).

[904] Schaffer M, Bonel H, Sroka R et al. Effects of 780 nm diode laser irradiation on blood microcirculation: Preliminary findings on time-dependent T1-weighted contrast-enhanced magnetic resonance imaging (MRI). J Photochemistry and Photobiology B: Biology. 2000; 54 (1): 55-60.

[905] Zhu Q, Yu W, Yang X et al. Photoirradiation improved functional preservation of the isolated rat heart. Laser Surg Med. 1997; 20: 332-339.

[867] Kitzes M, Twigg G, Berns M W. Alteration of membrane electrical activity in rat myocardial cells following selective laser microbeam irradiation. J Cell Physiology. 1977; 93: 99-104.

[868] Laakso L, Richardson C, Cramond T. Quality of light - is laser necessary for effective photobiostimulation? Australian Journal of Physiotherapy. 1993; 39 (2): 87-92.

[869] Tang X M, Chai B P. Effect of CO_2 laser irradiation on experimental fracture healing: a transmission electron microscopy study. Laser Surg Med. 1986; 6: 346-352.

[870] Horvath J, Tanos E. The situation of low level laser therapy in Hungary. Proc. 3rd Congress of the World Ass for Laser Therapy, Athens, Greece 2000. Poster, p. 118.

[871] Woodruff L D, Bounkeo J M, Brannon W M, Dawes Jr K S et al. The efficacy of laser therapy in wound repair: a meta analysis of the literature. Photomed Laser Surg. 2004; 22 (3): 241-248.

[872] Enwemeka C S, Parker J C, Dowdy D S et al. The efficacy of low-power laser in tissue repair and pain control. A meta-analysis study. Photomed Laser Surg. 2004; 22 (4): 323-329.

[873] Sattayut S, Bradley P F. Low intensity laser therapy (LILT) for TMD myofascial pain: results from a pilot study. 1998. Proc. 6th Int Congr Lasers in Dentistry. University of Utah Press. Ed: J Frame. ISBN 0-87480-606-2, p. 152-156.

[874] Bjorne A, Berven A, Agerberg G. Cervical signs and symptoms in patients with Ménière's disease: a controlled study. J Cranomandib Practice. 1998; 16 (3): 194-202.

[875] Wong E, Lee G, Mason D T. Temporal headaches and associated symptoms related to the styloid pro-cess and its attachments. Annn Acad Med Singapore. 1995; 24: 124-128.

[876] Cheng Z Y, Zhao C X, Zhang Y H, et al. Superficial acupuncture combined with He-Ne laser radiation in the treatment of facial spasm. Int J Clin Acupunct 1991; 2 (1): 95-7.

[877] Danhof S. Laser treatment and smoking cessation. Dissertation. Dutch Medical Acupuncture Assn. 2000.

[878] Fong K. Bronchial asthma treated by He-Ne laser radiation on ear points. Chin J Acupunct Moxibustion 1990 ; 3 (4): 272-273.

[879] Hirsch D, Leupold W. [Placebo-controlled study on the effect of laser acupuncture in childhood asthma]. Atemwegs Lungenkr. 1994; 20 (12): 701-705.

[880] Hoffmann B, Bar T. [The reactions of the skin surface temperature - a comparison between real and placebo laser acupuncture stimulation of LI 4]. Dtsch Z Akupunkt 1994; 37 (2): 28-32.

[881] Jia Y K, Luo H C, Zhan L, Jia T Z, Yan M. A study on the treatment of schizophrenia with He-Ne laser irradiation of acupoint. J Tradit Chin Med 1987; 7 (4): 269-272.

[882] Litscher G, Wang L, Wiesner-Zechmeister G. Specific effects of laserpuncture on the cerebral circulation Lasers Med Sci. 2000; 15 (1): 57-62.

[883] Morton A R, Fazio S M, Miller D. Efficacy of laser-acupuncture in the prevention of exercise-induced asthma. Ann Allergy 1993; 70 (4): 295-298.

[884] Odud A M, Potapenko P I. [The effectiveness of laser puncture in hypertension patients]. Vrach Delo. 1990; (6): 19-21. (In Russian)

[886] Odud A M, Potapenko P I. [The use of laser puncture for managing hypertensive crises]. Vrach Delo. 1991; (7): 34-36. (In Russian)

[886] Pothman R, Yeh HL. The effects of treatment with antibiotics, laser and acupuncture upon chronic maxillary sinusitis in children. Am J Chin Med. 1982; 10 (1-4): 555-558.

[887] Tan C H, Sin Y M. The use of laser acupuncture point for smoking cesssation. American J Acupuncture. 1987; 15: 137-141.

[845] Orchardson R, Whitters C J. Effect of HeNe and pulsed Nd:YAG laser irradiation on intradental nerve responses to mechanical stimulation of dentine. Laser Surg Med. 2000; 26: 241-249.

[846] Cassone M C, Lombard A, Rossetti V, Urciuoli R, Rolfo P M. Effect of in vivo HeNe laser irradiation on biogenic amine levels in rat brain. J Photochem Photobiol B. 1993; 18 (2-3): 291-294.

[847] Loginov A S, Sokolova G N, Trubitsyna I E et al. [Biogenic amines and cyclic nucleotides in the laser therapy of long-term nonhealing stomach ulcers]. Vrach Delo 1991; (1): 24-27. (In Russian)

[848] Loginov A S, Sokolova G N, Sokolova S V et al. [The content of biologically active substances in the margin of a stomach ulcer being treated with a copper-vapor laser]. Ter Arkh. 1991; 63 (8): 75-78. (In Russian)

[849] Mandel A Sh, Dunaeva L P. [Effect of laser therapy on blood levels of serotonin and dopamine scleroderma patients.] Vestn Dermatol Venerol. 1982; (8): 13-17. (In Russian)

[850] Miles V, Klein, Optics. John Wiley & Sons Inc. New York. Chapter 10.3, p. 507-520.

[851] Lowe A et al. Effect of low intensity monochromatic light therapy (890 nm) on a radiation-impaired, wound healing model in murine skin. Lasers Surg Med. 1998; 23: 291-298.

[852] Klima H, Haas O, Roschger P. In: Photoemission from Biological Systems (Ed J. Slavinski, B. Kochel) World Publishing House, Singapore, 1987.

[853] Allan R C, Stjernholm R L, Steele R H. Biochem. Biophys. Res. Commun. 1972; 47: 679.

[854] Nelson R D, Mills E L, Simmons R L et al. Infect. Immun., 1975; 14: 29.

[855] Rosen H S, Klebanoff S J. Federal Proceedings, 1976; 35: 1391.

[856] Andersen B R, Brendzdel A M, Lint T F. Infect. Immun. 1977; 17: 62.

[857] Reznikov, Leonid. Personal communication, Dec 1998.

[858] Jankiewicz Z, Zajac A. Detection of laser radiation in biological experiments. Proc. SPIE. 1995; Vol 2203; 148-161. (Laser Technology IV: Applications in Medicine, Wieslaw Wolinski; Tadeusz Kecik; Eds.)

[859] Shear J B, Xu C, Webb W W. Multiphoton-excited visible emission by serotonin solutions. Photochem Photobiol 1997; 65 (6): 931-936.

[860] Maiti S, Shear J B, Williams R M et al. Measuring serotonin distribution in live cells with three-photon excitation. Science 1997; 24; 275 (5299): 530-532.

[861] Delibasi E, Turan B, Yucel E. The quantitative investigation of infrared laser effects on the levels of copper and zinc in various tissues. Clin Phys Physiol Meas. 1988; 9: 375-377.

[862] Haberland U, Blazek V, Schmitt H. Chirp Optical Coherence Tomography of Layered Scattering Media. Journ. Biomedical Optics. 1988; 3 (3): 259-266.

[863] McMeeken J, Stillman B. Perceptions of the clinical efficacy of laser therapy. Australian J Physiotherapy. 1993; 39 (2): 101-105.

[864] Gamaleja N F, Polischuuk E I. The experience of skin tumours treatment with laser radiation. Panminerva Med. 1975; 17: 238-240. In Enwemeka, C.S. 1988, 'Laser Biostimulation of healing wounds: Specific effects and mechanisms of action'. The Journal of Orthopaedic and Sports Physical Therapy, 9 (10): 333-338.

[865] Gabel C P. Does Laser enhance bruising in acute sporting injuries? Aust. J. Physio. 1995; 41 (4): 267-269.

[866] Kramer J F, Sandrin M. Effects of Low-Power Laser and white light on sensory conduction rate of the superficial radial nerve. Physiotherapy Canada. 1993; 45 (3): 165-170.

[824] Nicola E M, Nicola H. Low-power CO2 laser in the treatment of chronic pharyngitis: a five-year experience. Proc. SPIE. 1994; Vol 2128: 85-87. (Laser Surgery: Advanced Characterization, Therapeutics, and Systems IV)

[825] Zhou, Chuannong; Song, Xuyan; Deng, Jinsheng; Liang, Junlin; Zhang, Hua; Huang, Wenjia; Liu, Tao; Ha, Xian-Wen Photodynamic effect of copper-vapor pumped-dye laser, HeNe laser, and noncoherent red light to the liver in normal mice. Proc. SPIE. 1993; Vol 1616: 239-245. (International Conference on Photodynamic Therapy and Laser Medicine, Jun-Heng Li; Ed.)

[826] Lerner L A. [Effectiveness of laser therapy in Bechterew's disease.] Terapevticheskii Arkhiv. 1988, 60 (4): 134-136. (in Russian)

[827] Wilson M et al. Bacteria in supragingival plaque samples can be killed by low-power laser light in the presence of a photosensitizer. J Appl Bacteriol 1995; 78 (5): 569-574.

[828] Bisht D et al. Effect of low intensity laser radiation on healing of open skin wounds in rats. Indian J Medical Research. 1994; 100: 43-46.

[829] Kleinman Y et al. Low level laser therapy in patients with venous ulcers: early and long-term out-come. Laser Therapy. 1996; 8 (3): 205-208.

[830] Ito A, Kakami K, Matsushita H, Fukaya M. Effects of Nd:YAG low power laser irradiation on the ulnar nerve. Aichi Gakuin Dent Sci. 1989; 2: 1-8

[831] Matsushita H, Kakami K, Ito A et al. Effect on the action potential of the low power Nd:YAG laser as irradiated directly to the nerve. Aichi Gakuin Dent Sci. 1989; 2: 19-28.

[832] Pyczek M, Sopala M, Dabrowski Z. Effect of low-energy laser power on the bone marrow of the rat. Folia Biol (Krakow). 1994; 42 (3-4): 151-156.

[833] Efendiev A I et al. [Increasing the scar strength after preventive skin irradiation with low-intensity laser.] Klin Khir. 1992; (1): 23-25. (in Russian)

[834] Iakovleva N E, Liapina L A, Novoderzhkina I S et al. [The effect of low-intensity laser radiation on the parameters of the blood anticoagulation system in the early postresuscitation period]. Anaesteziol Reanimatol. 1997; (4): 36-38. (in Russian)

[835] Jimbo K, Noda K, Suzuki K, Yoda K. Suppressive effects of low-power laser irradiation on bradykinin evoked action potentials in cultured murine dorsal root ganglion cells. Neurosci Lett. 1998; 240 (2): 93-96.

[836] van Rensburg S D, Wiltshire W A. The effect of soft laser irradiation on fluoride release of two fluoride-containing orthodontic bonding materials. J Dent Assoc S Afr. 1994; 49 (3): 127-131.

[837] Hicks M J et al. Root caries in vitro after low fluence argon laser and fluoride treatment. Compend Contin Educ Dent. 1997; 18 (6): 543-548.

[838] Hsu J et al. Combined effects of laser irradiation/solution fluoride ion on enamel demineralization. J Clin Laser Med Surg. 1998; 16 (2): 93-105.

[839] Shi K, Lu R, Xu X. Influence of low energy HeNe laser on the regeneration of peripheral nerves. Chung Kuo Hsiu Fu Chung Chien Wai Ko Tsa Chih. 1997; 11 (1): 14-8. (In Chinese)

[840] Mikhailov V A et al. The immunomodulating action of low-energy laser radiation in the treatment of bronchial asthma. Vopr Kurortol Fizioter Lech Fiz Kult. 1998; (4): 23-25.

[841] Okamoto H, Iwase T, Morioka T. Dye-mediated bactericidal efffect of HeNe laser irradiation on oral microorganisms. Laser Surg Med. 1992; 12 (4): 450-458.

[842] Wilson M, Pratten A. Lethal photosensitisation of Staphylococcus aureus in vitro: effect of growth phase, serum, and pre-irradiation time. Lasers Med Surg. 1995; 16 (3): 272-276.

[843] CRA Newsletter. 1997; 21 (4). Clinical Research Associates, Provo, Utah, USA.

[844] Walter Wintsch, Switzerland, personal communication

[801] Rao M L, Muller-Oerlinghausen B etv al. The influence of phototherapy on serotonin and melatonin in non-seasonal depression. Pharmacopsychiatry. 1990; 23 (3): 155-158.

[802] Partonen T, Vakkuri O, Lönnqvist J. Suppression of melatonin secretion by bright light in seasonal affective disorder. Biol Psychiatry. 1997; 42 (6): 509-513.

[803] Salinas E O, Hakim-Kreis C M et al. Hypersecretion of melatonin following diurnal exposure to bright light in seasonal affective disorder: preliminary results. Biol Psychiatry. 1992; 32 (5): 387-398.

[804] Checkley S A, Murphy D G, Abbas M et al. Melatonin rhythms in seasonal affective disorder. Br J Psychiatry. 1993; 163: 332-337.

[805] Rice J, Mayor J, Tucker H A, Bielski R J. Effect of light therapy on salivary melatonin in seasonal affective disorder. Psychiatry Res. 1995; 56 (3): 221-228.

[806] Rao M L, Muller-Oerlinghausen B, Mackert A et al. Blood serotonin, serum melatonin and light therapy in healthy subjects and in patients with nonseasonal depression. Acta Psychiatr Scand. 1992; 86 (2): 127-132.

[807] Lewy A J, Bauer V K, Cutler N L et al.. Morning vs evening light treatment of patients with winter depression. Arch Gen Psychiatry. 1998; 55 (10): 890-896.

[808] Deltito J A, Moline M et al. Effects of phototherapy on non-seasonal unipolar and bipolar depressive spectrum disorders. J Affect Disord. 1991; 23 (4): 231-237.

[809] Lam R W, Terman M, Wirz-Justice A Light therapy for depressive disorders: indications and efficacy. Mod Probl Pharmacopsychiatry. 1997; 25: 215-234.

[810] Wirz-Justice A. Beginning to see the light. Arch Gen Psychiatry. 1998; 55 (10): 861-862. Review.

[811] Light therapy for winter depression. Health News. 1998; Nov 20; 4 (14): 6.

[812] Light therapy. Health News. 1998; 4 (3): 5.

[813] Tolle R. Psychotherapy of depressive disorders: on the theoretical background and its clinical relevance. Nervenarzt. 1997; 68 (7): 602-605.

[814] Avery D H. A turning point for seasonal affective disorder and light therapy research? Arch Gen Psychiatry. 1998; 55 (10): 863-864. Review.

[815] Melges F T. Efficacy of therapies for depression. Am J Psychiatry. 1981; 138 (11): 1513.

[816] Haffmans J et al. Suicide after bright light treatment in seasonal affective disorder: a case report. J Clin Psychiatry. 1998; 59 (9): 478.

[817] Ash J B, Piazza E, Anderson J L. Light therapy in the clinical management of an eating-disordered adolescent with winter exacerbation. Int J Eat Disord. 1998; 23 (1): 93-97.

[818] Kripke D F. Light treatment for nonseasonal depression: speed, efficacy, and combined treatment. J Affect Disord. 1998; 49 (2): 109-117.

[819] Wetterberg L. Light and biological rhythms. J Intern Med. 1994; 235 (1): 5-19.

[820] Grzesiak-Janas, Grazyna A A. Low-power-laser therapy in Costen's syndrome. Proc. SPIE. 1996; Vol 2781. 1996: 126-128. (Lasers in Medicine)

[821] Strupinska E. Low-power-laser therapy used in tendon damage. Proc. SPIE. 1996; Vol 2781: 177-183. (Lasers in Medicine)

[822] Eduardo C P et al. Benefits of low-power lasers on oral soft tissue. Proc. SPIE. 1996; Vol 2672: 27-33. (Lasers in Dentistry II)

[823] Gao Yun-Qing, Liu Song-Hao, Zhang You, Liu T C. 367 cases of CO_2 laser therapy on facial acne. Proc. SPIE. 1996; Vol 2887: 60-62. (Lasers in Medicine and Dentistry: Diagnostics and Treatment)

[780]   Antipa C et al. Laser biostimulation (He-Ne and Ga-As) effects as compared to the conventional therapy in several pelvic inflammatory diseases. Proc. SPIE. 1993; Vol 1879: 15-22. (Lasers in Urology, Gynecology, and General Surgery)

[781]   Xu Yong-Qing et al. Experimental study of the effects of helium-neon laser radiation on repair of injured tendon. Proc. SPIE. 1993; Vol 1616: 598-604. (International Conference on Photodynamic Therapy and Laser Medicine)

[782]   Jarry G, Debray S, Perez J, Lefebvre J P, de Ficquelmont-Loizos M, Gaston A. In vivo transillumination of the hand using near infrared laser pulses and differential spectroscopy. J Biomed Eng. 1989; 11 (4): 293-299.

[783]   Tsang D, Yew D T, Hui B S. Further studies on the effect of low-dose laser irradiation on cultured retinal pigment cells of the chick. Acta Anat (Basel). 1986;125 (1): 10-13.

[784]   Yu W, Naim J O, McGowan M, Ippolito K, Lanzafame R J. Photomodulation of oxidative metabolism and electron chain enzymes in rat liver mitochondria. Photochem Photobiol. 1997; (6): 866-871.

[785]   Murphy P J, Campbell S S. Enhanced performance in elderly subjects following bright light treatment of sleep maintenance insomnia. J Sleep Res. 1996; 5 (3): 165-172.

[786]   Campbell S S, Murphy P J. Extraocular circadian phototransduction in humans. Science. 1998; 279 (5349): 396-399.

[787]   Bylesjö E I, Boman K, Wetterberg L. Obesity treated with phototherapy: four case studies. Int J Eat Disord. 1996; (4): 443-446.

[788]   Thalén BE, Kjellman BF, Mörkrid L, Wetterberg L. Melatonin in light treatment of patients with seasonal and nonseasonal depression. Acta Psychiatr Scand. 1995; (4): 274-284.

[789]   Wikner J, Andersson D E, Wetterberg L, Röjdmark S. Impaired melatonin secretion in patients with Wernicke-Korsakoff syndrome. J Intern Med. 1995; 237 (6): 571-575.

[790]   Thalén B E, Kjellman B F, Mörkrid L, Wibom R, Wetterberg L. Light treatment in seasonal and nonseasonal depression. Acta Psychiatr Scand. 1995; 91 (5): 352-360.

[791]   Wetterberg L. [Light and biological rhythms]. Läkartidningen. 1992; 89 (37): 2915-2918. (In Swedish)

[792]   Wetterberg L. Light therapy of depression; basal and clinical aspects. Pharmacol Toxicol 1992;71 Suppl 1: 96-106.

[793]   Wetterberg L et al. [Light therapy of depression]. Läkartidningen. 1991; 30; 88 (5): 310-312. (In Swedish)

[794]   Wetterberg L. [The importance of light for health and well-being]. Läkartidningen. 1991; 88 (5): 295-296. (In Swedish)

[795]   Petterborg L J, Kjellman B F, Thalen B E, Wetterberg L. Effect of a 15 minute light pulse on nocturnal serum melatonin levels in human volunteers. J Pineal Res. 1991; 10 (1): 9-13.

[796]   Wetterberg L. [The significance of lighting for health and wellbeing]. Nord Med. 1991; 106 (3): 90-91. (in Swedish)

[797]   Wetterberg L. Lighting. Nonvisual effects. Scand J Work Environ Health. 1990; 16 Suppl 1: 26-28.

[798]   Wu J, Sanchez de la Pena S, Hallberg F et al. Chronosynergistic effects of lighting schedule-shift and cefodizime on plasmacytoma growth and host survival time. Chronobiologia. 1988; 15 (1-2): 105-128.

[799]   Wetterberg L. Melatonin and affective disorders. Ciba Found Symp. 1985; 117: 253-265.

[800]   Illnerova H, Vanecek J, Krecek J, Wetterberg L, Sääf J. Effect of one minute exposure to light at night on rat pineal serotonin N-acetyltransferase and melatonin. J Neurochem. 1979; 32 (2): 673-675.

[761] Fagnoni V et al. Considerazioni clinico terapeutiche sull'ieffetto della luce laser di bassa potenza nell Herpes Simple Labiale. Laser Abstracts. 1984; 1: 28-33.

[762] Fagnoni V, Fontolan D. Importanza della laser-terapia di bassa potenza per la riduzione dei tempi di guarigione dopo interventi di chirurgia parodontale. Laser Abstracts. 3 (2): 25-33.

[763] Fagnoni V et al. Il laser di bassa potenza come coadiuvante nella terapia della sindrome algico-dizfunzionale dell'í articolazione temporo-mandibulare. Laser Abstracts. 1985; 3: 16-26.

[764] Fagnoni V et al. Study of behaviour of dental enamel in acid solution after treatment with fluorine combined with low power laser. Laser Abstracts. 2 (1): 30-34.

[765] Fagnoni V et al. Verifica sperimentale delle variazioni degli opoioidi endogeni plasmatici in pazienti affetti da nevralgie trigeminali e trattati con laser di bassa potenza. Laser Abstracts. 1985: 3 (2): 35-42.

[766] Fagnoni V et al. Studio sulla guarigione di ferite chirurgiche della mucosa di coniglio precedentemente irradiate con laser I.R. a dosaggi diversi. Laser Abstracts. 1985; 3: 32-37.

[767] Fagnoni V et al. Verifica sperimentale sulle variazioni termiche nella cavità pulpare di denti humani estratti, durante irraggiamento con laser di bassa potenza. Laser Abstracts, 1985; 3 : 27-31.

[768] Fagnoni V et al. Su di un caso di emangioma della mucosa orale trattato mediante irraggiamento con laser di bassa potenza. Minerva Stomatologica. 1983; 32 (5): 701-703.

[769] Antipa C et al. Pulsed-laser therapy (GA-As) in combined treatment of post-traumatic swellings and some dermatological disorders.In: Medical Applications cf Lasers. Proc. SPIE. 1994; Vol 2086: 371-377.

[770] Johnson D, Bertini J E, Harris J M, Hawkins J H.et al. Low-level laser therapy for Peyronie's disease. Proc. SPIE. 1995; Vol 2395: 108-110.

[771] Kapinosov I K et al. Reaction of lymphoid organs to laser radiation with different pulsation rates. Proc. SPIE. 1996; Vol 2678: 530-533. (Optical Diagnostics of Living Cells and Biofluids)

[772] Kucerová H et al. Modulatory frequency of lasers in connectior to laser beam therapeutic effect Proc. SPIE. 1998; Vol: 191-195. (Lasers in Dentistry IV)

[773] Kucerová H. et al. Effect of laser modulatory frequency on the secretion of IgA and albumin levels after the extraction of human molars in the lower jaw. In: Progress in Biomedical Optics, Proc. of Low-power Light on Biological Systems. Proc SPIE. 1997; Vol 3198: 98-101.

[774] Pavlova R N, Gomberg V G, Boiko, V N et al. Effects of low-energy laser isolation upon the development of postradiation syndrome. Proc. SPIE. 1996; Vol 2769: 78-81. (Laser Optics '95: Biomedical Applications of Lasers)

[775] Antipa C et al. Low-energy laser treatment of rheumatic diseases: a long-term study Proc. SPIE. 1995; Vol 2391: 658-662. (Laser-Tissue Interaction VI)

[776] Telfer J, Filonenko N, Salansky N M. Leg ulcer plastic surgery descent by laser therapy. Proc. SPIE. 1994; Vol 2086: 258-263. (Medical Applications of Lasers)

[777] Marchesini R, Dasdia T, Melloni E, Rocca E. Effect of low-energy laser irradiation on colony formation capability in different human tumor cells in vitro. Laser Surg Med. 1989; 9 (1): 59-62.

[778] Burns T, Wilson M, Pearson G J Killing of cariogenic bacteria by light from a gallium aluminium arsenide diode laser. J Dent 1994; 22 (5): 273-278

[779] Gross A J, Jelkmann W. Helium-neon laser irradiation inhibits the growth of kidney epithelial cells in culture. Laser Surg Med. 1990; 10 (1): 40-44.

[740] Bjordal J M, Greve G. What may alter the conclusions of reviews? Physical Therapy Reviews. 1998; 3: 121-132.

[741] Exner K. Sitzber Akad Wiss, Wien 76II, 522 (1877).

[742] Gabor D. Laser Speckle and Its Elimination. IBM Journal of Res, Sept. 1970.

[743] Hode L, Biedermann K. Observation of surface deformation in real time using laser speckles. Proc Conference in Physics, Lund, Sweden, June 12-14. 1972.

[744] Ragnarsson S-I. Vision Research. 1972; 12: 411.

[745] Hode L. [Elektronisk bildbehandling för speckelinterferometri i reell tid]. Proj. 1006. Institutet för Optisk Forskning, Kungl. Tekniska Högskolan. October 1973. (in Swedish).

[746] Burch J M. Interferometry with Scattered Light. Optical Instruments and Techniques. J. Home, Dickson ed. (Reading Conf. 1969) p. 213. Oriel Press, New Castle upon Tyne 1970.

[747] Carniel R. The 780 laser and the CO2-laser in chronic achilles tendinitis: Different methods compared. Proc. 2nd Congress World Assn for Laser Therapy, Kansas City, Sept 1998; p. 40-42.

[748] Gaydess E et al. The effects of laser stimulation on cell and bacterial growth in a cell culture wound model. Proc. 2nd Congress World Assn for Laser Therapy, Kansas City, Sept 1998; p. 72-73.

[749] Ribeiro M S, Zezell D M, Fontenele J D et al. Incorporation of [3H]-Proline in the Dermis of Mice Following He-He Polarized Laser Radiation in the Wound Healing Process. A preliminary Study. Proc. 2nd Congress World Assn for Laser Therapy, Kansas City, Sept 1998; p. 13-15. Also: Histological study on wound healing in rats following He-Ne and GaAlAs laser irradiation. Proc. SPIE. 1998; Vol 3569: 50-55.

[750] Nicola J H, Nicola E M D, Simões M, Paschoal J R. Role of polarization and Coherence of Laser Light on Wound Healing. Laser Tissue Interaction V (1994), S.L. Jacques, ed., Proc SPIE. 1994; 2134A: 448-450.

[751] Ivanov A S et al. [The morphofunctional status of the synovial membrane of the temporomandibular joint under exposure to helium-neon laser]. Morfologia. 1996; 109 (3): 59-63. (in Russian)

[752] Lee G et al. New concepts in pain management in the application of low-power laser for relief of cervicothoracic pain syndromes. Am Heart J. 1996; 132 (6): 1329-1334.

[753] Klima H, Haas O, Roschger P. In Photon emission from Biological Systems (Ed. J. Slawinsky, B. Kochel), World Publishing House, Singapore, 1987.

[754] Skinner S M, Gage J P, Wilce P A, Shaw R M. A preliminary study of the effects of laser radiation on collagen metabolism in cell culture. Aust Dent J 1996; 41 (3): 188-192.

[755] Valiente-Zaldivar C et al. Laserterapía en la neuralgía trigeminal. Informa preliminar. Rev Cubana de Estomat. 1990; 2 (22): 166-171.

[756] Valiente-Zaldivar C et al. Lasers en estomatología. Rev Cubana de Estomat. 1989: 26: 336-343.

[757] Machnikowski I et al. [Application of therapeutic laser in treatment of the selected chronic illnesses of the oral cavity]. Protet Stomatol. 1989; 39 (3): 147-150. (in Russian)

[758] Bernardini U D, Longo L. Terapia laser nella nevralgia del trigemino. Proc. Atti dell'VIII Congresso Nazionale A.I.S.D., Verona. 1985: 80-81.

[759] Fagnoni V et al. Studio sulla guarigione di ferite chirurgiche eseguite sulla mucosa orale di coniglio trattata con soft-Laser. Int Congress on Laser in Med and Surg, Bologna June 1985, p 269.

[760] Fagnoni V et al. Laser therapy in dentistry and stomatology. Observations on 200 cases treated, Medical Laser Report 1984; 1: 36-40.

[719] Ohno T. [Pain suppressive effects of low power laser irradiation. A quantitative analysis of substance P in the rat spinal dorsal root ganglion]. Nippon Ika Daigaku Zasshi. (J Jap Med School) 1997; 64 (5): 395-400. (in Japanese with English abstract))

[720] Gupta A K et al. The use of low-energy photon therapy in the treatment of leg ulcers - a preliminary report. J Dermatol Treat. 1997; 8 (2): 103-108.

[721] Nicolopoulos N, Dyson M et al. The use of laser surgery in the subtotal meniscectomy and the effect of low-level laser therapy on the healing potential of rabbit meniscus: an experimental study. Lasers Med Sci. 1996; 11 (2): 109-115.

[722] Karpen M. Low-level laser therapy in trials for urologiclal applications. J Clin Laser Med Surg. 1995; 13 (4): 293-294.

[723] Itoh T et al. The protective effect of low power HeNe laser against erythrocytic damage caused by artificial heart-lung machines. Hiroshima J Med Sci. 1996; 45 (1): 15-22.

[724] Barabash A G et al. [Experience in treating patients with lichen ruber planus by using a helium-neon laser]. Stomatologiia; 1995; 74 (1): 20-21. (in Russian)

[725] Reddy G K et al. Biochemistry and biomechanics of healing tencon: Part II. Effects of combined laser therapy and electrical stimulation. Med Sci Sports Exerc. 1998; 30 (6): 794-800.

[726] Gum S L et al. Combined ultrasound, electrical stimulation, and laser promote collagen synthesis with moderate changes in tendon biomechanics. Am J Phys Med Rehabil. 1997; 76 (4): 288-296.

[727] Karu T I. Depression of the genome after irradiation of human lymphocytes with HeNe laser. Laser Therapy. 1992. 4 (1): 5-24

[728] Reznikov L L et al. Biomechanism of low-energy laser irradiation is similar to a general adaptive reaction. Proc. SPIE. 1994; Vol 2086: 380-449.

[729] Pavlova R N. et al. Soft-laser radiation bioeffect: is laser a physical adaptogen? Proc. SPIE. 1993; Vol 1922: 225-229

[730] Reznikov L L et al. Similarity between the mechanisms of soft-laser radiation and chemical adaptogen action. Proc. SPIE. 1993; Vol 1883: 91-98.

[731] Funk J O et al. Helium-Neon laser irradiation induces effects on cytokine production at the protein and the mRNA level. Experimental Dermatology. 1993; 2: 75-83.

[732] Bjordal J M. Low level laser therapy in shoulder tendinitis/bursitis, epicondylalgia and ankle sprain. A critical review on clinical effects. Master thesis in Physiotherapy Science, Div Physiotherapy Science, Univiersity of Bergen, Norway. 1997.

[733] Mester E, Szende B, Tota J. Die Wirkung der Laser-Strahlen auf den Haarwuchs der Maus. Radiobiol. Radiother. 9: 621-626. Original paper: Mester E, Szende B, Tota JG. Effect of laser on hair growth of mice. Kiserl Orvostud. 1967; 19: 628-631.

[734] Mester E et al. Effect of laser-rays on wound healing. Am J Surg. 1971; 122 (4): 532-535.

[735] Conlan M J et al. Biostimulation of wound healing low-energy laser irradiation. A review. J Clin Periodontol. 1996; 23 (5): 492-496.

[736] Saunders L. The efficiacy of low-level laser therapy in supraspinatus tendinitis. Clin Rehab. 1995; 9: 126-134.

[737] Vecchio P et al. A double-blind study of the effectiveness of low level laser treatment of rotator cuff tendinitis. Br J Rheum. 1993; 32: 740-742.

[738] Heussler J K et al. A double blind randomized trial of low power laser treatment in rheumatoid arthritis. Annals Rheum Diseases. 1993; 52: 703-706.

[739] Tabau C. Contributions from Midlaser in the treatment of lateral ankle sprain. Medical Laser Report. 1984; 1: 29-32.

[699] Melnichenko E M et al [The clinico-experimental validation of the use of low-intensity laser radiation for the treatment of exacerbated recurrent herpetic stomatitis in children]. Stomatologiia. 1992; (2): 76-78. (in Russian)

[700] Sitnikov V P et al. [Use of helium-neon lasers in the treatment of postoperative wounds of the phar-ynx]. Vestnik Otorinolaringologii. 1989; (5): 46-49. (in Russian)

[701] Hubacek J et al. Lymphocyte reaction in the palatine tonsils after use of the HeNe laser. Ceskoslov Gastroenterol a Vyziva. 1983; 37 (8): 467-471.

[702] Ben-Dov N, Shefer G, Irinitchev A et al. Low energy laser irradiation affects satellite cell proliferation and differentiation in vitro. Biochem Biophys Acta. 1999; 1448: 372-380.

[703] Thorsen H. [Low energy laser treatment-effect in localized fibromyalgia in the neck and shoulder regions.] Ugeskrift for Laeger. 1991; 17; 153 (25):1801-1804. (in Danish)

[704] Sinev I V et al. [The local treatment of chemical burns of the esophagus via an endoscope by means of laser therapy and adhesive application.] Vestnik Khirurgii Imeni i - i - Grekova 1990; 145 (11): 62-64. (in Russian)

(705] Yamaguchi M et al. [Clinical study on the treatment of hypersensitive dentine by GaAlAs laser diode using the double blind test.] Aichi Gakuin Daigaku Shigakkai Shi - Aichi-Gakuin Journal of Dental Science 1990; 28 (2): 703-707 (In Japanese).

[706] Trelles M A, Rotinen S. He/Ne laser treatment of hemorrhoids. Acupuncture & Electro-Therapeutics Research. 1983; 8 (3-4): 289-295.

[707] Matouskova I. [Reaction of the palatal tonsils after the application of a HeNe laser]. Acta Universitatis Palackianae Olomucensis Facultatis Medicae. 1984;107: 315-320.

[708] Millson C E, Wilson M et al. The killing of Helicobacter pylori by low-power laser light in the presence of a photosensitiser. J Med Microbiol 1996; 44 (4): 245-252

[709] Simunovic Z, Trobonjaca T. Soft tissue injury during sport activities and traffic accidents - treatment woth low level laser therapy: a multicenter double blind, placebo controlled clinical study on 132 patients. Proc. IXX Annual Congress of ASLMS, Orlando, Florida. April 1999.

[710] Shesterina M V. [Effects of laser therapy on immunity in patients with bronchial asthma and pulmonary tuberculosis.] Probl Tuberk. 1994; 5: 23-26. (in Russian)

[711] Myrhaug H. [The theory of otosclerosis and Morbus Ménière (Labyrintine vertigo) being caused by the same mechanism: physical irritants, an otognathic syndrome.] Bergmanns Boktrykkeri A/S, Bergen, Norway. 1981. (In Norwegian)

[712] Mischenkin N V et al. [Effects of helium-neon laser energy on the tissues of the middle ear in the presence of biological fluids and drug solutions]. Vestn Otorinolaringol. 1990; 5: 18-21. (in Russian)

[713] Bogomilskii M R et al. [Effects of low-energy laser irradiation on the functional state of the acoustic analyzer.] Vestn Otorinolaringol. 1989; 2: 29-34. (in Russian)

[714] Dcabrowska E et al. [Intravital treatment of the pulp with simultaneous laser biostimulation] Rocz Akad Med Bialymst. 1997; 42 (1): 168-176. (in Polish).

[715] Bhagwanani N S et al. Low level nitrogen laser therapy in pulmonary tuberculosis. J Clin Laser Med Surg. 1996; 14 (1): 23-25.

[716] Agaev F F. [Endobronchial laser therapy in the surgery of tuberculosis]. Probl Tuberk. 1998; 1: 33-36. (in Russian)

[717] Kipshidze N N et al. Photoremodeling of arterial wall reduces restenosis after balloon angioplasty in an atherosclerotic rabbit model. J Am Coll Cardiol. 1998; 31 (5): 1152-1157.

[718] Barberis G et al. In vitro synthesis of prostaglandin E2 by synovial tissue after helium-neon laser radiation in rheumatoid arthritis. J Clin Laser Med Surg. 1996; 14 (4): 175-177.

[678]   Soriano F. GaAs laser treatment of venous ulcers. Proc. 2nd Congress World Assn for Laser Therapy, Kansas City, September 1998; p. 128-130.

[679]   Bucek M et al. Morphology of epithelizing varicose ulcers following HeNe laser therapy. Acta Uni-versitatis Palackianae Olomucensis Facultatis Medicae. 1991; 131: 303-316.

[680]   Ditrichova D. Application of biostimulative effects of HeNe laser in the therapy of crural ulcers. Ultrastructural findings in irradiated tissue. Acta Universitatis Palackianae Olomucensis Facultatis Medicae. 1988; 119: 337-346.

[681]   Gomberg V G et al. Endolymphatic laser therapy in management of acute nonspecific epididymitis. Proc. 2nd Congress World Assn for Laser Therapy, Kansas City, Sept 1998; p. 27

[682]   Reznikov L L et al. Urol Nefrol. 1991; 2: 45-49.

[683]   Ocaña-Quero J M, Gomez-Villamandos R, Moreno-Millan M, Santisteban-Valenzuela J M. Biological effects of helium-neon (He-Ne) laser irradiation on acrosome reaction in bull sperm cells. J Photochem Photobiol. B - Biol. 1997; 40 (3): 294-298.

[684]   Kovalev E V. [The effect of low-intensity laser irradiation on spermatogenesis in men]. Voprosy Kurortol, Fizioter Lechebnoi Fizicheskoi Kultury. 1990; (5): 33-36.

[685]   Tsushima T et al. Effects of two-point linear polarised near-infrared irradiation in difficult temporomandibular joint disorders. Proc. 2nd Congress World Assn for Laser Therapy, Kansas City, September 1998; p. 29-30.

[686]   Shiomi Y et al. Efficacy of transmeatal low power laser irradiation on tinnitus: a preliminary report. Auris Nasus Larynx. 1997; 24: 39-42.

[687]   Shiomi Y et al. [Effect of low power laser irradiation on innear ear.] Pract Otol (Kyoto). 1994; 87: 1135-1140. (in Japanese)

[688]   Palchun V T et al. [Low-energy laser irradiation in the combined treatment of sensorineural hearing loss and Ménière's disease]. Vestnik Otorinolaring. 1996; (1): 23-25 (in Russian).

[689]   Ribari O et al. [Closure of tympanic perforations with low-energy HeNe laser irradiation]. Acta Chir Academ Scient Hungaricae. 1980; 21 (3): 229-238. (in Hungarian with English abstract)

[690]   Bykov V L et al. [Low-energy laser irradiation in the complex treatment of patients with ear diseases.] Voprosy Kurortologii, Fizioterapii i Lechebnoi Fizicheskoi Kultury. 1985; (2): 60-62. (in Russian)

[691]   Hashimoto T, Kemmutso O, Otsuka H et al. Efficacy of laser irradiation on the area near the stellate ganglion is dose-dependent: a double-blind crossover placebo-controlled study. Laser Therapy. 1997; 9 (1): 7-12.

[692]   Kemmotsu O et al. Laser therapy for pain attenuation. Proc. 2nd Congress World Assn for Laser Therapy, Kansas City, September 1998; p. 7-8.

[693]   Wahl G, Bastianer S. Soft laser in postoperative care in dentoalveolar treatment. ZWR. 1991; 100 (8): 512-515.

[694]   Tiukhin N S et al. [Laser therapy in patients with inflammatory pleural exudates]. Problemy Tuberkuleza. 1997; 4: 38-40. (in Russian)

[695]   Sudoh A et al. Effect of low power laser irradiation on experimental tooth movement. J Dent Res 74 (IADR Abstracts). 1995; p. 457. abstr. 453.

[696]   Hashieh I A et al. Helium-neon laser irradiation is not a stressful treatment: a study on heat-shock protein (HSP70) level. Laser Surg Med. 1997; 20 (4): 451-460.

[697]   Kats A. [Treatment of erosive-ulcerative forms of lichen planus with low-energy laser irradiation]. Vestnik Khirurgii Imeni i - i - Grekova 1990 144 (4): 121-123. (in Russian)

[698]   Velizhanina I A et al. [The laser therapy of hypertension patients in the initial stages.] Voprosy Kuror Fizioter Lecheb Fizches Kult. 1998; 1: 9-11. (in Russian)

[659] Onac I et al. Histological study regarding the effects of HeNe (632.8 nm) laser biostimulation upon the tegument of Cavia Cobaia as compared with that of monochromatic red light (618 nm). Proc. 2nd Congress World Assn for Laser Therapy, Kansas City, September 1998; p. 52-53.

[660] Asagai Y et al. Application of low reactive-level laser therapy (laser therapy) in the functional training of cerebral palsy patients. Proc. 2nd Congress World Assn for Laser Therapy, Kansas City, September 1998; p. 99-100.

[661] Naeser M A. Treatment of carpal tunnel syndrome: research and clinical studies with laser acupuncture and microamps TENS. Proc. 2nd Congress World Assn for Laser Therapy, Kansas City, September 1998; p. 145-146.

[662] Katsuyama I et al. Suppressive effect of diode laser irradiation on picryl contact sensitivity. Laser Therapy 1998, 10 (3): 117-122.

[663] Taguchi Y. Clinical experiences of laser applications in physical therapy. Proc. 2nd Congress World Assn for Laser Therapy, Kansas City, September 1998; p. 106.

[664] Piller N B, Thelander A. Treatment of chronic postmastectomy lymphoedema with low level laser therapy: A 2.5 year follow-up. Lymphology. 1998; 31: 74-86.

[665] Amaral A C et al. HeNe laser action in the regeneration of the tibialis anterior muscle of mice. Proc. 2nd Congress World Assn for Laser Therapy, Kansas City, September 1998; p. 18-19.

[666] Kobayashi M et al. Studies of the diode laser therapy on blood supply in the rat model. Proc. 2nd Congress World Assn for Laser Therapy, Kansas City, September 1998; p. 70-71.

[667] Bibikova A et al. Enhancement of angiogenesis in regenerating gastrocnemius muscle of the toad (Bufo viridis) by low-energy laser irradiation. Anatomy & Embryology. 1994; 190 (6): 597-602.

[668] Takahashi Y, Hitomi S, Hirata et al.. Neovascularization effect with HeNe laser in the rat trachea. Thoracic & Cardiovascular Surgeon. 1992; 40 (5): 288-291.

[669] Samoilova K, Snopov S. A key role on whole circulating blood modification in therapeutic effects of ultraviolet and visible light. Proc. 2nd Congress World Assn for Laser Therapy, Kansas City, September 1998; p. 92-94.

[670] Gasparyan L. Investigations of sensations, associated with laser blood irradiation. Proc. 2nd Congress World Assn for Laser Therapy, Kansas City, September 1998; p. 87-88.

[671] Dillon K. Healing photons. Scientia Press, Washington D.C. 1998. ISBN 0-9642976-5-5.

[672] Longo L et al. Laser treatment of induratio penis plastic: advantages and limitations. Proc. 2nd Congress World Assn for Laser Therapy, Kansas City, September 1998; p. 104-105.

[673] Hall G et al. Effect of low level energy laser irradiation on wound healing. An experimental study in rats. Sw Dental J. 1994; 18 (1-2): 29-34.

[674] Schindl A et al. Increased dermal neovascularization after low dose laser therapy of chronic radiation ulcer determined by a video measuring system. Proc. 2nd Congress World Assn for Laser Therapy, Kansas City, September 1998; p. 34

[675] van der Ven Ph et al. The influence of IR-laser on the proliferation of fibroblasts: an in-vitro study. Proc. 2nd Congress World Assn for Laser Therapy, Kansas City, Sept 1998; p 120-122.

[676] Hrnjak M et al. Stimulatory effect of low-power density HeNe laser radiation on human fibroblasts in vitro. Vojnosanitetski Pregled. 1995; 52 (6): 539-546.

[677] Lichtenstein D. Morga B. Laser therapy in ambulatory patients with venous stasis ulcers. Proc. 2nd Congress World Assn for Laser Therapy, Kansas City, September 1998; p. 31-32.

[639] Alstergren P et al. Interleukin 1ß in the arthritic temporomandibular joint fluid and its relation to pain, mobility and anterior open bite. Swedish Dent J. 1998; 2: 247.

[640] Abramovici A, Roisman P, Hirsch A, Segal S, Fischer J. HeNe laser irradiation accelerate healing process of open gingival wounds in cats. In: Anderson R R, ed. Laser surgery: advanced characterization, therapeutics, and systems. IV. Proc. SPIE. Vol 2128: 248-256.

[641] Miyajima K, Yoshida K, Iwata T, et al. Effects of HeNe laser irradiation on gingival fibroblasts. Aichi-Gakuin Dent Sci. 1994; 7: 1-5.

[642] Nissan J, Binderman I. Effect of soft laser on bone healing of surgical defect in rat mandible. J Dent Res. 1993; 72 (4) :776, Abstract 53.

[643] Young J M, Altschuler B R. Laser holography in dentistry. J Prosthet Dent. 1977; 38 (2): 216-225.

[644] Groth E B. Treatment of dentine hypersensitivity with low power laser of Ga-Al-As. J Dent Res. 1995; 74 (3): 794, Abstract 163.

[645] Thaweboon B, Sa-Nguansin S, Thaweboon S, Buajeeb W. In vitro enhanced neutrophils phagocytosis by Ga-Al-As diode laser. J Dent Res. 1995; 74 (Spec Issue): 570, Abstract 1354.

[646] Yoshida K, Kato M, Ishida S, Arao M, Fukaya M. The management of the facial palsy patients using lower power output laser irradiation. 4th International Congress on Lasers in Dentistry, Singapore, 1994: 39.

[647] Simunovic Z. Low level laser therapy with trigger points technique: a clinical study on 243 patients. J Clin Laser Med Surg. 1996; 14 (4): 163-167.

[648] Mortiz A Irradiation of infected root canals with a diode laser in vivo. Results of microbiological examinations. Laser Surg Med. 1997; 21: 221-226.

[649] Mozgunov V N et al. [Method of treatment of common warts with low-energy laser irradiation.] Vestnik Dermatologii i Venerologii. 1985; (2): 55-56.

[650] Balaban P et al. HeNe laser irradiation of single neurons. Laser Surg Med. 1992; 12 (3): 329-337.

[651] Kosilov K V. [The treatment of neurogenic hyperreflexic bladder dysfunctions in girls with low-intensity laser radiation.] Urol Nefrologiia. 1995; (2): 16-19. (in Russian)

[652] Sakihama I. Effect of a helium-neon laser on cutaneous inflammation. Karume Medical J. 1995; 52 (4): 299-305.

[653] Parizotto N A, Baranauskas V. Structural analysis of collagen fibrils after HeNe laser photostimulated regenerating rat tendon. Proc. 2nd Congress World Assn for Laser Therapy, Kansas City, September 1998; p. 66.

[654] Eliseeva E V, Shusterov I A, Vakhrushev B N. [Intravasal laser irradiation of autologous blood in the treatment of eye diseases]. Vestn Oftamol. 1994; 110 (2): 23-24.

[655] Kólarová H et al. Effect of HeNe laser irradiation on phagocytic activity of leukocytes in vitro. Acta Universitatis Palackianae Olomucensis Facultatis Medicaee. 1991; 129: 127-132.

[566] Croley T. Laser treatment of fibroconnective tissue scarring. Proc. 2nd Congress World Assn for Laser Therapy, Kansas City, September 1998; p. 35-39.

[656] Basford, J R, Sheffield C G , Cieslak K R. Laser therapy: a randomized, controlled trial of the effects of low intensity Nd:YAG laser irradiation on lateral epicondylitis. Arch Phys Med Rehabil. 2000; 81 (11): 1504-1510.

[657] Reddy G K et al. The effects of laser stimulation on wound healing in diabetic rats. Proc. 2nd Congress World Assn for Laser Therapy, Kansas City, September 1998; p. 124-125.

[658] Landau Z. Topical hyperbaric oxygen and low energy laser for the treatment of diabetic foot ulcer. Archives of Orthopaedic & Trauma Surgery. 1998; 117 (3): 156-158.

[618] Thomasson T L. (Facial Pain/TMJ Centre, Denver, CO). Effects of Skin-Contact Monochromatic Infrared Irradiation on Tendonitis, Capsulitis and Myofascial Pain. 1995. 19th Annual Scientific Meeting, American Academy of Neurological & Orthopaedic Surgeons.

[619] Gou Jing-Zhen. Effects of HeNe regional irradiation on 53 cases in the field of pediatric surgery. In: Lasers in Dermatology and Tissue Welding. 1991. Proc. SPIE.Vol 1442: 9-.

[620] Moritz A et al. Advantage of a pulsed CO2 laser in direct pulp capping. A long-term in vivo study. Laser Surg Med. 1998; 22: 288-293.

[621] Mika T et al. [Infrared laser radiation in the treatment of low back pain syndrome]. Wiad Lek. 1990; 43 (11): 511-516. (in Polish)

[622] Iruzubieta J N. Effects of soft laser (HeNe) irradiation on corneal wound healing. An experimental study in the rabbit. Chibret Int J Ophthalm. 1991; 8: 25-33.

[623] Mikhailova R I et al. [The laser therapy and laser acupuncture of patients with chronic recurrent aphtous stomatitis.] Stomatologiia (Moscow). 1992; 3-6: 27-28.

[624] Hoteya K et al. Effects of a 1 W GaAlAs diode laser in the field of orthopedics. In: Meeting Report: The first Congress of the International Association for Laser and Sports Medicine. Tokyo, 1997. Laser Therapy 1997; 9 (4): 185.

[625] Kunin A A. et al. Biological effects caused by low power laser light in the treatment of the dentition, parodontium and mucosa of the oral cavity and lip diseases. Proc. SPIE. 1997. Vol 3198: 37-47.

[626] Schwartz F et al. Effect of low energy laser irradiation on cytokines secretion from skeletal muscle cells - involvement of calcium in the process. Proc SPIE. 1997. Vol 3198: 48-54.

[627] Cieslar G, Sieron A, Adamek M et al. Effect of low-power laser radiation in the treatment of the motional system overloading syndromes. Proc SPIE. 1997; Vol 3198: 76-82.

[628] Sagalovich E E. Secretory immunity changes in patients with acute and chronic herpetic stomatitis by laser therapy. Clin Immunol Immunopathol. 1995. 1 (7): 385.

[629] Noro S. Semi-conductor laser application for pain attenuation in the temporo-mandibular joint following facial contusion and facial fracture. Meeting report from the 1st Congr of the IALSM 1997. Laser Therapy. 1997; 9 (4): 184.

[630] Saito K. Effects of 830 nm diode laser irradiation on superficial blood circulation in college sumo wrestlers. Meeting report from the 1st Congr of the IALSM 1997. Laser Therapy. 1997; 9 (4): 187.

[631] Ciuchita T. Low-energy laser in the treatment of alopecia of the scalp. Proc. SPIE. 1997; Vol 3198: 116-126.

[632] Al-Watban F. Stimulation and inhibtion effects of Kr. laser for wound management. Laser Surg Med. 1998; Suppl 10: 5.

[633] Kulikova N G. [The effect of low-intensity infrared laser therapy on the endocrine function of patients with climacteric disorders.] Vopr Kurortol Fizioter Lech Fiz Kult. 1996; 5: 25-26.

[634] Conti P C. Low level laser therapy in the treatment of temporomandibular disorders (TMD): a double-blind pilot study. Cranio. 1997; 15 (2): 144-149.

[635] Pinheiro A L et al. Low-level laser therapy in the management of disorders of the maxillofacial region. J Clin Laser Med Surg. 1997; 15 (4): 181-183.

[636] Longo L, Simunovic Z, Postiglione M, Postiglione M.. Laser therapy for fibromyositic rheumatism. J Clin Laser Med Surg. 1997; 15 (5): 217-220.

[637] Cambier D C et al. Low-level laser therapy: the experience in Flanders. Eur J Phys Med Rehab. 1997; 7: 102-105.

[638] Giavelli F et al. [Low-level laser therapy in osteoarticular diseases in geriatric patients]. Radiol Med (Torino). 1998; 5 (4): 303-309. (in Italian)

[597] Soriano F et al. Low level laser therapy response in patients with chronic low back pain. A double blind study. Laser Surg Med. 1998. Suppl 10, p. 6.

[598] de Castro e Silva Júnior O, Zucoloto S, Menegazzo L A G et al. Laser enhancement in hepatic regeneration for partially hepatectomized rats. Laser Surg Med. 2001; 29: 73-77.

[599] Belkin M, Schwartz M. Ophthalmic effects of low-energy laser irradiation. Survey of Ophthalmology. 1994; 39 (2): 113-122.

[600] Naveh N et al. Low-energy laser: a new measure for suppression of arachidonic acid metabolism in the optic nerve. J Neurosci Res. 1990; 26: 386-389.

[601] Schwartz M et al. Effect of low-energy HeNe laser irradiation on posttraumatic degeneration of adult rabbit optic nerve. Lasers Surg Med. 1987; 7: 51-55.

[602] Yew D T et al. Low dose laser and the developing retina. A histochemical and scanning electronmicroscopic study. Acta Morphol Neerl Scand. 1982; 20: 57-63.

[603] Yew D T et al. Responses of astrocytes in culture after low dose laser irradiation. Scand Microscopy. 1990; 4: 151-159.

[604] Yamamoto Y, Kono T, Kotani H, Kasai S, Mito M. Effect of low-power laser irradiation on procollagen synthesis in human fibroblasts. J Clin Laser Med Surg. 1996; 14 (3): 129-132.

[605] Johannsen F et al. Low energy laser therapy in rheumatiod arthritis. Scand J Rheumatol. 1994; 23 (3): 145-147.

[606] Voronin I. [The use of laser therapy for restoring the fertilizing capacity of the ejaculate in men with chronic genital inflammation.] Vopr Kurortol Fizioter Lech Fiz Kult. 1994; 2: 24-26.

[607] Simunovic Z, Trobonjaca T, Trobonjaca Z. Treatment of medial and lateral epicondylitis - tennis and golfer's elbow with low level laser therapy: a multicenter double blind, placebo-controlled clinical study on 324 patients. J Clin Laser Med & Surg. 1998; 16 (3): 145-151.

[608] Longo L et al. Laser therapy of La Peyronie's syndrome: a review. Abstr. Laser Florence '97. European Medical Laser Assn. P. 18.

[609] Ortutay J, Koo E, Mester A. Psoriatic arthritis treatment with low power laser irradiation. A double blind clinical study. Lasermedizin - Laser in Med Surg. 1998; 13 (3-4): 140-144.

[610] Gelskey S C, White J M, Pruthi V K. The effectiveness of the Nd:YAG laser in the treatment of dentinal hypersensitivity. J Can Dent Assoc. 1993; 59 (4): 337-386.

[611] Barasch A et al. Helium-neon laser effects on conditioning-induced oral mucositis in bone marrow transplantation patients. Cancer. 1995; 76 (12): 2550-2556.

[612] Lundeberg T, Malm M. Low power HeNe laser treatment of venous leg ulcers. Ann Plast Surg. 1991; 27 (6): 537-539.

[613] Malm M, Lundeberg T. Effect of low power gallium arsenide laser on healing of venous ulcers. Scand J Plast Reconstr Hand Surg. 1991; 25 (3): 249-251.

[614] Moritz A et al. Irradiation of infected root canals with a diode laser in vivo: results of microbiological examinations. Laser Surg Med. 1997; 21: 221-226.

[615] Webb C et al. Stimulatory effect of 660 nm low level laser energy on hypertrophic scar-derived fibroblasts. Possible mechanisms for increase in cell count. Laser Surg Med. 1998; 22 (5): 294-301.

[616] Shefer G, Oron U, Irintchev A et al. Skeletal muscle cell activation by low-energy laser irradiation: a role for the MAPK/ERK pathway. J Cellular Physiology. 2001; 187: 73-80.

[617] Stelian J, Gil I, Habot B et al. Improvement of Pain and Disability in Elderly Patients with Degenerative Osteoarthritis of the Knee Treated with Narrow-Band Light Therapy. 1992. J Am Geriatr Soc; 40: 23-26.

[578] Amano A et al. Histological studies on the rheumatoid synovial membrane irradiated with a low energy laser. Laser Surg Med. 1994; 15 (3): 290-294.

[579] Tsai CL et al. Effect of CO2 laser on healing of cultured meniscus. Laser Surg Med. 1997; 20 (2): 172-178.

[580] Sato H. The effects of laser light on sperm motility and velocity in vitro. Andrologia. 1984; 16 (1): 23-25.

[581] Schindl L et al. Effects of low power laser-irradiation on differential blood count and body temperature in endotoxin-preimmunized rabbits. Life Sci. 1997; 60 (19): 1669-1677.

[582 Campaña V R, Moya M, Gavotto A, Soriano F et al. The relative effects of HeNe laser and meloxicam on experimentally induced inflammation. Laser Therapy. 1999; 11 (1): 36-41.

[583] Walsh L J. The use of lasers in implantology: an overview. J Oral Implantol. 1992; 18: 335-340.

[584] Yu H S et al. Low energy helium-neon laser irradiation stimulates interleukin-1 alpha and interleukin-8 release from cultured human keratinocytes. J Invest Dermatol. 1996; 107 (4): 593-596.

[585] Inoue K et al. Altered lymphocyte proliferation by low dosage laser irradiation. Clin Exp Rheumatol. 1989; 7 (5): 521-523.

[586] Yu W et al. The effect of laser irradiation on the release of bFGF from 3T3 fibroblasts. Photochem Photobiol. 1994; 59 (2): 167-170.

[587] Bibikova A, Oron U. Regeneration in denervated toad (Bufo viridis) gastrocnemius muscle and the promotion of the process by low energy laser irradiation. The Anatomical Record. 1995; 241: 123-128.

[588] Bjordal J M, Couppè C, Chow R T, Tunér J, Ljunggren A E. A systematic review of low level laser therapy with location-specific doses for pain from chronic joint disorders. Australian J Physiotherapy. 2003; 49: 107-116.

[589] Laor Y et al. The pathology of laser irradiation of the skin and body wall of the mouse. 1965; 47 (4): 643-662.

[590] Yu W et al. Improvement of host response to sepsis by photobiomodulation. Lasers in Surg Med. 1997; 21: 262-268.

[591] Xijing Wu et al. Observations on the effect of HeNe laser acupoint radiation in chronic pelvic inflammation. J Trad Chin Med. 1983; 7 (4): 263-265.

[592] Lubart R et al. Changes in calcium transport in mammalian sperm mitochondria and plasma membranes caused by 780 nm irradiation. Lasers in Surg Med. 1997; 21: 493-499.

[593] Crespi R et al. Periodontal tissue regeneration in beagle dogs after laser therapy. Lasers Surg Med. 1997. 21: 395-402.

[594] Schaffer M et al. Biomodulative effects induced by 805 nm laser light irradiation of normal and tumor cells. J Photochem Photobiol B:Biol. 1997; 40: 253-257.

[595] Eckerdal A. Kliniske erfaringer fra et 5-års icke-kontroleret studie af low power laser-behandling af periorale neuropatier. [Clinical experiences from a 5 year non-controlled study of low power laser treatment of perioral neuropatias]. In Danish). Tandlægebladet. 1994; 98 (11): 526-529.

[596] Cohen N, Lubart R, Rubenstein S et al. Laser irradiation of mouse spermatozoa enhances in vitro fertilization and Ca^{2+} uptake via reactive oxygen species. Proc. SPIE. 1996; Vol 2929: 27-37. Also: Cohen N, Lubart R, Rubinstein S, Breitbart H. Light irradiation of mouse spermatozoa: Stimulation of in vitro fertilization and calcium signals. Photochem Photobiol 1998; 68: 407-413.

[558] Georgadze A K et al. [Treatment of non-healing wounds and trophic ulcers by low-intensity laser irradiation in an outpatient clinic] Khirurgiia (Mosk). 1990; 12: 93-96. (in Russian)

[559] Soriano F. Venous leg ulcers healed with GaAs laser. Argentine experience. Proc Congr Int Soc Laser Surg Med, Bangkok 1993, p. 35.

[560] Santoianni P et al. Inadequate effect of helium-neon laser on venous leg ulcers. Photodermatology. 1984; 1: 245-249.

[561] Rochkind S, Barr-Nea L, Bartal A et al. New method of treatment of severely injured sciatic nerve and spinal cord. An experimental study. Acta Neurochirurgica. 1988; Suppl 43: 91-93.

[562] Lindholm A, de Mitri N, Swensson U. Clinical effect of non-focused CO_2 laser on traumatic arthritis in horses. Lasers Med Surg. Supplement 12, 2000: 51.

[563] Göran Renström, M D, Borlänge, Sweden. 1993; private communication.

[564] Mikhailov V A, Denisov I N. Activation of the immune system by low level laser therapy (laser therapy) for treating patients with stomach cancer in advanced form. Laser & Technology. 1997; 7 (1): 31-44.

[565] Funk J O, Kruse A, Kirchner H. Cytokine production after helium-neon laser irradiation in cultures of human peripheral blood mononuclear cells. J Photochem Photobiol B. 1992; 16 (3-4): 347-355.

[566] Koslov V I et al. [The microcirculation of patients with arterial ischemia of the lower extremities during laser therapy.] Fiziol Zh SSSR Im I M Sechenova. 1991; 77 (6): 55-67. (in Russian)

[567] Dudenko G I et al. [Treatment of acute trombophlebitis of the lower limbs with laser irrradiation.] Khirurgiia (Mosk). 1989; 9; 97-99. (in Russian)

[568] Gärtner C. Low reactive-level laser therapy (laser therapy) in rheumatology: a review of the clinical experience in the author's laboratory. Laser Therapy. 1992; 4 (3): 107-115.

[569] Saito S, Shimizu N. Stimulatory effects of low-power laser irradiation on bone regeneration in midpalatal suture during expansion in the rat. Am J Ortod Dentofac Orthop. 1997; 11 (5): 525-532.

[570] Buliakova N V et al. [Effects of helium-neon laser on regeneration capacity of skeletal muscles of adult guinea pigs.] Biull Eksp Biol Med. 1992; 113 (4): 411-414.

[571] Podelinskaia L V et al. [Effects of low-intensity laser irradiation on several parameters of microcirculation in the bulbar conjunctiva of patients with scleroderma.] Vestn Oftalmol. 1995; 111 (2): 10-12.

[572] Gassler N et al. Clinical data and histological features of trans-myocardial revascularuzation with CO_2 laser. Eur J Cardiothorac Surg. 1997; 12 (1): 25-30.

[573] Smithdeal C D et al. Carbon dioxide laser-assisted hair transplantation. The effect of laser parameters on scalp tissue - a histological study. Dermatol. Surg. 1997; 23 (9): 835-840.

[574] Umetov M A. [Effects of laser therapy on psychophysiological parameters and arterial blood pressure in drivers with hypertension]. Med Tr Prom Ekol. 1996; 8: 10-12. (in Russian)

[575] Cowen D et al. Low energy helium neon laser in the prevention of oral mucositis in patients undergo-ing bone marrow transplant: results of a double blind randomized trial. Int J Radiat Oncol Biol Phys. 1997; 38 (4): 697-707.

[576] Beckerman H et al. Efficacy of physiotherapy for musculoskeletal disorders: what can we learn from research? Br J Gen Pract. 1993; 43 (367): 73-77.

[577] Kurumada F. A study on the application of Ga-As semiconductor laser to endodontics. The effects of laser irradiation on the activation of inflammatory cells and the vital pulpotomy. Ohu Daigaku Shigakushi. 1990; 17 (3): 233-244.

[538] Weintraub M I. Noninvasive laser neurolysis in carpal tunnel syndrome. Muscle Nerve. 1997; 20 (8): 1029-1031.

[539] Wong E et al. Successful management of female office workers with "repetitive stress injury" or "carpal tunnel syndrome" by a new treatment modality - application of low level laser. Int J Clin Pharmacol Ther. 1995; 33 (4): 208-211.

[540] King C E et al. Effect of helium-neon laser auriculotherapy on experimental pain threshold. Phys Ther. 1990; 70 (1): 24-30.

[541] Kruchinina I et al. [Therapeutic effect of helium-neon laser on microcirculation of nasal mucosa in children with acute and chronic maxillary sinuitis as measured by conjunctival biomocroscopy]. Vestn Otorino-laringol. 1991; 3: 26-30. (in Russian with English abstract)

[542] Kruchinina I et al. [Effect of laser therapy on the local synthesis of class A immunoglubulin in children with acute and chronic maxillary sinuitis]. Vestn Otorinolaringol. 1988; 2: 19-21. (in Russian with English abstract)

[543] Pluzhnikov S M et al. [Use of intracavitary low-energy laser therapy in the complex treatment of inflammatory diseases in the sphenoid sinus]. Vest Otoringolaringol. 1986; 4: 72-73. (in Russian with English abstract)

[544] Toscani A, Bombelli G. [Laser therapy in post-extraction alveolitis]. Dent Cadmos. 1987; 55 (9): 73-74. (In Italian)

[545] Kim Jin Wang, Lee Joung Ok. Double blind cross-over clinical study of 830 nm diode laser and 5 years clinical experience of biostimulation in plastic surgery & aesthetic surgery in Asians. Laser Surg Med. 1998; Suppl 10: 59.

[546] Reddy G K et al. Laser photostimulation of collagen production in healing rabbit achilles tendons. Lasers in Medicine and Surgery. 1998; 22: 281-287.

[547] Axelsen S M, Bjerno T. [Laser therapy of ankle sprain]. Ugeskr Læger. 1993; 155 (48): 3908-3911. (in Danish)

[548] Darrre E M et al. [Laser treatment of achilles tendonitis]. Ugeskr Læger. 1994; 156 (45): 6680-6683. (in Danish)

[549] Winther A, Laserklinikken, Copenhagen, Denmark. 1997. Personal communication.

[550] Lievens P, Lippens E. The influence of low level infra red lasertherapy on the regeneration of cartilage tissue. Laser Surg Med. 1998; Suppl 10: 5.

[551] Gruszka M et al. Effect of low energy laser therapy on herniated lumbar discs. Laser Surg Med. 1998; Suppl 10: 6.

[552] Schindl A, Schindl M, Schön H, Knobler R, Havelec L, Schindl L. Low intensity laser irradiation improves skin circulation in patients with diabetic microangiopathy. Diabetes Care. 1998; 21 (4): 580-584.

[553] Skoric T et al. Laser biostimulation: application of the gallium-arsenide laser in the therapy of ulcus cruris. Laser Surg Med. 1998; Suppl 10: 7.

[554] Konstantinovic L et al. [Combined low-power laser therapy and local infiltration of corticosteroids in the treatment of radial-humeral epicondylitis.] Vojnosanit Pregl. 1997; 54 (5): 459-463. (in Croatian)

[555] Tulebaev R K et al. [Indicators of the activity of the immune system during laser therapy of vasomotor rhinitis]. Vestn. Otorinolaringol. 1989; 1: 46-49. (in Russian)

[556] Sugrue M E et al. The use of infrared laser therapy in the treatment of venous ulceration. Ann Vasc Surg. 1990; 4 (2): 179-181.

[557] Rakcheev A P et al. [Experimental and clinical substantiation of laser therapy of wounds and throphic ulcers] Ortop Travmatol Protez. 1989; 10: 66-70. (in Russian with English abstract)

[518] Ortutay J, Mester A. Laserstimulation therapy in the rehabilitation medicine. Proc. Laser Florence '97, 5th Congr EMLA, p. 22.

[519] Tsuchiya K et al. Diode laser irradiation selectively diminishes slow component of axonal volleys to dorsal roots from the saphenous nerve in the rat. Neuroscience Letters. 1993; 161: 65-68. Also: Tsuchiya K, Kawatani M, Takeshige C, et al.Laser irradiation abates neuronal responses to nociceptive stimulation of rat-paw skin. Brain Res Bull. 1994; 34 (4): 369-374

[520] Carney S A et al. The effect of light from a ruby laser on the metabolism of skin in tissue culture. Biochem Biophys Acta. 1967; 148: 525-530.

[521] Lievens P, Mohebbian M. The effect of IR-laser irradiation on the regeneration of muscle fibres. In: Laser Therapy in Dentistry and Medicine. Prima Books in Sweden AB. Eds Jan Tunér and Lars Hode. 1996, p. 164-179.

[522] Ozawa Y, Shimizu N, Abiko Y. Low-energy diode laser irradiation reduced plasminogen activator activity in human periodontal ligament cells. Laser Surg Med. 1997; 21: 456-463.

[523] Ohtsuka H et al. [Low recative-level laser therapy near the stellate ganglion for postherpetic facial neuralgia]. (in Japanese). Masui. 1992; 41 (11): 1809-1813.

[524] Petrek M et al. Immunomodulatory effects of laser therapy in the treatment of chronic tonsillitis. Acta Univ Palacki Olomuc Fac Med. 1991; 129: 119-126.

[525] Colvard M, Kuo P. Managing aphtous ulcers: laser treatment applied. J Am Dent Assoc. 1991; 122 (7): 51-53.

[526] Zubkova S T. [The use of helium-neon laser radiation in the treatment of trophic disorders in patients with diabetes mellitus]. Klin Khir. 1992; 3: 47-49. (in Russian with English abstract)

[527] Grubnik V V et al. [Combined laser therapy of diabetic gangrene of the lower limbs]. Klin Khir. 1994; 7: 20-22. (in Russian with English abstract)

[528] Yu W et al. Effects of photostimulation on wound healing in diabetic mice. Laser Surg Med. 1997; 20 (1): 56-63.

[529] el Sayed S O, Dyson M. Effect of laser pulse repetition rate and pulse duration on mast cell number and degranulation. Laser Surg Med. 1996; 19 (4): 433-437.

[530] Ibañez J C, Medico R O. [Laser therapy in temporomandibular dysfunction]. Rev Fac Odont Univ Nac (Córdoba). 1989; 17 (1-2): 21-30. (in Spanish)

[531] Howell R M et al. The use of low energy laser therapy to treat aphtous ulcers. Ann Dent. 1988; 47 (2): 16-18.

[532] Bertolucci L E, Grey T. Clinical analysis of Mid-laser versus placebo treatment of arthralgic TMJ degenerative joints. J Craniomandib Practice. 1995; 13 (1): 26-29.

[533] Buliakova N V. [Regereration of the x-ray irradiated gastrocnemius muscle in old rats after stimulation]. Biull Eksp Biol Med. 1989; 108 (7): 123-126. (in Russian with English abstract)

[534] Pekli F F, Kruchinina I L. [Physiological functions of the nose befroe and after laser treatment of acute and chronic maxillary sinusitis in children]. Vestn Otorinolaringol. 1988; (3): 53-55.

[535] Nissen L R et al. [Low-energy laser therapy in medial tibial stress syndrome]. Ugeskrift Læger. 1994; 156 (49): 7329-7331. (in Danish)

[536] Luger E J, Rochkind S et al. Effect of low-power laser irradiation on the mechanical properties of bone fracture healing in rats. Laser Surg Med. 1998; 22 (2): 97-102.

[537] Wollman Y et al. Low power laser irradiation enhances migration and neurite sprouting of cultured rat embryonal brain cells. Neurol Res. 1996; 18 (5): 467-470.

[497] Haina D et al. Temperature of the skin during application of softlaser. Laser in Medicine and Surgery. 1988; 4 (1): 26-29.

[498] T W Marín V. Experimental wound healing with coherent and non-coherent radiation. Laser & Technology. 1992; 2 (3): 121-134.

[499] Labajos M et al. ß-endorphine levels modification after GaAs and HeNe laser irradiation on the rabbit. Comparative study. Investigación clínica láser. 1988; 1-2: 6-8.

[500] Fructuoso F J G, Moset J M. Randomized double blind study on the biostimulatory effect of laser irradiation of the parotid gland in patients suffering of Sjögren syndrome. Invest y Clinica Laser. 1987; 1: 18-25. In Sp with E abstr. Also published in Centro Documentación Láser. 1987: 4 (13): 4-.

[501] Kotani H. Effects of low power laser stimulation on wound healing in rats. Lasermedizin - Laser in Med Surg. 1995; 11 (2): 25- .

[502] Rossetti V et al. Experimental studies on the in vivo effects of HeNe laser irradiation in rat brain. Lasermedizin - Laser in Med Surg. 1995; 11 (2): 24- .

[503] Glinkowski W et al. Sprained ankles treatment with use of laser therapy. Lasermedizin - Laser in Med Surg. 1995; 11 (2): 42-.

[504] Véles-Gonzáles M A. Absorción subcutaneo del salicilato de dietilamina tras la irradiación laser. Boletín CDL. 1987; 4 (12): 4-8.

[505] Juri H et al. Efectos del láser HeNe sobre las concentraciones de fibrinogeno en el plasma de ratas en lesiones tistulares. Boletín CDL. 1986; 10: 5-6.

[506] Padulles J et al. [Laser treatment of spinal pinching due to discal hernias in dogs]. Boletín CDL. 1986; 2: 11-14. (in Spanish)

[507] Kaiser C, Manso F, Zaragoza J R. Estúdio en doble ciego randomizado sobre la eficacia del HeNe en el tratamiento de la sinuitis maxilar aguda: en pacientes con exacerbación de una infección sinusal crónica. (Double blind randomized study on the effect of HeNe in the treatment of acute maxillary sinuitis: in patients with exacerbation of a chronic maxillary sinuitis). Boletín CDL. 1986; 9: 15-17.

[508] van den Brande P. Effect of HeNe - IR laser on cutaneous microcirculation in vascular patients. Proc. Lasertherapy III, Vrije Universiteit Brussel, October 1987.

[509] Fagnoni V et al. Trattamento delle nevralgie trigeminali con laser di bassa potenza. Laser Abstracts. 1985; 2: 23-36

[510] Yamada K. Effect of low power laser irradiation on osteoblastic cell growth. Surgical and Medical Lasers. 1989; 2-3 (2): 67 (abstract)

[511] Nicola J H et al. The role of coherence in wound healing stimulation by non-thermal laser radiation. Surgical and Medical Lasers. 1989; 2-3 (2): 70 (abstract)

[512] Karu T I. Mechanisms of interaction of monochromatic visible light with cells. Proc. SPIE. 1995; Vol 2630: 2-9

[513] Friedmann H, Lubart R. Competition between activayting and inhibitory processes in photobiology. Proc. SPIE. 1995; Vol 2630: 60-64.

[514] Martelli M R A. A clinico statistical investigation of laser effect in the treatment of pain and dysfunction of temporo-mandibular joint (T.M.J.). J Dental Proth. 1990; (18): 31-36.

[515] Marei M K. Effect of low-energy laser application in the treatment of denture-induced mucosal lesions. J Prosthet Dent. 1997; 77 (3): 256-264.

[516] Kim K-S, Kim J-K, Kim S-W et al. Effects of low level laser irradiation (LLLI) with 904 nm pulsed diode laser on osteoblasts: a controlled trial with the rat osteoblast model. Laser Therapy. 1996; 8 (4): 223-232.

[517] Popov B. [Trigeminal neuralgia with local laser irradiation and laserpuncture]. Stomatologiia Bulgaria. 1986; 68: 25-29.

[478] Schindl L et al. Topical low power laser irradiation shows a systemic increase in blood flow in conditions of disturbed microcirculation. Laser Therapy. 1996; 8 (1): 58. (abstract)

[479] Kubota J, Ohshiro T. The effect of diode laser laser therapy on flap survival: measurement of flap microcirculation with the laser specle method. Laser Therapy. 1996; 8 (4): 241-246.

[480] Amir A et al. The influence of low energy Helium-Neon laser irradiation on the viability of skin flaps of the rat. Laser Therapy. 1996; 8 (1): 59. (abstract)

[481] Koukoui L M et al. The differential approach to the application of laser, ultraviolet and roentgenological auto-blood irradiation for the correction of homeostatis. Laser Therapy. 1996; 8 (1): 60. (abstract)

[482] Samoilova K A, Kukui L M . Photochemotherapy in clinical and veterinary medicine: therapeutic effects and mechanisms. Laser Therapy. 1996; 8 (1): 62. (abstract)

[483] Kirichuk V F et al. Influence of low power laser radiation on platlet aggregation in pathological stress. Laser Therapy. 1996; 8 (1): 63. (abstract)

[484] Peláez A et al. Growing cartilage after IR laser radiation - utlrastructural study. Proc SPIE. 1993;. Vol 2086: 356-364. Also in: Peláez A, Vidal L, Vargas I. Quantitative study of the morphological changes in the thyroid gland following IR laser irradiation. Lasers Med. Sci.1989; 5: 77-80.

[485] Antipa C et al. Use of pulsed laser therapy (Ga-As) in combined treatment of posttraumatic swellings and some dermatological disorders. Proc SPIE. 1993; Vol. 2086: 371-377.

[486] Fagnoni V et al. Use of HeNe soft-laser in 32 cases of mouth aphta. Laser Abstracts (Rivista Europea di Laser Terapia Medica e Chirurgia). 2 (2): 25-29.

[487] Smith R J et al. The effect of low-energy laser on skin-flap survival in the rate and porcine animal models. Plastic and Reconstruct Surg. 1992; 89 (2): 306-310.

[488] Kasai S et al. Effects of low-power laser irradiation on impulse conductions in anaesthetized rabbits. J Clin Laser Med Surg. 1996; 14 (3): 107-109.

[489] Ulrich M et al. Influence of laser light (830 nm) on the growth kinetics of rat rhabdomyosarcomas. University of Hamburg, Department of Accident Surgery. Part of M.D. thesis

[490] Longo L, Evangelista S, Tinacci G, Sesti A G. Effects of diodes-laser silver Arsenide-Aluminium (Ga-Al-As) 904 nm on healing of experimental wounds. Laser Surg Med. 1987; 7 (5): 444-447.

[491] Makk A, Pollera M. Multicenter study related to laser treatment of TMJ syndrom. Proc. Internat Congress LASERMED, Munich, 1995, p. 104.

[492] Lubart R et al. Changes in calcium transport in mammalian sperm mitochondria and plasma membrane due to 630 nm and 780 nm laser irradiation. Proc. LASERMED Munich 1995, p. 104

[493] Rosner M, Caplan M, Cohen S et al. Dose and temporal parameters in delaying injured optic nerve degeneration by low-energy laser irradiation. Laser Surg Med. 1993; 13 (6): 611-617.

[494] Hoffman B, Bär Th. Reaktionen der Hautoberflächentemperatur - ein Vergleich zwischen Verum- und Placebo-Laserstimulation am Akupunkturpunkt Di 4. Dtsch. Zschr. Akup. 1994; 37 (2): 28.

[495] Mayordomo M M et al. Laser in painful process of locomotor system: our experience. 1985. Proc. of Laser Bologna 1985. Monduzzi Editore, Bologna.

[496] Choi J et al. A comparison of electroacupuncture, transcutaneous electrical nerve stimulation and laser photobiostimulation on pain relief and glucocorticoid excretion. Int J Acupunct Electrotherp Res. 1986; 11: 45-51.

[456] Chio Chung-Chin, Lin S-J, Kao M-C. Cytogenic effects of low level laser irradiation of human leukocytes. Laser Therapy. 1990; 2 (3): 111-116.

[457] Severtsev A N et al. The preliminary results of the immunomodulatory effects of HeNe-laser irradiation in human mixed lymphocytes culture. Laser Surg Med, Suppl 5. 1993; 10.

[458] Yamaya M, Shiroto C, Kobayashi Mechanistic approach to GaAlAs diode laser effects on production of reactive oxygen species from human neutrophils as a model for therapeutic modality at cellular level. Laser Therapy. 1993; 5 (3): 111-116.

[459] Tunér J. The Cochrane analyses - can they be improved? Laser Therapy. 1999; 11 (3): 138-143.

[460] Maeda T et al. Histological, thermographic and thermometric study in vivo and excised 830 nm diode laser irradiated rat skin. Laser Therapy. 1990; 2 (1): 32. (abstract)

[461] Masse J-F et al. Effectiveness of soft laser treatment in periodontal surgery. Int Dent J. 1993; 43: 121-127.

[462] Lyons R et al. Biostimulation of wound healing in vivo by a helium neon laser. Annals Plastic Surg. 1987; 18 (1): 47-50.

[463] Enwemeka C et al. Corrective ultrastructural and biomechanical changes induced in regenerated tendons exposed to laser photostimulation. Laser Surg Med. 1990; (Suppl 2): 12-19.

[464] Lim Hong Meng et al. A clinical investigation of the efficacy of low level laser therapy in reducing orthodontic postadjustment pain. Am J Orthod Dentofac Orthop. 1995; 108: 614-622.

[465] Oudoff H A F, van der Kuiji P. Inquiry about the application of low reactive level laser therapy in dental clinics in The Netherlands. Laser Therapy. 1996; 8 (1): 42. (abstract)

[466] Akai M et al. Laser's effect on bone and cartilage change induced by joint immobilization: an experiment with animal model. Laser Surg Med. 1997; 21 (5): 480-484.

[467] Halevy S et al. 780 nm low power laser therapy for wound healing - in vivo and in vitro studies. Laser Therapy. 1996; 8 (1): 20. (abstract)

[468] Schaffer M et al. Mitotic rate of normal mouse fibroblast cells and human tumor cells after diode laser irradiation. Laser Therapy. 1996; 8 (1): 23. (abstract)

[469] Mrowiec J et al. The antinociceptive effect of infrared laser radiation in experimental animals. Laser Therapy. 1996; 8 (1): 25. (abstract)

[470] Radelli, J et al. Metabolism and insulin-glycemic balance in rats. Laser Therapy. 1996; 8 (1): 26. (abstract)

[471] al-Watban F. Laser acceleration of open skin wound closure in rats and its dosimetric dependence. Laser Therapy. 1996; 8 (1): 27. (abstract)

[472] Kipshidze N N. Our experience in the use of a low intensity HeNe laser in the treatment of acute myocardial infarction. Laser Therapy. 1996; 8 (1): 28. (abstract)

[473] Horowitz I et al. Infrared spectroscopy analysis of the effect of low power laser irradiation on calvarial bone defect healing in the rat. Laser Therapy. 1996; 8: 29. (abstract)

[474] Wilden L, Dindinger D. Treatment of chronic diseases in the inner ear with low level laser therapy (laser therapy): pilot project. Laser Therapy. 1996; 8 (2): 209-212.

[475] al-Watban F, Zhang X Y. Comparison of the effects of laser therapy on wound healing using different laser wavelengths. Laser Therapy. 1996; 8 (2): 127-136.

[476] Moore K C. Postherpetic neuralgia as a complication of malignant disease and its treatment using a GaAlAs diode laser. Laser Therapy. 1996; 8 (1): 49. (abstract)

[477] Kleinman Y, Simmer S, Braksma Y et al. Low power laser therapy in pateints with diabetic foot ulcers: early and long term outcome. Laser Therapy. 1996; 8 (3): 205-208.

[435] Bradley P F, Rebliini Z. Low intensity laser therapy (LILT) for temporomandibular joint pain: a clinical electromyographic and thermographic study. Laser Therapy. 1996; 8 (1): 47 (abstract)

[436] Bradley F G, Reynolds P A. Low reactive level laser therapy in Oral and Maxillofacial Surgery. Review of 100 cases. Laser Therapy. 1994; 6 (1): 67. (abstract)

[437] Lomnitski I. [The mechanism of stimulation of reparative osteogenesis with laser radiation]. Stomatologiia (Mosk). 1983; 5: 18-20.

[438] Lomnitski I. [Clinical X-ray characteristics of the healing of mandibular fractures following the use of HeNe laser radiation]. Stomatologiia (Mosk). 1985; 3: 38-40.

[439] Urazalin Zh B et al. [Laser therapy in the combined treatment of mandibular fractures]. Stomatologiia. 1983; 62: 34-.

[440] Supiev T K. [Action of laser radiation on the course of an inflammatory process in the maxillofacial area]. Stomatologiia (Mosk). 1984; 5: 17-19.

[441] Önal B et al. Preliminary report on the application of pulsed CO_2 laser radiation on root canals with AgCl fibers: a scanning and transmission electron microscopic study. J Endodontics. 1993; 19 (6): 272-276.

[442] Moritz M D et al. The advantage of CO_2 treated dental necks, in comparison with a standard method: Results from an in vitro study. J Clin Laser Med Surg. 1996; 14 (1): 27-.

[443] Flöter T, Rehfisch H P. Pain treatment with laser: a double blind study. Proc. of the 4th Internat Symposium. Acup & Electroteher Res. 1988; 13 (4): 236-237.

[444] Simunovic Z. Curing stomatological and maxillo-facial diseases with MID laser therapy. 1984. QLT; 1.

[445] Smesny D B. Acupuncture laser in treating headache pain. 1989. Proc. SPIE.Vol 1353: 234-237.

[446] Belkin M, Schwartz M. Evidence for the existence of low-energy laser bioeffects on the nervous system. Neurosurg Rev 1994; 17 (1): 7-17.

[447] Onac I, Pop L, Onac I. Implications of low power He-Ne laser and monochromatic red light biostimulation in protein and glycoside metabolism. Laser Therapy. 1999; 11 (3): 130-137.

[448] Ryabykh T, Karu T I. Action of pulsed visible and near IR laser radiation on oxidative metabolism of cells evaluated by chemiluminescence measurement. Proc SPIE. 1995; Vol 2630: 12-21.

[449] Zarkovic J et al. Use of HeNe laser for treatment of soft tissue trauma: evaluation by Gallium-67 citrate scanning. J Orthop and Sports Physical Therapy. 1986; 8 (2): 93-96.

[450] Labbe R F et al. Laser photobioactivation mechanisms: in vitro studies using ascorbic acid uptake and hydroxyproline formation as biochemical markers of irradiation response. Laser Surg Med. 1990; 10: 201-207.

[451] Gerschman J A, Ruben J, Gebart-Eaglemont J. Low Level Laser for dentinal tooth hypersensitivity. Australian Dent J. 1994; 39 (6): 353-357.

[452] Eckerdal A, Lehmann Bastian H. Can low reactive-level laser therapy be used in the treatment of neurogenic facial pain? A double-blind, placebo controlled investigation of patients with trigeminal neuralgia. Laser Therapy. 1996; 8 (4): 247-252.

[453] Miyagi K. Double-blind comparative study of the effect of low-energy laser irradiation to rheumatoid arthritis. In: Current awareness of Excerpts Medica. Amsterdam. Elsevier Science Publishers BV. 1989; 25: 315. Also: J Jap Assoc Physical Med Balneol & Climatol. 1989; 52 (3): 117-126.

[454] Tunér J, Hode L. It's all in the parameters: a critical analysis of some well-known negative studies on low-level laser therapy. J Clin Laser Med Surg. 1998; 16 (5): 245-248.

[455] Lindén L-Å .Enhanced curing of dental lasers. Swedish Dental J. 1997; 6: 242-.

[413] Motomura K et al. Effects of various laser irradiation on callus formation after osteotomy. J Jpn Soc Laser Med. 1984; 4: 195-196.

[414] Yamada K. Biological effects of low power laser irradiation on clonal osteoblastic cells (MC3T3-E1). Nippon Seikeigeka Gakkai Zasshi (J Jpn Orthop Assn). 1991; 65: 787-799.

[415] Rigau J, Trelles M A. Effects of the 633 nm laser on the behaviour and morphology of primary fibroblast culture. Proc SPIE.Vol 2630. 1995: 38-42.

[416] Michels H. Erfahrungen mit dem HeNe Laser bei Herpes Erkrankungen. Proc. 7th Int Congr Laser 1985. Edit. W Waidelinch. 1986; 116-119. Springer-Verlag (Berlin).

[417] Brill G et al. Influence of HeNe laser irradiation on giant chromosomes. Proc.SPIE. Vol 2630. 1995; 51-59.

[418] Yamada H, Ogawa H. Comparative study of 60 mW diode laser therapy and 150 mW diode laser therapy in the treatment of postherpetic neutralgia. Laser Therapy. 1995; 7 (2): 71-74.

[419] Bolton P, Young S, Dyson M. The direct effect of 860 nm light on cell proliferation and on succinic dehydrogenase activity of human fibroblasts in vitro. Laser Therapy. 1995; 7 (2): 55-60.

[420] Glinkowski W, Rowinski J. Effect of low incident levels of infrared laser energy on the healing of experimental bone fractures. Laser Therapy. 1995; 7 (2): 67-70.

[421] Otsuka H, Numasawa R, Okubo K et al. Effects of helium-neon laser therapy on herpes zoster pain. Laser Therapy. 1995; 7 (1): 27-32.

[422] Calderhead G. Meeting report: International low power laser symposium, Vienna, Austria, October 7th-8th, 1994. Laser Therapy. 1995; 7 (1): 39.

[423] Otsuka K et al. Low reactive level laser therapy near the stellate ganglion for postherpetic facial pain. Jpn J Anaesthes. 1991; 41: 1809-1813. (Abstr. in English)

[424] Villaplana L A, Sarti M A, Trelles NM A et al. Changes in albino rat testicle interstitial cells after pituitary stimulation in vivo with HeNe laser. Laser Therapy. 1995; 7 (1): 19-22.

[425] Gomez-Villamandos R J. HeNe laser therapy by fibroendoscopy in the mucosa of the equine upper airway. Laser Surg Med. 1995; 16: 184-188.

[426] Oron U, Yaakobi T, Oron A et al. Low energy laser irradiation reduces formation of scar tissue following myocardial infarction in dogs. Circulation. 2001; 103 (2): 296-301.

[427] Mester A et al. Irradiation of arthritis with 820 and 830 nm diode lasers. Laser Therapy. 1996; 8 (1): 33. (abstract)

[428] Lubart R et al. Photosensitized biostimulation of fibroblasts by low energy visible light. Laser Therapy. 1996; 8 (1): 16. (abstract)

[429] Gürsoy B, Bradley P F. Penetration studies of low intensity laser therapy (laser therapy) wavelengths. Laser Therapy, 1996; 8 (1): 18. (abstract)

[430] Yaakobi T, Oron U. Enhancement of bone repair in the rat tibia by low energy laser irradiation. Laser Therapy. 1996; 8 (1): 19. (abstract)

[431] Bibikova A, Oron U. Attenuation of the process of skeletal muscle regeneration by low energy laser irradiation. Laser Therapy. 1996; 8 (1): 19. (abstract)

[432] Mrowiec J et al. Analgesic effect of low-power infrared laser radiation in rats. Proc SPIE. 1997; Vol 3198: 83-89.

[433] Neuman I, Finklestein Y, Lubart R. Low energy phototherapy in allergic rhinitis and nasal polyposis. Laser Therapy. 1996. 1: 37 (abstract)

[434] Götte S et al. Doppelblindstudie zur überprüfung der Wirksamkeit und Verträglichkeit einer niederenergetischen Lasertherapie bei Patienten mit aktiver Gonarthrose. Jaros Orthopädie. 1995. 1: 30-34

level laser treatment on maxillary arch dimensions after palatal surgery on beagle dogs. J Dent Res. 1991; 70 (11): 1467-1470.

[392] Fitz-Ritson D. Low energy laser therapy efficacy in the extension neck muscle recovery after whiplash injury. Laser Surg Med. 1993; 13: 9. (abstract)

[393] Friedman S, Liu M, Dörscher-Kim J, Kim S. In situ testing of CC2 laser on dental pulp function: Effects on microcirculation. Laser Surg Med. 1991; 11: 325-330.

[394] Assia E, Rosner M, Belkin M, Solomon A, Schwartz M. Temporal parameters of low energy laser irradiation for optimal delay of post-traumatic degeneration of rat optic nerve. Brain Research. 1989; 476: 205-212.

[395] Berki T, Németh, Hegedüs J. Effect of low-power continous-wave HeNe laser irradiation on in vitro cultured lymphatic cell lines and macrophages. Stud Biophys. 1985; 105: 141-.

[396] Kaneps A, Hultgren B, Riebold T, Shires G. Laser therapy in the horse: Histopathologic response. Am J Vet Res. 1984; 45 (3): 581-.

[397] Obata J et al. Clinical effects of total laser irradiation for the control of disease activity of chronic rheumatoid arthritis. Surgical and Medical Lasers. 1990; 3 (3): 140. (abstract)

[398] Sato K, Kaseno S, Takigawa C et al. A double blind assessment of low power laser therapy in the treatment of postherpetic neuralgia. Surgical and Medical Lasers. 1990; 3 (3): 134. (abstract)

[399] Filho W, Nogueira T et al. Effects of irradiation with a HeNe laser on the healing of the hard tissue. Surgical and Medical Lasers. 1989; 2-3 (2): 71-.

[400] Calderhead G. Watt's A Joule?: On the Importance of Accurate and Correct Reporting of Laser Parameters in Low Reactive-Laser Therapy and Photobioactivation Research: Laser Therapy 1991; 3 (4): 177-182.

[401] Cheetham M J, Young R S, Dyson M. Histological effects of 820 nm laser irradiation on the healthy growth plate of the rat. Laser Therapy 1992; 4 (2): 59-64.

[402] Ito A et al. Studies of Nd:YAG low power laser irradiation on stellate ganglion. In: Lasers in dentistry. Ed. H Yamamoto. 1989; p. 271. Elsevier Science Publishers B.V.

[403] Kato M et al. Clinical studies of low power density HeNe laser irradiation on stellate ganglion. Jpn J Oral Maxillofac Surg. 1987; 33 (12): 1-11.

[404] Moore K. Laser therapy in post herpetic neuralgia. Laser Therapy. 1996; 8 (1): 48. (abstract)

[405] Inoue K et al. Suppressed tuberculine reaction in guinea pigs following laser irradiation. Laser Surg Med. 1989; 9: 271-275.

[406] Yamamoto H et al. Pain clinic. 1987; 8: 43-48. (In Japanese)

[407] Waylonis G W, Wilke S, O'Toole D et al. Chronic myofascial pain: management by low-output helium-neon laser therapy. Arch Phys Med Rehab. 1988; 69 (12): 1017-1020.

[408] Yaakov N, Bdolah A, Wollberg Z et al. Recovery from sarafotoxin-b induced cardiopathological effects in mice following low energy laser irradiation. Basic Research Cardiology. 2000; 95: 385-389.

[409] Escola R et al. Beitrag zur ultrastrukturellen Untersuchung von Zahnfleischbeweben mit dem Soft-Laser. Zahnarztpraxis. 83: 110-115.

[410] Kazmina S et al. Laser prophylaxis and treatment of primary caries. Proc. SPIE.Vol 984; 1994: 231-233.

[411] Chen M et al. [Application of a pain alleviating effect of low power laser irradiation to patients in orthodontic treatment]. J Jpn Soc Laser Med. 1933; 14: 5-11 (in Japanese).

[412] Yoshida T et al. Pain reduction effect of soft laser in orthodontic therapy. Proc. Annual Meeting Jpn Orthodont Soc. 1992: 69-.

[371]   Soldo I et al. Effects of GaAs laser combined with radiotherapy on murine sarcoma depends on tumor size. Laser Surg Med. 1989; Suppl 1: 40.

[372]   Dima F V, Vasiliu V, Ionescu M D, Dima S V. Studies on some biological functions of macrophages activated by HeNe laser photodynamic treatment as compared to coryne-bacterium parvum and interferon activation. Laser Therapy. 1993; 5 (3): 117-124.

[373]   Takaduma K. Possible application of the laser in immunobiology. Keio J Med. 1993; 42 (4): 180-182.

[374]   Lubart R, Rochkind S, Sharon U, Nissan M. A light source for phototherapy. Laser Therapy. 1991; 3 (1): 15-18.

[375]   Friedman H, Lubart R. Nonlinear photobiostimulation: the mechanisms of visible and infrared laser-induced stimulation and reduction of neural excitability and growth. Laser Therapy. 1993; 5 (1): 39-42.

[376]   Friedman H, Lubart R. Towards an explanation of visible and infrared laser induced stimulation and damage of cell cultures. Laser Therapy. 1992; 4 (1): 39-42.

[377]   Friedman H et al. A possible explanation of laser-induced stimulation and damage of cell cultures. J Photochem Photobiol B Biol. 1991; 11: 87-95.

[378]   Passarella S et al. Increase in the ADP/ATP exchange in rat liver mitochondria irradiated in vitro by helium-neon laser. Biochem Biophys Res Commun. 1988; 156 (2): 978-986.

[379]   Lukashevich I G. [HeNe laser in facial pain]. Stomatologiia. 1985; 64: 29-31.

[380]   Roumeliotis D, Emmanouilidis O, Diamantopoulos C. C.W. 820nm 15mW 4J/cm^2, laser diode application in sports injunes. A double blind study. Proc. Fifth Annual Congress, 28-30 January 1987. British Medical Laser Association.

[381]   Malta J et al. The influences of Low Level Laser Therapy on Wound Healing after Palatinal Surgery in Beagle Dogs. EOS. 1990; 122: 82.

[382]   Manteifel V, Andreichuk T, Karu T I, Chelidze p, Zelenin A. Activation of transcription in lymphocytes after exposure to a HeNe laser. Mol.Biol. 1990; 24: 860-867.

[383]   Manteifel V, Andreichuk T, Karu T I. Reaction of the mitocondrial apparatus of the lymphocytes to irradiation by a HeNe laser and to the mitogen phytohema-glutinin. Mol.Biol. 1991; 25: 229-235.

[384]   Lowe A, Baxter D, Walsh D, Allen J. Effect of low intensity laser (830 nm) irradiation on skin temperature and antidromic conduction latencies in the human median nerve: Relevance of radiant exposure. Laser Surg Med. 1994; 14: 40-46.

[385]   Lowe A S, Baxter G D, Walsh D M et al. Low-intensity laser irradiation of the human median nerve: effect of energy density upon conduction and skin temperature. Abstracts 'London Laser 1992', Second Meeting of the International Laser Therapy Association, p. 56.

[386]   Abergel P, Lyons R, Castel J, Dwyer R, Uitto J. Biostimulation of wound healing by laser: Experimental approaches in animal models and in fibroblast cultures. J.Dermatol. Surg. Oncol. 1987; 13: 127-133.

[387]   Anders J J, Borke R, Woolery S, Van De Merwe W. Low power laser irradiation alters the rate of regeneration of the rat facial nerve. Laser Surg Med. 1993; 13: 72-82.

[388]   Bolton P A, Young S R, Dyson M. Macrophage responsiveness to light therapy. A dose response study. Laser Therapy. 1990; 2 (3): 101-106.

[389]   Bolton P A, Dyson M, Young S R. The effect of polarised light on the release of growth factors from the U-937 macrophage-like cell line. Laser Therapy. 1992; 4 (1): 33-42.

[390]   Bosatra M, Lucci A, Olliaro P, Quacci D, Sacchi S. In vitro fibroblast activation by laser irradiation at low energy. Dermatologica. 1984; 168: 157-162.

[391]   in de Braekt M M H et al. Effect of low level laser therapy of wound healing after palatal surgery in beagle dogs. Laser Surg Med. 1991; 11 (5): 462-470. Also: The effect of low-

[349] Obata J et al. The pain relief of low energy laser irradiation on rheumatoid arthritis. Pain Clin. 1987; 8: 18-.

[350] Schindl L et al. Influence of low-power laser irradiation on "arthus phenomenon" induced in rabbit cornea. Laser Therapy. 1994; 6 (1): 23. (abstract)

[351] Palmgren N et al. Low Level Laser Therapy of infected abdominal wounds after surgery. Laser Surg Med. 1991; Suppl 3:11.

[352] Lievens P. Infrared lasertherapy and bedsores. Laser Surg Med. 1992; Suppl 4: 11.

[353] van Breugel H et al. Low energy HeNe laser irradiation effects proliferation and laminin production of rat Schwann cells in vitro. Laser Surg Med. 1991; Suppl 3:10.

[354] Mulligan S et al. The effect of low energy HeNe laser irradiation on the neurite elongation in vitro. Laser Surg Med. 1991; Suppl 3: 10.

[355] Ben-Dov N, Shefer G, Irintchev A et al. Low energy laser irradiation affects cell proliferation and differentiation in vitro. Biochemica and Biophysica Acta. 1999; 1448: 372-380.

[356] Rezvani M et al. Prevention of x-radiation induced dermal necrosis in pig skin by monochromatic light. Laser Surg Med. 1991; suppl 3: 11.

[357] Palma J et al. Blockade of inflammatory signals by laser radiation. Laser Surg Med. 1991; Suppl 3: 11.

[358] Tardivo J P et al. Effect of low power laser over cells infected by herpes simplex virus (HSV). Laser Surg Med. 1989; Suppl 1: 31.

[359] Kamikawa K. Studies on low power laser therapy of pain. Lasers in Dentistry. 1989; p. 29-38. Elsevier Science Publisher B.V. Amsterdam

[360] Vélez-Gonsalez M et al. Treatment of relapse in Herpes Simplex on labial & facial areas and of primary herpes simplex on genital areas and "area pudenda" with low power laser (HeNe) or Acyclovir administred orally. Proc SPIE. 1995; Vol 2630: 43-50.

[361] Khullar S M, Brodin P, Barkvoll P et al. Preliminary study of low-level laser for treatment of long-standing sensory aberrations in the inferior alveolar nerve. J Oral Maxillofac Surg. 1996; 54 (2): 2-7.

[362] Snyder-Mackler L, Bork C, Bourbon B et al. Effect of Helium-Neon Laser on Musculoskeletal Trigger Points. Physical Therapy. 1986; 66 (7): 1087-1090.

[363] Kalivradzhiyan E et al. Usage of low-intensity laser radiation for the treatment of the inflammatory processes of the oral cavity mucosa after applying removable plate dentures. Proc SPIE. 1995; Vol 1984: 225-230.

[364] Sokolova I et al. Low-intensity laser radiation in complex treatment of inflammatory diseases of parodontium. Proc SPIE. 1995; Vol 1984: 234-237.

[365] Mamedova F M et al. Microbiological estimate of parodontitis laser therapy efficiency. Proc SPIE. 1995; Vol 1984: 247-249.

[366] Podolskaya E et al. Radiation damage of lips and its treatment by low-intensity laser irradiation. Proc SPIE. 1995; Vol 1984: 245-246.

[367] Kolomiyets L A et al. Mechanism of treatment effect of low-energy laser irradiation. Proc SPIE. 1996; Vol 2728: 63-67.

[368] Kozlov V et al. Lasers in diagnostics and treatment of microcirculation disorders under parodontitis. Proc SPIE. 1995; Vol 1984: 253-264.

[369] Ozawa Y et al. Stimulatory effects of low-power laser irradiation on bone formation in vitro. Proc SPIE. 1995; Vol 1984: 281-288.

[370] Shimizu N et al. Prospect of relieving pain due to tooth movement during orthodontic treatment utilizing a GaAlAs diode laser. Proc. SPIE.. 1995; Vol 1984: 275-280.

[327] Mester A. Biostimulative effect in wound healing by continous wave 820 nm laser diode double-blind randomized cross-over study. Lasers in Med Science, abstract issue July 1988.

[328] Henderson A R. Laser radiation hazards. Optics and Laser Technology, 1984; 2: 75-

[329] Moore K, Hira N, Broome I J, Cruikshank J A. The effect of infra-red diode laser irradiation on the duration and severity of postoperative pain. A double-blind trial. Laser Therapy. 1992; 4 (4): 145-150.

[330] Palmieri B. A double blind stratified cross over study of amateur tennis players suffering from tennis elbow using infrared laser therapy. Medical Laser Report. 1984; 1: 3-4.

[331] Soriano F. The analgesic effect of 904 nm gallium arsenide semiconductor low level laser therapy (laser therapy) on osteoarticular pain: a report on 938 irradiated patients. Laser Therapy. 1995; 7 (2): 75-80.

[332] Pöntinen P et al. Comparative effects of exposure to different light sources (He-Ne laser, InGaAl diode laser, a specific type of noncoherent LED) on skin blood flow for the head. Acupunct Electrother Res. 1996; 21 (2): 105-118.

[333] Scudds R A et al. A double-blind crossover study of the effectiveness of low-power gallium arsenide laser on the symptoms of fibrositis. Physiotherapy Canada. 1989; 41: (suppl 3) 2.

[334] Molina Soto J J, Moller I. La laserterapia como coadyuvante en el tratamiento de la A.R. (Artritis Reumatoidea). Bol. C.D.L. 1987; 14: 4-8.

[335] Taghawinejag M, Fricke R. Laser Therapie in der Behandlung kleiner Gelenke bei chronischer Polyarthritis. Z Phys Med Baln Med Klin. 1985; 14: 402-408.

[336] Tsurko V V, Muldiyarov P Y, Sigidin Y A. [Laser therapy of rheumatoid arthritis. A clinical and morphological study]. Terap Arkh. 1983; 55: 97-102. (in Russian)

[337] Walker J. Temporary suppression of clonus in humans by brief photo-stimulation. Brain Research. 1985; 340: 109-113.

[338] Mazo V. Transrectal laser therapy in prostatic problems' management.Proc. X Internat Congr Soc Laser Surgery and Medicine, Bangkok. 1993, p. 153.

[339] Garkavoy D V et al. Use of the Helium-Neon laser in the treatment of ulcer disease. Proc X. Internat Congr Soc Laser Surgery and Medicine, Bangkok 1993; p. 160.

[340] Vasilotta A. I.R. laser: a new therapy in rhino-sino-nasal bronchial syndrome with asthmatic component. Proc X. Internat Congr Soc Laser Surg Med, Bangkok 1993, p. 161.

[341] Kovács L. The stimulatory effect of laser on the physiological healing process of portio surface. Lasers in Surgery & Medicine 1981; 1 (3): 241-52

[342] Frugoni P. Shoulder calcified periarthritis recovery with low power laser therapy. Proc X Internat Congr Soc Laser Surg Med, Bangkok 1993, p. 200.

[343] Hall J et al. Low level laser therapy is ineffective in the management of rheumatoid arthritic finger joints. British J Rheumat. 1994; 33: 142-147.

[344] Kipshidze N N et al. Treatment of acute myocardial infarction with a low-intensity Helium-Neon laser. Proc X Internat Congr Soc Laser Surg Med, Bangkok 1993, p. 309.

[345] Castronuovo G et al. The skin role during a low level laser therapy. Laser Bologna '92, p. 19. Monduzzi Editore S.p.A., Bologna, Italy.

[346] Kamikawa K et al. Essential mechanisms of low power laser effects. Laser Bologna '92, p. 11. Monduzzi Editore S.p.A., Bologna, Italy.

[347] Herbert K E et al. Effect of laser light at 820 nm on adeonsine nucleotide levels in human lymphocytes. Lasers Life Sci. 1989; 3: 37.

[348] Verbruggen L A et al. Low-power laser therapy in chronic rheumatic diseases: Western and Soviet experiences. Phys Med Rehab. 1991; 1: 101-.

[306]   Olivier J, Plath P. Combined low power laser therapy and extracts of Gingo Biloba in a blind trial of treatment for tinnitus. Laser Therapy. 1993; 5 (3): 137-140.

[307]   Galletti G. Low-Energy Density CO2 Laser as Deep Tissue Stimulator: A Comparative Study. J Clin. Laser Medicine & Surg. 1991; 9 (3): 179-184.

[308]   Martin D et al. Effect of laser pulse repetition rate upon peripheral blood flow in human volunteers. Laser Surg Med. 1991; Suppl 3: 83.

[309]   Ponnudurai R N et al. Hypoalgesic effect of laser photobiostimulation shown by rat tail flick test. Intern J Acup and Electrother Res. 1987; 12: 93-100.

[310]   Ivanov A S et al. [Effect of Helium-Neon laser radiation on the course of temporomandibular joint arthritis and arthrosis]. Stomatologiia (Mosk). 1985; 64: 81-82.

[311]   Jensen H et al. Is infra-red laser effective in painful arthrosis of the knee? (In Danish) Ugeskr Laeger 1987; 149: 3104-3106.

[312]   Fursinn G et al. Effects of Nd:YAG laser irradiation on human cartilage cell metabolism. Proc of Laser-81, Opto-Elektronik. München 1981. Abstr 200.

[313]   Airaksinen O et al. Effects of infra-red laser irradiation at the trigger points. Scand J of Acup & Electrotherapy. 1988; 3: 56-61.

[314]   Atsumi K et al. Biostimulation effect of low-power energy diode laser for pain relief. Laser Surg Med. 1987; 7: 77-.

[315]   Ceccherelli F et al. Diode laser in cervical myofascial pain: A double blind study versus placebo. The Clinical J Pain. 1989; 5: 301-304.

[316]   Emmanoulidis O et al. CW IR low-power laser application significantly accelerates chronic pain relief rehabilitation of professional athletes. A double blind study. Laser Surg Med. 1986; 6: 173.

[317]   Kovács I, Mester E, Görög P. Stimulation of wound healing with laser beam in the rat. Experientia. 1974; 30 (11): 1275-1276.

[318]   Hopkins G O et al. Double blind cross over study of laser versus placebo in the treatment of tennis elbow. Proc Internat Congr in Laser, "Laser Bologna". 1985; p 210. Monduzzi Editore S.p.A., Bologna.

[319]   Kamikawa K, Kyoto J. Double blind experiences with mid-Lasers in Japan. 1985. Int Congr on Lasers in Med and Surg, Bologna June 1985, 165-169. Moduzzi Editore S.p.A., Bologna

[320]   Ohshiro T. To publish, or not to publish. Editorial. Laser Therapy. 1989; 1 (2): 61-62.

[321]   Basford J R et al. Low-energy Helium Neon laser treatment of thumb osteoarthritis. Arch Phys Med Rehab. 1987; 68: 794-797.

[322]   McAuley R et al. Soft laser: A treatment for osteoarthritis of the knee. Arch Phys Med Rehab. 1985; 66: 553-554. (abstract)

[323]   Kemmotsu M D at al. Laser therapy for pain attenuation - the current experience in the pain clinic. In: Progress in Laser Therapy. 1991: 197-200. John Wiley & Sons, Chichester, Engl. ISBN 0-471-93154-3.

[324]   Kreczi T, Klinger D A. A comparison of laser acupuncture versus placebo in radicular and pseudoradicular pain syndromes as recorded by subjective responses of patients. Acupunct Electrotherap Res. 1986; 11: 207-216.

[325]   Lonauer G. Controlled double blind study on the efficacy of HeNe-laser beams versus HeNe- plus Infrared-laser beams in the therapy of activated osteoarthritis of finger joints. Clin Experim Rheuma. 1987; 5 (suppl 2): 39. Also in Laser Surg Med. 1986; 7: 172.

[326]   Mach E S, Tursrko V V, Lebedeva O et al. Helium-Neon (Red Light) Therapy of Arthritis. Rhevmatologia, 1983; 3: 36-.

[284]	Ohshiro T. Treatment techniques to achieve superficial and intermediate laser therapy irradiation. Laser Therapy. 1989; 3 (1): 153-155.

[285]	Hernández L C, Santisteban P, del Valle-Soto M E et al. Changes in mRNA of thyryglobulin, cytoskeleton of thyroid cells and thyroid hormone levels induced by IR-laser radiation. Laser Therapy. 1989; 1 (4): 203-208.

[286]	Humzah M D, Diamantopoulos C, Dyson M. Multi-wavelength low reactive-level laser therapy (laser therapy) as an adjunct in malignant ulcers; case reports. Laser Therapy. 1993; 5 (4): 149-152.

[287]	Yasuda, Kubota J, Ohshiro T. The effects of diode laser low reactive-level laser therapy (laser therapy) on musculocutaneous flaps. Laser Therapy. 1993; 5 (4): 159-163.

[288]	Yoo C, Lee W K, Kemmotsu O. Efficacy of polarized light therapy for musculoskeletal pain. Laser Therapy. 1993; 5 (4): 153-157.

[289]	Bliddal H et al. Soft laser therapy of rheumatoid arthritis. Scand J Rheuma. 1987; 16: 225-228.

[290]	Siebert W et al. What is the efficacy of "soft" and "mid" lasers in therapy of tendinopathies? Arch Ortop and Traum Surg. 1987; 106: 358-363.

[291]	Bolton P, Young S, Dyson M. Macrophage responsiveness to light therapy with varying power and energy densities. Laser Therapy. 1991; 3 (3): 105-112.

[292]	Baxter G D. Therapeutic Lasers. 1994; p 148. Churchill Livingstone. ISBN 0-443-04393-0

[293]	Tasaki et al. Application of low power laser therapy in closed lock temporomandibular joint dysfunction. Laser Surg Med. 1992; Suppl 4: 84.

[294]	Chernoff W G et al. Cutaneous Laser Surfacing. Operative Techniques in Otolaryngology - Head & Neck Surgery. 1994; 5: 281-284.

[295]	Chernoff W G. Cutaneous Laser Resurfacing. Clinical Laser Monthly. December 1994.

[296]	Bellina J H. Laser in gynecology. Excerpts from Leventhal, J.M. et al (eds.): Current Problems in Obstetrics and Gynecology. Year Book Medical Publishers, Inc., Chicago. 1981.

[297]	Armino L, Forvc he effect of I.R laser irradiation on the vasomotricity of the lymphatic system. Lasers in Medical Science. 1991; 6: 189-191.

[299]	Lievens P C. The effect of a combined HeNe and I.R. laser treatment on the regeneration of the lymphatic system during the process of wound healing. Lasers in Medical Science. 1991; 6: 193-199.

[300]	Labajos M et al. Effect of the irradiation of GaAs diode laser on intestinal absorption: in vitro and in vivo studies. Lasers in Medical Science. 1986; 1: 21-25.

[301]	Miro L et al. Estudio capilaroscópico de la acción de un laser AsGa sobre la microcirculación. Investig Clínica Láser. 1984; 1/2: 9-14.

[302]	Airaksinen O et al. Effects of HeNe-laser irradiation on the trigger points of patients with chronic muscle tension in the neck. Scand J of Acup & Electrotherapy. 1989; 4: 63-65.

[303]	Zhong X et al. Correlation between endogenous opiate-like peptides and serotonin in laseracupuncture analgesia. Am J Acupunct. 1989; 17: 39-43.

[304]	Calderhead R G. Simultaneous low reactive-level laser therapy in laser surgery: the "alpha-phenomenon" explained. In: Progesss in Laser Therapy. 1991. John Wiley & Sons. P. 209-213.

[305]	Fine S, Klein E, Nowak W, Scott R E, Laor Y et al.. Interaction of laser irradiation with biological systems. I. Studies on interaction with tissues. Fed Proc 1965; 24, Supplement 14: 40.

[263] Mayayo E, Trelles M A, Calderhead R, Santafe M, Tomas J, Rigau J. Short term ultrastructural changes in soft tissue (Endomysium) after laser therapy Helium-Neon laser treatment. Laser Therapy. 1989; 1 (3): 119-126.

[264] Dyson M. Cellular and subcellular aspects of low level laser therapy. Progress in Laser Therapy. Eds. T. Ohshiro and R.G. Calderhead, John Wiley & Sons, Eng and. 1991, p. 221.

[265] Kubasova T, Kovács L, Somosy Z, Unk P, Kókai A. Biological effect of HeNe laser: Investigations on functional and micromorphological alterations of cell membranes, in vitro. Laser Surg Med. 1984; 4 (4): 381-388.

[266] Martin J L, Migus A, Poyart C, Lecarpentier Y, Antonetti A. Ultra-fast events in biological systems. Laboratoire d'Optique Appliquee INSERM U275. Ecole Polytechnique-ENSTA, Palaiseau, France. p. 218.

[267] Karu T I. Photobiology of low-power laser effects. Health Physics. 1989; 56 (5): 691-704.

[268] Boulton M et al. HeNe-Laser Stimulation of Human Fibroblasts and Attachment in vitro. Lasers in Life Sciences. 1986; 1 (2): 125-.

[269] Vulliez C et al. Éffet du Laser Infra Rouge a Diode sur le Tissue Conjuctif. Innov. Tech Biol. Med. 1990; 11 (1): 143-.

[270] Trelles M A, Mayayo E, Miro L, Rigau J, Baudin G, Calderhead G. The action of low reactive level laser therapy (laser therapy) on mast cells. Laser Therapy. 1989; 1: 27-30.

[271] el Sayed S et al. The Effect of Low Level Laser Irradiation on Mast Cell Degranulation. Proc 7th Ann Meeting of Am Soc Laser Med Surg 1987.

[272] Fenyö M et al. Theoretical and experimental basis of biostimulation by laser irradiation. Optics and Laser Technology. 1984: No 4: 209-.

[273] Ohta A, Abergel P, Uitto J. Laser modulation of human immune system: Inhibition of lymphocyte proliferation by a gallium-arsenide laser at low energy. Laser Surg Med. 1987; 7 (2): 199-201.

[274] Zheng H, Qin J, Xin H, Xin S. The activation action of low level Helium Neon laser radiation on macrophages in the mouse model. Laser Therapy. 1992; 4 (2): 55-58.

[275] Karu T I. Low Intensity Laser Light Action Upon Fibroblast and Lymphocytes. Progress in Laser Therapy, Eds. T. Ohshiro and R.G. Calderhead, John Wiley & Sons, England. 1991 p. 175.

[276] Weiss N, Oron U. Enhancement of muscle regeneration in the rat gastrocnemius muscle by low energy laser irradiation. Anat Embryol. 1992; 186: 497-503.

[277] Bibikova A, Oron U. Attenuation of the process of muscle regeneration in the toad gastrocnemius muscle by low energy laser irradiation. Laser Surg Med. 1994; 14: 355-361.

[278] Hall G, Anneroth G, Schennings T et al. Effect of low level energy laser irradiation on wound healing. An experimental study in rats. Swed Dent J. 1994; 18: 29-34.

[279] Kats A G et al. [Remote results of the complex treatment of chronic sialadenitis with the use of helium-neon lasers.] Vestnik Khirurgii Imeni i-i- Grekova. 1985; 135: 39-42.

[280] Morselli M et al. Effects of very low energy-density treatment of joint pain by CO_2 laser. Laser Surg Med. 1985; 5 (5): 150-153.

[281] Baxter G D et al. Low level laser therapy: Current clinical practice in Northern Ireland. Physiotherapy 1991; 3: 171-178.

[282] Iijima K, Shimoyama N, Shimoyama M et al. Effect of repeated irradiation of low-power Ne-He laser in pain relief from postherpectic neuralgia. Clin J Pain. 1989; 5 (3): 271-274.

[283] Kim K-S, Kim S-K, Lee P-Y et al. Effects of low incident energy levels of infrared laser irradiation on the proliferation of candida albicans. Part 1: A long term study on the pulse types. Laser Therapy. 1994; 6 (3): 161-166.

[243] Juri H et al. Effects of Nd:YAG laser radiation on PGE2 level in experimental arthtitis. Proc X Internat Congr Soc Laser Surg Med, Bangkok 1993, p. 314.

[244] Lopez V J. El láser en el tratiamento de las disfunciones de ATM. Revista de Actualidad de Odontoestomatologica Española. 1986; (Jun): 35-.

[245] Calderhead R G, Inomata K. A study of the possible haemorrhagic effects of extended infrared diode laser irradiation on encapsulated and exposed synovial membrane articular tissue in the rat. Laser Therapy. 1992; 4 (2): 65-74.

[246] Vizi E, Mester E, Tisza S, Mester A. Acetylcholine releasing effect of laser irradiation on Auerbach's plexus in guinea-pig ileum. J. Neural Transmission. 1977; 40: 305-308.

[247] Mizokami T, Aoki K, Iwabuchi S et al. Laser therapy (Low Reactive Level Laser Therapy) - a clinical study: relationship between pain attenuation and the serotonergic mechanism. Laser Therapy. 1993; 5 (4): 165-168.

[248] Ataka I et al. Studies of Nd:YAG Low Power Laser Irradiation on Stellate Ganglion. Lasers in Dentistry. 1989; page 271. Elsevier Science Publisher B.V. Amsterdam.

[249] Meyers A, Joyce J, Cohen J. Effects of low-watt Helium Neon laser radiation on human lymphocyte cultures. Laser Surg Med. 1987; 6 (6): 540-542.

[250] Lievens P. The Influence of Laser Irradiation on the Motricity of Lymphatical System and on the Wound Healing Process. Proc Int Congr on Laser in Med and Surg. Bologna, June 26-28, 1985; p. 171.

[251] Karu T I, Tiphlova O. Stimulation of E. Coli growth by laser and incoherent red light. Nuovo Cimento. 1983; 2 (4): 1138-.

[252] Lubart R, Friedmann H, Peled I, Grossman N. Light effect on fibroblast proliferation. Laser Therapy. 1993; 5 (2): 55-58.

[253] Laakso E L, Cramond T, Richardson C, Galligan J P. Plasma ACTH and ß-endorphin levels in response to low level laser therapy for myofascial trigger points. Laser Therapy. 1994; (6) 3: 133-142.

[254] Mester E, Mester A F, Mester A. The biomedical effects of laser application. Laser Surg Med. 1985; 5 (1): 31-39.

[255] Toya S, Motegi M, Inomata K, Ohshiro T. Report on a computer-randomized double blind clinical trial to determine the effectiveness of the GaAlAs (830 nm) diode laser for pain attenuation in selected pain. Laser Therapy 1994; 6 (3): 143-148.

[256] Klima H. Effect of Weak Laser Light and Oxygen Activation in Open Biological Systems. LASER - Journ Eur Med Laser Ass. 1988; 1 (No 2): 16-.

[257] Gaudel Y et al. Pico second study of free radical reactions in organized assemblies: Kinetics of univalent reduction of b-NAD+. Laboratoire d'Optique Appliquee INSERM U275. École Polytechnique-ENSTA, Palaiseau. p 219-.

[258] Chen Ji-wei, Zhou Yo-cheng. Effect of low level carbon dioxide laser radiation on biochemical metabolism of rabbit mandibular bone callus. Laser Therapy. 1989; 1 (2): 83-88.

[259] Parshad R, Sanford K. Proliferative response of human diploid fibroblasts to intermittent light exposure. J Cell Physiol. 1977; 92: 481-.

[260] Iijima K, Shimoyama N, Shimoyama M, Mizuguchi T. Red and green low-powered HeNe lasers protect human erythrocytes from hypotonic hemolysis. J Clin Laser Med Surg. 1991; 9 (5): 385-389.

[261] Labbe R, Skogerboe K, Davis H, Rettmer R. Laser photobioactivation mechanisms: In vitro studies using ascorbic acid uptake and hydroxyproline formation as bio-chemical markers of irradiation response. Laser Surg Med. 1990; 10 (2): 201-207.

[262] Trelles M A, Mayayo E. Mast cells are implicated in low power laser effect on tissue. A preliminary study. Lasers in Medical Science. 1992; 7: 73-.

[223]   Donko Z. Possible ab-initio explanation of laser "biostimulation' effects. Laser Applications in Medicine and Surgery. G. Galletti et al, Eds.: Proc 3rd World Congr - Int Soc Low Power Laser Appl in Medicine.: 1992: 57. Monduzzi Editore S.p.A., Bologna.

[224]   Spanner D C. The active transport of water under temperature gradient. Symp. Soc. Exp. Biol. 1954; 8: 76-.

[225]   Hort O, Vanpel T. Die verteilung von Na+ und K+ unter dem Einfluss von Temperaturgradienten. Pflügers Arch. 1971; 323: 158-.

[226]   Lögdberg-Andersson M, Mützell S, Hazel Å. Low Level Laser Treatment of Tendonitis and Myofascial Pains - a Randomized, Double-Blind Study. Laser Therapy. 1997; 9 (3): 79-86.

[227]   Plog F. Biophysical application of the laser beam. 1980. In Koebner H K: Lasers in Medicine. John Wiley, New York.

[228]   van Breugel HH, Bär PR. Power Density and Exposure Time of HeNe Laser Irradiation Are More Important Than Total Energy Dose in Photo-Biomodulation of Human Fibroblasts in Vitro. Laser Surg Med. 1992; 12 (5): 528-537.

[229]   Nivbrant B, Friberg S. Therapeutic Laser Treatment in Gonarthroses. Acta Orthop Scand. 1989; 60 (suppl 231): 33.

[230]   Lundeberg T, Haker E, Thomas M. Effect of laser versus placebo in tennis elbow. Scand J of Rehab Med. 1987; 19: 135-138.

[231]   Haker E, Lundeberg T. Laser treatment applied to acupuncture points in lateral humeral epicondylalgia. A double-blind study. Pain. 1990; 43: 243-247.

[232]   Sasaki K, Calderhead R G, Chin I, Inomata K. To examine the adverse photothermal effects of extended dosage laser therapy in vivo on the skin and subcutaneous tissue in the rat model. Laser Therapy. 1992; 4 (2): 69-74.

[233]   Greguss P. Biostimulation of tissue by laser radiation. Lasers and Medicine. 1989; 1353: 79-.

[234]   Greguss P. Interaction of optical radiation with living matter. Optics and Laser Technology. 1985; 3: 151-.

[235]   Greguss P. Letter to the editor. Biological effects of low power laser radiation. Optics and Laser Technology. 1985; 3: 161.

[236]   Rossman J A. Current research using the CO2 laser in guided tissue regeneration: animal studies. Proc Second Annual Advanced Application Seminar. Luxar Corp, USA., 1993.

[237]   Israel M. Current research using the CO2 laser in guided tissue regeneration. Clinical studies. Proc Second Annual Advanced Application Seminar. Luxar Corp, USA. 1993.

[238]   Takashi K. Clinical evaluation of a GaAlAs semiconductor unilaser irradiation on solitary aphta erosion and hypersensitive dentine. Shikwa Gauko. 1987; 87 (2): 295-.

[239]   Landthaler M et al. Behandlung von Zoster, postzosterischen Schmerzen und Herpes simplex recidivans in loco mit Laser-Licht. Fortschr. Med. 1983; 101 (22): 1039-1041.

[240]   Beck-Friis J, Borg G, Wetterberg L. Rebound increase of nocturnal melatonin levels following evening suppression by bright light exposure in healthy men: relationship to cortisol levels and morning exposure. In: The Medical and Biological Effects of Light. Wurtman RJ, ed. Ann. NY Acad Sci. 1985; 453: 371-375.

[241]   Sasaki K, Ohshiro T. Role of Low Reactive-Level Laser Therapy (laser therapy) in the Treatment of Aquired and Cicatricial Vitiligo. Laser Therapy. 1989; 1 (3): 141-146.

[242]   Gudmundsen J, Vikne J. Laserbehandling av epicondylitis humeri og rotatorcuffsyndrom. Dobbelt blindstudie - 200 pasienter. Telemark Sentralsjukehus, Norge. ["Laser Treatment of Epicondylitis Humeri and Rotator Cuff Syndrome. A Double-Blind Study - 200 Patients."] (In Norwegian.) Norsk Tidskrift for Idrettsmedisin 1987; 2: 6-11.

[204] Kana J, Hutschenreiter G, Haina D, Waidelich W. Effect of low-power density laser radiation on healing of open skin wounds in rats. Arch Surg. 1981; 116: 293-296.

[205] Shiroto C, Sugawara K, Kumae T et al. Effects of diode laser radiation in vitro on activity of human neutrofils. Laser Therapy. 1989; 1 (3): 135-140.

[206] Bezuur N J, Hansson T L. The effect of therapeutic laser treatment in patient with cranomandibular disorders. J Cranomandib Disorders. 1988; 2: 83-86.

[207] Midamba E D, Haanaes H R. Low reactive-level 830 nm GaAlAs diode laser therapy (laser therapy) successfully accelerates regeneration of peripheral nerves in human. Laser Therapy, 1993; 5 (3): 125-130.

[208] Haker E, Lundeberg T. Is Low-Energy Laser Treatment Effective in Lateral Epicondylalgia? J Pain Symptom Managment. 1991; 6 (4): 241-246.

[209] Ruffolo P et al. Impiego della Laser-terapia nelle leucoplachie del cavo orale. Int Congress on Laser Med and Surg, Bologna June 1985, p. 279. Monduzzi Editore S.p.A., Bologna, Italy.

[210] Obata J, Yanse M. Evaluation of the effects of low power laser therapy on rheumatoid arthritis joints by roentgenographic survey. Laser Bologna '92, p. 41. Monduzzi Editore S.p.A., Bologna, Italy.

[211] Parascandolo S et al. Azione della Laser-terapia nella nevralgia essenziale del trigemino. Int Congress on Laser in Med and Surg, Bologna June 1985, p 317. Monduzzi Editore S.p.A., Bologna, Italy.

[212] Cassese M et al. Laser-terapia nelle sindromi algico-disfunzionali delle articolazioni temoporo-mandibolari. Int Congress on Laser in Med and Surg, Bologna June 1985, p 337. Monduzzi Editore S.p.A, Bologna, Italy

[213] Kusakari H, Orikasa N, Tani H. Effects of low power laser on wound healing of gingiva and bone. Laser Bologna '92, p. 49-55. Monduzzi Editore S.p.A., Bologna, Italy.

[214] Konchugova T V et al. [The enhancement of immune supression by local laser irradiation in rats exposed to cyclophosphane.] Eksp Klin Farm. 1993; 56 (2): 42-43.

[215] Abe M et al. Role of 830 nm low reactive level laser on the growth of an implanted glioma in mice. Keio J Med 1993; 42 (4): 177-179.

[216] Fernando S et al. A randomised double blind comparative study of low level laser therapy following surgical extraction of lower third molar. Br J Oral Maxillofac Surg 1993; 31 (3): 170-172.

[217] Shiroto C. Clinical results of pain relief with low lever laser therapy. Laser Bologna '92, p. 25. Monduzzi Editore S.p.A., Bologna, Italy.

[218] Kaneko M et al. The application of Nd:YAG laser for low energy laser therapy in the intraoral region. Laser in Dentistry. Proceedings of the Intern Congr of Lasers in Dentistry, Tokyo, August 1988. p 131-136. Excerpta Medica, Elsevier Science Publishers, Amsterdam.

[219] Castro D J, Abergel R P, Johnston K et al. Wound healing: biological effects of Nd:YAG laser on collagen metabolism in pig skin in comparison to thermal burn. Ann Plast Surg. 1983; 11: 131-140.

[220] Castro D J, Abergel R P, Meweker C et al. Effects of the Nd:YAG laser on DNA synthesis and collagen production in human skin fibroblast cultures. Ann Plast Surg. 1983; 1 (3): 214-222.

[221] Boussignac G et al. Thermal effects of semiconductor lasers in men. Proc 6th Congress of The Internat Soc for Laser Surg Med. 1985; 77.

[222] Manne J. Le laser arséniure de gallium 6 watts, étude clinique en odonto-stomatologie. Le Chirurgien Dent de France 1985; 284: 15-.

[185]   Obata J et al. Evaluation of acute pain-relief effects of low power laser therapy on rheumatoid arthritis by thermography. Laser Therapy. 1990; 2 (1): 28. (abstract)

[186]   Murakami F, Kemmotsu O, Kawano Y et al.. Diode low reactive level laser therapy and stellate ganglion block compared in the treatment of facial paralysis. Laser Therapy.1993; 5 (3): 131-135.

[187]   Wu Wen-hsien, Ponnudurai R, Katz J et al. Failure to confirm report of light-evoked response of peripheral nerve to low power helium-neon laser light stimulus. Brain Research. 1987; 407-408.

[188]   Honmura A et al. Analgesic Effect of Ga-Al-As Diode Laser Irradiation on Hyperalgesia in Carrageenin-Induced Inflammation. Laser Surg Med. 1993; 13: 463-469.

[189]   Taguchi T et al. Thermographic Changes Following Laser Irradiation for Pain Relief. J Clin Laser Med Surg. 1991; 9 (2): 143-.

[190]   Wakabayashi H et al. Effect of Irradiation by Semiconductor Laser on Responses Evoked in Trigeminal Caudal Neurons by Tooth Pulp Stimulation. Laser Surg Med. 1993; 13 (6): 605-610.

[191]   Walker J B et al. Laser Therapy for pain of trigeminal neuralgia. Pain. 1987; 29: 585-.

[192]   Yu I. Low Power Laser Therapy for carpal tunnel syndrome.Proc X Internat Congress Int Soc Laser Surg Med, Bangkok 1993, p. 197.

[193]   Walker J B et al. Laser therapy for pain of rheumatoid arthritis. Laser Surg Med. 1986; 6: 171.

[194]   Avila R et al. Histological effects of HeNe laser on chick embryo. Proc X Internat Congress Int Soc Laser Surg Med, Bangkok 1993, p. 164.

[195]   England S, Farrell A J, Coppock J S. Low power laser therapy of shoulder tendonitis. Scand J Rheumatology. 1989; 18 (6): 427-431.

[196]   Dong-Sheng Zhan et al. The effect of postoperative irradiation of Low Level CO_2 laser on the skin flap survival and its mechanism. Laser Therapy, (ILTA Okinawa Congr Abstr Issue). 1990; 2 (1): 36.

[197]   Wasserman I, Rabau M Y, Shoshan S. Collagen metabolism in lowpower CO_2 laser welded intesitinal anastomosis in rats. Proc Ninth Congress of the International Society for Laser Surgery and Medicine, Anaheim, Cal., 2-6 November 1991.

[198]   Korytny D L. [Use of Helium-Neon laser in therapeutic stomatology]. Stomatologiia (Mosk). 1978; 57 (5): 5-21.

[199]   Gärtner C. Analgesy by low power laser (LPL): a controlled double blind study in ankylosing spondarthritis (SPA). Laser Surg Med. 1989; Suppl 1: 30.

[200]   Gáspar L et al. Oral lesions induced by scalpel, electrocautery and CO_2 laser compared with light scanning and electron microscopy. J Clin Laser Med Surg October 199; 9: 349-. Also: [Comparative light microscopic, scanning-electron microscopic and electron microscopic studies of the effect of experimental interventions by surgical scalpel, electrocautery and CO_2-laser beam in the oral cavity]. Fogorv Sz. 1992. 85 (2) :39-44. Review. In Hungarian

[201]   Kayano T. Effect of Er:YAG laser irradiation on human extracted teeth. J Clinical Laser Med Surg 1991; 9 (2): 147-.

[202]   Kawamura M, Watanabe H, Yamamoto H, Ishikawa I. Effect of Nd:YAG and diode laser irradiation on periodontal wound healing. Innov. Techn. Biol. Med. 1990; 11 (1) : 113-127.

[203]   Kim, Dong-Won. The healing effects of low power density laser to the experimental periodontitis; histopathologic study. Thesis for M.S., Dept. of Dentistry, Dankook University, Korea. Advisor: Prof. Chung, Chin-Hyung. 1993.

[164] Kim K et al. Study on the effect of low power laser irradiation in treating gingival inflammation. Clinical, microbiological, histological study. J Korean Acad Oral Med. 1987; 12: 5-16.

[165] Kim K et al. An experimental study on the effects of low power density laser (GaAs) on the wound healing of rat tongue and skin. J Korean Acad Oral Med. 1985; 10: 91-104.

[166] Armino L, Longo L. Effects of laser treatment on vulvar dystrophy. LASER. Journ Eur Med Laser Ass.; 1991: 4 (1-2): 10-14.

[167] Porteder H. Einsatz des Helium-Neon-Lasers zur Förderung der Wundheilung. Z Stomat. 1983; 80: 333-339.

[168] Horch H et al. Erfahrungen mit der Laserbehandlung oberflächlicher Mundschleimhauterkrankungen. Dtsch Z Mund-, Kiefer- u Gesichtschir. 1983; 7: 31-35.

[169] Kopf K et al. Endothelregeneration nach Laserbestrahlung - tierexperimentelle Untersuchungen an Kaninchen. Fortschr Kiefer u Gesichtschir. 1983; 28: 140-142.

[170] Senda A, Gomi A et al. A clinical study of Soft Laser 632, a Helium-Neon low energy medical laser. 1st report. The effect in releiving pain just after irradiation. Aichi-Gakuin J Dent Sci. 1985; 23 (4): 773-780.

[171] Lutsyk L et al. [Use of a helium-neon laser in the combined treatment of oral mucosa diseases in children]. Stomatologiia (Mosk). 1981; 60 (6): 15-16.

[172] Luomanen M. A comparative study of healing of laser and scalpel incision wounds in rat oral mucosa. Scand J Dent Res. 1987; 95 (1): 65-73.

[173] Hatit B Y, Lammens J P. Laser therapy with 10 600 nm defocused CO_2 laser. Laser Therapy. 1992; 4 (4): 175-178.

[174] Longo L, Tamburini A, Monti A et al. Treatment with 904 nm and 10 600 nm laser of acute lumbago - double blind control. LASER. Journ Eur Med Laser Ass. 1988; 1 (3): 16-20.

[175] Bahn J. Biostimulation laser: reality and perspectives. LASER. Journ Eur Med Laser Ass. 1988; 1 (1): 17-22.

[176] Kats A et al. [Use of laser in nonspecific inflammatory processes of the temporomnadibular joint]. Stomatologiia (Mosk). 1983; 62: 42-45. (in Russian)

[177] Kim, Ki-Suk and Kim, Young-Ku. Comparative study of the clinical effects of splint, laser acupuncture and laser therapy for temporomandibular disorders. J Dental College, Seoul Nat Univ. 1988: 1 (12): 195-.

[178] Lee P, Kim Kibeom and Kim Ki-Suk. Effects of low incident energy levels of infrared laser irradiation on healing of infected open skin wounds in rats. Laser Therapy 1993; 5 (2): 59-64.

[179] Lomnitski I, Bibiashevski E V. [Substantiation of the optimal exposure to monochromatic red light for stimulating osteogenesis]. Stomatologiia (Rus). 1982; 2 (61): 14-.

[180] Karu T I, Andreichuck T, Ryabykh T. Supression of human blood chemi-luminescence by diode laser irradiation at wavelengths 660, 820, 880 or 950 nm. Laser Therapy. 1993; 5 (3): 103-110.

[181] Shefer G, Halevy O, Cullen M, Oron U. Low level laser irradaition shows no histopathological effects on myogenic satellite cells in tissue culture. Laser Therapy. 1999; 11 (3): 114-118.

[182] Yarita T et al. Effect of low power laser on gingival microcirculation. Proc. X Internat Congress Int Soc Laser Surgery and Medicine, Bangkok 1993, p 235.

[183] Iijima K, Shimoyama N, Shimoyama M, Mizuguchi T. Evaluation of Analgesic Effect of Low Power HeNe laser on Postherpetic Neuralgia Using VAS and Modified McGill Pain Questionaire. J Clin Laser Med Surg . 1991; 9 (2): 121-126.

[184] Iijima K et al. [Evaluation of analgesic effect of low-power laser for outpatients in pain clinic]. J Jpn Soc Med Lasers. 1988; 9: 3-10. (in Japanese)

[144] Umeda Y et al. Blood pressure controlled by low reactive level diode laser therapy (laser therapy). Laser Therapy. 1990; 2 (2): 59-64.

[145] Schindl L, Kainz A, Kern H. Effect of Low Level Laser Irradiation on Indolent Ulcers Caused by Bürgers Disease. Laser Therapy. 1992; 4 (1): 25-32.

[146] Uchida K et al. Treatment of chronic prostatitis and prostatodynia with low reactive laser. Laser Therapy. (ILTA Okinawa Congr Abstr Issue) 1990; 2 (1): 36.

[147] Popova M et al. [Effect of Helium-Neon laser beam in regeneration of irradiated transplanted skeletal muscle]. Biull Exp Biol Med. 1978; 80: 333. (Russian with English abstract)

[148] Asencio-Arana F et al. Endoscopic Enhancement of the Healing of High-Risk Colon Anastomoses by Low-Power Helium-Neon Laser. Dis Colon Rectum. 1992; 35 (6): 568-573.

[149] Dimitriadis V et al. Effect of HeNe Laser on the Midgut Cells of Drosophila Auraria Larvae and its Correlation with Acupuncture. Acup & Electro-Therap Res. Int J. 1985; 10: 67-.

[150] Abergel P et al. Non Thermal Effects of Nd:YAG Laser on the Biological Functions of the Human Skin Fibroblasts in Culture. Laser Surg Med. 1984; 3 (4): 379-384.

[151] Herman J et al. In vitro Effects of Nd:YAG Laser Radiation on Cartilage Metabolism. J Rheum. 1988; 15 (12): 1818-1826.

[152] Goldman J, Chiapella J, Bass N et al. Laser Therapy of Rheumatoid Arthritis. Lasers Surg Med. 1980; 1 (1): 93-101.

[153] Loevscall H. The Application of Low Level Laser in Dentistry - A Critical Review. Dept of Oral Pathology, Royal Dental College, Aarhus University, Vennelyst Boulevard, DK-8000 Aarhus C, Denmark. 1992.

[154] Saperia D, Glassberg E, Lyons R F et al. Demonstration of elevated type I and type III laser. Biochem and Biophys Res Communic. 1986; 138 (3): 1123-1128.

[155] Clokie C et al. The effects of helium-neon laser on postsurgical discomfort: A pilot study. Canadian Dent Ass Journal. 1991; 7 (57): 584-586.

[156] Bernal, G. Helium Neon and Diode Laser Therapy is an effective adjunctive therapy for facial paralysis. Laser Therapy. 1993; 5 (2): 79-87.

[157] Maier M, Haina D, Landthaler M. Effect of Low Energy Laser on the Growth and Regeneration of Capillaries. Lasers in Medical Sciences. 1990; 5: 381-.

[158] Rochkind S, Nissan M, Lubart A. A single Transcutaneous Light Irradiation to Injured Peripheral Nerve: Comparative Study with Five Different Wavelengths. Lasers in Medical Sciences. 1989; 4: 259-263.

[159] Parrado C, Carrillo de Albornoz F, Vidal L et al. A quantitative investigation of microvascular changes in the thyroid gland after infrared (IR) laser radiation. Histol Histopathol. 1999; 14 (4): 1067-1071.

[160] Ben Hatit Y. The Nd:YAG Laser in Dentistry. LASER. Journ Eur Med Laser Ass. 1991; 4 (1-2): 17-20.

[161] Mokhtar B et al. A double blind placebo controlled investigation of the hypoalgesic effects of low intensity laser irradiation of the cervical roots using experimental ischaemic pain. ILTA Congress, London 1992, abstracts p 61.

[162] Mokhtar B et al. The possible significance of pulse repetition rate in laser-mediated analgesia: a double blind placebo controlled investigation using experimental ischaemic pain. ILTA Congress, London 1992, abstracts p 62.

[163] Taube S, Piironen J, Ylipaavalniemi P. Helium-neon laser therapy in the prevention of postoperative swelling and pain after wisdom tooth extraction. Proc Finn Dent Soc 1990; 86: 23-27.

[123] Li X H. Laser in the Department of Traumatology. With a report of 60 cases of soft tissue injury. Laser Therapy. 1990; 2 (3): 119-122.

[124] Enwemeka C et al. Effect of HeNe photostimulation on tendon fibroblast protein synthesis: preliminary report. Proc Ninth Congress of the International Society for Laser Surgery and Medicine, Anaheim, Calif, USA: 2-6 Nov 1991.

[125] Tasaki E et al. Application of low power laser therapy for relief of of low back pain. Proc Ninth congress of the International Society for Laser Surgery and Medicine, Anaheim, California, USA: 2-6 November 1991.

[126] Terashima H et al. Low Energy Laser Irradiation for Lateral Humeral Epycondylitis and de Quervains Disease. Laser Therapy. (ILTA Okinawa Congr Abstr Issue) 1990; 2 (1): 27.

[127] Vasseljen O et al. Low Level Laser versus placebo in the treatment of tennis elbow. Scand J Rehab Med. 1992; 24: 37-42. Also in Physiotherapy;. 1992; 78 (5): 329-334.

[128] Verplanken M. [Stimulation of wound healing after tooth extraction using low intensity laser therapy] (in French). Revue Belge de Medecine Dentaire. 1987; 42: 134-138.

[129] Maeno N, Kameya T,Yamada H, Abe N. Effects of laser therapy, Using Helium-Neon Laser on Infectious Bovine Keratoconjunctivitis. Laser Therapy. 1989; 1 (2): 79-82.

[130] Yamada H, Kameya T, Abe N, Miyahara K. Low Level Laser Therapy in Horses. Laser Therapy. 1989; 1 (2): 31-36.

[131] Antikatzides T G. Soft Laser Treatment of Muskuloskeletal and Other Disorders in the Equine Athlete. Equine Practice. 1986; 8 (2): 24-30.

[132] McKibbin L, Paraschak D A Study of the Effects of Lasering on Chronic Bowed Tendons at Whitney Hall Farm Limited, Canada. Laser Surg Med. 1983; 3 (1): 55-59.

[133] Wang L-S, Kameya T, Yamada H. A Review of Clinical Applications of Low Level Laser Therapy in Veterinary Medicine. Laser Therapy. 1989; 1 (4): 183-190.

[134] Kerns T. HeNe Lasers Show Promise in Treating Equine Injuries. Lasers & Applications. 1986; 39-42.

[135] Basko I. A New Frontier. Laser Therapy. California Vet. 1983; 10: 17-.

[136] Lee Chang Woo, Kim, Ki Suk. Study on the Effect of Low Denisty Power Laser Radiation in Treating Gingival Inflammation. Clinical, Microbiological, Histological Study. J Korean Acad Oral Med 1987; 1 (12).

[137] Changjun C et al. The Preoperative Period of the Veterinary Anaesthesia by Laser. Sichuan Agricultural College, Sichuan. Acupuncture Res. 1984; 9 (1): 16-.

[138] Antikas T. Low Power Laser Treatment of Musculoskeletal Disorders and Body Measurements of the Equine Athlete. Proc. SPIE. 1989; Vol 1353: 92-. (Lasers in Medicine)

[139] McKibbin L. Low Level Laser Therapy in Veterinary Practice on Standardbred Horses. In: Low Level Laser Therapy. A Practical Introduction, Eds Ohshiro & Calderhead. John Wiley & Sons. 1988: 77-80.

[140] Passarella S et al. Increase of proton electrochemical potential and ATP synthesis in rat liver mitochondria irradiated in vitro by helium-neon laser. FEBS Letters. 1984; 175 (1): 95-99.

[141] Hasan P, Rijadi S A, Purnomo S, Kainama H. The possible application of low reactive laser therapy (laser therapy) in the treatment of male infertility. Laser Therapy. 1989; 1 (1): 49-50.

[142] Deng Q Z, Han Z Y. Therapy of female infertility under defocused CO_2 and HeNe laser acupoint irradiation. Laser Therapy. 1990; 2 (3): 117-118.

[143] Takac S. Treatment of menstrual pain with GaAs-laser therapy. Novi Sad, Yugoslavia. 1992. (personal communication)

[103] Moustsen P et al. Laserbehandling af bihulebetændelse i almen lægepraxis vurderet ved en dobbelt-blind kontrolleret undersøgelse. [Laser Treatment of Sinuitis in General Medical Praxis Evaluated in a Double Blind Study] (In Danish). Ugeskrift Læger. 1991; 153 (32): 2232-2234.

[104] Roshal L. Application of Low-Level Laser in Pediatry and Pediatric Surgery in the USSR. In: Progress in Laser Therapy. Editors: Ohshiro & Calderhead. John Wiley & Sons. 1991, p. 112.

[105] Vélez-Gonzáles M et al. Activation of the subcutanus absorbtion of drugs previous laser irradiation. Proc. Ninth Congress of the International Society for Laser Surgery and Medicine, Anaheim, California, USA: 2-6 November 1991.

[106] Nagasawa A. Application of laser therapy in Dentistry. In: Low-Reactive Laser Therapy - Practical Application. Ed: T. Ohshiro. John Wiley & Sons. 1991: 76-85.

[107] Nagasawa A, Negishi A, Kato K. Clinical Applications of laser therapy in Dental and oral Surgery in the Urawa Clinic. Laser Therapy. Laser Therapy. 1991; 3 (3): 119-122.

[108] Trelles M A et al. Bone Fracture Consolidates Faster With Low-Power Laser. Laser Surg Med. 1987; 7: 36-45.

[109] Paschoud Y et al. Effet du soft-laser sur la néofromation d'un pont dentinaire après coiffage pulpaire direct de dents humaines à l' hydroxyde de calcium. Rev Mens Suisse Odont-Stomatol. 1988; 98 (4): 345-356.

[110] Takeda Y. Irradiation effect of low-energy laser on alveolar bone after tooth extraction. Experimental study in rats. Int J Oral Maxillofac Surg. 1988; 17: 388-391.

[111] Yo-Chen, Zhou. Practical Applications of Non-contact laser therapy in Various Fields. In: Low Level Laser Therapy. A Practical Introduction, Eds. Ohshiro & Calderhead. John Wiley & Sons. 1988: 71.

[112] Kats A et al. [Laser therapy in fracture of the mandible.] Vestn Kir. 1986; 136: 93 (in Russian with English abstract)

[113] Takeda Y. Irradiation effect of low-energy laser on rat submandibular salivary gland. J Oral Pathol. 1988; 17: 91-94.

[114] Mezawa S et al. The possible analgesic effect of soft-laser irradiation on heat nociceptors in the cat tounge. Ach Oral Biol. 1988; 33 (9): 693-694.

[115] Zhou Y C. Effect of HeNe laser irradiation of acupoint on analgesia and met-enkephalin contents in different regions in the rat. Laser Journal. 1986; 7: 41- (in Chinese with English abstract)

[116] Zhou Y C. An Advanced Clinical Trial with Laser Acupuncture Anaesthesia for Minor Operations in the Oromaxillofacial Region. Laser Surg Med. 1984; 4: 297-303.

[117] Bradley P. Thermographic Evaluation of Response to Low Level Laser Acupuncture. Proc. Second Meeting of the International Laser Therapy Association, London Sept 1992. p 32.

[118] Jackeviciute I. Low power laser treatment for bronchial asthma and chronic bronchitis. Proc. Scand Soc for Laser Therapy. 3rd Congress, Örebro, Sweden. Oct 2-4, 1991.

[119] Barnes J et al. Electronic Acupuncture and Cold Laser Therapy as Adjuncts to Pain Treatment. J Cranomandibular Pract. 1984; 2 (2): 148-152.

[120] Wong E et al. Efficacy of Low Power Laser Therapy in the Pain Relief of Migraine Headaches. Proc Ninth Congress Soc Laser Surgery and Medicine, Anaheim, California, USA: 2-6 November 1991.

[121] Kusakari H. The use of lasers to dental implant. Proc X Internat Congr Soc Laser Surg Med, Bangkok, 1993, p 332.

[122] Ohshiro T. Alleviating Sport-relating pain with the diode laser. J Jap Soc Laser Med Surg. 1985; 5 (3): 221-.

[83]   Walker J et al. Laser Therapy for pain of Rheumatoid Arthritis. The Clinical Journal of Pain. 1987; 3 (53): 54-59.

[84]   Carrillo J, Calatayud J, Manso F J et al. A randomized double-blind clinical trial on the effectiveness of helium-neon laser in the prevention of pain, swelling and trismus after removal of impacted third molars. Internat Dent Journal. 1990; 40: 31-36.

[85]   Hansson T. Infrared laser in the treatment of craniomandibular disorders, arthrogenous pain. J Prosthetic Dentistry. 1989; 61: 614-617.

[86]   Nagasawa A et al. Fundamental studies in reactive histological changes in pulp tissue of lased teeth. J Jap Soc Laser Med Surg. 1989.

[87]   Yaakobi T et al. Promotion of bone repair in the cortical bone of the tibia in rats by low energy laser (He-Ne) irradiation. Calcif Tissue Int. 1996; 59 (4): 297-300.

[88]   Midamba E D, Haanaes H. Effect of low level laser therapy (laser therapy) on inferior alveolar, mental and lingual nerves after traumatic injury in 15 patients. A pilot study. Laser Therapy. 1993; 5 (2): 89-94.

[89]   Walker J B, Akhanjee L K. Laser-induced somatosensory evoked potentials: evidence of photosensitivity in peripheral nerves. Brain Research. 1985; 344: 281-285.

[90]   Tsai J-C, Kao M-C. The Biological Effects of Incident Low Power Density Laser Irradiation on Cultivated Rat Glial and Glioma Cells. Laser Therapy. 1989; 1 (4): 191-202.

[91]   Asanami S, Shiba H, Ohtaishi M et al. The Activatory Effect of HeNe laser therapy Irradiation of Hydroxy-apatite Implants in the Rabbit Mandibular Bone. Laser Therapy. 1993; 5 (1): 29-32.

[92]   Lievens P. Effects of Laser Treatment on the Lymphatic System and Wound Healing. LASER. Journ Eur Med Laser Ass. 1988; 1 (2): 12-15.

[93]   Røynesdal A et al. The effect of soft-laser application on postoperative pain and swelling. A double-blind, cross-over study. J Oral Maxillofac Surg. 1993; 22: 242-245.

[94]   Zhang D, Zhou Y, Xiao B, Li G. The effect of postoperative irradiation with low incident levels of CO2 laser irradiation on skin flap survival and the possible mechanisms. Laser Therapy. 1992; 4 (2): 75-80.

[95]   Kiyoizumi T. Low Level Diode Laser Treatment for Hematomas under Grafted Skin and its Photobiological Mechanisms. Keio J Med. 1988; 37: 415-.

[96]   Honmura A et al. Therapeutic effect of GaAlAs diode laser irradiation on experimentally induced inflammation in rats. Laser Surg Med. 1992; 12: 441-449.

[97]   Palmgren N, Jensen G F, Kaae K et al. Low-Power Laser Therapy in Rheumatoid Arthritis. Lasers in Medical Science. 1989; 4: 193-196.

[98]   Asada K, Yutani Y, Shimazu A. Diode Laser Therapy for Rheumatoid Arthritis: A Clinical Evaluation of 102 Joints Treated with Low Reactive-level Laser Therapy (laser therapy). Laser Therapy. 1989; 1 (3): 147-152.

[99]   Oyamada Y et al. Trials in treatment of RA-related diseases by HeNe-laser. Surg Med Lasers. 1989; 2: 18. Also in: Oyamada Y, Satodate R, Nishida J et al. Estudio en double ciego del efecto del laser de baja potencia HeNe en la artritis reumatoidea. Bol. CDL. 1988; 17: 8-12.

[100]   Trelles M A, Rigau J, Sala P et al. Infrared Diode Laser in Low Reactive-Level Laser Therapy (laser therapy) for Knee Osteoarthroses. Laser Therapy. 1991; 3 (4): 149-154.

[101]   Kim K S, Hun L D, Kun K S. Effects of Low Incident Energy Levels of Infrared Laser Irradiation on the Proliferation of Streptococcus Mutans. Laser Therapy. 1992; 4 (2): 81-86.

[102]   Gilioli G et al. Studio ultrastrutturale di colture cellulari "vero" infettate con virus Herpes Simplex e sottoposte all'azione Laser. Int Congress on Laser Med and Surg, Bologna June 1985, p 207. Monduzzi Editore S.p.A, Bologna, Italy. Also in: Medical Laser Report 1985; 3: 28-31.

[63]   Herman J, Khosla R. Nd:YAG laser modulation of synovial tissue metabolism. Clinic Exp Rheumatol. 1989; 7: 505-512.

[64]   Guang Hua Wang et al. A study on the analgesic effect of low power HeNe-laser and its mechanism by electrophysiological means. In: Lasers in Dentistry. Excerpta Medica. Elsevier Science Publishers, Amsterdam. 1989: p. 277.

[65]   Kaihøj P. Low Level Lasers Effekt på Følsomme Tandhalse - en klinisk pilottest. ["The Effect of Low Level Lasers on Sensitive Toothnecks - a Clinical Pilot Study"] (In Danish). Odont Pract. 1991; 6 (2): 229-300.

[66]   Wakabayashi H et al. Treatment of dentine hypersensitivity by GaAlAs soft laser irradiation. J Dent Research. 1988; 67: 182-186.

[67]   Kami T, Yoshimura Y, Nakajima T et al. Effect of low-powered diode lasers on flap survival. Ann Plast Surgery. 1985; 14 (3): 278-283.

[68]   Riendeau F. An in vivo study of the effects of Helium-Neon laser on the breaking force and histological characteristics of wound. Proc Int Congr of Lasers in Dentistry, Tokyo, August 5-6. 1988: p 20.

[69]   Soudry M et al. Action d' un laser hélium-néon sur la croissance cellulaire: étude in vitro sur fibro-blastes gingivaux humains. J Biol Buccale. 1988; 16: 129.

[70]   Chomette G, Auriol M, Zeitoun R et al. Effet du soft-laser sur le tissu conjunctif gingival. I - Effet sur les fibroblastes. Étude d'histoenzymologie et de microscopie eléctronique. J Biol Buccale. 1987; 15: 45-50.

[71]   Chomette G, Auriol M, Zeitoun R et al. Effet du soft-laser sur le tissu conjunctif gingival. II - Effet sur la cicatrisation. Étude en microscopie optique, histoenzymologie et microscopie électronique. J Biol Buccale. 1987; 15: 51-57.

[72]   Gretzinger H et al. An in vivo study of the effect of helium-neon laser on human fibroblast migration. Proc Int Congr of Lasers in Dentistry, Tokyo, August 5-6. 1988: p 23.

[73]   Mousques T. Étude en double aveugle des effets du traitment unilateral au laser hélium-néon lors de chirurgies parodontales bilàterales simultanés. Quest Odontostomatol. 1986; 11: 245-251.

[74]   Enwemeka C. Laser biostimulation of healing wounds: specific effects and mechanisms of action. J Orthop Sports Physical Therapy. 1988; 9: 333-.

[75]   Loevschall H, Arneholt-Bindslev D. Low Level Laser Irradiation of Human Oral Mucosa Fibroblast in Vitro in Cultures of Human Oral Fibroblasts. Laser Surg Med. 1994; 14: 347-354.

[76]   Loevschall H Effects of low level diode laser irradiation in cultures of human oral mucosa. Proc. Second Meeting of the Internat Laser Theapy Assn., London, Sept 1992; p. 55.

[77]   Iwase T, Saito T, Nara Y, Morioka T. Inhibitory effect of HeNe laser on dental plaque deposition in hamsters. J Periodont Research. 1989; 24: 282-283.

[78]   Schenk P et al. Elektronenmikroskopische Untersuchungen von oralen Schleimhautepithelien nach Bestrahlung mit dem Helium-Neon-Laser. Dtsch Z Mund Kiefer Gesichts Chir. 1985; 9: 278-281.

[79]   Wafa F et al. A clinical study of laser therapy in fixed prosthodontic pain control after tooth preparation to receive a crown. 1990; 2 (2): 83-88.

[80]   Gomi A et al. A clinical study of soft Laser 632 Helium Neon low energy medical laser. 2nd report. The effects in the relieving the pain of hypersensitive dentine and the pain during seating inlay. Aichi Gukuin J Dent Sci. 1986; 24 (3): 390-399.

[81]   Harazaki M, Isshiki Y. Soft laser irradiation effects on pain reduction in orthodontic treatment. Bull Tokyo Dent Coll. 1997; 38 (4): 291-295.

[82]   Haimovici N et al. Clinical use of antiinflammatory action of the laser in activated osteoarthritis of small peripheral joints. LASER. Journ Eur Med Laser Ass. 1988; 1 (2): 4-11.

[40] Montesinos M. et al. Experimental Effects of Low Power Laser in Encephalin and Endorphin Synthesis. LASER. Journ Eur Med Laser Ass. 1988; 1 (3): 2-7.

[41] Anneroth G, Hall G, Rydén H, Zetterqvist L. The effect of Low-energy infrared laser radiation on woundhealing in rats. Brit J Oral & Max Surg. 1988; 26: 12-17.

[42] Rydén H, Persson L Preber H, Bergström J. Effect of low-energy laser on gingival inflammation. Swedish Dent J. 1990; 14: 47.

[43] Hedner E. Herpes simplex virus type 1 and intraoral wound healing (In Swedish). J of the S D A, 1994, 1: 8-10.

[44] Tamachi Y. Enhancement of antitumor chemotherapy effect by low level laser irradiation. Tokyo Medical College Newsletter; 1991: 888-893.

[45] Lundeberg T, Hode L, Zhou J. A comparative study of the pain-relieving effect of laser treatment and acupuncture. Acta Physiol Scand. 1987; 131 (1): 161-162.

[46] Pourreau-Schnedier N et al. Soft-Laser Therapy for Iatrogenic Mucositis in Cancer Patients Receiving High-Dose Fluorouacil: A preliminary report. J Nat Cancer Inst. 1992; 84 (5): 358-359.

[47] Ciais G et al. La laserthérapie dans la prévention et la traitement des mucities liées à la chimothérapie anticancéreuse. Bull Cancer. 1992; 79: 183-187.

[48] Sapiera D et al. Demonstration of elevated type I and type III procollagen mRNA levels in cutaneous wounds treated with helium-neon laser. Biochem Biophys Res Com. 1986; 3 (138): 1123-1128.

[49] Hatano Y. Lasers in the diagnosis of the TMJ problems. In: Lasers in dentistry. Eds. Yamamoto Y et al. 1989; p. 169-172. Elsevier Science Publishing B.V, Amsterdam

[50] Braverman B et al. Effect of Helium-Neon and Infrared Laser Irrradiation on Wound Healing in Rabbits. Laser Surg Med. 1989; 9: 50-58.

[51] David L, Abergel P. Laser for Cosmetic Surgery. Laser Surg Med. 1989; Suppl 1: 32.

[52] Nara Y et al. Stimulative effect of HeNe laser irradiation on cultured fibroblasts derived from human dental pulp. Lasers in the Life Sciences. 1992; 4 (4): 249-256.

[53] Shiroto C et al. Retrospective study of diode laser therapy for pain attenuation in 3635 patients: Detailed analysis by questionnaire. Laser Therapy. 1989; 1 (1): 41-48.

[54] Mizokami T et al. Effect of diode laser for pain: A clinical study on different pain types. Laser Therapy. 1990; 2 (4): 171-174.

[55] Hansen H, Thorøe U. Low power laser biostimulation of chronic orofacial pain. A double-blind placebo controlled cross-over study in 40 patients. Pain. 1990; 43: 169-179.

[56] Maricic B et al. Analgetic effect of laser in dental therapy. Acta Stomat Croat. 1987; 21 (4): 291-297.

[57] Moore K, Hira N, Kumar. Ohshiro T. Double blind crossover trial of low level laser therapy in the treatment of post herpetic neuralgia. Laser Therapy. 1988; (pilot issue): 7-10.

[58] McKibbin L et al. Treatment of post herpetic neuralgia using a 904 nm (infrared) low energy laser: A clinical study. Laser Therapy. 1991; 3 (1): 35-40.

[59] Hong J N, Kim T H, Lim S D. Clinical trial of low reactive-level laser therapy in 20 patients with postherpetic neuralgia. Laser Therapy. 1990; 2 (4): 167-170.

[60] Hachenberger I. Laserstrahlen bei Herpeserkrankungen. Ärztliche Kosmetologie. 1981; 11: 142-144.

[61] von Ahlften U et al. Erfahrungen bei der Behandlung aphtöser und herpetiformer Mundschleimhauterkrankungen mit einem neuen Infrarotlaser. Die Quintessenz. 1987; 5: 927-933.

[62] Abergel P. Laser treatment of acne scars. Laser Surg Med. 1992; Suppl 4: 70.

[19] Oulamara A et al. Biological activity measurement on botanical specimen surfaces using a temporal decorrelation effect of laser speckle. Journal of Modern Optics. 1989; 36 (2): 165-.

[20] Cherry R. Measurement of Protein Rotational Diffusion in Membranes by Flash Photolysis. Methods in Enzymology. 1978; (54): 47-61.

[21] Lubart R, Wollman Y, Friedman H, Rochkind S, Laulicht I. Effects of visible and near-infrared lasers on cell cultures. J. Photochem. Photobiol. B. 1992; 12: 305-310.

[22] Karu T I. Photobiological Fundamentals of Low Power Laser Therapy. IEEE Journal of Quantum Electronics. 1987; 23 (10): 1703-.

[23] Mester E et al. Auswirkungen direkter Laserbestrahlung auf menschliche Lymphozyten. [Effects of direct laser radiation on human lymphocytes]. Arch Dermatol Res. 1978; 263 (3): 241-245.

[24] Dougherty T J. Photosensitizers: Therapy and detection of malignant tumors. Photochem Photobio. 1987; 45 (6): 879-889.

[25] Dougherty T J. Photodynamic therapy. In: Innovations in Radiation Oncology. Withers H, Peters L, eds. Berlin/Heidelberg, Springer-Verlag, 1988, p. 175.

[26] Bossy J et al. In Vitro Survey of Low Energy Laser Beam Penetration in Compact Bone. Faculté de Médecine et CHRU de Nimes, BP 26, 3000 Nimes, France (1985).

[27] Svaasand L. Biostimulering med lav-intensitetslasere. Fysikk eller metafysikk? ["Biostimulation with low intensity laser: Physics or metaphysics?"] Nordisk Medicin. 1990; 103 (3): 72- .(in Norwegian)

[28] Derr V E, Klein E, Fine S. Free radical occurrence in some laser-irradiated biologic materials. Federal Proc. 1965; 24 (No 1, Suppl 14): 99-103.

[29] Lubart R et al. A possible Mechanism of Low Level Laser - Living Cell Interaction. Laser Therapy. 1990; 2 (2): 65-68.

[30] Kudoh Ch et al. Effects of 830 nm Gallium Aluminium Arsenide Diode Laser Radiation on Rat Saphenous Nerve Sodium-Potassium-Adenosine Triphosphatase Activity: A Possible Pain Attenuation Mechanism Examined. Laser Therapy. 1989; 1 (2): 63-67.

[31] Nasu F, Tomiyasu K, Inomata K, Calderhead R G. Cytochemical Effects of GaAlAs Diode Laser Radiation on Rat Saphenous Artery Calcium Ion Dependent Adenosine Triphosphatase Activity. Laser Therapy. 1989; 1 (2): 89-92.

[32] Rochkind S, Nissan M, Razon N et al. Electrophysiological Effect of HeNe Laser on Normal and Injured Sciatic Nerve in the Rat. Acta Neurochir. (Vienna). 1986; 83: 125-130.

[33] Karu T I et al. Biostimulation of HeLa-cells by Low-Intensity Visible Light. Nuovo Cimento. 1982; 1D (6): 828-.

[34] Mester E et al. The Biostimulating Effect of Laser Beam. Proc. Laser - 81, Opto-Elektronik, Munich 1981.

[35] Kovács I et al. Laser-Induced Stimulation of the Vascularization of the Healing Wound. Separatum Experientia. 1974; 30: 341-346.

[36] Lederer H et al. Influence of Light on Human Immunocompetent Cells In Vitro. Proc of Laser -81, Opto-Elektronik. Munich, 1981.

[37] Pourreau-Schneider N et al. Helium-Neon Laser Treatment Transforms Fibroblasts into Myofibroblasts. Am J Pathol. 1990; 137: 171-178.

[38] Walker J. Relief from Chronic Pain by Low Power Laser Irradiation. Neuroscience Letters. 1983; 43: 339-344.

[39] Rochkind S et al. Systemic Effects of Low-Power Laser Irradiation on the Peripheral and Central Nervous System, Cutaneous Wounds and Burns. Laser Surg Med. 1989; 9: 174-182.

14.1 Numeric references referred to in the book.

[1] Dima F V et al. Doserelated immunological and morphological changes observed in rats with Walker-256 carcinosarcoma after photodynamic therapy: a controlled study. Laser Therapy. 1991; 3 (3): 159-168.

[2] Skobelkin O K, Michailov V A, Zakharov S D. Preoperative activation of the immune system by low reactive level laser therapy (laser therapy) in oncologic patients: A preliminary report. Laser Therapy. 1991; 3 (4): 169-176.

[3] Mikhailov V A , Skobelkin O K, Denisov I N, Frank G A, Voltchenko N N. Investigations on the influence of Low Level Diode Laser irradiation of the growth of experimental tumors. Laser Therapy. 1993; 5 (1): 33-38.

[4] Steinlechner C, Dyson M. The effect of low level laser therapy on the proliferation of keratinocytes. Laser Therapy; 1993; 5 (2): 65-74.

[5] Dyson M, Young S. Effect of Laser Therapy on Wound Contraction and Cellularity in Mice. Lasers in Medical Science. 1986; (1): 125-129.

[6] Pedrola M et al. Acute cervical pain relieved with gallium arsenurio (GaAs) laser irradiation. A double blind study. Laser Surg Med. 1995, suppl 7, p. 10.

[7] Walsh D et al. The effect of low intensity laser irradiation upon conduction and skin temperature in the superficial radial nerve. Double blind placebo controlled investigation using experimental ischaemic pain. Proc. Second Meeting of the International Laser Therapy Association, London. Sept 1992.

[8] Abergel P, Meeker C A, Lam T et al. Control of connective tissue metabolism by lasers: Recent developments and future prospects. J Am Acad Dermatol. 1984; 11: 1142-1150.

[9] Saldo I et al. Effects of GaAs-laser combined with radiotherapy on murine sarcoma depends on tumor size. Laser Surg Med. 1989; Suppl. 1:40.

[10] Mester E. et al. Untersuchungen über die hemmende bzw. fördernde Wirkung der Laserstrahlen. [Studies on the inhibiting and activating effects of laser beams]. Langenbecks Arch Klin Chir. 1968; 322: 1022-1027.

[11] Mester Andrew, Mester Adam. Scientific background of laser biostimulation. LASER. Journ Eur Med Laser Ass. 1988; 1 (1): 23-29.

[12] King P. Low Level Laser Therapy: A Review. Lasers in Medical Science. 1989; 4: 141-.

[13] Bihari I, Mester A. The biostimulative effect of low level laser therapy of long-standing crural ulcer using Helium Neon laser, Helium Neon plus infrared lasers and noncoherent light: Preliminary report of a randomized double blind comparative study. Laser Therapy. 1989; 1 (2): 97-102.

[14] Kubota J, Ohshiro T. The effects of diode laser low reactive-level laser therapy (laser therapy) on flap survival in a rat model. Laser Therapy. 1989; 1 (3): 127-134.

[15] Berki T et al. Biological Effect of Low-power Helium-Neon (HeNe) Laser Irradiation. Lasers in Medical Science. 1988; 3: 35-38.

[16] Muldiyarov P et al. Effect of Monochromatic Helium-Neon Laser Red Light on the Morphology of Zymosan Arthritis in Rats. Biull Eksp Biol Med. 1983; 1: 55-.

[17] Haina D, Brunner R, Landthaler O et al. Animal Experiments on Light-Induced Woundhealing. Biophysica, Berlin. 1973; 35 (3): 227-230.

[18] Calderhead G. Meeting report: Proc Ninth Congress of the International Society for Laser Surgery and Medicine, Anaheim, California, USA: 2-6 November 1991. Laser Therapy. 1992; 4 (1): 43.

Chapter 14
References - Abbreviations

13.8 Laser phototherapy journals

Photomedicine and Laser Surgery. Mary Ann Liebert, Inc., New York, USA. Journal of the World Association for Laser Therapy and The North American Association for Laser Therapy. www.walt.nu, www.naalt.org

Lasers in Surgery and Medicine. The American Society for Laser Medicine and Surgery. Wiley-Liss, Inc. New York, USA. www.aslms.org

Lasers in Medical Science. Springer-Verlag London Ltd, London, UK. Journal of the World Federation for Laser Dentistry and the British Medical Laser Association. www.springer.com/medicine/journal/10103

SPIE - The International Society of Optical Engineering, Bellingham, WA, USA. Large numbers of proceedings reports from conferences, several on medical laser applications. www.spie.org

Journal of Oral Laser Applications. Journal of the International Society for 0ral Laser Applications. www.sola-int.org/content/journal/journal_frame.htm

Pöntinen P. (1988). LASER Lääketieteellisenä hoitomuotona. ISBN 952-90050-9-1. Invarmex OY, Finland.

Kert J, Rose L. (1989). Klinisk laserbehandling. ISBN 87-983204-0-8. Scandinavian Medical Laser Technology. Copenhagen, Denmark.

Pöntinen P. (1991). Lågeffektslasern som medicinsk vårdform. 91-7736-267-4. Prima Books, Sweden. (in Swedish)

Tunér J, Hode L. (1995). Lågeffektslaser inom odontologin. ISBN 91-971969-1-6. Swedish Laser-Medical Society, Stockholm, Sweden.

Tunér J, Hode L, Diklic S. (1996). Osnove primene lasera u medicini. Irradia DOO, Gavrila Principa 53, Sremska Kamenica, Yugoslavia.

Brugnera Junior A, Luiz B Pinheiro A. (1998). Lasers na Odontologia Moderna. ISBN 85-86266-09-4. Pancast Editora, São Paulo, Brazil.

Teixeira H. Laser Médico. A face Colorida do Laser. (2000). Clinica Medilaser Lda, Coimbra, Portugal.

Genovese W J. Laser de baixa intensidade. Aplicaçoes Terapeuticas em Odontologia. (2000). ISBN 85-85274-62-X. Editora Lovise Ltda, São Paulo, Brazil.

Brugnera Jr A et al. (2003). Laserterapia Aplicada à Clínica Odontológica. Santos Livraria Editora, São Paulo, Brazil.

Lizarelli R. (2005). Protocolos clínicos odontológicos - uso do laser de baixa intensidade. 2 ed. Ed. 99 pp. Ed. Suprema, São Carlos, Brazil.

Rezvan F, Farsani F, Araqi B, Kamrava K. (2005). Laser Therapy, Basic and Clinical Practice of Low Level Laser. ISBN 964-399-029-X. Iranian Medical Laser Association, Tehran, Iran. (in Farsi)

Tunér J, Hode L. (2006). Laser therapy - clinical practice and scientific background. In Korean. ISBN 89-8085-301-7.

Martínez Arizpe H. (2007). Odontología Láser. Editorial Trillas, S.A. de C.V., México D.F. ISBN 968-24-7773-5.

Tunér J, Hode L. (2008). Laser therapy - clinical practice and scientific background. Greek translation. ISBN 978-960-89805-6-3.

Füchtenbusch A, Bringmann W. Laser therapy and laser puncture.

Bringman W. Lasertherapie - Licht kann heilen. (2008). ISBN 978-3-00-022302-0.

Eghbali F, Fekrazad R. Applying Low Level Laser Therapy in Dentistry (in Farsi). (2009). ISBN 978-964-237-017-7.

Vintage books can in some cases be obtained through Prima Books. www.prima-books.com.

principles). English and Italian text. ISBN 88-85037-99-2. Cortina International, Verona, Italy

de Cuyper H. Het Gebruik van Laser in de Fysiotherapie. 90-352-1008-5.

Danhof G. (1994). Lasertherapie in de tandheelkundige praktijk. (in Dutch) ISBN 90-6523-08-0. Uitgeverij Stubeg bv, Hoogezand, The Netherlands.

Popp F A. Biologie des Lichtes. 3-489-61734-7.

Bahn, Klima, Bischko. Laser und. Infratorstrahlen in der Akupunktur. 3-7760-0962-4.

Lievens P C. Laser-Thérapie. Théorie et applications pratiques. 2-87671-037-4. Editions Frison-Roche, Paris, France.

Redureaux D. Le Laser. Application en physiothérapie. 2-224-01100-8.

Nogier R. Précis Pratique de Lasertherapie en Odontostomatologie.

Coche P. (1985). L'energie douce face à la doleur. ISBN 2-905692-00-6. Ateim, 8, rue Reyer, Toulouse, France.

Pöntinen P. Laser in der Akupunktur. 3-7773- 1019-0. Hippokrates Verlag GmbH, Stuttgart, Germany.

Danhof G. Lasertherapie in der Sportmedizin und Orthopädie. 3-921988-52-7.

Ambronn G. Laser- under Magnetfeld-terapie in der Tiermedizin. 3-334-60855-7.

Iliev E. (1988). Soft-laser in der Dermatologie. Edition Svesa, München, Germany. ISBN 3-927406-00-7.

Elias J. Akupunktur und Lasertherapie für die Praxis. 3925367-53-5.

Elias J. Laserakupunktur. (1996). 3-541-50101-4. Urban Fisher Verlag, Berlin, Germany.

Koebner K. LASER - von tödlichen zum heilenden Strahl. 3-921608-59-7.

Danhof G. (1991). Lasertherapie in der Allgemeinmedizin. WBV Biologisch-Medizinische Verlagsgesellschaft mbH & Co KG. DE-7060 Schorndorf, Germany. ISBN 3-921988-50-0

Danhof G. (1995). Lasertherapie in der Zahnheilkunde. ISBN-3-921988-54-3. WBV Biologisch-Medizinische Verlagsgesellschaft Schorndorf.

Bringman W. (2002). Laser Therapie. 2. erweiterte und überarbeitete Auflage.

Pöntinen P. (1998). Laser in der Akupunktur. 3-7773-1320-3. Hippokrates Verlag GmbH, Stuttgart, Germany.

22 Simunovic Z, ed. Lasers in Medicine, Surgery and Dentistry. (2003). Locarno, Switzerland. ISBN 953-99344-0-0.

23 Bjordal J M, Johnson M I, Couppè C. (2001). Clinical Electrotherapy. Your guide to optimal treatment. Høyskoleforlaget. Norwegian Academic Press. ISBN 82-7634-320-1.

24 Biomedical Photonics Handbook. Tuan Vo-Dinh. ISBN 0849311160.

25 Tunér J, Hode L. (2004). The Laser Therapy Handbook. Prima Books AB. ISBN 91-631-1345-7.

26 Brugnera Jr A, dos Santos A E, Bologna E D, Ladalardo T C. (2006) Laser therapy applied to clinical dentistry. Quintessence Editora Ltda. ISBN 85-87425-69-2.

27 Litscher G, Schikora D. (2005). Laserneedle-Acupuncture. PABST Science Publishers, Vienna. ISBN 3-89967-199-6.

28 Brugnera J et al. (2006). Atlas of Laser Therapy Applied to Clinical Dentistry. Quintessence Editora Ltda, Sao Paulo. ISBN 85-87425-69-2.

29 Gutknecht N, ed (2007). Proceedings of the 1st International Workshop of Evidence Based Dentistry on Lasers in Dentistry. Quintessenz Verlags-GmbH. ISBN 978-1-85097-167-2.

30 Karu T I. (2007). Ten Lessons on Basic Science of Laser Phototherapy. Prima Books AB. ISBN 978-91-976478-0-9.

31 Kahn F. (2008). Low Intensity Laser Therapy - The New Therapeutic Dimension. Meditech International, Toronto, Canada. ISBN: 978-0-9817701-1-6.

32 Simunovic Z, ed. (2009). Lasers in Medicine, Science and Praxis. Lasermedico, Switzerland.

13.7 Books in other languages, with ISBN.

Colls J. La Terapía Láser Hoy. 84-398-1811-4.

Trelles M A. Láser para la salud y la estética. 85667-02-6.

Trelles M A. Soft Láser Terapía. 84-300-7068-0.

Cisneros J L, Trelles M A. (1987). Laser y Terapeutica en Medicina y Cirugía Cutanea. 7717.000.2

Matura L. Lasertherapia - esperienze cliniche riabilative. 88-7449-137-9.

Longo L. Terapia Laser. 88-03-00185-9.

Fornezza U. (1986). Il laser in terapia e chirurgia - principi teorici e applicativi (Lasers in therapy and surgery. Theoretical and practical

7 Goldman L. (1991). Laser Non-Surgical Medicine: New Challenges for an Old Application. ISBN 87762-792-4. Technomic Publishing Co, USA.

8 Wolbarsht M L. (1991). Laser Applications in Medicine and Biology. Vol 5. (See espec. chapter 1). ISBN 0-306-43753-8 (v. 5). Plenum Press. NY, USA.

9 Ohshiro T. (1991). Low Reactive-Level Laser Therapy: Practical Application. ISBN 0-471-92845-3. John Wiley & Sons, Chichester, England.

10 Ohshiro T, Calderhead R G. (1991). Progress in Laser Therapy. Selected Papers from the October 1990 ILTA Congress. ISBN 0-471-93154-3. John Wiley & Sons, Chichester, England.

11 Galletti G. (1992). Laser Applications in Medicine and Surgery. Monduzzi Editore S.p.A, via Ferrarese 119/2, IT-40128 Bologna, Italy.

12 Pöntinen P. (1992). Low level laser therapy as a medical treatment modality. ISBN 951-96632-0-7. Art Urpo Ltd, Tampere, Finland. www.prima-books.com.

13 Baxter G D. (1994). Therapeutic Lasers. Theory and practice. ISBN 0-443-04393-0. Churchill Livingstone, England.

14 Hajder D. (1994). Acupuncture and Lasers. 2nd ed. ISBN 86-81979-17-6. DaDa, Sredacka 11, Belgrad, Yugoslavia.

15 Tunér J, Hode L (1996). Laser Therapy in dentistry and medicine. ISBN SE 91-630-4078-6. Prima Books AB.

16 van Breugel H. (1997). Laser Therapy in medical practice. ISBN 90-6523-048-3. Van den Boogaard Publishing, Oisterwijk, The Netherlands.

17 Karu T. (1998). The science of low power laser therapy. ISBN 90-5699-108-6. The Gordon and Breach Publishing Group.

18 Tunér J, Hode L. (1999) Low Level Laser Therapy, clinical practice and scientific background. Prima Books AB. ISBN 91-630-7616-0.

19 Simunovic Z, ed. (2000). Lasers in Medicine and Dentistry. Basic science and up-to-date clinical application of low energy-level laser therapy, laser therapy. Locarno, Switzerland. ISBN 953-6059-30-4.

20 Simunovic Z, ed. Lasers in Surgery and Dentistry. (2001). Locarno, Switzerland. ISBN 953-6059-46-0.

21 Low-intensity laser therapy of various diseases. Buylin V A, Moskvin S V. Moscow "Technika" Firm, Ltd., 2001, ISBN 5-89337-029-5;

13.5 Can you trust your laser?

In order to reach the medical results we want, it is necessary to be aware of reasonable dosage intervals. However, in order to know that those intervals are reached, we also need to know the output of our equipment. Unfortunately, this is not always possible. Few laser machines have built-in power meters and even so, the dose with vary with the temperature and the age of the diode. And even if there is a power meter, can we trust it? WALT has performed test measurements for a GaAs laser used in several published papers. These are the results:

4 diode cluster probe with lens, power per diode:
7000 Hz 0.18 mW; 5000 Hz 0.14 mW; 2000 Hz 0.07 mW

Without lens, single probe:
7000 Hz acc. to built-in power meter: 16.8 mW. Acc. to professional power meter: 20.55 mW
2000 Hz acc, to built-in power meter: 4.8 mW. Acc. to professional power meter: 8.57 mW

In the first case too low output for practical use, in the other case much more than indicated by the built-in power meter. This kind of lack of control of the basic parameters is a threat to LPT science.

13.6 English language books on LPT:

1. Wolbarsht M L. (1977). Laser Applications in Medicine and Biology. Vol 3. 4.3. ISBN 0-306-37163-4 (v. 3). Plenum Press. New York, USA.

2. LASER. (1986). Proceedings of the International Congress on Laser in Medicine and Surgery. Bologna June 26-28, 1985. Edited by G. Galletti. Monduzzi Editore S.p.A, via Ferrarese 119/2, IT-40128 Bologna, Italy.

3. Ohshiro T, Calderhead R G. (1988). Low Level Laser Therapy: A Practical Introduction. ISBN 0-471-91956-X. John Wiley & Sons, Chichester, England.

4. Colls J. Laser Therapy Today. 84-398-6137-0.

5. Kert J, Rose L. (1989). Clinical Laser Therapy. ISBN 87-983204-1-6. Scandinavian Medical Laser Technology, Copenhagen, Denmark.

6. Karu T. (1989). Photobiology of Low-Power Laser Therapy (Laser Science and Technology. ISBN: 3718649705. Harwood Academic Publ.

13.4 Poor documentation – compared to what?

It is sometimes claimed that LPT has a rather poor scientific documentation. While this may be a valid point to some extent, it is surprisingly common for generally used treatment modalities to have a poor documentation without being questioned. It is interesting to compare the widely used ultrasound modality with LPT. In the book "Clinical electrotherapy – your guide to optimal treatment", Bjordal [1187] has compared the documentation found in the randomised studies on LPT and ultrasound in physiotherapy.

	LPT	Ultrasound
Strong evidence of effect	Tendinopathy Osteoarthritis	None
Moderate evidence of effect	Myofascial trigger point syndrome	None
Weak evidence of effect	Rheumatoid arthritis Soft tissue injuries	Tendinopathy Soft tissue injuries Wounds

Table 13.12 LPT - ultrasound

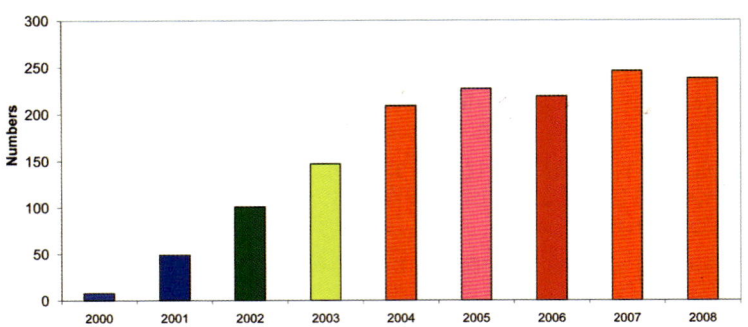

The post-millennium documentation has increased considerably and so has the quality of the papers published. In a survey by Bjordal, the following numbers of LPT studies were listed on PubMed 2000-2008.

What can be done to improve future studies?

The World Association for Laser Therapy has published dosage recommendations for musculoskeletal conditions (www.walt.nu) and is working on a similar document for wound healing and mucositis. The association has also published Standard for conduct of randomized controlled trials and Standard for conduct of systematic reviews and Meta-analyses [12] Although these so far concern musculoskeletal conditions, much can be applied to other conditions. The Scientific Secretary of WALT is also available for advice.

References:

C1. Tunér J. The Cochrane analyses - can they be improved? Laser Therapy. 1999; 11 (3): 138-143.

C2. Tunér J, Hode L. The Cochrane analyses - can they be improved? (http://www.laser.nu/lllt/lllt_editorial7.htm)

C3. Bjordal J M. Can a Cochrane review in controversial areas be biased? A sensitivity analysis based on the protocol of a systematic Cochrane review Low Level Laser Therapy in Osteoarthritis. Photomed Laser Surg. 2005; 23 (5):453-458.

C4. Flemming K, Cullum N. Laser therapy for venous leg ulcers. Cochrane Database Syst Rev 2000; (2):CD001182.

C5. Brosseau L, Welch V, Wells G et al. Low level laser therapy (classes I, II and III) for treating rheumatoid arthritis. In: The Cochrane Library. Issue 4, 2000. Oxford: Update Software.

C6. Brosseau L, Welch V, Wells G et al. Low level laser therapy (classes I, II and III) for treating oesteoarthritis. In: The Cochrane Library. Issue 4, 2000. Oxford: Update Software (Withdrawn)

C7. Bjordal J M, Greve G. What may alter the conclusions of reviews? Physical Therapy Reviews. 1998; 3: 121-132.

C8. Lanzafame R J, Stadler I, Coleman J, Haerum B, Oskoui P, Whittaker M, Zhang R Y. Temperature-controlled 830-nm low-level laser therapy of experimental pressure ulcers. Photomed Laser Surg. 2004; 22 (6): 483-488.

C9. Hode L, Tunér J. Wrong parameters can give just any result. Laser Surg Med. 2006; 38: 343 (Letter to the editor).

C10. Bjordal J M, Couppe C, Ljunggren A. Low level laser therapy for tendinopathies. Evidence of a dose-response pattern. Physical Therapy Reviews. 2001; 6 (2): 91-100.

C11. Bjordal J M, Couppè C, Chow R T, Tunér J, Ljunggren A E. A systematic review of low level laser therapy with location-specific doses for pain from chronic joint disorders. Australian J Physiotherapy. 2003; 49: 107-116.

C12. Consensus agreement on the design and conduct of clinical studies with Low-Level Laser Therapy and Light Therapy for musculoskeletal pain and disorders. Photomed Laser Sur. 2006. 24 (6): 759-762.

C13. al-Watban F, Zhang X Y. Comparison of the effects of laser therapy on wound healing using different laser wavelengths. Laser Therapy. 1996; 8 (2): 127-136.

C14. Bjordal J M, Johnson M I, Iversen V, Aimbire F, Lopes-Martins R A. Photoradiation in acute pain: a systematic review of possible mechanisms of action and clinical effects in randomized placebo-controlled trials. Photomed Laser Surg. 2006; 24 (2): 158-168.

The scarce reporting of parameters in this paper does not offer an opportunity for evaluation.

Pressure ulcers

Malm and Lundeberg, 1991 GaAs. Disqualified study because of the exposure of Lundeberg as a scientific cheater and for serious flaw in reporting of parameters.(http://www.laser.nu/lllt/pdf/Scientific_fraud_in_lasers.pdf)

Lucas, van Gemert and de Haan, 2003, 904 nm (pressure). A good study, 1 J/cm^2 on stage III pressure ulcers. Possible negative features; same irradiation over wound and skin, stage III pressure ulcers very difficult to treat in general, low dose.

Lucas, Coenen,and De Haan, 2000
904 nm, 1 J/cm^2 stated. 12 x 8 mW, 125 s (12 J) spread over a standard area of 30 cm = 0.4J/cm^2 . Spread over 30 J/cm^2 irrespective of wound size. 0.4 J/cm^2 , 904 nm for open wound is fair, over skin too low. For pressure wound the dose is generally too low.

As can be seen from the above:
- 6 studies should not have been included because of unavailable information or because they were not laser studies.
- 3 acceptable studies for crural ulcers. 2 different wavelengths.
- 2 acceptable studies for pressure ulcer, one wavelength.
- No dosage analysis has been performed or discussed
- No treatment technique difference has been addressed

Conclusions:

Three conclusions can be drawn from the above:

a) Even with a better and more updated selection of studies and a proper evaluation of these, LPT for crural and pressure ulcers would still not lead to the conclusion that the documentation is at an acceptable level.
b) The material of the study is not sufficient for a Meta analysis
c) From the Blue Cross study one would get the impression that the lack of effect of LPT for the conditions is confirmed by the chosen studies. Such a conclusion cannot be drawn. The present documentation does not confirm the effectiveness of LPT for these conditions, nor does it disprove it. It simply shows that there at not enough qualitative studies for the time being. Future and better designed studies are needed before any definite conclusions can be made and it is not yet time to throw out the baby with the bathing water.

And further to that, all wavelengths are put into the same basket. Each wavelength has a different therapeutic window.

The search for studies is not too impressing. A number of studies are listed as excluded from the study, and for very good reasons, since they are not at all related to the studied topic (tooth extraction, muscle injuries, etc). If high standard LPT studies in general were to be identified, the list would look quite different. Papers using the dose analysis concept are e.g. [C10, C11]

Let us look at the eleven studies:

Crural ulcers

Franek, Krol, and Kucharzewski, 2002. (810 nm), 4 J/cm^2. No serious objections.

Bihari and Mester, 1989. HeNe, HeNe/830, 4 J/cm^2.
This early positive study does have shortcomings in design and reporting. It is interesting to not that this positive is the only study using HeNe, beside Santoianni, which is the best wavelength for wound healing [C13] but not for pain relief.

Santoianni, Monfrecola, Martellotta et al., 1984. HeNe
Appears as a sound study but a confirmation on the used dosage cannot be extracted from the text.

Lundeberg and Malm, 1991 GaAs. Disqualified study
We have previously criticised these studies for complete lack of dose control and other shortcomings. Lundeberg has been exposed as a scientific cheater. This study is not qualified for any evaluation

Iusim, Kimchy, Pillar, et al., 1992. Not a laser study
The instrument used here is not a laser but an incoherent light source.

Lagan, McKenna, Witherow, et al., 2002. Crural. Not only laser.
This is a combined laser/LED study (660-950 nm) and should therefore be excluded.

Nussbaum, Biemann, and Mustard, 1994. Not laser
The authors used a combination of 820 nm laser and an array of 30 LED:s of three different wavelengths. Thus, again, this is not a laser study.

Crous and Malherbe, 1988.

[B22] Tunér J: What is in the LLLT literature? In (Simunovic Z, ed): Lasers in Medicine and Dentistry, European Medical Laser Assn. 2000; pp 217-226. ISBN 953-6059-30-4.

[B23] Vlassov V V, Pechatnikov L M, MacLehose H G. Low level laser therapy for treating tuberculosis. Cochrane Database Syst Rev. 2002; (3): CD003490.

13.3 An evaluation of the evaluators

As pointed out in several sections in this book, it takes a combined knowledge of medicine, scientific methods and physics to evaluate (or to perform) a study of the therapeutic laser modality. This combination is not always seen, and it can lead to incorrect conclusions. Such incorrect analyses are sometimes the basis for governmental authorities in charge of funding clinical studies and reimbursement.

The basic problem of several negative evaluations is a lack of understanding of laser parameters. For a correct outcome of a study, the researchers must have complete control (and understanding) about the dosage windows and the different properties of the wavelengths. Positive results from laser studies are found within "therapeutic windows" of dosage. If negative and positive studies are carefully scrutinised, it is obvious that the vast majority of negative results is due to low dosage or, rarely, over dosage. This window is fairly wide but most negative reports do not fall within its frame. It is also very important to be able to make an independent analysis of the dosage claimed. It is not uncommon that the dosage is miscalculated.

It has previously been found [C1,C2,C3] that the first three Cochrane evaluations of the effect of LPT [C4,C5,C6] are of little value. The critical comments on [4] is available on the Cochrane home page, but obviously not observed by the several authors, since they do make a reference to the wound healing analysis, but without any of the critical comments. Re-evaluations of negative Meta analyses of LPT for musculoskeletal conditions have turned out positive [C7] if an analysis of the dosage has been included in the study.

As and example of the situation, we have here chosen a report named *Wound-Healing Technologies: Low-Level Laser and Vacuum-Assisted Closure prepared for: Agency for Healthcare Research and Quality, U.S. Department of Health and Human Services*, and prepared by The Blue Cross and Blue Shield Association Technology Evaluation Center Evidence-based Practice Center (EPC) Chicago, Illinois. Year of publication is 2004.

The authors have identified 11 studies meeting the inclusion criteria. Reading the manuscript one can see that the authors are very qualified in the field of medicine and scientific methodology, but still lacking adequate knowledge about the field they are about to evaluate. Pressure ulcers and crural ulcers are "put in the same basket" but do not have same pathology and require different treatment parameters. The main problem with pressure ulcers is that the patient continuously is exposed to the pressure and the possibilities for healing are lower than for crural ulcers. If laser is used and the pressure is removed, healing is faster than for conventional therapy alone [8].

References:

[B1] Flemming K, Cullum N: Laser Therapy for venous leg ulcers (Cochrane review). In: The Cochrane Library, 4, 2000.

[B2] Brosseau L, Welch V, Wells G et al: Low level laser therapy (Classes I, II and III) for treating osteoarthritis. The Cochrane Library. Issue 4, 2000.(Withdrawn)

[B3] Brosseau L, Welch V, Wells G et al: Low level laser therapy (Classes I, II and III) for treating rheumatoid arthritis. The Cochrane Library. Issue 4, 2000.

[B4] Lundeberg T and Malm M: Low power HeNe laser treatment of venous leg ulcers. Annals of Plastic Surgery. 1991; 27: 537-539.

[B5] Malm M and Lundeberg T: Effect of low power gallium arsenide laser on healing of venous ulcers. Scandinavian Journal of Plastic Reconstruction and Hand Surgery. 1991; 25: 249-251.

[B6] Crous L and Malherbe C: Laser and ultraviolet light irradiation in the treatment of chronic ulcers. Physiotherapy. 1988; 44: 73-77.

[B7] Bülow P M, Jensen H and Danneskiold-Samsoe B: Low power GaAlAs laser treatment of painful osteoarthritis of the knee. Scandinavian Journal of Rehabilitation Medicine. 1994; 26: 155-159.

[B8] Basford JR, Sheffield C G, Mair S D, Ilstrup D M: Low-energy helium neon laser treatment of thumb osteoarthritis. Archive of Physical and Medical Rehabilitation. 1987; 68: 794-797.

[B9] Jensen H, Harreby M and Kjær J (1994): Infrared laser – effekt ved smertende knae-arthrose? Ugeskrift for Laeger, 149: 3104-3106.

[B10] Stelian J, Gil I, Habot B et al: Improvement of pain and disability in elderly patients with degenerative osteoarthritis of the knee treated with narrow band light therapy. Journal of the American Geriatric Society. 1992; 40: 23-26.

[B11] Walker J: Relief from chronic pain by low power laser irradiation. Neuroscience Letters. 1983; 43: 339-344.

[B12] Marks R, de Palma F: Clinical efficacy of low power laser therapy in osteoarthritis. Physiotherapy Research International. 1999; 4 (2): 141-147.

[B13] Johannsen F, Hauschild B, Remvig L et al: Low energy laser therapy in rheumatoid arthritis. Scandinavian Journal of Rheumatology. 1994; 23: 145-147.

[B14] Heussler J K, Hinchey G, Margiotta E et al: A double blind randomised trial of low power laser treatment in rheumatoid arthritis. Annals of the Rheumatic Diseases. 1993; 52: 703-706.

[B15] Walker J, Akhanjee L K, Cooney M M et al: Laser therapy for pain of rheumatoid arthritis. Clinical Journal of Pain. 1987; 3: 54-59.

[B16] Hall J, Clarke AK, Elvins DM, Ring EFJ: Low level laser therapy is ineffective in the management of rheumatoid finger joints. British Journal of Rheumatology. 1994; 33: 142-147.

[B17] Goats G C, Flett E, Hunter J A, Sterling A: Low intensity laser and phototherapy for rheumatoid arthritis. Physiotherapy. 1996; 82 (5): 311-320.

[B18] Seichert N: Physiotherapy: Controlled trials and facts. In (Schlapbach P, Gerber NJ eds): Rheumatology. 1991; p. 205-217.

[B19] Gam A N, Thorsen H and Lonnberg F: The effect of low-level laser therapy on musculo-skeletal pain: a Meta-analysis. Pain. 1993; 52: 63-66.

[B20] Bjordal J M, Greve G: "What may alter the conclusions of reviews?". Physical Therapy Reviews. 1998; 3: 121-132.

[B21] Tunér J, Hode L. It´s all in the parameters – a critical analysis of some well-known negative studies on low-level laser therapy. J Clin Lasers Med Surg. 1998; 16 (5): 245-248.

noses, which vary widely in pathology, tissue involved and prognosis. Added to this are all the inadequate treatment procedures and doses that have been employed in clinical LPT trials. Under such circumstances the majority of these trials will find no effect of active treatment. Therefore, we should be very careful when viewing all the trial results together to see if they add up to an effect significantly better than placebo. Future reviews are suggested to analyse the positive studies in order to find out what parameters seem to work. Subgroup analyses are of particular importance. Dosage analysis cannot be limited to the groups "high" and "low" because of the great variations in dosage. Neither can any wavelength be put into the "high" or "low" basket. 2 J HeNe for a finger joint may be "high" while 20 J HeNe for lumbar problem may be "low". GaAs requires lower doses than GaAlAs etc.

So what have these new Cochrane reviews brought us? Two distinct steps of progress can be identified. In the rheumatoid arthritis review, attempts have been made to evaluate effects separately for high and low dose. And secondly, they even give a (qualified) recommendation: "Low level laser therapy could be considered for treatment of rheumatoid arthritis for its short term effect and lack of side effects".

Future directions

Both laser researchers and reviewers have common responsibilities in enhancing our understanding of LPT The three mentioned Cochrane reviews on laser therapy have drawn some conclusions, to which we can comment that the literature on the evaluated indications was ambiguous at the time of publiction, the average quality of the studies is not very high and the number of relevant studies is rather low. It can therefore be postulated that there was still insufficient scientific support for the general use of Laser Therapy for the three indications reviewed by the Cochrane evaluators and that only moderate and short-term effects could be confirmed. However, the review methodology should include valid criteria for dose and target for laser irradiation (e.g. synovia, triggerpoints, acupuncture points, peripheral nerves, etc). Furthermore, the effect calculations could be performed for subgroups of different doses, treatment frequencies and laser types. There is also still room for improvement of the literature search. Further, reviewers must make their own dosage calculations, not taking the doses quoted in the studies for granted. Too many of the negative laser therapy studies contain serious flaws [B21], and such flaws must be firmly investigated when evaluating laser therapy studies.

In a recent Cohrane analysis of laser therapy Vlassov [B23] found no effect of laser therapy on tuberculosis. Owing to the incoherent literature on the subject, no dosage analyses could be performed in this study.

formed but the wide gap in dosages does not justify a subgroup analysis of merely two groups.

Hall [B16] and Goats [B17] used combined coherent and non-coherent light. Combined single wavelength coherent light and multi-wavelengths non-coherent light is a poorly studied area and there is no ground for postulating that they produce the same biological effects when used in various combinations or alone.

The Meta analysis by Gam [B19] (one of the Cochrane co-authors) is referred to. This analysis did not find any effect of LPT for musculoskeletal pain. The re-evaluation of the same studies made by Bjordal [B20] found a clear effect when an analysis of the dosage and therapeutic techniques was included. This latter Meta-analysis is not mentioned. Critical comments on the Cochrane reviews are supposed to be continuosly included. Bjordal writes:

"Gam et al made a firm statement that LLLT has no effect in musculoskeletal disorders. As already indicated, this review is highly sensitive to changes in inclusion criteria and demonstrates cirtical errors in data synthesis, which calls for considerable caution in making any conclusions at all. The statistical pooling in this review cannot be regarded as valid because of the large variation of trial designs, treatment procedures, dosage and diagnoses. In all, the conclusion of this review was assessed as invalid, because it did not adhere strictly to the available evidence, especially for subgroups."

Conclusions

The evaluators of the Cochrane groups have been successful in finding many of the relevant studies in the literature. Several interesting observations have been made and a skilful analysis of the design parameters has been performed. Evaluation of effects is a universal problem for all empirically developed therapies, where consensus of a clearly defined optimal dose range and adequate treatment procedure is lacking. For clinicians practicing LPT it is hard to understand why the reviewers have neglected some important factors, e.g. body area treated, size of area and dose. The methodology used seems to be that of drug studies. But drugs and LPT are quite different. Oral intake of a drug is the universal procedure. LPT can be applied in several ways, such as local irradiation, trigger point irradiation, acupuncture irradiation and irradiation over peripheral nerves. All these methods must be evaluated separately.

The biggest problem has been the fact that most of the reviews have "put into the same basket" a variety of doses, energy densities and treatment procedures. New treatment methods are often subject to trials where clinicians include all their non-responding patients, and the early laser literature is no exception. Flaws in LPT studies are not uncommon [B21]. The laser literature in the year 2000 included about 100 positive and 40 negative double blind trials [B22] on a heterogeneous sample of more than 20 different diag-

(see Rheumatoid arthritis below) used a dose above the generally accepted dosage window. In retrospect, the Bülow trial has been criticised for overlooking a significant short-term effect of active laser treatment by only testing the statistical significance at follow-up. Stelian used 55 times more energy than Jensen for knee osteoarthritis! The Jadad quality scale is applied correctly to the studies. But without inclusion of the laser parameters in the scale, evaluation tends to become a "study design beauty contest" instead of an evaluation of therapeutical significance.

In a re-evaluation of the Cochrane OA report Bjordal [1506] summarizes:

"This Cochrane review of LLLT for osteoarthritis contained possible data errors and trial omissions which were crucial for the direction of the conclusion. The review also lacked transparency in data selections for main results calculations and the review did not adhere to the study protocol for subgroup analyses. Our sensitivity analysis showed that the negative review conclusion could be altered to a positive conclusion without changing the criteria of the review protocol by including omitted data. Performance of lacking subgroup-analyses also revealed a highly significant dose-dependent effect from LLLT. Identification of 18 possible omissions, errors and equivocal data interpretations, revealed that 17 of these questionable selections supported the review conclusion. These findings challenge the assumption that Cochrane reviews are always reliable and unbiased. In areas of controversy, extra care must be taken to maintain validity and reliability of SRs. Thorough sensitivity analyses seem to be the most effective tool for testing how robust review conclusions really are. Transparency is needed to improve methods and reduce subjective preferences in reviews from controversial areas."

This paper [2] has been now been withdrawn by the Cochrane Collaboration.

3. Rheumatoid arthritis

Eight of 191 articles met the inclusion criteria; five were Randomised Controlled Trials. Five further studies are waiting assessment pending answers from the authors.

Comments:

Johannsen [B13] (negative outcome) used 11.9 J GaAlAs laser per finger joint, which is a high dose, maybe too high.
Heussler [B14] (negative outcome) used 1.5 J GaAlAs laser per finger joint.
Walker [B15] (positive outcome) used less than 1 mW of HeNe laser. Although Johannsen used a dose 1700 times higher than Walker, both studies are "put in the same basket". A low/high dose evaluation is actually per-

thus receive 0.6 J/cm² and the largest wound 0.046 J/cm², not the 1.96 J/cm² stated by the authors. Energy densities as well as dose for larger wounds is thus low. Treatment technique is not indicated. The report states that: "the laser was held perpendicular to the surface of the wound". This is not a sufficient description of the treatment method. There is a great difference between following the outer border of the wound (active healing area) and spreading the beam over the open wound area. The distance between diode and wound is not indicated. It is furthermore of interest to know that one of the authors have been exposed as a scientific cheater.

In summary, the energy level said to be applied in these studies must be questioned. The Cochrane evaluators have not observed the essential contradiction between the actual dose and the dose indicated by the authors. Further, in one of the four studies [6] the laser wavelength and dose are not stated in the original paper. This makes an evaluation impossible.

2. Osteoarthritis

Five trials were included out of 142 potentially relevant articles. Six abstracts are awaiting assessment after the authors have been contacted for further details. In the meantime, some comments on the analysis follows:

Bülow [B7] (negative outcome) is a good study using a reasonable energy level (GaAlAs laser 22.5 J/session) for painful knee osteoarthritis. However, see discussion below about chosen outcome measurements.

Basford [B8] (negative outcome) used HeNe laser 0.007 J per point for thumb arthritis. The dose used is virtually meaningless since it is too low.

Jensen [B9] (negative outcome) used GaAs laser, 0.2 J in total, for painful knee arthrosis. Here, too, the dose used is very low and below the dose levels that have been reported to be effective.

Stelian [B10] (positive outcome) used GaAlAs laser around 11 J per session, twice daily, amounting to 22 J per knee per day, 10 consecutive days. This study has a dose that is acceptable even in the light of today's experience, although it was published as early as 1992. The outcome of this study stands in contrast to the rather similar study by Bülow. The dose is the same, and the number of sessions is almost the same (10/9). However, Bülow applied the treatment 2-4 times a week, Stelian twice daily.

Walker [B11] (positive outcome) is a classic positive study, but the use of a HeNe laser of less than 1 mW throws doubt on this study. In our opinion it should not be used as anything but a purely historical reference.

The crucial criticism of the evaluation of the studies above is that there is no discussion about dosage! On the Jadad quality scale (1-5), Basford is given 3 and Bülow 2. However, Basford used a non-significant dosage for a finger joint while Bülow has a reasonable dose for knee osteoarthritis. Johannsen

13.2 The Cochrane LPT analyses – can they be improved?

The aim of the international Cochrane collaboration is to continuously evaluate new and old medical therapies. The basis for the systematic reviews is the recognition of Randomised Controlled Trials as the "gold standard" for scientific evaluation of small and moderate effects from treatment. A thorough search is made for the available literature and the most "qualified" studies are analysed. The purpose of the analysis is to find out whether or not there is any solid support for a specific medical treatment modality. Such analyses are published in medical journals and extended versions are quarterly updated in the Cochrane Library. Since the Cochrane reviews are influential, it is important that the persons performing them possess a thorough knowledge of all aspects of LPT.

Introduction

Five systematic reviews on the effectiveness of LPT have been published in the Cochrane Library. Three reviews have evaluated the effect of LPT for Venous ulcers [B1] Osteoarthritis [B2] and Rheumatoid arthritis [B3]. However, the Cochrane style of reviewing has been criticised [B20] for not taking into account the variability of diagnoses, treatment procedures and dosages of the included trials. The impact of the Cochrane Library in the field of medicine is profound. It is therefore essential to "evaluate the evaluation", to find out whether or not these analyses can live up to the prestige of the Cochrane Library. The following text is a critical "analysis of the analyses".

1. Venous ulcers

Four trials are analysed: two comparing laser with placebo, one comparing laser with non-coherent light and one comparing laser with ultraviolet light. Two studies comparing laser with placebo were reported by the same investigators [B4, B5]. In the first report a 6 mW HeNe laser was used. 4 J/cm^2 was said to be given to the ulcers. Ulcer size ranged from 3-32 cm^2. Treatment technique was not stated. Regardless of technique, it would take between 36 minutes and 6 hours to achieve the stated dose per wound and session. Using a sweep technique with a focused beam, the power density would be around 0.15 W/cm^2. If a defocused beam were used to cover the entire largest wound (32 cm^2), energy density would be around 0.00019 W/cm^2, which is extremely low, lower than the energy density of the normal illumination in a medical clinic. A dose miscalculation is probable but the authors of the study have been reluctant to reveal the parameters used. In the absence of such parameters, this study cannot be properly evaluated, but very low power density is a probable reason for its negative results. In the second study [B5] on venous ulcer, GaAs was employed. 4 mW was used for 10 minutes on ulcers ranging from 4 to 52 cm^2, regardless of ulcer size. The 4 cm^2 wound would

[A30] Lundeberg T, Malm M: Low power HeNe laser treatment of venous leg ulcers. Ann Plast Surg. 1991; 27: 537-539.

[A31] Hall J et al: Low level laser therapy is ineffective in the management of rheumatoid arthritic finger joints. Br J Rheuma. 1994; 33: 142-147.

[A32] Beckerman H et al: The efficacy of laser therapy for mucoskeletal and skin disorders: a criteria-based Meta-analysis of randomized clinical trials. Physical Therapy. 1992; 7 (72): 483-.

[A33] Gam A N et al: The effect of low-level laser therapy on musculo-skeletal pain: a Meta-analysis. Pain. 1993; 52: 63-66.

[A34] Baxter C D: Therapeutic lasers. Theory and practice. 1994. Churchill Livingstone.

[A35] Karu T: Photobiological Fundamentals of Low Power Laser Therapy. IEEE Journal of Quantum Electronics. 1987; QE23(10): 1703-1717.

[A36] Yamamoto Y et al.: Effect of low-power laser irradiation on procollagen synthesis in human fibroblasts. J Clin Laser Med Surg. 1996; 14 (3): 129-132.

[A37] Malm M, Lundeberg T.: Effect of low power gallium arsenide laser on healing of venous ulcers. Scand J Plast Reconstr Hand Surg. 1991; 25: 249-251.

[A38] Lundeberg T et al: Low power laser irradiation does not affect the generation of signals in a sensory receptor. Am J Chinese Med. 1998; 16 (3-4): 87-91.

[A39] Siebert W et al: What is the efficacy of "soft" and "mid" lasers in therapy of tendinopathies? A double-blind study. Archives of Orthopaedic & Traumatic Surgery 1987; 106 (6): 358-63.

[A40] Mulcahy D. et al: Low level laser therapy: a prospective double blind trial of its use in an orthopaedic population. Injury. 1995; 26 (5): 315-317.

[A41] Bjordal J M, Greve G : "What may alter the conclusions of reviews ?". Physical Therapy Reviews. 1998; 3: 121-132.

[A42] Lundeberg T, Hode L, Zhou J: A comparative study of the pain-relieving effect of laser treatment and acupuncture. Acta Physiol Scand. 1987; 131: 161-.

[A43] de Bie RA, de Vet HC, Lenssen TF, van den Wildenberg FA, Kootstra G, Knipschild PG: Low-level laser therapy in ankle sprains: a randomized clinical trial. Arch Phys Med Rehabil. 1998; 79 (11): 1415-1420.

[A44] Bounkeo J M, Brannon W M, Dawes Jr K S et al: The efficacy of laser therapy in the treatment of wounds: a Meta analysis of the literature. Proc. 3rd Congress of the World Ass for Laser Therapy, Athens, Greece, 2000, page 79.

[A45] Parker J, Dowdy D, Harkness E et al: The effects of laser therapy on tissue repair and pain control. A Meta analysis of the literature. Proc. 3rd Congress of the World Ass for Laser Therapy, Athens, Greece, 2000, page 77.

[A46] Kaiser C et al: Estudio en doble ciego randomizado sobre la eficacia del HeNe en el tratamiento de la sinuitis maxilar aguda: en pacientes con exacerbación de una infección sinusal crónica. [Double blind randomised study on the effect of HeNe in the treatment of acute maxillary sinusitis; in patients with exacerbation of a chronic maxillary sinuitis]. Boletín CDL. 1986; 9: 15. Also in Av Odontoestomatol. 1987; 3 (2): 73-76.

[A47] Bjordal J M, Couppé C, Ljunggren A E: Low level laser for tencinopathy. Evidence of a dose-response pattern. Physical Therapy Reviews. 2001; 6: 91-99.

[A48] Kopera D, Kokol R, Berger C, Haas J. Does the use of low-level laser influence wound healing in chronic venous ulcers? J Wound Care. 2005; 14 (8): 391-394.

[A9] Basford J R et al: Low-energy Helium Neon laser treatment of thumb osteoarthritis. Arch Phys Med Rehab. 1987; 68: 794-797.

[A10] Taube S, Piironen J, Ylipaavalniemi P: Helium-neon laser therapy in the prevention of postoperative swelling and pain after wisdom tooth extraction. Proc Finn Dent Soc 1990; 86: 23-27.

[A11] Lundeberg T, Haker E, Thomas M: Effect of laser versus placebo in tennis elbow. Scand J of Rehab Med. 1987; 19 (3): 135-138.

[A12] Masse J-F et al: Effectiveness of soft laser treatment in periodontal surgery. Int Dent J. 1993; 43: 121-127.

[A13] Smith R J et al: The effect of low-energy laser on skin-flap survival in the rat and porcine animal models. Plastic and Reconstruct Surg. 1992; 89 (2): 306-310.

[A14] Klein R et al: Low-energy laser treatment and exercise for chronic low back pain: a double-blind controlled trial. Arch Phys Med Rehabil. 1990; 71: 34-37.

[A15] Krikorian D et al: Use of HeNe laser for treatment of soft tissue trauma: evaluation by Gallium-67 Citrate scanning. J Orthop Sports Phys Ther. 1986; 8 (2): 93-97.

[A16] Zarkovic N et al: Effect of semiconductor GaAs laser irradiation on pain perception in mice. Lasers in Surgery and Medicine. 1989; 9: 63-66.

[A17] Jarvis D et al: Electrophysiologic recording and thermodynamic modelling demonstrate that Helium-Neon laser irradiation does not affect peripheral A - or C-fiber nociceptors. Pain. 1990. 43: 235-242.

[A18] Hansen H, Thorøe U: Low power laser biostimulation of chronic orofacial pain. A double-blind placebo controlled cross-over study in 40 patients. Pain. 1990; 43: 169-.

[A19] Moustsen P et al: Laserbehandling af bihulebetændelse i almen lægepraxis vurderet ved en dobbeltblind kontrolleret undersøgelse. (In Danish). Ugeskrift Læger. 1991; 153(32): 2232-. [Laser Treatment of Sinuitis in General Medical Praxis Evaluated in a double blind study].

[A20] Braverman B et al: Effect of Helium-Neon and Infrared Laser Irrradiation on Wound Healing in Rabbits. Lasers in Surgery and Medicine. 1989; 9: 50.

[A21] Rochkind S. et al: Systemic Effects of Low-Power Laser Irradiation on the Peripheral and Central Nervous System, Cutaneous Wounds and Burns. Lasers in Surgery and Medicine. 1989; 9: 174.

[A22] Airaksinen, O et al: Effects of laser irradiation at the treated and non-treated trigger points. Proc. 4th Intern Symposium. Acupunc & Electrother Res. 1988; 13 (4): 238-239.

[A23] Inoue K et al: Suppressed tuberculine reaction in guinea pigs following laser irradiation. Lasers in Surgery and Medicine, 1989; 9: 271-275.

[A24] Schindl L et al: Influence of low-power laser irradiation on "arthus phenomenon" induced in rabbit cornea. Laser Therapy. 1994; 1; 23. (abstract)

[A25] Rydén H, Persson L Preber H, Bergström J: Effect of low-energy laser on gingival inflammation. Swedish Dental Journ. 1994; 18: 35-41.

[A26] Kusakari H, Orikasa N, Tani H: Effects of low power laser on wound healing of gingiva and bone. Laser Bologna '92, p. 49. Monduzzi Editore S.p.A., Bologna, Italy.

[A27] Kozlov V et al: Lasers in diagnostics and treatment of microcirculation disorders under parodontitis. Proc SPIE. 1995; Vol 1984: 253-264.

[A28] Steinlechner C, Dyson M: The effect of low level laser therapy on the proliferation of keratinocytes. Laser Therapy. 1993; 5 (2): 65.

[A29] van Breugel H et al: Power density and exposure time of HeNe laser irradiation are more important than total energy dose in photo-biomodulation of human fibroblasts in vitro. Lasers in Surgery and Medicine. 1992; 12: 528-.

- Conclusions: Neither high nor low-dose LPT is effective in the treatment of lateral ankle sprains

Our comments

de Bie et al came to the conclusion that LPT has no effect on ankle sprains. This is an obvious misinterpretation of the presented results. Instead the laser treatment had a clear NEGATIVE effect on all studied parameters. There are several studies showing that LPT, on the indication chosen and with the parameters used, had no better effect than placebo. However, among the 2500 studies known to us, no study has reported such a clear negative effect of LPT, except for a few studies using doses clearly in the inhibiting dose range. Further, irradiating one single small area for ankle sprain does not appear to be optimal.

Conclusion

In studying the therapeutic effects of laser light, there are many pitfalls along the way, and many researchers have fallen in. Unfortunately, their work is still cited as evidence that LPT does not work. In fact, many of these older studies should be disregarded in future discussions on this subject, since they are clearly irrelevant.

Meta-analyses, too, may also prove meaningless unless pitfalls of this type can be avoided. In our analysis we have criticised a number of well-known negative studies, and it would be right to insist that a number of positive studies should be subjected to critical scrutiny as well. Positive studies have, however, been the subject of critical comment for many years, whereas only Baxter [A34] and Bjordal [A41] [A47] have hitherto made a detailed analysis of the parameters of negative studies.

Litterature:

[A1] Walker J: Relief from Chronic Pain by Low Power Laser Irradiation. Neuroscience Letters. 1983; 43: 339-344.

[A2] Snyder-Mackler L et al: Effect of helium-neon laser irradiation on skin resistance and pain in patients with trigger points in the neck or back. Physical Therapy. 1989; 69: 336-341.

[A3] Snyder-Mackler L et al: Effect of helium-neon laser on musculoskeletal trigger points. Physical Therapy. 1986; 66: 1087-1090.

[A4] Mester E et al: Effects of laser rays on wound healing. Am J Surg. 1971; 122: 532-535.

[A5] Kana J S et al: Effect of low-power density laser radiation on healing of open skin wounds in rats. Arch Surg. 1981; Vol 116: 293-.

[A6] Waylonis G W et al: Chronic myofascial pain: management by low-output helium-neon laser therapy. Arch Phys Med Rehab. 1988; 69: 1017-.

[A7] Jensen H et al: Infrarød laser - effekt ved smertende knæartrose? Ugerskr Læger. 1987; 149-.

[A8] Seichert N et al: Wirkung einer Infrarot-Laser-Therapie bei weichteilrheumatischen Beschwerden in Doppel-blindversuch. Terapiwoche. 1987; 37: 1375-1379.

when several persons are involved in a study, it is not unlikely that mistakes occur. This may or may not be the case in the following study by de Bie [A43]:

Author:	de Bie et al Ref no: [A44]
Title:	Low-level laser therapy in ankle sprains: a randomized clinical trial
Published in:	Arch Phys Med Rehabil 1998 Nov;79(11):1415-20
Laser type:	GaAs
Output:	Not stated
Pulsing:	Pulsed
Pulse repetition rate:	500, 5 000 Hz
Dose:	0.5 and 5 J/cm^2 "on skin"
Power density:	Not stated
Treatment distance:	Not stated
Laser model:	Not stated
Treated area:	1 cm^2
Treatment time:	Not stated
No. of patients:	217
No. of sessions:	12
Time between sessions:	2-3 days

Table 13.11 de Bie et al

The investigators obtained the following results:

- Function was significantly better in the placebo group at 10 days ($p = 0.01$) and 14 days ($p = 0.03$).
- Placebo group performed significantly better on number of days of sick leave ($p = 0.02$) and at some points of hindrance in daily life activities and pressure pain.
- Placebo group performed significantly better on subjective recovery ($p=0.05$).
- Total number of days of absence from work and sports was remarkably lower in the placebo group than in the laser group, the difference being 3.7 to 5.3 and 6 to 8 days, respectively.
- The total number of relapses at 1 year in the laser group ($n = 35$) was significantly higher than in the placebo group ($n = 13$).

studied. The stretch receptor of Astacus fluviais (crayfish) was mounted over a glass platform. HeNe 1.56 mW and GaAs 0.07 mW, 73 Hz, was used, dose not indicated. Dissecting and mounting the stretch receptor was done under the microscope, using very bright broadband light. This disturbing factor must be taken into account when evaluating similar trials.

10. Premature conclusions

Some researchers have used titles or conclusions such as "laser therapy is ineffective in...". This is an unscientific approach, since these reports have only investigated a few of the many possible parameters. The language used reflects an unscientific bias. An example [A42] of this is: "Our results indicate that the analgesic effects reported in humans with similar modes of laser therapy might be due to placebo" (comparison of response time on tail-flick between laser acupuncture, morphine and electrical stimulation).

11. Meta-analyses

Several Meta-analyses [A32, A33, A41, A44, A45] of the clinical effects of LPT have been performed. In one, various studies were graded by points on the basis of a number of quality criteria. By this means, a negative study may achieve a high grade even if one of the parameters is entirely wrong, though it may be essential to the result of the study. In Beckerman's work [A32], for example, Basford's study [A9] has been given the highest score (18 out of a possible 25) in spite of the fact that the dose used is not actually therapeutic. A comparison might be made with a chain: it is no use having 19 perfectly sound links if the 20th is open. By dividing the studies into two groups - studies with low and with reasonable dosage - Bjordal [A41], found a higher validity for the same studies than Gam [A33] did. Regarding the Beckerman study, Bjordal writes:

> "Beckerman et al. concluded that LLLT seemed to be efficient for three diagnoses (myofascial pain, rheumatoid arthritis or post-traumatic joint disorders). However, this conclusion is based on only a single trial (of acceptable standard) for each diagnosis; it would therefore appear that more caution should be called for in this case, as the conclusion is not supported by replication of trial results and sufficient statistical power."

12. Confusion between groups

One of the authors (LH) took part in a double-blind study several years ago. When the code was to be broken, the investigator entrusted with the envelope could not find it. There was certainly a significant difference between the two groups. However, it is not ethical to decide which group is supposed to be the placebo group just by looking at the outcome of the study, so the whole study had to be cancelled. Knowing how easy it is for codes to be mixed up, for documents to be mixed up and for misunderstandings to arise

If a defocused beam were used to cover the entire wound of 32 cm^2, energy density would be around 0.00019 W/cm^2, which is extremely low, lower than the energy density of the normal illumination in an operating theatre. A dose miscalculation is probable, but the authors of the study have been reluctant to reveal the parameters used. In the absence of such parameters, this study cannot be properly evaluated, but very low power density is a probable reason for its negative results. In another study on venous ulcers by Malm [A37] and Lundeberg, GaAs was employed. 4 mW was used for 10 minutes on ulcers ranging from 4 to 52 cm^2, regardless of ulcer size. The 4 cm^2 wound would thus receive 0.6 J/cm^2 and the largest wound 0.046 J/cm^2, not the 1.96 J/cm^2 stated by the authors. Energy densities as well as dose for larger wounds are thus low. Treatment technique is not indicated. "The laser was held perpendicular to the surface of the wound". This is not a sufficient description of the treatment method. There is a great difference between following the outer border of the wound (active healing area) and spreading the beam over the open wound area. It is also important to know the shape of the invisible GaAs beam. The distance between diode and wound is not indicated.

8. Mixed parameters

A study by Hall [A31] is confidently entitled "Low level laser therapy is ineffective in the management of rheumatoid arthritic finger joints". Such a title suggests that all reasonable parameters (wavelengths, doses, pulsing, etc.) have been checked and are kept properly under control. One of the probes used is a so-called cluster probe having a 15 mW GaAlAs laser diode surrounded by 30 non-coherent light-emitting diodes of three different wavelengths. Which wavelength was effective, which was ineffective, and did any particular wavelength have a detrimental effect on the overall result?

Blending coherent and non-coherent light while giving therapy with light of different wavelengths may possibly result in some clinical improvement but may also result in less improvement than if the therapy had been more exactly controlled. Karu, for example, has showed that in cell cultures first irradiated with laser light and showing a clearly demonstrable biological effect, the effect is reduced practically to zero if the cells are then irradiated with broad-band (non-monochrome, incoherent) light [A36]. The main objection to mixed parameters in research is that they do not result in unequivocal new knowledge.

9. The influence of ambient light

The influence of ambient light is not a clinical problem. In the laboratory, however, it may influence the outcome of a study. As mentioned above, Karu [A35] has shown that the effect of laser light may be partly or completely washed out by broadband light. In a study by Lundeberg [A38] the effect of HeNe and GaAs laser on the generation of signals in a sensory receptor was

ing an ischemic area. The ischemia will increase the penetration of the laser beam.

5. Systemic effects

The systemic effect of therapeutic laser light has been described by many researchers, such as Braverman [A20], Rochkind [A21], Airaksinen [A22], Inoue [A23] and Schindl [A24]. Essentially, a systemic effect is one where treatment of a given complaint at one site will also tend to affect a similar complaint elsewhere. It is therefore important to observe caution in interpreting the results of studies in which one part of the body of a test person/animal has been treated by laser and another part of the same body has been used as a control, especially in studies on small animals.

6. Tissue condition

Rydén [A25] observed no effect on angiogenesis in a study of experimental human gingivitis. Although this finding is confirmed in a study by Kusakari [A26], this author does report LPT as causing an increased flow of blood, which was not studied in Rydén's work. Both studies, however, are marred by the fact that healthy humans/animals were used as test subjects. Gingivitis was, in these studies, induced in young, perfectly healthy individuals whose immune system was in excellent order. A study by Kozlov [A27] reports that LPT had a moderate effect on slight periodontitis, a good effect on more manifest periodontitis, and little effect on advanced periodontitis. The immunological condition of the tissue and of the individual is a significant factor in the effectiveness of LPT, and a "genuine" clinical condition cannot be achieved in a study based on healthy volunteers. This may explain the discrepancy sometimes noted between clinical work and scientific tests.

The significance of the condition of the tissue can clearly be seen in an experiment by Steinlechner [A28] in which keratinocytes, present in 1% and 5% solutions of fetal calf serum, were irradiated with laser light. The cells in the less nutritious solution were more highly stimulated. The same observation has been made by Yamamoto [A36], irradiating human fibroblasts. There is reason to believe that the outcome of many *in vitro* studies has been just as influenced by the nutrient conditions of the cells as by the laser parameters.

7. Power density

According to a study by van Breugel [A29], power density appears to be more important than total dose in wound healing. Lundeberg [A30] used a 6 mW HeNe laser to treat venous leg ulcers. 4 J/cm^2 was said to be applied to the ulcers. Ulcer size ranged from 3-32 cm^2. Treatment technique is not stated. Regardless of technique, it would take between 36 minutes and 6 hours to achieve the stated dose per wound and session. Using a sweep technique with a focused beam, the power density would be around 0.15 W/cm^2.

laser produced an output of 6.5 mW. One group was given GaAs + HeNe, another HeNe with the GaAs diodes switched off (the placebo group). As both the "verum group" (0.258 J/cm^2) and the "placebo group" (0.134 J/cm^2) were actually treated by laser, there is in fact no control group here. The comparison made is not between laser and placebo but between a combination GaAs + HeNe laser and a HeNe laser.

In the study by Kopera [A48] a 685 nm InGaAlAs laser of 200 mW was used in a group of 44 patients with chronic venous ulcers. The outcome of the study is negative. Let us look at some possible reasons for the negative outcome. First of all, the only information given about dose and treatment technique is that the dose was 4 J/cm^2 and it is stated that the laser equipment calculated this dose acc. to the size of the wound. The accuracy of this cannot be estimated due to the lack of information about applied energy per point, total energy, continuous or pulsed, spot size and power density. As for treatment technique we do not know if the wound area was treated or the periphery of the wound (where healing is initiated) or both and, if so, at what fluences. In the placebo group an incoherent polychromatic commercial LED light source with a red glass window was used. No information is given about wavelength or power of the LED:s. It is known that LED:s can be used for superficial tissues such as wounds [1503, 1513, 1541, 1593, 1594], so the use of an LED array cannot be dismissed as a "placebo" light. In fact, the study quotes Gupta [720] as a laser study on wound healing, but it is in fact a LED study. The possibility of getting a clinical effect from the LED unit used as placebo is further underlined by the fact that this group had a better mean outcome than the control (traditional therapy) and laser group. The patients were treated during a period of 28 days. It is well known that venous ulcers are difficult to treat and require an extended therapy time. In short, this study leaves the reader much in the dark.

4. Therapeutic technique

Moustsen [A19] did not find any effect of LPT in sinuitis. Using 830 nm, four skin points close to the nose were irradiated, 3 J per point. This is a fair dose for reducing the mucosal oedema in the nostrils and opening the communication with the sinuses. However, in order to influence the actual inflammation inside the sinuses, intraoral irradiation [A46] is necessary. 4-6 J over 3-4 points over the palatinal bony wall plus 4-6 J over two points from the buccal side is recommended. Irradiation over the ethmoidal frontal sinuses is also recommended.

When using LPT the actual target site must always be understood and the approximate dose in the target area must be estimated. "One joule" at the surface with light skin contact may be utterly useless while "one joule" with pressure over the actual target area may be quite effective. With pressure, the probe comes physically closer to the target and blood is forced away, creat-

method) and rating on a pain scale for resting pain, movement pain, and pressure pain before treatment, after treatment, and 2 weeks after conclusion of therapy, as well as infrared thermography, served to check therapy. After the end of therapy, a significant reduction ($P = < 0.001$) of 50% was shown for resting pain as well as reductions of 30% for movement and 30% for pressure pain. This result was identical in the therapy group and in the placebo group. There was also no indication of a different result of therapy between the therapy and placebo groups with regard to the thermographic control and the extent of movement. The breakdown of the data in terms of age, sex, and duration of disease did not provide any indications of different results for placebo or therapy. It was striking that the patients who reported sensations during or after the treatment (irrespective of whether pleasant or unpleasant) had a greater reduction of pain than the patients without sensations. This laser therapy thus did not show any effect above and beyond that in the untreated group".

Baxter: "Despite being highly critical of the standard of previous laser research, these investigators employed a non-contact technique in their trial, irradiating the patients' skin from a distance of 10 cm. Given the beam divergence of clinical laser therapy apparatus, the use of such a distance would appear to be inappropriate, producing minimal power and energy densities on the irradiated tissue. This, coupled with the apparent inaccuracies in calculation of dosage (by a factor of 10), casts serious doubts upon the reliability and validity of the reported findings".

2. Inclusion criteria

In a study by Hansen [A18], 40 patients suffering from various "chronic orofacial pains" were laser treated. The pain had on average lasted 4.9 years (0.5 - 42 years). Twenty-eight patients suffered from "burning mouth syndrome" (oral dysesthesia), five from toothache in one single tooth, three from tension headaches, etc. There were no objective pathological findings. X-ray examination had revealed nothing. In the headache group, acrylic splints had proved ineffective. A painful tooth was vital and normal on X-ray. A GaAs laser was used, and the initial dose of 2.4 J/cm^2 was increased to 4.8 J/cm^2 if no effect was observed initially. According to the literature (quoted in the study), Burning Mouth Syndrome is considered to be either multi-factorial, psychosomatic or purely psychogenic. It is therefore safe to assume that the tissue treated for this study was healthy in every respect. That no pain relief was obtained, and that there was an absence of 5-HIAA in the patients' urine, is therefore only to be expected.

3. Lack of proper control groups

Seichert [A8] (see above) used a combined GaAs/HeNe laser in a study of patients suffering from various rheumatic complaints. The probes contained five GaAs diodes producing an output of 1.2 mW per diode, while the HeNe

Author:	Mulcahy D et al　　　　　　　　Ref no: [A41]
Title:	Low level laser therapy: a prospective double blind trial of its use in an orthopaedic population.
Published in:	Injury. 1995; 26 (5): 315-317.
Laser type:	Not stated
Output:	35 mW
Pulsing:	Not stated
Pulse repetition rate:	Not stated
Dose:	1 J/cm^2 "of skin"
Power density:	Not stated
Treatment distance:	Not stated
Laser model:	Not stated
Treated area:	Not stated
Treatment time:	Not stated
No. of patients:	20
No. of sessions:	8
Time between sessions:	2-4 days

Table 13.10 Mulcahy D et al

Our comments: Very little is known about the parameters, such as wavelength, pulsing/continuous and treatment technique. The indications are plantar fasciitis, trochanteric bursitis, tendinitis, lateral epicondylitis, knee pain, cervical pain and lumbar pain. If applied in the compressive mode, 1 J/cm^2 may be a reasonable dose (though on the low side) for some of the indications but is certainly subclinical for indications such as cervical pain and lumbago. The list could be made much longer. For example, Krikorian [A15] used a HeNe laser and a dose of 0.05 J/cm^2 to study wound healing in rats. Zarkovic [A16] used a GaAs laser and a dose of 0.0004 J/cm^2 to study pain perception in mice. Using a HeNe laser and a dose of 0.004 J/cm^2, Jarvis [A17] could (naturally) find no evidence of stimulation of thermoreceptors in humans.

It is interesting to quote the abstract of the negative study by Siebert [A40] and then compare it to the analysis made by Baxter [A35].

Siebert: "The efficacy of "athermic" lasers (HeNe/GaAs) in the treatment of tendinopathies was investigated in a randomised double-blind study. On 10 consecutive days, 64 patients (32 therapy, 32 placebo) were treated for 15 minutes each with a switched-on or switched-off laser under otherwise identical conditions. The extent of movement in involved joints (neutral 0

Author:	Seichert N. et al: Ref no: [A8]
Title:	Wirkung einer Infrarot-Laser-Therapie bei weichteilrheumatischen Beschwerden ...
Published in:	Therapiewoche, 1987; 37: 1375-1379.
Laser type (1):	GaAs-laser (904 nm)
Output: (each of 5 diodes):	1.2 mW average power
Pulsing:	Yes. 200 ns pulse width
Pulse repetition rate:	1200 Hz
Laser type (2):	HeNe-laser (633 nm)
Output:	6.5 mW
Pulsing:	Continuous
Pulse repetition rate:	-
Dose:	Not specified
Power density:	Not specified
Treatment distance:	15 cm
Laser model:	Space Laser MIX 5
Treated area:	Circular area, 6 cm diameter = 28 cm^2
Treatment time:	10 min = 600 sec
No. of patients:	18
No. of sessions:	5
Time between sessions:	

Table 13.9 Seichert N et al

Our comments: Although the author claims that his instrument is a GaAlAs laser, it is clear from the wavelength (as from the brand) that it is actually a GaAs laser. The dose is not explicitly stated, but for the GaAs laser can be calculated as $600 \times 0.0012 \times 5/28 = 0.128$ J/cm^2. On top of this comes the HeNe dose, which is more or less the same (0.139 J/cm^2). See below for the purported double-blind procedure.

Author:	Klein R G et al Ref no: [A14]
Title:	Low-energy laser treatment and exercise for chronic low back pain: double-blind controlled trial.
Published in:	Arch Phys Med Rehab. 1990; 71: 34-37
Laser type:	GaAs (904 nm)
Output:	10 diodes, each 0.4 mW
Pulsing:	Pulsed
Pulse repetition rate:	1000 Hz
Dose:	Stated: 1.3 J/cm^2 per point. Calculated: 0.1 J/cm^2
Power density:	Not specified
Treatment distance:	Not specified
Laser model:	Omniprobe
Treated area:	L4-L5, L5-S1 apophyseal capsules, ligaments
Treatment time:	4 min per point
No. of patients:	20
No. of sessions:	12
Time between sessions:	Three times per week

Table 13.8 Klein R G et al

Our comments: The authors state that a GaAs laser was used to produce a point dose of 1.3 J/cm^2, the indication being the heterogeneous diagnosis of "low back pain". However, an analysis of the parameters given shows that the dose was in fact only 0.1 J/cm^2 ($P_d = 2W \times 2 \times 10^{-7}$ sec $\times$ 1000 Hz = 0.4 mW average power. For t = 240 sec, the dose becomes $P_d = P \times t = 0.1$ J/cm^2) and that the total dose was 5 J. In our experience, this recalcitrant indication calls for at least 4-6 J/cm^2. The low power density of a 0.4 mW laser diode is questionable for a target such as columna lumbalis, located some 30 mm below the skin surface.

Author:	Smith R J et al Ref no: [A13]
Title:	The effect of low-energy laser on skin-flap survival in the rat and porcine animal model
Published in:	Plastic and Reconstructive Surgery, 1992; 89 (2): 306-309
Laser type (1):	HeNe-laser (633 nm)
Output:	2.75 mW
Pulsing:	Continuous
Pulse repetition rate:	-
Dose:	Not specified
Power density:	310 mW/cm^2 at probe tip
Treatment distance:	1 mm
Laser model:	Biostim 2000
Treated area:	Four dorsally based skin flaps with distal demarcation of necrosis
Treatment time:	30 sec/cm^2
No. of patients:	82
No. of sessions:	5
Time between sessions:	24 hours

Table 13.7 Smith R J et al

Our comments: This study specifies just about everything but the dose, although this may be calculated as being 0.0825 J/cm^2 per day. Five sessions of treatment were given before the skin flaps were prepared, and five afterwards. Therapeutic treatment carried out before surgical invasion of healthy tissue is probably of questionable value. The total dose per flap will therefore be 5 × 0.0825 J/cm^2 = 0.4125 J/cm^2. This dose is quite low. The control procedure may also be called into question since symmetrical flaps were prepared on the right and left sides of the animal and only one side was irradiated. This procedure ignores the systemic effects of laser treatment (see below).

Author:	Masse J-F et al Ref no: [A12]
Title:	Effectiveness of soft laser treatment in periodontal surgery
Published in:	Internat Den J. 1993; 43: 121-127.
Laser type (1):	HeNe-laser (633 nm)
Output:	0.27 mW
Pulse repetition rate:	Continuous
Pulse repetition rate:	
Laser type (2):	GaAs-laser (904 nm)
Output:	0.8 mW
Pulsing:	Pulsed, 200 ns pulse width
Pulse frequency:	47.5-3040 Hz
Dose:	Not specified
Power density:	Not specified
Treatment distance:	1 mm
Laser model:	Stomalaser, independent power measurement
Treated area:	Not specified
Treatment time:	2 min 30 sec
No. of patients:	28
No. of sessions:	1
Time between sessions:	

Table 13.6 Masse J-F et al

Our comments: In this report, the authors studied the effect of combined HeNe/GaAs therapy on bilateral free autogenous gingival grafts and, commendably, performed independent measurements of the output specified by the manufacturer. The HeNe output, specified as 4 mW, proved actually to be 2 mW and a mere 0.27 mW after sustaining heavy losses in the fibre-optic rig. The maximum peak power output of the GaAs laser, given as 2 watts, was found to be only 0.8 watts. The size of the area treated is not specified, but assuming it was 1 cm², the dose will be 0.0022 J/cm^2 GaAs, plus 0.04 J/cm^2 HeNe, that is, a total dose of 0.0422 J/cm^2. Further, a single application is not likely to give significant results.

Author:	Lundeberg T, Haker E, Thomas M Ref no: [A11]
Title:	Effect of laser versus placebo in tennis elbow
Published in:	Scand J Rehab Med. 1987; 19: 135-138.
Laser type (1):	HeNe-laser (632.8 nm)
Output:	1.56 mW
Pulsing:	Continuous
Pulse repetition rate:	-
Laser type (2):	GaAs-laser (904 nm)
Output:	0.07 mW
Pulsing:	Pulsed
Pulse frequency:	73 Hz
Dose:	0.09 J/point (HeNe), 0.004 J/point (GaAs)
Power density:	Not specified
Treatment distance:	1 mm
Laser model:	Model was not specified, nor whether fiberoptics were used
Treated area:	10 different acupuncture points through a 1 mm transparent plastic disc
Treatment time:	60 sec per point
No. of patients:	82
No. of sessions:	10 per point
Time between sessions:	

Table 13.5 Lundeberg T, Haker E, Thomas M

Our comments: The doses are so low that significant effects can hardly be expected. This is a study on laser acupuncture and not on actual LPT.

Author:	Taube S et al: Ref no: [A10]
Title:	Helium-neon laser therapy in the prevention of postoperative swelling and pain after wisdom tooth extraction.
Published in:	Proc. Finn Dent Soc. 1990 (86) 1: 23-27
Laser type:	HeNe-laser (633 nm)
Output:	8 mW (tube)
Pulsing:	Pulsed
Pulse repetition rate:	50 Hz
Dose:	Not specified
Power density:	Not specified
Treatment distance	Not specified
Laser model:	Biotronical Laser MC-8
Treated area:	Not specified
No. of patients:	17
Treatment time:	120 sec before suturing and day 2
No. of sessions:	2
Time between sessions:	24 hrs

Table 13.4 Taube S et al

Our comments: Assuming a 50% fibre loss and a 50% pulsing loss, the total dose will be 2 mW x 120 sec x 2= 0.48 J. This is indeed a very low total dose for such major surgery. The number of sessions is also low.

Author:	Basford J R et al: Ref no: [A9]
Title:	Low-energy Helium Neon laser treatment of thumb osteoarthritis.
Published in:	Arch Phys Med Rehab. 1987; 68: 794-797.
Laser type:	HeNe-laser (633 nm)
Output:	0.9 mW
Pulsing:	Continuous
Pulse repetition rate:	-
Dose:	Not specified
Power density:	Not specified
Laser model:	Dynatronics (model not specified), via fiberoptics
Treated area:	4 different points around 3 joints (altogether 12 points)
Treatment time:	15 sec per point
No. of patients:	
No. of sessions:	9
Time between sessions:	

Table 13.3 Basford J R et al

Our comments: Assuming that the fibre loss is about 50%, the dose will here be 15 sec x 0.9 mW x 0.50 = 0.007 J per point. No obvious effect can be expected from such a low dose. This was a single-blind study

- 2 J per acupuncture point and 1 - 4 J per trigger point, it is hardly surprising that no significant effect was observed. And since the instrument used can be pulsed, the dose and the effect may actually have been reduced still further. The study is said to have been double-blind, although there is no description of how this was achieved. This would, in fact, have been valuable information, since double-blind studies are normally quite difficult to carry out with HeNe lasers - they use red, visible light that is immediately distinguishable from conventional red light by its characteristic laser speckles.

Author:	Jensen H. et al: Ref no: [A7]
Title:	Is Infrared laser effective in painful arthroses of the knee?
Published in:	Ugeskr Læger. 1987; 149: 3102-3106.
Laser type:	GaAs-laser (904 nm)
Output:	0.3 mW
Pulse repetition rate:	Yes. 200 ns pulse width
Pulse frequency:	190-250 Hz
Dose:	Not specified
Power density:	Not specified
Treatment distance:	Not specified
Laser model:	Space Laser IR CEB
Treated area:	All together 4 points per knee
Treatment time:	180 sec per point
No. of patients:	29
No. of sessions:	5
Time between sessions:	1 day

Table 13.2 Jensen H et al

Our comments: Although the dose is not explicitly stated, approximate figures may be calculated from other data. The power output is given as 0.3 mW, although in Space's instruments (as in many other GaAs lasers), the output is directly proportional to the pulse frequency. At 1000 Hz, these Space instruments usually produce an output of 1 mW. The pulse frequency interval is stated as being 195 - 250 Hz. On the basis of the power output stated, the dose may be estimated as 0.0003 W x 3 x 60 sec = 0.054 J. Four points were treated on each knee, giving a total dosage per session of 0.2 J. This dose is totally inadequate for a part of the body as large as the knee. This was a double-blind cross-over study

13.1.5 Pitfalls

1. Low outputs

In the following we review some of the studies in which a low dose can plainly be identified as the most significant negative factor. We have also listed the parameters that we consider should always be specified in studies of this nature. It is not unusual for an author to criticise previous studies for inadequate specification of parameters and then be guilty himself of the same sort of omission.

In the following examples, the parameters are summarised in tabular form. It should be noted that the power output is here to be understood as mean output on pulsing, since this is the figure required in order to calculate the dose.

Author:	Waylonis G.W. et al: Ref no: [A6]
Title:	Chronic Myofascial Pain: Management by Low-Output Helium-Neon Laser Therapy.
Published in:	Arch Phys Med Rehab. 1988; 69: 1017-1020.
Laser type:	HeNe-laser (633 nm)
Output:	Not specified
Pulse repetition rate:	Not specified
Pulse frequency:	Not specified
Dose:	Not specified
Power density:	Not specified
Treatment distance:	Not specified
Laser model:	Dynatron (model 1120), with fiberoptics
Treated area:	Altogether 12 acupuncture points
Treatment time:	15 sec per point
No. of patients:	62
No. of sessions of treatments:	2 x 5 (6 weeks between courses)
Time between sessions:	Not specified

Table 13.1 Waylonis G W et al

Our comments: This study is frequently quoted. No dose is specified. However, other sources state that the tube output of the HeNe laser (Dynatron 1120) is less than 1 mW. Assuming that losses in the fibre-optic set-up reduce this to 0.5 mW, and given an irradiation time per point of 15 seconds, the dose will be 0.5 mW x 15 sec = 0.0075 J. Since a normal dose today is 0.5

from the manufacturers or agents, while over-optimistic, ignorant salesmen often laid traps that would ensnare both themselves and the researchers.

Many studies will come in for criticism in the following paragraphs, although the researchers involved need not always take this to heart. As often as not they pioneered new territory, seeking either to retain an open mind towards the examination of new methods or reacting to what they perceived as a lack of objectivity. The purpose of our criticism is described in the Introduction - we wish to draw the reader's attention to the fact that many negative studies are poorly structured and are therefore largely irrelevant, even though they constantly feature in bibliographies and reading lists and are cited as "evidence" that LPT does not work. Few people appear to have actually read them. As we see it, it is high time they were weeded out so that they can no longer function as traveler's tales in the future.

13.1.4 Dose development

A number of early positive reports on the clinical effects of very weak HeNe lasers suggested that there was cause for some optimism - and skepticism, too. Among them are Walker (1983) [A1] (calculated at approx. 0.005 J per point) and Snyder-Mackler (1988) [A2, 3] (calculated at approx. 0.01 J per point), reporting on the effect of very weak HeNe lasers.

It must be remembered that Mester had been working with doses of around 1 J as far back as the late sixties. Later, in an article published in 1971 [A4] he recommended a dose of 1.5 J as conducive to wound healing. The first laser he used was a ruby laser. When he and his group used HeNe laser, it had an output of 25 mW from the tube. The beam was taken directly from the tube without losses in a fiber optic. For a long time Mester's papers attracted little attention in the West, since they were published in relatively unknown journals. Later, in 1981, Kana [A5] published a study on the healing of open skin wounds, in which he presented an analysis of the biological effects of 4, 10 and 20 J therapy, finding 4 J optimal. The instrument used was a HeNe laser with an output of 25 mW from the laser tube. Mester's and Kana's experience of doses suitable for wound healing still holds good today. Although HeNe lasers with a power output of 25 mW were extremely expensive at the time, it cannot be said that information on suitable doses was not then available. It should be noted, too, that the treatment of pain requires larger doses than does the healing of open wounds. It seems that a large proportion of the negative studies concentrated mainly on testing the reliability of studies such as [A1, 2 and 3] without regard to the existing knowledge of reasonable doses.

In the following analysis of the available literature, we have chosen to analyse those studies that were unable to demonstrate the effectiveness of LPT. Although priority was given to double-blind studies, non-double-blind studies were also included in typical cases. Certain studies were also included merely on the grounds that they are among the most frequently cited.

13.1.1 "I heard it through the grapevine"
A recognisable pattern is often distinguishable in the bibliographies accompanying scientific reports. The manner in which these patterns arise goes something like this: Researcher A is the man or woman behind some pioneering achievement and is therefore extensively quoted by researcher B, as well as by C, D, E and several others. Researcher K, however, is content to read what E has written about A and B, while researcher Z treats the work of A and B as a simple historical reference point previously described by researcher P. And, like a rumour, the word spreads: everyone knows about A, B and C, but no one has actually read their published work. Although generally known, therefore, older studies are not always relevant and it may sometimes be rewarding to go back and review them in detail. Often, especially in the light of new findings, the impression given is quite unlike that suggested in later, second-hand reports.

13.1.2 Positive from negative
Having previously concentrated on studies positive to LPT, we found ourselves over the last years becoming more and more interested in studies with a negative view. Provided they have been properly carried out, they may be able to show us which parameters do not appear to work. Naturally, negative reports must always be taken seriously, but the fact that a given study has been unable to demonstrate the effectiveness of LPT does not necessarily mean that the method studied is incapable per se of producing results for the indication in question. All that it shows is that the parameters selected for the study were not sufficiently effective. Therefore, it is illogical to conclude that LPT is ineffective simply because no effect was reported in that particular study. A number of studies reporting negative results are marred by such startling illogicality.

13.1.3 Negative from negative
LPT is a relatively young science that has only just emerged from its *Sturm und Drang* period, and it might perhaps be unfair to criticise the earlier negative studies. Many medical researchers then had - and indeed still have - a rather diffuse knowledge of physics, and advanced books on the physics of LPT were long in appearing. In many cases, the only information available to researchers on doses, methods of treatment and suitable indications came

In this chapter we aim to discuss the LPT literature in more depth. Much more work should be done in the evaluation of the available literature, which consists of more than 5000 studies. Since LPT is a fairly new treatment modality, many of the early studies were non-controlled and provided little information on the parameters used. Negative as well as positive studies must therefore be subjected to an objective analysis in the search for the optimal parameters. Some of the studies will have to be transferred to the wastebasket. The most striking general feature in the negative studies is the use of very low dosages. Similarly, most analyses of the literature are characterized by a lack of an evaluation of the connection between positive results and reasonable dosage on the one hand, and negative result and low dosage on the other hand. However, negative studies and poorly performed positive studies are not without interest. Negative studies, if performed correctly, are of great value. Positive studies may, even if poorly designed, stimulate further research in an interesting direction. In general, it is clear that the average methodological quality of the pre-millennium LPT literature is not very high An analysis of papers published between 2007 and 2009 still show that 70% of the papers still lack the type of dose-related information needed to permit a reasonable comparison of studies [2026]. However, the quality is higher than for widely used methods such as ultrasound [1187].

13.1 Are all the negative studies really negative?

An analysis of a number of frequently cited studies on the effects of LPT has been performed by the authors of this book. In many of these studies, analysis uncovered one or more reasons for the negative findings reported, the most common being the use of extremely low doses. Other reasons were: unsuitable inclusion criteria, inaccurate control group definition, ineffective methods of therapy, inadequate attention to systemic effects and tissue condition, and low power density. A weakness often encountered in these studies is their failure to provide sufficient data on laser parameters. Since negatively inclined studies are often quoted as "proof" of the ineffectiveness of LPT, it is important that they be subjected to a proper critical analysis. 1400 articles were scanned for this analysis, the emphasis being on double-blind studies. Of the 151 localised double-blind studies, scanned in the year 2000, 109 reported positive findings.

Although important, the critical examination of scientific literature is decidedly unglamorous. It involves hours and days of searching through a wide variety of different sources, and all information is by no means yet available on-line. There are numerous pitfalls, too, especially for those who opt to read abstracts only - criticism of sources is impossible unless an article can be studied in its entirety. Basing an opinion on abstracts obtained from Pubmed is risky. In addition, only a minority of the early LPT research reports are available from the major databases.

Chapter 13
The laser phototherapy literature

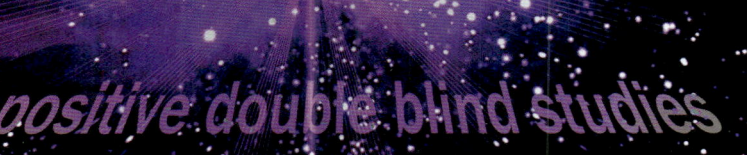

positive double blind studies

Meta-analyses

The Cochrane analyses

12.2.4 Recommendations of WALT - The World Association for Laser Therapy

The World Association for Laser Therapy (WALT) has published recommendations to guide scientists and researchers. These can be found on the WALT website www.walt.nu and are:

Consensus agreement on the design and conduct of clinical studies with low level laser therapy and light therapy for musculoskeletal pain and disorders.

Standard for the design and conduct of systematic reviews with low level laser therapy for musculoskeletal pain and disorders.

Laser dosage table for musculoskeletal disorders using 904 nm pulse lasers.

Laser dosage table for musculoskeletal disorders using 780 - 860 nm lasers.

The recommendations of the World Association for Laser Therapy can be found here:
http://www.walt.nu/dosage-recommendations-and-scientific-guidelines.html

Conclusion
One of the reasons for the lack of general acceptance of laser therapy among medical doctors and dentists is the overall quality of research. Lack of quality control has produced negative results in some studies and criticism of many of the positive studies. Ironically enough, the major failure in many laser therapy studies has been lack of attention to the therapeutic tool itself. By improving the design as well as the reporting of all the variables used in trials, we believe that laser therapy will become as well a recognised entity as laser surgery.

6) Pre-, parallel- or post-medication

Sometimes it is of interest to compare the effects of laser therapy with effects of medication. If parallel medication is prescribed, one group with medication only, one with laser only and one with a combination of laser and medication could be considered. Synergistic effects can be expected in many cases. A drug intake diary will be a valuable indirect clue to the effect of the laser therapy.

7) Treated with other methods before

Many times the patients have tried many other treatment modalities like physiotherapy, acupuncture, ultrasound, electro-stimulation and pharmaceuticals. This information is of interest, since a favourable outcome of laser therapy would indicate the severity of the condition to be overcome.

8) Drop-out rate

This information is of importance since it will give a clue on patients' compliance and researchers' control of the protocol.

9) Follow up

While the effect of laser therapy may be immediate for some problems, it may also take a long time to surface in other conditions. It may have a long lasting effect or be of short duration only. Therefore, short-time as well as long-time follow up is valuable.

10) Outcome measures

Visual Analogue Scale and other subjective outcome measures are useful, but to obtain more objective outcome measures methods such as thermography, blood analysis, microdialysis, MRI, etc., are recommended.

11) Statistical Analysis

A statistical evaluation of the study is necessary and it is advisable to consult an expert before the final design of the study is determined. Students t-test, Mann Whitney U-test, Chi-square test are examples of methods used and they should be selected according to the type of study outlined.

12) Economy

In order to be able to follow the specifications above, good research funding is necessary. This is seldom the case. Laser manufacturers of today are not too profitable and the outcome of a study cannot be patented, like a pill. The above list can therefore be seen as the list given to Santa Claus before Christmas - you must expect to receive less. The main thing is to be aware of "the ideal situation" and to explain why limitations have been made.

stated if it can be calculated from the number of points treated and the number of joules/point.

9) Frequency of treatment sessions
The intervals between sessions should be stated. Treatment once a week may be inappropriate for an acute condition but may be appropriate for a chronic condition. The pathology will determine the frequency of treatment. It is rather common to start a treatment series with two or three sessions per week and after some time go down to one treatment per week - this should be described. In the clinical situation, the intervals can be related to the patient's response, but in a scientific set-up the schedule must be rigid.

12.2.3 Closer description of the medical parameters
1) Description of the problem to be treated
It is important that the problem to be treated is well defined and that the treatment situation is as equal as possible for all the patients. In other words, we must have a correct diagnosis. One of the most important issues is to find out the history of disease for each patient. Also, it may be of interest how the diagnosis was reached - the tools used; X-rays, ultrasound scanning, thermal mapping, etc.

2) Patients (number, age, sex)
In the description we need to state parameters as number, age and sex. But things like skin type may also be of interest, as dark skin absorbs light much more than white skin.

3) Exclusion criteria
Typical exclusion criteria may be pregnancy, high blood pressure, epilepsy, etc. - also extremes (e.g. when treating ulcers, too large and too small ones can be excluded).

4) Inclusion criteria
In selecting the patient population to be treated within the trial, appropriate inclusion and exclusion factors should be used to obtain as homogeneous a group as possible. The diagnosis, e.g. tendinitis or myofascial pain, should be as clear as possible. The particular pathology of the patient being treated should, if possible, conform to standard diagnostic criteria such as those of the International Society for Pain or other appropriate international bodies.

5) Condition of patient
Diabetes or other diseases may influence the reaction to laser therapy treatment. Acute and chronic conditions should be differentiated. The dose of laser may need to be adjusted according to the type of pathology.

6) Treatment distance (spot size), type of movement, scanning

In some studies, the light from a laser aperture is spread out to cover the whole area to be treated (e.g. a leg ulcer). This results in a low power density. An alternative is to use a narrow beam and scan it over the surface - by hand or mechanically. This will give a higher power density and a better result. Whatever the method, it should be described in detail.

7) Sites of treatment

The anatomical entity that is treated should be explicitly described. This will differ depending on the condition or site being treated as well as the site of the pathology. A schematic picture would be desirable.

Anatomical sites should be described as well as sites of muscle insertions or ligaments. For example, in the treatment of lateral epicondylitis, the lateral epicondyle itself would be treated. But tender/trigger points in the extensor muscles of the forearm and their insertions may also be treated, as well as tender points in the neck relating to the myotome of the affected muscles. The position of the arm/leg will affect the distance to the patholgy in several conditions.

Where possible, a quantitative estimate of the depth of a site being treated should be performed, by ultrasound, CT scan or MRI, to help assess whether or not an appropriate dose has been applied to that area.

Acupuncture points should be described, using the WHO nomenclature for acupuncture points. It is also appropriate to describe the rationale for the point selection. Trigger points should be described according to the muscle in which they are located, a diagram being used where possible, and the rationale for their selection should be explained.

If the light is brought in by means of fibre optics or endoscopes, this should be described in detail. Output power should be measured at the aperture of the transfer system.

It is only when an explicit description of the treated sites is given that the study will be reproducible. It will then be possible to gauge whether or not the laser light has been able to reach the target tissue and an appropriate dose applied.

8) Number of treatment sessions

The total number of treatment sessions given in the course of treatment needs to be stated. Three or four sessions for laser acupuncture may be totally inadequate when a course of ten is regarded as usual.

It is also of interest to state if all patients receive treatment on the same number of occasions and whether all sessions are equal. Maybe a smaller dose is given per session as the surface of an ulcer decreases.

The total number of joules per treatment session should also be stated. If 10 contact points are treated at a rate of 1 joule/point, the total dose will be 10 joules per session. This may have relevance in terms of the condition treated as well as potential side effects. This may not need to be explicitly

1) Treatment area

It is of course important to clearly specify the treatment area - if it is one area or several, if it includes areas over deep or shallow problems, as well as acupuncture and trigger points.

2) Dose: Energy density

In the absence of clearly defined protocols in the current literature, decisions about dosage need to come from clinical experience, case series and reports as well as from secondary sources of information such as books and manufacturers' manuals. Energy density of penetrating radiation falls off exponentially in the tissues - much higher doses at skin surface are needed to achieve the desired dose at deeper sites. Too low doses are certainly one of the reasons why many studies are reported as having negative outcomes. However, when treating over a vein or artery with low or no probe pressure, a marked fraction of the light affects the blood cells. This is of importance for systemic effects and general effects on the immune defence.

3) Dose per treatment and total dose

There are many methods of treatment and the description of treatments is essential. The description should include dose per treatment session, whether different doses are given to different areas, such as open wound area and wound edges (acupuncture or trigger points included) as well as the total dose for the whole series of treatment for each patient.

4) Intensity: Power density

The power density of the machine is a function of the power of the laser and the spot size of the area being treated. When in contact with the skin, the spot size will be the area under the probe tip. It is a measure of the potential thermal effects of the laser beam. Very often the power density at skin surface is determined by the aperture of the laser probe (the aperture is the area of the beam as it leaves the probe. When treating in contact, it is also the area of light penetration into the skin/tissue). For small apertures it is suggested that the power density be given in watts or milliwatts/point and for larger areas (<0.5 cm^2) in watts or milliwatts/cm^2.

5) Treatment method

A description of whether the laser is to be used in a scanning mode or in contact with the surface of the skin must be given. Also, it should be specified whether pressure is applied and if the probe area is flat or if the aperture(s) protrude(s), (which will give a higher local pressure, resulting in a larger blood-free volume under the contact area). Doses will vary according to which technique is used. In some cases, manufacturers might be able to indicate the appropriate distance from the skin surface used to achieve a particular dosage, as calculation of the dose is dependent on the particular characteristics of the machine. Some machines will calculate doses and energy densities depending on the technique used.

8) Power density at probe aperture

Power density at the probe aperture is not always important, because it is the power density in the actual problem volume that is the essential parameter. However, this is usually not known in detail and normally we chose a surface dose that is sufficiently high to obtain at least a reasonable dose at the depth of the problem to be treated. However, in order to make it possible to repeat a study, power density at the probe aperture is essential to know. Also, when some parameters are missing in a published study, this can be helpful to know. Power density is stated in mW/cm^2. It is also important to specify the area and shape of the aperture.

The most common treatment technique is to put a hand-held laser probe in contact with the skin or mucosa under which there is a problem to treat. In this case, the treated area is equal to the aperture size. If the aperture is small (5 mm diameter or less) the treated area can be regarded as a point and we can regard the power distribution across the treated area as a constant (in reality it is practically never constant, but with small treated areas it will not make any difference in the three-dimensional power distribution deep in tissue if the power density across the aperture is constant or not).

9) Calibration of the instrument

The output power of an instrument is often not the same as stated in the brochure. It is recognised that, as a laser diode heats up during use, its power tends to fall off unless the machine has an appropriate cooling device. The power of the laser should be measured, preferably by an independent source, before the beginning of the trial as well as at appropriate intervals within the trial and on completion of the trial, in order to determine that the laser power has remained constant throughout. It also happens that a laser diode or some electronic part breaks, leading to loss of most or all of the energy - in the worst case, maybe the whole trial is thus invalidated.

The power meter (or equivalent) should be specified (type of detector, wavelength sensitivity, make and producer). Some instruments have a built-in power meter, which may often be inaccurate. The user of an instrument needs to know if the laser source loses power over time and correct measurements are essential in scientific work.

12.2.2 Closer description of the treatment parameters

Among these parameters we find the two most essential ones: the energy density (dose) and the power density (intensity). These parameters are more closely described in chapter 1.2.13 "Power density" on page 17, chapter 3.3.1.4 "Power density" on page 69, chapter 3.3.1.5 "Energy density" on page 70 and chapter 10 - "The difficult dose and intensity" on page 311.

The combination and permutation of laser therapy variables for the treatment of different conditions is practically infinite and it can be very difficult to make decisions about what is an optimal dose for a particular pathology when the primary evidence is equivocal.

frequencies give different biological responses, even when all other parameters are kept constant. Furthermore, there is a connection between penetration depth, power density and output power (peak and average output power).

However, there are many ways to pulse light (often the term "modulate" is used). This is described in: chapter 1.2.10 "Continuous and pulsed lasers" on page 16, chapter 1.2.12 "Average power output" on page 17 and Figure 1.7 "Different types of pulsing" on page 18. It is, of course, important to specify not only whether the light is pulsed or not, but also the duty cycle.

The most important parameter for a pulsed laser is the pulse repetition rate. This means the number of laser pulses per second and is measured in Hz. In some instruments, programmes control the pulse repetition rate so that at first one pulse repetition rate is used, and after some seconds the pulse repetition rate is changed. There are even examples of devices where the pulse repetition rate is gradually changed from low to high and back again. In the case of pulsing with pulse trains, it is necessary to specify exactly how the pulsing is done.

In the literature there are many examples showing that different pulse frequencies give different biological effects - (See chapter 3.3.1.13 "Pulse repetition rate" on page 78.) However, although research clearly shows that pulsing is of importance, there is very little knowledge about the clinical implication of a specific pulse repetition rate. And chopping of a continuous laser and true pulsing of a GaAs laser is probably not the same, even if the pulse repetition rate happens to be the same. The author should explain the reason for the choice of the pulsing mode.

7) Output power

The output power of a laser should be stated in watts or milliwatts per source. If the laser is pulsed, the situation becomes a bit more complicated. Then the following parameters must be clearly described:

A Pulse repetition rate. One or several frequencies used?

B Type of pulsing (chopping/switching, super-pulsing, modulation, e.g. pulse trains)

C Duty cycle

D Peak power

E Pulse shape, pulse energy.

F Average output power

There is also the following relation between average power and energy per pulse: average power = energy per pulse multiplied by the pulse repetition rate.

wavelengths for the HeNe laser are 543, 594 and 612 nm, although the 632.8 nm wavelength can give the highest output power).

Furthermore, two laser types can have the same wavelength but still give different biological results due to different coherence lengths. An InGaAlP-laser, for instance, can have the same wavelength as a HeNe-laser (632.8 nm). But a HeNe laser has a higher degree of coherence and a narrower bandwidth. (See chapter 1.5.1 "The Helium-Neon laser (HeNe)" on page 40 and chapter 11.1.2 "Comparisons between coherent and non-coherent light" on page 335.

The wavelength of the laser is an essential parameter. A certain wavelength may hence be more appropriate for a certain condition than other wavelengths. The wavelength should be given in nanometres or in micrometers. It is not sufficient just to describe the laser as "visible" or "infrared", though this can be added.

3) Laser beam characteristics
A laser beam is not just a laser beam. Typical characteristics are polarised or non-polarised light, divergent light, collimated or even focused light. Furthermore, the distribution of intensity within a beam of light can be very different from one laser to another. A semiconductor laser often has a fan-shaped beam.

4) Number of sources
It is not uncommon to have more than one laser source in a single instrument. A multi-probe has more than one light source. In this case, it is important to describe the situation carefully - how many sources, their spatial distribution and orientation and sometimes also different wavelengths. Always describe the outline of the diodes of a multi-probe by means of a photo or a drawing of the end of the laser probe - a picture says more than a thousand words!

N.B! Sometimes light emitting diodes (LEDs) are used as the active source/sources together with laser diodes. It is of importance to describe this and to specify the wavelength, bandwidth, power and power density of each source. If LEDs are used as light indicators only, this should be specified.

5) Beam delivery system
Laser systems can look very different and, depending on the beam delivery system, the distribution of the light on the surface of the tissue and inside the tissue can vary considerably. The light can be transported by fibre optics (which usually eliminates polarisation), or it may come from a hand-held probe. It may be defocused to cover a larger area, or a focused beam may be moved across a determined surface using a scanner.

6) Pulsed or continuous emission
It is important to specify whether a laser is pulsed or not, as well as the method of pulsing. One reason is that it has been shown that different pulse

7　Treatment distance (spot size), type of movement, scanning

8　Sites of treatment (leg, knee, internal via fibre etc.)

9　Intended tissue target (synovia, cartilage, ganglion etc) and its approximate distance from the skin surface.

10　Number of treatment sessions (is it the same for all patients?)

11　Frequency of treatment sessions (e.g. 2 per week for 3 weeks, then 1 per week)

Medical parameters

1　Description of the problem to be treated (history of disease)

2　Patients (number, age, sex)

3　Exclusion criteria (pregnancy, high blood pressure, epilepsy etc)

4　Inclusion criteria (how is the diagnosis defined?)

5　Condition of patients (acute, chronic, diabetics, other diseases)

6　Pre- parallel- or post-medication

7　Treated with other methods before (acupuncture, ultrasound, pharmaceuticals)

8　Dropout rate

9　Follow up (short- and long term)

12.2.1　Closer description of the technical parameters

Many of these parameters have been described previously and are well known to workers in the field. Some are less well described, however, and it is essential to understand them in order to know how a laser is best used in a particular trial.

1) Name of instrument (producer)

In many studies, where many parameters are lacking, it can be helpful to know the name (and producer) of the laser instrument. This makes it at least possible to get some information afterwards. It may also be useful to know the year of manufacture.

2) Laser type and wavelength

Traditionally a certain wavelength has been typical of a certain laser type, but with the development of semiconductor laser, groups of possible wavelengths for a certain laser type have appeared. The GaAlAs laser can be mentioned as an example; it can have more or less any wavelength in the region 730 to 890 nm. Tuneable lasers are also becoming more frequent. Even a HeNe laser does not necessarily have a wavelength of 632.8 nm (possible

6 *Cross-over study*. Sometimes it is necessary to use a reference group that gets no laser treatment, even in the case of suffering people (or animals). In this case a so-called crossover study is acceptable. This means that after the treatment sessions have been completed, only a short-time evaluation is done and the groups are then switched, so that the laser group gets placebo and vice versa. This method can also be used in blinded studies.

Much has been written about designing trials which are methodologically sound, and we will not further dwell on these matters. In order to make a trial reproducible, it is necessary to describe in considerable detail the parameters and mode of application of the laser, as outlined below.

12.2 Parameters

The parameters can be separated into three categories: Technical parameters that are related to the equipment used, treatment parameters that are related to the treatment situation, and medical parameters that are independent of the instrument used.

Technical parameters

1. Name of instrument (producer), production year.
2. Laser type and wavelength (e.g. 632.8 nm, HeNe laser)
3. Laser beam characteristics (polarised, divergent, collimated)
4. Number of laser sources (source distribution spatially)
5. Beam delivery system (fibre optics, hand held probe, scanner)
6. Pulsed or continuous emission (pulse repetition rate, type of pulsing and duty cycle)
7. Output power (peak power / average power / energy per pulse)
8. Power density (mW/cm^2) at probe aperture (aperture size)
9. Calibration of the instrument (external, internal, meter type)

Treatment parameters

1. Treatment area (size and number of sites and/or number of treated points)
2. Dose: Energy density (described in detail) in J/cm^2 and/or J/point.
3. Total dose per treatment session and total dose for the entire course of treatment.
4. Intensity: Power density (at the treated surface) in mW/cm^2
5. Rationale for chosen dosage
6. Treatment method (contact, pressure, distance illumination)

Five studies based on sound methodology but using very low dosages, resulting in five negative studies with high scores. Another five studies, methodologically less sound but using realistic dosages, resulting in five studies showing positive effects but low scores. In this case a summing up of the average score leads to the conclusion that laser therapy has no significant effect.

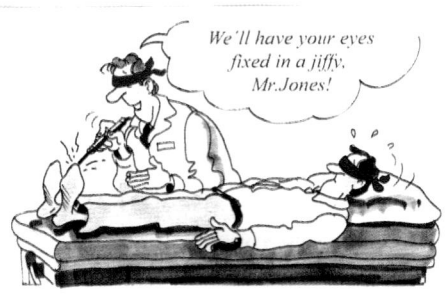

12.1 Methodology of a trial

After selecting a medical indication, consider the following points:

1 *Type of trial.* Do you want to make a pilot study, a single or double-blind study, a randomised or maybe a multi-centre study? A literature study or a meta-analysis? What resources do you have and how much time can you spend? Are there other studies published within your selected field?

2 *Preparations.* It is not unusual that the author(s) have not studied the literature well enough. Study articles - both positive and negative ones. Do not confine your literature search to Medline. Make independent evaluation of references.

3 *Selection of patients.* Remember that the effects of laser treatment on healthy tissue are much lower (if any) than on pathological or disturbed tissue.

4 *Blinding* In the case of treating people (contrary to treating cells and animals), attention must be paid to the blinding of the observer and the patients. Observer blinding has priority. Blinding procedures when visible lasers are used are difficult.

5 *Randomisation.* It is important that the randomisation occurs in such a way that a patient has an equal chance of being in the placebo group or the control group. Care must be taken to ensure that there is true randomisation rather than pseudo-randomisation. Therapists should be unaware of which group the patients have been randomised into.

probe to skin or contact; (7) mono-laser or multi-laser; (8) treatment time and pulse repetition rate; (9) probe position to skin - angular or perpendicular; (10) miscellaneous - plastic foil used for hygienic reasons, alcohol use, etc.

H   Three points if a comparison is used with a study group receiving a placebo treatment only.

I   Three points if a comparison is made between two or more existing interventions.

J   One point if co-interventions are comparable between the groups; three points if co-interventions are standardised or avoided in the study design.

K   One point if blinding of patients was attempted. Three additional points if the blinding proved to be successful.

L   One point if blinding of therapists was attempted. Three additional points if the blinding proved to be successful.

M   Points for assessed outcome measure: Two points for pain; four points for global measure of improvement (decreased wound surface area) and one point for adverse reactions.

N   Points for every blindly assessed outcome measure: One point for pain; two points for global measure of improvement (decreased wound surface area), and one point for adverse reactions.

O   Three points if the timing of effect measurement is identical for all study groups. Two additional points if final effect measurement was made at least three months after randomisation.

P   Two points for intention-to-treat analysis. One point if data for most important outcomes measure on the most important moments of effect measurements are adequately presented (frequencies, mean, standard deviation). One additional point for an adequate analysis with adjustments for dropouts, loss-of-follow up, missing values, non-compliance and co-interventions if appropriate.

Q   Two points for having adequate corrections for confounding variables.

As can be seen from this list, some 95% of the points concern methodology and 5% concern description of parameters, while no points concern the realism of parameter values. Hence, there are studies that receive a lot of points - i.e. are methodologically very well done - but are still more or less worthless because the laser parameters are badly chosen. For instance, if the dose chosen is so low that it can be regarded as "homeopathic", the study is bound for failure. To include such a study in a meta-analysis can lead to incorrect conclusions. An example:

Designing a clinical trial is part science, part art. You need a sense of what works and the commitment to stick to it. The acceptance of a new method of medical treatment or medication must be based on good scientific research. In chapter 13 "The laser therapy literature" on page 379 in this book we will look at the laser therapy literature. We have found that many of the published articles are of low scientific value. However, this is not typical only of the positive studies. In the following chapter we suggest some guidelines for scientific work with laser therapy. Basically, laser therapy should be subject to the same standards of evaluation as other physical methods but must be combined with a knowledge of the special parameters of this method. Without this it will not become the valuable therapeutic tool in medicine that it has the potential to become. It is not uncommon to find a trial that is methodologically sound but not reproducible on the basis of the information supplied.

If you are going to perform a study and want to publish it, it is worth taking a look at how a study can be evaluated in a meta-analysis. Then you can allocate points to different criteria, such as the following, taken from the thesis by Lucas [1184].

A One point each if selection criteria are clearly described, restriction to a homogenous population with respect to diagnoses, duration of complaint, previous treatments and contra-indications for the laser treatment.

B Five points if randomisation procedure is described and is a procedure which excludes bias.

C Five points if smallest group is larger than 25 patients immediately following randomisation; ten points if larger than 50 patients and fifteen points if larger than 75 patients.

D Two points each if the study groups are comparable at baseline for (1) duration of complaint; (2) age; (3) baseline scores for outcomes measured; (4) recurrence status; (5) previous treatment of complaint.

E Five points if there are no dropouts after randomisation. Two points if there are dropouts, with the number of dropouts given for each study group. Three additional points if the reason for withdrawal after randomisation is given for each study group.

F Loss-to-follow up: 1 minus (the number of patients at the main moment of effect measurement / the number or patients at randomisation) x 100 %. One point if loss-to-follow up is less than 20% in each group. Four points if it is less than 10% in each group.

G Points are given to a description of the treatment. One point each for: (1) type of laser used; (2) wavelength and repetition rate [pulse repetition rate]; (3) duty cycle; (4) power; (5) irradiation [intensity]; (6) distance of

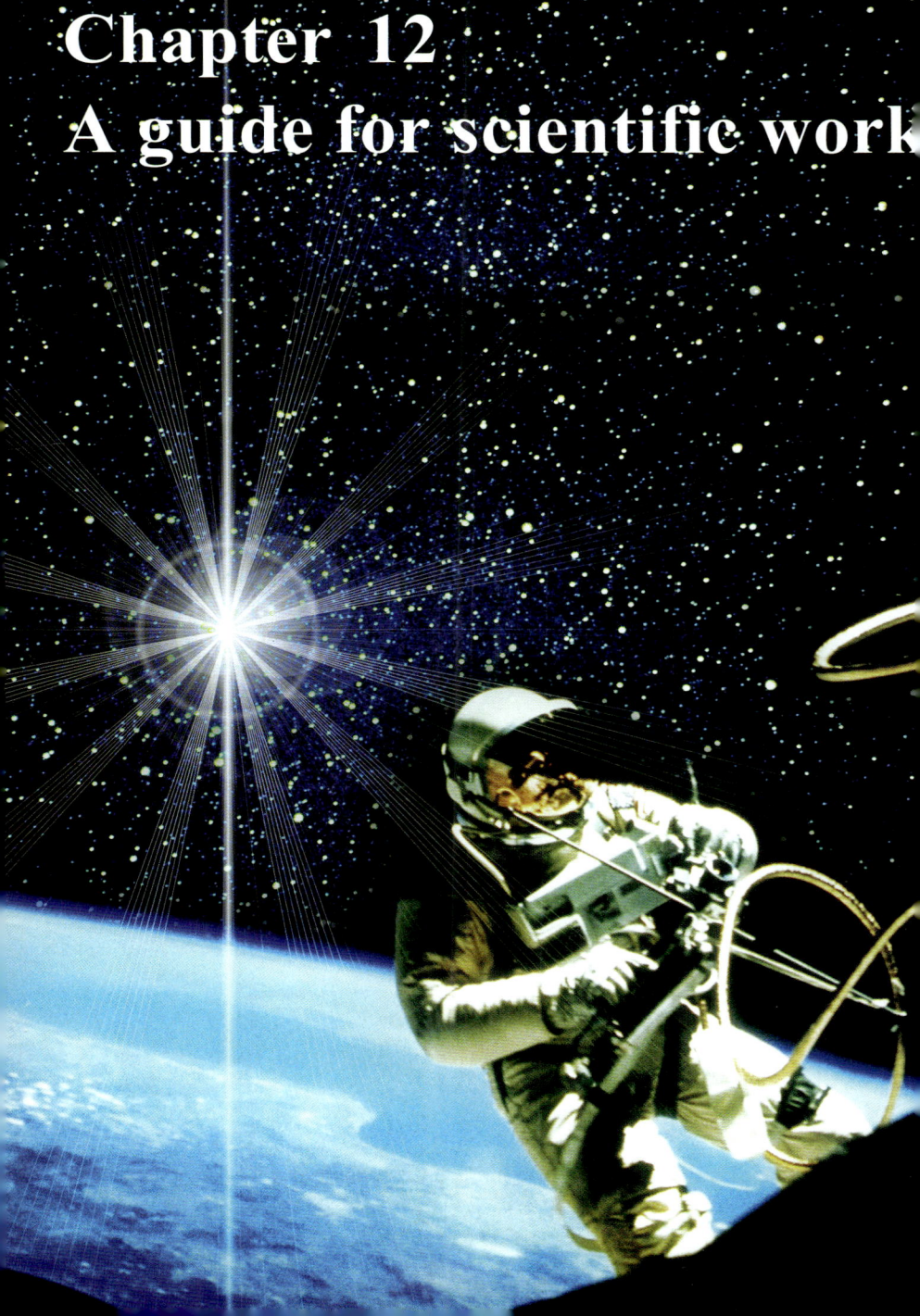

Chapter 12
A guide for scientific work

lengths below 340 nm and between 550 and 700 nm. Furthermore, fluorescence of M. tuberculosis indicated the presence of porphyrins and HPLC analysis of sonicated M. marinum showed that coproporphyrin III was present, which highly justified that porphyrins were present in M. tuberculosis. Production of singlet oxygen through adiation of porphyrins with light of e.g. 400 nm seems to be a most plausible explanation why Finsen's therapy worked in spite of the lack of shortwave ultraviolet radiation, which Finsen believed was the most effective radiation for treating skin tuberculosis. Finsen was therefore a PDT pioneer without knowing it.

Literature: [24, 25, 825]

11.7 Other medical uses of lasers

The critics of laser therapy have repeatedly claimed that coherence disappears when laser light is scattered in tissue. If this were correct, optical coherence tomography [862] would not work.

A useful application of laser technique is the Laser Doppler Velocimeter that can be used to measure arterial, venous and lymph microcirculation. Speckle Interferometry can be used to measure intracellular movements.

Laser spectroscopy can be used for quantitative analysis of e.g. frozen skin biopsies for calcium, arsenic and gold. This technique has also found its application in forensic medicine. With the Laser Doppler Spectrometer, spermokhinezymetry can be performed.

Laser microscopy exists in many different forms, such as Laser Microscopic Masonic Analyzer (LAMMA) and Laser Fluorescent Microscopy.

Laser cytofluorometry utilises the argon laser for scanning single stained cells and has achieved utilisation in mass examination programs for Pap-smear determinations. The same technique is used in a cell sorting system that is now important in monoclonal antibody determination in hybridoma technology.

Lasers can also be used in laser particle size measurement techniques, and laser nephelometry for determination of immunoglobulin classes and autoantibodies such as rheumatoid factors.

Examples of other techniques are transillumination by lasers (diaphanography), laser retinoscopy and holography

Laser-based methods have also been used to study air pollution involving carcinogens in occupational exposures and for the detection of narcotic drugs.

11.5 Diagnostics with Therapy Lasers

In Chapter 7 - "Veterinary use" on page 279, we have mentioned that horses are more sensive to laser light than humans. High local power density - and superpulsing - brings about a reaction (sometimes including a pain reaction) when the probe enters the vicinity of an injury or problem area. This is particularly true of GaAs lasers and at high pulse-train frequencies. It can therefore be used to locate an injury.

Another possibility of using a laser therapy instrument to locate a problem is to use a focused GaAlAs-laser with a sufficiently high output. If 100 - 500 mW is focused or concentrated on a surface in the order of 1 mm^2, most patients will feel some kind of sensation when this "light needle" hits a place connected to a problem. This can be used as a diagnostic aid.

In dentistry, laser has been used to make a differential diagnosis in cases of pulpitis of uncertain origin. By irradiating over the apex of the suspected teeth, microcirculation will increase, intra-pulpal pressure will rise and the "guilty" tooth will react with a pain attack. The longer the duration of the attack, the more compromised is the pulp.

11.6 Photodynamic Therapy - PDT

A method for detecting and destroying cancer tumours, is photodynamic therapy. It is often performed in two steps: detection and destruction. Detection is based on the following. HPD (hematoporphyrin derivate = a selectively retained photosensitive dye, at a dose of 10 mg/kg), or Photofrin, photosan etc, labelled with an antibody specific to the kind of tumour in question, is injected in the patient intravenously 24 hours prior to light irradiation. By irradiating the patient with green light and looking at the irradiated area through red bandpass filters, fluorescence can be seen. Fluorescence will occur at areas with higher concentrations of the dye, indicating the presence of a tumour. By irradiating the tumour area with laser light with a wavelength around 630 nm, the dye will split, releasing toxic agents in the tumour area, possibly killing the tumour. It has been established [24, 25] that the depth of laser light penetration is sufficient to obtain a biological response (necrosis) as far down as 10 mm in the tissue.

In 1903, Niels Ryberg Finsen was awarded the Nobel Prize for his invention of light therapy for skin tuberculosis (lupus vulgaris). The mechanism of action has not been shown; thus, Möller et al [1510] wanted to elucidate the mechanism of Finsen's light therapy. They measured radiation that could be transmitted through his lens systems and absorption of the stain solution filters in the lamps, and related the obtained results to the possible biological effects on Mycobacterium tuberculosis. Judged from transmission characteristics all tested lens systems were glass lenses (absorbing wavelength < 340 nm). The tested filters likewise absorbed wavelengths < 340 nm. The methylene blue solution used to absorb heat, blocked out wave-

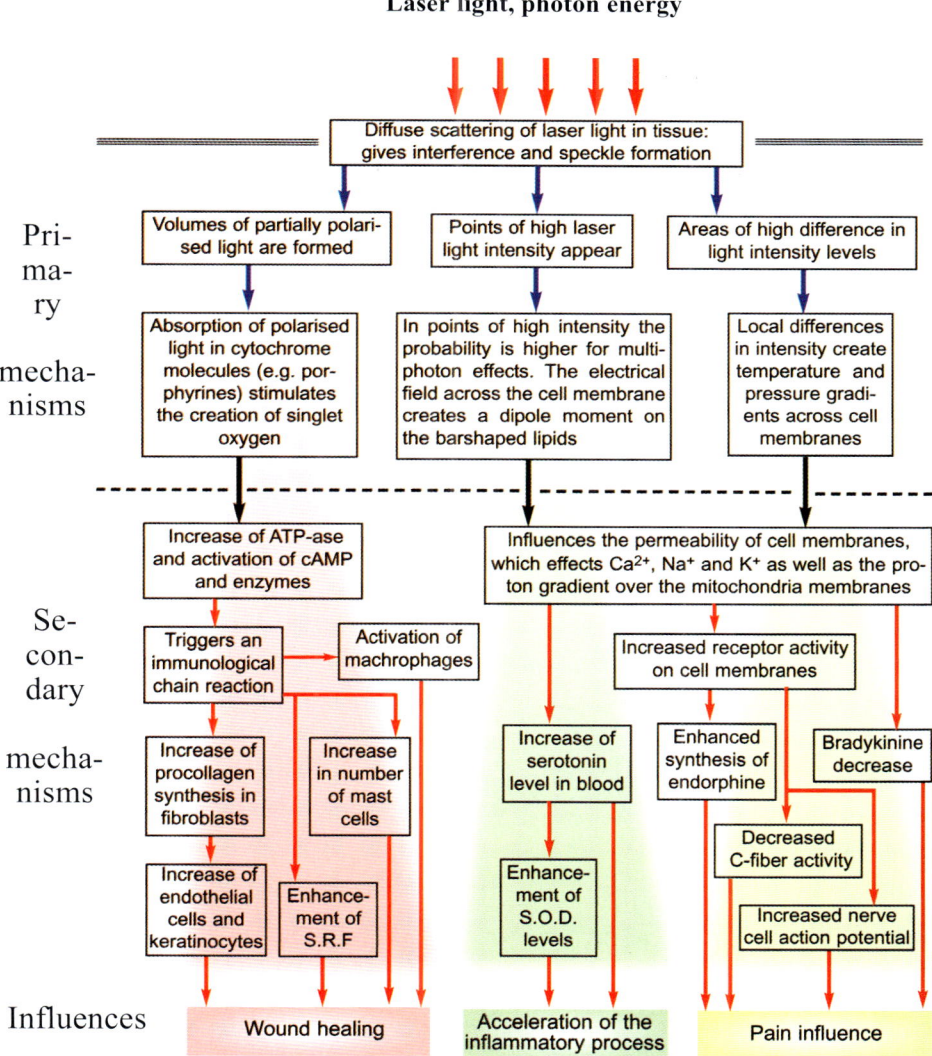

Figure 11.8 The mechanism of laser therapy

* Visible and infrared light affect biomodulation in different ways - visible light elicits photochemical changes, whilst infrared can only produce physical changes. However, the end result may - in some cases - be the same.
* The biological response to laser stimulation can be significantly different according to the sequence in which different wavelengths are applied, and even non-existent if two or more wavelengths are used simultaneously.

Further literature:
The stimulation of ATP synthesis [140, 149, 241, 257, 378, 590, 946, 1258]
DNA replication [21, 22, 33, 75, 121, 181, 220, 249, 251, 510, 587, 675, 754, 947, 948, 950].

11.4 Summary of mechanisms

In an effort to summarise the mechanisms to some degree, in the manner we believe we understand them, and in accordance with other researchers we have contacted, we have created the block diagram shown below. There is, of course, a lot more published about the details in the different stages of the diagram, but including all these beyond the scope of this book.

uncommon. There is not any physical agent besides laser light which we never experienced evolutionary - radiation, gravity, temperature, light, pressure, CO_2 or O_2 saturation, etc. Because of multiple exposures to changes of those conditions (effectors) during the evolution, listed effectors may induce stress only if they are approaching to damage (hazardous) range. The real therapeutic effect related to stress/adaptation, however, may be expected only if the effector does not add its own hazardous effect. Among all known cases it is possible only if laser light is applied at the low dose. Why?

Unlike other physical factors, the light with narrow spectral band is absolutely unusual for our nature. There is no situation where bio-organisms on Earth could be exposed to this kind of light and develop unresponsiveness to that during evolution. Because of that, we believe that the most important for laser effects is not the wavelength but the monochromatic nature, especially with narrow spectral band.

If we will excuse ourselves from the discussion on differences in light absorption and energy of photons (the important aspect of optimisation in laser therapy) and will focus on the induction of adaptive reaction: the more "odd" light we are exposed to, the more response we can expect. If the light's bandwidth increases, the effector loses power to induce adaptive reaction (even if this light still is considered monochromatic, at some degree, it may be not so unique evolutionary as the light with less band-width).

In other words, extreme monochromatic light (such as laser light) exposure was not experienced evolutionary. As such, it is a stimulus that is unique to the experience of the organism. The more unique the light, the more the organism is required to resort to adaptive mechanisms, to resolve the stimulus. For this reason, laser light is considered a unique adaptogen, generating adaptive reactions. The less band-width of the light, the more unique the light is to the experience of organism resulting in greater efficiency of laser therapy."

In the book "The science of low-power laser", Karu pinpoints some typical features of laser therapy, based on extensive in vitro studies:

*   Patient response to laser therapy depends upon their physiological status;
*   Laser therapy effects are truly dosage and wavelength dependent;
*   Biological responses may be maximised within certain "action spectra". A number of action spectra may apply for a particular biological response, and the response may be maximised at a specific wavelength within each action spectrum.
*   The biological responses of cells to pulsed laser therapy can be different (but not necessarily better or worse) from responses to continuous wave, and there is a strong dependence on pulse repetition rate, pulse duration and duty cycle, as well as dosage and wavelength.

11.3.3 Stimulatory and regulatory mechanisms

In 1981 Mester [34] presented an article in which he summarised the research his group in Budapest had published: "The following model is proposed in order to explain the stimulating effects of polarised light (100% from a laser, 75% from a thermal light source): the electrical field intensity from the linearly polarised light changes the conformity of the double lipid layer in the cell membrane by means of electron polarisation of the lipids' electrical dipoles. One of the consequences of this is a change in the distribution of charge on the surface of the cell membrane, which can lead to changes in the lipid-protein bonds. Because the membrane acts as a biological amplifier, changes in the cell membrane affect every process associated with the cell membrane: the cell's energy production, its immunological processes, enzyme reactions, transport factors, etc."

11.3.4 Effects on the immune system

In the same article by Mester, the effects on the immune system were presented. In a study of the changes of the immune defence components by means of measurements before and after laser treatment, e.g. the alpha-I-lipoprotein content increased by 120%. The effect of laser therapy on macrophages is an indication of this claim [291].

Literature:

Dima [372] compared the activation of macrophages using HeNe laser, interferon and corynebacterium parvum. All three methods activated an intense phagocytic activity of the macrophages.

Yamaya [458] found that 904 and 830 nm laser enabled a rapid activation of the superoxide system, NADPH-oxidase.

Stadler [1031] irradiated human whole blood with 660 nm laser by using fluences between 0.1 and 5 J/cm^2. The lymphocytes were isolated after irradiation of the whole blood. As a control experiment, lymphocytes were first isolated and then irradiated with the same fluences. Lymphocyte proliferation was significantly higher in samples irradiated in the presence of whole blood compared with lymphocytes irradiated after isolation from whole blood. Free radical and lipid peroxide production also increased significantly when samples were irradiated in the presence of red blood cells. Thus, the reaction of light with haemoglobin seems to be one of the keys in biostimulation.

Further literature: [1, 2, 214, 262, 273, 373]

11.3.5 Other interesting possibilities

An interesting hypothesis about the effect of laser therapy has been put forward by Reznikov and Pavlova, based on three separate studies [728, 729, 730]. Reznikov [857] gives the following description:

"Laser light could be considered as a trigger of an adaptive reaction because during evolution, this kind of "irritator" (stresser) is unusual,

role as an extracellular neurotransmitter. With non-linear process, we do not mean non-linear optical effects as described in, (See chapter 11.2.8 "Non linear optical effects" on page 557.)

In another study [377], the same author suggests a mechanism of stimulation of damaged cell cultures: Laser irradiation is assumed to intensify the formation of a trans-membrane electrochemical proton gradient in mitochondria. This enhances ATP production, which activates the Ca^{2+} pumps, depleting the Ca^{2+} concentration in the cytoplasm and increasing the Ca^{2+} concentration gradient of the surrounding medium relative to the cytoplasm. This triggers enhanced Ca^{2+} influx into the cells via the Ca^{2+} ion channels of the cell membrane. In addition, with sufficient irradiation, the proton-motive force (pmf), due to the proton gradient, causes more Ca^{2+} to be released from the mitochondria by an "antiport" process. The additional calcium transported into the cytoplasm, together with other factors controlled by the pmf triggers mitosis and enhances cell proliferation. At higher doses, too much Ca^{2+} is released. This causes hyperactivity of Ca^{2+} ATP-ase and exhausts the ATP reserves in the cell.

Brill [999] suggests the system of guanilate cyclase - cyclic guanosin monophosphate - NO-synthase as a primary photoacceptor.

Further literature: [1014]

11.3.2 Effects on blood circulation

Thermographic studies have shown that laser therapy can indirectly cause a higher temperature in the tissue, which is due primarily to an increased blood flow [170, 189]. In a number of studies [109, 190, 221], this rise in temperature has been measured in tissue irradiated with laser light, with the result that the temperature can rise by an average of 0.9 degrees over the area, and up to four degrees at certain points [14].

Literature:

Miro [301] has measured the effect of laser therapy on blood circulation in the nail bed and the mesenteric capillary flow. The increased blood flow continued for 20 minutes after the cessation of the laser treatment, even when the tissue was cooled.

Meada [460] measured the thermic changes after laser therapy using thermographic and thermometric methods. Excised skin in rats showed an increase of 0.4 °C, which remained constant during 30 minutes and was noted equally on both the irradiated side and on the unirradiated contra lateral dorsum. There was no change in histology.

Haina [497] reports a maximum temperature rise of 1 °C in human skin after HeNe irradiation of a density of 600 mW/cm^2, spot size 2 mm.

Sato [398] measured an increase in regional body temperature of 0.7 °C in a group of patients receiving active laser treatment for postherpetic neuralgia. Interestingly enough, there was no increase of temperature in the placebo group.

Serotonin production was found to be enhanced when rat brains were irradiated with HeNe laser. In this study by Rossetti [502], the rats were exposed to stress. In both irradiated and control animals the enzymes aspartate transferase (AST), both cytosolic and mitochondrial, glutamate dehydrogenase (GIDH), and total superoxide dismutase (SOD) were monitored spectrophotometrically. In the brain of the irradiated rats there was a marked increase of total SOD, together with an appreciable decrease of cytosolic AST, and insignificant variations in mitochondrial AST and GIDH. In rats exposed to stress alone, the SOD decreased and the cystolic AST increased.

Montesinos [40] has shown that laser light affects the production of endorphins.

Honmura [188], by blocking opiates with naloxone, has been able to demonstrate that the pain-relieving effects of laser therapy do not depend solely on endorphins.

In a study on rabbits, Labajos [499] found an increase of ß-endorphine levels when a pain stimulus was given simultaneously with GaAs or HeNe laser.

Wakabayashi [190] has demonstrated that GaAlAs laser has a suppressive effect on injured tissue by blocking the depolarisation of C-fibre afferents.

Vizi [246] has demonstrated that ruby laser can enhance the release of acetylcholine.

A study by Mrowiec [432] indicates that nitric oxide is involved in the mechanism of laser therapy-induced analgesia. The analgesic effect of GaAs laser light in rats was prevented by an injection of I-NAME, an inhibitor of nitric oxide syntheses.

As mentioned earlier, Lubart [29] has demonstrated that singlet oxygen is produced in cells irradiated by HeNe laser. Singlet oxygen, in small amounts, is very important in biochemical processes and may be important in biostimulation. It is proposed that singlet oxygen is photo-produced by the natural porphyrins in the cells.

According to Lubart, only red (632 nm) and green (540 nm) light has an effect on the Compound Action Potential of the nerve. 904 nm laser light failed to produce this effect, supporting the theory that light with a wavelength in this region activates enzymes in the cell membranes while porphyrins act as photoreceptors in the visible range of the spectrum.

Friedman [375] reports that non-linearity in photo-biostimulation is a process where linear optical absorptions produce active chemicals such as cytoplasmatic H^+ and Ca^{2+}. These chemicals participate in chemical reactions, the rates of which depend on non-linearity of the concentration of these photoproduced chemicals, thus allowing very sensitive light control of non-linear biological reactions. Important contributions to neural excitability and growth include photostimulation of ATP production, which fuels the action potential and fills the synaptic ATP vesicles. ATP plays an important

therapy. In particular, the CO_2-laser biostimulatory effect is very difficult to explain as the light is absorbed so superficially and also has such low photon energy. The wide-band action of tissue working as a dye laser can also make it easier to understand why biostimulation occurs for so many different wavelengths. Wide-band radiation, such as that from the sun, exhausts a lot of excited levels, thus inhibiting the effect of the laser therapy. Such sunlight induced extinction will only occur at depths that can be reached by that light. Secondary effects caused by laser treatment cannot be extinguished by sunlight or light from other sources.

11.2.8 Non linear optical effects

Theoretically, it is possible that non-linear optical effects can also occur in tissue. An example of a non-linear optical effect is the KTP (Kalium Titanyl Phosphate) crystal in the KTP laser (frequency-doubled Nd:YAG with 532 nm wavelength) which causes harmonic overtones, of which the first is used (532 nm is half the wavelength of the pumping light, in this case, Nd:YAG laser light - 1064 nm).

In order to achieve non-linear effects, high power density is needed. How high depends on the matter in question. We regard it as theoretically possible, but unlikely, that such phenomenon will take place in tissue. But if so, it is most likely to occur if lasers with high peak power, such as the GaAs laser is used, further intensified in bright speckle points due to interference.

11.2.9 Opto-acoustic waves

If intense light pulses are absorbed, acoustic waves may occur. In chapter 7 "Veterinary use" on page 465, we have noted that horses can "feel" GaAs laser light. It is possible that this is due to opto-acoustic waves.

11.3 Secondary mechanisms

11.3.1 Effects on pain

Pain is very complex in its nature. Since we are not specialists in this field, we have chosen to show that laser therapy influences many of the transmitter signal substances that we know are involved, such as endorphines, nitric oxide, bradykinine, serotonine etc, and also direct effects on nerves, e.g. C-fibres.

Literature:

Mizokami [247] has studied the change of serotonin in plasma in 63 patients with chronic pain. He used a GaAlAs laser, 830 nm, 60 mW output power. Patients achieving good pain relief from laser therapy were selected. On the first day of therapy, the change rate of plasma serotonin had a stable tendency to give a positive ratio. The treatment was applied every other day, resulting in a negative ratio from the tenth day of treatment.

photon excitation. A minimum bound for the two-photon emission action cross-section was observed at 830 nm.

Maiti [860] measured serotonin distribution in live cells with three-photon excitation. Three-dimensionally resolved images were made along with measurements of the serotonin concentration from about 50 mM and up.

These investigations and many others, show that serotonin works as an optical target, especially for high photon density light pulses. With laser light (coherent) in particular, it is possible to achieve extra high intensity peaks due to interference.

11.2.7 Lasing effects in tissue

According to what is known as " First Law of Photo Chemistry", light must be absorbed before photochemistry can occur. This is true if we are talking about energy transfer. But this does not mean that light cannot influence matter/tissue unless it is absorbed, since light can act as a catalyst. The existence of the laser is a proof of that. Lasing occurs when an excited atom is stimulated to emit a photon before emission occurs spontaneously. This takes place when a photon of the right energy (wavelength) enters the electromagnetic field of the excited atom: the incident photon triggers the electron energy shift and the energy difference is converted into electro-magnetic radiation and released by means of an identical second photon.

And **nota bene:** the trigger photon is not absorbed.

For a laser to work - i.e. to emit more photons of a certain energy than comes in, we must have an inverted population. In normal matter this is never the case. Living matter, however, has a very complex structure with a multitude of continuously ongoing chemical reactions where any conceivable level of energy is found. There are constantly excited molecules at every level of energy and it is not too unlikely for them to be triggered by incoming photons to release energy in the form of a photon while the triggering photon continues as it does in a laser. Hence, it seems possible that stimulated emission (laser action) can take place in tissue and that tissue itself can act more or less like a dye-laser.

There are currently thousands of different types of laser, and these produce light, UV or IR radiation of various wavelengths. Though a laser usually has one characteristic wavelength, it is sometimes possible to choose within a range of wavelengths. There are tuneable lasers where the wavelength can be changed, even during operation. Dye-lasers have a lasing medium that can be liquid and has a broadband amplification profile. Rhodamin, for example, has an amplification profile between 560-650 nm which covers both the wavelength of the HeNe laser and the InGaAlP lasers. Rhodamin is similar to porphyrin in optical property - it can easily cause fluorescence.

So, it is not unlikely that excited molecules in the tissue act like the medium in a dye laser and that this is triggered by the laser therapy. This could perhaps be part of the explanation of the rather deep effects of laser

11.2.5 Fluorescence - luminescence

Most people have at some time seen fluorescence. In discotheques, for instance, a UV-lamp is often set up to illuminate the guests. When the ultra-violet light hits our white shirt or our teeth, the invisible ultra-violet light is converted to visible light by means of fluorescence. Nice, bright porcelain crowns could suddenly "disappear", to the dismay of the owners. Modern ceramics have now adjusted to this embarrassing situation. In the old type of alarm clock, light energy from the bed lamp excited the phosphor molecules and the energy from the light was then stored for minutes or more and slowly emitted in the form of greenish light. This long-term storage is called phosphorescence.

Many animals have the ability to convert chemical energy into light energy - a process called luminescence. From this it is clear that light can change not only chemical processes in our bodies, but also that our cells can create light by a variety of different processes. It is also known that cells can communicate with each other by means of emitted and absorbed photons [753, 852].

Allan [853] discovered in 1972 that polymorphonuclear leukocytes emit photons during phagocytosis with a spectral maximum close to 600 nm. Nelson [854] found in 1976 that macrophages also emit light. Rosen [855] found experimentally that singlet oxygen is involved in the process; and Andersen [856] compared the emission spectrum from singlet oxygen with the spectrum from polymorphonuclear leukocytes in 1977 and found that they were more or less identical.

Part of the mechanisms of biostimulation can include fluorescence, phosphorescence or luminescence as possible means of communication between cells in different places.

Further literature: [448, 1000, 1001]

11.2.6 Multi-photon effects

Multi-photon effects are today more and more used in PDT, see chapter 11.6 "Photodynamic Therapy - PDT" on page 564 and in two-photon laser scanning microscopy by using a Ti:sapphire laser (superpulsed like the GaAs laser).

One possible explanation of the efficiency of the GaAs laser is action through multi-photon effects. The photon energy of the HeNe laser is 50% higher than the photon energy of the GaAs laser. However, in the extreme pulses of the GaAs laser, the photon density is very high, which is necessary for multi-photon action.

Literature

Shear [859] studied non-linear excitation of the neurotransmitter serotonin by means of Ti:sapphire laser light pulses. The results indicate that serotonin is photochemically transformed as a consequence of four-photon absorption to a photoproduct that then emits in the visible region via two-

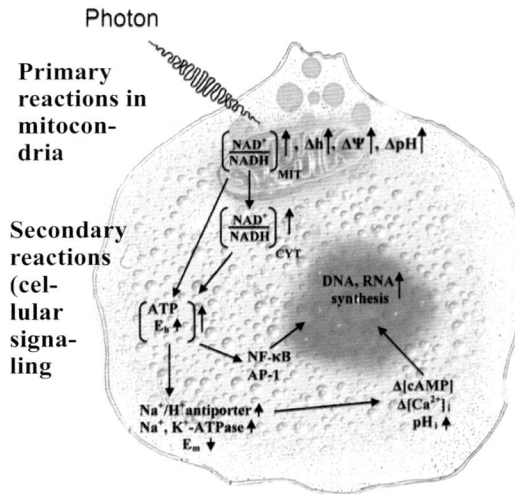

Primary reactions in mitochondria

Secondary reactions (cellular signaling)

Cytochrome-c-oxidase and flavoproteins like NADH in the respiratory chain in the mithocondria can act as photoreceptors. This can cause a short time activation of the respiratory chain and oxidation of NADH pool leading to changes in the redox state of both mitochondria and cytoplasm, changes in pmf (proton motive force), $\Delta\Psi$, Δph and leading to extra synthesis of ATP. Also a rise of Na^+/H^+ antiporter in the cytoplasmic membrane which causes a short term increase in pH_i and causing a change in the redox state of the cytoplasm, i.e. the redox state in the whole cell.

Figure 11.7 This figure is from Karu 1988. The process as described is of course simplified, but all steps are verified through experimental work.

These processes have been further verified. Yaou Zhang et al. [1416] used the cDNA microarray technique to investigate the gene expression profiles of human fibroblasts irradiated by low-intensity red light. Proliferation assays showed that the fibroblast HS27 cells responded differently to different doses of low-intensity red light irradiation at a wavelength of 628 nm. An optimal dose of 0.88 J per cm^2 was chosen for subsequent cDNA microarray experiments. The gene expression profiles revealed that 111 genes were regulated by the red light irradiation and can be grouped into 10 functional categories. Most of these genes directly or indirectly play roles in the enhancement of cell proliferation and the suppression of apoptosis (see also Rubinov, chapter 11.2.3 "Mechanical forces" on page 549). Two signaling pathways, the p38 mitogen-activated protein kinase signaling pathway and the platelet-derived growth factor signaling pathway, were found to be involved in cell growth induced by irradiation of low-intensity red light. Several genes related to antioxidation and mitochondria energy metabolism were also found to express differentially upon irradiation. This study provides insight into the molecular mechanisms associated with the beneficial effects of red light irradiation in e.g. the acceleration of wound healing by laser therapy.

excitation energy is inevitably converted to heat, which causes a local transient increase in the temperature of absorbing chromophores.

The first two processes are of Redox type and the next two give rise to reactive oxygen species (ROS). The belief that only one of these reactions occur when a cell is irradiated and excited electronic states are produced is groundless. Rather, it is likely that more or less all of them take place. The question is, which mechanism is decisive?

Also; it is quite possible that all the mechanisms mentioned above lead to a similar result - a modulation of the redox state of the mitochondria (a shift in the direction of greater oxidation). However, depending on the light dose and intensity used, some of these mechanisms can prevail significantly. Experiments with *E. coli* provided evidence that, at different laser-light doses, different mechanisms were responsible - a photochemical one at low doses and a thermal one at higher doses. [1413]

11.2.4.2 Secondary reactions due to cell signalling

After the primary reactions in the mitochondria, a scheme of cellular signalling cascades (secondary reactions) occur in a mammalian cell. In the figure below, from Tiina Karu, E_h ↑ means a shift of the cellular redox potential to more oxidized direction. Further, the arrows ↑ and ↓ indicate increase or decrease of the respective values, brackets [ ] indicate the intracellular concentration of the respective chemicals.

results demonstrate that the salutary effects of laser therapy on wound healing are temperature independent in this model.

The temperature increase in tissue of black as well as white mice was investigated by Stadler [1457]. Irradiation at 830 nm and 5.0 J/cm² fluence induced a small temperature increase at the surface and at 1 mm in depth. The smaller effects seen in white mice might be due in part to reflection. This suggests that the thermal effects of colour should be considered, particularly at higher fluences.

Further literature: [398, 460, 497, 1257, 1547]

11.2.4.1 Primary reactions due to excitation

There are several such possible primary reactions. When a photon is absorbed, it can transfer its energy to an electron. If the photon energy is high enough, it can change the energy state of the electron, e.g. from level S_0 to S_1. Also triplet states can be involved. It has also been shown that excitation can occur by means of multiple photon action.

The mechanisms that have been proposed are:

1. Changes in redox properties and acceleration of electron transfer. ("Redox properties alteration hypothesis" [1349]. Photo-excitation of certain chromophores in the cytochrome-*c*-oxidase molecule (like Cu_A and Cu_B or hemes *a* and a_3 [1351] influences the redox state of these centers and, consequently, the rate of electron flow in the molecule. [1349]

2. NO release from catalytic center of cytochrome *c* oxidase. ("NO hypothesis") [1369]. It is thought that laser irradiation and activation of electron flow in the molecule of cytochrome-*c*-oxidase could reverse the partial inhibition of the catalytic center by NO and in this way increase the O_2-binding and respiration rate.

3. Superoxide generation. ("Superoxide anion hypothesis"). It has been suggested [1411] that activation of the respiratory chain by irradiation would also increase production of superoxide anions and that the production of $^-O_2$ primarily depends on the metabolic state of the mitochondria. [1412]

4. Photodynamic action. ("Singlet oxygen hypothesis") [1367]. Certain photo-absorbing molecules like porphyrins and flavoproteins (some respiratory-chain components belong to these classes of compounds) can be reversibly converted to photosensitisers.

5. Changes in biochemical activity induced by local transient heating of chromophores. ("Transient local heating hypothesis") [1374]. When electronic states are excited with light, a noticeable fraction of the

3 In a comparison between light of different kinds, cell cultures with T- and B-lymphcytes were irradiated with (a) polarised HeNe-laser light, (b) polarised narrow band incoherent light and (c) non-polarised narrow band incoherent light – all three with the same wavelength and dose. If the effect of the laser light (a) is set to 100%, the polarised narrow band incoherent light (b) gave 81% and the non-polarised narrow band incoherent light gave less than 1% effect [23].

4 Even polarised broadband light [272, 1284] has a clear effect on cell cultures and also affects open wounds and certain skin problems; however, it is not as effective as polarised laser light.

5 Under certain power density conditions, non-polarised broadband light can also have an influence on cells in cultures [252, 374]. Biostimulative effects have been noticed after treatment with so-called IPL devices (Intensive Pulsed Light, originally used for hair removal) with a spectrum limited to 600-1200 nm, power densities of 20-50 J/cm^2 and peak power density in the order of 1 kW/cm^2. This can indicate that multi photon actions may be of importance. (See chapter 11.2.6 "Multi-photon effects" on page 555.)

Karu [33] has demonstrated stimulating biological effects in cell cultures from monochromatic incoherent light. However, she has also shown that cell cultures which are first irradiated with laser light, and have consequently exhibited biological effects, and which are then irradiated with broadband (that is, non-monochromatic and incoherent) and laser light simultaneously, subsequently have their laser-produced biological effects reduced to almost nothing [22]. This indicates that there are more mechanisms at work here than simply the excitation of polarisation-sensitive chromophores.

It is important to understand the purely optical difference between irradiating tissue, which spreads light very diffusely, and a thin transparent cell layer in culture. If a thin layer of cells in culture is irradiated with polarised light, the polarisation is maintained right through the whole layer. This means that the cells are entirely surrounded by polarised light. Mester has shown that leukocytes in culture are affected by both polarised laser light and polarised incoherent light, but not by unpolarised incoherent light [23]. Our opinion is that many of the phenomena that hundreds of research scientists around the world have been able to establish as a result of laser irradiation of cells and tissue, are laser-specific in vivo, and that this is due to the coherence and/or narrow-band nature of the light, but not always laser specific in vitro.

11.2.2 The effect of heat development in the tissue

It has occasionally been asserted that the "possible" effects of laser therapy are due to the laser heating the tissue, and that one could just as well use a blanket, hot shower or a heat-lamp. Heat can of course be valuable many times, but in this context we have to look a bit closer into the matter.

11.2.2.1 Macroscopic heating

A heat-lamp has an output of 50-100 watts, while a therapeutic laser often has an output of 5-100 milliwatts (one milliwatt is a thousandth of a watt), that is, thousands of times weaker. All light that is absorbed by tissue is converted to heat, but it is not the heat itself that is of importance here. A blanket, hot shower or a heat lamp causes macroscopic heating of the skin and tissue - a rather even and smooth temperature distribution. Therapeutic lasers cause no perceptible heating, which heat-lamps obviously do and still there is a clear biostimulative effect, also on chilled tissue. So if it were just a question of heating the tissue, heat-lamps would give just as good or even better therapeutic results! It is true that a GaAlAs laser in the >100 mW range can cause sensations of heat on sensitive areas such as the lip, and on pigmented areas, but more than 95% of the laser therapy described in the literature is performed with lasers in the <100 mW range.

11.2.2.2 The microscopic heat effect

However, the uneven, speckled light distribution in tissue causes local temperature differences. These have been calculated by Horvath [223]. Such temperature differences lead to local gradients in certain concentrations of substances, which in turn bring about transport of materials in the tissue in the manner described by Fink's equations. In other words, when tissue is irradiated with laser light, a microcirculation will be initiated, which is not the case during irradiation with non-coherent light sources, such as LEDs for example. Spanner [224] has shown that a temperature difference across a cell membrane of 0.01 °C causes a difference in pressure of 1.32 atmospheres, and this can mean that the distribution pattern of Na^+ and K^+ can be considerably influenced [225]. The local transient rise in temperature of absorbing biomolecules may cause structural (e.g., conformational) changes and trigger biochemical activity (cellular signaling or secondary dark reactions). [1373], [1374]

11.2.3 Mechanical forces

A very interesting experiment has been performed by Rubinov [1417]. He brings about a new approach to the understanding of biological activity caused by low-intensity laser radiation, in which coherence is a factor of paramount importance. This is based on the dipole interaction of gradient laser fields with cells, organelles and membranes. The laser intensity gradients in an object arise due to the interference of the light scattered by the tissue with the incident light beam (speckle formation). Apart from speckles, different types of light spatial modulation can be created deliberately, using different schemes for beam interference. It is shown that gradient laser fields may cause spatial modulation of the concentration of particles and increase their "partial temperature". Rubinov presents the results of experimental observation of trapping of different types of particles, including human lymphocytes, in the interference fields of the HeNe laser. The sweep-net effect on particles of different sizes when moving the laser field is demonstrated and crystal-like self-organisation of particles in the laser gradient field is observed. The influence of gradient laser fields on erythrocyte rouleaus, on the apoptosis of human lymphocytes as well as on their chromosome aberrations is demonstrated.

It may be concluded from the experimental studies that the influence of an interference laser field with a correctly chosen period can stimulate the repair system of a cell, increasing its viability.

Rubinov concludes further: *"Illumination of biological tissue by coherent laser light unavoidably leads to strong intensity gradients of the radiation in the tissue due to speckle formation. This causes the appearance of inter- and intracellular gradient forces whose action may significantly influence the paths and speeds of biological processes. In contrast to the photochemical action of light, which is accompanied by absorption of quanta and has a specific character (i.e. is characterized by a specific spectrum of action), the action of the gradient field is of non-resonant type. It is not accompanied by photon absorption and has a universal character, i.e. it depends weakly on the radiation wavelength, but requires a high degree of coherence. The use of different schemes of interference allows us to obtain different configurations and periods of spatial modulation of the laser light intensity. The application of such interference fields opens new possibilities for controlling fundamental biological processes and may lead to new technologies in laser therapy."*

No doubt that these effects of gradients are very essential. However, they can not be the only important effects occurring in laser illuminated tissue. Also photon absorption and other photon energy specific effects occur, see e.g. the reference [1279] below, but the effects of field gradients are laser specific and can also be (at least part of) the explanation of why so many different laser types (wavelengths) give similar biologic effects. The more we learn about this, the more we realize that the mechanisms behind laser biostimulation are very complex and the authors of this book doubt that we will ever know all details. Why are for instance about 10% of humans and animals resistant to laser therapy?

11.2.4 Excitation effects

The most obvious photochemical and photo-biological effects are due to excitation of photon absorbing molecules. In this field, a lot of work has been done by professor Tiina Karu. In the following section, we have, with her permission used some of her material and ideas.

Literature:

The stimulation of cellular ATP production has been suggested as one of the most important effects of laser therapy. In a study by Mochizuki [1279] the effect of 830 nm laser irradiation on the energy metabolism of the rat brain was observed. A diode laser was applied for 15 min with an irradiance of 4.8 W/cm^2. Tissue adenosine triphosphate (ATP) content of the irradiated area in the cerebral cortex was 19% higher than that of the non-treated area, whereas the adenosine diphosphate (ADP) content showed no significant difference. Laser irradiation at another wavelength (652 nm) had no effect on either ATP or ADP contents. The temperature of the tissue was increased by 4.4 - 4.7 °C during the irradiation of both wavelengths. These results suggest that the increase in tissue ATP content did not result from the thermal effect, but from a specific effect of the laser operated at the 830 nm wavelength.

Karu [2019] irradiated a monolayer of HeLa cells with an He-Ne laser (632.8 nm, 100 J m^2, 10 s) and the amount of adenosine triphosphate (ATP) was measured by the luceferin-luciferase bioluminescent assay technique at different times (5-45 min) after irradiation. The amount of ATP in the log phase of cultured cells remained at the control level (0.79 +/- 0.09) x 10(-15) mol per cell) during the first 15 min after irradiation; it then increased sharply and, after reaching a maximum (170.8%) 20 min after irradiation, decreased slowly to the control level. The ability of monochromatic red light to induce an increase in the cellular ATP level was found to depend on the growth phase of the culture, being insignificant in the lag phase of cultured cells, increasing in the log phase of cultured cells and reaching a maximum (about 190%) in cells at the late logarithmic and early plateau phase.

The negligible effect of the presence of heat in laser therapy has been well demonstrated by Lanzafame [1447]. Pressure ulcers were created in mice by placing the dorsal skin between two round ceramic magnetic plates for three 12-h cycles. Animals were divided into three groups (n = 9) for daily light therapy, 830 nm, 5.0 J/cm^2 on days 3-13 post ulceration in both groups A and B. A special heat-exchange device was applied in Group B to maintain a constant temperature at the skin surface (30 degrees C). Group C served as controls, with irradiation at 5.0 J/cm^2 using an incandescent light source. Temperature of the skin surface, and temperature alterations during treatment were monitored. The wound area was measured and the rate and time to complete healing were noted. The maximum temperature change during therapy was 2.0 +/- 0.64 degrees C in Group A, 0.2 +/- 0.2 degrees C in Group B and 3.54 degrees C +/- 0.72 in Group C. Complete wound closure occurred at 18 +/- 4 days in Groups A and B and 25 +/- 6 days in Group C. The percentage of the wound closure at 14 days was 75. 4 +/- 7.2% and 77.7 +/- 5.6% for Groups A and B, respectively (NS differences). However, animals in Group C demonstrated a wound closure of 36.3 +/- 4.8%. These

negative effect on cells already stimulated). The light would directly encounter the cells in the wound, where there is no overlying skin to reduce or eliminate the polarisation. The positive effect of polarisation has been shown by Bolton [1284]. When macrophages were irradiated by visible 95% polarised light the fibroblast proliferation was greater than when irradiated with 14% polarised light.

Now, accepting that laser light gives rise to areas of polarised light in tissue (as earlier described), we might also ask the question: what is there in the body/tissue/cells that reacts to the light's polarisation? Are there polarisationsensitive elements?

Yes, there are. It is known that matrix-fixed chromophore molecules (e.g. the body's porphyrins) possess absorption dipoles and both absorb and emit (e.g. through fluorescence) linearly polarised light [20] of a determined polarity. Porphyrins are just one of the elements in the mitochondria's respiratory chain and are the molecules chiefly responsible for the absorption of blue and red light. The polarisation in the speckles created by laser light is significant here, and this could explain why the studies mentioned above showed different results with lasers and incoherent light sources. Some persons have the opinion that the respiratory chain is at the base of all effects that laser therapy might have. However, there are effects of e.g. HeNe laser irradiation on red blood cells in which there are no mitochondria [987]. As the cytochrome system in the mitochondria is influenced by photons [1312], it is logical to assume that other chromophores in the cell could be influenced by photons as well.

The conditions we have described above are in no way a complete list. We simply want to show, by looking at the physical conditions in more depth, that it is inappropriate (in the way chosen by some authors) to try to prove that laser therapy cannot work. It is reminiscent of the well-known proof, as deduced by mathematicians and physicists, that a bumblebee cannot fly because its wings are too small in relation to its body weight.

11.2.1.3 Cell cultures and tissue have different optical properties

In a number of studies in which the biological effects of monochromatic light from various sources have been compared, the following has been found:

1 In cell cultures (low scattering medium) laser light gives almost the same effect [33] as incoherent light (i.e. colour-filtered light from a light bulb or an LED of the same wavelength).

2 When tissue (highly scattering medium) is irradiated, laser light gives a stronger effect than incoherent light in all the studies so far conducted. In some of the studies, certain effects were also achieved with LEDs, but the studied LED-light-influenced phenomena were not as clear as with laser light of the same wavelength and the same dose. It should be noted that in four of these studies, adverse effects from LED light were seen [332, 493, 659, 825].

11.2.1.1 What characterises the light in a laser speckle

The phenomenon of speckles is a form of optical noise. It was observed long before the laser arrived. As early as 1877 Exner [741] reported granulations in filtered mercury lamp light. When the first lasers came, the speckles became not only much more noticed but also a problem. Dennis Gabor, the "father of holography", published an article in 1970 with the title: "Laser Speckle and Its Elimination" in which he described different ways to get rid of speckles.

Speckles can be real or virtual. The three-dimensional structure of real speckles is manifest not only in an apple but also in a patient's tissue during irradiation with laser light. It arises as a result of interference between different beams with a random direction, amplitude and phase. In laser speckles, (See Figure 1.5 "Laser speckles" on page 15.), which have a higher intensity than the surrounding environment, the light is linearly polarised, or partially polarised (a mathematical description of partially polarised light is found in reference [850]), because the higher intensity has come about as a result of constructive interference, which occurs only if the interfering waves have the same polarisation. In this way, islands of polarised light appear in the tissue with an average size of a few tenths of a millimetre, that is, generally larger than the cells they surround. Interestingly enough, these islands occur regardless of whether the irradiating laser emits polarised or unpolarised light.

Literature:

Hode [743, 745] investigated 1972-1973 the possibility of using the inherent information in speckle fields to observe surface movements and deformation in real time.

Horvath [223] has actually measured the light distribution in tissue when illuminated with coherent and incoherent light. He used a small detector and could verify that there is a three-dimensional speckle structure of the light in the tissue if illuminated by laser light but not by incoherent light. This proves that the laser light, after penetration of tissue, is spatially coherent.

Literature: [744, 746]

11.2.1.2 Porphyrins and polarised light

If polarisation is important, can we not simply use polarised normal light? The answer is yes and no. If we illuminate cell cultures, the polarisation remains unchanged throughout the thin layer of cells. However, in the case of a highly scattering medium, such as living tissue, the polarisation is lost after a penetration of a millimetre or so. Therefore, if we polarise light from a pocket torch and use it to irradiate skin, the polarisation will disappear before it encounters the deeper-lying tissues. However, we could use polarised normal (broadband incoherent) light to treat open wounds and improve healing [272] (if we filter off all wavelengths shorter than 600 nm, since these have a

Wavelength in nm	Culture type	Measured activity	Stimulation dose, J/cm²	Inhibition dose, J/cm²	References
632.8	HeLa	Clonogenicity	0.01 ~ 0.1	>1	Karu [1228]
632.8	Mouse mast cells	Cell granule release	2 - 4		Trelles [1227]
660	Hypertrophic scar-derived fibroblasts	Proliferation	2.4 - 4		Webb [615]
660	Human neutrophils	Bacteria killing	2.4 -4.8		Yu [1231]
694.3	Murine melanoma cells	Growth rate	< 0.01	> 0.2	Carney [520] Hardy [1226]
812	Human buccal fibroblasts	Proliferation	0.45		Loevschall [75]
860	Human fibroblasts	Succinic dehydrogenase activity	2	16	Boulton [419]
904	Keratinocytes	Proliferation	0.25 - 4		Steinlechner [4]

Table 11.3 Examples of different dose levels in vitro

11.2.1 Polarisation effects

One important property of light is the polarisation. Any kind of light can be made polarised, simply by letting it pass a polarisation filter. It is easy to show that when non-coherent polarised light is penetrating and being scattered in tissue, the degree of polarisation rapidly decreases as a function of penetration depth.
(In a non scattering medium the polarisation can be kept high, see chapter 11.2.1.3 "Cell cultures and tissue have different optical properties" on page 547) When tissue (or any scattering medium) is illuminated with coherent light, polarised light will occur due to the formation of laser speckles (se below). This is independent of whether the incident light is polarised or not. If the incident coherent light (laser light) is polarised, this polarisation is evenly distributed. This degree of polarisation rapidly decreases as a function of penetration depth, but instead, laser speckles are formed by interference and then an uneven polarisation distribution has occured.

It has been documented that ordinary broadband non-coherent polarised light can give biostimulative effects on superficial problems like wounds and ulcers, but not deeper down in tissue. The Bioptron lamp is such a device. This further supports that some of the mechanisms are laser specific. See chapter 11.2.1.2 "Porphyrins and polarised light" on page 546.

Loginov [847] investigated the effect of copper vapour laser therapy (578 nm) on the content of biogenic amines - serotonin and histamine and the state of the adenylcyclase (AC) system (content of cAMP, cGMP and AC activity) at the edge of a gastric ulcer. Direct effect of laser radiation (single dose 10-15 J.) produced a significant increase of serotonin, histamine, cAMP, AC activity and an insignificant increase of cGMP. Healing of the ulcerative defect after 5-6 laser therapy sessions was followed by a reduction of the content of serotonin and an increase of histamine, cAMP and AC activity. Loginov discusses the biostimulative effect of laser radiation by influencing the inflammatory-proliferative processes in the epitheliocytes in prolonged non-healing gastric ulcers.

11.2 Possible primary mechanisms

In order to facilitate an understanding of the mechanisms of laser therapy, we have chosen to separate what we call the primary mechanisms and the secondary mechanisms. The primary mechanisms relate to the interactionbetween photons and molecules in tissue, while the secondary mechanismsrelate to the effect of the chemical changes induced by the primary effects.

The fact that the biostimulative effects are dose dependent indicates that there may be thresholds involved in different mechanisms - a certain photon density is needed. There can be many reasons for this, one of which may be multiple photon action. If the effects simply were due to electron excitation and ionisation, there would be no thresholds - single photons would do the job. The table below shows examples of dose levels for different cell types and different wavelengths in vitro.

Wavelength in nm	Culture type	Measured activity	Stimulation dose, J/cm^2	Inhibition dose, J/cm^2	References
633	Chinese hamster	cAMP	0.01		Karu [F16]
630-633	Chinese hamster fibroblasts	Proliferation	0.1		Abdvakhitova [1230]
632.8	Human embryonic foreskin fibroblasts	Proliferation	0.01		Boulton [268]
632.8	Red blood cells	Deformability	-	>1	Yova [1229]

Table 11.3 Examples of different dose levels in vitro

BLT literature:	Our comments:
Thalén [790]: Ninety patients with major depressive disorders were treated with a luminance of 350 cd/m² (approximately 1500 lux) at **eye level**. Depressed patients with a seasonal pattern improved significantly more than those with a non-seasonal pattern.	In this report, too, we can see that the author believes that the effects are due to retinal illumination. Spectrum, bandwidth, coherence, pulsing, different areas to treat, treatment interval, etc., remain to be investigated.
Lewy [807]: Morning light was more anti-depressant than evening light.	Thalén [790]: There were no significant differences between morning and evening BLT.
Kripke [818]: Light therapy can be combined with standard therapies for treating non-seasonal depressions and appears synergistic.	Laser therapy also acts synergistically with other therapies.

Table 11.2 BLT literature

11.1.7 Similarities and differences

Both laser therapy and BLT are non-invasive, safe and painless light treatment methods. Most of the laser therapy effects have been known for 30 years. BLT has been used for less than 19 years (2002) and the mechanism is not yet known - just recently it was discovered that it does not only work through retinal effects.

Our belief is that BLT and laser therapy act in similar ways and may use the same mechanisms. We think that maybe a "laser solarium", using laser light in the visible red part of the spectrum, might be more efficient than BLT. It also seems that ordinary solariums have an anti-depressive "side-effect" and that this may be one of the reasons that they still are so popular in spite of all the alarming reports of their danger.

BLT increases serotonin levels [787, 800, 801, 806] and laser therapy increases serotonin levels [191, 247, 303, 496, 846, 847, 848, 849].

Literature:

Cassone [846] studied the metabolic modifications induced in rat brain by low power HeNe laser irradiation in vivo. Both the variations in the biogenic amine levels in cortex, striatum and hippocampus were studied. Noradrenaline (NA), dopamine (DA) and serotonin (5-HT) were evaluated by HPLC-EC on irradiated rats, untreated rats (controls) and rats that had undergone restraint stress (stressed). The results showed that irradiation caused a strong increase in serotonin (5-HT) in striatum and hippocampus and a small but significant decrease in NA in cortex, while DA levels were not significantly affected.

ture and melatonin concentrations throughout the circadian cycle before and after light pulses presented to the popliteal region (behind the knee). A systematic relation was found between the timing of the light pulse and the magnitude and direction of the circadian phase shifts. These findings challenge the belief that mammals are incapable of extra-retinal circadian photo-transduction.

The literature is, as always, to some extent contradictory. We find the following:

BLT literature:	Our comments:
Rao [801]: Light treatment increases blood serotonin throughout the day. This increase is seen in all patients and healthy subjects after bright (2500 lux) as well as dim (50 lux) light. These results suggest that the influence of light is more pronounced on serotonin than melatonin metabolism. Treatment 2 hours daily.	Main influence on serotonin. This is also typical of laser therapy. It is surprising that the light intensity is not of greater importance. Maybe saturation is reached due to illumination of a large body area.
Rice [805] compared 2 weeks of light therapy with full spectrum white light with cool white light. Both treatment methods reduced depression scores, advanced the timing of the melatonin rhythm, and increased melatonin concentrations	Full spectrum white light also has a great deal of infrared radiation which cool light has not. Maybe the infrared part of the spectrum is of less importance. What about narrow band treatment or even laser light?
Wetterberg [819] writes "Light may be used to treat depression, sleep disorders, menstrual dysregulations and other illnesses with disturbed circadian and seasonal rhythms".	Treatment of menstrual dysregulations with laser therapy has successfully done by Takac [143]
Bylesjö [787]: Three of the 4 women reduced their net weight (1.5-2.4 kg) and improved in mood. 1500 lux.	It was actually popular to treat overweight with laser therapy in Sweden. We don't know how successful these treatments were. Maybe it works ...

Table 11.2 BLT literature

11.1.6 Bright Light Phototherapy

It has been known for many years that daylight influences seasonal depressions. As early as in 1990 Rao [801] investigated the circadian profiles of melatonin in serum and serotonin in blood before and after 7 days of artificial light treatment in 30 patients with non-seasonal depression and 12 healthy subjects. Patients and volunteers were allocated at random to either dim (50 lux) or bright light (2500 lux) for 2 hours daily. Light treatment was found to marginally modify the circadian melatonin profiles of depressed patients and healthy subjects. However, it increased blood serotonin throughout the day. This increase was seen in all patients and in healthy subjects after bright as well as dim light. These results suggest that the influence of light is more pronounced on serotonin than on melatonin metabolism.

In 1991 Deltito [808] treated patients with either 400 or 2500 lux phototherapy for 2 hours on seven consecutive days. Unexpectedly, the result was the same regardless of the intensity of the light. The changes were judged to be quite clinically significant. All patients showing a response were noted to have maintained their response at a 3-month follow-up.

The same year [795] Petterborg examined the effects of a single exposure to a brief burst of bright light on serum melatonin in groups of healthy human volunteers of both sexes. They were treated with a 15-minute dose of bright light (350 cd/m^2) early in the evening during the winter months. Serial blood samples were collected from each person and the effect of the light dose on serum melatonin and cortisol levels was determined. Melatonin levels were significantly but only transiently suppressed by the light dose, while cortisol levels were not affected. These results demonstrate that short duration bright light treatment can influence the melatonin rhythm generating system in humans.

From these studies, it seems to be clear that it is the serotonin level that is mainly influenced, and to some extent the melatonin level as well.

It has been the general belief that mammals are not influenced by light except in the retina. Wetterberg [796] writes (1991): "The light which reaches the eye affects us both visually and non-visually. New results of treatment for depression show that strong artificial light has physiological effects on man ... "

Our opinion is that this is wrong. If it were only a question of sending light to a person's eyes, it would not be necessary to sit in a room with high intensity light - it would be quite easy to make "light goggles" with small built-in lamps. Among the "laser therapy society" it has been known for more than 30 years that our cells (other than those in the retina) and our tissue react to light and especially laser light!

However, in 1998 it also became clear to the non-laser therapy society, from the following experiment, that this opinion was wrong: Campbell and Murphy [786] investigated, in a randomised controlled trial, the effect of light irradiation on physiological and behavioural rhythms. The response to extraocular light exposure was monitored by measurement of body tempera-

Absorption coefficient 17 mm^{-1}
Scattering coefficient 0.0 mm^{-1}
Intensity as a function of depth in pure water $I = I_0 \times e^{-17 \times d}$

Depth in mm	Intensity in %
0.0	100.0
0.1	18.0
0.2	3.3
0.3	0.6
0.4	0.1
0.5	0.02

Table 11.1 Absorption

This means that, at the depth of 0.5 mm, 99.98% of the radiation is absorbed. As tissue does not consist of 100% water - rather, it contains between 70-90% - the penetration will be somewhat higher, but the difference is not so large since organic matter also strongly absorbs this wavelength.
(See chapter 1.5.5 "The defocused strong lasers" on page 46.)

Literature:

Gürsoy [429] made comparisons between 660 and 830 nm laser penetration in tissue, using CCD camera, radiometer and isotropic detectors. A 200 mW 830 probe could give a depth of 3.5 cm with a lateral spread of 2.7 cm. Both wavelengths were scattered widely regardless of the collimation. Attenuation in skin and muscle was equivalent. Less attenuation was observed in bone and salivary tissue.

Kolárová [959] also used CCD camera technique to establish the penetration of 50 mW, HeNe laser light, 633 nm and 21 mW diode laser 675 nm. In the thickest skin sample (19 mm with epidermis + dermis + subcutaneous fat from regio abdominalis) approximately 0.3% of the HeNe and 2.1% of the diode laser light penetrated. In granular tissue the penetration was about 2.5 times higher.

Jarry [782] performed in vivo dual wavelength differential spectrography on the hand of an adult male, using a collimated transillumination device. A pulsed laser with sufficiently high peak power and sufficiently low energy was employed so that transillumination could be realised without thermal damage. Spectrochemical analysis based on the absorbance of oxygen transporting molecules (OTM), i.e. haemoglobin in blood vessels and myoglobin in muscles, was performed along a 70 mm scanning line within the near-red infrared range. The two wavelengths used (675 and 800 nm) were chosen on the basis of the absorption spectrum of haemoglobin. In other words, so much light penetrates the hand of an adult person that it is possible to measure the spectrum of the transmitted light!

Further literature: [1254]

11.1.5 How deep does light penetrate into tissue?

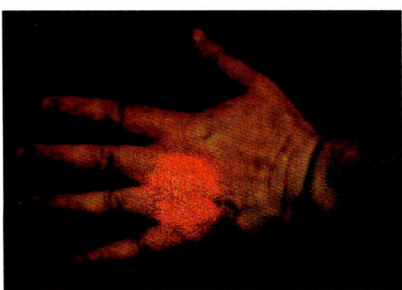

Figure 11.6 Transilluminated hand

It is easy to establish that the light penetrates deeper than 1-2 mm in tissue. If you hold your hand in front of a pocket torch, you can see that the light penetrates your fingers, and they are generally thicker than 1-2 mm. You will also note that the light which penetrates is red, so it is the red light in particular which penetrates, while the blue, green and yellow are absorbed. Infrared light is not visible, but it is easy to demonstrate that it penetrates deeper than visible light. Therapeutic lasers emit red or infrared light.

The depth of penetration of the red light has been studied in conjunction with a technique called PDT (photodynamic therapy) by which HPD (hematoporphyrin derivate), for example, is injected in the tumour area and then irradiated with laser light with a wavelength of 630 nm. It has been established [24, 25] that the depth of penetration is enough to get a biological response (necrosis) as far down as 10 mm in the tissue.

With the above mentioned definition, [37% =1/e of the intensity on the surface, where e = 2.71828 - (See chapter 11.1.4 "Moonlight" on page 537.)] - the depth of penetration becomes totally independent of the laser's output, which means that the same depth value is achieved no matter how weak (or strong) the laser. The definition in question specifies, in actual fact, the <u>relative penetration,</u> while the decisive factor for the biological effect is the beam's momentary <u>absolute value</u> and, as has been mentioned, the <u>absolute penetration</u>. This is decisive for the intensity of the electric field across the cell membranes deep in the tissue.

Our understanding and experience, based on 20 years of experiments and practical work, is that laser therapy achieves direct biological effects at a depth of 1 - 4 cm in tissue, depending on the type of laser used, the laser's output, and other parameters. Further, systemic effects due to circulation of blood and of other forms of communication in the tissue, such as the transport of transmitters or signal substances occur at much deeper levels and, as a matter of fact, throughout the entire body.

If poor penetration would indicate that therapeutic lasers just could not work (according to Greguss and King), it would be even less logical for CO_2 lasers to have an effect. The penetration of CO_2-laser light is considerably poorer than that of the conventional therapeutic lasers. The calculation below shows the penetration of CO_2-laser light (wavelength 10600 nm) into pure water:

has calculated that at the depth inside the body of, for example, a shoulder joint, laser treatment gives a light intensity equal to that of moonlight. This is probably correct. However, laser therapy is not a case of broadband moonlight, but of highly monochromatic and, at least partially, polarised, coherent laser light, which even at low levels can impart interference effects. And what light intensity does it have to be? Would perhaps starlight level be enough? In theory, one single photon can actually start a chain reaction.

Let us make a little calculation: A fully adapted human eye can see about 10^{-9} lux. This corresponds to about 1.5×10^{-17} watts of visible power or about 30 photons per second of energy through the pupil of an eye. This little energy flow can create a minute nerve signal.

In a dark room, a 10 mW HeNe-laser can transilluminate a hand. A GaAlAs laser (820 nm) has even better transmission but its longer wavelength cannot be seen by the naked eye. It has to be measured by instruments. 2 cm down in tissue, only between 0.1% and 0.01% of the incident power remains. Suppose that we use the lower transmission value. Assume that the laser probe has an output power of 60 mW (0.060 watt) which is a power level often referred to in the literature. Assume further that said 60 mW laser light is concentrated to a 3×3 mm surface, i.e. gives a power density of 660 mW/cm². This means that 2 cm down in tissue the laser power is as low as $0.0001 \times 0.660 = 6.6 \times 10^{-5}$ watt/cm², i.e. 66 microwatts per cm². The rest of the power has been absorbed, been transmitted or, after scattering, been reflected away. An interesting question is now: How many photons per second (N) passing through the surface of 1 cm², equals 66 microwatts/cm²?

$N = 6.6 \times 10^{-5}$ watt / photon energy (hv) =
$= 6.6 \times 10^{-5}$ watt / 3×10^{-19} joules =
$= 2.2 \times 10^{14}$ photons / second =
$= 220\ 000\ 000\ 000\ 000$ photons / second

That is a tremendous amount of photons!

Let's look even deeper into the tissue: At a depth of 4 cm (thickness of an arm), the laser power is as low as 0.006 microwatts, with the same chosen absorption factor. This corresponds to 22 000 000 000 photons per second and cm², also a very large number. This is about 700 million times more than the 30 photons per second that it takes to produce the chemical reaction needed to create a nerve signal that we can notice.

At 6 cm depth we get 2 200 000 photons per cm² per second, which is 70 000 times more than the 30 photons per second that are capable of stimulating a nerve signal in a human eye. So, even at such large depths, theoretically, there is enough laser light energy to give rise to chemical reactions and secondary chain reactions.

Nils Abrahamsson, at The Swedish Royal Institute of Technology in Stockholm, observed these speckles through a microscope and was probably the first to notice that the speckles on the surface of an apple move. He could relate this movement to particle movement within the cells of the apple.

The phenomenon has since been surveyed by French scientists [19], who studied the movement of the laser speckles and could differentiate two different forms of particle movement in the interior of the apple cells. As this is not possible with light sources other than laser, it is fairly obvious that there is a great difference in quality between laser light and incoherent light and that the coherence of laser light is not lost.

Kamikawa [359] shows in his article "Studies on low power laser therapy of pain" a picture of a finger that is transilluminated by a diode laser of 1 mW. The light from the laser passes through the finger and shows, on the opposite side, interference fringes. When the same experiment was done with an LED, no interference fringes appeared. This experiment also shows that coherence is not lost when laser light is diffusely scattered in tissue.

Enlarged real laser speckles recorded on a black and white film. Bright parts correspond to areas (volumes) with higher intensity than average.

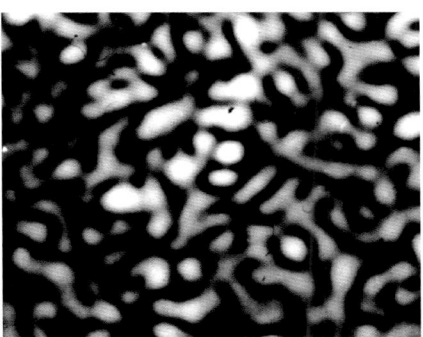

Figure 11.5 Enlarged real laser speckles
Photo: Lars Hode

11.1.4 Moonlight

King and Greguss also assert that, for example, the light from a HeNe laser (red visible light) only penetrates 1-2 millimetres into the skin and laser therapy can therefore have no effect, except for a very superficial one. They define the penetration as "the depth where the light intensity has dropped to 37% (=1/e of the intensity on the surface, where e = 2.71828...) of the intensity on the surface".

Svaasand [27] has tried to lead the way in proving that the reported effects of laser therapy on tissue would contradict the laws of physics. He

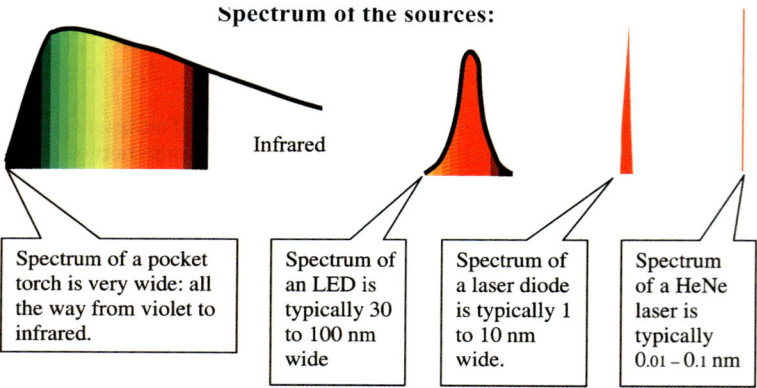

Figure 11.4 Different light sources have different spectra

Even though the laser diode has a much shorter coherence length than the HeNe-laser, the speckles are very pronounced in both laser spots. The LED has such a short coherence length that no speckles can be seen. The coherence length of a light source is more or less inversely proportional to its spectral bandwidth. This means that lamp light has a very short coherence length (in the order of nanometres) while a gas laser can have a coherence length of several metres.

We have noticed that in the treatment of ulcers, herpes and some other skin and mucous problems, a higher dose is needed when a diode laser is used than when a HeNe laser is used. This is most probably due to the difference in coherence length between those two sources.

11.1.3 Abrahamsson's apple

This is an other experiment showing that the coherence of laser light does not disappear when spread diffusely.

If we direct a narrow beam from a HeNe laser at an apple, we can see a halo with a diameter of 1-2 cm around the intense target point. This halo occurs because the laser light is spread and reflected in all directions in the tissue of the apple, and consequently, some of it is also, after scattering, reflected out of the apple. If we look at the halo, we also see laser speckles (virtual speckles), which shows that the laser light retains its coherence after its passage through the tissue of the apple. Furthermore, the coherence of the laser light is much greater than the coherence of light from a red LED, for example, which does not exhibit clear speckles when directed towards the apple. The distribution of the laser light inside the apple is not homogeneous but grainy, due to interference, i.e. it consists of a three-dimensional speckle structure (real speckles).

We can draw the following conclusions from this experiment:

A. Both light spots are red after their passage through the meat. This shows that red light has the best penetration of the visible light wavelengths. Measurements using instruments show that infrared radiation penetrates even better.

B. The coherence of the laser light does not disappear. The laser speckles can be clearly seen, and it is obvious that there is a difference between laser light and the light from a torch. This physical difference characterising the light after its passage through tissue can explain at least some of the research results mentioned above.

C. The HeNe laser beam is narrow and parallel (collimated) when it encounters the minced beef. After its passage through the meat, it is scattered considerably. If we use a laser with visible and highly divergent light (e.g. a diode laser) and place it close to the surface of the meat, we get the same light image on the back as with the collimated laser.

light image on the back as with the collimated laser. The collimation therefore has no significance for the light image in tissue [429].

It is easy to extend this experiment by including a red light LED. This gives the following result:

11.1.2.3 Hode's big burger

At the European Medical Laser Association 2nd International Meeting in Florence, October 28-31, 1999, L Hode presented an extended version of the same experiment using four light sources - HeNe laser, InGaAlP diode laser (650 nm), a cluster of 7 red LEDs (660 nm) and a normal small pocket torch. Two of the four red light spots showed laser speckles and two of them did not - guess which one!

These nice and simple experiments can be performed by anyone who has a laser and a pocket light. Anyone can see the difference between the laser light and the non-coherent light after penetration of the tissue (meat). It is essential that one has a stable set-up so that movements do not distort the speckle pattern.

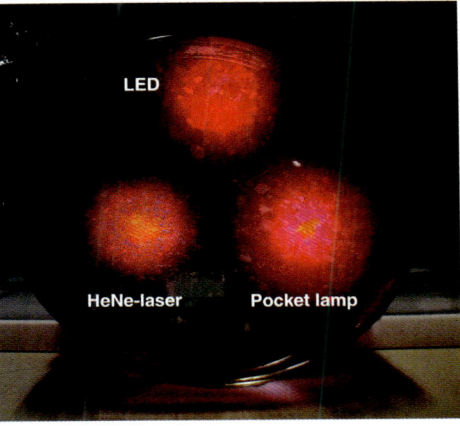

Figure 11.3 Extended set-up

11.1.2.2 Hode's hamburger

The literature gives no support to King's and Greguss' assumption that the coherence of laser light is lost when it penetrates tissue. We maintain that coherence is not lost.

It is, however, well known that the coherence length decreases in the event of diffuse reflection, but it does not drop to zero. We can firmly establish this by means of the following experiment, first demonstrated by L. Hode at The Ninth Congress of the International Society for Laser Surgery and Medicine in Los Angeles in 1991. Anyone with a HeNe laser can conduct this experiment.

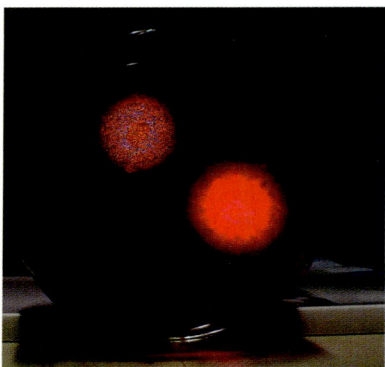

Figure 11.1 Hode's hamburger

1. Press newly minced fresh beef, e.g. raw hamburger meat, between two glass plates so that you have a 5 - 10 mm thick slab of minced beef.

2. Aim the light from a 5 - 10 mW HeNe or InGaAlP-laser (red visible light with a wavelength of 633 nm) at the glass plates with the minced beef slab as shown in the figure. You can see a red spot on the back of the minced beef where the light has penetrated.

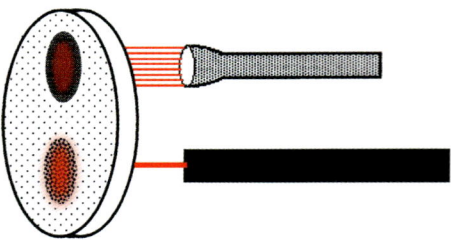

Figure 11.2 Set-up for Hode's hamburger experiment

3. Next, place a small penlight torch beside the laser and put its front end against the surface of the glass. The torch emits normal white light. This light also penetrates the minced beef and forms a light spot beside that caused by the laser. The spot from the penlight torch is also red, even though the torch emits white light. This is because the white light's blue, green and yellow colour components are absorbed, and only the red component penetrates.

4. Now study both the red light-spots on the back of the slab from a distance of a few metres. The laser light spot shows clear laser speckles which you can see if you slowly move your head. The spot from the torchlight has no laser speckles.

tigated. The laser parameters used indicated that all clinical variables improved as well as some of the laboratory variables. In that first study one side of the mouth was treated with laser and the opposite side was used as control. In spite of the possibility of systemic effects, the clinical and laboratory findings suggested that the model could be a base for a study on the importance of the length of coherence.

In the second study a HeNe laser was used on one side of the mouth and an InGaAlP laser on the other side of the mouth. The output power of both lasers was 3.0 mW. The round aperture had a diameter of 4.0 mm, giving an aperture area of 0.122 cm^2. Supposing that the light intensity distribution is equal over the aperture area, the power density was 3.0 mW / 0.122 / cm^2 = 24 mW/cm^2. If instead the average intensity (power density) over 1 cm2 including and surrounding the aperture (held in contact with the tissue) is calculated, we have 3.0 mW/1 cm^2 = 3.0 mW/cm^2. The lasers used were a custom made 3 mW HeNe laser (632.8 nm) and a diode laser (650 nm), equally of 3 mW. Both lasers had the same size of the aperture, allowing for equal power densities. The outputs of the lasers were controlled weekly using analogue power metres provided by the manufacturers. The lasers were selected in spite of the low output because they had identical features.

Treatment time was 180 seconds per point, resulting in a dose value in the aperture area of 180 sec × 24 mW/cm^2 = 4.3 J//cm^2. On the other hand, with the more common definition of dose, using averaging over 1/cm^2 rather than over the area of the aperture, results in a dose of 180 × 3 mW/cm^2 = 0.54 J/cm^2.

Laser therapy started one week after baseline with one session every week for six weeks. Each buccal papilla of the teeth 13, 14, 15, 16, 17, 23, 24, 25, 26, 27 and in addition the lingual papillae of 16 and 26 were irradiated for three minutes each, representing an energy of 0.54 J per point, total energy per quadrant 3.24 J. Final measurements were performed one week after the last laser session. The irradiation was performed in light contact with the tissue.

The difference between the two lasers was obvious, in spite of the possible systemic effect. It is therefore suggested that the length of coherence is an important parameter in laser therapy. It is possible that increased dose from the diode laser could compensate for its shorter length of coherence but this is still an open field for research.

sessions, excepting weekends. 40% of the laser treated patients recovered fully, while in the non-coherent group no patients recovered fully.

In a further study, Simunovic and Trobonjaca [709] compared the efficiency of laser therapy on lateral epicondylitis (tennis elbow) in 120 patients with:
   a) transcutaneous electro-neural stimulation (TENS),
   b) visible, incoherent polarised light (VIP) and
   c) placebo "treatment" with a non working laser unit.

The number or treatment sessions per patient was twelve. The laser dosage was 4 J/point and the VIP-light dosage was 4 J/cm^2. The results demonstrated that the laser therapy gave the highest percent of pain relief (>45% of lased patients reported 90-100% pain relief), TENS gave the second best pain relief. None of the patients in the VIP group reported 90-100% pain relief. The worst result was reported by the placebo group (<20% of average pain relief).

We wish to underline that the studies above do not indicate that non-coherent light therapy for suitable indications and with sufficient energy densities is inefficient. It only shows that whenever compared, coherent light has come out on top. But indeed, the effect of non-coherent light therapy has been verified [1074], even in double blind studies [433, 941, 1232]. However, in these studies, non-coherent light was not compared with coherent light.

11.1.2.1 What is the importance of the length of coherence?

One of the first therapeutic lasers in the red spectrum was the helium-neon laser with a wavelength of 632.8 nm. In recent years red laser diodes in the range 630-660 nm (InGaAlP) have been replacing the HeNe laser. There are many advantages with diode lasers compared to gas lasers - smaller size, low voltage power supply, not fragile and much lower price. Lately, the red diodes can also offer higher power than most HeNe lasers. However, a HeNe laser has a spectral width of 0.01 nm compared to about 1 nm for a diode laser of the same wavelength. Correspondingly, a HeNe laser typically has a much longer coherence length - several centimetres and possibly up to meters - than diode lasers. In many therapeutic instruments using a HeNe laser, the light is transported through an optical fibre. This reduces the length of coherence considerably but anyway remains longer than that of a typical red laser diode.

Most therapeutic HeNe lasers are in the range 1-10 mW. Higher output is available but becomes expensive. Still the HeNe lasers have been successful during the years, in spite of their low power. Could it be that the superior length of coherence has something to do with it?

The aim of the study by Qadri [1606] was to investigate whether or not the length of coherence has any clinical significance. The study design was copied from a previous study by the authors [1185]. In that clinical split mouth study the effect of laser light on the gingival inflammation was inves-

doses cause focal epidermic hypertrophy. Thus, the therapeutic window seems to be narrower for monochromatic non-coherent light.

Nicola [750] investigated the role of polarisation and coherence of laser light on wound healing in rats. There were four groups of wounds:
#1 was treated with coherent and polarised HeNe laser light (633 nm).
#2 was treated with non-polarised, coherent HeNe laser light (633 nm).
#3 was treated with polarised, low degree coherent light (633 nm).
#4 was untreated and served as control.

After the fourth treatment, lesions #1 had healed completely; lesions #2 had not healed completely but showed a more advanced healing process than lesions #3. The lesions #4 showed a poor degree of cicatrisation as compared to lesions #1, #2 and #3.

One investigation that unexpectedly strengthens our hypothesis that most treatments in vivo are laser specific, was published by Zhou [825]. The study concerns PDT (Photo dynamic therapy) using three light sources: a) copper-vapour pumped-dye laser, b) HeNe laser, and c) non-coherent red light (filtered from a halogen lamp), when irradiating the liver in normal mice. The mice (each group containing 18 - 20 mice) received hematoin derivative in a dose of 10 mg/kg intravenously, 24 hours prior to light irradiation. The mice livers were directly irradiated with different types of red light at a dose of 5, 10, 25, 50, or 100 J/cm^2, respectively. Forty-eight hours later the mice were killed and the depth of liver necrosis was measured using a computerised image-analysis system. No necrosis was found in the control liver irradiated with 500 J/cm^2 alone. The depth of photodynamic necrosis showed a light dose-dependent response. The mean depth of necrosis of all groups was compared statistically. The Cu-dye laser showed the best effect, while the non-coherent light showed the poorest. There were significant differences between non-coherent light and laser-irradiated groups but not between Cu-dye and HeNe laser groups. The results indicate that of the light sources examined, the Cu-dye laser is most suitable to photodynamic therapy (PDT) of tumours. However, the halogen lamp with a special filter device may still be occasionally used as a light source in PDT if needed.

In a study by Paolini [940], 99 patients with shoulder tendinitis were divided into three groups. One received HeNe laser irradiation, one LED 660 nm irradiation and one anti-inflammatory medication. 25 sessions with either laser or LED were given. The outcome of the laser group was better than the pharmacological group and much better than the LED group.

Antipa [1077] compared the effect of: 1) GaAlAs laser, 720 nm 3 mW, 2) non-coherent light at 750 nm, 9 mW, and 3) placebo irradiation. 74 patients with sciatic problems were treated. The positive results were 66.6% for the laser group, 52% for the non-coherent group and 36.4% for the placebo group.

Simunovic [1134] compared the effects of 830 nm laser light with broadband, non-coherent, polarised light in the treatment of epicondylitis. Both groups of patients (n = 20) received 4 J/cm^2, 12 consecutive treatment

Haina [17] compared the effects of HeNe-laser and incoherent light of the same wavelength. Experimental wounds were punched out in the muscle fascias of 249 Wistar rats. In the HeNe groups, the granulation tissue increased 13% at 0.5 J/cm^2 and 22% at 1.5 J/cm^2. The increase in the incoherent group was less than 10%.

Rochkind [158] compared five different wavelengths, giving a single transcutaneous irradiation to injured peripheral nerves. HeNe laser prevented the drop in functional activity following crush injury. 830 nm laser was less effective, 660 nm incoherent light was even less effective, and 880 and 950 nm incoherent light was completely ineffective.

Laakso [253] studied the relationship between laser therapy and opioids. In a double blind study, 56 selected patients with chronic pain conditions were treated with 820 nm laser therapy 25 mW, 670 nm laser therapy 10 mW, or 660 nm LED 9.5 mW. ACTH and β-endorphin levels were significantly elevated in the laser therapy groups but not in the LED group.

Pöntinen [332] compared the effect of laser light (633 and 670 nm) and light from a LED-source (with 660 nm wavelength) on head skin blood flow in 10 healthy men, using laser doppler technology. Doses were from 0.1 to 1.36 J/cm^2. Skin blood flow was measured before, immediately after and 30 minutes after each treatment session at 4 sites on the scalp. The conclusion was that 670 nm laser induced a temporary vasodilatation and increased blood flow when the dose given was in the range of 0.12 - 0.36 J/cm^2. The non-coherent visible monochromatic irradiation with doses between 0.68 and 1.36 J/cm^2 decreased blood flow for at least 30 minutes after irradiation.

Lederer [426] found that "irradiation with coherent HeNe laser light affected leukocytes in migration inhibition assays. Incoherent light of the same wavelength and power density showed no influence."

Rosner [493] evaluated the ability of HeNe laser to delay posttraumatic optical nerve degeneration in rats. The optical nerve was crushed and irradiated through the eye. Interestingly enough, irradiation immediately before the injury was as effective as irradiation beginning soon after it. Non-coherent infrared light was ineffective or had an adverse effect. However, the non-coherent light had a wavelength of 904 nm, which makes comparisons difficult.

Nicola [511] developed a technique of causing highly reproducible inflammatory lesions on the skin of rats. HeNe laser with a dose of 1 J/cm^2 produced an acceleration of the healing process. Incoherent light of the same wavelength and dose was less favourable.

Onac [659] compared the effect of HeNe laser and monochromatic light at 618 nm. The intact skin of guinea pigs was irradiated with different doses. He not only compared the two different light sources but also compared them at different doses (from 0.63 J/cm^2 and up to 38.1 J/cm^2) and came to the following conclusion: Non-coherent monochromatic red light irradiation leads to tegument trophicity at 4.96 J/cm^2 (but less than a HeNe-laser); lower doses have no effect (the HeNe laser does) whereas higher

Firstly: There have been quite a number of studies conducted on both people and laboratory animals [13, 14, 15, 16, 17, 158, 204, 205, 253, 332, 426, 493, 511, 659, 750, 851, 940, 1077, 1105, 1233] - even blind studies - in which the effect of laser light was compared with the effect of light from other sources, such as LED's. A significant effect was observed with lasers, which was not achieved with the other, less narrow-band light sources Conclusion: Either all the investigators who conducted this research were mistaken, or the effects are specific to laser light.

Secondly: The coherence of laser light is not lost in tissue due to the phenomenon of scattering. Light is neither coherent nor incoherent but is more or less coherent (see the term "coherence" as explained above).

Thirdly: There is no "normal light" with the same optical properties as a laser, although if one did exist, it would of course produce the same biological effects as a laser.

Fourthly: The penetration of light into tissue is not minimal. This will be discussed later. (See chapter 11.1.5 "How deep does light penetrate into tissue?" on page 539.)

11.1.2 Comparisons between coherent and non-coherent light

In the literature there is good support for the hypothesis that at least some of the biostimulative effects in vivo are laser specific. In fact, we have not yet found even one single study indicating that non-coherent light is as efficient as coherent light for anything but for superficial structures. This does not mean that non-coherent light is not useful for therapy, only that it is less efficient and probably mainly useful on superficial structures.

Literature:

Bihari [13] treated three groups of patients with long-standing crural ulcers with HeNe, HeNe/GaAs and non-coherent unpolarised red light, respectively. Groups 1 and 2 demonstrated excellent healing, with group 2 slightly better than group 1, compared to group 3, which had a low effective percentage.

Kubota [14] found that a 830 nm GaAlAs laser increased flap survival area in a rat model. Laser treated flaps had better perfusion, a greater number of larger blood vessels and significantly enhanced flow rates. There was no difference between control and LED 840 nm groups.

Berki [15] used a HeNe laser to stimulate activation of cells in vitro. These effects (increased phagocytic activity, immunoglobulin secretion) were not seen when irradiating the cell cultures with normal monochromatic light of the same wavelength and doses.

Muldiyarov [16] used a HeNe laser on arthritis in rats and found that the laser exerted an evident therapeutic effect. Analysis of the cases where the rats were treated with ordinary red light revealed no essential differences from the control group.

11.1 Are the biostimulative effects laser specific?

All forms of light affect the living organism. It has been shown that white light in certain doses influences seasonal depression conditions [240], see chapter 11.1.6 "Bright Light Phototherapy" on page 541. It is also known that it shows stimulating effect on collagen production in skin that can be used for treatment of wrinkles.

It is essential to clarify whether or not the biological effects obtained with laser therapy will appear only if the light source is a laser - that is, if the effects are laser specific. This is not just of theoretical interest. If one could just as well use a light bulb with a polarisation filter, so called Visible Incoherent Polarised light (VIP) - or ordinary Light Emitting Diodes (LED) of a certain colour or infrared light (such as in remote controls) - it would be considerably less expensive to manufacture therapeutic instruments. Some producers of therapeutic instruments claim that treatment with LEDs is as effective as laser treatment. Some producers even claim that LEDs are more efficient than lasers. They often make references to laser research in their marketing, obviously due to lack of support for LED effects.

We will discuss this problem closely in this chapter and the reader will, hopefully, feel more enlightened on the subject after having read this part of the book.

Furthermore, we will try to look into the mechanisms behind the healing laser light. But first we will take a look at the arguments advanced by some "non-believers".

11.1.1 Is it possible to prove that laser therapy doesn't work?

New knowledge and treatment modalities within medicine have not always been well received. When Louis Pasteur claimed that there are small microscopic beings that make meat decay, his contemporary colleagues scorned him. "But," said he, "have a look for yourselves in my microscope!" His colleagues laughed and said they would certainly not do that.

It is an interesting phenomenon that physicists have entered the debate in an attempt to prove that laser therapy just cannot work. As an example of this, we have chosen to discuss an article by King [12] who, like Greguss [233, 234, 235] before him, maintains that therapeutic lasers cannot work because it would be contrary to the laws of physics. King and Greguss claim that:

(A) In terms of their biological effect, lasers may just as well be replaced by a "normal light" with the same optical characteristics, due to the laser light's loss of coherence through scattering in tissue, and
(B) Laser light can have no medical effect, due to its minimal penetration in tissue.

We consider this to be a mistake, on the basis of the following:

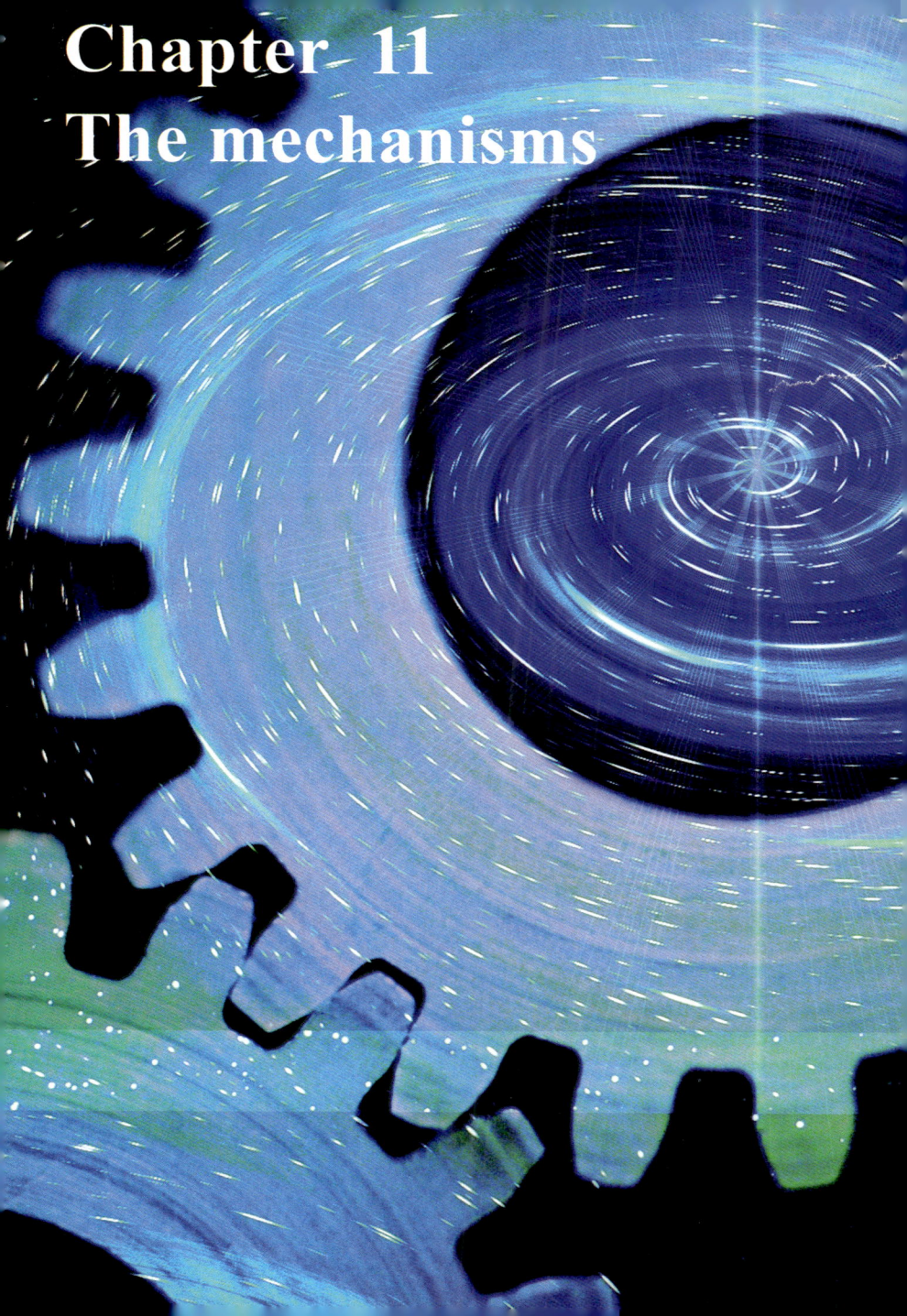

Chapter 11
The mechanisms

Chapter 10 The difficult dose and intensity

Technique and expertise mean a lot. This is shown clearly in a study by Ortutay [518]. The outputs of 13 different laser wavelengths (604-1219 nm) were compared in medical rehabilitation applications. The same pain alleviation effects were achieved regardless of wavelength or pulsing if the dose was controlled. The minimum dose for skin was 4 J/cm^2, but the location of the target in the tissue was always taken into account. It was sometimes necessary to increase the dose up to 20 J/cm^2 to compensate for absorption. If the target was deep, only infrared wavelengths were used in order to increase penetration. There is generally no point in increasing the dose if the wavelength has a low penetration factor; the penetration of the particular wavelength must be taken into account. However, as mentioned before, pain treatment needs higher doses than e.g. wound healing.

This study clearly shows that a "joule" is very much a relative concept. The dose recommendations in this book make the assumption that the joule is delivered in a more or less optimal manner. This means, in most cases of local treatment, that it is delivered as close to its anatomical target as possible.

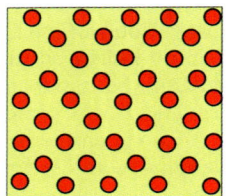 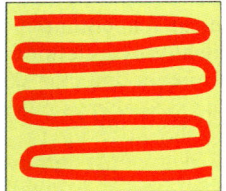 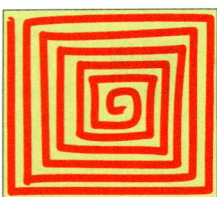

Figure 10.14 Treatment technique

The question at hand is not how many joules are delivered during a treatment session - that information may in fact be entirely irrelevant. The question is how many joules actually reach the diseased tissue. The two figures may be widely divergent.

When treating a known anatomical point located just beneath the skin, there are large dose differences depending on whether the light is delivered from a distance with a narrow collimated beam, from a distance with a divergent beam (spread out over a larger area), in contact with the skin, or in contact with added pressure. The difference between remote, contact and pressure treatment is great. The amount of energy (number of photons) reaching the inflamed tissue may vary a lot. Saying that "3 joules per point" were delivered may be meaningless for purposes of comparison. One therapist may end up delivering a dose (and/or power density) 100 times greater than that delivered by a colleague, although the same "dose" was given! Or, even if the dose is the same, taken as an average over a certain area, the power density can differ very much, giving different treatment results.

If the diseased tissue is deeper still, a new problem arises: where in the tissue is the treatment target?

Another important factor which comes into play is the skill of the therapist. If the diagnosis is correct, it is easier to know which tissue to irradiate. If the therapist has a good knowledge of anatomy, he or she will also know how to reach the tissue with the lowest possible energy loss. It may be necessary to place the patient in a particular position so that intervening muscles move out of the way and reveal the target. In such situations, the dose delivered by a qualified therapist may exceed that delivered by an unqualified colleague by a thousand-fold. Comparing the number of "joules delivered" in such a case is meaningless. It may very well be the case that therapist number one has found the right point and applied pressure to ensure minimum power loss. Therapist number two has irradiated from a distance, through an intervening layer of muscles, covering the target area by chance and luck. If therapist number two thinks that lasers are ineffective, we can understand why.

Diagrammatically this may appear as below:

If this is one square centimetre (1 cm²) and 1 joule of energy is applied equally over its total area, then the energy density is 1 J/cm² in every point over the total area.

100 mW x 10 sec/1 cm² = 1 J/cm²

If the round spot shown in the figure is the area of light from a laser probe applied in contact with the skin, held still during the exposure time and having an area of 0.1 cm², then the energy density is 10 J/cm² in every point over the spot area if 1 joule of energy is applied.

100 mW x 10 sec /0.1 cm² = 10 J/cm²

However, the average over the whole 1 cm², is 1 J/cm².

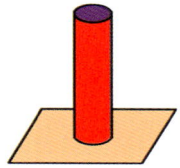 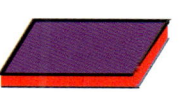

Unevenly distributed light = unevenly distributed dose

Evenly distributed light = evenly distributed dose

Figure 10.13 Distributed light

Point treatment is used in the treatment of trigger points and in laser acupuncture. (See chapter 3.3.3 "Treatment method parameters" on page 95.) A suitable dose for a trigger or acupuncture point is one to four joules.

10.11 More about treatment technique

When treating a certain area, different techniques may be used. Some therapists use the "spot" technique, meaning that they hold the probe still, move it slightly, hold it still, etc. Others use a scanning technique, slicing the probe over the skin. Different figures can be used and it does not really matter what technique you use as long as you have a good idea about the doses you give. Whether one treats clockwise or anti-clockwise is of no relevance

per "apple" at different depths. (See Figure 3.4 "Apple ready reckoner" on page 84.)

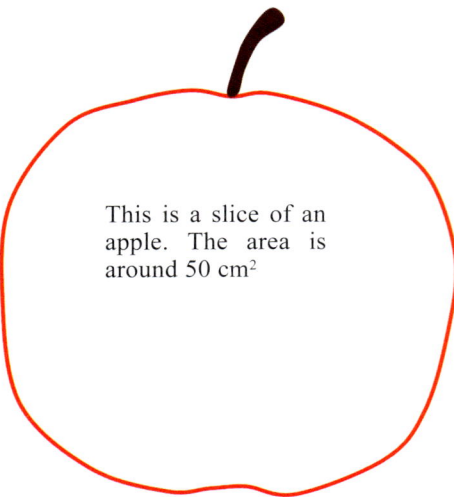

Figure 10.12 Apple

Example 1: For an area the size of an apple using a GaAs-laser probe with an average output power of 60 mW at the chosen treatment frequency (N.B.: in many GaAs-lasers, the output power is frequency dependent) and a deep problem, you should treat for a minimum of 3 minutes. Is the area larger than an apple - e.g. the size of 4 apples - treat for 4 × 3 minutes as a minimum. Maximum treatment time: Choose twice the minimum value.

10.10 Dose per point

In the treatment of trigger points and acupuncture points the dose is often said to be a number of joules per "point", the assumption being that a point is something small. We have defined a "point" as an area that is 5 mm in diameter (= 0.2 cm^2) or less. This means that if we hit the skin with the light concentrated to this small area and administer 1 joule, we have given 1 J "per point", and if this "point" is 0.2 cm^2, the dose value is 5 J/cm^2 .

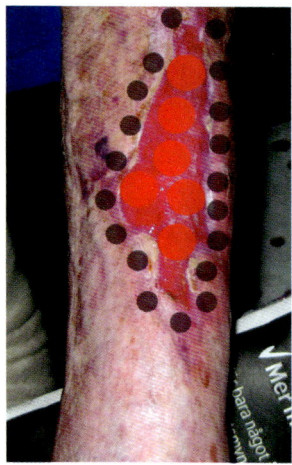

Figure 10.11 Illustration of technique for wound healing. Low intensities in non contact over the open wound, higher intensities in contact over adjacent skin areas.

1. We can use a treatment distance such that the beam covers the entire ulcer (as in figure 10.9), or ...

2. ... we can choose a short treatment distance (higher power and energy density) for the ulcer edges and a longer distance for the open parts of the ulcer (as in figure 10.10).

When treating an open wound, almost all the energy delivered reaches the intended target. The wound is naked and easily inspected, and the laser light goes directly into the relevant tissue without first passing through covering layers of skin, which, through absorption, diffusion, and reflection, remove a large percentage of the light. If the laser light is collimated (parallel light that does not spread en route from the source to the target), it makes no difference if it is delivered from a distance, since air does not absorb the light. If the laser light is not collimated, however, it should be delivered close to the surface to achieve proper power density and to avoid unnecessary complications in calculating the light intensity in the tissue.

Ready-reckoner.

For most people, mathematical formulas give negative associations. For the common therapist, it is, however, not necessary to use a calculator for every treatment. We have made the process easy. For the treatment of large areas, such as back, neck, shoulders, arms, knees, etc., we use "apples". If you cut an apple in two halves, the cut surface has an area of about 50 cm^2. Supposing that you know the laser type you have and its output power, you simply look up your laser in the table below and enter the depth of the problem: Is it deep or superficial? The table will show you the treatment time in minutes

different distances from the laser diode, the power density varies considerably. Just outside the glass covering of the laser diode (or end of a fibre) the power density is very high; it then decreases rapidly with the distance (inversely proportional to the square of the distance from the source).

If we want to treat a circular leg ulcer with a diameter of 3 cm (area 10 cm^2) we can choose the following alternatives:

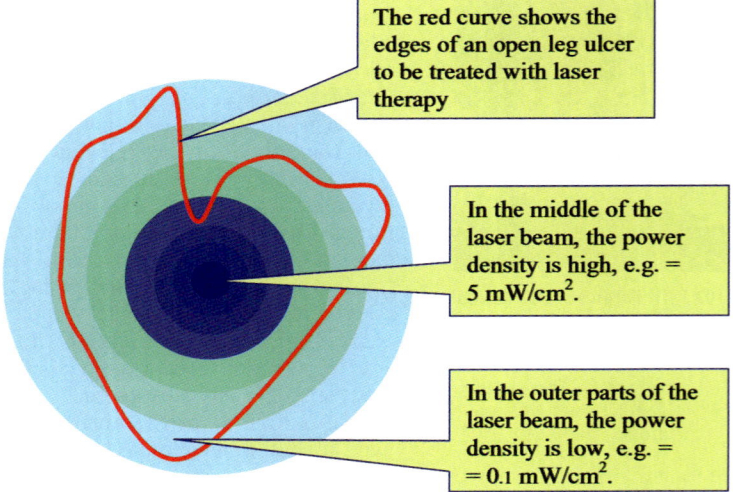

Figure 10.10 Treatment of an open leg ulcer

However, this is not necessarily a problem as long as the tissue in those volumes is healthy - the laser light is not harmful to healthy tissue even at very high doses.

In an attempt to illustrate how the dose is distributed in treated tissue, we have shown a typical situation for two lasers with different wavelengths, one being less absorbed in tissue than the other. .

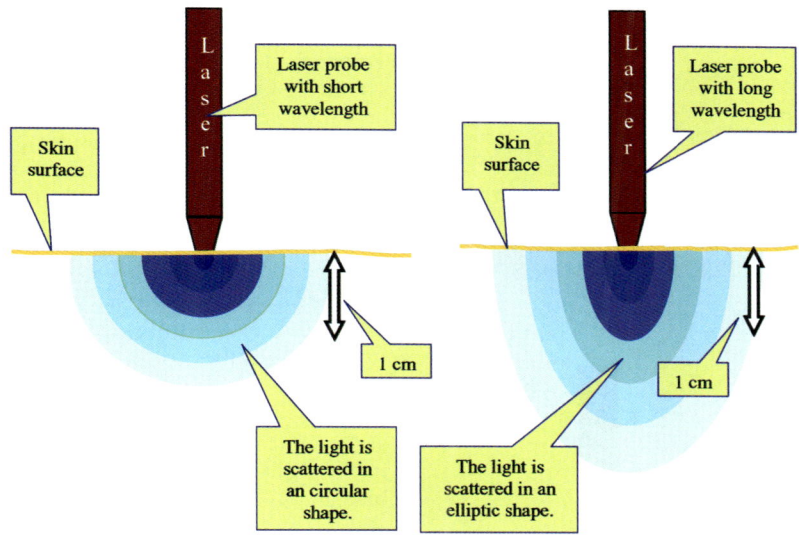

Figure 10.9 Lasers on skin, short - long wavelength

Two examples of treatment: Short wavelength light (wavelengths up to about 700 nm) is scattered more than long wavelength (700 to 1100 nm) light, resulting in different shapes of the "light ball" in the tissue underneath the skin surface. This is also the reason for the deeper penetration of most of the infrared lasers.

10.9 The dose does not depend on the intensity

What is not obvious is that with one and the same laser, dose and intensity are independent, even without changing the output power. To simplify the situation, we assume that the light from the laser diode is divergent and that the light cone is circular, (See Figure 10.1 "Typical beam from laser diode without collimator" on page 508.), and not elliptical and that, within the circle, it gives an even distribution of light all over the area hit by the beam. At

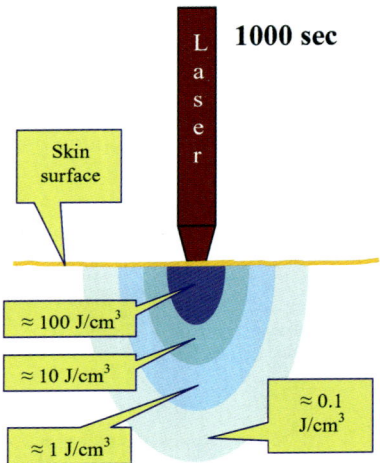

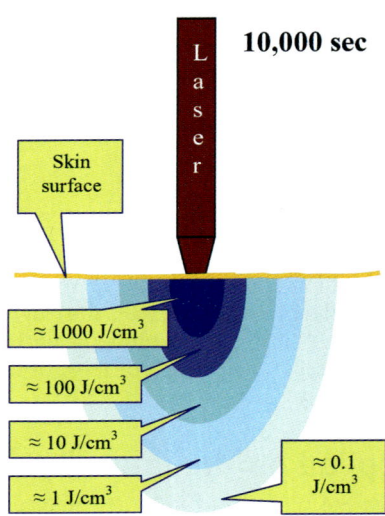

Figure 10.8 Lasers on skin

When we previously talked about dose, we always used the unit J/cm^2. But the observant reader has already noticed that in the figures shown here, the dose is expressed in joules per volume, e.g. J/mm^3 or J/cm^3. In reality this is a more correct way of expressing the energy density in a volume and in most cases we do treat volumes. Only in the treatment of cell cultures can the volume be regarded as so small that joules per surface unit may be acceptable. Even when we treat a superficial ulcer we also, in reality, treat a volume rather than a surface.

In the figures to the left, the different colours represent different dose levels. The darker the colour the higher the dose (of course there are no such sharp edges in reality - it is a smooth and gradual change). In the volume in the figure to the left, the darkest blue area is shown as receiving about 1000 J/cm^3, but this does not mean that the shown volume is 1 cm^3, nor does it mean that it is the same dose everywhere in the volume; it is an average value.

In the bottom figure the difference in dose between the darkest and the lightest volume is in the order of 10 000 times. This may mean that no stimulatory effect, or even an inhibiting effect, may occur in the volumes receiving the highest doses.

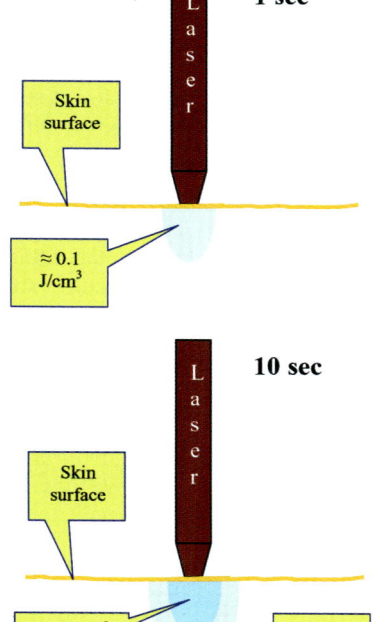

When you hold the laser probe against the skin for **one second** and the laser probe has an output power of 100 mW, 0,1 joule enters into the tissue. The distribution of that energy is usually egg shaped as can be seen in the figure to the left. In the gray area a biostimulative dose within the therapeutic window will occur.

If we keep this set-up unchanged and keep the probe in the same position, with the same output power, for **ten seconds** instead of one second, we have put ten times more energy into the tissue and we will get a larger volume of tissue receiving doses within the therapeutic window. Also note that the dose decays exponentially from the area right beneath the probe and out against the outer regions.

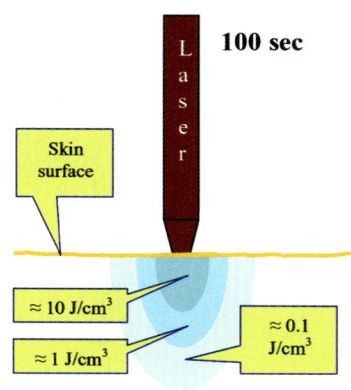

In order to illustrate this further, let us assume that we keep this set-up unchanged and increase the time, holding the probe still and in skin contact for **one hundred** seconds instead of ten seconds. Now we have administered ten times more energy into the tissue, i.e. one hundred times more energy of laser light than in the case shown in the top figure. We will then get an even larger volume of tissue receiving doses within the therapeutic window.

Figure 10.7   Laser on skin

way down from the surface to the problem volume. In a large volume, the light will be "diluted" in a manner of speaking. In reality, the light intensity decreases approximately exponentially with the distance from the surface. However, to use an exponential function in the calculation leads to complicated calculations and is not necessary because of the variations in tissue, type of indication and physical variations of the patient (skin, pigmentation, blood, bone etc) and the use of different treatment methods, see chapter 3.3.3 "Treatment method parameters" on page 95.

It would, however, be wrong not to take into account the rapid decrease of light intensity. Therefore, we suggest the use of a linear compensation as in the formula below (suggested by L. Hode in the original edition of "Laser som läker" [Laser that Heals], 1987). In this formula, which is simple to use, we have added the term (1+d) where d stands for the depth in centimetres and is limited to 1 = 0 to 4 cm.

$$t = \frac{D \times A}{P} \times (1 + d) \quad [\sec]$$

N.B.! The correct units to be used are: P in watts (not milliwatts), D in J/cm^2, the area A in cm^2 and the depth d in cm. The treatment time will then be expressed in seconds. Values 1 - 4 of the parameter d are only applicable to the infrared laser types (GaAs laser and GaAlAs lasers). For CO2, HeNe and InGaAlP-lasers, use value d=0. For problems situated deeper than 4 cm in tissue, the dose is so low (even at long treatment times) that only systemic effects will do the job.

When laser therapy was in its infancy in the early seventies, leading researchers such as Mester used doses in the range of 0.5 - 1.5 J for the treatment of wounds. They had access to 25 mW HeNe lasers, which were extremely expensive at the time - undoubtedly much too expensive to be used by anyone other than researchers and a handful of enthusiasts. It is nevertheless surprising that in the early eighties many companies introduced HeNe lasers with output powers of less than 1 mW and asserted that they were clinically useful. After fibre-optic losses, these instruments could deliver 0.1 mW or even less. This had a negative effect on clinical results, research and confidence in laser therapy. The joule suddenly disappeared from the landscape, its place being taken by the milli-joule. (See 13.1 "Are all the negative studies really negative?" on page 582.)

Generally, the dose is the amount of energy administered to a surface area of tissue. This is the same as the intensity multiplied by the time the illumination goes on and can be written:

$$D = I \times t \quad [\text{J/cm}^2] \qquad \text{where} \qquad I = \frac{P}{A} \quad [\text{W/cm}^2]$$

This equation tells us that if the intensity (I) is constant and t is the treatment time, then the administered dose is proportional to these factors. It also says that if we treat for a certain time (e.g. for 10 seconds) and we increase the intensity, then the dose is changed in proportion. So, we can give a certain dose using a strong laser for a short time or a weak laser for a longer time. Will then these two cases give the same result? Not necessarily there is a difference - the power density is different! With a ten times stronger laser we often get a better result (historically, therapy lasers have had a fairly low power density, far from the optimal value). The literature supports the hypothesis that higher power density yields better clinical results.

In pointing this out, it is not our intention to encourage therapists with low-powered instruments to scrap them in favour of newer, more powerful instruments. Their instruments will continue to be useful clinical tools if they are used with a proper understanding of the relevant facts. But remember this when it is time to buy a new laser.

Further, the dose D can be calculated as:

$$D = \frac{P \times t}{A} = \frac{E}{A} \quad [\text{J/cm}^2]$$

where P is the laser's output power in watts, t is the treatment duration in seconds, E is the energy, and A is the area treated in cm². If the laser is pulsed, then the average output power in watts is to be used. P x t is the energy produced by the laser with output P, emitted over the time t. This can be written as E.

To make the equation part more complete, we add the treatment time formula from, see chapter 3.3.1.9 "Calculation of treatment time for a desired dose" on page 82. The most common situation in laser therapy is that we want to administer a certain dose D to a specified area A with our laser, having an output (or average output) power P, and we need to find the treatment time t for the laser probe at hand. We can look at two cases: superficial treatment or deeper treatment. For treatment of the skin, the following equation can be used:

$$t = \frac{D \times A}{P} \quad [\text{sec}]$$

If, however, the problem to treat is situated at a deeper level (e.g. 1 cm or more) we have to compensate for the scattering and absorption losses on the

ten times as long, we have an energy density (i.e. dose) that is ten times higher at every point reached by the light.

10.8 Treatment dose

Again, the treatment dose (or the fluence) is the same as the energy density. We will mainly use the term dose. The dose is the most important treatment parameter. Dosage refers to the amount of energy per unit area applied to tissue surface or cell culture surface.

Biostimulatory effects of laser are governed by the arndt-Schulz law of biology, i.e. weak stimuli excite physiological activity, strong stimuli retard it. Many therapists have the feeling that the more energy the better the result. But as can be seen from the diagram below, what was originally a stimulating laser dose may become an inhibitory dose if you continue the irradiation beyond the optimal value. The optimal dose for biostimulation, based on current clinical experience, is 0.5 - 1 J/cm^2 in an open wound and 2 - 4 J/cm^2 when treating through overlaying skin. Dosage should also be adjusted according to individual response.

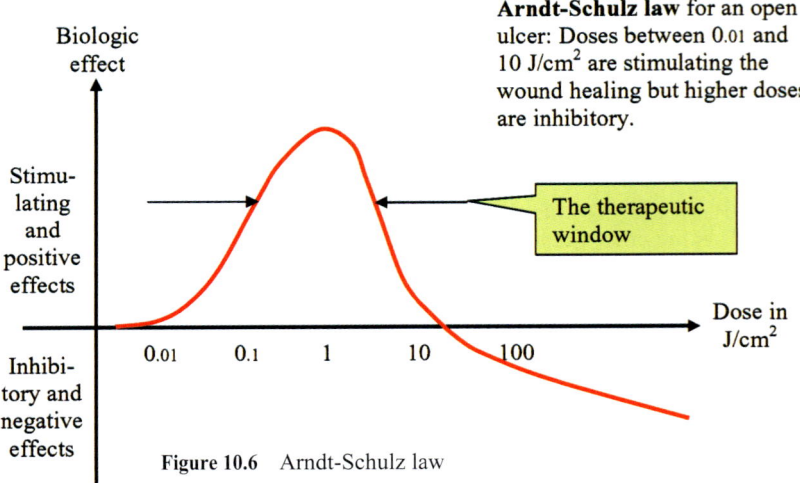

Figure 10.6 Arndt-Schulz law

Dosage and treatment intervals can only be specified schematically. This is because the various laser wavelengths and different treatment conditions mean that different doses must be given. People are receptive to laser treatment to varying degrees - some can "feel the laser right down to their toes", others are entirely impervious. It is appropriate to begin with a low dose for a new patient to ensure that you do not enter a biosuppressive dose range on the first treatment.

point itself it can be extremely high (See Figure 10.2 "Laser with focusing lens" on page 509.)

g.   A laser probe can have more than one source, in which case it is usually called a multiprobe. Multiprobes can have the laser diodes unprotectedly mounted at the end, (See Figure 7.2 "Laser probe for veterinary use." on page 470.), or mounted inside in a multiprobe. In a multiprobe, the laser diodes are usually spaced over an area.

h.   Combination probes where different types of lasers are mixed (e.g. visible and non- visible wavelengths, pulsed with non-pulsed etc). In this case it has not been shown that simultaneous treatment with two or more laser types is advantageous.

i.   Combination probes where one or several laser diodes are mixed with LEDs (here we don't mean LEDs which work solely as indicator lights). These require more research before we can safely accept them as useful. (See 11.1.2 "Comparisons between coherent and non-coherent light" on page 529.

10.6 Pulsed lasers

These have been discussed in, chapter 1.2.10 "Continuous and pulsed lasers" on page 16. A matter previously not commented on is the fact that if the laser is pulsed the power density is a function of time and can be divided into two figures: The peak power density (which in itself is not constant over the illuminated surface) and the average power density (with the same spatial distribution).

Specifically looking at the GaAs-laser, the peak power density is extremely high. Assume, for example, that the peak power of a GaAs-laser diode is 10 watts and that the diode is held in skin contact. Then, typically, the light is concentrated over a very small surface, e.g. 1 mm^2. This means that the power density in this small area is in the order of 10 W/mm^2 = 1000 W/cm^2. However, the average power density is of course much lower.

10.7 Energy density

Energy density is also named "dose" or "fluence". The difference between power density and energy density is simply the time. As mentioned above, the power density is measured in watts per cm^2. The energy density is measured in watt-seconds per cm^2, which is the same as joules per cm^2. For calculation of energy density. (See chapter 3.3.1.7 "Calculation of doses" on page 78.)

Looking at a specific situation with laser light penetrating into tissue, we will have points and areas with high power density and other areas with low power density. If this distribution of light is held constant over a certain time, we will have an energy distribution that, at every point, is exactly proportional to the power distribution. If we keep the same situation going for

10.5 The laser probe

In a practical situation, we have to look at our particular kind of laser probe (hand piece). There are many ways to design a probe:

a. In a gas laser (HeNe, Argon) a fibre is often used. It usually has a small diameter and ends at the top of the probe.

b. For diode lasers, the laser diode is usually situated inside the probe itself. In some probes the laser diode is unprotected and mounted at the very end of the probe in such a way that the glass surface of the diode is in contact with the skin during treatment. When irradiating from a distance, the light is divergent, which is advantageous from the point of view of eye hazards. But when the laser diode glass surface is in direct contact with the skin, we have a very small "light-spot" (typically in the order of one mm^2) which gives a very high power density. Further, the probe can be pressed against the skin, leading to tissue compression, which in turn causes the blood to move away from the beam. This will on the one hand increase the penetration depth and on the other lead to less effective treatment of blood cells than if the probe is not compressing the tissue.

c. In other probes the laser diode is mounted at some distance from the probe-end and there will be a distance (air) between the glass aperture of the laser diode and the skin. Depending on the distance and the angle of divergence of the laser light, the "light-spot" may be small or big with correspondingly high or low power density.

d. In some probes, the light from the laser diode is collimated by means of a collimator (lens system), resulting in a parallel and usually narrow beam. This gives us a choice of two options. In the first case, the glass surface of the collimator is at the extreme probe-end, making contact possible between skin and glass surface (compare point b). Here the cross section of the beam is usually larger than in case b. A typical cross section of such a collimated beam is in the order of 2×5 mm = 10 mm^2 = 0.1 cm^2. Remember that a collimated beam can be dangerous to the eyes, especially if it is invisible.

e. In the second case, the glass surface of the aperture can be situated at some distance from the probe-end with no possibility of skin contact. Instead of pressing against the skin with a glass surface, we often get a ring-shaped contact area. A consequence of this can be that some blood is trapped inside the ring, preventing penetration into the tissue. In this case the collimated beam can be dangerous to the eyes of patient and therapist, especially if it is invisible and carelessly aimed.

f. Another option is focusing the light from the laser diode through a lens. This focus can be placed inside the probe at the very end of the probe (possibly equipped with a glass surface) or slightly outside the end of the probe. Between the lens and the focal point the beam is convergent and after the focal point the beam is divergent, which is favourable from the point of view of risk to the eyes. The advantage of a focused beam is also that at or in the neighbourhood of the focal point the power density is high - at the focal

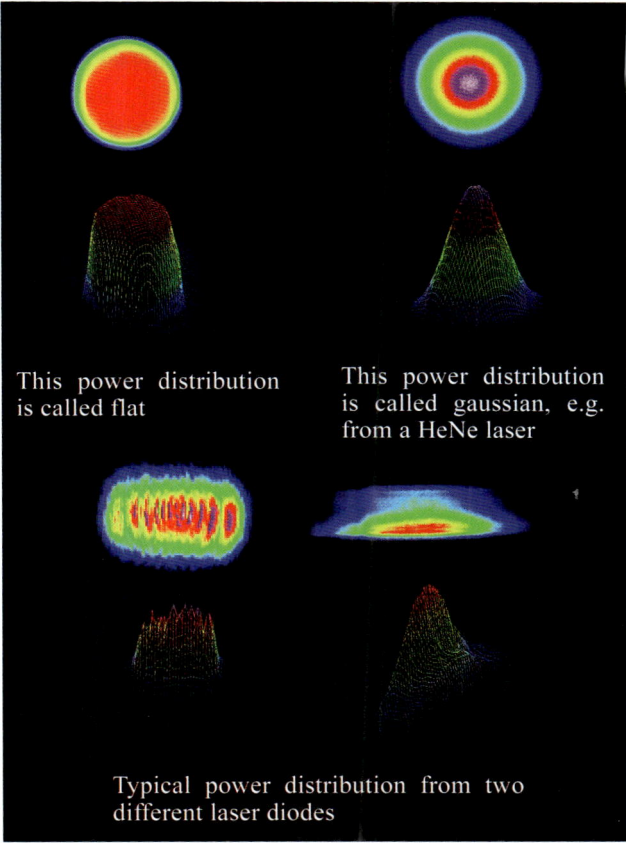

In this figure we show two ways to demonstrate the power distribution in a laser aperture. Top figures in colour coded two dimensional picture and below each figure, the corresponding three dimensional picture.

Figure 10.5 Measured power distribution in typical probe apertures
Courtesy James Carroll

The intensity distribution within the aperture is mainly of interest in scientific work, such as *in vitro* treatment, because in the treatment of tissue the light is strongly scattered. (See Figure 3.10 "Depth of penetration, direct contact" on page 119.) If, however, the beam is spread out over a larger surface (one or several square centimetres), then the intensity distribution is of importance.

10.4 The laser beam

The opening or glass surface through which the light comes out is called the "aperture". The beam from a laser tube or a laser probe does not usually have the same intensity in all parts of the aperture.

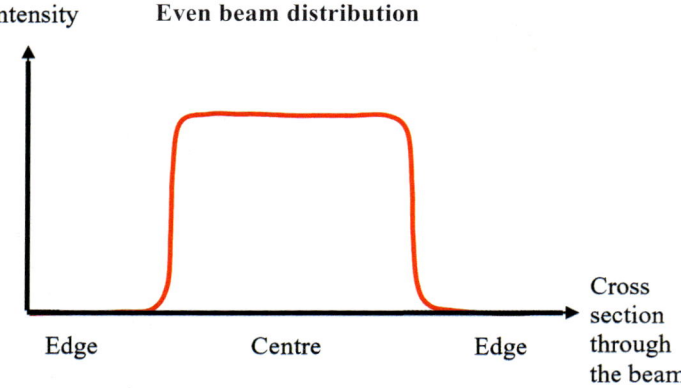

Figure 10.3 Even beam distribution

Usually it is stronger in the middle than at the edges. This often takes the shape of a so called Gaussian distribution (see the figure below).

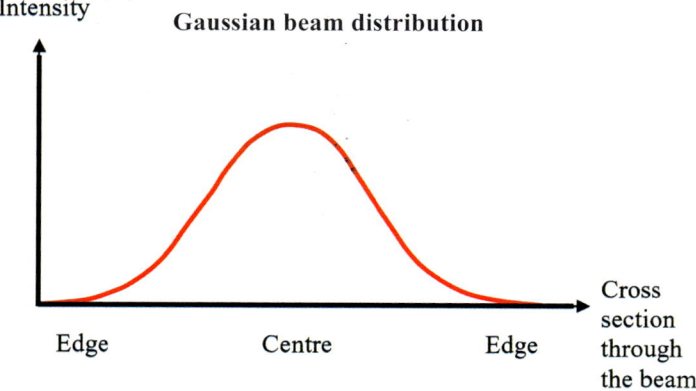

Figure 10.4 Gaussian beam distribution

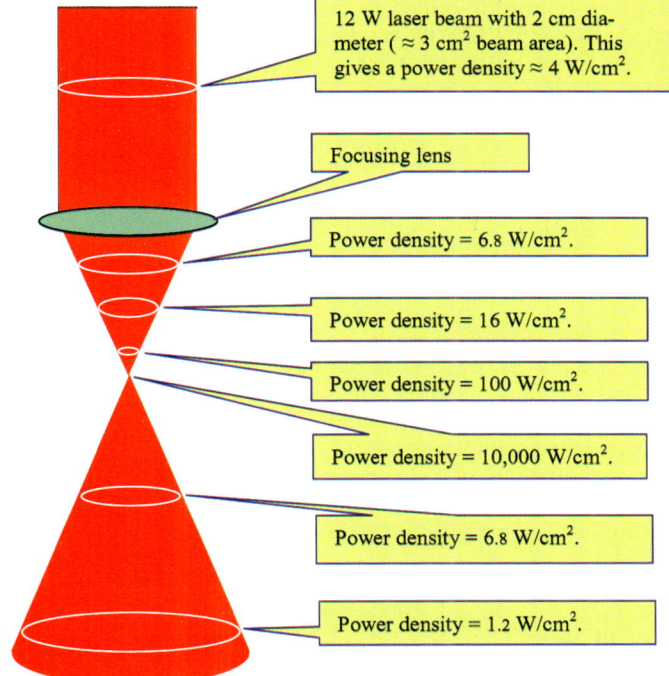

Figure 10.2 Laser with focusing lens

We have already mentioned that there are probes with focused light. When a surgical laser is used to cut tissue, this takes place near the focus point. Again: Looking at a specific situation with laser light penetrating into tissue, we will get scattering of the light, points and areas with high power density and other areas with low power density will occur. If this distribution of light is held constant for <u>one</u> second, we will have an energy density distribution that, in every point, is exactly the same number of joules as the number of watts in power distribution. If we keep the same situation going for ten seconds, we have an energy density (i.e. dose) that is ten times higher in every point reached by the light.

Like the power density, the energy density is not constant - it has a two-dimensional distribution over a surface (this is also true for the area hit by the laser light when a treatment probe is held in skin contact) and has a three-dimensional distribution in the treated tissue volume. (See chapter 3.4 "Other considerations" on page 118.)

10.3 Power density

Power density is briefly described in chapter 1.2.13 "Power density" on page 18 and in chapter 3.3.1.4 "Power density" on page 77. It is more or less the same as the "intensity" of the light and is measured in watts per cm² or milliwatts per cm² (in some literature watts per m²). Intuitively we understand that if we spread out the light over a large area we will get a lower light intensity than if we concentrate it to a smaller surface. The power density (I) can be calculated as

$$I = \frac{P}{A} \quad [\text{W/cm}^2]$$

From this equation we can see that with constant output power from the laser (P), the power density (I) is inversely proportional to the surface (A) that it illuminates. In a practical situation, the power density is not constant over the illuminated surface - it has a two-dimensional distribution over the surface (even when a treatment probe is held in contact with the skin) and has a three-dimensional distribution inside the treated tissue.

In the picture below, we illustrate how the power density varies with the distance from the source in a divergent beam of a diode laser.

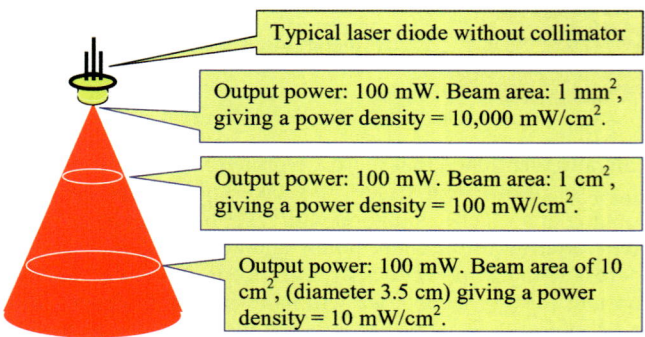

Figure 10.1 Typical beam from laser diode without collimator

Before leaving this subject, we illustrate the situation when a beam is focused - at the focal point we have an extremely high power density.

Another example of energy conversion is when potential energy of the water in a water dam is first converted into the kinetic energy of moving water in a waterfall, which in turn is converted into electrical energy by means of a turbine connected to an electric generator. Even matter itself is a form of energy - *material energy* - following the famous equation

$$E = mc^2$$

formulated by Albert Einstein. In a nuclear reactor, matter is converted to thermal energy.

10.2 Output power

When you work with a laser, there are two fundamental things you need to know:

- Your laser type and its wavelength
- Its output power (for pulsed lasers - average and peak power)

If you don't know the output power of your laser, then you have no idea about the doses you administer - maybe you are just giving "homeopathic" doses or maybe you are giving too large doses.

Power is measured in watts, which is the same as joules per second, which is an energy flow. A strong laser has a high output power and a weak laser has a low output power. Power is in some way synonymous with "strength". However, power is not the same as intensity (see power density in next paragraph).

We have pointed out earlier that it is important to find out the real output of your instrument, which often is not what your brochure or manual claims. Output can decrease by ageing or by dirt in the aperture. The laser diode may even be broken (especially if it is infrared and invisible). The best precaution is to have a power meter, either built into the instrument or as a separate device.

We have previously pointed out that this book is not intended to be a tutorial in physics. However, we want to clarify some definitions in order to better understand the problems of dose and power density.

10.1 Basics about energy

For many people, the word energy means something else than it does for a physicist. A healer may say that he transfers "energy" to the patient. But that "energy" cannot be measured in the scientific sense. In this book, we will stick strictly to the form of energy that can be measured in joules (J). One of our most fundamental laws, valid in the entire universe, is the so called "principle of energy". This law says:

Energy can never be created and never be destroyed.

Energy can occur in many forms. It was traditionally synonymous with "work". Climbing up a hill takes a lot of work/energy. If my body weights 75 kg and I transport it from one level and up to a level 10 meters higher, I have performed an amount of work and increased my *potential energy* by

75 kg × 10 m × 9.81 m/s2 = **73 600 joules** = potential energy

Where 9.81 m/s^2 is the earths gravity constant
In this case I convert *chemical energy* in my body into potential energy. If I fall down from this height, I will convert that potential energy into kinetic energy.
If I travel with the speed of 10 m/s (36 km/hour) and my weight is 75 kg, then I have a *kinetic energy* of

0.5 × 75 kg × (10 m/s)^2 = **37 500 joules** = kinetic energy

If I heat water with my electric heater and use 220 volts and 5 amperes for 100 seconds, then I have consumed *electrical energy* from the electric mains supply.

220 volt × 5 amp × 100 sec = 110 000 Ws = **110 000 joules** = electric energy

In this heater, this amount of energy is converted into the same amount of *thermal energy* which we can feel in the form of heat in the water.

A **laser** (or other radiation source) emits *radiation energy* in the form of a flow of photons, each with a well-defined energy. If its output power is 250 mW (= 0.25 W) and it is kept radiating for 2 minutes (= 120 sec), its emitted energy will be

0.2 W × 120 sec = 24 Ws = **24 joules** = radiation energy

Chapter 10
The difficult dose and intensity

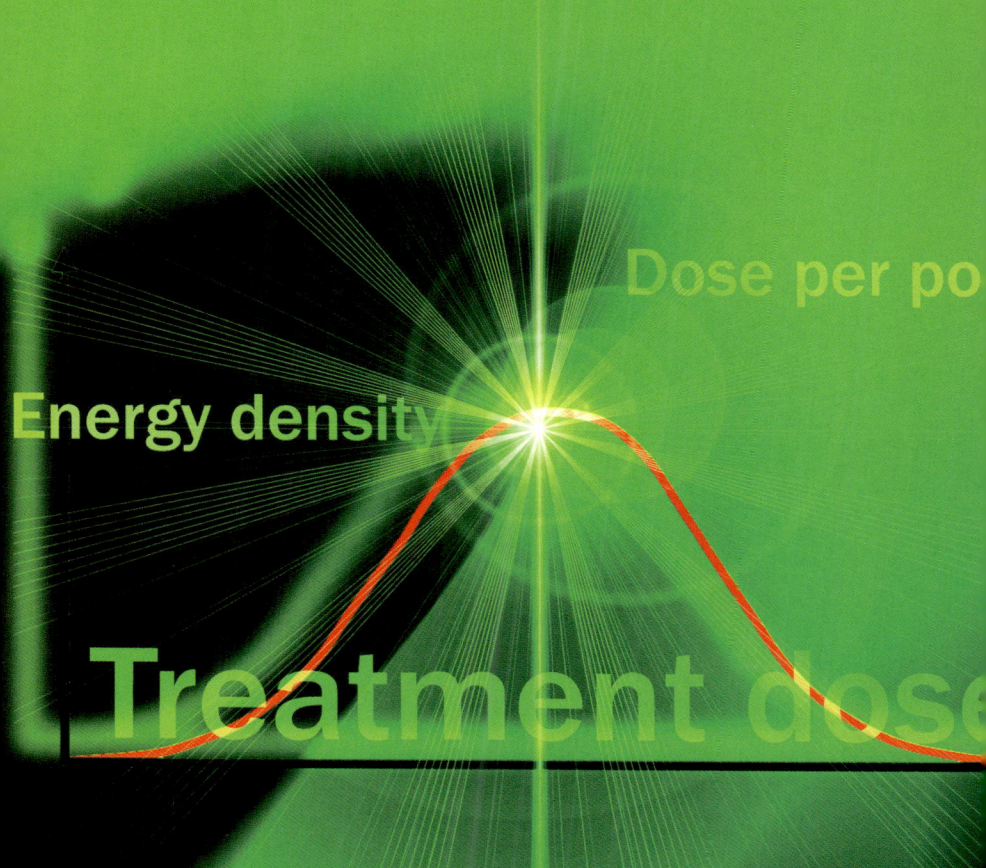

My answer is: I don't know if it is physically possible. But I think it is technically impossible and also economically impossible. I would be very interested in studying the technical solution in such a laser instrument claiming the existence of solitons waves.
Lars

Experiments are reported where solitary waves consisting of matter wave coupled with counter propagating light waves which propagates through the periodic media containing films with metallic nanoparticles (or quantum dots, nanoagregates with nonlinear dielectric properties) resonant to the light waves, alternating with dielectric layers.
Solitons moving without emitting radiation do not exist, at least in the small-amplitude limit. It has been shown that when a soliton is moving at a general speed it will experience radiative deceleration until it either stops and remains pinned to the lattice.

Some relevant literature:

L. Hocking and K. Stewartson, Proc. R. Soc. Lond. A 326, 289 (1972);
N. Pereira, L. Stenflo, Phys. Fluids 20, 1733 (1977);
K. Nozaki and N. Bekki, J. Phys. Soc. Jpn. 53, 1581 (1984).
M. C. Cross and P. C. Hohenberg, Rev. Mod. Phys. 65, 851 (1993);
F. Martin, Microwave and Millimeter Wave Technology, 485, (2000)
I. S. Aranson and L. Kramer, Rev. Mod. Phys. 74, 99 (2002)
D. N. Christodoulides, F. Lederer, and Y. Silberberg, Nature 424, 817 (2003);
N. K. Efremidis and D. N. Christodoulides, Phys. Rev. E 67, 026606 (2003).
J. W. Fleischer, M. Segev, N. K. Efremidis, and D. N. Christodoulides, Nature 422, 147 (2003).
K. Hizanidis, S. Droulias, I. Tsopelas, N. Efremidis, and D. N. Christodoulides, Phys. Scr.T107, 13 (2004).
C. Rotschild, M. Segev, Z. Xu, Y. V. Kartashov, L. Torner, and O. Cohen, Opt. Lett. 31, 3312 (2006).
Y. V. Kartashov, V. A. Vysloukh, and L. Torner, Opt. Express 15, 9378 (2007).

Another aspect of this: Assume that we could say that optical soliton waves - like in water, do exist - what would you do to the laser/light source or to the beam to create them? Research is going on using erbium doped nonlinear optical fibers. But after leaving the fiber end, they disperse and disappear. And even if we knew what soliton light waves were, why would it mean a deeper light penetration into human tissues? Should they follow the general optical laws - if not, what laws would they follow?

If certain producers of therapeutic lasers have solved the above mentioned problems with instability and with detectable soliton power and proved that this means a deeper light penetration in tissue - in my belief, it would be a scientific sensation and hardly remain unpublished.

Now, back to your question: Is it physically possible to use so-called Soliton Wave technology in a soft/cold laser, for the purpose of achieving deeper laser light penetration into human tissues, or not?

Interesting question. I made some research and found that this was shown in an experiment performed in the institution of neurology at the Karolinska Institute in Stockholm during 2001. In that experiment, all the test persons were subjected to painful heat. Some of the test persons was given pain relive in the form of opioides before they were subject to the painful heat and other test persons did only receive placebo pills and at further occasions they got no medicine at all.

The patients' brain activity pattern was investigated by means of positron emission-tomography (PET). Comparison between the patients brain activities showed that the anterior cortex of cingulum was active in connection with pain relief. Surprisingly it was also active for the persons who thought that they got pain relief, but not for the persons who neither got, nor thought that they got a pain-relieving drug. The investigators, Predrag Petrovic and Ingvar, also found that the activity in the anterior cortex of cingulum was coupled to activities in deeper areas of the brain, especially in pons. I don't know if there is a difference between negative and positive placebo.
Lars

9.2.10 Soliton waves
I have a question: Is it physically possible, to use so-called Soliton Wave technology, in a soft/cold laser, for the purpose of achieving deeper laser light penetration into human tissues, or not?
Johan

Soliton waves were first observed in water and especially in boat channels, acting as wave guides. A soliton is a fundamental nonlinear/discrete phenomenon. It is one of a number of phenomena that are shown to be universal and relevant for many non-optical systems, as localized voltage drops in ladders of the Josephson junctions, localized modes in the antiferromagnetic crystals, or localization of matter waves in the Bose - Einstein condensates. In optical systems we are usually speaking about "soliton like" phenomena. Some attention is devoted to the discrete intrinsic localized modes like discrete solitons and breathers which are candidates for guiding, steering, and switching of light beams in some nonlinear optical lattices. There are studies of properties of moving localized structures in lattices with different type of nonlinearity. Soliton-like phenomena in nonlinear media exist in a variety of forms and shapes. There exist stationary states with complex spatial shapes, including multiple light spots, or states with nontrivial topological structures, such as vortex solitons. However, in local uniform media such complex patterns tend to be unstable. The study of discrete or periodic optical systems and solitons has recently attracted attention due to the possible potential for all-optical switching applications.

spective purchasers because they are actually able to do, safely and effectively, much or all of what is claimed of them.

In short, the 'laser war' is not really about the devices but about the sometimes huge discrepancies between what their purveyors' marketing claims and what they are truly capable of doing. There is enough high-quality evidence available to support a wide range of very valid claims about lasers and laser therapy, so there is no need whatsoever to resort to such wild and patently false claims except to deliberately mislead a largely uninformed market. Misleading marketing is NOT a tactic that an honest and ethical company with a quality product will employ.

Keep this in mind when choosing a laser instrument for your practice and, most importantly, your patients.

Peter

NB: Another important consideration for US purchasers/users, especially professional medical/health practitioners, is whether the device is FDA-cleared. Many devices, including some mentioned above, are marketed illegally for use in human medicine and healthcare and yet are not cleared by the FDA for such use.

FDA-clearance has no real bearing upon whether a device will or will not be an effective therapeutic tool, but it is a legal requirement, and one must question the integrity of any device manufacturer/marketer who would knowingly and willingly break the law to sell their product. Statements like 'practitioner-assembled', or 'FDA-registered facility' are warning signs that should cause one to ask for proof of FDA-clearance.

9.2.9 HeLa cells

I have seen the name HeLa cells. What are they?

Eva

Hi Eva, I made some research and found out that HeLa cells stands for **Hen**rietta **La**cks. She died, 31 year of age 1951. Before she died, a sample of cervical cancer cells was taken from her cervix. The sample of the HeLa cell culture survived and multiplied so well in culture, that they were soon being shipped to research labs around the world for study. Although Henrietta Lack is dead, her cells live on in research labs around the world! In fact, some biologists believe that HeLa cells are no longer human at all and consider them to simply be unique and should rather be celled microorganisms!

Lars

I recently heard that the placebo effect now can be measured. Then I don't mean statistically from tests with active and placebo group, but physically in the brain. But how about positive and negative placebo, can that be verified too?

Alex

be linear at 5% per mm of tissue for infrared lasers. For red HeNe laser we postulate that further energy loss is 10% per mm of tissue." Bjordal J, Couppe C, Chow R, Tunér J, Ljunggren E. A Systematic Review of Low Level Laser Therapy With Location-Specific Doses for Pain From Chronic Joint Disorders. Aust J Physiother. 2003;49(2):107-116.

So, according to this, and given the wavelength(s) and operating mode of the K-Laser (and other Class IV devices), approximately 80% or more of the incident energy is 'lost', primarily through absorption in the skin.

We know that energy which is absorbed doesn't simply disappear, it can only be transformed.

If one is delivering light energy to the tissue, and some 80+ percent is being absorbed, some of this absorbed light energy will be transformed into chemical energy but the majority will be converted to heat energy - and laser therapy is NOT a thermal modality.

If one uses an appropriately-powered device, most of the energy absorbed in the skin will be transformed into chemical energy, and very little will be converted into heat. That heat that is generated will be sufficiently low that it is dissipated before it can appreciably increase the local tissue temperature.

However, if the rate of energy delivery is sufficiently high, the heat generated will increase at a rate higher than that at which it can be dissipated, leading to an increase in local tissue temperature. At the rate at which the K-Laser and deliver energy (some 6-10 Watts per second), the local tissue temperature will increase to uncomfortable and potentially injurious levels very quickly.

Ok, so what is my point again?

It is not that some lasers are incapable of producing results and so shouldn't be purchased. It is, however, that anyone considering the purchase and use of a laser therapy device should look very closely and critically at the claims made by ALL marketers of therapeutic laser devices, and also consider what their particular use will be for a laser device, and then make the best-informed decision they can.

If a laser can only, realistically, achieve 10-20% of what is claimed for it, then it is probably not a very wise purchase - this marketing technique alone calls the integrity of the manufacturer/marketer into question.

If, however, a device is capable of achieving 70, 80, 90%+ of what is claimed, and if what it can do is useful to you, then it is more likely to be better value and backed by a company with greater integrity.

Such companies, and there are many of them, have no need to rely upon excessive marketing hype or psuedo-scientific mumbo-jumbo to differentiate themselves, but instead rely upon the understanding and application of good, solid, science and demonstrated, repeatable results.

Many of these companies produce very high-quality laser devices at reasonable prices, and which would seem to offer much better value to pro-

claim this constitutes "a lack of adequate evidence of effectiveness of Class III 'low-level' (under 500mW) laser therapy".

Dose is only related to power through time! A low dose can be increased by increasing the emission time, or by increasing the laser power. So claiming that negative outcomes due to low doses constitute a lack of evidence of effectiveness of Class III lasers is simply wrong: NEGATIVE OUTCOMES DUE TO LOW DOSES ARE ONLY DUE TO THE USE OF DOSES TOO LOW FOR THAT PARTICULAR STUDY/CONDITION!

Could this be related to the use of too low a power?
Yes.
Is it support for the use of higher powers?
Sometimes.
Is it a mandate for the use of Class IV lasers?
Absolutely not!

The type, power and wavelength of the device used, AND the irradiation time, AND the application technique, are all important factors that contribute to the success or failure of any particular study.

In the third point, above, they have blatantly misrepresented a statement by Tunér & Hode.

A final example of a deliberately misleading inference drawn by K-Laser is:

o High powers are necessary because most of the energy is absorbed before reaching the damaged tissue being treated. Bjordal places the range of laser energy absorption (joules) by the skin and subcutaneous tissue to be in the range of 50%-90%.

In the context used this is intended to 'prove' the case for Class IV lasers, whereas in fact it is simply a statement that 50-90% of energy is absorbed in the skin.

Of course, if you want to treat deeper tissues you must take these losses into account when calculating your irradiation time, and it certainly helps by using a wavelength and power that is appropriate for the condition being treated.

Taking the apparent, yet simplistic, logic of K-Laser's argument (that a Class IV laser will deliver more energy into the entire tissue mass, thereby making more energy available to deeper tissues), we still have to account for the 80%+ of the delivered energy that is absorbed in the skin, how that energy is transformed, and the rate at which it is delivered.

The actual passage from Bjordal et al: "A systematic review...", states:

"We postulate that energy loss due to the skin barrier for continuous HeNe (632nm) laser is 90%, for continuous GaAlAs (820nm) and Nd:YAG (904 nm) lasers, 80% and for GaAs (904 nm) infrared pulse laser, 50%. Further energy loss is, according to the porcine penetration model, postulated to

o Pegasus (vet);
o Companion (vet);
o Avicenna;

Certain wavelengths, such as 980nm, are used in laser surgery because they DON'T PENETRATE as deeply as others, yet 980nm is the wavelength of choice for some of the Class IV laser manufacturers whose marketeers claim it penetrates to unrealistic depths (10 inches, in one such case!).

The worst offender in this 'misleading and exaggerated marketing claims by Class IV laser marketeers' bunch is K-Laser USA. The claims they make about the so-called inadequacies of Class 3B laser devices are very clever, and deliberately misleading.

In one example, for instance, on one of their web sites they claim that:

"Higher Power Reduces Treatment Time
How long will it take for a 6-Point (72 Joule) Carpal Tunnel Treatment?
With K-Laser it takes just 11 seconds, to treat ALL 6 points!"

Yes, with the K-Laser it will take 11 seconds to deliver 72 Joules. However, this is unlikely to produce as good a result as, say, a 450mW laser device delivering the same energy. To achieve similar results with the K-Laser (or any Class IV device) you would most likely need to deliver much higher energy doses to the tissue, and there is much evidence to support the failure of reciprocity (the Bunsen-Roscoe Law) in vivo. This is borne out by the pre-programmed protocols that come with the K-Laser, and other similar devices, which typically require treatment times of 2-8 minutes and so deliver doses upwards of 700-5000 Joules, some tens or hundreds of times higher than those required by lower (yet appropriately) powered devices.

A few other examples of deliberately misleading statements from the same site:

o Recently published reviews of the literature have concluded that there is a lack of adequate evidence of effectiveness of Class III "low-level" (under 500 mW) laser therapy for treatment of musculosceletal [sic] disorders, arthritis and pain due to extremely low dosages.
o Tunér and Hode have performed an analysis of a number of frequently cited studies on the effects of (Class III) "low-level" laser therapy. The authors state: "In many of these studies, analysis uncovered one or more reasons for negative findings, the most common being the use of low doses."
o "It would appear that "high-powered" therapeutic lasers will be able to further expand the scope of laser therapy."

Firstly, regarding the first two statements, they take the correct conclusion of a number of reviewers that "extremely low dosages" contribute to poor outcomes in clinical studies, and then misleadingly (and incorrectly)

o Q1000 (soliton waves);
o Scalar Wave Laser (scalar waves);
o and, no doubt, others...

Again, these devices are probably capable of achieving some therapeutic benefit, but are any such results likely to be optimal?
No.
Are any such results in any way related to the claimed 'scalar' or 'soliton' waves?
No!
Have these devices ever been demonstrated to produce - or are they even physically capable of producing - the claimed waveforms?
ABSOLUTELY NOT!!
These claims, patented or not, are simply a marketing gimmick that uses pseudo-scientific language to pull wool over the eyes of the gullible! There is NO FACTUAL BASIS WHATSOEVER for these claims!
Ok, now we come to the likes of many LED device marketeers who rely heavily upon making reference to research conducted using lasers (primarily Class 3B devices) to lend credibility to their particular claims, but then in the same breath go on to tell you that lasers are unnecessary because 'light is light'. There are too many LED devices out there using laser research as a basis for their claims to even create a short-list of the worst ones.
That said, however, there are also some very good LED device manufacturers which make no such (or, at least, few) embellished or exaggerated claims and simply rely upon scientifically-valid statements in support of their products, such as that LEDs can be effective in treating superficial tissues (where photon absorption is the primary stimulus and the deep-tissue effects of laser speckles are of no concern).
In a similar vein, purveyors of Class IV lasers find it suits their purposes to refer to 'low-level laser therapy' studies (mostly undertaken using laser devices which fall within the Class IIIB range) as evidence of laser therapy's effects and benefits (largely because there has as yet been very little research into the effects and efficacy of 'high-power laser therapy'), but then go on to claim that Class 3B lasers are obsolete and that they've been surpassed by Class IV devices.
Another common, yet incorrect, claim by Class IV laser marketers is that increasing the output power to many Watts will increase the penetration depth of the laser radiation - almost regardless of wavelength (which we know is simply not true!) - and overcome all the supposedly 'negative' things about Class 3B lasers. Let's now look at why such claims are tremendously exaggerated, at best, and, in some cases, simply not true.

Some of the culprits:
o K-Laser;
o LiteCure;

It is not that these devices are incapable of producing therapeutic effects. They are. It is that they are simply NOT capable of delivering upon many (in some cases, most) of the claims that are made about them, whether those claims be about the range of treatable indications, therapeutic outcomes, depth of penetration, speed of treatment, method of application, or patented waveforms, etc..

Some of the worst offenders are those that sell very low-powered visible red lasers, multi-emitter/multi-wavelength 'patented wave-producing' devices, and Class IV lasers.

Let's start with the very low powered visible red devices:

o Erchonia;
o GRT-Lite (an Erchonia-like device);
o LazrPulsr (another Erchonia-like device);
o Excaliber (yet another Erchonia-like device);
o and other similar devices...

Given the very low power of these devices, and given what we know about the achievable depths of penetration of visible red light, it is clear that the treatment of any conditions other than very superficial ones must rely solely upon the systemic effects generated by absorption in very superficial tissues (and only if that light is incident upon the tissue, not applied to clothing...).

There is nothing wrong with relying upon systemic effects, as long as you - the purchaser and user of the device - are aware that this is the case. Applied correctly, these devices are fine for the treatment of wounds and mucosa. If that is primarily what you treat, and you can justify paying the inflated prices charged for many of these devices, then make your purchasing decision accordingly. Keep in mind, however, that visible red LED devices, such as the one developed in conjunction with NASA, will produce similar results. If you already own one of these devices you should perhaps understand that although they may produce results for deeper-tissue conditions, those results are likely to be somewhat less-than-optimal.

The take-home message here is that, if considering the purchase of a laser device, one should keep in mind that there are many other devices out there which can not only treat superficially, but which also offer powers & wavelengths that successfully can reach deeper tissue structures directly and can therefore also irradiate larger volumes of tissue, potentially creating better outcomes overall through both improved local and systemic effects.

We then have the incredible 'patented-wave' producing multi-wavelength/multi-emitter type devices:

is a difficult issue for the Agency since we can only take an action, usually a Warning Letter telling company to cease such advertising when we have a specific complaint or we ourselves become aware of this. Continually monitoring such advertising is difficult and manpower intense and we do not usually have staff sufficient to do this.

Richard

The way I understand it NO MEDICAL DEVICE can be legally marketed in the USA for use on humans without either a PMA or a 510(k) unless it is a preamendment device (one marketed in the U.S. before May 28, 1976) since preamendments products were exempted (grandfathered). I should qualify that by saying class III and most class II devices. Which includes LLLT / LED therapy devices.

James

Since no laser therapy devices have to be approved for marketing in the US no claims can be made since these device would be considered unapproved devices and therefore cannot be legally marketed. The only way a laser therapy device can be marketed in the US is as an investigational device being used in an Institutional Review Board (IRB) approved clinical study.

Richard

Ah, but where do we stand on the sale and use of LED devices. Diomedics make an LED device, which they claim has FDA approval (under the old 510(k) for Infra-red heating lamps) and I'll bet you they are interpreting the term LLLT as Low Level Light Therapy. So how do their claims stand in view of the above? They are openly selling it and making all kinds of claims.

Melyni

This clearance was not granted for a Low Level Laser Therapy device, the clearance was based on the fact the device created heat at a level and duration that would make the device equivalent to heat lamps, which have this indication. There are no Low Level Laser Therapy devices approved/cleared for marketing that use non-thermal biostimulation mechanisms for their claimed benefit. The decision to find the Light Force Therapy device equivalent was based on comparison to Infrared Lamps which would mean evidence was provided that the system generate heat to result in a specific increase in skin temperature. This clearance was not based on any claim of photostimulation.

Richard

Todd, I think you've touched upon one of the biggest concerns many of us have about Erchonia (and about the producers/marketers of other laser devices, too), which is the huge discrepancy between what their laser devices CAN conceivably do, and what they CLAIM they can do!

super-pulsing (like GaAs) does not give the same tissue reaction as the on/off type pulsing of continuous lasers. Anybody who has experience in this would be welcome to tell me.
Lars

I find that on very fresh trauma, the higher frequencies are sometimes uncomfortable, Its is mostly with the 904 nm units and the higher powered (1W) 810 probes. I am still not entirely sure whether it's the frequency or the wavelength that is the culprit here. But in terms of effectiveness, as in whether one frequency has better results than another, I am not sure that there is any real difference.

I agree that are some very sensitive horses out there who really don't like the higher-powered probes/dosages. I find the best way to overcome this is to keep the probe moving around slightly so it isn't stationary. That isn't the best technique but it seems to alleviate the discomfort.

On myself when I treat a fresh trauma there is a degree of discomfort with the laser probe, not with the LED cluster. After a few treatments or even later in the same session, the discomfort goes. But that's only on me, and I am hardly a statistically valid number!
Melyni

9.2.8 FDA approval
Does anyone have any experience regarding what kind of marketing claims can be made of laser therapy in the USA as is allowed by the FDA?
David

FDA regulates the sale and marketing of devices and thus regulates what a manufacturer may or may not say in promoting their device. The issue of what a physician/healthcare professional says to their patients is more difficult and is really a grey area. The risk a user takes in promoting a device, which has not received FDA permission to market, is the risk something adverse will occur or the claimed benefit will not occur.

What the user cannot do is to publicly adverse the specific device for any claims. Again this becomes the issue of advertising unapproved devices for unapproved uses. What you tell an individual patient is between you and them, what you say publicly either in print or by Internet can become a FDA issue.
Richard

Does this mean that a physician cannot mention their thoughts/ results on what it can to for their patients?
David

Any claim other than as a heat source would be considered advertising of unapproved uses. It appears that a number of companies are doing this. This

site. If advertising is used on this site, it will soon vanish. The Producers contribution is a pure advertisement. To the best of my knowledge, it is not even a laser but a LED equipment.

The main problem with laser therapy for tinnitus is the diagnosis. Since many cases of tinnitus are related to muscular tensions, irradiation directed into the cochlea only will not be helpful in these particular cases. The temporomandibular joint will benefit somewhat, but it is necessary to irradiate all muscles involved, quite often in the neck and in the lateral pterygoid. These cases generally require TMD therapy, sometimes physical therapy and often relaxation programmes. Without a differential diagnosis the outcome of laser therapy will be guesswork. More information is available at www.laser.nu/tlc.

Jan

9.2.7 Pulse frequencies

My own take on frequency of pulsation is that it is irrelevant. This I must point out is a totally non-scientific personal observation based on my limited experience I have no measurement whatsoever to back the statement up!

Melyni

That's interesting. My experience with horses is that higher frequencies are more analgesic - if they are tolerated. Have had a few very sensitive animals that would clearly object to high frequencies or continuous but would tolerate low frequencies on the laser, or LED instead - same dosage. My husband has three partially herniated discs in his lumbosacral spine. Same thing happened with him. Couldn't tolerate the high frequencies - even gave him radicular pain shooting all the way to his foot. I ruthlessly experimented on him during that treatment session, sneaking back to the higher frequency again with exactly the same result and he had no idea what I was doing.

Eleanor

I can confirm Swedish experiences with GaAs-laser (904 nm) on horses. That laser type can almost be used as a diagnosing tool. If set on a high pulse frequency, e.g. 5000 Hz, the horse will clearly react when the light reaches the painful area. This will not happen (at least not as noticeable) if the pulse frequency is low. It happens, though not so often, that also human patients can feel the difference. However, it must be observed that this only holds true if the laser is a super pulse type (very high peak power and preferably also pulse-train regulated laser = same output over all frequencies). In many GaAs lasers the average power is reduced in proportion to the frequency. Then it would only be an effect of reduced dose. We have not been able to find the same phenomenon using a GaAlAs laser that is "chopped" with the same frequency. The subject of frequencies is intriguing. What is obvious from research is that different frequencies produce different effects. And

Ed

Well, for the information of more serious persons on this list, here are a few comments:
- In all (about 20) studies comparing lasers and LED, laser has come out on top. LED often effective, but less, but sometimes not at all and sometimes negative effect.
- The argument that cluster LED probes can have many wavelengths is devious. Every pill (wavelength) must have a meaning and interactions must be considered. Same thing goes with wavelengths.
- I doubt that laser manufacturers earn more money than LED manufacturers, but certainly LED's are cheaper. But what matters is not price but efficiency.
- Laser clusters are available as well but are only advantageous when treating large areas. Therapy must often be pinpointed. Laser therapy is not a hit-and-run story.
- I am not against the use of LED, it is a useful therapy if used in selected indications. But I am against those trying to fool people into believing that lasers and LED's are the same and using the laser scientific studies as references, trying to imply that what goes with lasers goes with LED's.

Jan

Thank you Jan. I was also bothered by that post from the Producer company. That piece of equipment is an LED device and no power or wavelength parameters were given making it less than useful!

The main problem with laser therapy for tinnitus is the diagnosis. Since many cases of tinnitus are related to muscular tensions, irradiation directed into the cochlea only will not be helpful in these particular cases. The temporomandibular joint will benefit somewhat, but it is necessary to irradiate all muscles involved, quite often in the neck and in the lateral pterygoid. These cases generally require TMD therapy, sometimes physical therapy and often relaxation programmes. Without a differential diagnosis the outcome of laser therapy will be guesswork.

That's my experience with muscle tension work too; it needs a wide application of area of treatment, most esp. the muscles of the neck and shoulder as well. While we are here, what experience does anyone have in treating corneal ulcers with either LED or laser? I have a client with a horse with a nasty corneal ulcer that is not responding to conventional treatment.

I have had some pretty good experiences with the LED cluster on corneal scratches and ulcers. I have to date only used the laser as an acupuncture treatment around the eye, I have never dared to use actually over the eye. What experience do others have with this?

Melyni

Stating the brand of the equipment we are using may be reasonable, but it would be better just to state wavelength and power. This is not a commercial

that irradiation reaching only the skin (like defocused CO_2 laser therapy) can have an effect on deeper structures. So there must be messenger metabolites involved. This means that LEDs might influence deep structures even though the actual light does not, in sufficient quantities. Lasers, on the other hand, can reach superficial and deep targets at the same time.

Future research will show what would happen if we apply paragraph 3 below (What about not like-for-like but rather the best LED parameters vs. the best laser parameters?). That would really be interesting.

I don't mind discussing LEDs on this list. This topic needs discussion since they are widely in use and still lacking good scientific support. So did lasers 10 years ago. So the main thing is that the discussion is based on facts, not on loud marketing.

Many years ago I visited The Voice of Free China in Taipei and talked to "The Dragon Man", a producer on the international service. He needed listeners' letters to keep his bosses happy, so when the letters were few, he intentionally said something stupid on the air. And the letters poured in. This discussion list really came to life.

Jan

It does not matter if it is a laser or and LED unit. Once it enters the skin it is scattered and is no longer a coherent collimated beam. The big advantage of the LED's is that the angle of the beam is already between 20-40 degrees so it covers a much larger area. With an LED cluster you can cover a much larger area in a shorter time and a LED unit has the ability to use several wavelengths in a single probe, which the laser cannot duplicate. Of course you could buy several lasers with different wavelengths but then you are still limited to the number of wavelengths available. I know the manufacturers would much rather sell the lasers because they make a lot more money and the cost to manufacture is not much more than the LED units.

LED instrument producer.

The Producer's contributions are NOT valuable, misleading and in violation of the marketing claims the company is allowed to make, given their intended use allowed them by the FDA. I suggest they be removed from the list.

JS

There are similar affects of a LED and a LLLT. But your conclusion is flawed. We do not know "scientifically" how either work. We know Light is a particle, we know Light is a wave. Therefore you conclude that 1: particle = wave, and 2: more is better. I am interested in not only HOW it works but WHY.

If the power density is known, the dose (energy density) is simply given by multiplying with the time. Example: if the power density is 1 mW/cm^2, in a particular point or area, and this illumination is going on for 30 seconds, then the dose 30 × 1 mW/cm^2, i.e. 30 mJ/cm^2 or 0.03 J/cm^2 is given.
Lars

9.2.6 Light emitting diodes (LED)
The machine I use has both LED and laser on it. In purely practical terms I find that the LED probe is best over open wounds and less uncomfortable when used over fresh trauma than the laser. You can definitely feel the laser go in, and certainly the horses can. With some of the higher-powered laser probes they can be quite unhappy with the laser beam if it is held on for too long.

The LED cluster is great for big amorphous areas, like bruises and kicks. Or when you are not quite sure exactly where the trouble comes from like sore backs. But for acupuncture work or for tendons etc you really need the pinpoint accuracy of the laser. And if I need to do specific areas like the navicular joint or stifle joint I get better results with the laser.

If I have deep work like the big muscles of the back, the LED just can't seem to get deep enough to effect a release, but it is useful for softening up the surface layers so you can feel the deeper knots and spasms.
Melyni

I believe the above is a good description of the different application possibilities for lasers and LED. But I suspect the horses would be just as happy with lasers, if these were multidiodes and at rather low power density. Not many such lasers are around, while this is a typical LED design.
Jan

There are few people who have studied LLLT that dispute that certain wavelength LED's delivering sufficient power, used for enough time do have physiological effects and that they are clinically effective.

The more debatable point is: could you get a better result with laser? Published work in this area so far suggests laser wins. Though I would like to argue how like-for-like the parameters were given the differing beam characteristics. www.laser.nu summarises 14 studies comparing laser and LED http://www.laser.nu/lllt/laser_discussion.htm But what about like-for-like cost? What about like-for-like treatment times? What about not like-for-like but rather the best LED parameters vs the best laser parameters?
Ars longa, vita brevis, as they used to say.
James

These three studies clearly show the benefit of LEDs, if within the therapeutic window with dosage and wavelength. But they are all on superficial structures. For deeper structures the laser is probably needed. However, we know

from the laser to the patient. However, depending on the geometry of the beam, you usually get a different power density when changing the distance (L).

Let us consider 3 situations. (**A**) you have a HeNe-laser without any optics or fibre. (**B**) You have a GaAlAs laser with direct output from the laser diode (no lenses or optics) and (C) you have a InGaAlP laser with a lens that collects the light into a focus 1 cm from the end of the probe. After the focus point, the light is divergent with a top angle of e.g. 20°. Let us further assume that all three lasers have an output of 10 mW.

(**A**) Such a laser has typically a circular beam with a divergence of only about 0.1 degree (1-2 mrad). Let us further assume that the laser has a circular symmetric beam with a gaussian distribution and a beam diameter of 3 mm at the aperture. This means that you get a spot with an effective area of around 7 mm^2 close to the aperture. If you treat a patient from a distance of one meter, you have approximately the same surface hit by the beam due to the small divergence, the same total power and the same power density.

(**B**) A semiconductor laser has a fan-shaped beam with large divergence (typically 30° to 60°) in one direction and a small divergence (typically 1° to 3°) perpendicular to the said direction. It means that when you hold the laser probe close to the skin, you get an image shaped like a "minus sign". This means that in the case of contact between skin and surface of the laser diode, all the light hits a 1 to 2 mm^2 area, giving a very high power density. But at e.g. 2 cm treatment distance, the power density is 100-fold lower. The total power is the same - it is always the same - but the power density is much lower! It is highest in the middle and then decreasing against the ends of the "minus sign".

(**C**) In this case, the focused light can be used to treat e.g. acupuncture points in the ear. In the focus, the power density is extremely high (for instance a 10 mW laser focused into a point with 0.1 mm diameter gives a power density higher than 100 watt/cm^2 assuming that the focusing lenses transmits 80% of the light from the laser diode). After the focus point, we get the following situation:

- At 1 cm distance away from the focus, the spot size is about 3.5 mm in diameter (spot area about 10 mm^2) which gives a power density of 100 mW/cm^2.
- At 10 cm distance away from the focus, the spot size is about 35 mm in diameter (spot area about 10 cm^2) which gives a power density of 1 mW/cm^2.
- At 100 cm distance away from the focus, the spot size is about 35 cm in diameter (spot area about 1000 cm^2) which gives a power density of 0.01 mW/cm^2.

This is the power density at the surface of the skin. Down in tissue, the situation is of course completely different. Power density at different depths depends on many factors, not least the wavelength but also power distribution at the surface, type of tissue, pigmentation, incident angel etc.

power is **on** during 50% of the time and **off**, rest of the time. In this case the average output power is 50% of the peak power (= continuous level). This is when the factor 2 (mentioned in your question) occurs. If the (less usual) duty cycle 25% is used, then the average output power is 25% of the peak power (i.e. the continuous wave situation). [To be correct, not even this is necessarily true. In the 25% case, the laser diode is not charged as much as if it had to run on CW and then it is often possible to increase the current through the laser diode above what is possible in the CW situation, as it often is the power dissipation that is limiting the maximum performance of the diode and that means that the possible CW output is lower than the possible peak power level. Hence the relation between average and continuous output power does not have to be equal to the duty cycle.] Chopping of the light is usually applied to HeNe lasers and switching of the current is usually applied to GaAlAs- and InGaAlP laser diodes.

In the case of super pulsing (**b**), we are usually talking about GaAs laser diodes, though some other laser types are possible to choose. This type of diode has a very high lasing threshold. This means that it is lasing only when the current through the semiconductor chip is very high. Such a semiconductor chip can have the dimensions $0.2 \times 0.5 \times 0.8$ mm and the current through, may have to be in the order of 25 - 50 amperes with e.g. 5 volts across, giving a momentary electric power surge of about 125 to 250 watt, resulting in a radiation peak power in the order of 5 to 25 watts. As the chip will burn up in less than a milli-second, this current is pulsed in the nano-second region, typically 100 - 200 nano-seconds, and producing light pulses in the same time domain. Hence the peak power output of a GaAs laser diode is typically in the order of watts and the average power output in the order of milli-watts. As an example, a GaAs-laser probe from Irradia (Sweden) with four GaAs laser diodes, set on 10 000 Hz pulse frequency and a pulse duration of 150 nano-seconds has 4×10 watt peak power output and 4×15 mW average power output. I am sure that you then also can see that the duty cycle for such a laser is very low - in this example, it is only 0.15 %. The advantage with this laser type is that the penetration through tissue is high - in the moments of laser light emission, the power is very high (many watts) and it is clear that strong light penetrates deeper than weak light. At this wavelength both absorption in melanin, most proteins and water is low.

Lars

Thanks Lars. Could you advise me on how to calculate laser power received by the patient. Means, if a laser output power is W, the distance between laser source to patient is L, then how is the power decay from the source to the patient

June

Hi again, First of all, normal air does not absorb light (you can see objects at many kilometres of distance). This means that you do not loose any power

Nicola J H et al. The role of coherence in wound healing stimulation by non-thermal laser radiation. Surgical and Medical Lasers. 1989; 2-3 (2): 70 (abstract)
Nicola J H, Nicola E M D, Simões M, Paschoal J R. Role of polarisation and Coherence of Laser Light on Wound Healing. Laser Tissue Interaction V (1994), S.L. Jacques, ed., Proc SPIE.1994; 2134A, 448-450.

The latter study showed that wound healing was better when the light was polarised. Lasers can be either polarised or non-polarised, but are generally non-polarised. But the light within the speckles is more or less polarised independently on the polarisation of the incident laser light. Lars can explain this better.

Jan

I have heard about an instrument named Bioptron. Is that laser or LED? It is not very expensive. What is it used to?

Caroline

The Bioptron has a very wide spectrum, more or less the whole visible spectrum. The light is made polarised by means of a polarisation filter. The polarisation of the light gives effects on blood samples, as shown by Samoilova et al. We know that the polarisation is gradually lost as the light enters the tissue, but maybe it still has some degree of polarisation when it reaches the arterioles, which could explain the effects. While Bioptron has its merits it would be interesting to know which wavelengths are optimal for different conditions rather than using all wavelengths available just to make sure one of them is included. To treat with all wavelengths at the same time is like when some GaAs laser instruments sweep the pulse frequency between max and minimum values, claiming that this is a good concept. I doubt it. Good medicine is refinement.

Jan

9.2.5 Laser power

How come that some laser therapy equipment has power in watts and some only in milli-watts? If the peak power value is 70 W, the average power should be 70 W / 2, i.e. shall be 35 W, instead of 35 mW. Is this correct?

June.

Hi June, This is a very good question. And it is not so easy to explain. It is like this: We separate between two types of pulsing: (**a**) the chopped (or switched) pulsing and (**b**) super pulsing.

In the case of (**a**), the constant output power is mechanically or electrically interrupted, meaning that you get a lower output than if you have a continuous output (CW). How much lower depends on the so called "duty cycle". The duty cycle can vary between 0% (no output at all) and 100% (continuous wave). Most common is a duty cycle of 50%, meaning that the

The photoreceptors seem to be different for different wavelengths. For example, Lubarts group has shown that porphyrin is a photoreceptor for red. The max. for porphyrin is below 633, so the absorption is reduced with longer wavelengths. But then there are other photoreceptors.
Jan

I have an article where they use the unit angstrom for wavelength. It says that the laser has a wavelength of 106 000 angstrom. What laser is that?
Nick

In older literature wavelengths may be given in Angstroms. This unit got its name from the Swedish physicist Anders Ångstöm (the unit of which is usually written A) where 1 Ångström = 1×10^{-10} metre. This means that 1 nm = 10 A. The laser you mention must then be a CO_2 laser having a wavelength of 10 600 nm, which is equal to 10.6 µm (microns).
Lars

9.2.3 Coherence
Jan, I remember the paper by you and Lars showing that the laser penetrated the tissue with no loss of coherence. Would hold true also for different tissues? E.g bone, connective tissue or tendon.
Melyni

Yes it does. The penetration, though, is different in different tissue; muscles are less transparent than bone (blood is major absorber).
Jan

Hi Melyni. Yes, it is said in many articles that the coherence is not lost when laser light is penetrating tissue. However, this is not correct. In fact its length of coherence is reduced, but it is coherent enough to form laser speckles through interference. In the laser speckles the light is polarised and that is one of the advantages with lasers compared to e.g. LED's. The light from LED's does not create speckles and hence no polarisation in the tissue and polarisation is shown to be of importance.
Lars

9.2.4 Polarisation
I am interested in the polarisation issue. Is polarisation in laser not lost too? And why is polarisation important, in terms of cellular response?
Melyni

Hi Melyni. I can recommended this literature:

be much less irritating, I can use a 200 mW, 660 nm probe with less problem than a 10 mW, 904 nm. With an active inflammation, wound, trauma, or joint, the red wavelengths also seem to be more effective. The biggest problem has been that until recently we just didn't have any very powerful probes emitting in the 600-700 nm range. So treatment times were long and often seemed ineffective on the deeper stuff. But I have recently purchased a 200 mW 660 and that seems to make a big difference. I have found especially useful on active arthritis.

Melyni

Quite apart from the problem of Laser and LED companies trying to advertise their products on this list, I am bothered more by the comparisons of the value of LED versus Laser, when no wavelength is mentioned. In general, it is the wavelength of light produced that is important, not the machine that produces the light. Yes, the different machines (LED and laser) do offer advantages for different situations, but the most import parameters are the wavelength of the light, and the dose, and dose rate of the light.

Sticking just with lasers for a moment, it is often found in the literature that for a particular therapy that a laser at 830 nm does not work, yet a laser at 632.8 nm does work, and vice versa. Again, it is the wavelength of the light, and the dose, and the dose rate of the light that is most important for a particular therapy. It is the absorption of a particular wavelength of light by specific target molecules within tissues that produces the therapeutic effect. If a given wavelength of light is NOT absorbed by target molecules that are essential for the particular therapy, then no matter how long you irradiate with the wrong wavelength, you will never obtain a therapeutic effect. THINK WAVELENGTH!

Kendric

I'd love to know more about the difference between the various wavelengths and their effect on different tissues.

Melyni

The studies by al-Watban have demonstrated that all wavelengths work for wound healing but that red is best and that dosage is not the same. Studies by Adam Mester have shown that all wavelengths work for arthritis but the dose has to be adapted to the type of joint. Red would just not work for a knee but would be fine for a finger. So infrared has to be used for the knee. Further, red at least used to be low powered and not practical in some situations. Low power cannot be compensated by long time. Energy density is important.

Since all wavelengths have at least some effect, very broadly speaking, it is ok to use whatever your equipment has to offer. Very few therapists can afford to have many lasers so we have to do the best we can with whatever is at hand. Certainly not always optimal, this is the clinical reality but not very scientific, of course.

9.1 Laser therapy on the Internet
LaserWorld, the home of the Swedish Laser Medical Society offers abstracts of the literature, questions and answers about laser therapy, guest editorials, links to congresses, associations, manufacturers, publishers and much more. The URL is www.laser.nu or www.laserworld.org.
Pub Med is an excellent and free source for scientific literature
www.ncbi.nlm.nih.gov/entrez/query.fcgi
Another excellent source is Scirus
http://www.scirus.com/

9.2 Internet discussion groups
The Internet is a rich source of information about laser therapy. Joining one of the discussion groups can be of great help. The members of these groups are therapists, doctors, dentists, manufacturers, physiotherapists, researchers, administrators etc. and everyone has a chance of extending his own knowledge. The following offers some examples of discussions. The quotations below are examples of questions and answers in such a forum, LLLT@topica.com.

9.2.1 Tinnitus
Can anyone comment on results of laser therapy for tinnitus? Who makes a unit for tinnitus? And does anyone in the US use one?
WS

I use a scanner (480/20 mW GaAlAs/HeNe) for tinnitus, vertigo and hearing loss in conjunction with chiropractic, allergy testing and nutritional support. As always: Sometimes the results are phenomenal, sometimes they are poor.
Dr. Z

Dear David, We have done a double-blind placebo controlled trial with 830 nm 150 mW GaAlAs diode laser on unselected tinnitus patients in a Private ENT practice. There was no statistical significant difference between the treated or untreated groups. There were, however, a few remarkable results - as most people will find if they utilise LLLT for tinnitus. One theory holds that cases with active Meniere's disease are more likely to benefit - this would fit in nicely with the anti-inflammatory effects of laser therapy. I am not aware at this stage of a study looking at this specific subset of patients. I am therefore not using it as routine therapy for the general tinnitus patient.
Neels

9.2.2 Wavelength
With regards to the red light (630 nm - 680 nm), I have a couple of observations. No matter the power or the frequency used those wavelengths seem to

Chapter 9
Laser therapy on the Internet

For further reading: (See chapter 4.1.17 "Diabetes" on page 223.)

8.10 Tatoos

Tatoos contain different pigments and even fairly low energies of laser light will be absorbed in these pigments. Depending on the type of pigment, a patient may experience heating or even pain when a therapeutic laser is used over a tattoed area. It is therefore prudent to start irradiation from a distance, then approaching the skin surface until the patient feedback decides to power density. Tatoos do not constitute a contraindication, but high intensities over tatoos will cause high absorption and may bring out a pain reaction.

There are no absolute contraindications for LPT, only relative ones and caveats. As can be seen from the above, some alleged contraindications are pure nonsense, others are rather caveats due to legal implications - which are often based upon the nonsense! But it pays to be on the safe side and to be careful with epileptics, pregnant women and patients with thyroid problems, unless you are performing research. Another caveat is patients with *coagulation disorders*, because we still do not know how LPT affects the coagulation mechanisms, only that it does.

tured cells were irradiated for various periods at two selected intensities and then stimulated with various mitogens. When stimulating cells after irradiation, significantly increased levels (biostimulatory effect) of all cytokines were detected after 30 minutes of irradiation (18.9 J/cm^2), whereas after 60 min of irradiation (37.8 J/cm^2), cytokine levels were found to be significantly decreased (bioinhibiting effect).

Mucositis (painful mucosal wounds in the oral and pharyngeal mucosa) is an effect of radiation therapy for head and neck cancer patients. It has been shown that red laser can not only reduce this severe side effect but also prevent it if irradiation is given before radiation therapy. (See chapter 4.1.9 "Cancer" on page 190.)

Further literature: [1034]

8.9 Diabetes

Diabetes has been suggested as a contra indication. However, we have not found any evidence that laser therapy could aggravate symptoms. Laser treatment increases blood flow and is effective in wound healing. Laser therapy should therefore, on the contrary, be recommended as an additional treatment modality, e.g. for diabetic foot problems, according to Kleinman [477].

Since the experimental model of using healthy rats for wound healing studies has been questioned, rats with genetic diabetes have been suggested as a better model. Wound healing studies using this model [986, 1275, 1423, 1455, 1755, 1863, 1877, 1887] are promising, as well as diabetic wounded cells [1864, 1871, 1927, 1926, 1927]. Far from being a contra-indication, LPT to handle the circulatory side effects in diabetics appears to be a very good indication!

Literature:

An experiment by Radelli [470] on rats, using 904 nm GaAs laser, did not confirm any influence on the insulin-glycemic balance.

In a thermographic study by Schindl [478] carried out on patients with microanginopathic disorders, the improvement of blood flow started 15 minutes after the onset of laser irradiation and persisted up to 45 min after stopping the irradiation. A maximal temperature rise of 2.5° C was measured.

Kotani [501] compared the wound-healing rate in three groups of rats: 1. normal rats, 2. rats with experimentally induced diabetes mellitus, and 3. rats treated with doxorubicin. Doxorubicin inhibits the proliferation of fibroblasts and is used as an anti-cancer agent in medicine. 5.4 J/cm^2 of HeNe laser light was applied daily. In the diabetic group, irradiated wounds healed faster than non-irradiated. In the low dose doxorubicin group, healing was comparable to the non-irradiated control. In the group of healthy animals, irradiated wounds healed slightly faster but not statistically better than control. This again illustrates the importance of the condition of the tissue - healthy individuals will not improve greatly from laser therapy.

Restraint stress per se led to a considerable decrease in 5-HT and DA in striatum and hippocampus, but did not significantly alter the NA levels.
Further literature: [502,1427, 1589, 1756, 1807, 1872, 1928]

8.8 Radiation therapy patients

Radiation therapy patients have been considered as contra-indicative for laser therapy. This is not entirely self-evident, in that the radiation they are subjected to has different characteristics from laser therapy. There are studies showing that laboratory animals receiving X-ray radiation made better progress if they received laser therapy first [147]. There are several studies in which effects on the immune system have been demonstrated. These effects have primarily been local. More and more studies are being published concerning laser treatment of circulating blood [180]. Changes in the components of the blood relating to the immune defence following laser treatment could obviously lead to effects in many other parts of the body, such as an improved defence against cancer. In fact, LPT appears to have a radioprotective effect on tissue, described by McGuff [1856] already in 1966 and confirmed by i.a. da Cunha [1812] 40 years later.

Literature:

Irradiation of a tumour with a low-level laser enhances the effect of chemotherapy. Tamachi [44], has studied the uptake of the cytotoxin 5FU in various experiments using rats. Laboratory rats that received 6 J/cm^2 of HeNe showed a greater uptake of 5FU than those who were given 5FU only. The irradiation causes blood vessels to dilate, allowing greater amounts of the anticancer drug to accumulate in the lesion. Hence laser therapy can minimize the required dose of the anticancer drug used.

Podolskaya [366] has used a HeNe laser on post-radiation reactions and injuries in lip skin and mucous membranes. The method has been more successful than previous medical treatments.

Kolomiyets [367] treated patients with precancerous changes in the gastric mucosa with a HeNe laser. Positive clinical and morphological effects were noted in 65% of the patients.

Soldo [371] studied the effect of GaAs laser radiation on murine sarcoma and found it to be anti-tumour on small tumours, probably due not to a direct effect on the tumour itself but rather to changes in the tumour-host relationship such as the immune defence.

Schaffer [468] irradiated mouse fibroblasts and human tumour cells with 805 nm laser. Both tissues received either 4 or 20 J/cm^2. With 4 J, an increase of mitotic activity in the healthy mouse cells could be registered, while at 20 J there was a slight decrease. The tumour cells were not stimulated by 4 J. 20 J, on the other hand, decreased the mitotic rate.

Funk [565] has investigated cytokine production following HeNe laser irradiation in cultures of human peripheral blood mononuclear cells. Cul-

ning 1 to 24 hours post embolisation. Behavioural analysis was conducted from 24 hours to 21 days after embolisation, allowing for the determination of the effective stroke dose (P50) or clot amount (mg) that produces neurological deficits in 50% of the rabbits. Using the RSCEM, a treatment is considered beneficial if it significantly increases the P50 compared with the control group. In the present study, the P50 value for controls were 0.97+/-0.19 mg to 1.10+/-0.17 mg; this was increased by 100% to 195% if laser treatment was initiated up to 6 hours, but not 24 hours post embolisation (P50=1.23+/-0.15 mg). Laser treatment also produced a durable effect that was measurable 21 days after embolisation. Laser treatment (25 mW/cm^2) did not affect the physiological variables that were measured. This study shows that laser treatment improved behavioural performance if initiated within 6 hours of an embolic stroke and that the effect of laser treatment is durable.

The aim of the study by Ilic [1590] was to investigate the possible short- and long-term adverse neurological effects of LPT given at different power densities, frequencies and modalities on the intact rat brain. In a previous study on the effect of laser therapy for stroke in a rat model [1589], an optimal dose had been confirmed and now served as baseline dose 118 rats were used in the study. Diode laser (808 nm, wavelength) was used to deliver doses of 7.5, 75, 750 mW/cm^2 transcranially to the brain cortex of mature rats, in either continuous (CW) or pulse (Pu) modes. Multiple doses of 7.5 mW/cm^2 were also applied. Standard neurological examination of the rats was performed during the follow up periods post laser irradiation. Histology was performed at the light and electron microscopy levels. Both the scores from standard neurological tests and the histopathological examination indicated that there was no long-term difference between laser-treated and control groups up to 70 days post treatment. The only rats showing an adverse neurological effect were those in the 750mW/cm^2 (about 100-fold optimal dose), CW mode group. In Pu mode there was much less, heating and no tissue damage was noted. Long-term safety tests lasting 30 and 70 days at optimal 10x and 100X doses, as well as multiple doses at the same power densities, indicate that the tested laser energy doses are safe under this treatment regime. Neurological deficits and histopathological damage to 750 mW/cm^2 CW laser irradiation are attributed to thermal damage and not due to tissue-photon interactions.

In order to elucidate the metabolic modifications induced in rat brain by low power He-Ne laser irradiation in vivo, the variations in the biogenic amine levels in cortex, striatum and hippocampus were studied. Noradrenaline (NA), dopamine (DA) and serotonin (5-HT) Cassone [846] evaluated by HPLC-EC on irradiated rats, untreated rats (controls) and rats which had undergone restraint stress (stressed). The results obtained on groups of four to eight rats assayed individually showed that irradiation caused a strong increase in 5-HT in striatum and hippocampus, a small but significant decrease in NA in cortex, and DA levels were not significantly affected.

irradiated knee joints, the untreated contralateral knee joint or those in the sham-irradiated control group.

Renström [563] has successfully treated 30 children aged 11-15 for Morbus Schlatter. He treated their knees and lower legs with 60 mW, GaAs laser light at 30 Hz, pulse train modulated, and 0.1 J/cm².

Mb Schlatter has also successfully been treated by Paolini [945]. 15 young patients were given 30 sessions of GaAs laser therapy and the end result was compared to 15 patients who underwent conventional therapy, including surgery. The best results were obtained with laser therapy.

Ailioe [985] has used visible diode laser light for the treatment of the peripheral nerve system in new-borns and infants.

Wollman [537] irradiated foetal brain cells in vitro using a HeNe laser. One single dose enhanced the appearance of brain cells around the treated aggregates. Two and three doses were correlated with 97% and 142% increases respectively. Rhodamine-labelled antibodies bound to receptors on cells indicated massive neurite sprouting and outgrowth of migrating brain cells in culture.

It is obvious that LPT dosage must be adapted to the weight of children but there is no indication in the litarature suggesting that children, including neonatal babies, should not benefit from LPT.

8.6 Cancer

Cancer, or suspected cancer, should never be treated by anyone who is not a specialist. This is not because laser therapy would not have a positive effect but because the law, quite sensibly, does not allow anyone but an expert to treat cancer. As a palliative treatment in terminal patients, LPT could still be a very viable option for pain control and general stimulation.

8.7 Irradiation of the brain

Based on the findings by Ilic, below, it seems safe to irradiate in brain areas. When it comes to use the brain as the actual target of LPT, much remains to be explored. However, the effects on stroke are encouraging. Whether or not the intellectual capacity can be stimulated by laser irradiation is not documented, but is a fascinating field for investigations. In the meantime, it is prudent to stick to whatever brain capacity you have. What can be postulated is that brain damage will not occur when areas over the skull are being treated, for one reason or the other, but actually targeting the brain is so far not recommended due to insufficient documentation.

Literature:

In a study by Lapchak [1427] the rabbit small clot embolic stroke model (RSCEM) was used to assess whether laser treatment (7.5 or 25 mW/cm²) altered clinical rating scores (behaviour) when given to rabbits begin-

roid gland. In a later recalculation of these doses, however, Azevedo [1625] shows that the actualy doses were 3.12 and 9.36 J/cm². but that the cumulative doses were still very high.

Mikhailov [982] reports on the use of 890 nm laser treatment of autoimmune thyroiditis. 42 patients were given ten applications at 2.4 J/cm². The irradiated areas were the thymus projection zones (area of the sternum at a level of the second edge), vascular junction (left axillary area) and thyroid gland. A control group of similar size was given L-thyroxin, 100 mg/day. The clinical effect in all laser patients was a decreased feeling of squeezing in the field of the thyroid gland and a decrease of the facial oedema. The gland became softer palpatively and its size was reduced according to the ultrasound examination. The number of patients catching cold during the winter decreased. The immunoregulatory index (Th/Ts) normalised from 7.5 to 4.2%. The laser effect was still noticeable in 78% of the patients 4 months after treatment. This index was only slightly changed in the control group.

Peláez [484] showed that laser irradiation stimulated the growth and maturation of thyroidal endothelial cells in young mice, while in adult mice, it could cause thickening of the endothelium and reduction of capillary lumen.

The purpose of the study by Azevedo [1625] was to assess whether there were alterations in the thyroidal hormone plasma levels under infrared laser irradiation, in the thyroid gland region. Sixty-five albino male mice were used and assigned to five groups (n=13), with differences in the times that they were sacrificed. Irradiation procedures consisted of a diode laser emitting at 780 nm, at 4 J/cm², in contact mode, point manner. Blood was collected before irradiation (group 1), and then at 24 h (group 2), 48 h (group 3) and 72 h (group 4), and 1 week (group 5) after the third irradiation. The collected material was used for clinical analysis to evaluate the T3 (triiodothyronine) and T4 (thyroxin) hormones. Five animals were used for light microscopy analysis. A statistically significant hormonal level alteration between the first day and 7 days after the last irradiation was found. There were no morphological changes.

Further literature: [1214, 1663, 1664, 1665]

8.5 Children

Children - should they be treated with laser therapy? What about the growth plates?

Literature:

Cheetham [401] irradiated the healthy growth plates in young rats. One knee joint of each animal in the experimental group was irradiated three times a week at an energy density of 5 J/cm². The animals were examined histologically after 6 and 12 applications. There was no difference between the

wavelengths and energy densities, laser irradiation is a novel and useful tool for the treatment of peripheral and central nervous system injuries and disorders. Adult male albino rats were divided into three groups: control rats, pilocarpinized rats (epileptic animal model), and pilocarpinized rats treated daily with laser irradiation (90 mW at 830 nm) for 7 d. The following parameters were assayed in cortex and hippocampus: amino acid neurotransmitters (excitatory: glutamic acid and aspartate; and inhibitory: gamma-aminobutyric acid [GABA], glycine, and taurine) by high-performance liquid chromatography (HPLC), glucose content, and the activity of alanine aminotransferase (ALT) and aspartate aminotransferase (AST), using a spectrophotometer. Significant increases in the concentrations of glutamic acid, glutamine, glycine, and taurine were recorded in the cortices of pilocarpinized rats, and they returned to initial levels after laser treatment. In the hippocampus, a moderate increase in aspartate accompanied by a significant increase in glycine were observed in the epileptic animal model, and these dropped to near-control values after laser treatment. In addition, a significant increase in cortical AST activity and a significant decrease in ALT activity and glucose content were obtained in the pilocarpinized animals and pilocarpinized rats treated with laser irradiation. In the hippocampus, significant decreases in the activity of AST and ALT and glucose content were recorded in the epileptic animals and in the epileptic animals treated with laser irradiation. Based on the results obtained in this study, it may be suggested that nearinfrared laser irradiation may reverse the neurochemical changes in amino acid neurotransmitters induced by pilocarpine.

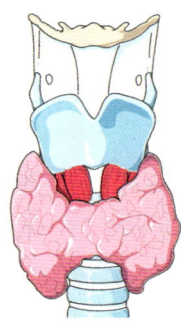

8.4 Thyroid gland

It has not been reported that LPT can cause irreversible damage, but because the thyroid is sensitive to light, it may be wise to avoid irradiating over this gland until further research has elucidated the matter. At the same time, this gland provides an interesting subject for research into hypo- and hyperthyroidism.The thyroid is often reported as a caveat but there are no studies confirming this and no such clinical experience.

Literature:

Hernandéz [285], using GaAs, reports that the decrease of T3 and T4 hormones after infrared laser irradiation might be explained by the changes in the cyto-skeleton and/or thyroglobuline synthesis.

Studies on mice by Parrado [159] indicate that the subject can suffer from disorders if irradiated with large doses.These authors irradiated for 15 consecutive days using GaAs, 46.8 and 140.4 J/cm². in the region of the thy-

Older literature on lasers often repeats certain alleged contra indications related to laser treatment. We have analysed some of these.

8.1 Pacemaker

As pacemakers are electronic and cased in metal they cannot be influenced by light, and this is therefore a misconception. Try influencing your CD player with a laser! This city tale can still be seen in some literature. It seems that safety regulations for lasers were, in many cases, simply transferred from safety regulations for electrical devices.

8.2 Pregnancy

Pregnancy is another alleged contra indication. In this case, normal medical judgement with respect to the effect on the foetus should prevail. Large doses over the abdomen should perhaps be avoided, but the foetus will certainly not be any the worse off for its mother being rid of a sensitive tooth neck or a herpes sore. Avila [194] has demonstrated cell damage in chicken embryos after irradiation with a HeNe laser through an opening in the egg. We should bear in mind that the small chicken embryo received 5 mW of laser light for five minutes from a short distance through more or less transparent tissue. To give a human embryo the same dose per kilo of body weight via the mother's skin, weeks of treatment would be needed! The problem with both pacemakers and pregnancy is that they have long been presented as contra indications. If a complication unrelated to the use of a laser arises during or shortly after laser treatment, it is easy to blame the laser and the therapist is left with the burden of proof. It pays, therefore, to be prudent. Acupuncturists should avoid the "forbidden" points with lasers as well as needles.

8.3 Epilepsy

Epilepsy is another alleged contra indication. Because pulsed visible light, particularly at pulse frequencies in the 5-10 Hz range can cause epileptic attacks, one should obviously be careful with instruments that use flashing visible light. It is rare, however, for therapeutic lasers to have pulsing visible light. Nothing is said in the literature on the subject of invisible pulsing light affecting epileptics, but some anecdotal accounts would suggest that it is best to be careful with GaAs when treating such patients. Simunovic [444] reports on GaAs treatment of an epileptic person who could only tolerate frequencies below 800 Hz.

On the other hand, the recent animal study by Radwan [2086] points into another direction - LPT might be a future treatment modality. The aim of the study was to investigate the effect of daily laser irradiation on the levels of amino acid neurotransmitters in the cortex and hippocampus in an epileptic animal model induced by pilocarpine. It has been claimed that at specific

Chapter 8
Contra indications

Cancer

Pacemaker

Pregnancy

Children

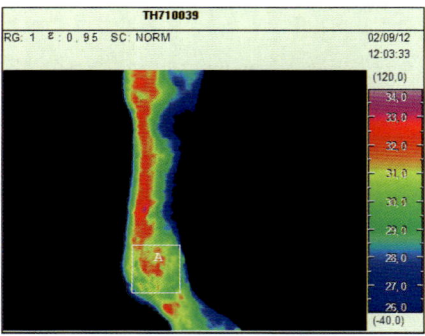

Courtesy: Lindströms Digital Infrared Thermal Imaging

It is amazing how quickly the inflamed tissue reacts. The fur is not cut or shaved off, hence the temperature difference is even higher on the skin under the fur.

Laser parameters: The average output power of the laser probe is measured to 62 mW (four GaAs-laser diodes, each with 13 watt peak power, 150 ns pulse duration, pulse train modulated with basic frequency 16 kHz, 50% duty cycle and envelop frequency 2500 Hz).

Treatment parameters: Treatment was done over the whole inflamed area. That area was about 5 × 40 cm (200 cm^2). Treatment time was 4 minutes. This gives a treatment dose of about 0.075 J/cm^2, which is rather normal for the GaAs-laser type.

For more information see "Thermography" on page 138.

The first picture shows the temperature distribution about 15 minutes before laser treatment.

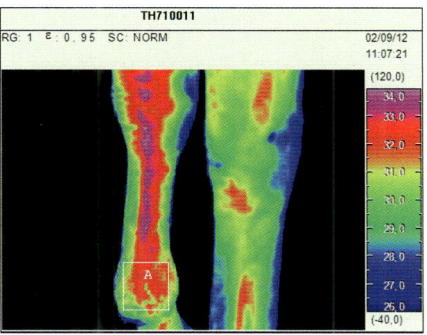

Within the square (marked "A") the maximum temperature is 32.9 °C. The average temperature is 31.5 °C. The following picture is taken 5 minutes after the treatment:

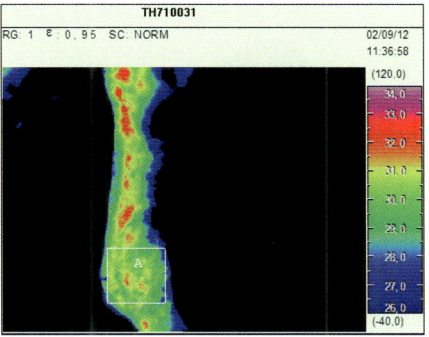

Within the square (marked "A") the maximum temperature is 31.8 °C. The average temperature is 30.0 °C. Next picture is taken 33 minutes after the treatment.

And what if the dog owner has an accident with his pet? Jih [1544] describes a case of a large linear atrophic dog-bite scar on the chin of greater than 2-year duration, treated for three sessions at 4- to 6-week intervals with a 1450 nm diode laser. Fifty to seventy-five percent improvement in the appearance of the scar resulted after three treatments with the 1450 nm diode laser. No adverse effects were noted from the treatment. The patient subjective rating of scar improvement was more than 50%. The 1450 nm diode laser may provide a non-invasive, non-ablative and effective alternative for the treatment of atrophic traumatic scars.

For animal breeding LPT can be quite valuable when artificial insemination is used, since LPT can improve the quality of sperm cells, documented by i.a. Corral-Baques [1269, 1557].

Further literature: [129, 130, 131, 132, 133, 134, 135, 137, 138, 139, 381, 391, 396, 425, 506, 1152].

Laser probe with eight protruding laser diodes for veterinary use

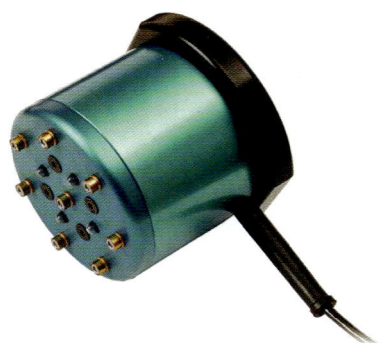

Figure 7.2 Laser probe for veterinary use.

Heat camera measurement

An interesting method is to use a heat camera in diagnostics. It can also be used to objectively study effects of laser treatment. In the following pictures a heat camera was used to follow the reaction after laser therapy of an oedema outside the fetlock joint caused by a hard blow.

doses were 12 mg of ßM, 20 mg of HA and 60 J/cm² of CO2-laser over the treated area, respectively. Convalescence before training was 21 days for both groups in the observer-blind study. In the prospective study, convalescence in the ßM/HA group was 21 days but was only 7 days for the laser-treated group. In the observer-blind study, three of five treated joints recovered in both cohorts. In the prospective study, the groups had significantly different recovery rates - 68% of the ßM/HA-treated joints and 80% of the carbon dioxide laser-treated joints. These results indicate that the defocused carbon dioxide laser should be an applicable mode of treatment of acute traumatic synovitis in horses.

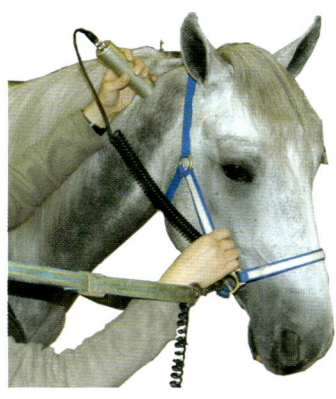

Although laser therapy has been very successfully used in treating horses, there are some studies showing little or no effect. In a study by Petersen [1153] GaAlAs laser was administered to full thickness skin wounds (3 × 3 cm) induced surgically on the dorsal aspect of the metacarpophalangeal joints of 6 crossbred horses in a randomised, blind, controlled study. Wounds that received a daily laser dosage of 2J/cm² were compared with nontreated control wounds on the opposite leg. There were no significant differences in wound contraction or epithelialisation between the laser treated and the control wounds. Laser therapy had no clinically significant effect on second intention wound healing.

Our comment on this is that it seems that the wounds were induced surgically on healthy individuals, which means that the tissue was healthy and the healing capacity therefore close to optimal. The immunological condition of the tissue and of the individual is a significant factor in the effectiveness of laser therapy. See further chapter 13.3: "Are all the negative studies really negative", under section 6: "Tissue condition". Furthermore, it is not an optimal situation with controls in the same individual due to the influence of possible systemic effects.

Gomez-Villamandos [425] induced duplicate pharyngeal mucosal ulcers in 12 horses. Using a fibroendoscope, one of the two injured sides was treated daily with a HeNe laser at 8 J/cm². On day 7, histological samples were taken from two horses. Irradiated lesions cicatrised after 10.5 days and non-irradiated lesions after 18. A histological study showed coagulation, necrosis and oedema at the control site. However, in the samples from the irradiated lesions, no inflammatory oedema, numerous active fibroblasts, connective tissue or intensive epithelial regeneration were observed.

three-layers of continuous suture pattern. Group B and D wounds were treated with 3.64 J/cm² of LPT using a helium-neon system continuous wave (632.8 nm) output of 8.5 nW. The teat wall in non-LLLT groups was significantly thicker than in LPT groups on day 7, 14 and 21. The mean blood flow differences between control and sutured sites in LPT groups were significantly lower than those in non-LPT groups. The morphology of the epidermis in LPT groups more closely resembled the normal epidermis than that of non-LPT groups. Collagen fibers in LPT groups were denser, thicker, better arranged and more continuous with existing collagen fibers than those in non-LPT groups. The mean tensile strength was significantly greater in LPT groups than in non-LPT groups.

These positive results could not be confirmed in the study by Stoffel [1004],

Laser therapy of mastitis has been successfully used for dairy cattle and Herzog [1002] reports good effects on 66 individuals, using 830 nm, 30 mW, 0.5-2 J per point. On the other hand, Stoffel [1004] reports that HeNe laser, 25 mW had no effect on bovine mastitis. However, the irradiation area of 7.5 cm in diameter produces a very low energy density.

Herman [151] has studied the effects, in vitro, of Nd:YAG laser therapy on articular cartilage in cattle and has shown bio-chemically that laser light influenced the healing process.

Rochkind [561] subjected 17 dogs to laminectomy and transection of the spinal cord at D12-L1. An autograft of the left sciatic nerve was then implanted into the injured area. Neurorrhaphy was performed on the right sciatic nerve. Seven dogs did not receive any additional treatment and served as a control. The other 10 were treated transcutaneously with 16 mW of HeNe laser light for 20 days (high doses) over the operated area. The 7 dogs in the control group became paralysed as expected. The 10 dogs that underwent the same operation but were immediately treated with a laser were able to stand after 7-9 weeks, and could walk a few steps after 9-12 weeks. The histological picture obtained from the dogs 21 days post operation showed no rejection and no prominent scar tissue at the site of contact between the spinal cord tissue and the transplanted nerve. Moreover, new axons and blood vessels originating in the spinal tissue extended into the graft. These were seen only in the laser treated group and not in the control group, in which scar tissue had developed at the site of transection.

The clinical effects of intra-articular betamethasone together with hyaluronic acid (ßM/HA) and treatment with a defocused carbon dioxide laser on acute traumatic arthritis of the fetlock joint were assessed in a study by Lindholm [1280]. The horses in these studies were selected using a thorough lameness examination, including intra-articular anaesthesia, abolishing the lameness. This investigation comprised an observer-blind study, including 10 sport horses (10 joints), and a prospective study, including 180 sport horses (333 joints). In both studies, the material was divided into two groups treated with either ßM/HA or a carbon dioxide laser. The treatment

When treating horses and dogs, it must be born in mind that their coat can be essentially impenetrable to light. By measuring light absorption in various types of coats, we have determined that between 50% (thin, light coat) and more than 99% (brown hair and the coat of an Icelandic pony) of the light is absorbed by hair and skin. This absorption is essentially independent of wavelength, which is not the case as regards penetration of tissue. Further, the skin (beneath the coat) may be more or less strongly pigmented, which also affects light penetration.

The negative effects of hair on light absorption can obviously be eliminated by shaving the areas to be treated. Horse owners do not always want it to be obvious that their horse is under treatment, and shaving entails certain difficulties as well. For these reasons, it is not uncommon to give laser treatment through the hair. This presents no problem if the laser instrument is designed to do so, in which case the light is carried down through the hair by optical fibres or the like - much as a comb contacts the skin under the hair. Unfortunately many instruments used for veterinary treatment are not intended specifically for that purpose, but rather for treatment of humans, and their efficacy is therefore often limited.

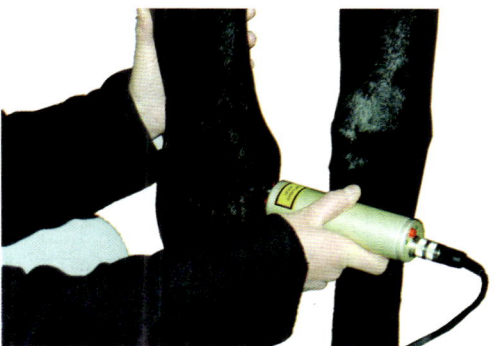

Figure 7.1   Treatment of joint inflammation

Literature:

Ghamsari [1120, 1121] made perforating wounds on 32 teats in eight diary cattle. Four different suture patterns were used and evaluated. Four of the eight groups were additionally treated with HeNe laser, 3.64 J/cm². It was found that wound healing was accelerated in the groups treated with laser. The epidermis in the laser groups more closely resembled normal epidermis and collagen fibres were denser, thicker and better arranged.

Ghamsari [1192] created full thickness wounds on the cranial surface of the teats. Teats were distributed into four groups; group A and B wounds were closed with a Gambee pattern, group C and D wounds were closed with

7.1 Veterinary use

Veterinary medicine is another field in which the laser enthusiast can find further uses for his or her laser. All the common laser types are effective, and GaAs is particularly good for deep-lying tissue.

The scientific documentation in the field of veterinary medicine is extensive, with over one thousand published studies on animals. In most cases, effects have been observed. Most of these studies have involved animals for whom a veterinarian would not ordinarily be called in the event of problems - rats, mice, rabbits, guinea pigs, etc. However, at the present time some documentation is also available on dogs and horses.

Fortune hunters and unscrupulous sales representatives managed to give the laser treatment of trotting horses a bad reputation during the 1980s. In the veterinary field, as in so many others, the reaction was to throw the baby out with the bath water. It is not the laser that is at fault, but often the deficient knowledge of the user and the poor quality of the equipment. A sound knowledge of equine medicine is necessary to achieve good results, in the same way as in human medicine.

Horses are more sensitive to laser light than humans. High local power density - and especially super pulsed lasers - bring about a reaction (including sometimes a pain reaction) when the light enters the vicinity of an injury or problem area. This is particularly true of GaAs lasers and at high pulse or pulse-train frequencies. If the horse reacts strongly, it is suitable to start with a low pulse frequency before going to the higher levels. This reaction in horses can also be used to locate a problem. In trotting and sport in general, the practitioners of laser therapy with the right training and the right equipment are enthusiastic about the results. The economic incentives are obvious. Dogs, cats and other household pets can also be treated with lasers with good results. As with pharmatecuticals, dosage must be adapted to the size of the animal and the type of fur.

Lindholm [562, 1280] has treated more than 500 horses with a defocused CO_2-laser. The results have been 80% positive in treatment of vertebral joint problems, but the treatment is significantly less effective for tendinitis. The clinical outcome of defocused CO_2-laser therapy for acute traumatic arthritis reveals at least an equal therapeutic effect compared with conventional therapy.

A common problem, and one that is even more pronounced in the treatment of race-horses because of the amounts of money involved, is, as we have discussed elsewhere, that laser treatment can radically alleviate pain after just one or two applications. In a couple of cases, when people without medical expertise have observed that the horse's limp has disappeared and ordered hard training, the result has been an exacerbation of the injury rather than a healing. This problem is to some extent associated with treatment of human athletes, too.

Chapter 7
Veterinary use

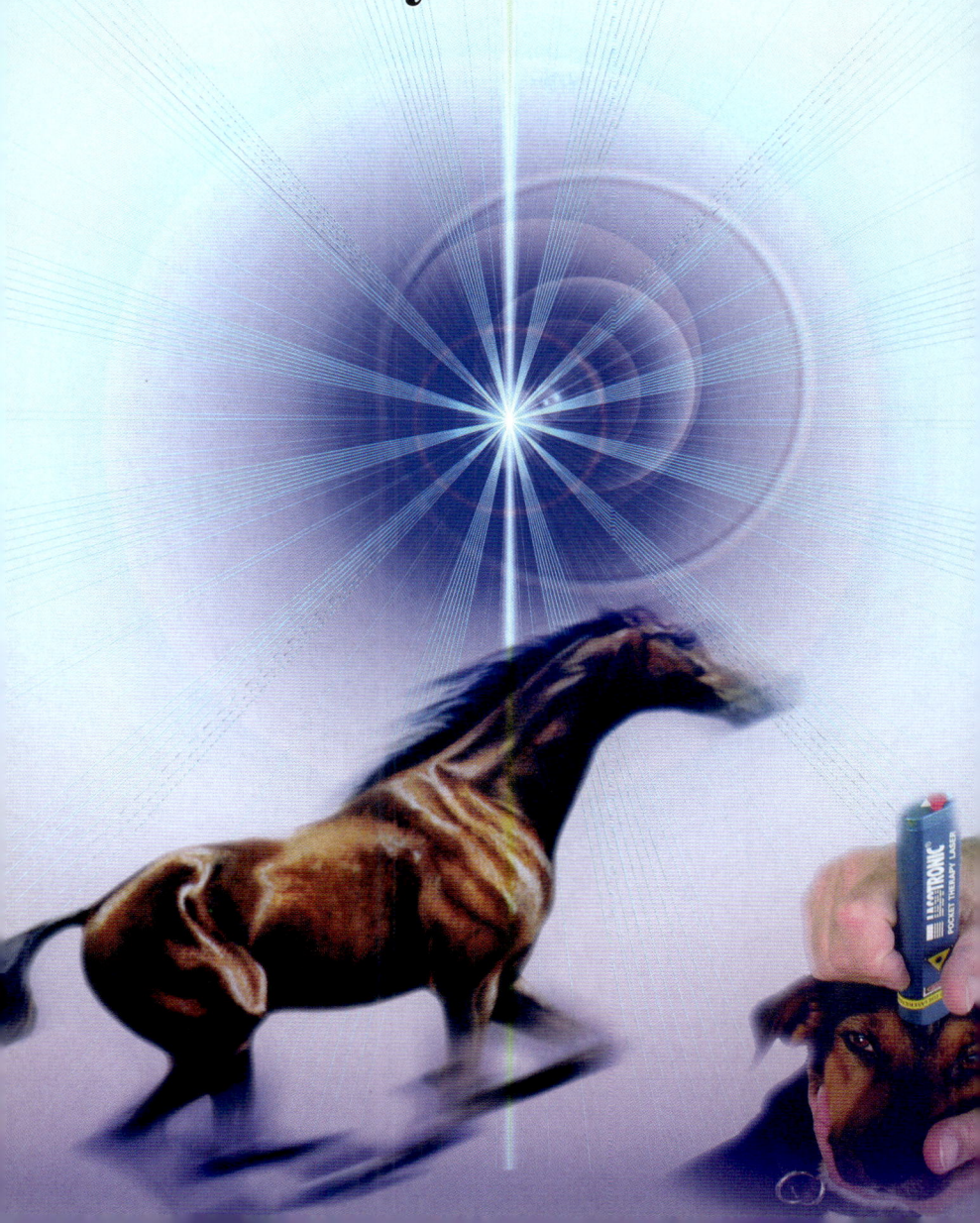

reported a >50% pain reduction. However, four noted minimal or no change and improvement did not reach statistical significance for the group as a whole. No statistically significant changes in autonomic function were noted. There were no adverse consequences. The irradiation was well tolerated. There is a suggestion in this small study that treatment is beneficial and that its benefits are not dependent on changes in sympathetic tone.

Otsuka [1578] performed linear polarised light irradiation near the stellate ganglion in a 55 year old female with Raynaud's sign. She was suffering from cold and numb pain in bilateral fingers for 1 year. Stellate ganglion block and laser therapy near the stellate ganglion were not sufficient to relieve this symptom. Polarised light irradiation near the stellate ganglion induced a sting stimulation and warm sensation in her hands. Thermograms revealed a remarkable increase in temperature of her hands. The results imply that ed light irradiation near the stellate ganglion increases blood flow of forearms and relieves Raynaud's sign.

Wajima [1577] evaluated the effect of linear polarised light irradiation around the stellate ganglion area on skin temperature and blood flow in healthy adult volunteers. The researchers carried out two experiments. In study I, they investigated one-sided irradiation around the stellate ganglion area or posterior neck on the skin temperature of the bilateral nasus externi and earlobes. In study II, they investigated one-sided irradiation around the stellate ganglion area or posterior neck on the skin temperatures of both hands and skinblood flow on the irradiated side. In study I, irradiation around the stellate ganglion area increased skin temperature on the irradiated sides of the nasus externi (wings of the nose), and in study II, skin temperature and blood flow were increased on the irradiated side of the hands. These results suggest that linear polarised light irradiation around the stellate ganglion area would be useful and beneficial in clinical therapy.

Further literature: [1686, 1687, 1688]

6.3 Broadband polarised light (VIP)

See references: [1611, 1612, 1613, 1614, 2030, 2031, 2032]

6.2 Linear polarised light

Shibata [1558] examined the anti-inflammatory effect of infrared linear polarised light irradiation on the MH7A rheumatoid fibroblast-like synoviocytes stimulated with the proinflammatory cytokine interleukin IL-1. Expression of messenger ribonucleic acids (mRNAs) encoding IL-8, RANTES (regulated upon activation, normal T cell expressed and secreted), growth-related gene alpha (GRO) and macrophage inflammatory protein-1 (MIP1) was measured using real-time reverse transcription polymerase chain reaction, and the secreted proteins were measured in the conditioned media using enzyme-linked immunosorbent assays. It was found that irradiation with linear polarised infrared light suppressed IL-1-induced expression of IL-8 mRNA and, correspondingly, the synthesis and release of IL-8 protein in MH7A cells. This anti-inflammatory effect was equivalent to that obtained with the glucocorticoid dexamethasone. Likewise, irradiation suppressed the IL-1-induced expression of RANTES and GRO mRNA. These results suggest that the irradiation of the areas around the articular surfaces of joints affected by rheumatoid arthritis (RA) using linear polarised light may represent a useful new approach to treatment.

There are reports of erythrocyte deformability improved by HeNe laser irradiation. In the study by Yokoyama [1573] human erythrocyte samples stored for three weeks were adjusted to 30% hematocrit. Erythrocyte deformability presented as the filter filtration rate was measured. There was no difference of the filter filtration rate between control group without irradiation and the group of 125 mJ/cm^2 exposure level at a wavelength of 830 nm. However, the groups of 625 and 1,250 mJ/cm^2 exposure levels at a wavelength of 830 nm showed higher filter filtration rates compared to the control group. Linearly polarised near-infrared irradiation in a range of 625-1,250 mJ/cm^2 exposure level at a wavelength of 830 nm improved the deformability status of human stored erythrocytes.

The study by Basford [1575] was designed to assess the physiological effects of irradiation on the stellate ganglion function in normal subjects and people with complex regional pain and to quantitate its benefits in people with upper extremity pain due to Complex Regional Pain Syndrome I (CRPS I, RSD). This was a two-part study. In the first phase, six adults (ages 18-60) with normal neurological examinations underwent transcutaneous irradiation of their right stellate ganglion with linearly polarised 0.6-1.6 microm light (920 mW, 88.3 J). Phase two consisted of a double-blinded evaluation of active and placebo radiation in 12 subjects (ages 18-72) of which 6 had upper extremity CRPS I and 6 served as "normal" controls. Skin temperature, heart rate (HR), sudomotor function, and vasomotor tone were monitored before, during, and for 30 minutes following irradiation. Analgesic and sensory effects were assessed over the same period as well as 1 and 2 weeks later. Three of six subjects with CRPS I and no control subjects experienced a sensation of warmth following active irradiation. Two of the CRPS I subjects

Al-Watban [1541] determined the effect of polychromatic light-emitting diodes (LED) in burn healing of non-diabetic and streptozotocin-induced diabetic rats. The polychromatic LED is a cluster of 25 diodes emitting photons at wavelengths of 510-543, 594-599, 626-639, 640-670, and 842-879 nm with 272 mW output power. Age-matched rats (n=30) were used. Streptozotocin was used for diabetes induction. Rat weight, hyperglycemia, and glycosuria were monitored for the first 3 days and weekly thereafter. Rats were anesthetized and shaved after 1 week of diabetes. Burn areas of $1.5 \pm .03$ cm^2 were created using a metal rod pre-heated up to $600°C$ that was applied for 2 sec. Diabetic and non-diabetic rats were randomized into the following treatment groups: control, 5, 10, 20, and 30 J/cm^2. Light treatment commenced after burn infliction and was repeated three times per week. Burn areas were measured daily. Burn healing was impaired significantly during diabetes by -46.17%. Polychromatic LED treatment using 5, 10, 20, and 30 J/cm^2 incident doses influenced healing by 6.85%, 4.93%, -4.18%, and -5.42% in the non-diabetic rats; and 73.87%, 76.77%, 60.92%, and 48.77% in the diabetic rats, relative to their controls, respectively. The effect of polychromatic LED in non-diabetic rats was insignificant; however, it simulated the trend of stimulation and inhibition seen using low-level lasers. Significant stimulation observed in the diabetic rats demonstrated the usefulness of polychromatic LED in diabetic burn healing.

Minatel [2123] tested the hypothesis that combined 660 and 890 nm LED phototherapy will promote healing of diabetic ulcers that failed to respond to other forms of treatment. A double-blind randomized placebo controlled design was used to study 23 diabetic leg ulcers in two groups of 14 patients. Group one ulcers were cleaned, dressed with 1% silver sulfadiazine cream and treated with "placebo" phototherapy twice per week. Group two ulcers were treated similarly but received 3 $J/cm2$ dose. At each of 15, 30, 45, 60, 75, and 90 days of healing, mean ulcer granulation and healing rates were significantly higher for group two than the "placebo" group. While "placebo" treated ulcers worsened during the initial 30 days, group two ulcers healed rapidly; achieving 56% more granulation and 79.2% faster healing by day 30, and maintaining similarly higher rates of granulation and healing over the "placebo" group all through. By day 90, 58.3% of group two ulcers had healed fully and 75% had achieved 90-100% healing. In contrast, only one "placebo" treated ulcer healed fully by day 90; no other ulcer attained > or =90% healing.

Further literature: [720]

wound healing. Polyvinyl acetal (PVA) sponges were subcutaneously implanted in the dorsum of mice. LED treatments were given once daily, and at the sacrifice day, the sponges, incision line and skin over the sponges were harvested and used for RNA extraction. The RNA was subsequently analyzed by cDNA array. The study revealed certain tissue regenerating genes that were significantly upregulated upon LED treatment when compared to the untreated sample. Integrins, laminin, gap junction proteins, and kinesin superfamily motor proteins are some of the genes involved during regeneration process. These are some of the genes that were identified upon gene array experiments with RNA isolated from sponges from the wound site in mouse with LED treatment.

The effects of infrared and red pulsed monochromatic non-coherent light, with varied pulsations and wavelengths, on the healing of pressure ulcers were evaluated in the prospective, randomized, controlled study by Schubert [1513]. Elderly patients (>or=65 years) with Stage 2 or 3 skin ulcers were enrolled and assigned to one of two groups. Both groups were given the same standard ulcer therapy. One group was also given phototherapy with pulsed monochromatic infrared (956 nm) and red (637 nm) light. Treatments lasted 9 min each time using a regimen with pulse repetition rates varied between 15.6 Hz and 8.58 kHz. Patients were followed for 10 weeks or until the ulcer was healed, whichever occurred first. The ulcer surface area was traced weekly. Patients treated with pulsed monochromatic light had a 49% higher ulcer healing rate, and a shorter time to 50% and to 90% ulcer closure compared with controls.

In view of promoting the wound-healing process in diabetic patients, a preliminary in vitro study by Vinck [1594] investigated the efficacy of green light emitting diode (LED) irradiation on fibroblast proliferation and viability under hyperglycemic circumstances. To achieve hyperglycemic circumstances, embryonic chicken fibroblasts were cultured in Hanks' culture medium supplemented with 30 g/L glucose. LED irradiation was performed on 3 consecutive days with a probe emitting green light (570 nm) and a power output of 10 mW. Each treatment lasted 3 min, resulting in a radiation exposure of 0.1 J/cm^2. A Mann-Whitney U test revealed a higher proliferation rate in all irradiated cultures in comparison with the controls.

In another study by Vinck [1593] cultured fibroblasts were treated in a controlled, randomised manner during three consecutive days, either with an infrared laser or with a LED light source emitting several wavelengths (950 nm, 660 nm and 570 nm) and respective power outputs. Treatment duration varied in relation to varying surface energy densities (radiant exposures). Statistical analysis revealed a higher rate of proliferation in all irradiated cultures in comparison with the controls. Green light yielded a significantly higher number of cells than red and infrared LED light and than the cultures irradiated with the laser; the red probe provided a higher increase than the infrared LED probe and than the laser source. However, the doses for LED:s and laser were not the same.

respectively, compared to untreated throat pain at about posttransplant day seven.

6.1.4.6 Nerve conduction

A randomised controlled study was conducted by Vinck [1592] through measuring antidromic nerve conduction on the peripheral sural nerve of healthy subjects (n=64). One baseline measurement and five post-irradiation recordings (2-min interval each) were performed of the nerve conduction velocity (NCV) and negative peak latency (NPL). Interventional set-up was identical for all subjects, but the experimental group (=32) received an irradiation (2 min at a continuous power output of 160 mW, resulting in a radiant exposure of 1.07 J/cm^2) with an infrared LED device, while the placebo group was treated by sham irradiation. Statistical analysis of NCV and NPL difference scores, revealed a significant interactive effect for both NCV and NPL. Further post hoc LSD analysis showed a time-related statistical significant decreased NCV and an increased NPL in the experimental group and a statistical significant difference between placebo and experimental group at various points of time. Based on these results, it can be concluded that LED irradiation at the wavelength and dosage used, applied to intact skin at the described irradiation parameters, produced an immediate and localized effect upon conduction characteristics in underlying nerves.

6.1.4.7 Retinal damage

The study by Eells [1504] was undertaken to test the hypothesis that exposure to monochromatic red radiation from light-emitting diode (670 nm) arrays would protect the retina against the toxic actions of methanol-derived formic acid in a rodent model of methanol toxicity. Using the electroretinogram as a sensitive indicator of retinal function, it was demonstrated that three brief (2 min, 24 s) 670 nm LED treatments (4 J/cm^2), delivered at 5, 25, and 50 h of methanol intoxication, attenuated the retinotoxic effects of methanol-derived formate. This study documents a significant recovery of rod- and cone-mediated function in 670 nm-treated, methanol-intoxicated rats. It is further shown that 670 nm irradiation protected the retina from the histopathologic changes induced by methanol-derived formate. These findings provide a link between the actions of monochromatic red to near-IR light on mitochondrial oxidative metabolism in vitro and retinoprotection in vivo. They also suggest that photobiomodulation may enhance recovery from retinal injury and other ocular diseases in which mitochondrial dysfunction is postulated to play a role.

6.1.4.8 Wound healing

The purpose of the study by Whelan [1503] was to assess the changes in gene expression of near-infrared light therapy in a model of impaired

6.1.4.3 Dermatology

Weiss [1605] describes the experience over the last 2 years using 590 nm LED photomodulation within a dermatologic surgery environment. Practical use of non-thermal light energy and emerging applications in 3,500 treatments delivered to 900 patients is detailed. LED photomodulation has been used alone for skin rejuvenation in over 300 patients but has been effective in augmentation of results in 600 patients receiving concomitant nonablative thermal and vascular treatments such as intense pulsed light, pulsed dye laser, KTP and infrared lasers, radiofrequency energy, and ablative lasers. LED photomodulation reversed signs of photoaging using a new non-thermal mechanism.

6.1.4.4 Hatching

The objective of the study by Yeager [1602] was to assess the survival and hatching success of chickens exposed in ovo to far-red (670 nm) LED therapy. Fertile chicken eggs were treated once per day from embryonic days 0-20 with 670 nm light at a fluence of 4 J/cm^2. In ovo survival and death were monitored by daily candling (after Day 4). The researchers observed a substantial decrease in overall and third-week mortality rates in the light-treated chickens. Overall, there was approximately a 41.5% decrease in mortality rate in the light-treated chickens. During the third week of development, there was a 68.8% decrease in the mortality rate in light-treated chickens. In addition, body weight, crown-rump length, and liver weight increased as a result of the phototherapy. Light-treated chickens pipped (broke shell) earlier and had a shorter duration between pip and hatch. These results indicate that 670 nm phototherapy by itself does not adversely affect developing embryos and may improve the hatching survival rate.

Further literature: [1503]

6.1.4.5 Mucositis

The purpose of a study by Whealan [1803] was to determine the effects of prophylactic near-infrared light therapy from light-emitting diodes in pediatric bone marrow transplant (BMT) recipients. 32 consecutive pediatric patients undergoing myeloablative therapy in preparation for BMT were recruited. LED therapy consisted of daily treatment at a fluence of 4 J/cm2 using a 670 nm LED array held to the left extraoral epithelium starting on the day of transplant, with a concurrent sham treatment on the right. Patients were assessed before BMT and every 2-3 days through posttransplant day 14. Outcomes included the percentage of patients with ulcerative oral mucositis (UOM) compared to historical epidemiological controls, the comparison of left and right buccal pain to throat pain, and the comparison between sides of the buccal and lateral tongue OMI and buccal pain. The incidence of UOM was 53%, compared to an expected rate of 70-90%. There was also a 48% and 39% reduction of treated left and right buccal pain,

6.1.4.1 Cytochrome c oxidase

Previous studies using 670 nm light-emitting diode arrays suggest that cytochrome c oxidase, a photoacceptor in the NIR range, plays an important role in therapeutic photobiomodulation. If this is true, then an irreversible inhibitor of cytochrome c oxidase, potassium cyanide (KCN), should compete with LED and reduce its beneficial effects. This hypothesis was tested on primary cultured neurons in a study by Wong-Riley [1499]. 670 nm treatment partially restored enzyme activity blocked by 10-100 micromol KCN. It significantly reduced neuronal cell death induced by 300 micromol KCN from 83.6 to 43.5%. However, at 1-100 mm KCN, the protective effects of LED decreased, and neuronal deaths increased. 670 nm significantly restored neuronal ATP content only at 10 micromol KCN but not at higher concentrations of KCN tested. Pretreatment with 670 nm enhanced efficacy of the irradiation during exposure to 10 or 100 micromol KCN but did not restore enzyme activity to control levels. In contrast, 670 nm was able to completely reverse the detrimental effect of tetrodotoxin, which only indirectly down-regulated enzyme levels. Among the wavelengths tested (670, 728, 770, 830, and 880 nm), the most effective ones (830 nm, 670 nm) paralleled the NIR absorption spectrum of oxidized cytochrome c oxidase, whereas the least effective wavelength, 728 nm, did not. The results are consistent the hypothesis that the mechanism of photobiomodulation involves the up-regulation of cytochrome c oxidase, leading to increased energy metabolism in neurons functionally inactivated by toxins.

6.1.4.2 Delayed Onset Muscular Soreness (DOMS)

Several studies have failed to observe an effect of LED therapy for this indication.

Douris [1745] performed a randomized double-blind controlled study with 27 subjects, assigned to one of three groups. The experimental group received 8 J/cm^2 of phototherapy each day for five consecutive days using super luminous diodes with wavelengths of 880 and visible diodes of 660 nm at three standardized sites over the musculotendinous junction of the bicep. The sham group received identical treatment from a dummy cluster. The controls did not receive treatment. The study was completed over five consecutive days: on day one baseline measurements of RANG and upper arm girths were recorded prior to DOMS induction. On days 2-5, RANG, girth, and pain were assessed using VAS and the McGill Pain Questionnaire. The experimental group exhibited a significant decrease in pain associated with DOMS compared to the control and sham groups based upon the VAS at the 48-h period. The McGill Pain Questionnaire showed a significant difference in pain scores at the 48-h period between the experimental and the sham groups. There were no significant differences day to day and between the groups with respect to girth and RANG.

Further literature: [1674, 1675]

enide laser source, 3 times a week. Energy used was 4.5 J/cm2. Ulcers in the control group received sham treatment. Healing of the ulcer, defined as the complete closure of the wound with healthy scar tissue, time taken for the ulcer to heal, and stage of the ulcer and Pressure Sore Status Tool score 14 days after last treatment. There was no significant difference in healing between the treatment and control groups. Eighteen ulcers in treatment group and 14 in control group healed completely. Mean time taken by the ulcers to heal was 2.45±2.06 weeks in the treatment group and 1.78±2.13 weeks in the control group. Time taken for stage 3 and 4 ulcers to reach stage 2 was 2.25±0.5 weeks in treatment group and 4.33±1.53 weeks in control group. Multi wavelength light therapy from a gallium-aluminum-arsenide laser source did not influence overall healing pressure ulcers. Limited evidence suggested that it improved healing of stage 3 and 4 pressure ulcers.*

The word "laser" is actually used in the abstract, but reading closely it is obvious that the equipment contains LED:s.

6.1.3 Lasers - better than LED:s?

The scientific documentation for laser phototherapy has been, and remains superior to that of non-coherent light sources. When coherent and non-coherent sources have been compared, the outcome has been in favour of the coherent sources, with very few exceptions. Admittedly, these studies have not succeeded well in using the same light parameters for coherent and non-coherent sources. So the situation is, for the time being, in favour of coherent light. A lot of reference is still used to *in vitro* studies, showing that it is the wavelength and energy density that counts. For the *in vitro* situation this is correct, and to some extent also for open wounds and mucosa. For bulk tissue, however, the situation is different. Unfortunately many manufacturers have been quoting *in vitro* studies as proof of a general equality between coherent and non-coherent light.

6.1.4 The come-back of the LED:s

In recent years a lot of very qualified research has been published in the field of LED light therapy. There is no longer any doubt about the efficacy of LED light therapy in itself. However, so far only superficial and transparent tissues have been documented, while deep tissue conditions such as DOMS have failed. And still today there is not one study comparing coherent and incoherent light for any deep tissue condition. However, the controversy over the LED:s has subsided and today coherent and incoherent light therapies can be used in their own right, within the documented fields of application. The aim of this chapter is to underline the "come-back" of the LED:s since research published after 2004, when our most recent book was published, has been more convincing. Other parts of this books deal with the different mechanisms between the two types of light more in depth.

Literature examples:

6.1 Light Emitting Diodes

6.1.1 The controversial LED:s

Already in the early years of phototherapy, equipment containing Light Emitting Diodes were marketed as being lasers. The LED:s in those years were very weak and so was the scientific documentation. However, LED companies offered long lists of scientific studies, containing laser phototherapy studies. The laymen were fooled. This unscrupulous marketing harmed not only LED light therapy but laser therapy as well. Later on cluster arrays appeared, containing LED:s and lasers together. The advantage of this set up is not obvious. No certain knowledge exists about the interaction between different wavelengths of coherent and incoherent light sources. A further disadvantage is that any positive documentation of such therapy can only be reproduced using an array of the very same configuration. And there are not two manufacturers producing identical arrays. These combination arrays are the opposite to what is looked for in medicine - to identify the active ingredient.

6.1.2 Confusion between lasers and LED

It has not been unusual for manufacturers of LED equipment to use references to laser studies, pretending LED and laser are the same. This confusion has also spread among investigators and it is not uncommon for LED studies to be misinterpreted as laser studies when referred to in other articles. A few examples are the studies by Gupta [720] and Iusim [1063]. Sometimes the title of a study or the abstract is inconclusive in this respect and in list of references LED studies can be found "disguised" as laser studies, even in meta analyses. One example is the study by Iusim . The title of the paper is "Evaluation of the degree of effectiveness of Biobeam low level narrow band light on the treatment of skin ulcers and delayed postoperative wound healing". The "low level narrow band light" is actually emitted by a LED unit, but the phrase can easily be mistaken for a laser source, owing to the "home made" definition by the author.

Here is another example from the study titled: Taly A B, Sivaraman Nair K P, Thyloth Murali T, Archana J. Efficacy of multiwavelength light therapy in the treatment of pressure ulcers in subjects with disorders of the spinal cord: A randomized double-blind controlled trial. Archives of Physical Medicine and Rehabilitation. 2004; 85 (10): 1657-1661.

In a study by Taly [1424] thirty-five subjects with spinal cord injury, with 64 pressure ulcers (stage 2, n=55; stage 3, n=8; stage 4, n=1), were randomized into treatment and control groups. Mean duration of ulcers in the treatment group was 34.2±45.5 days and in the control group, 57.1±43.5 days. Treatment group received 14 sessions of multi wavelength light therapy, with 46 diodes of different wavelengths from a gallium-aluminum-ars-

Chapter 6
Non-coherent light sources

Linear polarised light

LED - Light Emitting Diodes

Broadband polarised light

Wound healing

10 J.K. A. 75 years old male has been skiing cross-country and now has two frozen and painful finger tips. No medical therapy had been offered, rather suggestions about the possibility of amputations. Indium over the finger tips removed the pain within an hour. Pain is back next day but is again removed with the laser. After 5 sessions pain is gone permanently and healing is taking place. The fingers were in the end completely healed.

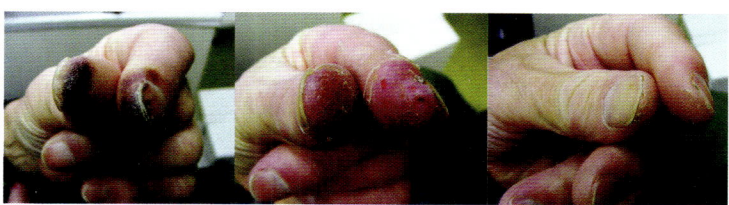

The few examples above are cases in which laser treatment has helped when it has been difficult to find other forms of treatment which work, bearing in mind the circumstances. The latter cases, which do not really come under the "dental laser treatment" heading, do nevertheless give some indication of the various conditions in which a dentist can have the opportunity to use the laser.

a week and immediately before a match increased the pain-free period by 100%.

7 M.D. A 49-year-old woman. At the age of 28, she had developed pains in the soles of her feet, which gradually spread to the palms of her hands. After a few years, the pain had spread throughout her skin. No certain diagnosis had been offered, despite many doctors' appointments. The patient had not taken the recommended pain-relief medication in order to avoid side effects. It was sometimes impossible for her to walk because of the pain. The problem came to the attention of the dentist when he touched the patient's cheek, at which she felt pain. 6 J of GaAs was administered over one side of the face. The patient experienced an obvious reduction in pain, and a new "itching" sensation in the cheek. When the patient came to the next appointment, she no longer had any pain in the side of her face treated with laser. The whole face was now treated, along with the palms of the hands and the soles of the feet, with a GaAs multiprobe. A total of 14 J was administered. At the next appointment, the patient reported a large, general reduction in pain. The arms and legs were also treated (20 J). At the following appointment, only mild pain in the part of the soles of the feet where the pain began remained. After six LPT applications, the patient no longer experienced pain and a few months later said she was enjoying her "best year in ages". After 7 years, there has been no recurrence.

8 J.S. A man in his 50s with shoulder pain since several years. Steroid injections had had a good but not long lasting, effect. Sleep was impaired, and he could not have his cameras hanging over his shoulder the way he was used to. After three treatments, he was able to sleep on the affected side, after six he was completely pain free. Full Range of Movement. A tennis elbow was cured in three sessions en passant.

9 A.M. This female patient had been suffering from pain in her neck and shoulders for about ten years. Due to the difficulties in moving her neck, GaAlAs laser treatment was administered prior to dental treatment, 10 J per point. This had a satisfactory effect. The patient said that the centre of her stiffness was in the right trapezius. As this part was treated the pain and stiffness were considerably reduced. At the following dental appointment the patient pointed out that her tinnitus on the right side had almost gone. This condition was not previously known by the therapist. Since there was some, although lighter, tinnitus on the left side as well, both sides of the body were treated, this time including the masticatory muscles. At the next appointment the tinnitus was almost gone in both ears, and the patient remarked: "my vertigo is much reduced!" This condition was also unknown to the therapist. Five follow up sessions were performed. The patient was almost free of problems at four months' checkup. After five months the problems started to reappear since the patient had continued the kind of work that initially caused the problems.

in the area on occasion, but this could be eradicated after one or more laser treatments.

3 F.Å. A 56-year-old woman with few teeth remaining in the lower jaw, full upper jaw prosthesis, and partial prosthesis in the lower jaw. She was encouraged by a doctor to seek the help of a dentist for her long-standing headaches. The prostheses were highly abraded, and new prostheses with a larger vertical dimension and better occlusal stability were made. The patient returned five days after the new prostheses were fitted for the treatment of a small decubital wound. The headaches remained. By way of an experiment, a GaAs multi-probe (19 Hz) was placed against the right temple. The patient immediately said that it "felt good". After three minutes' irradiation (11 J), mainly on the most painful side, the patient said that most of the pain was gone. Out of scientific curiosity, the pulse repetition rate was increased to 5000 Hz, at which the patient experienced a sensation of pressure. At 6 Hz, the patient did not feel anything in particular. The changes in pulse repetition rate were made without the patient's knowledge, but she could tell immediately when it "felt good" and when it "tightened". At a new appointment the next day, the headache had disappeared completely. 8 J was administered, and the patient was still able to notice differences in pulse repetition rate. At a check-up after three months, the patient was still untroubled by headaches.

4 B.S. A 43-year-old woman with "fibromyalgia" as a preliminary diagnosis. The patient was in need of dental care, but lying in a dentist's chair even for as little as ten minutes increased her pain considerably. She could be treated in a sitting position, but this would make the planned treatment, involving porcelain inlays, more difficult. GaAs irradiation along the spine and on the trigger points of the back once a week and immediately before treatment made a 45-minute treatment session possible, and the patient experienced a much improved pain situation for one to three days after each laser treatment.

5 L.J. A 34-year-old man who needed emergency treatment for a fractured upper incisor. His usual dentist did not have the time to treat him. On the same day, the patient had injured his left hand and the tips of three fingers had been cut off. He arrived via the hospital's casualty department with bandaged fingers and in great pain, and would not take analgesics on principle. During the dental treatment, the patient held a GaAs multiprobe against the palm of his left hand and soon noticed a pleasant sensation. After four minutes (14 J) the pain had disappeared, leaving the patient both pleased and surprised.

6 T.D. A 23-year-old male football player. The patient noticed the LPT equipment in the dentist's surgery and wondered whether it might help his periostitis. He could play football for only 30 minutes or so without the pain in his legs becoming unbearable. Scanning laser treatment with HeNe once

This wavelength happens to be the peak wavelength in LED-based curing lights!

5.4.3 Tooth bleaching

Argon (488 nm), GaAlAs, Nd:YAG and CO_2 lasers as well as blue LED:s are used in combination with in-office tooth bleaching. The laser is marketed to make bleaching faster, but will not bleach teeth better than at-home bleaching or bleaching without laser [843]. The laser/LED is said to excite the hydrogen peroxide molecule in the bleaching gel. The short wavelength and the higher photon energy of the argon laser would then make it a first choice. Halogen lamps, plasma-arch lamps and other heat lamps emit short wavelengths as well as longer invisible infrared thermal wavelengths and are more likely to create unfavourable pulpal responses.

5.4.4 Caries detection

Laser fluorescence can be used to detect occlusal caries. A diode of 655 nm has been successfully used to diagnose hidden occlusal caries.

5.5 Case reports

Case reports are of limited scientific value and are often referred to condescendingly as "anecdotal accounts". Of course, case reports should not be seen as anything other than treatment effects observed in particular cases, and perhaps by only a few therapists. They can, however, serve as useful guides for the clinician and as examples of what can be attempted. They are the kind of stories you might relate to a colleague during a coffee break between lectures but would not consider mentioning in the lecture itself. They are, in any event, the cases you sometimes remember most clearly, and are useful from a practical point of view. Below is a more readable rounding-off of this chapter - some case reports from the author's experience.

1. A.B. A 20-year-old woman with pain in the maxillary joint and who was grinding acutely. She could not open her mouth more than 17 mm with deviation. GaAs laser light was administered bilaterally (8 J) over the joint area and the immediately surrounding tissue, after which the patient could open her mouth 22 mm with greatly reduced pain and deviation. An imprint for a bite splint could be taken without any problems.

2. I.C. A 54-year-old man suffering from painful candida-infected leukoplakia bilaterally under the tongue. HeNe laser light had a good, but only temporary, pain relieving effect. After surgical removal of the leukoplakia, HeNe was administered on the side where the postoperative pain was greatest. This side healed more quickly. The patient later experienced pain

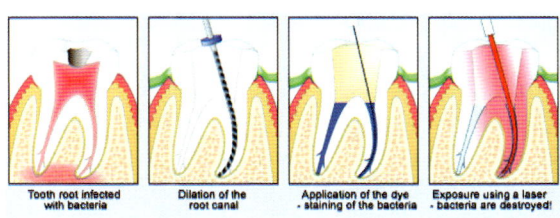

Figure 5.12 Photo Activated Disinfection. After scaling the pocket is filled with the dye and irradiated with red laser light.
Courtesy: HELBO

Literature:

Further literature: [708, 778, 827, 841, 842, 930, 1115, 1239, 1709, 1710, 1711]

5.4.2 Composite curing

A common wish among dentists is to be able to cure dental composite material quicker and more thoroughly. Experiments in curing have been conducted with argon lasers (488 nm), nitrogen lasers and HeCd lasers (443 nm). There are commercial systems based on argon lasers, but the high price is a disincentive to general use. The argon laser is capable of curing a layer of 2 mm within 10 seconds, compared to the recommended 20 seconds with traditional blue halogen curing light. Laser curing will improve the physical properties of the resins. It can, however, increase shrinkage and brittleness [455]. With the advent of plasma arch and LED-based curing lights, laser curing seems to have lost its appeal.

The intense curing light is likely to have biological effects but this phenomenon has not been studied. The LED curing lights are more narrow-banded than the halogen lights are even more likely to affect the irradiated cells.

Soukos [1502] has shown that broadband light in the range 380-520 nm rapidly and selectively kills oral black-pigmented bacteria in pure cultures and in dental plaque samples obtained from human subjects with chronic periodontitis. Cultures of Prevotella intermedia and P. nigrescens were killed by 4.2 J/cm^2, whereas P. melaninogenica required 21 J/cm^2. Exposure to light with a fluence of 42 J/cm^2 produced 99% killing of P. gingivalis. In dental bleaching procedures the dosages of blue light are high.

Enwemeka [2108] has demonstrated that 470 nm light has a strong bactericidal effect on MRSA (Meticillinresistent Staphylococcus aureus).

Further literature: [83, 100, 176, 206, 212, 218, 310, 491, 514, 530, 618, 629, 635, 751, 820, 932, 1108, 1329, 1418, 1886]

5.4 Other dental laser applications

5.4.1 Dental photo dynamic therapy

Laser light at LPT levels has been shown to activate the bactericidal effect of different dyes, such as toluidine blue (TBO). This combination therapy could have important advantages in the treatment of caries and periodontal disease. The commercial names are aPDT (antimicrobial Photo Dynamic Therapy) and PAD (Photo Activated Disinfection).

LED is likely to work just as well as laser in these superficial tissues. aPDT/PAD has been suggested as a suitable therapy for periodontal pockets, root canal disinfection, carious disinfection and periimplantitis [1709, 1710, 1711]. Apart from the antimicrobial effect, there is of course a stimulating effect from the laser itself. An interesting possibility is pointed out by Bisland [1685], suggesting that laser phototherapy can "prime" cancer cells to become more sensitive to PDT.

Literature:

The purpose of the study by Zanin [1571] was to evaluate the antimicrobial effect of toluidine blue O (TBO), in combination with either HeNe laser or a light-emitting diode on the viability and architecture of Streptococcus mutans biofilms. Biofilms were grown on hydroxyapatite discs in a constant depth film fermentor fed with artificial saliva that was supplemented with 2% sucrose four times a day, thus producing a typical 'Stephan pH curve'. Photodynamic therapy was subsequently carried out on biofilms of various ages with light from either the HeNe laser or LED using energy densities of between 49 and 294 J/cm^2. The LED system works with a spectrum ranging from 620 to 680 nm with a peak close to 633 nm. Significant decreases in the viability of S. mutans biofilms were only observed when biofilms were exposed to both TBO and light, when reductions in viability of up to 99.99% were observed with both light sources. Overall, the results showed that the bactericidal effect was light dose-dependent and that older biofilms were less susceptible to photodynamic therapy. Confocal laser scanning microscopy images suggested that lethal photosensitization occurred predominantly in the outermost layers of the biofilms.

of the condylar position. This was performed twice per week, for a total of eight sessions. A Visual Analogue Scale and a colorimetric capsule method were employed. Data were obtained three times: before treatment (Ev1), shortly after the eighth session (Ev2), and 30 days after the first application (Ev3). Statistical tests revealed significant differences at one percent (1%) likelihood, which implies that superiority of the active group offered considerable TMJ pain improvement. Both groups presented similar masticatory behavior, and no statistical differences were found. With regard to the evaluation session, Ev2 presented the lowest symptoms and highest masticatory efficiency throughout therapy.

In a study by da Cunha [1989] the sample consisted of 40 patients, divided into an experimental group (G1) and a placebo group (G2). The treatment was done with an infrared laser (830nm, 500mW, 20s, 4J/point) at the painful points, once a week for four consecutive weeks. The patients were evaluated before and after the treatment through VAS and the Craniomandibular Index (CMI). The baseline and post therapy values of VAS and CMI were compared by the paired T-test, separately for the placebo and laser groups. A significant difference was observed between initial and final values in both groups. Baseline and post-therapy values of pain and CMI were compared in the therapy groups by the two-sample T-test, yet no significant differences were observed regarding VAS and CMI. After either placebo or laser therapy, pain and temporomandibular symptoms were significantly lower, although there was no significant difference between groups. **The actual energy is 500 x 20 seconds = 10 J/point. The two studies above appear to be rather similar, but the one delivering positive results treated twice a week, the negative study once a week. The longer time used in the positive study may also be of importance, even though the energy per point was lower than in the negative study.**

Myofacial pain dysfunction syndrome (MPDS) is the most common reason for pain and limited function of the masticatory system. The aim of a study by Shirani [1995] was to evaluate the efficacy of a particular source producing 660 nm and 890 nm wavelengths that was recommended to reduce of the pain in the masticatory muscles. This was a double-blind and placebo-controlled trial. Sixteen MPDS patients were randomly divided into two groups. For the laser group, two diode laser probes (660 nm, 6.2 J/cm^2, 6 min, CW and 890 nm, 1 J/cm^2, 10 min, 1,500 Hz were used on the painful muscles. For the control group, the treatment was similar, but the patients were not irradiated. Treatment was given twice a week for 3 weeks. The amount of patient pain was recorded at four time periods (before and immediately after treatment, 1 week after, and on the day of complete pain relief). A visual analog scale was selected as the method of pain measurement. In each group the reduction of pain before and after the treatment was meaningful, but, between the two groups LPT was more effective.

cally significant improvements were also detected between the two groups regarding reduction in the number of tender points.

The clinical trial by Nuñez [1759] was performed in 10 patients, 18-56 years old, diagnosed with TMD of multiple causes. All patients received both methods of treatment in two consecutive weeks. Laser was delivered via a 670 nm diode laser, output power 50 mW, fluence 3 J per site/4 sites (masseter muscle, temporal muscle, mandibular condyle, and intrauricular). TENS therapy was applied with a two-electrode machine at 20 W, maximum pulse repetition rate of 60 Hz, adjusted by the patient according to their sensitivity. The amplitude of mouth opening was recorded before treatment and immediately after using a millimeter rule; the measurements were performed from the incisal of the upper incisors to the incisal of the lower incisors. A paired t-test was applied to verify the significance of the results. A significant improvement in the range of motion for both therapies was observed immediately after treatment. Comparing the two methods, the values obtained after laser were significantly higher than those obtained after TENS. Both methods are effective to improve mouth opening. Comparing the two methods, laser was more effective than TENS applications.

The objective of the study by Emshoff [1818] was to assess the effectiveness of LPT in the management of temporomandibular joint (TMJ) pain in a random and double-blind research design. TMJ pain patients, randomly assigned, received 2 to 3 treatments per week for 8 weeks of active LPT (632.8 nm, 30 mW) (n = 26) or sham LPT (n = 26). Measures of TMJ pain during function were evaluated at baseline and weeks 2, 4, and 8 after the first LPT session. At the 8-week point, within-group improvements were present for TMJ pain during function, for both the active and sham LPT groups. Between-group differences were not highly evident.

In a study by Fikackova [1870] the active group of 61 patients was treated with 10 J/cm^2 or 15 J/cm^2, and the control group of 19 patients was treated with 0.1 J/cm^2. LPT was performed by a 830 nm laser with output of 400 mW, in 10 sessions. The probe with an aperture of 0.2 cm^2 was placed over the painful muscle spots in the patients with myofascial pain. In patients with TMD arthralgia the probe was placed behind, in front of, and above the mandibular condyle, and into the meatus acusticus externus. Changes in pain were evaluated by self-administered questionnaire. Application of 10 J/cm^2 or 15 J/cm^2 was significantly more effective in reducing pain compared to placebo, but there were no significant differences between the energy densities used in the study group and between patients with myofascial pain and temporomandibular joint arthralgia. Results were most obvious in those with chronic pain.

Carrasco [1988] selected fourteen patients and divided them into two groups (active and placebo). Infrared laser (780 nm, 70 mw, 60s, 4.2 J/point, 105 J/cm^2) was applied precisely and continuously into five points of the temporomandibular joint (TMJ) area: lateral point (LP), superior point (SP), anterior point (AP), posterior point (PP), and posterior-inferior point (PIP)

cases placebo laser, (4) Chronic cases J/cm², (5) J/cm², and (6) Chronic cases placebo laser. Evaluation of the condition was performed before LPT, directly after LPT, one week and 30 days after LPT. Decrease in pain intensity and increase in average amplitude of all mandibular movements was found in all laser groups, as compared to the placeo groups.

de Medeiros [1618] examined the effects of LPT on the contraction force of the masseter muscle in patients with neuromuscular discomfort. Fifteen patients of both genders, ages 19-29, suffering from pain in the masseter muscle, were exposed to InGaAlP laser irradiation, applied from a 2-mm distance. Laser parameters were 670 nm, 15 mW, 2 J per each cm^2 irradiated, covering the whole projection of the masseter muscle. All patients showed improvement in muscle contraction strength of about 2.51-3.01 kgf on both sides.

The aim of the study By Makihara [1659] was to evaluate the facial thermographic changes before and after low-level laser irradiation applied to the temporomandibular joint in normal subjects. Nine healthy subjects underwent irradiation using the continuous wave setting of a CO_2 laser with a power output of 1.0 W. The laser tip was positioned 10 cm above the skin over the right TMJ area for 10 min. The actual fluence on the facial surface was 7.64 J/cm². Variation of the facial temperature was evaluated by using thermography. The facial temperature 10 min after stopping irradiation was higher than that after 10 min of irradiation applied to the opposite side. The warmer area was found not only over the TMJ area but also over the temporal area, forehead area, and eyelid area on both sides.

A study by Venancio [1737] aimed to evaluate the effectiveness of LPT in 30 patients presenting temporomandibular joint (TMJ) pain and mandibular dysfunction in a random and double-blind research design. The sample, divided into experimental group and placebo group, was submitted to the treatment with infrared laser (780 nm, 30 mW, 10 s, 6.3 J/cm², 0.3 J per point, total of 0.9 J per session) at three TMJ points. The treatment was evaluated throughout six sessions and 15, 30 and 60 days after the end of the therapy, through visual analogue scale, range of mandibular movements and TMJ pressure pain threshold. The results showed a reduction in VAS but through the ANOVA with repeated measures it was observed that the groups did not present statistically significant differences.

In a study by Cetiner [1758] thirty-nine patients with myogenic TMD-associated orofacial pain, limited mandibular movements, chewing difficulties, and tender points were included. Twenty-four of them were treated with therapeutic laser (830 nm, 7 J/cm²) for 10 daily sessions, excluding weekends, as test group, and 15 patients with the same protocol received placebo laser treatment as a control group. These parameters were assessed just before, just after, and 1 month after the treatment. Maximal mouth-opening improvement and reductions in pain and chewing difficulty were statistically significant in the test group when compared with the control group. Statisti-

received placebo laser, one was treated with a 60 mW GaAlAs laser (4 J per point) and the third with a 300 mW GaAlAs laser (20 J per point). Energy densities were 20 and 100 J/cm^2, respectively. Assessment before and after the three treatment sessions was made by algometry of trigger points in masticatory muscles. Statistically significant increases in pressure point threshold and electromyographic amplitude recorded from voluntary triple clenching compared with placebo were seen in the high-energy group but not in the low-energy group, although a trend towards improvement was seen. A significantly greater number of patients recovered from myofascial pain and TMJ arthralgia as assessed clinically in the high-energy group compared to the placebo group.

The inter-relation between TMD and tinnitus has been addressed by i.a. Myrhaug [711]. The influence of n. trigeminus and n. facialis in TMD is well recognized by dentists. These two nerves also govern m. tensor tympani and m. stapedius, respectively. Treating the TMD could therefore also influence these two muscles in the middle ear. Reducing the tonus of the masticatory muscles would also relax the two middle ear muscles.

The relation between Menière's disease and problems in the masticatory muscles (the lateral pterygoid in particular), the atlas and the axis has been discussed by Bjorne [874, 1227, 1228]. Laser treatment of these muscles has so far had a promising clinical result.

Wong [875] stresses the fact that the styloid process and its attachments are often overlooked in the treatment of oro-facial pain. No less than 11 pains and symptoms have been identified from this structure, among them tinnitus. A GaAlAs laser directed at this site could relieve the symptoms.

The purpose of this study by Farina [1468] was to analyse the effects of LPT associated or not to occlusal splints in patients with TMD. Pain, mouth opening, muscular functions and bite force were measured. Ten patients were selected and divided into three groups: laser (GL), laser + occlusal splint (GLO) and occlusal splint (GO). In the first visit, the patients answered a Mc.Gill's short form. In each visit, mouth opening ability was measured, and the patients filled a Visual Analogue Scale (VAS) form. Electromiography (EMG) in both sides of masseter and temporal muscles was performed in the first visit, and one week later. For EMG and the bite force measurements, an occlusal splint was positioned over the tooth in both arcades and then a transducer was positioned for the tasks. The EMG was measured with 0% (relaxed), 25%, 50%, 75% and 100% of maximum voluntary contraction (MVC). The LPT was performed during 4 sessions with an interval of 48 h. The laser used was a continuous wave GaAlAs, 780 nm. The dose was 25 J/cm^2, in three points of TMJ, 15J/cm^2, in two points of masseter muscle as well as in three points of the temporal muscle and in one point of pterygoid muscle. Patients from GLO showed a higher mouth opening ability and higher pain relief than other groups.

Lizarelli [1554] divided 60 patient with acute or chronic TMJ disorders into six groups: (1) Acute cases 5 J/cm^2, (2) Acute cases J/cm^2, (3) Acute

Gray [1040] performed a clinical study where the effects of shortwave diathermy, megapulse, ultrasound and laser were compared in TMD therapy. There was no significant difference in success rate between the four therapies but all were better than placebo. The laser used was Space IRCEB-Up, 904 nm, and the reported dose was 4 J/cm^2, 3 minutes application, 3 times weekly for 4 weeks. There is no information in the text making a verification of this dose possible. This laser typically had 4 mW of power in contrast to pamphlet values and only at maximum pulsing. Nor is there any information on the therapeutic technique for either arthritis/arthrosis or myosis. This makes an evaluation of the laser part of the study difficult.

Bertolucci [532] compared two groups of patients (16+16) receiving physical therapy for mandibular dysfunction. One group received sham irradiation, the other GaAs laser over three weeks. The results were as follows (treatment group/placebo group): change in pain 40.25/1.56; change in vertical opening 1.35/-0.05; change in left and right deviation 3.78/0.62.

Cho [1183] performed a double blind study on the pressure pain threshold in patients with TMD. 19 dental students with TMD and 20 with no TMD were treated with LPT or placebo laser. There was a significant reduction in pain indexes in the laser group.

Conti [634] performed a double blind study on the effect of GaAlAs on two small groups of patients suffering from arthrogenous and myogenous problems respectively. Using a 100 mW laser, 4 J of energy was applied over the lateral joint surface in the arthrogenous group. In the myogenous group the same energy was applied to the most painful muscle point. The patients received three doses once a week. There was no statistical difference between placebo and laser groups. The lack of success in the study can probably be attributed to the low dose in the myogenic group, too few sessions, too long intervals between sessions and the fact that only a single myogenic pain point was irradiated. The arthrogenous group (5 + 5 patients) had very diverse diagnoses. 4 J for arthrogenous pain is a reasonable level, while for myogenous pain much higher doses are needed and more painful points must be irradiated, the lateral pterygoid not to be forgotten. The author himself also suggests the need for higher doses and more therapy sessions. The importance of higher doses and indeed higher energy densities is illustrated in the following studies.

The improved outcome of LPT, if higher doses are given, is documented in the study by Sanseverino [1224]. 10 patients with pain and limitation of movements of the jaw were treated by 785 nm GaAlAs laser, dose 45 J/cm^2. The joint and tender points in the masticatory and muscles otherwise involved were applied three times per week over three weeks. A control group of 10 patients was given sham LPT. The evaluation was performed through subjective pain assessment and measurement of the movements of the jaw. There was a significant improvement in the laser group only.

Sattayut [873] performed a double blind study on 30 patients. These patients had had their TMD problems for more than 6 months. One group

cular effects which locally resemble the vascular effects achieved with needle acupuncture, although it takes more time for laser stimulation to achieve an effect. Both forms of acupuncture were more effective on known acupuncture points than on randomly chosen points. St 6 was used throughout as a "known acupuncture point".

Kim [177] divided a group of 36 patients with maxillary joint problems into three therapy groups. The patients were treated either with bite splints, GaAlAs laser treatment or laser acupuncture. The treatment results were compared after two and four weeks with a check on status before treatment. The following conclusions were drawn. The patients' subjective discomfort was reduced in both the bite splint and laser treatment groups. The improvement in the laser group was much greater than in the bite splint group. Clinically noticeable symptoms showed a significant reduction in all groups, but the group treated with laser light responded faster to treatment than the other groups. EMG (electromyogram) activity gradually decreased in all groups, without any great difference between groups. Laser treatment had more beneficial effects than bite splints, while laser acupuncture produced the poorest results.

Kim [1119] found improvement in maximum mouth opening and increase in the pressure pain threshold after irradiating tender points in the masseter and trapezius. Laser was more effective than ultrasound.

Lopez [244] treated a group of 168 patients with problems related to TMJ disorders by using a combination of bite splints and HeNe laser light. An obvious improvement could be observed in 52 of the patients after a single application of treatment. After ten applications, 90% of the patients had improved. No further improvement was brought about in the other 10% by administering further treatment. The laser treatment was given directly over the maxillary joint - 6 mW for five minutes. The extent of healing was inspected using a tomographic X-ray before treatment and after six months. At that point, healing had advanced to a stage usually seen after 12 to 18 months when only a bite splint is used. In a group of 88 patients with pain in the jaw muscles, pain was alleviated for up to six hours, but without lasting results. The author concluded that HeNe lasers are effective as a complementary method to bite splints when treating arthrosis and arthritis, but that this wavelength is not optimal for myogenic pain.

Frugoni [342] also used X-rays to confirm the recovery rate in patients affected by calcification problems, using GaAs and HeNe lasers. In this particular study, the shoulder joint was studied.

Hatano [49] used a GaAlAs laser to study the effect on palpation pain in 15 patients with TMJ problems. A 30 mW laser was used for 3 minutes in the area of one temporo-mandibular joint. The other side served as control. Palpation score was estimated directly after irradiation and 20, 40 and 60 minutes after irradiation. There was a significant decrease in palpation pain with better results after 20, 40 and 60 minutes than directly after irradiation.

occipital muscles should be palpated since they are often involved. If tender, stretching of these muscles in combination with laser can temporarily lead to the reduction or even the elimination of tinnitus. This is an important diagnostic finding. The relation between muscular tension and tinnitus has been explained by Shore [1229] who found a connection between the sensory part of n. trigeminus and the ventral auditory nucleus in the brain stem. (See chapter 4.1.52 "Tinnitus, vertigo, Ménière´s disease" on page 330.)

Literature:

Interleukin-1ß in the synovial fluid is associated with TMD pain [639]. In a study by Shimizu [370], GaAlAs laser light influenced the production of this substance.

Hansson [85] studied the effects of GaAs laser on arthritis of the temporo-mandibular joint. He stresses that lasers are not an alternative to conventional treatment, but that it seems possible to reduce healing periods and to reduce inflammation more quickly.

Bezuur and Hansson [206] treated a group of 27 patients suffering from long-term problems related to TMJ (temporo-mandibular joint) disorders with a GaAs laser. The treatment was administered over the joint on five consecutive days. 80% of the 15 patients with arthrogenous pain experienced total pain relief. The maximum jaw-opening ability increased during the treatment period and continued to increase during the year that the group was monitored. The group suffering from myogenic problems also improved both in terms of pain and jaw-opening ability. The effect here was, however, much lower. As the muscles were not treated, it is assumed that this group also had undiagnosed arthritis. The reduction of joint sounds may possibly have been due to an increase of metabolism in articular cell structures, e.g. an activation of the synovial membrane, producing more synovial fluid.

Eckerdal [595] reports on the clinical experience of a 5-year non-controlled study of perioral neuropathias. The treated diagnoses were trigeminal neuralgia, atypical facial pain, paraesthesias and TMD pain. Of these diagnoses, the TMD pain group was the most successful one. At the end of treatment, 73% of the patients (N = 40) had a good response, at six months the number was still 73%, and at one year 70%. 10 J/cm^2 was applied to the joint over 4-8 sessions.

In a study comprising 75 cases, Bradley [435] found LPT effective as a monotherapy when treating acute joint pain (of less than eight weeks duration). In more chronic cases, without bone changes noticeable on X-ray, LPT was used as an adjunct to splints and the like. In osteoarthritic cases, LPT can be almost as useful as intra-articular steroids.

Bradley [117] used GaAs laser acupuncture when treating a small group of patients suffering from TMJ pain dysfunction syndrome who had not responded to treatment with a bite splint or psychotropic medicine. Needle acupuncture was used in a comparative group. Both types of acupuncture can be studied with thermography. Biostimulation was observed to yield vas-

5.3.29 Temporo-mandibular disorders (TMD)

Lasers can be of benefit in various ways for problems relating to temporo-mandibular disorders. As with any treatment, a correct diagnosis is essential to obtain a satisfactory result. In a number of conditions, i.e. occlusal adjustment and taking impressions for a splint, the pain itself prevents conventional treatment. By irradiating the joint and tender points, pain relief can be achieved, musculature is relaxed, and treatment can begin. Recent clinical experience and clinical studies indicate that rather high doses are needed for myogenic conditions and that the energy density itself is of importance. The inconsistent success reported in older studies seems to be related to this fact.

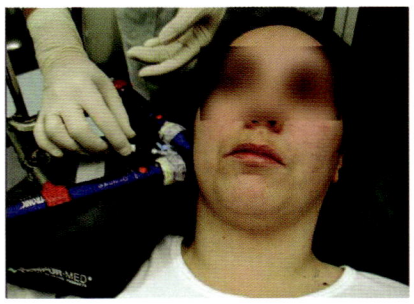

Evaluation of microcirculation in tender points in the m. masseter, using active and placebo laser.

Figure 5.11 Evaluation of microcirculation in tender points
Courtesy: Marie Tullberg

In cases of trismus [293], tender points and muscle attachments are treated. 6-10 J per point is usually a good start, but higher energies are sometimes required. Make a note of the maximum jaw-opening ability before treatment starts, then measure it again afterwards. During subsequent treatment, even more peripheral muscle attachments (e.g. the sternocleidomastoid) are palpated and irradiated. The treatment in TMD patients should not be discontinued as soon as pain disappear, but should be continued at longer intervals. Two to three applications in the first week, then once a week, can be sufficient for myoses. Arthritis/arthrosis requires lower energies due to the superficial location; 4-6 J per session is suggested. LPT is almost as effective as intra-articular steroids for joint pain [435].

Additional irradiation of the stellate ganglion [691, 692, 685, 1053] in pain patients has been effective in several studies and can be recommended for TMD treatment as well.

Dentists should be aware of the potential connection between tinnitus/vertigo and TMD (somatosensory tinnitus). Occlusal adjustment and/or splints will be very helpful in this group of patients. LPT reduces palpation tenderness and improves microcirculation in the tense muscles, thus leading to more rapid success. Tinnitus patients are over-represented among TMD sufferers [1488, 1722, 1723, 1724]. There is also an overrepresentation of TMD problems in persons with sensorineural hearing loss [1633].

Typical findings in these patients are premature contacts in the lower incisives and crossbite. Apart from tender points in the masticatory muscles (dominated by m. pterygoidalis lateralis, always on the tinnitus side), the

The aim of a study by Simunovic-Soskic [2116] was to monitor therapeutic response by determining the level of proinflammatory cytokines TNF-alpha and IL-6 in whole unstimulated saliva in patients with denture stomatitis (DS), before and after laser phototherapy (LPT). A sample consisting of 40 consecutive subjects was selected on a voluntary basis from patients who presented for the diagnosis and treatment of DS. A clinical examination was performed according to the standard clinical criteria. Lesions described as palatal inflammation were diagnosed as Newton type II denture stomatitis. The patients were randomly assigned to either an experimental group (20 patients receiving real LPT) or a control group (20 patients receiving inactive/placebo laser treatment). Following treatment with LPT for 4 wk, the levels of TNF-alpha and IL-6 decreased and were significantly different from controls.

Further literature: [79, 80, 66, 363]

5.3.28 Secondary dentine formation

Being able to stimulate secondary dentine formation with LPT would be of great benefit to the dental practitioner eager to preserve as much as possible. There are signs that this may be possible, but we do not yet know the optimum wavelengths and dosages.

Literature:

Nagasawa [106, 107] reported strong secondary dentine formation when rat teeth received Nd:YAG laser treatment at dosages within the biostimulating range. These results have recently been confirmed on human teeth.

In a pig experiment Prezotto [1466] found that 12,8 J/cm^2 (10 mW during 10 secs) stimulated secondary dentine formation when checked at 7 days post irradiation, while 89,7 J/cm^2 (70 mW during 10 secs) delayed formation as compared to control. At 45 days after irradiation there was no difference between low dose/high dose or control group.

ing. Treat the wound with a laser and polish the adjusted area. It should now be possible to bite hard. The laser has stopped the wound from being painful and keeps the patient free from symptoms during the time it takes for the oedema to disappear. The healing process is also shortened.

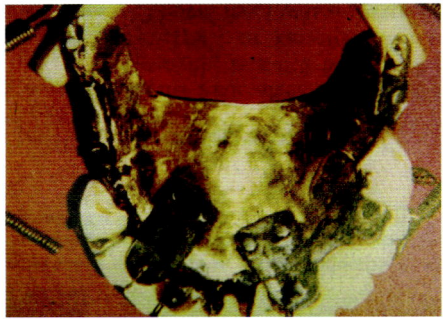

Figure 5.10 Upper denture once worn by George Washington

Literature:

Marei [515] divided 18 male denture wearers with mucosal lesions into three groups of six according to the treatment applied: denture removal, relining dentures with temporary tissue, or application of laser while continuing to wear the dentures. Clinically and histologically, the laser group healed best. Furthermore, the bone underlying the lesions showed an increase in optical density.

A study by Ferreira [1882] investigated the biomodulatory effect of the 670 nm laser in pulp cells on reactional dentinogenesis, and on the expression of collagen type III (Col III), tenascin (TN), and fibronectin (FN) in irradiated dental tissues and controls (not irradiated). Sixteen human premolar teeth were selected (after extraction due to orthodontal reasons) and divided into irradiated and control groups. Black class V cavity preparations were accomplished in both groups. For the irradiated group, laser (670 nm, 50 mW) with an energy density of 4 J/cm^2 was used. Soon after, the cavities were restored with a glass ionomer and the extractions made after 14 and 42 days. Histological changes were observed by light microscopy; less intense inflammatory reaction in the irradiated group was found when compared to the controls. Only the irradiated group of 42 days exhibited an area associated with reactional dentinogenesis. After immunohistochemical analysis, the expression of Col III, TN, and FN was greater in the irradiated groups. : These results suggest that a laser with energy density of 4 J/cm^2 and wavelength of 670 nm causes biomodulation in pulp cells and expression of collagen, but not collagen of the extracellular matrix, after preparation of a cavity.

a LPT for the treatment of deep intra-bony defects. This study was an intra-individual longitudinal test of 12 months' duration conducted using a blinded, split-mouth, placebo-controlled and randomized desig, and the same type of laser as above. In 22 periodontitis patients, one intra-bony defect was randomly treated with EMD+LPT, while EMD alone was applied to the contra-lateral defect site. LPT was used both intra- and post-operatively. Clinical measurements were performed by a blinded periodontist at the time of surgery, in the first week and in the first, second, sixth and 12th month. Visual analogue scale (VAS) scores were recorded for pain assessment. The results showed that the treatment of intra-bony defects with EMD alone or EMD+LPT leads to probing depth reduction and attachment-level gain. In addition, EMD+LPT had resulted in less gingival recession less swelling and less VAS scores compared with EMD alone.

More reading: chapter 5.3.12 "Implantology" on page 411 and chapter 4.1.8 "Bone and cartilage regeneration" on page 174.

Further literature: [1106, 1225, 1307, 1314, 1320]

5.3.27 Prosthetics

Opening the gingival pocket with retraction cord in conjunction with the taking of impressions can cause postoperative discomfort. Electrosurgery can cause even greater distress, especially if the electrocoagulator comes in contact with bone. 2-3 J in each proximal space eases pain and should be given prophylactically before the anaesthetic has worn off.

When trying in a crown on a vital tooth, the patient is often reluctant to anaesthetise again, particularly in the front of the upper jaw. 2-3 J on the exposed dentine raises the pain threshold enough to test the crown. The same applies to cementing, in which cleaning, drying and exposure to the cement can cause postoperative discomfort. If you have not administered treatment prophylactically, postoperative problems can be dealt with after cementing by irradiating over the apex. The dosage depends on the position of the root apex. If vital dentine is irradiated directly, a brief pain reaction can arise. This passes quickly, so pause for a while before continuing the laser treatment.

The preparation of vital teeth is traumatic for the pulp, although this is a trauma that most teeth can cope with. 1-2 J to stimulate the pulp and reduce any postoperative difficulty is recommended.

Transient pain reactions in the pulp can be the result of vigorous occlusal adjustment. The laser here presents an excellent source of immediate help for the patient. 3-4 J over the apex of each involved root is the normal dosage.

If a dental prosthesis chafes, superfluous acrylic must be ground away. Because the decubital wound is sensitive and swollen, an overadjustment of the surface of the prosthesis is required in order to relieve all symptoms. Recommended treatment for the dentist equipped with a laser is as follows: adjust only until the patient is free from symptoms when lightly bit-

Lai [1916] evaluated the adjunctive effect of a HeNe laser in the non-surgical periodontal treatment of patients with moderate to advanced chronic periodontitis. Sixteen patients with probing pocket depth (PPD) >/ =5 mm and comparable bone defects on both sides of the mouth were recruited. Supragingival plaque (PL), bleeding on probing (BOP), PPD, and probing attachment level (PAL) were recorded at baseline and at 3, 6, 9, and 12 mo, while gingival crevicular fluid (GCF) samples and standardized intra-oral radiographs for digital subtraction radiography were taken at baseline and at 1, 3, 6, 9, and 12 mo. After non-surgical mechanical peri-odontal treatment, the test sites were selected randomly and irradiated with a HeNe laser (output power 0.2 mW) for 10 min for a total of eight times in the first 3-mo period, while the control sites received no additional treatment. PL percentage (83-16%) and BOP percentage (95-34%) decreased significantly after 12 mo. Statistically significant changes in reductions of PPD and GCF volume, gain in PAL, and increase in recession were seen in both test and control sites when compared to baseline. No statistically significant differences in any clinical parameters or radiographic findings were found between the test and control sites. Changes in GCF volume were significant only at 3 mo in the test sites. **The energy delivered by a 0.2 mW laser during 10 minutes is 0.12 J and the total energy applied during eight sessions was less than 1 J. The negative outcome of this study is therefore to be anticipated.**

Twenty patients with inflammatory gingival hyperplasias on their symmetrical teeth were included in a study by Ozcelik [1822]. After gingivectomy and gingivoplasty, a diode laser (588 nm) was randomly applied to one side of the operation area for 7 days. The overall energy density per irradiation of 5 min. was 4 J/cm^2. During irradiation, the tip of the laser probe was placed on both the buccal and the lingual side of the periodontal defect area (5 min. for each). The flaps were then replaced and sutured with modified internal mattress sutures. LPT was again applied for 10 min. from the outer buccal and lingual surfaces (again for 5 min. for each) of the flaps immediately after suturing for the test sites. The surgical areas were disclosed by a solution to visualize the areas in which the epithelium is absent. Comparison of the surface areas on the LPT-applied sites and controls were made with an image-analysing software. Despite the prolonged time needed for application, patients have tolerated LPT well. While there were no statistically significant differences between the stained surface areas of the LPT applied and the control sites immediately after the surgery, LPT-applied sites had significantly lower stained areas compared with the controls on the post-operative third, seventh and 15th day. Within the limitations of this study, the results indicated that LPT may enhance epithelisation and improve wound healing after gingivectomy and gingivoplasty operations.

The aim of another study by Ozcelik [1921] was to evaluate the immediate post-operative pain, wound healing and clinical results after the application of an enamel matrix protein derivative (EMD) alone or combined with

Damante [1443], however, could not find that 670 nm accelerated the healing of the oral mucosa after gingivoplasty. 4 J/cm² was applied to each point in one single session.

In the study by Ribeiro [1906] ten patients were selected and submitted to measurement of six sites per tooth, four teeth per hemiarch (960 sites in all). All patients then received subgingival scaling and root planing. Besides periodontal treatment, the test side was also submitted to laser application. The analysis comprised measurement of probing depth, clinical attachment level, and gingival index. Laser energy was applied at a wavelength of 780 nm (35 J/cm², 70 mW, 20 sec per site) for preoperative analgesia, and scaling and root planing were performed with application of laser energy at a wavelength of 780 nm (35 J/cm², 70 mW, 20 sec) for analgesia, and at a wavelength of 630 nm (8.8 J/cm², 35 mW, 10 sec) for healing. The patients filled out a visual analogue scale to assess the pain they felt during the procedure. After 24 and 48 h, the laser was again applied at the wavelength of 630 nm, and the patients were re-evaluated after 3 days. There was a reduction in gingival inflammation, yet without a statistically significant difference between the study and control sides, both in clinical aspects and evaluation of pain during the procedure. **While the therepeutic dose was well within the therapeutic window, the presumed energy of 1.4 J per point is well below the pain relieving energy.**

The study by Aboelsaad [1913] aimed to investigate the influence of 830 nm, CW, 40 mW and 4 J/cm² on the healing of surgically created bone defects in rats treated with bioactive glass graft material. Surgical bone defects were created in the mandibles of 36 Wistar rats divided into two groups, each consisting of 18 rats. Group I was treated with bioactive glass plus laser irradiation. Group II was treated with graft material only. The animals were killed at 4 weeks, 8 weeks and 12 weeks postoperatively for histological examination. Laser irradiation had significantly accelerated bone healing at 4 weeks and 8 weeks in comparison with that at the sites not irradiated. However at 12 weeks, complete healing of the defects had occurred with no difference detected.

In a following clinical study [1914] Aboelsaad aimed to investigate the same procedure in a clinical setting, with total energy density of 16 J/cm² on the healing of human infra-bony defects treated with bioactive glass graft material. Twenty patients with chronic periodontitis and bilateral infra-bony defects were included. Using a split mouth design, the group treated 20 defects with bioactive glass plus laser irradiation during surgical procedures and on days 3, 5, 7 postoperatively; 20 contra-lateral defects were treated with bioactive glass only. Clinical probing pocket depths, clinical attachment levels and standardized periapical radiographs were recorded at baseline and at 3 months and 6 months postoperatively. At 3 months there was a statistically significant difference between the laser and non-laser sites in the parameters investigated. However, at 6 months, no difference was observed.

the other side, after the teeth having been debrided. 635 nm diode laser 0.9 J was applied at the base of the interdental papilla and GaAlAs 3.5 J at the projection of the alveolar bone margin. The results were as follows (laser side/placebo side): gingival index 0.54/1.4, plaque index 0.26/0.68, pocket reduction 0.92/0.16. The gingival exsudate was reduced on the laser side, 0,04 µl vs. 0.14 µl. The metalloproteinase-8 (MMP-8) was slightly reduced on the laser side and elevated on the placebo side. There was no difference in elastase activity or of the amount of IL-1β, nor any significant changes in microbiology.

The aim of another study by Qadri [1634] was to study whether or not the length of coherence is of importance in phototherapy. Laser light is coherent but the length of coherence of gas lasers such as a HeNe laser is much greater than that of a diode laser of the same wavelength. The biological significance of the length of coherence has hitherto not been investigated. 20 patients with light to moderate periodontitis were selected. After instruction about oral hygiene, scaling and root planing (SRP), one side of the upper jaw of each patient was randomly selected for HeNe (632.8 nm, 3 mW) or InGaAlP (650 nm, 3 mW) laser irradiation, using the same power and dose, irradiating once of week during six weeks. One week after the SRP the following parameters were measured: pocket depth, gingival index, plaque index, GCF volume, MMP-8, IL-8 and microbiology in the pocket. The irradiation (180 seconds per point, $0.54 J/cm^2$) was then performed by a dental hygienist and the selection of side was blinded to the evaluators. After six weeks renewed measurements revealed that all clinical parameters had improved significantly better on the HeNe side. MMP-8 was more reduced on the HeNe side while there was no difference for IL-8 or pathogens. Coherence is an important factor in phototherapy but even the length of the coherence appears to be of importance.

The aim of the work of Kiernicka [1629] was to evaluate the influence of LPT on the periodontal pocket depth after routine conservative periodontal treatment with or without additional use of LPT; in two groups of pockets: above and below 5 mm. The laser was an 830 nm probe of 200 mW. 4 Joules were applied on the papilla every day or every two days for seven days. In six patients having periodontitis 613 sites were submitted to statistic analysis (290 treated conservatively only, including 251 with the depth 2-5 mm and 39 above 5 mm as well as 323 with the use of LPT including 297 shallow pockets and 26 deep pockets). The initial values of Proximal Plaque Index, Plaque Index, Sulcus Bleeding Index, Periodontal Pocket Depth (PPD) and their changes in the course of the treatment were registered. During each control appointment the patients subjectively estimated periodontal pain occurrence. In both groups a statistically essential decrease of the evaluated parameters was obtained. Reinforcing the conventional treatment with LPT shortened the healing time and led to elimination of pain faster than with the use of conservative treatment only. The changes of the PPD index were statistically higher in the laser group, especially in relation to deep pockets.

pockets, SIgA-level in saliva, and R-protein level in gingival blood. LPT shortened healing time considerably.

Mamedova [365] used ultraviolet and HeNe lasers in combination in the treatment of a group of 90 persons suffering from parodontitis. The optimal doses for the antimicrobic effect on the pocket microorganisms were assessed.

Mousques [73] carried out simultaneous periodontal operations in two quadrants, treated on one side with HeNe laser, and compared the results in terms of healing. Several parameters were studied using a double-blind technique, and all showed better results in the laser group.

Masse [461] reports no effect on periodontal flap surgery using a combined HeNe/GaAs laser. However, independent measurement of the output, initiated by the researchers, showed 0.27 mW for the HeNe from the fibre (4 mW stated) and 80 mW peak power for the GaAs (2 watts stated). The dosage is not reported but is calculated to be 0.04 J/cm^2, which predisposes the study to fail.

Conlan [735] has performed a literature study and come to the conclusion that LPT has no place in dentistry. Interestingly enough, not one dental study is listed among the references.This paper is from 1996 and an updated review would come to different conclusions.

An investigation by Efanov [1721] was made of applying pulsed 890 nm laser radiation in the treatment for early diagnosed periodontitis. The investigation was made on 65 patients (47 patients constituted the experimental group and 18 patients constituted a control group affected by periodontitis). Clinical and functional tests revealed that LPT produced a strong effect on the course of the illness. It reduced bleeding, inflammation, and pruritus. Biomicroscopic examinations and periodontium rheography revealed that the gingival blood flow became normal after the course of LPT. The capillary permeability and venous congestion decreased, which was confirmed by the increased time of vacuum tests, raised gingival temperature, reduced tissue clearance, and increased oxygen tension. Apart from that, LPT subsided fibrinolysis, proteolytic tissue activity, and decreased the exudative inflammation of the periodontium.

The effect of LPT in periodontal surgery has been reported by Silveira [1241]. 20 patients with periodontal disease were subjected to gingivectomies. Gingival biopsies were taken from a non-mineralised wall of a suprabony periodontal pocket. The first sample was taken before laser irradiation, the second after 785 nm laser irradiation and the third after 688 nm laser irradiation (50 mW, 8 J/cm^2). After biopsy the samples were fixed, cut and stained. Both laser wavelengths promoted mast cell degranulation as compared to control and there was no statistical difference between the two wavelengths.

In the study by Qadri [1185] a combination of 635 nm diode laser and GaAlAs laser were used to treat gingivitis and periodontal disease. 17 patients received laser on one side of the upper arch and placebo laser on

were observed clinically and histomorphologically. The amount of regeneration was highest in group 3 but the difference between group 2 and 3 was not statistically significant. The height of the regenerated bone was higher in groups 2 and 3 as compared to control, but the difference was just in the limit of significance .

The aims of the study by Silveira [1907] were to investigate the effect of laser irradiation on the total number of mast cells as well as the percentage of degranulation in human gingiva. Blood vessel dilation was also evaluated. In periodontal tissue, mast cells may influence either the destructive events or the defense mechanism against periodontal disease via secretion of cytokines and through cellular migration to improve the healing process. Mast cells play an important role in the inflammatory process. Twenty patients with gingival enlargement indicated for gingivectomy were selected. Gingival fragments were obtained from each patient and divided into three different groups before surgery. One fragment was removed without any irradiation. The two others were submitted to punctual irradiation with either 688 or 785 nm, with an energy density of 8 J/cm^2 at an output power of 50 mW at 36 Hz for 36 sec before gingivectomy. Non-degranulated and degranulated mast cells were counted in five areas of the gingival fragment connective tissue. Major and minor diameters of the blood vessels were also measured. Both red and infrared radiation promoted a significant increase in mast cell degranulation compared to controls; however, no statistically significant differences were observed between the irradiated groups. No significant differences among the groups were observed regarding blood vessel size.

The aim of a study by Garcia [2079] was to compare LPT as adjuvant treatment for induced periodontitis with scaling and root planing (SRP) in dexamethasone-treated rats. One-hundred twenty rats were divided into groups: D group (n = 60), treated with dexamethasone; ND group (n = 60) treated with saline solution. In both groups, periodontal disease was induced by ligature at the left first mandibular molar. After 7 days, the ligature was removed and all animals were subjected to SRP and were divided according to the following treatments: SRP, irrigation with saline solution (SS); SRP + LPT, SS and laser irradiation, 660 nm; 24 J; 0.428 W/cm2. Ten animals in each treatment were killed after 7 days, 15 days and 30 days. The radiographic and histometric values were statistically analyzed. In all groups radiographic and histometric analysis showed less bone loss in animals treated with SRP + LPT in all experimental periods. **The dose used in this study is much higher than expected for stimulation.**

Clinical studies

Sokolova [364] studied 60 patients with parodontitis (ages 25-55), divided into two equal groups. Conventional treatment was given in both groups, but one group also received therapeutic laser treatment. Healing was studied using periodontal index, hygiene index, bacterioscopy of the gingival

The aim of an investigation by Gerbi [1471] was to assess histologically the effect of LPT (830 nm, 40 mW, CW, area diameter approximately 0.6 mm, 16 J/cm^2 per session) on the repair of surgical defects created in the femur of the Wistar Albinus rat. The defects were filled to lyophilized bovine bone associated or not to GTR. Surgical bone defects were created in 42 animals divided into five groups: Group I (control, 6 animals); Group II (Gen-ox, 9 animals); Group III (Gen-ox + Laser, 9 animals); Group IV (Gen-ox + Gen-derm, 9 animals); Group V (Gen-ox + Gen-derm + Laser, 9 animals). The animals on the irradiated group received 16 J/cm2 per session divided into four points around the defect (4 J/cm^2) being the first irradiation immediately after surgery and repeated seven times at every 48 h. The animals were humanly killed after 15, 21, and 30 days. The results of the present investigation showed histological evidence of improved amount of collagen fibers at early stages of the bone healing (15 days) and increased amount of well organized bone trabeculae at the end of the experimental period (30 days) on irradiated animals compared to non irradiated ones.

The aim of the investigation by Torres [1905] was to histologically assess the effect of laser photobiomodulation (LBPM) on the repair of autologous bone grafts in a rodent model. A major problem in modern dentistry is the recovery of bone defects caused by trauma, surgical procedures, or pathologies. Several types of biomaterials have been used to improve the repair of these defects. These materials are often associated with procedures of guided bone regeneration (GBR). In the present study twenty four animals were divided into four groups: group I (control); group II (LPBM of the bone graft); group III (bone morphogenetic proteins [BMPs] + bone graft); and group IV (LPBM of the bed and the bone graft + BMPs). When appropriate, the bed was filled with lyophilized bovine bone and BMPs used with or without GBR. The animals in the irradiated groups received 10 J/cm^2 per session, divided over four points around the defect (4 J/cm^2), with the first irradiation immediately after surgery, and then repeated seven times every other day. The animals were humanely killed after 40 d. The results showed that in all treatment groups, new bone formation was greater and qualitatively better than the untreated subjects. Control specimens showed a less advanced repair after 40 d, and this was characterized by the presence of medullary tissue, a small amount of bone trabeculi, and some cortical repair. It is conclude that LPBM has a positive biomodulatory effect on the healing of bone defects, and that this effect was more evident when LPBM was performed on the surgical bed intraoperatively, prior to the placement of the autologous bone graft.

Fekrazad [1551] performed an experimental clinical trial in 5 healthy dogs. A square lesion was made in the exposed periodontal bone. The lesions were divided into three groups: (1) Control group, where the flap was closed an sutured. (2) Flap was closed and sutured with a resorbable membrane inserted in the bony defect. (3) As with group 2 but followed by 890 nm daily irradiation during two week., 0.01 J/cm^2. After two months the specimens

In a study by Kubota [1116], a 1000 mW, 830 nm laser was used to treat skin ulcers. The power density was 669 mW/cm^2 and the dose 6.3 J/cm^2. Less postoperative pain, better coagulation, better bone regeneration, increased tensile strength and enhanced angiogenesis can be expected.

Zhang [94] carried out an experiment similar to Kubota's, but using a defocused CO_2 laser at a power density of 300 mW/cm^2, in a rat model. Mean survival length of the flap was 5.83 cm in the LPT group and 3.60 cm in the control group.

The "surgical" lasers can, at advantage, be defocused and used as biostimulators, as demonstrated by Pourzarandian [1606].

Schenk [78] studied the effects of a HeNe laser on gingiva and sublingual mucous membrane in dogs. The preparation was produced with 60 and 120 seconds' exposure, and sub-cellular changes were studied. An increased number of vesicles, vacuoles, enlarged mitochondria and dilation of the endoplasmic reticulum were observed. The investigators consider that the morphological changes confirm the hypothesis about the stimulating effect of HeNe laser on various cell systems.

Kawamura [202] studied the effects of Nd:YAG and GaAlAs lasers on epithelium downgrowth in the pocket after a flap operation. Flaps with root scaling and iatrogenic bone defects were given to 54 hamsters. One group received irradiation (as much as 80 J/cm^2) once, immediately after the operation. Another group was given laser treatment once a week. Unacceptable necrosis could be seen in the Nd:YAG group. Of the GaAlAs groups, the group that received a single dose of laser showed a reduced downgrowth of pocket epithelium when inspected during week 1. This difference had disappeared by week 3. The group that underwent three laser treatments was no different from the control group when inspected in week 3, but by week 5 exhibited better bone regeneration and reduced downgrowth of epithelium in the pocket. Some stimulation of fibroblasts could be established.

Kim [203] studied the effects of GaAs laser treatment on experimentally produced parodontitis in dogs. The experiment consisted of four groups: 1. An experimental parodontitis group treated with a laser; 2. A control group with experimentally produced parodontitis, not treated with a laser; 3. An experimental parodontitis group on which a flap operation was performed and laser treatment was administered; and 4, as 3, but without laser treatment. Laser groups 1 and 3 received laser treatment on five consecutive days. The histopathological findings were: reduced pseudoepitheliomatous proliferation and a reduced degree of inflammation could be observed in group 1. This group also exhibited increased formation of periodontal ligaments, and the infiltration of newly formed collagen could be observed. Group 3 exhibited a reduced degree of inflammation and osteoclast activity, further capillary proliferation, and reduced pseudoepitheliomatous proliferation. By MT coloration, newly formed collagen in periodontal ligaments and alveolar bone was also observed in group 3.

cytokines and through cellular migration to improve the healing process. Mast cells play an important role in the inflammatory process. In a study by Silveira [1907] twenty patients with gingival enlargement indicated for gingivectomy were selected. Gingival fragments were obtained from each patient and divided into three different groups before surgery. One fragment was removed without any irradiation. The two others were submitted to punctual irradiation with an energy density of 8 J/cm^2 at an output power of 50 mW at 36 Hz for 36 sec before gingivectomy. Nondegranulated and degranulated mast cells were counted in five areas of the gingival fragment connective tissue. Both red and infrared radiation promoted a significant increase in mast cell degranulation compared to controls; however, no statistically significant differences were observed between the irradiated groups.

Animal studies

Kami [67] has studied how GaAlAs laser light affects flaps, and observed that the frequency of success, measured in area, was greater in the LPT group than in the control group. Microvascular flow was greater in the LPT group. Hypovascularised zones, with reactive surrounding vasodilatation, could be seen in the laser probe's contact zones, observed one hour after the irradiation. This effect disappeared after 48 hours, although a greater occurrence of blood vessels could be seen in the irradiated flaps.

Kubota [14] performed a similar experiment in which he treated a group of animals with LED light of the same dosage and wavelength as the LPT group. The LPT group exhibited 45% better vascularisation of the flap than the LED and control groups when measured with fluorescent angiography. More flaps survived in the LPT group than in the other two groups. The failure of LED may be dose-dependent. The use of LED, by the way, is controversial, but LEDs are not totally ineffective

Yoo [288] reports effects on musculoskeletal pain using polarised LED light at 1800 mW. Such high power led to first and second degree burns, however.

Kami's and Kubota's experiments were performed with a GaAlAs laser. Kubota also used GaAlAs laser in a clinical study together with Yasuda [287] and Ohshiro involving patients where musculo-cutaneous flaps were indicated following surgery related to circulatory disorders. There was a significant rise in blood flow and volume following LPT.

Kubota [479] has also checked flap survival and microcirculation using the laser speckle method. 4 J was given at the centre of the flap. After five days, the survival area of the laser diode-irradiated flaps was greater than in the control group. A noticeable improvement in microcirculation was observed following LPT.

Amir [480] used HeNe laser for the same kind of study on rats. The treated animals healed faster and the flaps showed tremendous capillary and fibroblast proliferation.

(bFGF), insulin-like growth factor-1 (IGF-1), and receptor of IGF-1 (IGFBP3) from human gingival fibroblasts (HGF). The number of all samples in the study were 30, and the samples were randomly divided into three equal groups; In the first group (single dose group), HGF were irradiated with laser energy of 685 nm, for 140 s, 2 J/cm^2 once, and in the second group, energy at the same dose was applied for two consecutive days (double dose group). The third group served as non-irradiated control group. Proliferation, viability, and bFGF, IGF-1, IGFBP3 analysis of control and irradiated cultures were compared with each other. Both of the irradiated groups revealed higher proliferation and viability in comparison to the control group. Comparison of the single-dose group with the control group revealed statistically significant increases in bFGF and IGF-1 but IGFBP3 increased insignificantly. When the double dose group was compared with the control group, significant increases were determined in all of the parameters. In the comparison of the differences between the two irradiated groups (one dose and two doses), none of the parameters displayed any statistically significant difference. In both of the laser groups, LPT increased the cell proliferation and cell viability. The results of this study showed that LPT increased the proliferation of HGF cells and release of bFGF, IGF-1, and IGFBP3 from these cells. LPT may play an important role in periodontal wound healing and regeneration by enhancing the production of the growth factors.

Porreau-Schneider [37] carried out an in vitro study of the effect of HeNe laser light on human fibroblasts, and found that the laser energy caused the fibroblasts to turn into myofibroblasts. Biopsies of gingiva were taken in conjunction with the removal of wisdom teeth in order to examine the clinical effect. After 48 hours, myofibroblasts could be found in the laser-treated biopsies, while the contralateral biopsies showed active or dormant fibroblasts. These findings have been confirmed by Rigau [415].

Smoking is a considerable risk factor in periodontal disease. The aim of the study by Fujimaki [1543] was to examine the effects of LPT on the production of reactive oxygen (ROS) species by human neutrophils. The laser device used was the infrared diode laser of 830 nm continuous wave (150 mW/cm^2). After irradiation, ROS production by neutrophils was measured using luminol-dependent chemiluminescence (LmCL) and expression of CD11b and CD16 on neutrophil surface was measured by flow cytometry. The LmCL response of neutrophils was reduced by laser irradiation at 60 min prior to the stimulation with opsonized zymosan and calcium ionophore. The attenuating effect of LPT was larger in neutrophils of smokers than non-smokers, while the amount of produced ROS was larger in neutrophils of smokers. Expression of CD11b and CD16 on neutrophil surface was not affected by LPT. Attenuation of ROS production by neutrophils may play a role in the effects of LPT in the treatment of inflammatory tissues. There is a possible usage of LPT to improve wound healing in smokers.

In periodontal tissue, mast cells may influence either the destructive events or the defense mechanism against periodontal disease via secretion of

shorten the duration of anaesthesia, thus reducing the risk of bite wounds in the lip, tongue, and cheek.

3. Before drilling takes place, 4-6 J at the tooth neck and the same amount of energy over the projection of the apex of a decidious tooth will in many cases produce complete anesthesia.

4. Trauma to the lips and front teeth is common in children. 3-4 J over a bleeding and swollen lip will reduce swelling and pain and allow dental treatment on the following day. 1-2 J around mobile teeth will improve healing and facilitate normal chewing.

5. 0.5-2 J as an additional treatment in pulp capping will improve the outcome of the treatment. Irradiate the exposed pulpal area before applying the capping agent. The same dose is given for pulpectomies.

5.3.26 Periodontics

A reduction of the inflammatory process has been demonstrated in many studies and makes LPT an excellent adjuvant treatment modality to conventional pepriodontal therapy. Good oral hygien after SRP is mandatory for good results, but the addition of the laser will not only reduce the inflammatory process but also lead to less postoperative pain and oedema.

According to some reports [202, 203], it is possible to reduce epithelial down-growth after flap operations. Laser treatment administered only at the time of the operation relieves postoperative discomfort and improves tensile strength after suturing. To achieve positive effects, repeated treatment is required. In addition to treatment of the operation area, each tooth neck can be treated with 2-3 J. This reduces postoperative sensitivity in the root surfaces. When the periodontal dressing is removed, the patient's root surfaces will be less sensitive (supplementary treatment can be administered after a check-up), and the patient will be able to heed the advice given regarding dental hygiene.

Another important aspect in periodontology is the regeneration of bone, also in combination with GTR and bone grafts.

HSV viruses are not uncommon findings in periodontal pockets [1942, 1943] and the well established effect of LPT on HSV1 and 2 may have an influence in this field.

The combination of dyes like TBO and LPT can have dramatic bactericidal effect [827] and this PDT-like therapy has a great potential in periodontics. Dortbudak [1709], Haas [1710] and Shibli [1711] have demonstrated the usefulness of this concept effective for peri-implantitis.

Literature:
In vitro studies

The aim of the study by Saygun [1842] was to determine whether laser irradiation can enhance the release of basic fibroblast growth factor

From the above studies it can be concluded that dosage is essential. Low dosage seems to stimulate orthodontic movement whereas high doses inhibit the speed of movement. As suggested by Goulart, low doses can be used during the orthodontic movement period and higher doses when the movement is finished. The higher bone density stimulated by higher doses would assist the moved tooth to remain in place. Infrared is recommended since it has a greater penetration and often higher power densities but the Chinese studies above indicate that even HeNe can be used.

Further literature: [411, 412, 1223, 1693, 1695, 1713]

5.3.23 Pain
(See chapter 4.1.42 "Pain" on page 293)

5.3.24 Mild dental pain
It is a part of the dentist's everyday work to cause patients mild forms of pain, which we dentists tend to think of as a trifling matter. It may be caused by wedging, depuration, intraligamental anaesthesia, proximal polishing, etc. This type of "petty pain" is so common and so undramatic that dentists (and patients to a certain extent) take it for granted as nothing to worry about. However, we believe this to be an erroneous point of view, stemming from the time when we did not have the facilities to prevent pain that we have today. We have gone from amalgam to ceramic laminates, so we should be able to improve quality to the same extent when it comes to dealing with pain. Patients may have resigned themselves to accepting these milder forms of pain, but don't imagine that they can't do without it! Rounding off routine treatment with 2-3 J of LPT can reduce or eliminate mild pain. The patient will experience this as improved quality of treatment, and the dentist will certainly receive many good references. Assisting staff can perform the treatment itself.

5.3.25 Paediatric dental treatment
Treating children with a therapeutic laser is no different from treating adults. However, a non-traumatic introduction to dentistry is very important, and will save future chair time and patient anxiety. To a child, a laser is not a threat; it's "cool", an attractive tool. Some suggested therapeutic uses are listed below:

1. The eruption of deciduous as well as permanent teeth is sometimes painful. A few joules over the painful area will alleviate the problem and avoid analgesics. Irradiating the lymph nodes in the area is recommended [915].

2. 2 J at the injection site has a brief anaesthetic effect in the mucosa, permitting an injection without pain if injected slowly with a 30g needle. 2-3 J over the anaesthetised area before dismissing the patient will

J/cm^2, on 4 days of each month. Data of the biometrical progress of both groups were statistically compared. All patients showed significant higher acceleration of the retraction of canines on the side treated with LPT when compared to the control. These findings suggest that LPT accelerates human teeth movement and could therefore considerably shorten the whole treatment duration.

The aim of a study by Youssef [1806] was to evaluate the effect of GaAlAs diode laser (809 nm, 100 mW) on the canine retraction during an orthodontic movement and to assess pain level during this treatment. A group of 15 adult patients with age ranging from 14 to 23 years was included. The treatment plan for these patients included extraction of the upper and lower first premolars because there was not enough space for a complete alignment or presence of biprotrusion. The orthodontic treatment was initiated 14 days after the premolar extraction with a standard 18 slot edgewise brackets. The canine retraction was accomplished by using prefabricated Ricketts springs, in both upper and lower jaws. The right side of the upper and lower jaw was chosen to be irradiated with the laser, whereas the left side was considered the control without laser irradiation. The laser was applied with 0-, 3-, 7-, and 14-day intervals. The retraction spring was reactivated on day 21 for all sides. The amount of canine retraction was measured at this stage with a digital electronic caliper and compared each side of the relative jaw (i.e., upper left canine with upper right canine and lower left canine with lower right canine). The pain level was prompted by a patient questionnaire. The velocity of canine movement was significantly greater in the lased group than in the control group. The pain intensity was also at lower level in the lased group than in the control group throughout the retraction period.

The purpose of a study by Tortamano [2117] was to clinically evaluate the effect of LPT as a method of reducing pain reported by patients after placement of their first orthodontic archwires. The sample comprised 60 orthodontic patients (ages, 12-18 years; mean, 15.9 years). All patients had fixed orthodontic appliances placed in 1 dental arch (maxillary or mandibular), received the first archwire, and were then randomly assigned to the experimental (laser), placebo, or control group. This was a double-blind study. LPT was started in the experimental group immediately after placement of the first archwire. Each tooth received a dose of 2.5 J/cm^2 on each side (buccal and lingual). The placebo group had the laser probe positioned into the mouth at the same areas overlying the dental root and could hear a sound every 10 seconds. The control group had no laser intervention. All patients received a survey to be filled out at home describing their pain during the next 7 days. The patients in the LPT group had lower mean scores for oral pain and intensity of pain on the most painful day. Also, their pain ended sooner. LPT did not affect the start of pain perception or alter the most painful day. There was no significant difference in pain symptomatology in the maxillary or mandibular arches.

nese female with an Angle Class I malocclusion and crowding in the mandible. Treatment consisted of extraction of maxillary and mandibular first premolars and use of the Edgewise technique. A GaAlAs diode laser was used to irradiate an area of 0.5 cm^2 at the labial and lingual gingival papilla between the canines. The time of exposure was 6 minutes for 3 days, carried out between the relevelling and en masse stages of movement. The total energy corresponding to 6 minutes of exposure varied from 1.90 J/cm^2. There was no further evidence of open gingival embrasure space, except at the mandibular central incisor. Further: an improvement in the gingival inflammation caused by a periodontal disease was observed, and periodontal pocket depth was maintained. These results suggest that laser irradiation may inhibit the incidence of open gingival embrasure space after orthodontic treatment.

A study by Rattanayatikul [1662] was a double blind, randomized placebo/control matched pairs clinical trial to test the efficacy of GaAlAs LPT on 12 young adult patients who required retraction of maxillary canines into first premolar extraction spaces using tension coil springs with fixed edgewise appliance. Laser was applied on the mucosa buccally, distally and palatally to the canine on the test side and using a sham laser on the placebo side. The laser was a 100 mW GaAlAs laser and the energy per point was 2.3 J, 5 points in total, 25 J/cm^2. Laser was applied immediately after placing the retraction and for the two following days. Dental impressions and casts were made at the commencement of the trial and at the end of the first, second and third months after starting the trial. Measurement of tooth movements was made on each stage model using a stereo microscope. There was no significant difference of means of the canine distal movement between the laser side and the sham side for any time periods

The objective a study by Turhania [1729] was to analyze the effect of a single laser irradiation on pain perception in patients having fixed appliance treatment. 76 patients enrolled in this single-blind study were assigned to 2 groups. The patients in group 1 received a single course of 670 nm, 75 mW for 30 seconds per banded tooth. The patients in group 2 received placebo laser. Pain perception was evaluated at 6, 30, and 54 hours after LPT by self-rating with a standardized questionnaire. Major differences in pain perception were found between the 2 groups. The number of patients reporting pain at 6 hours was significantly lower in G1 (n = 14) than in G2 (n = 29), and the differences persisted at 30 hours (G1, n = 22; G2, n = 33). At 54 hours, no significant differences were seen between the number of patients reporting pain, although the women had a different prevalence between G1 and G2.

Eleven patients were recruited for a 2-month study by Cruz [1432]. One half of the upper arcade was considered control group (CG) and received mechanical activation of the canine teeth every 30 days. The opposite half received the same mechanical activation and was also irradiated with a diode laser emitting light at 780 nm, during 10 seconds at 20 mW, 5 J/

osteoclast precursor cells was detected at an early stage (day 2 and 3) in the irradiation group. In conclusion, these findings suggest that LPT stimulates the velocity of tooth movement via induction of RANK and RANKL.

The objective of the study by Kim [2099] was to investigate the combined effects of Corticision and LPT on the tooth movement rate and paradental remodeling in beagles. The maxillary second premolars (n=24) of 12 beagles were randomly divided into four groups (n=6 per group) based on the treatment modality: group A, only orthodontic force (control); group B, orthodontic force plus Corticision; group C, orthodontic force plus LPT; group D, orthodontic force plus Corticision and LPT. Ratios of second premolar-to-canine movement were greater by 2.23-fold in group B and 2.08-fold in group C, but 0.52-fold lesser in group D than in group A. The peak velocity was observed at an earlier stage of tooth movement in group B but at a later stage in group C during the 8-week treatment period. At week 8, both tartrate-resistant acid phosphatase (TRAP)-positive osteoclasts on the compression side and proliferating cell nuclear antigen (PCNA)-positive osteoblasts on the tension side increased significantly in group C but decreased in group D. Histomorphometric analysis revealed that the mean apposition length of newly formed mineralized bone during the 8 weeks of treatment significantly increased in both group B (2.8-fold) and group C (2.2-fold). In group D, the labeling lines on lamina dura were thin and discontinuous, but intratrabecular remodeling and lamellation were found to be active.

Clinical studies

The effect of LPT on reduction of pain while undergoing orthodontic treatment was examined by Harazaki [81]. The patients were randomly separated into 3 groups: non-treated control group (CG), blind irradiation group (BG), and GaAlAs laser irradiated group (LG). The effect of laser irradiation on reduction in pain was analysed by a questionnaire given to patients who had been wired with an edgewise appliance of a multi-bracket system for orthodontic therapy. Just after application of the initial wire, LG patients were irradiated with the laser from the labial and lingual sites for a total of one minute. A delay in the pain appearance was noted as compared to the other two control groups.

In a study by Lim [464], 39 patients had elastomeric separators placed at the proximal contacts of one premolar in each quadrant to induce orthodontic pain. 830 nm, 30 mW laser light was applied for 15, 30 and 60 seconds and one placebo treatment of 60 seconds with each patient for a period of 5 days. Patients were asked about pain levels after each session. Analysis of the VAS scores showed that pain was less after laser treatment but not statistically significant.

The purpose of the study by Meguro [1660] was to investigate the inhibitory effect of LPT on an incidence of open gingival embrasure space after orthodontic treatment. The patient was a 20-year, 7-month-old Japa-

placed between the first molar and the second premolar for stabilisation purpose. Group I was irradiated with a dosage of 5.25 J/cm^2 on the right side, whereas the left side was used as the control group. Group II was submitted to the same procedure, but was irradiated with a dosage of 35.0 J/cm^2. Irradiations were done every 7 days, for a total of nine irradiations. The orthodontic space was measured every 21 days. The 5.25 J/cm^2 dosage accelerated orthodontic movement during the first observation period, from 0 to 21 days, whereas the 35.0 J/cm^2 dosage retarded the orthodontic movement in the treated group when compared with the control group, during both the first and second observation periods, from 0 to 42 days. The results suggest that LPT may accelerate orthodontic movement at a dosage of 5.25 J/cm^2, whereas a higher dosage, 35.0 J/cm^2, may retard it.

However, the experimental study by Seifi [1671] has come to the opposite conclusion. The study was conducted on 18 male albino rabbits divided into three equal groups: Laser 1 (5 mW peak power, 850 nm wavelength, 3 minutes per session, pulsed, pulse repetition rate of 3000 Hz, duration of pulse 100 nsec, total energy in experiment 2.43 J) and Laser 2 (10 mW, continuous, wavelength 630 nm, 5 minutes per session, total energy in experiment 27 J), and a non irradiated group. The first mandibular molars, in all groups were under a four ounce tension using NiTi-Closed coil springs. The control group was not irradiated but the laser groups were irradiated for nine days. After sixteen days, following the termination of therapeutic regime; samples were sacrificed. The distance between the distal surface of the first molar and the mesial surface of the second molar was measured with 0.05 mm accuracy. The mean orthodontic tooth movements of the first mandibular molars were 1.7±0.16 mm in control group, 0.69±0.16 mm in Laser 1 group and 0.86±0.13 mm in Laser 2 group. These results indicate that the orthodontic movement velocity can be modulated with the energy density or the total energy applied.

The receptor activator of the nuclear factor-kB (RANK) / RANK ligand (RANKL)/osteoprotegerin (OPG) system is essential and sufficient for osteoclastogenesis. A study by Fujita [1917] was designed to examine the effects of LPT on expressions of RANK, RANKL, and OPG during experimental tooth movement. To induce experimental tooth movement in rats, 10 g of orthodontic force was applied to the molars. Next, a GaAlAs laser was used to irradiate the area around the moved tooth and the amount of tooth movement was measured for 7 days. Immunohistochemical staining with RANK, RANKL, and OPG were performed. Real time PCR was also performed to elucidate the expression of RANK in irradiated rat osteoclast precursor cells in vitro. In the irradiation group, the amount of tooth movement was significantly greater than in the non-irradiation group by the end of the experimental period. Cells that showed positive immunoreactions to the primary antibodies of RANKL and RANK were significantly increased in the irradiation group on day 2 and 3, compared with the non-irradiation group. In contrast, the expression of OPG was not changed. Further, RANK expression in

histological observation under a light microscope, the osteoclasts and osteoblasts on the experimental side remained more active than those of the control side. There is significant difference in amount of osteoclasts between the experimental and the control sides, 3, 5 or 7 days after the treatment.

The purpose of yet another study by Sun [1780] was to investigate the effect of HeNe irradiation on the expression of transforming growth factor beta1 (TGF-beta1) during experimental tooth movement in rabbits. Thirty-five rabbits were used. The animals were randomly divided into 7 groups equally: normal group and experimental (1, 3, 5, 7, 14, 21 days) groups, 5 rabbits in each group. An orthodontic appliance, consisting of a coil spring was ligated to the bilateral first maxillary molar and connected to an orthodontic wire ligated onto the incisors, and exerting a force of approximately 80 g. The left side was used as control, and the right side was designed as irradiated side. The animals from each group were sacrificed at the time discontinued. The histological sections were proceeded with immunohistochemical staining of TGF-beta1. Then it was analyzed by Computer Image Analyzing System and statistically processed. The expression of TGF-beta1 was demonstrated in the area of tension and pressure of periodontium tissue in both of the irradiated and control sides. The TGF-beta1 staining in the pressure area of the irradiated side decreased significantly at 1 day compared with the control side. TGF-beta1 staining increased significantly at 3 to 5 days in the pressure area. But in the tension area of the irradiated side, TGF-beta1 staining was significantly increased at 3 to 7 days. The peak value of the area of tension and pressure both appeared at the same time of the 5th day.

The purpose of the study by Zhu [1661] was to investigate the effects of LPT on basic fibroblast growth factors (bFGF) expression in periodontal tissue during tooth movement. 18 white rabbits were randomly divided into 6 groups with 3 rabbits in each group, including groups of 1, 3, 5, 7, 14 and 21 days. Under an anesthesia condition by 2% pentobarbital sodium, stainless coil springs were fixed between the first maxillary molar and the incisor producing the force of 80 g. The right side of maxilla was considered as the experimental group under the irradiation of laser, with the left side as the control groups. The expression of bFGF was investigated half-quantitatively through immunohistochemical analysis. The expression of bFGF in periodontal tissue with irradiation of laser was higher than the control side. There were significant differences among the 5, 7, and 14 day groups. In the tension area of the experimental side, the expression of bFGF in the osteoblastic surface of alveolar bone was characteristically greater than that of the control side. Thus, LPT promotes the expression of bFGF in the periodontal tissue and alveolar bone remodelling.

The aim of a study by Goulart [1689] was to evaluate, through a double-blind study, the effect of GaAlAs laser irradiation on the speed of orthodontic movement in canine premolars. Eighteen dogs were divided into two groups, and their third molars were extracted. An orthodontic device was

C. In conclusion, the irradiation may directly promote osteoblast proliferation and differentiation, and indirectly inhibit osteoclast differentiation, by downregulating the RANKL:OPG mRNA ratio in osteoblasts.

Animal studies

Saito [569] expanded the midpalatal suture in rats. A 100 mW GaAlAs laser was used to influence bone regeneration. Irradiation during the two first postoperative days was effective, showing an acceleration at 1.2 to 1.4-fold as compared to the control group. Irradiation in the late period (days 4 to 6) was not effective, nor one single irradiation.

Kawasaki [917] applied 10 g of orthodontic force to rat molars to cause experimental tooth movement. Irradiation was performed daily for ten days, 54 J per session. Increased osteoclast activity was observed on the pressure side in the laser group as well as increased rate of cellular proliferation on the tension side. Tooth movement was increased 1.3-fold.

Sudoh [695] applied a load of 100 g to maxillary canines in 15 cats. GaAlAs laser irradiation was performed daily over the area for two weeks. At day 7 and 14 the moving distance was measured and the animals sacrificed for histological examination. At two weeks the moving distance was larger in the laser group than in the control group. In the laser group a prominent new bone deposition with marked osteoblastic activity was seen on the alveolar bone on the tension side. On the compressed side, bone resorption with an increased number of tartrate resistant acid phosphatase-positive osteoclasts took place at the inner aspect of the alveolar bone adjacent to the hyalinized zone. Morphometric analysis demonstrated that the area of both newly formed bone and bone cavity and the number of TRAcP-positive osteoclasts were significantly larger in the irradiated area as compared to control.

The aim of a study by Sun [1779] was to investigate effects of LPT on experimental tooth movement and the remodeling of alveolar bone in rabbits. A total of 42 white rabbits were chosen and randomized into one control group and six experimental groups, with 6 rabbits in each group. After anesthesia orthodontic appliances consisting of a coil spring connected bilaterally the upper first molar with the upper incisor by using a ligature wire. The force exerted at the time of insertion was approximately 80 g. The left side served as the control side, and the right side was the experimental side treated by receiving irradiation of laser. The treatment periods of different groups lasted separately for 1, 3, 5, 7, 14, 21 days respectively. The displacement extent of teeth was measured by employing the computer image analyzing system. The results were analyzed statistically. Through HE staining, the histomorphological character of tissue around first molar was also investigated, and numbers of osteoclasts were counted. The displacement extent of teeth on the experimental side, which was irradiated by laser, was more obvious than that of the normal control side. The difference was statistically significant 1, 3, 14, 21 days after the beginning of the treatment. Through

GaAs laser multiprobe extraorally, at least 12 J for pain and oedema (in particular). The good results observed by the authors and other clinicians remain to be verified scientifically. The right parameters for GaAlAs laser on this indication are not yet known.
More information in 5.3.8
Further literature: [773, 1180]

5.3.22 Orthodontics

After the insertion of any orthodontic apparatus, a few days of noticeable pain follow in the areas subjected to stress. Lasers used directly after treatment delay the onset of pain and reduce its intensity. LPT also appears to be able to increase the speed of tooth movement and the bony remodeling. Most studies indicate a faster process of tooth movement but since one paper has come to the opposite conclusion, the effect of laser here is, as always, dose dependent.

Literature:
In vitro studies

Shimizu [370, 1012] studied the effect of GaAlAs laser light on prostaglandin E2 and interleukin-1β production in stretched human periodontal ligament (PDL) cells in vitro at varying intervals and doses. The PDL cells showed a marked elevation of prostaglandin and interleukin in response to mechanical stretching. PGE2 production was significantly inhibited by LPT in a dose-dependent manner. IL-1β production was also reduced, but only partially under these conditions. It is therefore possible to propose a mechanism whereby pain relief and bone resorption activity could be modulated through LPT.

Ozawa [522] suggests that LPT may reduce collagen breakdown around the PDL, associated with traumatic occlusion. Stretched healthy human PDL cells were irradiated with GaAlAs laser light. Plasminogen activator (PA) activity was elevated in cells subjected to stretching. LPT reduced this activity in a dose-dependent manner, between 55% and 86%.

A study by Xu [1915] aimed to investigate the effect of 650 nm, 2 mW irradiation on mRNA expression of receptor activator of NF-kappaB ligand (RANKL) and osteoprotegerin (OPG) in rat calvarial cells. Cultured cells were treated with LIPL irradiation of 1.14 J/cm^2 (group A) or 2.28 J/cm^2 (group B), and non-irradiated cells (group C) were used as controls. The changes in cell numbers, alkaline phosphatase (ALP) activity, RANKL, and OPG mRNA expression in the three study groups was determined using MTT, UV/VIS spectrophotometry, and RT-PCR analyses. The cell numbers in groups A and B increased significantly (7.52% and 8.80%, respectively), as did ALP activity (71.95% and 88.20%, respectively), compared with group C. RANKL and OPG mRNA expression in group A were 51.06% lower and 3.35 times higher, respectively, than those seen in the controls and the RANKL:OPG mRNA ratio in group A was 81.82% lower than that in group

few minutes, although the influence on the healing process could not be firmly established. Extractions of an identical number of teeth were performed on 12 patients at the same treatment session in two separate quadrants. One quadrant was treated with a laser every day for seven days, while the other served as a control. Better healing was observed in eight cases treated with laser, and in the other four the healing was as advanced as in the control group. Pain was estimated as lower on the laser-treated side, and no alveolitis occurred in the treatment quadrants. No difference in swelling could be observed.

Clokie [155] studied the effects of HeNe laser treatment in conjunction with the extirpation of impacted teeth. Patients with double sets of similarly impacted teeth were given HeNe laser light (5.4 mW at fibre tip, total dose approx. 1 J) on one side after the operation, and placebo "laser" on the other. Postoperative pain on the day of the operation and the day after was lower in the laser group.

Taube [163] selected symmetrically impacted wisdom teeth in 17 patients. Both the wisdom teeth in the lower jaw were surgically removed on the same occasion and the effects on postoperative pain and swelling were studied. Irradiation was carried out during the operation and one day after the operation. The total dosage was less than 2×0.3 J of HeNe laser light. No effect on pain or swelling was observed.

Pinheiro [635] treated 172 patients with 633, 670 or 830 nm laser light. The diagnoses were TMJ pain, trigeminal neuralgia, muscular pain, aphthae and tooth hypersensitivity. 127 patients became asymptomatic, 25 improved considerably and 20 did not improve.

LPT in conjunction with the removal of wisdom teeth is a well studied dental LPT indication. It is also one of fields where the reports are least favourable. Interestingly, the two HeNe reports (Carillo, Clokie) found effects on pain and trismus. This is a bit surprising. Trismus would be better treated with GaAlAs or GaAs [293]. Using HeNe laser (Carrillo) in the alveolus, on the base of the flap, and on the suture line is recommended for faster and better healing of the superficial wound. However, removing an impacted wisdom tooth is a major trauma, as is obvious when we see the patient the day after the operation! Such trauma requires high doses, since the tissues are filled with blood and therefore less transparent. The pain after elevating, incising, burring in the bone, etc., is considerable, and high doses should be expected.

Núñez [1475] found that 670 nm laser, 3 J/cm² was more effective than TENS for trismus in TMD patients.

Fernando [216] applied 4 J from an IR laser directly into the extraction socket and found no positive effect on pain or swelling.

Røynesdal [93] used 6 J GaAlAs laser pre- and postoperatively distributed over the operation area, but found no effect on swelling and pain.

The authors of this book use HeNe laser over the sutures (tensile strength) and in the alveolus (osteoblastic stimulation), about 0.5 J/cm², then

5.3.18 Nausea

A common complication in dentistry is nausea and gagging. Some patients are very sensitive to operations behind the premolars and taking impressions may be very difficult. In these cases, the laser can be applied to the sulcus mento-labialis in the contact mode. 2-3 J will reduce nausea in a great number of cases. If not successful, the acupuncture point P6 on the wrist can be used. The effect will arise a couple of minutes post irradiation.

Literature: [892]

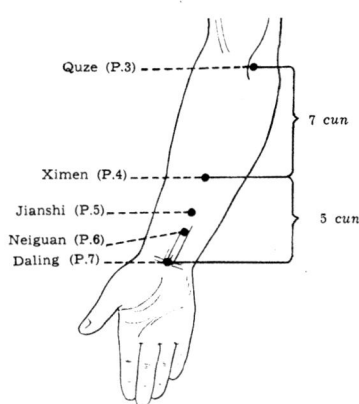

Figure 5.9   Location of the P6 point

5.3.19 Nerve injury

Damaged nerves heal slowly. Feared complications in odontology are damage to n. alveolaris inferior and n. lingualis. It is not uncommon for a patient to be afflicted by lengthy or permanent paraesthesia as a result of oral surgery. General practice dentists can also cause paraesthesia through trauma from hypodermic needles, the use of elevator of the lingual side of the lower jaw, and other causes. LPT is the only available treatment in these cases. An indication of the effects of LPT is the patient's unspecified sense of emerging anxiety in the area treated with laser. Dentists have carried out a great deal of successful research in this field.

(See chapter 4.1.39 "Nerve regeneration and function" on page 272)

5.3.20 Oedema

(See chapter 4.1.40 "Oedema" on page 285)

5.3.21 Oral surgery

The term "oral surgery" is so broad that the references below could easily be put under entirely different headings, such as oedema or pain. However, we describe some studies within the field of oral surgery under this heading. In our experience, HeNe laser is not ideal in oral surgery, bearing in mind its relatively shallow penetration and the low level of mW that HeNe lasers generally emit.

Literature:

Porteder [167] describes the results of treating a number of indications with HeNe laser light. When herpes simplex was treated in its early stage, no sores appeared. Aphthae were rendered much less painful after a

5.3.16 Lip wounds

Angular cheilitis caused by a low vertical dimension can be successfully treated with LPT but will reappear if the fundamental cause is not dealt with. Wounds on lips usually heal quickly with LPT in cases of trauma and mechanical/chemical irritation. Lip fissures are well worth treating. A typical symptom is that they begin to bleed after having been very dry - this is the beginning of the healing process. HeNe or small doses of GaAlAs laser are recommended.

Literature: [1201]

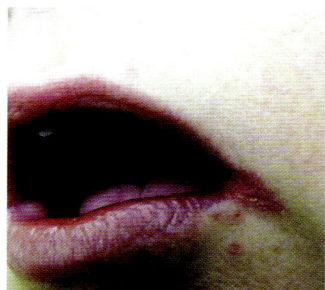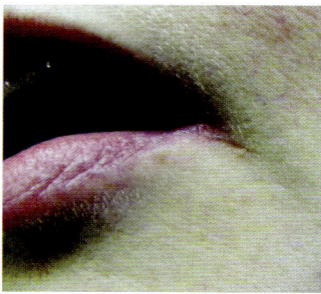

Figure 5.8 Non-healing angular chielitis after one week of daily red laser therapy

5.3.17 Mucositis

(See chapter 4.1.9 "Cancer" on page 190.)

Considering bone area within the threads, no significant difference was found for treatment, e.g., with or without laser. In conclusion, LPT did not affect the area of bone formed within the threads, but it may improve BIC in rabbit tibiae.
Further literature: [91, 121, 213, 583, 931, 1218, 1219, 1607, 1608]

5.3.13 Jaw fractures

Fractures of the facial skeleton are treated locally over the fracture itself every other day for one to two weeks.

Literature:

Kats [112] studied the effects of a HeNe laser (30-480 mJ/cm^2) on fractures of the jaw. In the trial group of 19 patients, quicker healing and a moderation of the inflammatory process were observed as compared with the control group of 27 patients.

Glinkowski [420] used GaAlAs, 830 nm and GaAs, 904 nm lasers in a study of standardised tibial fractures in mice. Bone radiographs were studied using a laser densitometer. Both wavelengths accelerated healing, but 904 nm was more successful.

Further literature: [108, 944] (See chapter 4.1.8 "Bone and cartilage regeneration" on page 174)

5.3.14 Leukoplakia

This condition does not always produce subjective symptoms. If the patient does have leukoplakia symptoms, they can be alleviated with LPT. Whether LPT can actually cure the condition has not been reported, but a stimulation of the immune system in the area affected is worth trying.

Literature: [209]

5.3.15 Lingua geographica (glossitis)

This condition is sometimes free of symptoms, sometimes associated with varying types of subjective discomfort. 3-4 J LPT over 5-6 points relieves the symptoms. Its effect on long-term healing is not clear, but there is no effective treatment of any other kind that can heal this condition.

Literature:

Mezawa [114] studied the effects of GaAlAs laser light on nociceptors in cat tongues. A decrease in nociceptor activity could be demonstrated after one minute's irradiation. No further change was noted in the 5-10 minute interval, and the authors drew the conclusion that a plateau was reached after five minutes.

Hubacek [1036] reports successful treatment of glossodynia using GaAlAs laser, 4-6 J/cm^2, 4-10 sessions.

phorus on the implant test surface after the tensile test. The mean tensile forces, measured in Newton, of the irradiated implants and controls were 14.35 (SD+/-4.98) and 10.27 (SD+/-4.38), respectively, suggesting a gain in functional attachment at 8 weeks following laser. The histomorphometrical evaluation suggested that the irradiated group had more bone-to-implant contact than the controls. The weight percentages of calcium and phosphorus were significantly higher in the irradiated group when compared to the controls, suggesting that bone maturation processed faster in irradiated bone.

In yet another study by Khadra [1439] the effect of LPT on attachment and proliferation of human gingival fibroblasts (HGF) cultured on titanium implant material. HGF were exposed to gallium aluminum arsenide diode laser at dosages of 1.5 or 3 J/cm and then cultured on commercially pure titanium discs. Cell profile areas were measured after 1, 3 and 24 h, using scanning electron microscopy and an automatic image analyzer. The results were expressed as percentage of attachment. In order to investigate the effect of LPT on cellular growth after 8 and 10 days, HGF were cultured on titanium discs for 24 h and then exposed to laser irradiation on 3 consecutive days. Colony-forming efficiency (CFE) and clonal growth rates (CGR) were measured. Cell viability was determined by Hoechst and prodidium iodide staining. Non-lased cultures served as controls. Morphologically, the cells spread well on all titanium surfaces, indicating good attachment by both irradiated and non-irradiated cells. Fibroblasts exposed to laser irradiation had significantly higher percentages of cell attachment than the non-exposed cells. CFE and CGR were also enhanced for the irradiated cells. Cell viability was high in the irradiated and control groups, without significant differences.

In the paper by Kim [1844] the author concludes: "From the above results, the expression of OPG, RANKL, and RANK during the osseointegration of the dental titanium implant was observed within bone tissue. The application of the LPT influenced the expression of OPG, RANKL, and RANK, and resulted in the expansion of metabolic bone activity and increased the activity of bone tissue cells."

A study by Pereira [2074] aimed to histometrically evaluate the influence of LPT treatment on bone healing around titanium implants placed in rabbit tibiae. Each tibia of 12 adult rabbits received a 3.3 x 6-mm titanium implant. The implants placed in the right tibiae were irradiated with a GaAlAs laser every 48 hours for 14 days postoperatively, and the left tibiae were not irradiated. After 3 or 6 weeks, the animals were sacrificed (six animals per period), and nondecalcified sections were obtained and analyzed for bone-to-implant contact (BIC) and bone area within the implant threads. BIC was significantly increased in the laser-treated group at both 3 weeks and 6 weeks. BIC did not increase significantly with time (3 weeks versus 6 weeks). Conversely, bone area within the threads was significantly increased with time (3 weeks versus 6 weeks), regardless of whether the laser was used.

Through near-infrared Raman spectroscopy (NIRS), Lopes [1444] studied the incorporation of hydroxyapatite of calcium (CHA) on the healing bone around dental implants submitted or not to low-level LPT. Fourteen rabbits received a titanium implant on the tibia; eight of them were irradiated with 830 nm laser (seven sessions at 48-h intervals, 21.5 J/cm^2 per session, 10 mW, 85 J/cm^2 treatment dose), and six acted as control. The animals were sacrificed at 15, 30, and 45 days after surgery. Specimens were routinely prepared for Raman spectroscopy. Twelve readings were taken on the bone around the implant. The results showed significant differences in the concentration of CHA on irradiated and control specimens at both 30 and 45 days after surgery.

The aim of the study by Khadra [1438] was to investigate the effect of LPT with GaAlAs on titanium implant healing and attachment in bone. This study was performed as an animal trial of 8 weeks duration with a blinded, placebo-controlled design. Two coin-shaped titanium implants with a diameter of 6.25 mm and a height of 1.95 mm were implanted into cortical bone in each proximal tibia of twelve New Zealand white female rabbits (n=48). The animals were randomly divided into irradiated and control groups. The LPT was used immediately after surgery and carried out daily for 10 consecutive days. The animals were killed after 8 weeks of healing. The mechanical strength of the attachment between the bone and 44 titanium implants was evaluated using a tensile pullout test. Histomorphometrical analysis of the four implants left in place from four rabbits was then performed. Energy-dispersive X-ray microanalysis was applied for analyses of calcium and phosphorus on the implant test surface after the tensile test. The mean tensile forces, measured in Newton, of the irradiated implants and controls were 14.35 and 10.27, respectively, suggesting a gain in functional attachment at 8 weeks following. The histomorphometrical evaluation suggested that the irradiated group had more bone-to-implant contact than the controls. The weight percentages of calcium and phosphorus were significantly higher in the irradiated group when compared to the controls, suggesting that bone maturation processed faster in irradiated bone.

The aim of another study by Khadra [1610] was to investigate the effect of LPT with GaAlAs on titanium implant healing and attachment in bone. This study was performed as an animal trial of 8 weeks duration with a blinded, placebo-controlled design. Two coin-shaped titanium implants with a diameter of 6.25 mm and a height of 1.95 mm were implanted into cortical bone in each proximal tibia of twelve New Zealand rabbits (n=48). The animals were randomly divided into irradiated and control groups. The laser was used immediately after surgery and carried out daily for 10 consecutive days. The animals were killed after 8 weeks of healing. The mechanical strength of the attachment between the bone and 44 titanium implants was evaluated using a tensile pullout test. Histomorphometrical analysis of the four implants left in place from four rabbits was then performed. Energy-dispersive X-ray microanalysis was applied for analyses of calcium and phos-

contact between the implant and bone with strong osteoblast activity and new formation of bone. A comparison of the calcium content of the bone around the implant showed a considerable difference between the experimental and control groups.

Guzardella [1305] placed cylindrical hydroxyapatite implants in both distal femurs of 12 rabbits. From postoperative day 1 and for 5 consecutive days, the left femurs of all rabbits were submitted to LPT of the following parameters: 830 nm, 1000 mW, 300 J/cm^2, 300 Hz, 10 minutes. The right femurs were sham irradiated. 3 and 6 weeks after implantation, histomorphometric and microhardness measurements were taken. A higher affinity index was observed at the HA-bone interface in the laser group at 3 and 6 weeks; a significant difference in bone microhardness was seen in the laser group as compared to the sham group.

Kusakari [121] studied the effects of GaAlAs 30 mW on implants in the lower jaws of dogs. The following are some of the findings: the collagen and RNA content of the gum reached its peak on the fifth day; no change in DNA content was observed; and the number of cell elements in the bone marrow had risen by day 3. By day 7, the amount of new-formed bone around the operation defect was greater on the side treated with laser than on the control side. LPT increased DNA synthesis in the osteoblasts without affecting morphology. LPT also increased the alkaline phosphate activity.

In an adult dog experiment by Monteiro Martins [970], 830 nm, 4.8 J/cm^2 was given around the implants three times a week for two weeks. SEM analysis 45 and 60 days after surgery showed better osseointegration with more compact and organised cancellous bone, with increased vascularisation in the irradiated group. These characteristics were more pronounced in the superior and median third of the implants.

Pinheiro [1128] made implants in five dogs with another five serving as control. The animals were sacrificed after 45 and 60 days. Transcutaneous irradiation was performed with a 40 mW, 830 nm laser, 4.8 J/cm^2, total energy 1.2 J per point. The specimens were analysed through SEM. The irradiated specimens showed better bone healing.

The effects of 680 and 830 nm lasers on osseointegration were studied by Blay [1220]. 30 adult rats were divided into three groups; two laser groups and one control. The rats in the two laser groups had pure titanium Frialit-2 implants implanted into each proximal metaphysis of their respective tibias, inserted with a 40 Ncm torque. The initial stability was monitored by means of a resonance frequency analyser. Ten irradiations were performed, 48 hours apart, 4 J/cm^2 on two points, starting immediately after surgery. Resonance frequency analysis indicated a significant difference between frequency values at 3 and 6 weeks, as compared to control. At 6 weeks the removal torque in the laser groups was much higher than in the control group.

ment of dentinal hypersensitivity. A total of 164 teeth from 30 patients with clinical diagnoses of dentinal hypersensitivity were selected for this randomized, placebo-controlled, double-blind clinical study. The teeth were randomized to three groups: GaAlAs laser, oxalate gel, and placebo gel. The treatment sessions were performed at 7 d intervals for four consecutive weeks. The degree of sensitivity in response to an air blast and tactile stimuli was assessed according to a visual analogue scale at baseline, immediately after the fourth application, and then 3 months after the fourth application. The reductions in dentinal hypersensitivity from baseline at the two follow-up assessments were evaluated as the main outcome. In both the active and control groups, there were statistically significant reductions in dentinal hypersensitivity immediately after and 3 months after the treatments, when compared with the hypersensitivity at baseline. No significant differences among the three groups could be detected in their efficacy at either the immediate or 3 month evaluations irrespective of the stimulus.

Further literature: [66, 1332]

5.3.12 Implantology

LPT can achieve good results on postoperative swelling and pain and shorten the healing period of an oral surgical wound [1151], as in implant work. There are also studies indicating that the integration of titanium implants is accelerated. "Early loading" of dental implants has been the new trend in implantology and preliminary studies indicate the potential of LPT here. (See chapter 4.1.8 "Bone and cartilage regeneration" on page 174)

Literature:

The aim of the study by Dortbudak [1440] was to determine the effect of continuous wave diode laser irradiation on osteoblasts derived mesenchymal cells. Three groups of 10 cultures each were irradiated 3 times (days 3, 5, 7) with a pulsed diode soft laser with a wavelength of 690 nm for 60 s. Another 3 groups of 10 cultures each were used as control groups. A newly developed method employing the fluorescent antibiotic tetracycline was used to compare bone growth on these culture substrates after a period of 8, 12 and 16 days, respectively. It was found that all lased cultures demonstrated significantly more fluorescent bone deposits than the non-lased cultures. The difference was significant in the cultures, examined after 16 days. Hence it is concluded that irradiation with a pulsed diode soft laser has a biostimulating effect on osteoblasts in vitro, which might be used in osseointegration of dental implants.

Asanami [91] placed hydroxyapatite implants in the lower jaws of rabbits. The laser group was treated with a HeNe laser (6 mW, 10 minutes). After three weeks, both groups were studied histologically. A macroscopically visible extrusion had arisen in the control group, while no such extrusion could be observed in the experimental group. Very little granulation tissue was observed in the experimental group. There was evidence of direct

cervical dentine hypersensitivity. Twelve patients, with at least two sensitive teeth were selected. A total of 60 teeth were included in the trial. Prior to desensitizing treatment, dentine hypersensitivity was assessed by a thermal stimulus and patients' response to the examination was considered to be a control. The GaAlAs laser (15 mW, 4 J/cm^2) was irradiated on contact mode and fluoride varnish was applied at cervical region. The efficiency of the treatments was assessed at three examination periods: immediately after first application, 15 and 30 days after the first application. The degree of sensitivity was determined following predefined criteria. Data were submitted to analysis and no statistically significant difference was observed between fluoride varnish and laser. Considering the treatments separately, there was no significant difference for the fluoride varnish at the three examination periods, and for LPT, significant difference was found solely between the values obtained before the treatment and 30 days after the first application. It may be concluded that both treatments may be effective in decreasing cervical dentinal hypersensitivity. Moreover, the low-level GaAlAs laser showed improved results for treating teeth with higher degree of sensitivity.

Rodrigues de Santana [1467] points out that LPT is a good indication for hypersensitivity in patients with amelogenesis imperfecta.

The survey by Mahdavi [1632] was undertaken in a randomized clinical trial. 34 vital teeth scheduled for posterior fixed prosthesis abutment were chosen for the survey. In all stages (temporary, framework, porcelain, primary and permanent cementation laser was used. In the control group the laser was used in the switched off mode. The applied GaAs laser had the following properties: 5 W, 80 Hz, 100 ns, 2 minutes per point. Irradiating over teeth which were sensitive after preparation showed that after the framework stage and onwards, pain decreased and the differences between laser and control group were significant.

The aim of study by Pesevska [2070] was to compare the effectiveness of laser irradiation to traditional topical fluoride treatment for treatment choices of dentinal hypersensitivity following scaling and root planing. The experimental group (15 patients) was treated with low-energy-level diode laser at each site of dentinal hypersensitivity following scaling and root planning. The control group (15 patients) received topical fluoride treatment (protective varnish for desensitization). All the patients were treated at baseline visit, and then at day 2 and 4 after the initial treatment; the pain was subjectively assessed by the patients as strong, medium, medium low, low, or no pain. Total absence of the dental hypersensitivity was reported in 26.66% of the examined group even after the second visit, compared to the control group where complete resolution of the hypersensitivity was not present after the second visit in any of the treated cases. Complete absence of pain was achieved in 86.6% of patients treated with laser and only in 26.6% in the fluoride treated group, after the third visit.

The study by Vieira [2107] evaluated the immediate and 3 month clinical effects of a GaAlAs laser and a 3% potassium oxalate gel for the treat-

Groth [644] treated 25 hypersensitive teeth with GaAlAs laser 790 nm, 30 mW, 7 J per treatment. The irradiation was repeated after 72 hours. Evaluation was performed during a period of 2-4 weeks and the results proved to be significant as compared to control teeth.

In a study by Brugnera [910] 300 human teeth were treated for hypersensitivity. Pulpal vitality was verified using thermal tests, and only reversible processes were treated. HeNe and GaAlAs lasers were used. All teeth received 4 J/session for up to 5 sessions. 79% of the patients were treated in 3 sessions with success; 8.6% were cured in 4 sessions; and 4.3% were successfully treated in 5 sessions, obtaining 92% success in total. In a more recent article [1127] Brugnera reports on the outcome of treating 1102 teeth and 338 patients. 40 mW GaAlAs was mainly used, 25 seconds per point, four points per tooth, total energy per tooth 4 J, dose 50 J/cm^2. A maximum of five treatments were given, but the therapy was always finished when the symptoms were gone. 36.7% of the patients required only one session, 23.14% needed two sessions, 16.1% three sessions, 9.7% four sessions and 5.35% five sessions. 8.71% did not respond.

In another study Brugnera [1127] evaluated the histological reaction of the pulp in rats after LPT. Thirty-two upper molars from albino rats with mechanically exposed occlusal pulps (~1 cm^2) were treated. The parameters of the laser were HeNe 6 mW, beam cross section 1.8 mm^2, and exposure time 240 s, 1.44 J/cm^2, in scanning mode. The animals were divided into four different groups, each with its own control group, and were given weekly applications. The results showed that irradiated animals presented an increased production of dentine and shutting of dentinal tubuli. On the other hand, non-irradiated subjects still showed signs of intense inflammatory reactions and even necrosis for the same experimental times. Irradiated teeth did not show cell degeneration. The irradiation was shown to be efficient in the stimulation of odontoblast cells, producing reparative dentin and closing dentin tubuli.

In the study by Marsilio [1509] 25 patients, with a total number of 106 cases of dentinal hypersensitivity (DH), were treated with GaAlAs LPT. 65% of the teeth were premolars; 14% were incisors and molars; 6.6% were canines. The teeth were irradiated with 3 and 5 J/cm^2 for up to six sessions, with an interval of 72 h between each application, and they were evaluated initially, after each application, and at 15 and 60 days follow-up post-treatment. The treatment was effective in 86 and 88% of the irradiated teeth, respectively, with the minimum and maximum energy recommended by the manufacturer. There was a statistically significant difference between DH and after a follow-up of 60 days for both groups. The difference between the energy maximum and minimum was not significant.

660 nm was found to be more effective than 830 nm in the study by Ladalardo [1295].

The aim of the study by Corona [1536] was to evaluate in vivo the use of GaAlAs laser and sodium fluoride varnish (Duraphat) in the treatment of

The patients are disappointed and some of them have to undergo endodontics. Such postoperative sensations can be eliminated or reduced by using LPT before cementing and filling. If post-operative problems appear, the laser could solve many of them in one or a few sessions. This is indeed much more profitable than free endodontics.

There are a great number of studies in this field. For a literature review, the article by Kimura [1055] is recommended. These studies also confirm the safety of the therapy.

Literature:

Kaihøj [65] treated 84 sensitive tooth necks with a GaAlAs laser. In 17 cases, there was no result, 12 showed some effect, 34 experienced good results, and 21 perfect results. Treatment was administered on days 1, 21, and 90, with a check-up three to six months after the last treatment. No supplementary treatment was undertaken.

Gomi [80] studied the pain-relieving effect of three types of laser in 130 cases of hypersensitive dentine (I) and 120 cases of pain during cementation of inlays (II). In experiment (I), HeNe laser treatment was effective in 71% of the cases in which it was administered once, in 79% of the cases in which it was administered twice, and in 100% of cases treated three times. The total effectiveness in experiment (II) was 71%.

Gerschman [451] studied the effect of 830 nm light on tactile and thermal dental hypersensitivity in a double-blind test. Both parameters responded favourably.

In another double-blind study, Gelskey [610] studied the effect of HeNe or HeNe + Nd:YAG on patients with dentine hypersensitivity on both sides. One was treated with HeNe laser (guide light, dose not stated) and one with a combination of HeNe and Nd:YAG. Surprisingly enough, HeNe reduced dentine hypersensitivity to air by 63% and to mechanical stimulation by 61% over three months. The HeNe + Nd:YAG treatment reduced sensitivity to air by 58% and to mechanical stimulation by 61%. All teeth remained vital with no adverse effects.

The effect of Nd:YAG could be confirmed by Orchardson [845], but not the effect of HeNe. Only the HeNe aiming beam of the Nd:YAG laser was used and no dosage is indicated.

A study by Yamaguchi [705] was conducted to evaluate the results of treating hypersensitive dentine with a GaAlAs laser, 30 mW, 790 nm, using a double blind technique. For this purpose, 66 teeth were examined. 30 of the teeth were treated with laser irradiation (active group), while the other 36 were not (dummy group). The following results were obtained: Two hours after laser irradiation, 40% of the active group and 13.9% of the dummy group showed effective results. After one day these values were 36.9% and 13.9%, and after 5 days 43.3% and 19.4%, respectively. An overall evaluation indicated these values to be 60.0% and 22.2% respectively.

dose, irradiating once of week during six weeks. One week after the SRP the following parameters were measured: pocket depth, gingival index, plaque index, GCF volume, MMP-8, IL-8 and microbiology in the pocket. The irradiation (180 seconds per point, 0.54 J/cm^2) was then performed by a dental hygienist and the selection of side was blinded to the evaluators. After six weeks renewed measurements revealed that all clinical parameters had improved significantly better on the HeNe side. MMP-8 was more reduced on the HeNe side while there was no difference for IL-8 or pathogens. Coherence is an important factor in phototherapy but even the length of the coherence appears to be of importance.

Further literature: [72, 76, 77, 164, 165, 166, 641, 1185]
For more studies, see "Periodontitis"

5.3.10 Herpes zoster
(See chapter 4.1.62 "Zoster" on page 372)

5.3.11 Hypersensitive dentine
Painful necks of teeth often respond well to laser treatment. Recent desensitising agents have greatly reduced the problem of hypersensitive dentine. While these products effectively reduce minor sensitivities, LPT is superior for cases with more profound pulpitis. The seriousness of the hypersensitivity decides the dosage and number of sessions needed. The tooth neck should be treated until the patient feels a distinct improvement (check with the air syringe). With GaAlAs/GaAs lasers and its greater penetration, it is possible to irradiate directly over the apex, through mucous membrane and bone. With HeNe laser it is only possible to use the tooth neck, except for the upper incisors. A combination irradiation over the coronary pulp, tooth neck and apex is recommended. A hypersensitive tooth that does not respond to 4-6 J per root in 2-3 sessions is a candidate for endodontics.

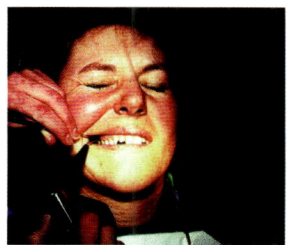
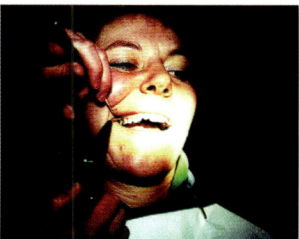

Figure 5.7 Patient's reaction to the air syringe before and after LPT.
Courtesy: Per Hugo Kristensen

With the advent of porcelain inlays/onlays and large composite fillings, the number of postoperative complaints has increased considerably.

A comparative study of the influence details of low-intensity pulse and continuous oscillation of laser radiation of red and infrared parts of spectrum upon microcirculation indices in comprehensive treatment of chronic parodontitis of light and middle severity was performed by Krechina [2011]. The predominantly activating influence upon microcirculation in gingival tissues of the pulsed laser radiation in the red part of spectrum was established.

The aim of a study by Igic [2010] was to determine the efficiency of a LPT in the therapy of chronic gingivitis in children. The study included 100 children with permanent dentition and suffering from chronic gingivitis. They were divided into two groups: group I-50 children with chronic gingivitis, who underwent the basic therapy; group II-50 children with chronic gingivitis, who underwent the basic therapy and also LPT. Evaluation of the condition of oral hygiene, the health of gingiva and periodontium was done using appropriate index before and after the therapy. For the plaque index (PI) following results were obtained: in the group I PI = 1.94, and in the group II PI = 1.82. After the therapy in both groups PI was 0. In the group I sulcus plaque index (SPI) was 2.02 before the therapy and 0.32 after the therapy. In the group II SPI was 1.90 before the therapy and 0.08 after the therapy. In the group I Community Periodontal Index of Treatment Needs (CPITN) was 1.66 before the therapy and 0.32 after the therapy, and in the group II CPITN was 1.60 before the therapy and 0.08 after the therapy. Chronic gingivitis in children can be successfully cured by the basic treatment but the use of LPT can significantly improve this effect.

In the study by Qadri [1185] a combination of 635 nm diode laser and GaAlAs laser were used to treat gingivitis and periodontal disease. 17 patients received laser on one side of the upper arch and placebo laser on the other side, after the teeth having been debrided. 635 nm diode laser 0.9 J was applied at the base of the interdental papilla and GaAlAs 3.5 J at the projection of the alveolar bone margin. The results were as follows (laser side/placebo side): gingival index 0.54/1.4, plaque index 0.26/0.68, pocket reduction 0.92/0.16. The gingival exsudate was reduced on the laser side, 0,04 μl vs. 0.14 μl. The metalloproteinase-8 (MMP-8) was slightly reduced on the laser side and elevated on the placebo side. There was no difference in elastase activity or of the amount of IL-1β, nor any significant changes in microbiology.

The aim of another study by Qadri [1634] was to study whether or not the length of coherence is of importance in phototherapy. Laser light is coherent but the length of coherence of gas lasers such as a HeNe laser is much greater than that of a diode laser of the same wavelength. The biological significance of the length of coherence has hitherto not been investigated. 20 patients with light to moderate periodontitis were selected. After instruction about oral hygiene, scaling and root planing (SRP), one side of the upper jaw of each patient was randomly selected for HeNe (632.8 nm, 3 mW) or InGaAlP (650 nm, 3 mW) laser irradiation, using the same power and

A study conducted by Yarita [182] found no change of morphology in the initial stages of gingivitis in humans. In a group that had received laser treatment, however, increased blood flow was observed.

Kozlov [368] has studied the microcirculation in patients with periodontal disease of various degrees, using biomicroscopic techniques and laser Doppler flowmetry. The intensified tissue blood flow observed after HeNe laser irradiation was caused by intensification of blood microcirculation and the activation of neovascularisation. Tissue blood flow stimulation was caused by precapillary dilatation and opening of "reserved" capillaries. Doses between 10 and 30 J/cm^2 had adverse effects. The best effect was observed in patients with moderate periodontal disease. The key to the four studies above is the condition of the tissue. Experimental gingivitis in healthy subjects reacts differently to LPT than a true disease would.

Lee [136] examined the gingivitis of 13 dental students. GaAlAs laser light was administered to one side of the jaw on days 1, 3, 5 and 7. A histological evaluation was carried out on day 4. The sulcus bleeding index decreased on the experimental side, but the pocket depth and plaque index were unchanged. On the side treated with laser, a reduction in motiles and spirochetes was observed, along with an increase in non-motiles. From a histological point of view, the inflammatory infiltration decreased in density and extent after LPT.

Amorim [1225] selected seven patients who were to undergo gingivectomy on both sides of the jaw. In these patients LPT (685 nm, 50 mW, 4 J/cm^2) was applied on one side only, the other side serving as control. The healing process was monitored clinically and biometrically, using photographs for a period of 35 days. The analysis was performed by three specialists in periodontology. Biometrical evaluation showed improvement of the healing for the period of 21 and 28 days in the laser group. Clinical evaluation showed better reparation mainly after the third day.

The aim of the split-mouth controlled clinical trial by Ozcelik [1822] was to assess the effects of LPT on healing of gingiva after gingivectomy and gingivoplasty. Twenty patients with inflammatory gingival hyperplasias on their symmetrical teeth were included in this study. After gingivectomy and gingivoplasty, a diode laser (588 nm) was randomly applied to one side of the operation area for 7 days. The surgical areas were disclosed by a solution to visualize the areas in which the epithelium is absent. Comparison of the surface areas on the LPT-applied sites and controls were made with image-analysing software. While there were no statistically significant differences between the stained surface areas of the LPT applied and the control sites immediately after the surgery, LPT-applied sites had significantly lower stained areas compared with the controls on the post-operative third, seventh and 15th day. Within the limitations of this study, the results indicated that LPT may enhance epithelisation and improve wound healing after gingivectomy and gingivoplasty operations.

the biopsy, (laser group) cicatrisation took place within 14 days, and in the control group (no gingivitis, no laser treatment) within 21 days. Even in the presence of gingivitis, the laser groups exhibited quicker and better cicatrisation.

Loevschall [75] examined the effects of GaAlAs laser on human oral fibroblasts. This study showed increased incorporation of thymidine in the fibroblasts, which suggests that LPT can stimulate DNA synthesis.

Kim [948] conducted an in vitro study of the GaAlAs laser's stimulating effect on gingival fibroblasts from human subjects. The cell cultures were treated daily for four days, and the treatment period in the three groups was 30, 60 and 90 seconds. The number of cells in the experimental group rose with increased exposure to laser irradiation, although the rise was not statistically significant in comparison with the control group. It was also found, when comparing the protein content of the different cultures, that a very significant increase had taken place in the experimental group treated with 90 seconds GaAlAs irradiation. In terms of DNA content, the only significant difference was in the group that had received 60 seconds GaAlAs irradiation.

In the study by Sakurai [1008] laser irradiation inhibited PGE_2 by LPS in hGF cells through a reduction of COX-2 mRNA level. The findings suggest that LPT may be of therapeutic benefit against the aggravation of gingivitis and periodontitis through bacterial infection

Animal studies

Kubota [479] measured the microcirculation in skin flaps using the laser speckle method. One minute after irradiation the perfusion was less, and 30 minutes later it was greater than in the control flap.

In a histopathological study, Abramovici [640] studied the effect of a HeNe laser on the healing process of open gingival wounds in cats. The irradiation initiated a massive inflammatory cell exudate together with an antioedematic effect after the second postoperative day. A substantial acceleration of the healing process was noted on the sixth day. The biostimulatory effect seemed to act photodynamically at both the intracellular and extracellular levels, thus promoting the proliferatory capacity of fibroblasts and the capillary bud formation necessary for a rapid differentiation of connective tissue.

Clinical studies

Rydén [42] studied the effect of a GaAs laser on experimental gingivitis in 10 healthy human volunteers. After three weeks plaque accumulation, one side was given a total dose of 1 J, divided between day 21 and day 24. The degree of gingivitis was examined by identifying the vessels in the area, using photography, on day 0, day 21, day 28 and day 42. No statistical difference was found between the laser group and the control group with respect to the number of vessels.

with red/infrared wavelengths and energy doses of 6 -7.5 Joules, is effective in reducing acute inflammatory pain.

The purpose of a study by Aras [2062] was to compare the effects of extraoral and intraoral LPT on postoperative trismus and oedema following the removal of mandibular third molars. Forty-eight patients who were to undergo surgical removal of their lower third molars were studied. Patients were randomly allocated to one of three groups: extraoral LPT, intraoral LPT, or placebo. In the study, 808 nm was used, and the laser therapy was applied by using a 1 x 3-cm handpiece. The flat-top laser beam profile was used in this therapy. For both of the LPT groups, laser energy was applied at 100 mW for a total of 120 s, 12 J. Patients in the extraoral-LPT group (n= 16) received 12 J, 4 J/cm^2, and the laser was applied at the insertion point of the masseter muscle immediately after the operation. Patients in the intraoral-LPT group (n=16) received 12J (4 J/cm^2 intraorally at the operation site 1 cm from the target tissue. In the placebo group (n = 16), the handpiece was inserted intraorally at the operation site and then was touched extraorally to the masseter muscle for 1 min at each site (120 s total), but the laser was not activated. The size of the interincisal opening and facial swelling were evaluated on the second and seventh postoperative days. At the second postoperative day, trismus and swelling in the extraoral-LPT group were significantly less than in the placebo group. Trismus in the extraoral-LPT group at the seventh postoperative day was also significantly less than in the placebo group. However, at the seventh postoperative day in the intraoral-LPT group, only trismus was significantly less than in the placebo group. This study demonstrates that extraoral LPT is more effective than intraoral LPT for the reduction of postoperative trismus and swelling after extraction of the lower third molar using these parameters.

Further literature: [1132, 1193, 1293]

5.3.9 Gingivitis

LPT can be used as supplementary treatment for gingivitis. In combination with conventional treatment, LPT quickens healing and reduces postoperative pain. The need for complete debridement and good oral hygiene must be emphasised. Preoperative LPT reduces pain associated with scaling.

Literature:
In vitro studies

Chomette [70] studied the histology of biopsies of human gingiva taken five minutes, 15 minutes, one hour and 24 hours after HeNe laser irradiation. As early as an hour after irradiation, the fibroblasts' enzymatic activity had increased. An increase of the number of fibroblasts and cell organelles was also reported, along with increased collagen production. No similar change was observed in the control biopsies.

Chomette [71] also studied the healing process in 14 patients from whom gingiva biopsies had been taken. In patients with no gingivitis before

local anesthesia was achieved with 0.5% bupivacaine plain or 2% lidocaine with 1:80.000 epinephrine. In the second part of the study, 90 patients undergoing lower molar surgical extraction with local anesthesia received postoperative laser irradiation (30 patients) and a preoperative single dose of 100 mg diclofenac (30 patients), or only regular postoperative recommendations (30 patients). The results of the first part of the study showed a strikingly better postoperative analgesic effect of bupivacaine than lidocaine/epinephrine (11 out of 12; 4 out of 12, respectively, patients without postoperative pain). In the second part of the study, LPT irradiation significantly reduced postoperative pain intensity in patients premedicated with diclofenac, compared with the controls. Provided that basic principles of surgical practice have been achieved, the use of long-acting local anesthetics and LPT irradiation enables the best postoperative analgesic effect and the most comfortable postoperative course after surgical extraction of lower molars.

The aim of another study by Markovic [1911] was to compare the effectiveness of LPT and dexamethasone after surgical removal of impacted lower third molars under local anaesthesia. There were 120 healthy patients divided into four groups of 30 each. Group 1 received LPT irradiation immediately after operation (4 J/cm^2, 50 mW, 637 nm); group 2 also received intramuscular injection of 4 mg dexamethasone into the internal pterygoid muscle; group 3 received LPT irradiation supplemented by systemic dexamethasone 4 mg i.m. in the deltoid region, followed by 4 mg of dexamethasone intraorally 6h postoperatively; and the 4th (control) group received only the usual postoperative recommendations (cold packs, soft diet, etc.). Laser irradiation with local use of dexamethasone (group 2) resulted in a statistically significant reduction of postoperative edema in comparison to the other groups. No adverse effects of the procedure or medication were observed.

The purpose of the literature study by Bjordal [1782] was to investigate if the observations about the anti-inflammatory and pain reducing effects of LPT found in the literature can be translated into clinical situations, like the classical model of third molar extraction. Systematic reviews of randomized controlled trials (RCT) with Meta-analysis of pain (continuous data) within 0-24 hours after surgery were gathered. Methodological assessments of trials were made according to Jadad's scale. Subgroup analyses were planned for wavelength, irradiance and energy dose. The literature search yielded 9 RCTs, of which 8 RCTs with acceptable quality and a total of 658 patients reported pain data within 0-24 hours after surgery. There was a significant pain reduction from all 8 RCTs combined at 7.8 mm measured on a 100 mm VAS. Subgroup analysis revealed no significant interaction between effect and wavelength (red/infrared) or irradiance. But in 3 trials administering low energy doses (0.37-0.96 Joules), the overall effect was not significantly different from placebo at 1.2 mm on VAS, while high energy doses (6-7.5 Joules) in 5 RCTs induced significant pain relief at 9.6 mm on VAS. In one RCT, there was no significant difference between high dose LPT and the anti-inflammatory drug diclofenac. In conclusion, LPT

coagulum, and postoperative pain and swelling were measured. The author summarised the results as follows: "We could observe a significant stimulation of the healing process as a result of LPT."

Wahl [693] was not able to find any effect of a 6 mW HeNe laser on the postoperative outcome after removal of the third molar.

Tay [1137] studied the effect of LPT following third molar surgery. 55 patients with bilateral and similarly impacted third molars were selected for surgery under general anaesthesia by one surgeon at one sitting. A 30 mW GaAlAs laser was used. The patients were divided into laser and placebo laser groups. The laser group received 10 J at four sessions during the first 24 hours postoperatively, a total of 40 J. The contralateral side served as control. There was a significant reduction of pain in the laser group, with the greatest reduction found after the initial dose of 10 J.

C-reactive protein plasma concentration can be monitored to evaluate the degree of inflammation in tissue. CRP plasma concentration is usually low, increases quickly at the onset of acute inflammatory processes and quickly falls when effective control of the process occurs. Freitas [1268] used this method to monitor the possible anti-inflammatory effect of 830 nm laser after the removal of impacted third molars. 12 patients were irradiated with 4.8 J per session 24 and 48 hours after surgery. A control group (n=12) was treated with sham laser. CRP values were more symmetric and better distributed for the irradiated group 48 hours after surgery but there was no statistical difference between the groups.

The aim of the study by Neckel [1597] was to evaluate the effect of LPT on the bony regeneration of extraction sockets. 40 extraction sockets of first mandibular molars were randomly selected into four test groups.
1. Control group: 10 sockets. No additional therapy
2. Test group I: 10 sockets: LPT immediately postoperative, 3 days, 6 days, 9 days and 12 days postoperatively; 24 mW, 150 sec, 7,5 J/cm².
3. Test group II: 10 sockets: LPT immediately postoperative, 3 days, 6 days, 9 days and 12 days postoperatively; 36mW, 150 sec, 11,3 J/cm².
4. Test group III: 10 sockets. LPT immediately postoperative, 3 days, 6 days, 9 days and 12 days postoperatively; 48mW, 150 sec, 15,1 J/cm².
Clinical and radiological re-evaluation took place after 8 weeks. Intraoral radiographs were compared in subtraction radiography and the changes in bone density evaluated. LPT showed statistically significant better results than the control group.

The aim of the study by Markovic [1766] was twofold: (1) to evaluate the postoperative analgesic efficacy, comparing long-acting and intermediate-acting local anesthetics; and 2 to compare the use of laser irradiation and the nonsteroid anti-inflammatory drug diclofenac, which are claimed to be among the most successful aids in postoperative pain control. A twofold study of 102 patients of both sexes undergoing surgical extraction of LTM was conducted. In the first part of the study, 12 patients with bilaterally impacted lower molars were treated in a double-blind crossover fashion;

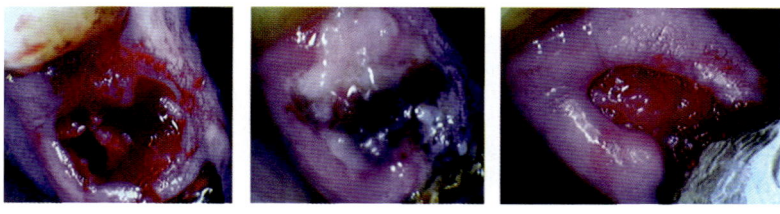

Figure 5.5 Tooth extraction directly postop, at 15 and at 30 days.

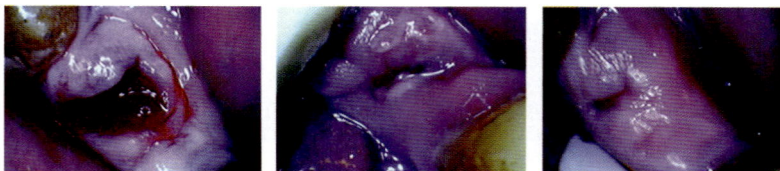

Figure 5.6 Same patient, contra-lateral side; with red laser treatment directly postop, at 15 and 30 days.

Courtesy: Talat Qadri

Literature:

Filho [399] extracted the upper left incisor of 24 rats. 12 of the extraction wounds were given HeNe laser with 3 J/cm^2. Clinically, the rats exposed to the laser beam showed a better healing rate than the unlased rats from the control group.

Takeda [110] studied the effects of a GaAs laser on tooth extraction. 24 rats were used in the experiment, in which irradiation was administered immediately after extraction. The wound was then studied under a microscope on days 0, 2, 4 and 7. Five minutes after the extraction there was no histological difference as compared with the control group. On day 2, fibroblasts had begun to proliferate from the remaining periodontal membrane in the clot. This proliferation was more pronounced in the laser group than in the control group. The ossification process was more advanced in the laser group on day 4, and on day 7 the laser group's trabeculae were thicker and greater in number.

Fernando [216] compared the effects of 830 nm laser light during the simultaneous extraction of two similarly impacted lower wisdom teeth. Postoperative pain and swelling were studied. 4 J was applied directly into the empty socket. In a double-blind study, no difference was observed between the treated and untreated sides.

Verplanken [128] treated 44 patients with GaAs laser immediately after tooth extraction, with a control group of 27 patients. The distance between the bucco-lingual and mesio-distal wound walls, the colour of the

laser group irradiation was performed 1, 3, and 7 days after surgery. In the placebo group, irradiation was performed without laser activation. In the control group, neither laser nor placebo therapy was used. Swelling, wound healing, and pain were evaluated by a blinded investigator 1, 3, and 7 days postoperatively. The laser had a wavelength of 680 nm, 75 mW, energy density 3-4 J/cm². The irradiated area was approx. 4 cm². No statistically relevant differences between the laser and the placebo groups were found. Patients in the control group reported statistically stronger pain.

Propopowisch [1553] treated a total of 120 teeth in 90 patients endodontically. The teeth were divided into three groups: (1) Simulated laser, (2) 2 J/cm² into the canal opening and 1 J/cm² over the apical area and (3) 2 Jcm²over the apical area only. After 24 hours and 7 days the degree of postoperative pain was evaluated. Group (2) had significantly less pain that the other two groups.

Further references: [1550]

5.3.8 Extraction

After extraction, the alveolus is irradiated along with the lingual and buccal bony wall. Faster coagulation, less postoperative discomfort and quicker healing can be expected. A normal consequence of using elevators during extraction is that neighbouring teeth become sensitive, which makes chewing difficult. 2-4 J over the apex usually reduces this discomfort, and the treatment can be administered prophylactically immediately after the extraction.

For reduction of oedema, relatively high doses of GaAs or GaAlAs light are needed on a large area around the wound. The laser decreases the permeability of the lymphatic vessels and induces dilatation of these vessels.

It has not yet been possible to determine the "best" wavelength, although a HeNe/InGaAlP laser seems to be the best option for coagulation, which is vital for continued healing. GaAlAs and GaAs lasers have more effect on postoperative pain and swelling than HeNe.

When removing impacted wisdom teeth, or after operations involving stress on the maxillary joint, 2-3 J over the joint directly after the operation is recommended. HeNe can be used here, even if the dosage is more quickly reached with GaAs/GaAlAs. For postoperative oedema and pain, energies of 15-25 J are needed locally and extraorally. The energy must be correlated with the amount of trauma.

gamma) and lipopolysaccharide (LPS), and stimulated by substances leached from an epoxy resin-based sealer (AH-Plus) and a calcium hydroxide-based sealer (Sealapex). Cytotoxicity was indirectly assessed by measuring mitochondrial activity. Macrophages were stimulated by the leached substances or not (controls), and the groups were then irradiated or not. The secretion of pro-inflammatory cytokines (TNF-alpha and MMP-1) was analyzed using ELISA. Two irradiations at 6-h intervals were done with 780 nm, 70 mW, spot size 4.0 mm², 3 J/cm², for 1.5 sec) in contact mode. The sealers were non-cytotoxic to macrophages. The production of TNF-alpha was significantly decreased by LPT, regardless of experimental group. The level of secretion of MMP-1 was similar in all groups. Based on the conditions of this study the authors conclude that in activated macrophages, LPT impairs the secretion of the pro-inflammatory cytokine TNF-alpha, but has no influence on MMP-1 secretion.

Liu [1114] confirms the pain-relieving effect of laser after post-endodontic filling pain.

The results of the study by Utsunomiya [1010] suggest that laser irradiation accelerates wound healing of the pulp and the expression of the lectins and collagens. Furthermore, D-glucose-, D-mannose-, N-acetyl-D-galactosamine-, and N-acetyl-neuraminic acid-binding sugars and type I, III, and V collagens play an important role in the healing of pulp.

The effect of bone repair in periapical lesions has been studied by Sousa [1238]. 15 patients with a total of 18 periapical lesions were divided into two groups. One group received endodontic treatment and/or periapical surgery. The patients in the other group were submitted to the same procedure and in addition the lesions were irradiated by GaAs laser, 11 mW average power, 9 J/cm². This therapy was performed during 10 sessions with an interval of 72 hours. Bone regeneration was evaluated through X-ray examination. The results showed a significant difference between the laser and the control group in favour of the laser group.

The aim of the study by Kreisler [1501] was to evaluate the effect of laser application on postoperative pain after endodontic surgery in a double blind, randomized clinical study. Fifty-two healthy adults undergoing endodontic surgery were included into the study. Subsequently to suturing, 26 patients had the operation site treated with an 809 nm GaAlAs laser at a power output of 50 mW and an irradiation time of 150 s. Laser treatment was simulated in further 26 patients. Patients were instructed to evaluate their postoperative pain on 7 days after surgery by means of a visual analogue scale (VAS). The results revealed that the pain level in the laser group was lower than in the placebo group throughout the 7 day follow-up period. The differences, however, were significant only on the first postoperative day.

Seventy-two endosurgery cases on incisors and premolars were included in a study by Payer [1616]. After PDT therapy over the dental apex regular LPT was performed over the sutured area. The cases were split randomly into a laser test group, a placebo group, and a control group. In the

Literature:

Paschoud [109] exposed pulp horns and studied the effects of HeNe laser light in direct pulp capping with three different pulp capping preparations, all based on calcium hydroxide. Pulp capping preparations only were used in three control groups. When capping with Pulpdent and Contrasil, a dentine bridge was developed over a shorter period by those treated with a HeNe laser than by the control group. No positive results were achieved in combination with Dycal.

The conclusions drawn were that calcium hydroxide preparations can create a dentine bridge during pulp capping, and that HeNe laser light further stimulates new formation of dentine. The properties of the preparation itself are central to the result. The intrapulpal temperature was also taken during this experiment. After two minutes it had increased by 0.5 °C, after which it increased no further.

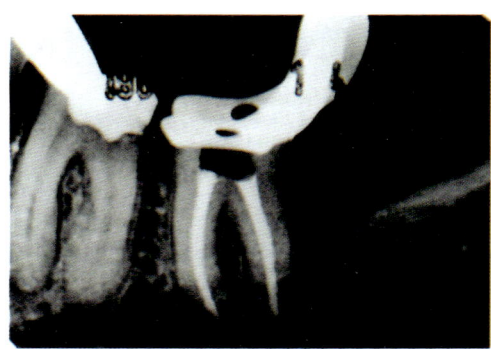

Figure 5.4   Endodontics

Dcabrowska [714] performed 30 pulp cappings or amputations in combination with calcium hydroxide and LPT. 36 teeth were treated with calcium hydroxide only. The laser treated group had a more favourable outcome.

Kurumada [577, 1549], on the other hand, used GaAs laser light without calcium hydroxide on vital pulpotomies. Laser irradiation induced enhancement of calcification in the wound surface and stimulated formation of calcified tissue.

Nagasawa [107] has observed that Nd:YAG and argon laser irradiation within LLL doses strongly stimulates the formation of secondary dentine.

Thwee [1118] performed pulpotomy in rats and exposed the open pulp to HeNe laser irradiation. After irradiation, the pulp was coated with a calcium hydroxide coating. A large amount of dentine-like calcified barrier was formed in the laser irradiated group.

Ohbayashi [1107] isolated human dental pulp cells and irradiated the cells with two doses of GaAlAs laser. In the laser groups there was an increased collagen production, increase in the calcified nodules and enhancement of osteocalcin and alkaline phosphate activity.

In a study by Sousa [2080] the aim was to analyze the effect of LPT on the secretory activity of macrophages activated by interferon-gamma (IFN-

visit. *After the irradiation, the cavities were filled with composite resin. The second group received the same treatment, except by the LPT. 28 days postpreparation, the teeth were extracted and processed for transmission electron microscopy analysis. Two sound teeth, without cavity preparation, were also studied. The irradiated group presented odontoblast process and all posterior occurrences of odontoblastic to odontoblast in higher contact with the extracellular matrix and the collagen fibrils and all posterior occurrences of fibres to fibrils appeared more aggregated and organised than those of the control group. These results were also observed in the healthy teeth. These findings suggest that laser irradiation accelerates the recovery of the dental structures involved in the cavity preparation at the predentine region.*

Further literature: [842, 1510, 1785]

5.3.6 Dentitio dificilis (pericoronitis)

Conventional treatment is supplemented with local LPT over the operculum, buccal and lingual bony wall and any tender points in the musculature. Complementary use of LPT leads to a much faster reduction of discomfort than conventional treatment on its own. LPT is also effective in alleviating pain during the eruption of deciduous teeth. The submandibular lymph nodes should be included in the treatment [915, 1470]. Herpes virus is suspected to be involved in the symptoms during eruption of deciduous teeth [1743], which would further explain the good effect of LPT. If the patient shows signs of an infection spreading down towards the neck areas, LPT should be postponed until full antibiotic protection is obtained, since LPT will open the circulatory system into an area where it is not supposed to go.

Literature:

Manne [222] treated 12 cases of juvenile pericoronitis with GaAs. In eleven cases, there were quick positive reactions, while one case was unsuccessful despite two applications within the space of 24 hours, and extraction was necessary.

5.3.7 Endodontics

A pain reaction can arise after over-instrumentation in root canals when treating both vital and non-vital pulp. This pain is short in duration but still causes the patient discomfort. 2-3 J over the apex eases the symptoms in most cases. This treatment can be administered prophylactically to some advantage when it is known that over-instrumentation has occurred.

In other respects, LPT can be recommended for pulp capping and pulp amputation of milk teeth. LPT appears to stimulate the odontoblast calcium and collagen production, leading to secondary dentine formation.

appeared to diminish the caries progression, laser irradiation did not present any additional benefit compared with acidulated phosphate fluoride on the prevention of induced-dental caries in rats.

A study by Ferreira [1882] investigated the biomodulatory effect of the 670 nm laser in pulp cells on reactional dentinogenesis, and on the expression of collagen type III (Col III), tenascin (TN), and fibronectin (FN) in irradiated dental tissues and controls (not irradiated). Sixteen human premolar teeth were selected (after extraction due to orthodontal reasons) and divided into irradiated and control groups. Black class V cavity preparations were accomplished in both groups. For the irradiated group, laser (670 nm, 50 mW) with an energy density of 4 J/cm^2 was used. Soon after, the cavities were restored with a glass ionomer and the extractions made after 14 and 42 days. Histological changes were observed by light microscopy; less intense inflammatory reaction in the irradiated group was found when compared to the controls. Only the irradiated group of 42 days exhibited an area associated with reactional dentinogenesis. After immunohistochemical analysis, the expression of Col III, TN, and FN was greater in the irradiated groups. : These results suggest that a laser with energy density of 4 J/cm^2 and wavelength of 670 nm causes biomodulation in pulp cells and expression of collagen, but not collagen of the extracellular matrix, after preparation of a cavity.

Kazmina [410] investigated the caries-preventive action of a HeNe laser. 350 children and 50 adults were divided into three groups. All groups were treated conventionally to restore oral health. Normal preventive measures were taken. The first group received no further treatment and the second group received additional treatment with a fluoride lacquer, three sessions, repeated twice a year. The third group had the same treatment as group two but had additional treatment with a HeNe laser twice a year. The laser employed had a power output of 17 mW (from a tube) and a bundle diameter of 5 mm and was thus able to irradiate the entire tooth. Each tooth was irradiated for one minute per session. At the four-year control the CFE index was used (Caries-Filling-Extraction). The index for the untreated group one was 1.0, indicating one new carious lesion per patient. The fluoride lacquer group had an index of 0.29 and the lacquer/LPT group had an index of 0.02.

Kunin [625] used a HeNe or GaAs laser in combination with fluoride lacquers. Percentual reduction in enamel solution rate was studied in four groups. Group 1 received fluoride varnish only, group 2 semiconductor laser treatment only, group 3 HeNe and varnish, group 4 semiconductor laser and varnish. The reductions were 12.7, 19.5, 27.2 and 23.8 respectively.

Two female volunteers with 8 premolars indicated for extraction for orthodontic reasons were recruited in the study by Godoy [1781]. Class I cavities were prepared and the teeth were randomly divided into two groups. The first group received treatment with a GaAlAs laser, 660nm, 30mW and energy dose of 2J/cm^2, directly and perpendicularly into the cavity in a single

Literature:

In an in vitro study, Hicks [837] evaluated the effect of combining low level argon laser treatment and acidulated phosphate fluoride treatment on caries initiation and progression in human root surfaces. The combination of laser and fluoride treatment increased the caries resistance of root surfaces when compared with no treatment and with laser irradiation treatment alone.

Therapeutic laser light doses also seem to have a positive effect on the bonding mechanisms between dental substances and composite bonding materials, according to Kunin [1103].

The enhancement of the fluoride effect when using LPT has also been noted by Liu [1104].

van Rensburg [836] used a GaAlAs laser with an energy of 5.45 J (30 mW for 180 seconds) and an energy density of 27.54 J/cm^2 to irradiate two fluoride containing orthodontic bonding materials. SEM evaluation showed that the laser irradiation had no superficial physical ultrastructural effects on either of the two materials. However, the fluoride release of one material could be enhanced for up to seven months by a sole application of laser. Fluoride release from the other material was also increased but was not statistically significant.

Okamoto [841] has demonstrated that cariogenic bacterias are sensitive to HeNe laser light, but only in the presence of various dyes, mainly phenylmethane dyes. There was a dose dependent suppressive effect on the bacteria and it is suggested that HeNe laser may be suitable for clinical applications in preventive dentistry.

Iwase [77] studied plaque build-up in 20 hamsters fed on a sucrose-rich diet. One molar in each of the animals was given HeNe laser treatment for two minutes, five times a week, for five weeks. Prior to this, plaque had been allowed to build up freely for four weeks. After a total of eight weeks, the amount of plaque around the treated tooth was measured and compared with the amount of plaque on the contralateral tooth. In 19 of the 20 cases, there was a smaller amount of plaque on the treated tooth, and in the last case a greater amount.

In a study by Müller [1847] dental caries were induced in molars of 40 rats divided into five groups: control group (CG), the teeth were not submitted to any treatment; laser group (LG), teeth were irradiated with a red laser, power of 30 mW and dose of 5 J/cm^2; fluoride group (FG), teeth were treated with topical acidulated phosphate fluoride (APF) 1.23% applied for 4 min; laser + fluoride group (LFG), teeth were irradiated with LPRL followed by APF; fluoride + laser group (FLG), teeth were treated with APF followed by LPRL. The animals were killed after 48 days, and the first and second molars were extracted to analyze the caries lesion area, microhardness, and calcium and phosphorus ratio. There were no statistical differences among FG, LFG, and FLG regarding to caries area and microhardness, although the caries area were smaller in LFG. Ca/P ratio did not show significant differences among all groups. Although laser irradiation before APF application

fibrinogen-heparin complexes but failed to increase the level of heparin in the postreanimation period.
Further literature: [106, 1448]

5.3.5 Caries

Every operation on the hard tissue of teeth involves trauma for the dental pulp. It is subjected to thermal variations, vibrations and then chemical influence from insulating and filling materials. The normally very short-term symptoms a patient experiences after an operation involving the hard tissue can be eliminated by administering 1-2 J per root and 2 J into the cavity, after the operation. 1-2 J can also be given over the papilla to eliminate postoperative irritation from wedging. This kind of prophylactic operation may seem trivial to the dentist - perhaps we ourselves should sit a little more often in the dentist's chair in order to feel more motivated to treat this "insignificant" discomfort that we cause.

Hyperaemia after composite fillings and the cementation of ceramic inserts is an all too common problem. In most cases, the problem is of a transitory nature, but who wants a hyperaemic tooth for several weeks? The majority of these problems can be avoided if the tooth is given 2-3 J per root immediately after filling/cementation. A number of telephone calls are also avoided. More serious hyperaemia should be treated repeatedly, but this is clearly preferable to root treatment on a tooth that was problem-free before we started to treat it!

Several studies have shown that CO_2 and various YAG lasers have the ability to decrease the solubility of enamel. Hsu [838] has shown that even rather low intensities of CO_2 laser (85-170 J/cm^2) can induce this effect and that it is dramatically increased in the presence of fluoride. The interesting question is - how low intensities are necessary? Early Russian studies indicate that HeNe laser in combination with a fluoride varnish will decrease the decay. Later studies in the USA and South Africa seem to confirm these findings.

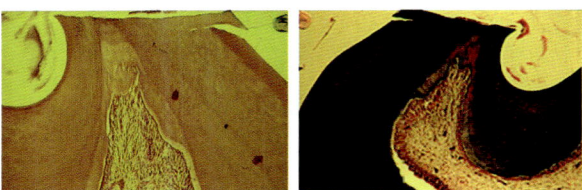

Figure 5.3 Pulp recation after drilling in rat molars with and without LPT.
Courtesy: Aldo Brugnera Jr.

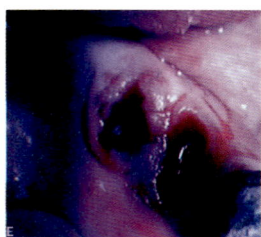 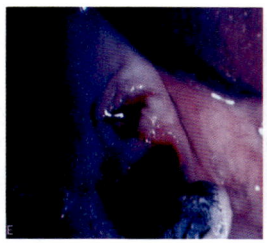 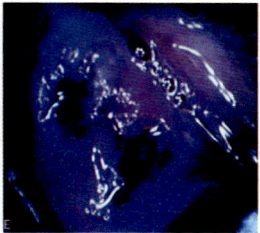

Figure 5.2 a) directly after extraction; b) after 3 minutes of HeNe irradiation; c) the following day.

Courtesy: Talat Qadri

Literature:

Brill [1083] suggests that HeNe laser irradiation inhibits platelet activation and aggregation through the involvement of intracellular secondary messengers – cGMP and/or NO.

Fine [305] studied the effect of ruby and Nd:YAG laser on the bleeding of heparinised mice. The tails of the animals were cut and the effect of laser irradiation on the bleeding was monitored. The bleeding stopped after a period between 10 seconds to 5 minutes in mice irradiated at 60 J, focused on a spot of 3-8 mm in diameter. The animals in the control group were exsanguinated.

Trelles [262] reports that vasodilatation of both arterioles and venules is one of the biological effects characterising the action of LPT on tissue. Vasodilatation does not occur immediately but a few minutes after irradiation and then continues even if the affected tissue is cooled.

Kubota [479] used the laser speckle method to measure the microcirculation in flaps. The blood flow rate was reduced immediately following one-minute irradiation with 830 nm. 30 minutes later the flap perfusion was greater than in the control flap.

Juri [505] summarises a rodent study as follows: It is concluded that HeNe laser radiation blocks the usual increment of plasma fibrinogen level after tissue injury, probably by interfering with the interaction of PGE1 + Bradykinin.

Iakovleva [834] studied the effect of HeNe laser exposure, power 1 mW, at the tip of the light-guide, on the blood anticoagulant system in narcotised mongrel dogs during the postresuscitation period after 4-min clinical death from massive blood loss. The anticoagulant system of the blood plasma was depleted during the reanimation period (the activities of plasmin and fibrinogen-heparin complexes and the level of heparin dropped). Intravascular laser exposure of the blood (for 30 min. during blood loss after drop of the mean arterial pressure to 40 mm Hg and at the beginning of the second hour of the postreanimation period) boosted the activities of plasmin and

mm of its outer border without using a clear and defined point of irradiation. In group (2) a well defined point beam of the laser was irradiated from a distance of 2 mm from the centre of the ulcer, in a helical fashion and covering up to 1 mm of the ulcer's outer border. In group (3) the HeNe laser was used as placebo at a long distance and not covering the aphte itself, while the Nd:YAG laser beam was off. In group (1) and (2) a significant reduction in pain was observed compared to group (3) The duration of pain and the duration of the recovery period were shortest in group (2).

Guerra [1420] used a 20 mW GaAlAs laser to treat apthae. In this observed blind and randomised study the laser group received 1.8 J altering days acc. to the evolution of the aphtae. The control group received Lidocaine 2% gel, analgesics and alimentary counselling. Cases were classified acc. to size and the two groups were almost identical in this respect. Total scarring within different time frames was as follows, with control group within brackets: <48 hrs 17(0), 48 hrs-4 days 8(0), 5-7 days 1(21), >7 days 0 (5). One ulcer of the large type healed with laser with in 4 days and another within 5 days while one case of herpetifom ulcer healed only after 7 days.

Further literature: [56, 525, 531, 623, 635, 1036]

5.3.4 Bleeding

A laser is useful in the treatment of postoperative bleeding. Although the mechanism behind this is unclear, the literature shows that LPT brings about an initial vasoconstriction, but that it is followed by a vasodilatation [44, 121, 152, 479, 630]. Logically speaking, this should lead to increased bleeding, but clinical experience shows the opposite, which is why other mechanisms must be involved. HeNe laser or InGaAlP radiation is absorbed better in haemoglobin than GaAlAs and GaAs and thus seems most suitable. The low power of most HeNe lasers is an obstacle, however. 3-4 J is administered in and around each alveolus directly after the extraction. GaAlAs has been shown to counteract the appearance of fibrin networks [96], which could be one reason why HeNe and InGaAlP laser have a better effect on this indication.

sions are often necessary to prevent any discomfort to the patient until the aphthae have disappeared. 4-6 J is a good "starting point".

Aphthae treated with Er:YAG laser, before and immediately after irradiation.

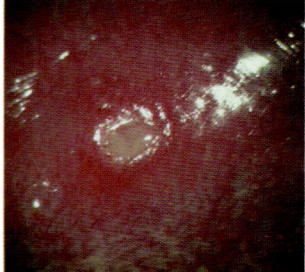 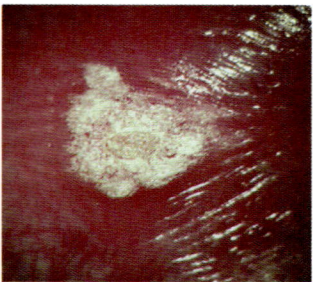

Figure 5.1 Aphthous ulcer
Courtesy: Continuum Lasers

Literature:

Guang Hua Wang [64] demonstrated a pain-alleviating effect when a HeNe laser was used on aphthous ulcers. A 1% and a 10% KCl solution were applied to the aphthous ulcer, after which the SRT (Shortest Response Time) was measured. The procedure was repeated three times, after which the SRT was 100%, i.e. an immediate response. The trial group (25 people) was irradiated with a HeNe laser immediately after the third application of KCl solution. The SRT increased markedly in the trial group but not in the control group. The application was repeated every five minutes for 45 minutes. The laser output was 25 mW, and the treatment time was ten seconds.

Manne [222] treated 12 cases of aphthae with a GaAs laser. In 11 cases the aphthae disappeared three days after a single treatment session, and in the last case five days after two sessions.

Fagnoni [486] treated 32 aphthae cases with a HeNe laser, 300 mJ/cm^2. Approximately 22% of the lesions healed within one day, 41% in two days and 31% in three days.

Takashi [238] reports the positive effect on aphthae using a HeNe laser.

The study by Fekrazad [1568] was performed as a clinical trial on 138 patients with aphtous ulcers. The patients were randomly assigned into three groups, as follows: (1) treatment with a focalised beam; (2) treatment with a non-focalised beam and (3) placebo treatment. The specifications of the laser treatment were as follows: Nd:YAG laser, power 3 W, energy 100 mJ, pulse repetition rate 30Hz, time 60 sec. A HeNe laser was used for marking the beam of the Nd:YAG area (power 5 mW). In group (1) the laser beam was administered from a distance of 6 mm from the centre of the ulcer and up to 1

pain threshold will be raised. The method can be used on co-operative patients. For pediatric restorative dentistry, 4-6 J at the gingival level and over the projection of the apex of the decidious tooth will very often be sufficient for pain-free drilling and filling.

An injection per se rarely causes complications, and the perforation of the mucous membrane is hardly noticed if thin 30 gauge hypodermic needles are used. 2-3 J over the injection area can further reduce the patient's awareness of the injection.

Unfortunately, we now and again hit a vessel with the needle, and in addition to the usual treatment with pressure and cooling, 6-8 J can reduce the oedema and the subsequent pain. Treatment is administered both extraorally and intraorally.

Intraligamental anaesthesia can lead to postoperative pain if the injection is given too rapidly. 3-4 J under the papilla reduces the pain. Prophylactic treatment before the anaesthesia wears off is recommended.

Literature:

Vélez-Gonzáles [105, 504] injected a salicylic solution subcutaneously in rats and compared absorption between irradiated and non-irradiated animals. Using HeNe laser with doses ranging from 1.9-4.9 J/cm^2, absorption was found to increase in a dose-dependent fashion.

Tamachi [44] administered HeNe to rats that had been given experimental cancer. The uptake of the cytotoxin 5 FU in the cancer cells was higher in the group treated with a HeNe laser than in the group that received only 5 FU.

Omura [1047] discusses the problem of insufficient drug uptake in some patients. The situation can, in the author's experience, be improved by using several treatment modalities, such as acupuncture, electrical stimulation and LPT.

Yang Li [1135] has observed that animals in wound healing studies frequently have reacted with a negative response if anaesthetics such as ketamine and ether have been used. It is speculated that there is some reagent competing against laser for the same receptor in the fibroblast.

Koultchavenia [1442] found that transcutaneous IR laser increased the uptake of the anti-tuberculosis drug isoniazid in the kidney. The concentration was confirmed by surgical PAD in the concomitant surgery and was compared to a group not receiving laser preoperatively.

5.3.3 Aphthae (canker sores)

Aphthae are not as easy to treat as herpes simplex. The symptoms of most patients can, however, be alleviated by laser treatment, and the healing period can be reduced. Carbon dioxide, Er:YAG and Nd:YAG lasers can also alleviate symptoms if a defocused beam is used. The dosage is determined by the patient's response to pain relief. When the patient feels a distinct reduction in pain, you are on the way to the "right" dosage. Several treatment ses-

The suggested dosages should be seen as average doses, and clinical judgement should always be the basis for dosage calculation. It should also be noted that most complaints require repeated treatment. This is often difficult from a practical point of view. The patient may not be motivated enough to visit every other or every third day, or the dentist may think it difficult to charge for such drawn-out treatment if assisting personnel are unable to administer it. In practice then, laser treatment often takes place in connection with the patient's ordinary appointments, in which case treatment is hardly ever optimised.

In spite of the higher cost of the Nd:YAG and Er:YAG lasers more dentists seem to be looking at these semi-surgical lasers rather than at the therapeutic lasers. It should be born in mind that all dental lasers have a biostimulative effect and can be adopted for biostimulation if the dosage is adjusted accordingly.

5.3.1 Alveolitis

LPT directly after extraction helps to prevent alveolitis. If alveolitis is already established, 4-5 J before and after the alveolus is debrided and plugged with medication is recommended. Irradiate the alveolus and the surrounding area directly. If the alveolitis is very painful, do not hesitate to use 15-20 J.The local lymph nodes can be irradiated at advantage [1470].

Literature:

A study by Hedner [43] has shown that 47% of patients with "dry socket" manifested a reaction of herpes simplex type 1 after the extraction of the third molar in the lower jaw. This raises an interesting hypothesis: does the alveolitis-preventive effect of LPT depend in part on the anti-viral effect of the laser?

Further literature: [106, 111, 116, 218, 544, 1943, 2027] (See chapter 4.1.26 "Herpes simplex" on page 241)

5.3.2 Anaesthetics

Some patients are difficult to anaesthetise. By administering 2-3 J over the apex, circulation is increased and the anaesthetic is more quickly absorbed. This also means, of course, that duration is reduced. The duration of the numbness in the lip after anaesthesia can therefore be reduced by LPT. This can be advantageous in pediatrics.

Teeth with a large volume of pulp can be successfully anaesthetised with a defocused surgical laser such as the argon, Nd:YAG and Er:YAG. Lasers with an output within the biostimulative power density range cannot give this full anaesthetic dosage but can still be used to raise the pain threshold. When treating caries in young teeth, the following method can be tested. The enamel should be drilled as usual - this does not usually present any problems as far as pain is concerned. The laser should then be applied into the cavity and 8-10 J administered. The pulp will not be anaesthetised but the

may even begin treating their patients for seemingly non-odontological problems, in which case they will appear to their patients as unusually skilled professionals, even if, by definition they are working outside their normal sphere of business. Experience also shows that many practitioners have too much respect for the new tool in the beginning. Remember that it is only light! Bearing the few contra indications in mind, a great new field is now opening up. Many dental conditions are not limited to the oral cavity and TMD certainly often extends way down to the trapezius. The upper trapezius and the neck would then be in the dental sphere.

In the following text, as well as in chapter 4, the indication of "dose" is sometimes joules, sometimes J/cm^2. This comes from the fact that we quote data from the literature, where sometimes energy (joules) and sometimes dose (J/cm^2) is indicated, not always both. In the clinical setting the use of "joule per point" is a convenient method, although not completely accurate.

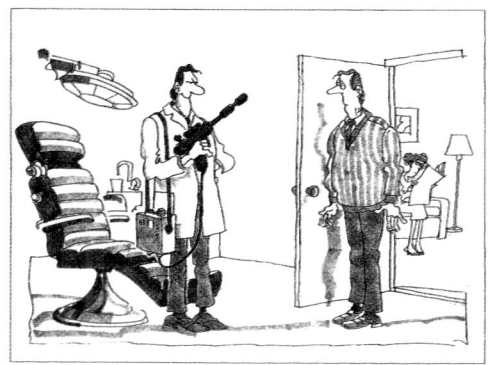

5.3 Dental indications

This chapter may seem like rather heavy reading, as it contains numerous short summaries of articles that discuss studies of different LPT fields. We prefer this structure, despite its drawbacks, as the aim of this book is not just to inform the dental profession about the uses of LPT but to show that there is a great deal more scientific documentation on the subject than most people realise.

The following is a body of information (in alphabetical order by subject) about a number of areas of use for LPT. The text is intended as a source of inspiration for the laser user, not a set of detailed treatment instructions. Several "dental" areas are to be found in chapter 4 as well as there is no defined boundary between medicine and dentistry.

The therapeutic laser is just one of many modern tools which we can use in our everyday work. It is also a fairly new tool which relatively few dentists have acquired yet. But in the not too distant future we may come to see it as a natural part of our equipment, no more unusual than the curing light or the ultrasonic scaler.

The mechanisms behind LPT are more complex and difficult to understand than those behind the curing light or the ultrasonic apparatus, however. More research needs to be conducted before we can fully understand all the important aspects of LPT. But the method has been in use for over 40 years without any reports of patients being harmed, so why make patients wait?

5.1 The dental laser literature

In a 2004 survey of the dental LPT literature, performed by the authors, nearly 400 studies were found. Studies were classified as dental if the indication studied was dental or if the researcher was a dentist. The studies originate from more than 100 faculties in 38 countries. The number of studies is not very high and the quality varies. However, more than 90% of these studies report positive effects, so it is still a good indicator for the efficacy of the therapy.

5.2 On which patients can LPT be used?

LPT can be used, with few exceptions, on all patients but we should remember that this form of treatment is no different from other forms of medical treatment. Not all patients react in the same way to LPT, and one patient may not always react the same way, depending on the condition of the tissue and immune system.

Let us look at anaesthetic injections by way of comparison. Some patients are thought to need double quantities of anaesthetic, while others need very little. In some cases, the effects disappear very quickly, in others they remain for an unusual length of time. Even a patient who normally finds it easy to be fully anaesthetised may suffer when the dentist treats his deep pulpitis - it may be that nothing helps.

In general terms, we can expect up to 80% of patients to respond positively to LPT. If a patient does not respond to treatment, bear in mind that the degree of success of the treatment is contingent on a number of parameters. A poor result can be due to too small a dosage, too great a dosage, incorrect diagnosis, too few treatment sessions, power density, etc. Remember: the more experienced the practitioner, the more success he or she will have with LPT.

Experience shows that practitioners use LPT not only on patients, but on themselves, on relatives, staff and on friends, and maybe even treat complaints outside their own domain. The next step could be that practitioners

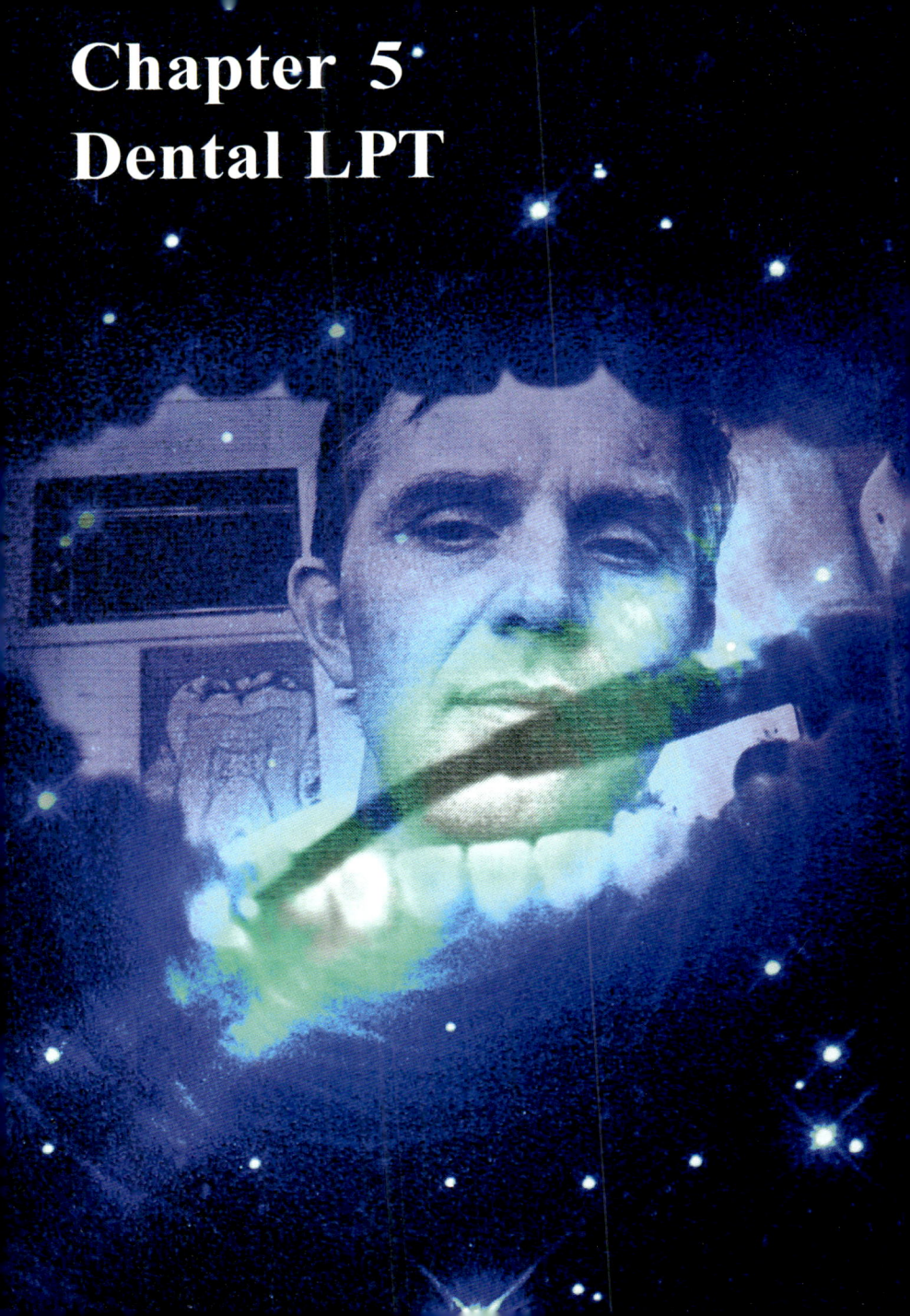

Chapter 5
Dental LPT

peeling and mechanical dermabrasion). There is no question that biostimulation is a decisive factor in the process.

This is even more strongly underlined in the recent reports about so called "non-ablative skin rejuvenation". Here, laser powers and fluencies have been used at levels that do not cause pain, and often not even a heat sensation. Examples of such lasers are: 590 nm pulsed dye-laser [1145], 1064 nm Nd:YAG-laser [1146], 1320 nm Nd:YAG-laser [1147] and 1540 nm Nd:glass laser [1146]. This is obviously a question of adjuvant biostimulation effects (See chapter 1.4.1.1 "Carbon dioxide lasers in surgery" on page 31).

Earlier studies show that one in three Swedish women suffer from menstrual pain. Although, analgesics may to some extent reduce the pain, the side effects of such treatments are not ignorable and thus other safe approaches must be sought. Twenty volunteer women suffering from painful menstruation participated in a pilot study by Kim [2105]. Every individual were treated 15 minutes per week for 8 weeks each time with a total of 200 joules energy using a GaAs multiprobe laser. Approximately 80% of treated individuals experienced milder pain during menstruation. The consumption of analgesics was considerably reduced during menstruation. This results show that laser therapy is efficient in reducing menstrual pain and may potentially replace analgesics.

Further literature: [143]

4.2.12 Withdrawal periods

In the study by Mirzaii-Dizgah [1901] the effects of LPT on naloxone-induced withdrawal signs of morphine-dependent rats were examined. A GaAlAs laser with a power density of 12.5 J/cm^2 was used. One-way ANOVA showed that the LPT applied immediately or 15 min prior to naloxone injection significantly decreased total withdrawal score (TWS). These results suggest that LPT prior to naloxone injection attenuates the expression of withdrawal signs in morphine-dependent rats.

4.2.13 Wrinkles

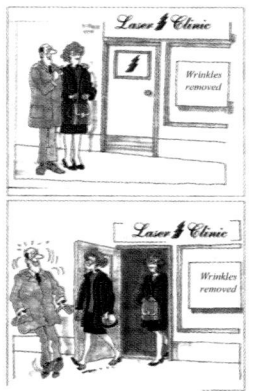

Wrinkles are the LPT critic's favourite subject. We have not been able to find the source of the assertion that therapeutic lasers can remove wrinkles. The assertion is probably as incorrect as the critic's explanation of the alleged effect: "The laser can possibly cause a local inflammatory reaction in the skin which leads to local oedema, which in turn temporarily flattens out the wrinkles". LPT does not cause any local inflammatory reaction in the skin. But the critics have obviously seen a temporary smoothing of wrinkles, as they are theorising about the underlying cause.

However, as mentioned previously (see chapter 3.5.1 "Laser therapy with carbon dioxide lasers" on page 126), it has been demonstrated that superficial burning ("laser peeling") with a CO_2-laser beam or an Er:YAG laser is effective in skin resurfacing for the treatment of wrinkles. Chernoff [294, 295] performed over 50 exfoliations to smooth out perioral, lip, and periorbital wrinkles and scars. The thermal damage depth was between 75 and 150 µm. The result is astonishing (far better than what can be achieved with chemical

in vivo irradiation were more pronounced than those observed in similar in vitro experiments.

It has been hypothesized that reduced axonal transport contributes to the degeneration of neuronal processes in Parkinson's disease (PD). Mitochondria supply the ATP needed to support axonal transport and contribute to many other cellular functions essential for the survival of neuronal cells. Furthermore, mitochondria in PD tissues are metabolically and functionally compromised. To address this hypothesis, Trimmer [2050] measured the velocity of mitochondrial movement in human transmitochondrial cybrid "cytoplasmic hybrid" neuronal cells bearing mitochondrial DNA from patients with sporadic PD and disease-free age-matched volunteer controls (CNT). The absorption of LPT by components of the mitochondrial electron transport chain (mtETC) enhances mitochondrial metabolism, stimulates oxidative phosphorylation and improves redox capacity. PD and CNT cybrid neuronal cells were exposed to near-infrared laser light to determine if the velocity of mitochondrial movement can be restored by LPT. Axonal transport of labeled mitochondria was documented by time lapse microscopy in dopaminergic PD and CNT cybrid neuronal cells before and after illumination with an 810 nm laser (50 mW/cm2) for 40 seconds. Oxygen utilization and assembly of mtETC complexes were also determined. The velocity of mitochondrial movement in PD cybrid neuronal cells was significantly reduced compared to mitochondrial movement in disease free CNT cybrid neuronal cells. For two hours after LPT, the average velocity of mitochondrial movement in PD cybrid neurites was significantly increased and restored to levels comparable to CNT. Mitochondrial movement in CNT cybrid neurites was unaltered by LPT. Assembly of complexes in the mtETC was reduced and oxygen utilization was altered in PD cybrid neuronal cells when compared to CNT cybrid neuronal cells. PD cybrid neuronal cell lines with the most dysfunctional mtETC assembly and oxygen utilization profiles were least responsive to LPT. The results from this study support the proposal that axonal transport is reduced in sporadic PD and that a single, brief treatment with near-infrared light can restore axonal transport to control levels.

4.2.11 Post-menstrual stress

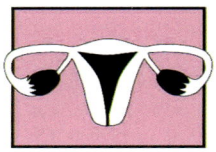

PMS is a problematic condition for many women. It can be treated with oestrogene but the side effects are potentially serious. The authors have limited but very positive experience of using a GaAs multiprobe over the projection of the ovaries. This therapy has reduced symptoms and in one case eliminated the need for hormones. Further indications related to women's health, reported by Behling [1939], are Endometriosis, Ovarian Cysts, Fibrocystic Breast conditions, Dysmenorrhea, Herpes - Genital and Oral, Infertility/Optimal Fertility, Fibromyalgia, Vulvadynia.

were restricted to the brown fatty tissue, in which a tendency was shown for multivacuolar cells to be transformed into the unilocular type. The number of cells which exhibited enlargement and fusion of small vacuoles was greater in the 4 J/cm^2 and 16 J/cm^2 groups. Increased vascular proliferation and congestion was another more evident finding in laser-treated animals compared to non-treated animals. Laser irradiation at therapeutic levels cause brown adipose fat droplets to coalesce and fuse. Additionally, it stimulated proliferation and congestion of capillaries in the extracellular matrix.

The aim of a study by Senhorino [1901] was to evaluate the influence of LPT on the morphometry of adipose cells in rats. The sample consisted of 20 rats randomized into four groups. The dorsal fat pads of the animals were exposed to the InGaAlP laser with fluencies of 2, 8, 16 and 0 J/cm^2 for L1, L2, L3 and L4 respectively. The average morphometry, in pixels, was: 3741 ±704.14, 3762 ±947.54, 3737 ±1076.92 and 4619 ±781.52 for L1, L2, L3 and L4, respectively, without any significant differences amongst the groups. The application of LPT with different fluencies did not influence the morphometry of white adipose cells differently.

A study by Mvula [2111] investigated the effects of LPT and epidermal growth factor (EGF) on adult adipose-derived stem cells (ADSCs) isolated from human adipose tissue. Isolated cells were cultured to semi-confluence, and the monolayers of ADSCs were exposed to low-level laser at 5 J/cm^2 using 636 nm diode laser. Cell viability and proliferation were monitored using adenosine triphosphate (ATP) luminescence and optical density at 0 h, 24 h and 48 h after irradiation. Application of low-level laser irradiation at 5 J/cm^2 on human ADSCs cultured with EGF increased the viability and proliferation of these cells. The results indicate that low-level laser irradiation in combination with EGF enhances the proliferation and maintenance of ADSCs in vitro.

4.2.10 Parkinson's disease

Several new indications for LPT are preliminary but deserve attention, even though the documentation still is scarce. Other indications, such as LPT for stroke, were just "investigational" some years ago. The papers below create an embryo for further research.

Komelkova [1851] studied the influence of LPT on the course of Parkinson's disease in 70 patients. This influence appeared adaptogenic both in the group with elevated and low MAO B and Cu/Zn SOD activity. LPT resulted in a reduction of the neurological deficit, normalization of the activity of MAO B, Cu/Zn-SOD and immune indices. There was a correlation between humoral immunity and activity of the antioxidant enzymes (SOD, catalase).

The effect of HeNe laser on the activity of MAO B, Cu/Zn-SOD, Mn-SOD, and catalase in blood cells from patients with Parkinson's disease was studied in vivo and in vitro by Vitreshchak [1852]. The effects of intravenous

Total energy values of 1.2 J/cm^2, 2.4 J/cm^2, and 3.6 J/cm^2 were applied on human adipose tissue taken from lipectomy samples of 12 healthy women. The tissue samples were irradiated for zero, two, four and six minutes with and without tumescent solution, and were studied using the protocols of transmission electron microscopy and scanning electron microscopy. Non-irradiated tissue samples were taken for reference. More than 180 images were recorded and professionally evaluated. All microscopic results showed that without laser exposure, the normal adipose tissue appeared as a grape-shaped node. After four minutes of laser exposure, 80% of the fat was released from the adipose cells; at six minutes of laser exposure, 99% of the fat was released from the adipocyte. The released fat was collected in the interstitial space. Transmission electron microscopic images of the adipose tissue taken at x60,000 showed a transitory pore and a complete deflation of the adipocytes. The laser energy affected the adipose cell by causing a transitory pore in the cell membrane to open, which permitted the fat content to go from inside to outside the cell. The cells in the interstitial space and the capillaries remained intact.

In a study by Brown [1428], this observation could not be confirmed. To explore published data on the effects of LPT on fatty tissue, Brown initiated a series of in vitro experiments on human preadipocytes in a porcine model. Using a 635 nm laser of 1.0 J/cm^2, these studies were designed to determine whether alterations in adipocyte structure or function were modulated after LPT. Cultured human preadipocytes after 60 minutes of laser irradiation did not change appearance compared with non-irradiated control cells. In the porcine model, LPT (30 minutes) was compared with traditional lipoplasty (suction-assisted lipoplasty) and ultrasound-assisted lipoplasty. From histologic and scanning electron microscopic evaluations of the lipoaspirates, no differences were observed between LPT-derived and suction-assisted lipoplasty-derived specimens. Using exposure times of 0, 15, 30, and 60 minutes in the presence or absence of superwet wetting solution and in the absence of lipoplasty, a power output of 0.9 mW was delivered to tissue samples at three increasing depths from each experimental site. No histologic tissue changes or specifically in adipocyte structure were observed at any depth with the longest LPT (60 minutes with superwet fluid). Three subjects undergoing large-volume lipoplasty were exposed to superwet wetting fluid infiltration 14 minutes before and 12 minutes after. Tissue samples from infiltrated areas were collected before suction-assisted lipoplasty and lipoaspirates from suction-assisted lipoplasty. No consistent observations of adipocyte disruptions were observed in the histologic or scanning electron microscopy photographs.

In a study by Medrado [1697], dorsal fat pads of normal adult rats were submitted to laser irradiation applied locally through intact skin with four different dose schedules (4, 8, 12 and 16 J/cm^2), with a further group being sham-irradiated. Histology, morphometry, immunofluorescence, and electron microscopy were all used to analyse irradiated tissues. Changes

Riboflavin improves energy efficiency in mitochondria and reduces oxidative injury. The purpose of a study by Moges [2085] was to examine the synergistic effect of LT and riboflavin on the survival of motor neurons in a mouse model of FALS. G93A SOD1 transgenic mice were divided into four groups: Control, Riboflavin, Light, and Riboflavin+Light (combination). Mice were treated from 51 days of age until death. A single set of LT parameters was used: 810 nm diode laser, 140 mW output power, 1.4 cm² spot area, 120 seconds treatment duration, and 12 J/cm² energy density. Behavioral tests and weight monitoring were done weekly. At end stage of the disease, mice were euthanized, survival data was collected and immunohistochemistry and motor neuron counts were performed. There was no difference in survival between groups. Motor function was not significantly improved with the exception of the rotarod test which showed significant improvement in the Light group in the early stage of the disease. Immunohistochemical expression of the astrocyte marker, glial fibrilary acidic protein, was significantly reduced in the cervical and lumbar enlargements of the spinal cord as a result of LPT. There was no difference in the number of motor neurons in the anterior horn of the lumbar enlargement between groups. The lack of significant improvement in survival and motor performance indicates study interventions were ineffective in altering disease progression in the G93A SOD1 mice. These findings have potential implications for the conceptual use of light to treat other neurodegenerative diseases that have been linked to mitochondrial dysfunction.

4.2.9 Obesity

Obesity has been reported to be affected by LPT. When treating a person with GaAs on an area of the abdomen, therapists have been able to observe a slight "depression" in the fat layer where the probe has been held - the laser has in some way affected the tissue. However, the patient has not lost any weight, and furthermore, where would all the fat have gone if no weight was lost?

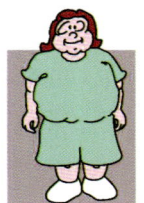

However, what we usually regard as "fat" is not just fat. The "fat" in a thigh contains only about 30% fat – the rest is water and glycogen. In some cases it can be regarded, more or less, as an oedema. As laser treatment of oedema can be very effective, local treatment of "fat" can appear to be effective as well.

The use of laser therpy prior to liposuction remains controversial, as can be seen from the different outcomes in the studies below.

Literature:

Support for the effect on fat cells is given by Neira [1317, 2025]. This study examined whether 635 nm lasers had an effect on adipose tissue in vivo and the procedural implementation of lipoplasty/liposuction techniques. The experiment investigated the effect of 635 nm, 10 mW diode laser radiation.

reduction in LDL levels without experiencing a reduction in HDL levels (or "good cholesterol"). Of the 20 participants, 60 percent demonstrated a reduction in triglyceride levels.

4.2.6 Eczema

Although no scientific papers on this indication can be found on PubMed, it doesn't mean that LPT is ineffective - just that the indication has not been investigated in a scientific setting. The photos below underline the fact that eczema is a good indication.

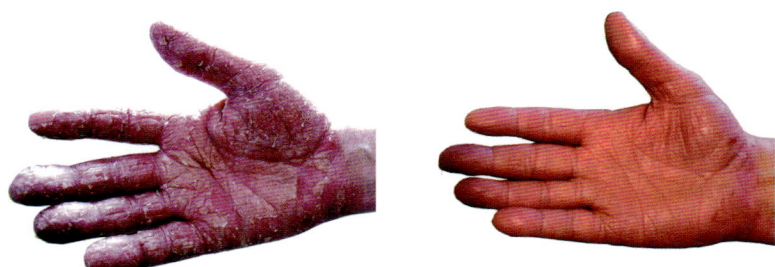

Courtesy: Chrisse Bäckström

4.2.7 Erectile dysfunction

A company has produced a laser especially designed for treatment of erectile dysfunction [1692]. All in all 44 volunteers were randomly assigned to treatment with placebo or 808 nm GaAlAs laser light. Altogether 39 patients completed all treatments and follow-up visits: 18 patients in the treatment group (A) and 21 in the placebo group (B). The treatments were delivered for 19 minutes, twice a week, with a total of six treatment sessions. The laser unit used has two rows of five treatment points each and the unit is applied on the dorsal aspect of the penis, every row corresponding to the corpus cavernosum of the penis. Treatment was given for 20 minutes, twice a week, six to eight times. Power of each diode was 150 mW. Questions three and four, as well as the Erectile Function Domain from the International Index of Erectile Function (IIEF), assessed the improvement in Erectile Dysfunction. The improvement duration on average was six months.

4.2.8 Familial amyotrophic lateral sclerosis (FALS)

Familial amyotrophic lateral sclerosis (FALS) is a neurodegenerative disease characterized by progressive loss of motor neurons and death. Mitochondrial dysfunction and oxidative stress play an important role in motor neuron loss in ALS. Light therapy (LPT) has biomodulatory effects on mitochondria.

used and the protocol consisted of irradiation of three points on the upper lid just above the levator, and one point on the corrugator muscle on each side in contact mode, with three sessions per week (890 nm, peak power 94 W, average power 28 mW, pulse duration 200 ns, spot size 3 mm, pulse repetition rate 3000 Hz, duration of irradiation 40 sec per point, energy per point 1.1 J, total energy per session 8.8 J, dose 16 J/cm^2). The result was complete recovery from ptosis after 10 sessions, but the cosmetic results persisted for several months.

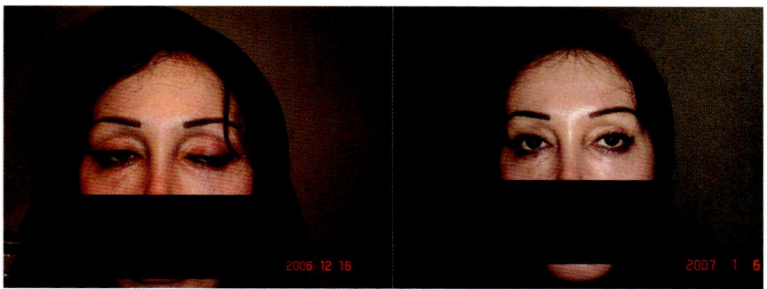

Figure 4.26 Rapid evolution of botox eylid prolaps.
Courtesy: Gholamreza Majlesi

4.2.4 Cellulites
LPT has a stimulating effect on various pathological skin conditions. Whether or not cellulitis is a pathological condition is open to discussion. No documented reports on the effects of LPT for this indication have been published, but red laser machines can be seen demonstrated on TV and in other media.

4.2.5 Cholesterol reduction
In a study by Maloney [2096] 20 volunteers between the ages of 18 and 65 participated in a non-controlled, non-randomized study. Participants received LPT treatments three times per week for two weeks, with each treatment session lasting approximately 40 minutes. Treatments were administered across the abdomen and waist area wrapping around the lower back, an area which generally contains the most concentrated pockets of subcutaneous fat. The laser therapy used was a 17.5 mW, 635 nm diode. 75 % of study participants demonstrated an overall reduction in cholesterol serum levels, with the reduction ranging from -1.0 to -31.0 mg/dL and an average reduction of -16.1 points. For those participants demonstrating an overall reduction in cholesterol serum levels, 93 percent experienced a reduction in LDL levels (commonly referred to as "bad cholesterol"), with 47 percent revealing a

by Go 6983 (specific inhibitor of PKC). Furthermore, LPT involved an increase in mRNA of the cell survival member bcl-xl and a decrease in the up-regulation of cell death member bax mRNA caused by A-beta(25-35). Further data shows that a low fluence of LPT could reverse the increased level of bax/bcl-xl mRNA ratio caused by A-beta (25-35) treatment. In addition, Go 6983 could inhibit the decreased level of bax/bcl-xl mRNA ratio. Taken together, these data clearly indicate that LPT inhibited A.beta(25-35)-induced PC12 cell apoptosis via PKC-mediated regulation of bax/bcl-xl mRNA ratio.

4.2.2 Bisphosphonate-induced osteonecrosis
The aim of the study by Scoletta [2097] was to detail the clinical efficacy of LPT for the management of bisphosphonate-induced osteonecrosis of the jaws (ONJ-BP). ONJ-BP is the term to describe a significant complication in a subset of patients receiving drugs such as zoledronic acid, pamidronate, and alendronate. No definitive standard of care has been set for ONJ-BP and no definitively agreed guidelines have been provided. There is currently no consensus on the correct approach to the issue. The investigators studied a prospective cohort of 20 patients affected by ONJ-BP, who received biostimulation with a pulsed GaAs laser Patients were exposed to 50 kHz, 28.4 J/cm^2 energy density, 40% duty cycle, spot size 0.8 cm. Outcome variables were the size of lesions, edema, visual analogue score of pain, presence of pus, fistulas, and halitosis. Preoperative results were compared with the postoperative outcome and statistically evaluated. Four weeks after LPT, a statistically significant difference was observed for reported pain, clinical size, edema and presence of pus and fistulas.

4.2.3 Botox failures
The widespread use of botulinum toxin type A (BTX-A) for aesthetic procedures in recent years has brought about some unwanted side effects that, though they are self-limited, cause inconvenience for patients. Injection of this paralytic toxin inactivates target muscle(s) for many months and unwanted facial movements will thus be prevented. Spreading of the toxin beyond the target muscles sometimes affects muscles necessary for other facial movements, such as the levator palpebrae, inactivation of which causes upper eyelid ptosis. Mild cases resolve after two to three weeks, but in severe cases the complication may last as long as the cosmetic results persist (three to four months), and until now there has been no medical intervention to accelerate healing.

Literature:

In an effort to achieve more rapid recovery from eyelid ptosis due to an overdose of BTX-A in the glabella, laser therapy was used by Majlesi [2024] in a 46-year-old woman with bilateral eyelid ptosis (partial on the right side and complete on the left) 12 d after injection. A GaAs laser was

had a similar effect. The same author also reports a stimulative effect from stellate ganglion irradiation in patients with Raynaud's disease.

Hashimoto and Kemmutso [691, 692] have also shown that even irradiation of the stellate ganglion alone can have an effect on pain. In a double-blind study, patients with postherpetic neuralgia were treated with either 150 mW GaAlAs, 60 mW GaAlAs or placebo laser. Laser affected VAS pain scores and regional skin temperature, but there was no change in the placebo group. The pain reduction was dose dependent. It is suggested that laser irradiation of the stellate ganglion is a good alternative to traditional blocks.

In a double-blind study on the effect of GaAlAs laser on postherpetic neuralgia, Sato [398] found that the regional body temperature in the laser group increased from 31.9 °C to 32.6 °C, while it did not change in the placebo group.

Further literature: [418, 421, 1051]

4.2 Indications in the pipeline

Many indications have been tested clinically but still lack scientific support. Some of these are minor indications such as insect stings, nonetheless, some are important, such as osteoporosis, PMS and strawberry haemangiomas.

At a meeting held at the University of Oslo in February 1999, Wintsch [844] reported on the treatment of allergic rhinitis with LPT. In the discussion afterwards, he was criticised and his report was regarded to be "anecdotal", as it was neither blinded nor controlled. Calderhead then pointed out that a single case report may be of low value, but when there are many case reports showing similar results, there may be something of interest behind them. Many important discoveries have started with case reports or even anecdotal reports. (Literature on rhinitis: [433, 555, 781, 985, 1052, 1070, 1318])

In every profession, unconfirmed reports and tales of pure fiction circulate. Let us look at some of the examples that now and again pop up in the therapeutic laser field.

4.2.1 Alzheimer's disease

Apoptosis is a contributing pathophysiological mechanism of Alzheimer's disease (AD). In a study by Zhang, [1992] the techniques of fluorescence resonance energy transfer (FRET) and real-time quantitative RT-PCR were used to investigate the anti-apoptotic mechanism of LPT. Rat pheochromocytoma (PC12) cells were treated with amyloid beta 25-35 (A-beta(25-35)) to induce apoptosis before LPT treatment. The cell viability assays and morphological examinations show that a low fluence of LPT (0.156 J/cm^2-0.624 J/cm^2) could inhibit the cell's apoptosis. An increase of PKC activation was dynamically monitored in the cells treated with PMA (specific activator of PKC), LPT only or A-beta (25-35) followed by five minutes LPT treatment, respectively. However, the effect of LPT activating PKC could be inhibited

patients. The placebo group experienced little improvement after the first four treatment sessions, but after four "real" laser applications they came very close to the results of the laser group. Pain intensity and spreading were measured. With 10 as a starting value for pain intensity, the average result was 2 and 3.3 respectively in the two groups. Pain distribution was initially set to 100, and the end result was 31 and 41. Of those treated, 15% experienced either little or no effect. When the experiment ended, the initial laser group had better scores than the second. This confirms the ongoing positive effect of LPT even after the end of a treatment period.

In a retrospective report covering 300 patients over nine years, Moore [404] summarises: cephalic zoster patients experienced less pain reduction (61%) than thoracic patients (78%), with an equivalent difference in pain recurrence of 22% and 33% respectively. In a cost-efficiency calculation, LPT was some 28% less expensive. The use of LPT in the acute phase greatly reduces the incidence of postherpetic neuralgia.

In another study by Moore [476], comprising 20 PHN patients with malignant disease, all patients obtained at least 50% pain reduction after 8-10 treatment sessions. This patient category often does not tolerate the usual medication for PHN due to the high incidence of side effects. Power density was $3W/cm^2$.

McKibbin [58] treated 39 PHN patients with a GaAs laser. Patients estimated pain on a VAS scale of 1 to 10, the average value for the whole group being 8.5. At the end of the treatment period, the average value was 3.3, and one year after treatment it was 2.8 (44% were entirely free from symptoms).

Hong [59] reports on the outcome of the treatment of 20 PHN patients who had not responded to conventional therapy. Sixty percent of the cases were deemed to be successful after a year. The laser used was a GaAlAs.

Hachenberger [60] irradiated 41 cases of postherpetic neuralgia, 93 herpes simplex patients and 3 herpes progenitalis patients. He observed that these related complaints all responded well to HeNe laser treatment. None of the 93 herpes simplex patients experienced a recurrence in the same place during the observation period of three years.

Iijima [183] treated 18 outpatients suffering from postherpetic neuralgia with a HeNe laser. Up to 50 doses were administered! Judged on a scale of one to four, the number of effective cases was 94.4%. VAS dropped from 6.2 to 3.6, and the total pain intensity from 100 to 44.6%. The results agreed with those of a previous study comprising 36 patients [184].

Otsuka [421] also reports positive results of HeNe (with GaAlAs as an adjunct in difficult cases) during the acute phase of zoster.

Epidural or stellate ganglion blocks have been used to ease postherpetic pain. Otsuka [423, 523] has also used LPT near the stellate ganglion and found effects similar to those of traditional injections. Thermograms illustrated a facial temperature increase. Irradiation near the carotid artery

In a triple-blind study on healthy persons, Hopkins [1486] found that non-irradiated wounds close to the actually irradiated wounds also healed better than control. **This is a typical sign of the "systemic effect".**

A case of a large linear atrophic dog-bite scar on the chin was treated for three sessions at four to six week intervals with a 1450 nm diode laser in a case study by Jih Ming [1544].The wound had been present for more than two years. A 50-75% improvement in the appearance of the scar resulted after three treatments. No adverse effects were noted from the treatment. The patient subjective rating of scar improvement was more than 50%. A 1450-nm diode laser may provide a non-invasive and effective alternative for the treatment of atrophic traumatic scars.

Chavantes [1478] reports success in treating tracheal stenosis in entubated patients; 685 nm, 35 mW, 8 J/cm^2 was applied on the tracheal lumen.

Further literature: [704, 828, 935, 975, 976, 1149, 1164, 1165, 1246, 1248, 1273, 1290, 1291, 1292, 1457, 1458, 1498, 1514, 1523, 1586, 1690, 1691, 1751, 1752, 1839, 2017]

4.1.62 Zoster

Zoster (shingles) is a much-feared condition, not only for the acute pain that it causes, but also because it can lead to longer periods of pain after objective healing. This "postherpetic neuralgia" (PHN) is most common in older patients. The Norwegian and Danish word for zoster is "fire of hell", which is rather apt. Laser has an effect both on the acute zoster outbreak and on the post-herpetic pain. Shingles affects not only the midriff but also, for example, the trigeminal nerve. This can make it impossible to close the eye, or cause motor control difficulties, sores in the throat and oral cavity, and pulpitis sensation. In general, LPT relieves the symptoms, and a series of treatments reduces the patient's suffering considerably. It has been shown [404] that treatment in the acute phase reduces the risk of PHN. Apart from the therapeutic effect when treated in the acute phase, the reduced risk of post herpetic neuralgia may be the best argument for using LPT. A rather low percentage of zoster patients do develop post herpetic neuralgia, but we do not know in advance which ones, and for the unfortunate ones it may become a life long "fire of hell". One of the suggested effects of LPT on zoster is that it restores the intraneural blood flow, preventing the death of larger nerve fibres and thus arresting the development of PHN [692]. Red laser is recommended in the acute phase, infrared in the chronic phase.

Literature:

Moore [57] treated 20 patients suffering from PHN for whom conventional treatment had failed and who had experienced pain and discomfort for at least six months. Altogether 10 patients were treated with a GaAlAs laser. Another 10 received placebo laser treatment followed by GaAlAs laser light (a "cross-over study"). The experiment could thereby be conducted in a double-blind fashion while still administering equivalent treatment to all

A cumbersome task in wound healing therapy is the changing of dressings. If a dressing could be transilluminated by laser light without losing too much of the light energy, the therapy would be much facilitated. Lilge [1066] has addressed this problem.

Guirro [1474] measured the transmission through different dressings using wavelengths of 670, 830 and 904 nanometers. The results showed that the PVC Film was the material that presented the least attenuation of transmissivity at any of the wavelengths analysed, being 90%, 88% and 97% for the wavelengths of 670, 830 and 904 nm, respectively. Following the sequence of the same wavelengths, there was the adhesive Band-Aid® (60%, 64% and 81%), Micropore (36%, 33% and 62%), Adhesive tape (9%, 8% and 28%), Sabiá® porous plaster (4%, 5% and 20%) and lastly, the Band-Aid® cushion (2%, 2% and 6%). The results showed that the transmission of low power laser depends on the irradiated material as well as on the wavelength

A systematic review of the literature by Lucas [1046] was limited to infrared studies. Only four randomised clinical trials were found and only one [13] showed any effect. A Meta analysis was performed for three of the studies and no significant effects could be found for decibitus ulcers, venous leg ulcers or other chronic wounds. **The dosage calculation inaccuracy for the study [613] was not observed. In two of the three studies, the light sources are not lasers. One study [1063] is a non-coherent light study. Another study [1064] was excluded because of a different definition of the outcome, making a comparison difficult. It should, however, not have been included in the first place, since it is not a laser study but a study of the effect of combined laser and LED.**

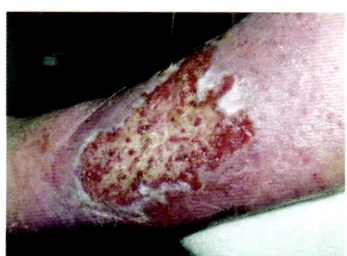
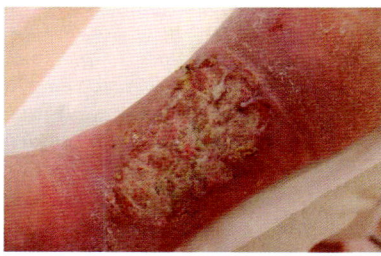

Figure 4.25 Non healing venous ulcer where "everything" had been tried, after initiation with LPT. Healing is slow but pain reduction is rapid.
Courtesy: Chrisse Bäckström

High powered lasers can easily be defocused and used within the regular therapeutic doses. In a study by Kubota [1116], a 1000 mW, 830 nm laser was used to treat skin ulcers. The power density was 669 mW/cm^2 and the dose 6.3 J/cm^2. Favourable results are reported.

infections during the treatment, 28 (60.86%) patients healed completely in an average time of 13.78 weeks, 6 patients healed partially (13.04%), and 12 (26.09%) did not heal. The pain was relieved completely in 33 patients (71.74%)

In the study by Kopera [1594], a 685 nm InGaAlAs laser of 200 mW was used in a group of 44 patients with chronic venous ulcers. The outcome of the study is negative. **Let us look at some possible reasons for the negative outcome. First of all, the only information given about dose and treatment technique is that the dose was 4 J/cm^2 and it is stated that the laser equipment calculated this dose acc. to the size of the wound. The accuracy of this cannot be estimated due to the lack of information about applied energy per point, total energy, continuous or pulsed, spot size and power density. As for treatment technique, we do not know if the wound area was treated or the periphery of the wound (where healing is initiated) or both and, if so, at what fluences. In the placebo group, an incoherent polychromatic commercial LED light source with a red glass window was used. No information is given about wavelength or power of the LED:s. It is known that LED:s can be used for superficial tissues such as wounds [1503, 1513, 1541, 1593, 1594], so the use of an LED array cannot be dismissed as a "placebo" light, unless very low powered. In fact, the study quotes Gupta [720] as a laser study on wound healing, but it is in fact a LED study. The possibility of getting a clinical effect from the LED unit used as placebo is further underlined by the fact that this group had a better mean outcome than the control (traditional therapy) and laser group. The treatment period consisted of 28 days. It is well known that venous ulcers are difficult to treat and require an extended therapy time.**

Marino [951] treated 34 geriatric patients suffering from bed sores with HeNe scanning, 7.3 mW, 0.024 – 0.054 J/cm^2. Photographic and planimetric evaluations were performed every 15 days. Daily sessions were performed until at least 80% of the initial area was reduced. The number of sessions needed was related to the general clinical condition of the patient, and higher doses were more successful. **Bed sores are normally difficult to heal, even with lasers, since the impetus of the pressure is not changed.**

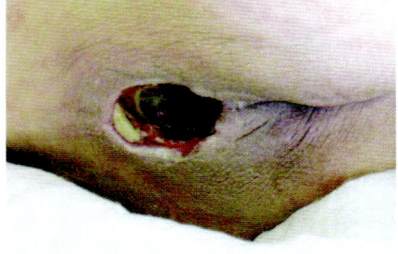 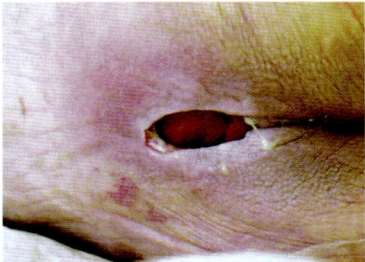

Figure 4.24 Improvement of bed sore after LPT.
Courtesy: Chrisse Bäckström

cebo group). The wound healing per day was 2.45 cm^2 in the laser group and 1.67 cm^2 in the placebo group.

In a study by Schaffer [907], three women with painful mastitis from irradiation after breast cancer with ionising radiation, and a male with a radiation ulcer, were treated with a GaAlAs laser 780 nm, 5 J/cm^2. The healing of the ulcers was controlled using MRI measurement before and after treatment. In all patients, a complete clinical remission was noted following LPT. The results were confirmed by a decrease in inflammatory changes as depicted in MRI imaging.

The same indication is reported by Schindl [967]. Three patients with radiation ulcers following breast cancer therapy were treated with HeNe laser, 30 J/cm^2, three times weekly. At the 36-month control no patient showed any recurrence of the radiation ulcers or any neoplasm.

Almeida-Lopes [969] divided 150 patients who had undergone maxillofacial surgical CO_2 laser treatment into three groups: one control without LPT, one with 688 nm LPT, and one with 830 nm LPT. The LPT groups were irradiated immediately after surgery, and on days 7 and 14 with a fluence of 2 J/cm^2. The results showed that the LPT groups healed quicker than the non-irradiated group. There was no statistical difference between the 688 and the 803 nm group.

In the study by Gaida [1429], 19 patients with burn scars were treated with a 400 mW 670 nm laser twice a week over eight weeks. In each patient a control area was defined, which was not irradiated. Parameters assessed were the Vancouver Scar Scale (VSS) for macroscopic evaluation and the Visual Analogue Scale (VAS) for pruritus and pain. Photographical and clinical assessments were recorded in all the patients. A total of 17 out of 19 scars exhibited an improvement after treatment. The average rating on the VSS decreased from 7.10±2.13 to 4.68±2.05 points in the treated areas, whereas the VSS in the control areas decreased from 6.10±2.86 to 5.88±2.72. A correlation between scar duration and improvement through laser could be found. No negative effects were reported.

Soriano [1473] prospectively protocolised the local treatment of vasculitis ulcers for 10 years, using a GaAs laser, 904 nm, peak power 20 W, average power 40 mW, divergency angle 6°, cooled by a Peltier system. Punctual technique was used with a point spread of 2 cm and a punctual dose of 3 J/cm^2, irradiating the outer border, internal border and ulcer bed. Irradiation frequency being three times a week during alternating days. The ulcer was covered by a vaseline coated bandage for protection. The patients had ambulatory freedom and if any infection was detected, they were treated with oral Ciprofloxacine. During the period of study, 46 patients were treated: 22 affected with systemic lupus, 14 rheumatoid arthritis, 3 scleroderma, 2 antiphospholipid antibody syndrome, 2 cryoblobulinemia, 1 mixed connective tissue disease, 1 lung neoplasia, 1 multiple myeloma. The majority showed multiple ulcers in both legs with intense pain and an average time of evolution of 38.86 weeks. All in all 6 (13.04%) patients suffered from local

gery. In the non-steroid laser-treated rats, significant acceleration of epithelization and collagen synthesis 2 days and 6 days after surgery were observed in laser-stimulated wounds. In steroid laser-treated rats, 2 days and 14 days after surgery, a decreased leucocyte/macrophage ratio and a reduction in the area of granulation tissue were recorded, respectively. LPT improved wound healing in the non-steroid laser-treated rats, but it was not effective after corticosteroid treatment.

A series of studies by al-Watban [2113] used 532-, 633-, 810-, 980-, and 10,600-nm lasers (visible to far infrared) and polychromatic LED clusters (510-872 nm, visible to infrared) as photon sources. Sprague-Dawley rats (n=893) were used. The improvements seen show that phototherapy with the 633 nm laser is quite promising for alleviating diabetic wound and burn healing, and exhibited the best results with 38.5% and 53.4% improvements, respectively. In this induced-diabetes model, wound and burn healing were improved by 40.3% and 45%, respectively, in 633 nm laser dosimetry experiments, and diabetic wound and burn healing was accelerated by phototherapy. This indicates that the healing rate was normalized in the phototherapy-treated diabetic rats. In view of these interesting findings, 633 nm laser therapy given three times per week at 4.71 J/cm2 per dose for diabetic burns, and three times per week at 2.35 J/cm2 per dose for diabetic wound healing are recommended as actual doses for human clinical trials, especially after major surgery in those with impaired healing, such as diabetics and the elderly.

A study by Al-Watban [2114] was designed to assess and compare the efficacy of accelerating burn healing in diabetic rats using low-power visible and invisible lasers. Male Sprague-Dawley rats were used in the study. Streptozotocin was given for diabetes induction. A burn wound was created on the shaved back of the animals using a metal rod heated to 600 degrees C. The study was performed using 532-, 633-, 670-, 810-, and 980-nm diode lasers. Incident doses of 5, 10, 20, and 30 J/cm2 and a treatment schedule of three times per week were used in the experiments. The percentage of burn healing on diabetic rats after LPT was 78.37% for the visible lasers and 50.68% for the invisible lasers. There was a significant difference between visible lasers and invisible lasers in the percentage of burn healing on diabetic rats after laser therapy.

Clinical studies

Guo [619] reports on the outcome of HeNe laser treatment in 53 cases of pediatric surgery. The results in children were better than in adults.

In a double-blind study, Palmgren [351] investigated the effect of LPT on infected abdominal wounds after surgery. A GaAlAs laser, 820 nm, 15 mW output, was used to treat nine patients, while nine patients were given sham irradiation. The dose was 1.6 J/cm^2. Healing time to half the wound size was significantly shorter in the laser group (6.8 days versus 14 days in the pla-

mens containing the whole wound area were removed and processed for histological analysis using conventional techniques. Serial cross-sections were analyzed to evaluate the organization of the dermis and epidermis as well as collagen deposition. The animals of groups LG, PS, LPS, and LPSG presented a higher collagen content and an enhanced re-epithelialization as compared to CG (control) and GB rats. Connective tissue remodelling was more evident in groups LPS and LPSG. The results clearly indicated a synergetic effect of light+photosensitizer+delivery drug on tissue healing. PDT did not cause any healing inhibition or tissue damage during the healing process.

The negligible effect of the presence of heat in LPT has been well demonstrated by Lanzafame [1447]. Pressure ulcers were created in mice by placing the dorsal skin between two round ceramic magnetic plates for three 12-h cycles. Animals were divided into three groups (n=9) for daily light therapy, 830 nm, 5.0 J/cm^2 on days 3-13 post ulceration in both groups A and B. A special heat-exchange device was applied in Group B to maintain a constant temperature at the skin surface (30 degrees C). Group C served as control, with irradiation at 5.0 J/cm^2 using an incandescent light source. Temperature of the skin surface, and temperature alterations during treatment were monitored. The wound area was measured and the rate and time to complete healing were noted. The maximum temperature change during therapy was 2.0 +/- 0.64 degrees C in Group A, 0.2 +/- 0.2 degrees C in Group B and 3.54 degrees C +/- 0.72 in Group C. Complete wound closure occurred on 18 +/- 4 days in Groups A and B and 25 +/- 6 days in Group C. The percentage of the wound closure on day 14 was 75. 4 +/- 7.2% and 77.7 +/- 5.6% for Groups A and B, respectively (NS differences). However, animals in Group C demonstrated a wound closure of 36.3 +/- 4.8%. These results demonstrate that the salutary effects of LPT on wound healing are temperature-independent in this model.

In a study by Silveira [1725], the researchers evaluated mitochondrial respiratory chain complexes II and IV and succinate dehydrogenase activities in wounds after irradiation with LPT. The animals were divided into two groups: group 1, the animals had neither local nor systemic treatment and were considered as control wounds; group 2, the wounds were treated immediately after they were made and every day thereafter with a GaAs for 10 days. The results showed that LPT improved wound healing. Besides, the results showed that LPT significantly increased the activities of complexes II and IV, but did not affect the succinate dehydrogenase activity.

In a study by Gál [2001], four round, full-thickness skin wounds were made on the backs of 48 rats that were divided into two groups (non-steroid laser-treated and steroid laser-treated). Three wounds were stimulated daily with a diode laser (daily dose 5 J/cm^2), each with a different power density (1 mW/cm2, 5 mW/cm2, and 15 mW/cm2), whereas the fourth wound served as a control. Eight animals from each group were killed and samples were removed for histological evaluation 2 days, 6 days, and 14 days after sur-

Steroids are known to delay wound healing. In a study by Pessoa [1455], 48 rats were used, and after execution of a wound on the dorsal region of each animal, they were divided into four groups (n = 12), receiving the following treatments: G1 (control), wounds and animals received no treatment; G2, wounds were treated with laser; G3, animals received an intraperitoneal injection of steroids, dosage (2 mg/kg of body weight); G4, animals received steroids and wounds were treated with laser. The laser emission device used was a 904 nm unit, in a contact mode, with 2.75 mW gated with 2.900 Hz during 120 sec. After a period of 3, 7, and 14 days, the animals were sacrificed. The results have shown that the wounds treated with steroid had a delay in healing, while laser accelerated the wound healing process. Also, wounds treated with laser in the animals receiving steroids presented a differentiated healing process with a larger collagen deposition and also a decrease in both the inflammatory infiltrated and the delay in the wound healing process. Laser accelerated healing, delayed by the steroids, acting as a biostimulative coadjutant agent, balancing the undesirable effects of cortisone on the tissue healing process.

The combination of steroids with LPT should therefore be avoided, if possible. This is confirmed in a study by Lopes-Martins [1456]. In this study, the classical experimental mice-model of carrageenan-induced pleurisy was used to investigate if the anti-inflammatory effect of low power LPT could be blocked by the steroid agent mifepristone. For the intervention group, mifepristone was injected into the pleural cavity an hour prior to the carrageenan injection. Pleurisy was then induced by an intrathoracic injection of carrageenan (0.5mg/cavity), or LPS from E. coli (250 ng/ cavity) in mice. Laser irradiation (650 nm) was then carried out three times with hourly intervals on the skin of the injection site for both groups. Laser was administered with a previously established optimal accumulated dose of 7.5 J/cm^2. While laser after four hours effectively reduced inflammation almost to pre-injection levels of neutrophil cell counts, the anti-inflammatory effect was blocked after pre-injection of mifepristone.

Yang Li [1135] has observed that animals in wound healing studies frequently have reacted with a negative response if anaesthetics such as ketamine and ether have been used. It is speculated that there is some reagent competing against laser for the same receptor in the fibroblast.

A promising concept of combining laser theraphy and PDT (Photo Dynamic Therapy) is reported by Silva [1529]. That study analyses the effect of InGaAlP (685 nm) radiation, either alone or combined with a phthalocyanine-derived photosensitizer (PS) in a gel base delivery (GB) system, on the healing process of cutaneous wounds in rats. The rats were divided into six groups: control (untreated) (CG), gel base (GB), photosensitizer (PS), laser (LG), laser+photosensitizer (LPS), and laser+photosensitizer in a GB (LPSG). Standardised circular wounds were made on the dorsum of each rat with a skin punch biopsy instrument. After wounding, treatment was performed once daily and the animals were killed on day eight. Tissue speci-

tion tissue. The vascular proliferation was most apparent when immunohistochemically sections marked for smooth muscle actin were examined. Fibroblast proliferation and collagen deposition accompanied vascular proliferation. Collagen fibres appeared more regularly organised (in densely packed parallel bands) in the laser groups. **This study seems to verify the common opinion that wounds in healthy tissue will heal in normal time, with or without laser. However, the symptoms of oedema and pain will be reduced. Apart from the reduction of post-accident symptoms, the scar tissue will improve, which may have implications in aesthetic surgery. It is also worth observing that one single irradiation immediately after accident/surgery has a positive but not optimal effect.**

The purpose of a study by Kawalec [1423] was to evaluate therapy with a high power 980 nm GaAlAs laser for wound healing. Using genetically diabetic and non-diabetic mice, two 6 mm wounds were created on the back of each mouse by using a punch biopsy. The mice were assigned to one of four subgroups for laser treatment at different fluences and frequencies: 5 W (18 J/cm^2) every 2 days, 5 W (18 J/cm^2) every 4 days, 10 W (36 J/cm^2) every 2 days, and 10 W (36 J/cm^2) every 4 days. In addition, control mice were used and the wounds were allowed to heal naturally. Wound healing was evaluated on days 5, 12, and 19 by percentage of wounds healed and percentage of wound closure. A maximum of five mice per subgroup were killed on days 7, 14, and 21, and histology was conducted on the wound sites. For diabetic mice receiving 5 W every 2 days, the percentage of wounds healed after 19 days was 100% versus 40% in the control group. Only 20% of wounds in the 10 W diabetic subgroups achieved healing during the same period. For the subgroups whose wounds did not completely heal, all but the 10 W every 2-days subgroup had an average closure of >90%. The 100% closure for the 5 W every 2-days subgroup was significantly greater than the other subgroups. For non-diabetic mice, 100% of the wounds in the 5 W every 4-days and control subgroups were completely healed, whereas 90% of the wounds from the 5 W every 2-days and the 10 W every 4-days subgroups were completely healed. In the latter 2 subgroups, wound closure was 99.4% and 98.8%, respectively. These differences were not significant. The histology results confirmed these findings.

The aim of the study by Grbavac [1750] was to assess the effects of LPT and its possible dose dependency on the healing of CO_2 laser surgical wounds. Circular surgical wounds were created on the dorsum of rats, which were separated into three groups (A, B, and C) Group A acted as control and had no additional treatment. Groups B and C were irradiated with 685 nm laser light, either with 20 J/cm^2 (Group B) or 40 J/cm^2 (Group C). Laser-irradiated groups showed a healing process characterized by a more prominent fibroblastic proliferation, with young fibroblasts actively producing collagen; no myofibroblasts were found. No statistically significant differences were observed when the different doses were compared.

turer's instructions. Treatments were repeated at 24-h intervals for seven days. The animals were sacrificed on days three, five and seven post-burn. The specimens were routinely cut and stained and analyzed by light microscopy using hematoxylin and eosin and Sirius red. The analysis of the results demonstrated that the damaged tissue was able to efficiently absorb and process the light at all tested wavelengths. LPBM at 660 nm showed better results at early stages of wound healing. However, the use of 780 nm laser light had beneficial effects throughout the experimental period, with the animals growing newly-formed tissue similar to normal dermis.

The aim of a study by Hemvani [1641] was to examine the effect of HeNe and nitrogen lasers on the apoptosis of polymorphonuclear cells (PMN) in normal versus burn patients. Inflammation is a major consequence of thermal injury, and PMN infiltration exacerbates the inflammatory process through the release of proinflammatory cytokines. The apoptotic death instead of necrotic death of PMN during the situation may help to resolve inflammation. Ten healthy volunteers and 10 burn cases (30-50% burn surface) were included in the study. The PMN was separated by dextran sedimentation and density gradient centrifugation before suspending in RPMI-1640 medium supplemented with autologous serum. The cell suspension aliquoted in microwells was exposed to nitrogen laser (wavelength of 337 nm, 3 mW) and HeNe (3 mW) lasers for 10 and 5 min. The wells not exposed to laser were used as controls. After 24-36 h of incubation, the apoptotic rates were measured. The percentage of apoptotic death increased from 32.9% in control PMN to 41.97% in PMN exposed to nitrogen laser for 5 min, and further increased to 62.7% with nitrogen laser exposure for 10 min. HeNe laser exposure for 10 min increased the apoptotic cell percentage to 41.9%. Increased apoptosis in PMN exposed to nitrogen laser was statistically significant both for PMN from healthy subjects and burn cases. It was significantly elevated ($p = 0.005$) only for PMN from healthy volunteers exposed to HeNe laser for 10 min, but not among HeNe exposed PMN from burn cases.

Although LPT of wound healing is best used for non-healing wounds, the study by Medrado [1270] suggests that the quality of the wound healing process in perfectly healthy tissue is still influenced by LPT. Cutaneous wounds were performed on the back of 72 rats. Altogether 24 rats received one single irradiation of 4 J/cm^2, another 24 received 8 J/cm^2 and 24 served as control. The wavelength was 670 nm, 9 mW, and continuous mode. The lesions were analysed after 24, 48, 72 hours and 5, 7 and 14 days. After 14 days, all wounds had healed in a similar morphological fashion. However, histology and immuno-histochemistry in the three groups were different. Both laser groups revealed improved healing parameters compared to the control group, and all parameters were best in the 4 J/cm^2 group. During the first days, signs of acute inflammation were less intense and subsided earlier in the laser treated animals. The degree of oedema, vascular congestion and the exudation of neutrophilic polymorphonuclear leukocytes were particularly affected. After 72 hours, the laser groups showed prominent granula-

third-degree burns in Wistar rats. Fifty-five animals were used in this study. A third-degree burn measuring 1.5 × 1.5 cm was created on the dorsum of each animal. The animals were divided into three subgroups according to the type of laser they received (wavelength of 660 or 780 nm, 35 mW, area diameter 2 mm, and 20 J/cm^2). In the animals receiving treatment, it was begun immediately post-burn at four points around the burn (5 J/cm^2) and repeated at 24-h intervals for 21 d. The animals were humanely killed after 3, 5, 7, 14, and 21 d by an intraperitoneal overdose of a general anesthetic. The specimens were routinely cut and stained, and then analyzed by light microscopy. The results showed more deposition of collagen fibers, larger amounts of granulation tissue, less edema, a more vigorous inflammatory reaction, and increased revascularization on all laser-treated animals. These features were more evident at early stages when the 660 nm laser was used, and were more evident throughout the experimental period for the animals receiving 780 nm LPT.

Mast cells have been shown to participate in the wound healing process. Bayat [1735] investigated the effects of LPT on mast cell numbers in the inflammation, proliferation, and remodeling phases of the wound healing process of experimental burns. Sixty rats subjected to third-degree burns were divided into four groups: two laser-treated, one control, and one nitrofurazone-treated group. In the two laser-treated groups, burned areas received LPT with a helium-neon laser at energy densities of 38.2 J/cm^2 and 76.4 J/cm^2, respectively. The effects on mast cell number and degranulation were assessed 7, 16, and 30 days postburn (inflammation, proliferation, and remodeling phases of wound healing, respectively). Intact and degranulated mast cells were counted. Five rats with no burns were used for baseline studies. On day 7 in the first laser group, the total number of mast cells was significantly higher than in the other groups. On day 16 in the nitrofurazone-treated group, the total number of mast cells was significantly higher than in the control, first laser, and normal groups. LPT on the experimental third-degree burns significantly increased the total number of mast cells during the inflammation phase of wound healing; also, topical application of 0.2% nitrofurazone ointment on the same burns significantly increased the total number of mast cells during the proliferation phase of burn healing.

In a study by Chagas-Oliveira [1903], this group of researchers compared the above findings with polarized light. The aim was to compare, by light microscopy, the effects of the use of laser photobiomodulation (LPBM) and polarized light (PL) on second-degree burns on rodents. Forty five rats were used in this study. A second-degree burn was created on the dorsum of each animal, and the animals were divided into four groups: PL (400-2000 nm, 40 mW, 2.4 J/cm^2/min); LPBM-1 (780 nm, 35/40 mW, area diameter 2 mm, 4 x 5 J/cm^2); LPBM-2 (660 nm, 35/40 mW, area diameter 2 mm, 4 x 5 J/cm^2); while untreated animals acted as controls. The treatment was started immediately post-burn at four points around the burned area (laser: 5 J/cm^2 per site). The illumination with PL was performed according to the manufac-

The effects of LPT on burns are described in [1029, 1048, 1049, 1050]. In a study by Schlager [1067], the effect of 635 and 690 nm on experimental burn wounds in rats was studied. There was no effect using the parameters of the study. **This study has been criticised by al-Watban [1068] for lack of information about the procedures and parameters.**

The paper by Bayat [1639] presents the results of a study on the effects of two different doses of LPT on healing of deep second-degree burns. Sixty rats were randomly allocated to one of four groups. A deep second-degree burn was inflicted in each rat. In the control group burns remained untreated; in two laser treated groups the burns were irradiated daily with a helium-neon laser with energy densities of 1.2 and 2.4 J/cm^2, respectively. In the fourth group the burns were treated topically with 0.2% nitrofurazone cream every day. The response to treatments was assessed histologically on days 7, 16 and 30 after burning, and microbiologically on day 15. The number of macrophages on day 16, and the depth of new epidermis on day 30, was significantly less in the laser treated groups in comparison with control and nitrofurazone treated groups ($P=0.000$). Staphylococcus epidermidis was found in 70% of rat wounds in the laser treated groups in comparison with 100% of rats in the control group. S. aureus was found in 40% of rat wounds in the nitrofurazone treated group, but was not found in either the wounds of laser treated groups or in control groups. It is concluded that LPT on deep second-degree burns caused a significant decrease in the number of macrophages and depth of new epidermis. In addition, it decreased the incidence of S. epidermidis and S. aureus.

A study by Vasheghani [2029] sought to investigate whether LPT with a HeNe laser would affect mast cell number and degranulation in second-degree burns in rats. Sixty-five rats were randomly allocated to one of five groups. A deep second-degree burn was inflicted on all rats except those in the control group. In the sham-exposed group burns remained untreated. In the two laser-treated groups, the burns were irradiated every day by LPT, with energy densities of 1.2 and 2.4 J/cm^2. In the fifth group the burns were treated topically with 0.2% nitrofurazone cream every day. The unburned skin of the rats in the control group was used for baseline study. The effects on mast cell number and degranulation were assessed by counting the number of intact and degranulated mast cells in sections fixed in formalin and stained with toluidine blue. On the 7th and 16th days post-burn, the type 1 mast cell count in the 2.4-J/cm^2 laser-treated group was significantly higher than that of the control group. On the 30th day, the total number of mast cells in the laser-treated groups was lower than those in the control and sham-exposed groups. In conclusion, LPT of deep second-degree cutaneous burns in rats significantly increased the number of intact mast cells during the inflammatory and proliferative phases of healing, and decreased the total number of mast cells during the remodeling phase.

The aim of an investigation by Meirelles [1880] was to compare by light microscopy the effects of laser at wavelengths of 660 and 780 nm on

experimental group and the control groups were sacrificed at 24, 48 and 72 hours after the procedure. At 24 hours, there was a dramatic increase in ATP production per mg of mitochondrial protein in the laser group. At 48 and 72 hours there was no difference. The quantification of the liver regeneration was estimated by counting the nuclei stained in the PCNA immunohistochemical assay. The increase in the labeling index for the laser treated group was remarkable after 24 hours, but the difference was small at 48 and 72 hours. This study illustrates the regenerative effect of LPT and also the need for repeated irradiation to keep the process going.

The long term effects of LPT can involve mechanisms connected with activation of migration of stem cells towards damaged areas. Migration of stem cells was tested by Gasparyan [1627] under influence of laser light alone, as well as in a case of a combined influence of light and stromal cell-derived factor-1 alpha (SDF-1 alpha). This cytokine plays an important role in stem cell homing. Cells in group 1 were the control group, cells in group 2 received red laser light irradiation, cells in group 3 had IR laser light irradiation, cells in group 4 were treated with SDF-1 alpha, cells in group 5 were irradiated with red laser light in addition to SDF-1 alpha, and cells in group 6 by IR laser light and SDF-1 alpha. The count of migrated cells was 1496,5±409 (100%) in case of control. Red and IR laser light increased migration activity of stem cells up to 1892±283 (126%) and 2255,5±510 (151%) accordingly. Influence of SDF-1 alpha was more significant, than effects of light irradiation alone 3365,5±489 (225%). Combined effects of light irradiation and SDF-1 were significantly stronger: 5813±1199 (388%) for SDF-1 alpha and red laser light, and 6391,5±540 (427%) for SDF-1 alpha and IR laser light.

Souza [1718] divided 60 amputated worms into three study groups: a control group and two other groups submitted to daily one and three minutes long laser treatment sessions at approximately 910 W/m^2 power density. A 685 nm diode laser with 35 mW optical power was used. Samples were sent for histological analysis on the 4th, 7th and 15th day after amputation. A remarkable increase in stem cell counts for the 4th day of regeneration was observed when the regenerating worms were stimulated by the laser radiation.

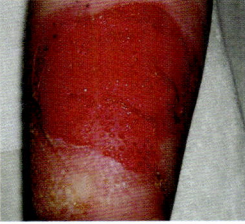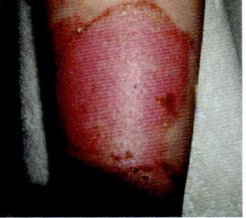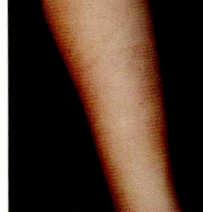

Figure 4.23 Scald injury treated with LPT. Note lack of post scarring at 4 months.

Courtesy: Chrisse Bäckström

logical changes such as the inflammatory degrees in gastric mucosa, the morphology and structure of parietal cells were observed, and the thickness of mucosa was measured by micrometer under an optical microscope. In the model control group, the secretion of gastric acid was small, and pathologic morphological changes in gastric mucosa such as thinner mucous, atrophic glands, notable inflammatory infiltration were found. After a 3.36 J/cm^2 dose of HeNe laser treatment for 20 d, the secretion of gastric acid was increased, the thickness of gastric mucosa was significantly thicker than that in the model control group, and the gastric mucosal inflammation cells were decreased. Morphology, structure and volume of the parietal cells all recuperated or were close to normal. A 3.36 J/cm^2 dose of HeNe laser has a significant effect on CAG in rats.

Morrone [921] reports that 780 nm LPT showed better qualitative and quantitative healing in traumatised muscles as compared with controls in a rabbit experiment.

Gomez-Villamandos [425] induced duplicate pharyngeal mucosal ulcers in 12 horses. Using a fibroendoscope, one of the two injured sides was treated daily with a HeNe laser at 8 J/cm^2. On day 7, histological samples were taken from two horses. Irradiated lesions cicatrised after 10.5 days and non-irradiated lesions after 18. A histological study showed coagulation, necrosis and oedema at the control site. However, in the samples from the irradiated lesions, no inflammatory oedema, numerous active fibroblasts, connective tissue or intensive epithelial regeneration were observed.

Anneroth [41] could not observe any beneficial effects of GaAs irradiation, 0.24 J (0.5 mW for 8 minutes), on the wound healing quality in punched wounds on the back of healthy rats. The effects were observed from day 1 until day 14.

The objective of a study by Mendez [1498] was to histologically compare the effect of GaAlAs (830 nm, 35 mW) and InGaAlP (685 nm, 35 mW) lasers, alone or combined, with doses of 20 or 50 J/cm^2 on cutaneous wounds in the dorsum of the rat. Sixty rats were divided into seven groups: Group I - control (non-irradiated); Group II - 685 nm, 20 J/cm^2; Group III - 830 nm, 20 J/cm^2; Group IV - 685 nm and 830 nm, 20 J/cm^2; Group V - 685 nm, 50J/cm^2; Group VI - 830 nm, 50 J/cm^2; and Group VII - 685 nm and 830 nm, 50 J/cm^2. The animals were sacrificed three, five and seven days after surgery. Light microscopic analysis using H&E and Picrosirius stains showed that, at the end of the experimental period, irradiated subjects showed an increased collagen production and organization when compared to non-irradiated controls. Inflammation was still present in all groups at this time. Group IV (830 nm and 685 nm, 20 J/cm^2) presented better results at the end of the experimental period.

The regeneration of the liver after partial hepatectomy, followed by LPT, is reported by Castro e Silva [598]. Seventy percent of the liver in rats was removed by scalpel. Before suturing, a dye laser of 590 nm, 50 mW/cm^2, was used for five minutes in the experimental group. The animals in both the

between the two groups were compared by histology, transmission electron microscopy, scanning electron microscopy and autoradiography three and seven days after operation. The laser treated experimental animals demonstrated thicker collagen fibers and an increased quantity of collagen at the junction of the anastomosis compared to control animals. An increased uptake of labelled proline was also evident in the laser treated animals. These observations all point to a possible enhancement of collagen synthesis triggered by laser irradiation.

In the study by Pugliese [1535] on extra-cellular matrix elements, cutaneous wounds were performed on the back of 72 rats and a GaAlAs laser was punctually applied with different energy densities. The animals were killed after 24, 48, 72 hours and 5, 7 and 14 days. Tissues were stained with hematoxilin-eosin, sirius red, fast green and orcein and then analyzed. It was observed that the treated group exhibited larger reduction of oedema and inflammatory infiltrate. The treated animals presented a larger expression of collagen and elastic fibres, although without statistical significance. Treatment with a dosage of 4 J/cm^2 exhibited more expressive results than that with 8 J/cm^2. In this study, the authors concluded that LPT contributed to a larger expression of collagen and elastic fibres during the early phases of the wound healing process.

The effects of low dose laser were studied by in vivo and in vitro systems by Mok [1598]. The experimental tissues that were used included bladders, tracheas and tongues as experimental tissues. Buddings (round surface projections) from the transitional epithelium of the bladder were frequently observed three days after laser treatment in both the in vivo and in vitro systems. The trachea and tongue were less affected. In both the in vivo and in vitro systems some epithelial cells of the trachea showed decreased microvilli and cilia three days after treatment, whereas the epithelial cells of the tongue revealed no response to laser treatment in either system. Low dose, however, appeared to promote the rate of healing of experimental tongue ulcer: healing occured about one day earlier in the laser treated animals compared to the non-treated animals, and vessel infiltration and epithelialisation were also detected earlier in the treated tissue.

Many Russian studies have reported a positive effect on gastric conditions, using an endoscopic technique. The effect has been confirmed in an experimental rat study by Shao [1754]. Sixty-three male adult rats were randomly divided into five groups, including a normal control group, a model control group and three groups treated with different dosages of HeNe laser. The chronic atrophic gastritis (CAG) model in rats was made by pouring medicine, which was a kind of mixed liquor including 2% sodium salicylate and 30% alcohol, down the throat for eight weeks to stimulate rat gastric mucosa, combined with irregular fasting and compulsive sporting as pathogenic factors; 3.36, 4.80, and 6.24 J/cm^2 doses of HeNe laser were used, respectively, for three different treatment groups, once a day for 20 d. The pH value of diluted gastric acid was determined by acidimeter, the histopatho-

Animal studies

In a rabbit study by Nicolopoulos [721], a subtotal meniscectomy of the medial meniscus was performed in 24 animals. In group A, the operation was performed with a surgical blade, and in group B and C with CO_2 laser. The animals in group C received GaAlAs laser, 48 J/cm^2 every day until sacrificed. It was concluded that: 1) less damage was produced by the CO_2 laser than by the surgical blade; 2) the healing potential of rabbit meniscus following laser resection was accelerated by the use of LPT post-operatively.

Krypton laser light (670 nm) is rarely used for biostimulation. However, al-Watban [632] reports the results of wound healing experiments in rats. The optimal wound healing effect of 30% was found at 20 J/cm^2, zero stimulation was found at 100 J/cm^2, and a maximum 14% deceleration was found at 260 J/cm^2. The more widely used lasers showed better results than Krypton laser in the range of 9-20%.

al-Watban [471], [475] used several wavelengths (442, 514, 632, 670, 780, and 830 nm) in a study of wound healing in rats. It was found that 633 nm had the best effect, but all wavelengths had a positive effect. The doses should be decreased with increasing wavelengths. Depending on wavelength, healing was accelerated from 15% to 29% in time, and from 32% to 50% in size reduction. Since wound healing in rodents is mainly through contraction, it is necessary to irradiate the entire wound with the beam, unlike in humans, where irradiation of the periphery is more important.

In a study by Bisht [897], linear skin wounds were produced on either side of the dorsal midline in rats and immediately sutured. Wounds on the left side were irradiated daily with a helium neon laser at 4 J/cm^2 for five minutes, while those on the right side were not exposed and served as controls. The mean time required for complete closure in the control group was seven days, while irradiated test wounds took only five days to heal. The mean breaking strength, as measured by the ability of the wound to resist rupture against force, was found to be significantly increased in the test group. Early epithelisation, increased fibroblastic reaction, leukocytic infiltration and neovascularisation were seen in the laser-irradiated wounds.

In an experiment on 218 white rats, Efendiev [833] established an effect on the site of a future incision with the infrared laser irradiation in continuous mode. Output power ranging from 1 to 150 mW (dosage between 0.06 and 9.3 J/cm^2) induced a pronounced stimulation of the processes of collagen formation and a significant increase in the strength of scars. When the power density was increased, the reparative processes in the wounds were slowed and disturbed.

The effect of low dose He-Ne laser on the healing of intestinal anastomosis in the albino rat was studied by Yew [1596]. A small piece of jejunum was removed from each rat and the ends sutured back with a simple interrupted pattern. In the experimental animal, the anastomosis was irradiated through an optic fiber with a HeNe laser (1 mW) for 15 minutes, whereas in the control animal, the anastomosis was not irradiated. The differences

were irradiated and a cell count was taken. The irradiated hypertrophic cells exhibited significantly higher cell counts than control on days one to four for HST and days one to three for NDT.

Hrnjak [676] irradiated human embryonic fibroblasts with 0.5, 1, 1.5 or 2 J/cm^2. A single HeNe laser irradiation exhibited a significant stimulation effect on the fibroblast proliferation.

In the important paper by Zhang [1416], the cDNA microarray technique was used to investigate the gene expression profiles of human fibroblasts irradiated by low-intensity red light. Proliferation assays showed that the fibroblast HS27 cells responded with a curve effect to different doses of low-intensity red light irradiation at a wavelength of 628 nm. An optimal dose of 0.88 J per cm^2 was chosen for subsequent cDNA microarray experiments. The gene expression profiles revealed that 111 genes were regulated by the red light irradiation and can be grouped into 10 functional categories. Most of these genes directly or indirectly play roles in the enhancement of cell proliferation and the suppression of apoptosis. Two signaling pathways, the p38 mitogen-activated protein kinase signaling pathway and the platelet-derived growth factor signaling pathway, were found to be involved in cell growth induced by irradiation of low-intensity red light. Several genes related to antioxidation and mitochondria energy metabolism were also found to react differentially upon irradiation. This study provides insight into the molecular mechanisms associated with the beneficial effects of red light irradiation in accelerating wound healing.

A study by Hawkins [1886] aimed to establish the behavior of wounded human skin fibroblasts (HSF) after HeNe laser irradiation using one, two, or three exposures of different doses, namely, 2.5, 5.0, or 16.0 J/cm^2 on each day for two consecutive days. Cellular responses to HeNe laser irradiation were evaluated by measuring changes in cell morphology, cell viability, cell proliferation, and damage caused by multiple irradiations. A single dose of 5.0 J/cm^2, and two or three doses of 2.5 J/cm^2, had a stimulatory or positive effect on wounded fibroblasts with an increase in cell migration and cell proliferation while maintaining cell viability, but without causing additional stress or damage to the cells. Multiple exposures at higher doses (16 J/cm^2) caused additional stress, which reduces cell migration, cell viability, ATP activity, and inhibits cell proliferation. The results show that the correct energy density or fluence (J/cm^2) and number of exposures can stimulate cellular responses of wounded fibroblasts and promote cell migration and cell proliferation by stimulating mitochondrial activity and maintaining viability without causing additional stress or damage to the wounded cells. Results indicate that the cumulative effect of lower doses (2.5 or 5 J/cm^2) determines the stimulatory effect, while multiple exposures at higher doses (16 J/cm^2) result in an inhibitory effect with more damage.

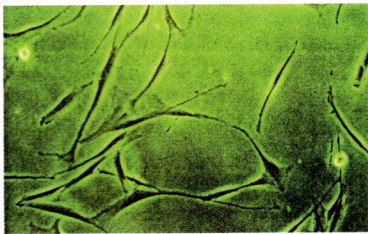 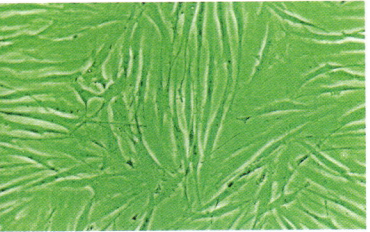

Figure 4.22 Fibroblasts in vitro before and after laser irradiation.
Courtesy: Luciana Almeida Lopes

Webb [911] investigated the effect of a 660 nm, 17 mW laser diode at dosages of 2.4 J/cm^2 and 4 J/cm^2 on cell counts of two human fibroblast cell lines derived from hypertrophic scar tissue and normal dermal tissue explants. Estimation of fibroblasts utilised the methylene blue bioassay. Post-660 nm-irradiated hypertrophic scar fibroblasts had very significantly higher cell counts than controls.

Hubacek [1036] summarises the outcome of experimental data on HeNe wound healing: "HeNe laser emission 1.5 J/cm^2 applied five times during the course of one week improves wound healing through fibroblast stimulation in a directly irradiated wound, as well as in a remote wound. After irradiation with 1.8 J/cm^2 during a week, the production of collagen differs depending on the phase of the healing wound. Early irradiation in the first week stimulates inflammatory type III collagen. Late irradiation in the third week inhibits the inflammatory reaction and improves deposition of type I collagen."

van der Veen [675] studied the effect of 904 nm laser on the proliferation of mice fibroblasts. At an average power density of 3 mW/cm^2 there was a proliferation effect on the cultivated fibroblasts as compared to control. The BrdU-labeling showed an increased DNA activity. There was also a perfect match between the increased number of fibroblasts and the DNA activity.

Yu [586] studied the effect of 660 nm LPT on the production of basic fibroblast growth factor (bFGF). Fibroblasts irradiated with 2.16 J/cm^2 demonstrated increased cell proliferation and enhanced production of bFGF. At 3.24 J/cm^2, no proliferation or production of bFGF could be detected.

Yu [584] found that HeNe laser irradiation of keratinocytes in vitro stimulated interleukin-1 alpha and interleukin-8 production and their respective mRNA expression. Both these cytokines play a profound role in the enhancement of keratinocyte proliferation.

Webb [615] wanted to test the claim that LPT could prevent or improve previously created hypertrophic scar tissue. A 17 mW 660 nm laser diode was used at dosages of 2.4 or 4 J/cm^2. Two cell lines derived from hypertrophic scar tissue (HST) and normal dermal tissue explants (NDT)

- Reduction of IL1-ß [188, 370, 1314, 1815, 1891]

Literature:
In vitro studies

In the work by Lilveria [1894], researchers evaluated mitochondrial respiratory chain complexes II and IV and succinate dehydrogenase activities in wounds after irradiation with laser. The animals were divided into two groups: group 1, the animals had no local nor systemic treatment and were considered as control wounds; group 2, the wounds were treated immediately after they were made and every day thereafter with a GaAs laser for 10 days. The results showed that LPT improved wound healing. Besides, the results showed that LPT significantly increased the activities of complexes II and IV, but did not affect succinate dehydrogenase activity. These findings are in accordance with other works, where cytochrome c oxidase (complex IV) seems to be activated by LPT. Moreover, researchers showed, for the first time, that complex II activity was also activated.

The aim of a study by Rigau [415] was to investigate the behaviour of the confluence monolayer fibroblast's culture when a central scratch of 0.4 - 1 mm and two irradiations are performed, by means of the study of the colony formation, haptotaxis (direction) and chemotaxis-chemokinesis (movement). An argon pumped DYE-laser, with a wavelength set at 633 nm, 2 J / cm^2 was used. The results indicate that all these phenomena appear sooner in the LPT cultures than in non-treated cultures.

In the study by Almeida-Lopes [906], human gingival fibroblasts were cultured in Petri dishes with different Fetal Bovine Serum concentrations, 5% or 10%. Four irradiations of 2 J/cm^2 were given at 12-hour intervals. Lasers with 670, 692, 780 and 786 nm were used. Cells in 5% FBS proliferated better than in all control groups, whereas the cells in the 10% FBS did not proliferate better than controls. The 670 and 692 nm visible lasers caused a higher improvement in cell proliferation than the infrared lasers. **This study confirms the fact that cells in a less-than-optimal stage react better to LPT than cells in an optimal nutritional stage. It also confirms that visible red is the best wavelength for superficial wound healing. The fibroblasts in the 10% solution did not proliferate better when irradiated. However, the irradiation caused a polarised cell pattern, forming bundles in different directions, a phenomenon also reported by Enwmeka [1161] and Tang [1162]. This may be a part of the explanation of the improved wound healing seen in laser surgery.**

exclusion criteria. In another Meta analysis on tissue repair [872], the outcome was +1.81. The number of studies was thirty-four.

LPT is an appreciated tool in cosmetic circles and one reason for that is the effects seen on the fibroblasts. When wounds are treated with LPT, the fibroblasts are distributed among organised, parallel collagen bundles [906, 1904], leading to a smoother skin surface.

While there are many studies, the overall methodological quality of the LPT literature for wound healing is low, according to a review by Lucas [1184] in 2000. The quality has since then improved considerably but the documentation is still insufficient on the clinical side.

An important caveat in wound healing studies is the precense of steroids. These are known to reduce the effect of LPT, as described elsewhere in this book. A recent example is [2001], described below.

Different wavelengths and different power densities will yield different results in LPT. Without a refined knowledge about optimal parameters, LPT will be a bit random. However, the "therapeutic window" is rather wide, and even without optimal parameters LPT usually improves wound healing. The delicate selection of optimal parameters is well illustrated in the study by Nascimento [1453]. Eighteen standardized wounds were surgically created on the dorsum of rats, which were subsequently divided into two experimental groups according to wavelengths used, 670 or 685 nm. Each group was divided into three subgroups of three animals according to the intensity of the applied irradiation (2, 15, or 25 mW). Twelve animals were used as untreated controls and were not irradiated. The irradiation was carried out for seven consecutive days. The animals were sacrificed eight days after surgery. For all laser groups, light microscopy showed a substitution repair process, chiefly associated with shorter wavelength and low power density. Remarkably, all of the six laser groups had slight variations in the healing process. **The results indicate that LPT improved cutaneous wound repair and that the effect is a result of an inversely proportional relationship between wavelength and intensity, with treatment being more effective when combining higher intensity with short wavelength or lower intensity with higher wavelength.**

Some of the observed effects of LPT in wound healing studies are:
- Upregulation of the growth factor TGF-ß, responsible for inducing collagen synthesis in fibroblasts [1149,1672]
- Increase of protein and mRNA levels of IL-1 alpha and IL-8 [584]
- Upregulation of cytokines responsible for fibroblast proliferation such as VEGF, bFGF, HGF and SCF [1673]
- Increase of platelet-derived growth factor (PDGF), transforming growth factor-ß (TGF-ß) and blood-derived fibroblast growth factor (bFGF) [1891].
- Transformation of fibroblasts into myofibroblasts [1270]
- Increase of prostaglandin E_2 production via the induction of cyclooxygenase-2 mRNA [1646]
- Reduction of PGE_2 [243, 357, 582, 718, 1008, 1276, 1461, 1560, 1800]

porcine models, dairy cattle models and humans all point in the same direction. It has also been argued that wound healing studies using healthy animals is not a suitable approach. The healing ability in healthy individuals can only be promoted slightly, whereas the best effect of LPT is shown in individuals with a less-than-optimal immune situation. Thus, diabetic rats have been used with greater success [922]. This, in itself, underlines the usefulness of LPT to treat the all too common circulatory complications in diabetic individuals. More about this in the chapter about diabetes.

Yet another drawback with early rat model wound healing studies is that bilateral wounds were studied, and the systemic effects in small animals are considerable. Certainly clear differences have been demonstrated in intra-individual studies, but for an accurate evaluation a non-irradiated control group is necessary.

Since wound healing in rats is mainly dependent on contraction, a different irradiation technique should be used in such studies. The entire wound should be covered by the laser beam, in contrast to the recommendations for humans, as described above. In the above study by Reddy [922], two circular wounds were created on either side of the spine. The left wound of each animal was treated with HeNe 1.0 J/cm^2 for five days a week until the wound was closed (three weeks). Measurements of the biomechanical properties of the laser treated wounds indicated that there was an increase in maximum load (16%), stress (16%), strain (27%), energy absorption (45%) and toughness (84%) compared to control wounds of diabetic rats. Biochemical assays revealed that the amount of collagen was significantly increased in laser treated wounds. Sequential extraction of collagen from healing wounds showed that laser treated wounds had significantly greater concentrations of neutral salt soluble (15%) and insoluble collagen (16%) than control wounds, suggesting accelerated collagen production in laser treated wounds. There was an appreciable decrease in pepsin soluble collagen (19%), indicating higher resistance to proteolytic digestion.

To avoid the many interacting parameters in wound healing studies, Houghton [1098] used experimental wounds in the separated limbs of fetal mice. GaAs doses of 0.23, 1.37, 2.75 and 3.66 J/cm^2 improved wound healing, while 4.8 J/cm^2 showed no improvement as compared to control. The best outcome was noted with the two lowest doses. The 4.8 J/cm^2 group actually showed the best wound size change at day three, but at day seven all the other groups showed better results. Collagen deposition in dermis and bone was enhanced in the 0.23, 2.75 and 3.66 J/cm^2 groups, but not in the 1.37 J/cm^2 group. The above well illustrates the problem of establishing a "good-for-everything" dose.

In a 2004 Meta analysis of the available literature of LPT for wound healing [871], the laser treatment modality was found to be highly significant (d=+2.22). Further sub-analyses revealed that the efficacy for animals was +1.97 and for humans +0.54. Twenty-four studies met the inclusion and

the contact method. Then sweep slowly over the open wound at a distance of 1 cm, with a dosage of 0.5 J/cm^2. The open wound receives a lower dosage than the skin-covered periphery, as the laser light is not reflected, scattered or absorbed by skin in the unprotected wound, and hence hits the uncovered cells directly. Treat daily for three to four days, then every other day, and evaluate the healing process. If no improvement has occurred, raise the dosage by 50%. Severe wounds with pus and exudates require higher doses. Varicose ulcers and bedsores are appropriate indications for LPT in combination with conventional therapies. In addition to improved wound healing, a considerable reduction in pain can be expected. The outcome of bedsore (pressure) wounds is less positive, except for pain scores [1424]. This may partly be due to the fact that the pressure is more or less permanent in these patients.

The above dosages apply to GaAlAs - for GaAs, about one-third of the above dosage should be given. HeNe has proved to be the best source for wound healing [471, 475], but the low outputs and high costs of HeNe lasers have been complicating factors. The advent of more high-powered and less expensive diode lasers in the 630-660 nm range will possibly solve this problem. Diodes require higher doses than HeNe, although the wavelength may be the same. This may be because of the superior length of coherence of the HeNe laser [1634]. LPT is always a supplementary method: wounds must be cleaned and dressed as usual. Infected wounds are sometimes mentioned as a caveat for LPT. It is true that the germs in the wound will be stimulated as well; however, the stimulation of the immune system and growth factors will be even greater. A reasonable caution could still be to treat the periphery of the wound only and to avoid irradiation over the open wound.

For all types of treatment where infection is present, it is further beneficial to stimulate the immune system by irradiating the involved lymph nodes [915] before treatment of the wound begins. A total of 1-2 J per point is a common dosage, then administering 0.5 J per point along the lymphatic vessels leading to the wound area.

It is not uncommon that a chronic wound initially appears to deteriorate, so the patient should be pre-informed about the possibility of a transient change for the worse.

If heat is used in combination with LPT, should the laser treatment come first? Heat will increase blood flow in the tissue, and by increased absorption of light in the blood, the penetration will be reduced. On the other hand, more blood will be irradiated which can lead to positive systemic effects. Penetration of the laser can be increased by using pressure technique over skin areas. If cooling (ice) is used, blood flow in the area will be reduced and the light will have a higher penetration rate after the application of cooling. For open wounds, contact technique is seldom used. However, if it is used, the area can be covered by e.g. a clin film

It has been argued that successful studies of rats cannot necessarily be extrapolated to apply to human skin. This is a point well taken, but studies on

repair of nerve injury. The purpose of the study by Wu [2013] was to evaluate the effectiveness and safety of HeNe lasers in treating SV, and determine the effects on the repair of sympathetic nerve dysfunction. Forty patients with stable-stage SV on the head and/or neck were enrolled in this study. He-Ne laser irradiation was administered locally at 3.0 J/cm^2 with point stimulation once or twice weekly. Cutaneous microcirculatory assessments in six SV patients were performed using a laser Doppler flowmeter. The sympathetic adrenoceptor response of cutaneous microcirculation was determined by measuring cutaneous blood flow before, during and after iontophoresis with sympathomimetic drugs (phenylephrine, clonidine and propranolol). All measurements of microcirculation obtained at SV lesions were simultaneously compared with contralateral normal skin, both before and after HeNe laser treatment. After an average of 17 treatment sessions, initial repigmentation was noticed in the majority of patients. Marked repigmentation was observed in 60% of patients with successive treatments. Cutaneous blood flow was significantly higher at SV lesions compared with contralateral skin, but this was normalized after HeNe laser treatment. In addition, the abnormal decrease in cutaneous blood flow in response to clonidine was improved by HeNe laser therapy.

4.1.61 Wound healing

Non-healing skin wound before and after two days of HeNe LPT

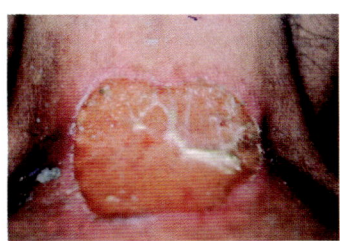

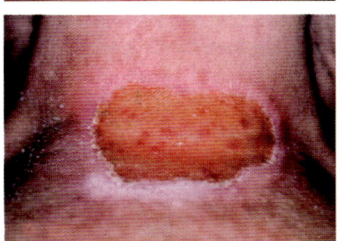

Figure 4.21 Skin wound
Courtesy: René-Jean Bensadoun

One of the most thoroughly studied areas in LPT is wound healing. In fact, this was one of the first indications reported, with studies by Mester and by Carney [520] as early as 1967. The first studies were done using healthy rats. This effect has been confirmed in the extensive animal studies by i.a. al-Watban [471, 475, 632]. However, the effect in a healthy individual is limited and the prime indication for LPT is for individuals or tissues in a compromised state. But it is not a good idea to wait and see whether or not a wound will heal, and then treat it with laser if it fails to heal. On the contrary, an evaluation of the actual state of the individual/tissue should be made in the first place and LPT applied if deemed favourable. We have touched upon this subject in the descriptions of various indications earlier in the book.

The suggested technique for extraoral wounds is as follows (for GaAlAs): start by administering 3-4 J/cm^2 on points along the periphery of the wound, using

Literature:

In a study by Yu [1321], the author sought to determine the theoretical basis and clinical evidence for the effectiveness of helium-neon lasers in treating vitiligo. Cultured keratinocytes and fibroblasts were irradiated with 0.5-1.5 J per cm^2. The effects of the laser on melanocyte growth and proliferation were investigated. The results of this in vitro study revealed a significant increase in basic fibroblast growth factor release from both keratinocytes and fibroblasts, and a significant increase in nerve growth factor release from keratinocytes. Medium from laser irradiated keratinocytes stimulated (3H)thymidine uptake and proliferation of cultured melanocytes. Furthermore, melanocyte migration was enhanced either directly by HeNe laser irradiation or indirectly by the medium derived from laser treated keratinocytes. Thirty patients with segmental-type vitiligo on the head and/or neck were enrolled in this study. Helium-neon laser light was administered locally at 3.0 J/cm^2 with point stimulation once or twice weekly. The percentage of repigmented area was used for clinical evaluation of effectiveness. After an average of 16 treatment sessions, initial repigmentation was noticed. Marked repigmentation (>50%) was observed in 60% of patients with successive treatments.

In a study by Lan [1771], the researchers investigated the physiologic effects of He-Ne laser irradiation on two MB cell lines: the immature NCCmelb4 and the more differentiated NCCmelan5. The intricate interactions between MBs with their innate extracelluar matrix, fibronectin, were also addressed. The results showed that He-Ne laser irradiation enhanced NCCmelb4 mobility via enhanced phosphorylated focal adhesion kinase expression and promoted melanogenesis in NCCmelan5. In addition, He-Ne laser decreased the affinity between NCCmelb4 and fibronectin, whereas the attachment of NCCmelan5 to fibronectin increased. The alpha5β1 integrin expression on NCCmelb4 cells was enhanced by He-Ne laser. In conclusion, it was demonstrated that He-Ne laser induced different physiologic changes on MBs at different maturation stages and recapitulated the early events during vitiligo repigmentation process brought upon by He-Ne laser in vitro.

Ataie [1322] treated vitiligo patches by using a 630 nm GaAlAs laser (20 mW, 1 J/cm^2), twice a week for a maximum of 24 treatments. Patients were followed for nine months and the effect of treatment was evaluated. Six patients were evaluated for the purposes of this analysis. Their ages ranged from 11 to 46 years. Decreases in surface area of depigmented lesions were seen ranging from 25% to 75%. Pigmented stippling within depigmented lesions occurred in all patients. In two patients, a repigmentation of previously depigmented hair was seen. Only one patient experienced arrest of progression of disease after 24 sessions of treatment.

Since segmental-type vitiligo lesions (SV) are resistant to conventional forms of therapy, its management represents a challenge for dermatologists. HeNe laser, wavelength 632.8 nm, has been employed as a therapeutic instrument in many clinical situations, including vitiligo management and

showed a difference between group 2 and 3 (most improved) after four weeks, reaching statistical significance after eight weeks.

The study by Chow [1702] was undertaken to test the efficacy of a 300 mW, 830 nm laser in a prospective double-blind, randomised, placebo-controlled trial in patients with chronic neck pain. Ninety patients were enrolled. Laser was applied using the contact method over tender areas in the neck musculature, twice a week for 7 weeks. The primary outcome measure was change in a 10 cm Visual Analogue Scale for pain. Other measures used included a Self-Reported Improvement in pain, measured by a VAS, Short-Form 36 Quality-of-Life Questionnaire, Northwick Park Neck Pain Questionnaire, Neck Pain and Disability Scale and the McGill Pain Questionnaire. Measurements were taken at baseline, at the end of 7 weeks of treatment and at 12 weeks from baseline. Patients in the treated group experienced a mean self reported improvement of 48.5% compared with 3.99% in the placebo group.

The aim of an article by Jensen [2100] was to summarise the existing evidence concerning interventions for non-specific neck pain. Neck-and-shoulder pain is commonly experienced by both adolescents and adults. Although the prevalence appears to vary among different nations, the situation is essentially the same, at least in the industrialised nations. Explanations for the wide variation in incidence and prevalence include various methodological issues. Back and neck disorders represent one of the most common causes for both short- and long-term sick leave and disability pension. Evidenced risk factors for the onset and maintenance of non-specific neck and back pain include both individual and work-related psychosocial factors. Based on the existing evidence different forms of exercise can be strongly recommended for at-risk populations, as well as for the acute and chronic non-specific neck pain patient. Furthermore, for symptom relief this condition can be treated with transcutaneous electric nerve stimulation, low level laser therapy, pulse electromagnetic treatment or radiofrequency denervation.

4.1.60 Vitiligo

Vitiligo is a type of hypopigmentation and is a result of lack of melanin production. There are two main causes for this condition. Either the epidermal melanocytes exist but are dormant, or they are failing to produce melanin granules as a result of an enzyme deficiency. Hypopigmentation is more difficult to treat than hyperpigmentation. Laser treatment of vitiligo was described already in 1988 by Ohshiro [978]. After first using an argon laser, Ohshiro tried the new GaAlAs laser, using 6 J/cm^2, four sessions. For the cicatrose type of vitiligo, the argon laser was used first since there are no melanocytes left in the scar area.

laser was used in a urethral approach (every third day, 8 sessions). More than 65% of the patients had symptom relief even after six months. Spermatic fluid was analysed before and after therapy. There was an increase in the total germinal cell count, and an improvement in motility and morphology. Prostate ultrasound showed a mean reduction of prostate volume from 29.9 cc to 21.9 cc, probably due to resolution of oedema.

Strada also reports that urethral strictures have been treated with GaAs laser, 10 sessions. Only patients with stricture diameters larger than 3 mm were treated. Five patients improved their micturation and flowmetry.

Male genital tract chronic inflammations were treated by Gasparyan [912] using combinations of transdermal, transrectal (prostate gland) and intravenous HeNe laser irradiation. The energy of a 2 mW HeNe laser was applied via a light guide into a vein. The projections of the male genital organ and the inguinal areas were irradiated with a 890 nm, 5W peak power cluster probe. For the transrectal prostate gland irradiation with a super-pulsed GaAs laser 890 nm, 15W peak power was used. In all 36 patients were given conventional medical therapy and another 36 were given LPT in combination with medical therapy. Clinical and laboratory findings were statistically better in the LPT group and relapse rate was lower. It is suggested that LPT increases the local circulation and thus also improves the effect of antibiotics.

Further literature: [142, 606, 684, 722, 920, 1202, 1647-1658]

4.1.58 Warts
LPT is widely used to treat common warts. The effect is not well documented and the results are inconsistent. The success rate in children is higher than in adults.

Further literature: [649, 1316]

4.1.59 Whiplash-associated disorders
In the experience of the authors, secondary muscular involvement can be successfully treated with LPT, whereas the primary problems will possibly require prolonged therapy. Reduced pain, improved sleep and reduced consumption of analgesics can be expected in most cases. Neck pain often has secondary consequences for masticatory dysfunction [2015], and LPT appears to be a promising and non-invasive method to approach these problems.

Literature:

Fitz-Ritson [392] compared three types of treatment for whiplash injury. The first group (17 patients) received joint manipulation and soft tissue therapy. The second group (18 patients) received the same treatment plus an exercise programme. The third group received the same treatment as group 2, plus InGaAlP laser light at 660 nm, 6 mW, and GaAlAs light at 880 nm, 8 mW **(possibly LED)**. *Extensor muscle strength was measured. The data*

lation and subpopulations of lymphocytes were evaluated. Endolymphatic irradiation was found to be more efficient than trans-scrotal LPT. The former required four procedures at intervals of 24 hours, whereas trans-scrotal irradiation required one to three days longer. Laser acupuncture was not effective.

Induratio penis plastica is a rare affection of the penis, even though occurrence is reported in 6 - 9% of the male population. The dual mechanism of the effect of laser treatment can be employed in implicating overproduction of fibrin (and its resorption), as well as in exerting a direct influence on inflammatory processes.

In a study by Prochazka [895], 40 patients were followed under a period of more than five years. Classic medicamentous techniques (colchicine, vitamin E) were combined with laser treatment of the following parameters: probes 200 and 300 mW, 50 J/cm^2 continuous mode + 50 J/cm^2 with the beam modulated to a 5 Hz pulse repetition rate in one therapy bout. The therapy was applied 20 times in succession, twice a week as an introductory series of procedures, followed by a maintenance series of three to five procedures 2 - 3 times a year. In combination with ultrasound, the total effect was very satisfactory.

Longo [608, 672] has treated some 100 cases of induration penis plastica with GaAs or defocused CO_2 laser. Circular and/or transversal plaque formation is a contra indication for LPT. In other milder forms, LPT can reduce pain, recurvatio, signs of inflammation and ecographic findings. The increase of elasticity during the erection is the first visible result of the treatment. Around 4 J per point has been used.

Johnson [770] reports the preliminary results of a non-randomised trial using a 30 mW GaAlAs laser to treat patients with symptomatic Peyronie's disease. All patients in the study had the disease, consisting of a well-defined fibrous plaque causing pain and/or curvature of the penile shaft when erected, which interfered with satisfactory sexual intercourse. 3 J per point was administered, beginning at the base of the penis and extending to the coronal sulcus over the dorsum of the penis at 0.5 cm intervals. An additional 3 J was delivered to each 0.5 cm of palpable plaque. The ability of the therapy to reduce the size of the fibrous plaque, the severity of the penile curvature, and the severity of pain associated with penile erection and the treatment's effect on the patient's quality of life were assessed for each patient at completion of therapy and six weeks later.

Strada [983] has treated nearly 300 patients with Peyronie's disease. GaAs laser treatment in combination with ultrasound was performed once a week for five weeks. All the patients showed pain reduction at the two-month control. A total of 60% reported a reduction of recurvatio penis. A group of patients underwent phlebocavernosometry, showing a disappearance of patches in 30% of the cases. Strada has also treated more than 200 patients with chronic abacterial prostatitis. A GaAs laser probe was used in an endorectal approach (every second day, 12 sessions) and a 30 mW GaAlAs

that low doses of laser light have a biostimulatory effect on the spermatogenesis and may provide benefits to the patients with oligospermia and azoospermia.

Corral-Baqués [1902] studied the effects on sperm motility of 655 nm continuous wave diode laser irradiation at different output powers with 3.34 J (5.97 J/cm^2). The second fraction of fresh dog sperm was divided into five groups: control, and four to be irradiated with an average output power of 6.8 mW, 15.4 mW, 33.1 mW and 49.7 mW, respectively. At 0 min and 45 min after irradiation, pictures were taken and a computer aided sperm analysis (CASA) was performed to analyse different motility parameters. The results showed that different output powers affected dog semen motility parameters differently. The highest output power showed the most intense effects. Significant changes in the structure of the motile sperm subpopulation were linked to the different output powers used.

Clinical studies

Hasan [141] used LPT on male infertility. The testicles of 25 childless men were irradiated with a combination of HeNe and GaAs light. Of these 25, 4 were azoospermic, 9 were highly oligospermic, and 7 were moderately oligospermic. No result was achieved in the azoospermic group, while in the oligospermic groups the sperm count increased by between 200% and 500%. Libido also increased in 15 of the oligospermic patients. Treatment was administered twice a week, a total of ten times. As sperm creation takes two to three months, the mechanism at work here is not known. LPT is, however, shown to be a supplementary method for subfertile men.

Kovalev [684] treated 55 men suffering from aspermatogenic sterility with HeNe laser. The results indicate a stimulating effect on the testicular function.

Uchida [146] treated 20 patients with chronic prostatitis or prostatodynia. GaAs laser was administered through the perineum or the rectum. In some cases, the acupuncture point Tsubo was used. In all 2 patients were freed from their symptoms completely, and 14 experienced good to average improvement. The soreness in the prostate disappeared in most of those who received irradiation through the rectum.

Mazo [338] has also reported on transrectal treatment of prostatic problems.

The effect of different approaches to LPT of acute non-specific epididymitis was studied by Gomberg [681]. In a previous study by Reznikov [682], trans-scrotal HeNe irradiation had proved beneficial. Gomberg compared trans-scrotal endolymphatic and laser acupuncture for the treatment of a group of 28 patients. The endolymphatic treatment was performed via a small quartz fibre inserted into the regional lymphatic node, 0.15 J in total. The transdermal dose used was at a maximum of 2.7 J. Laserpuncture (Hegu and Zusanli) was performed using a maximum of 30 J per point. The clinical outcome as well as the polymorphonucleocyte/lymphocyte index, main popu-

in bull sperm cells. It is concluded that the application of HeNe laser at doses from 2 to 16 J/cm^2 induced the acrosome reaction and decreased the bull sperm cell mortality percentage in vitro significantly better than the other capacitation agents, and as compared to the control group.

Sperm motility depends on energy consumption. Laser irradiation increases adenosin triphosphate (ATP) production and energy supply to the cell. The aim of a study by Corral-Baqués [1557] was to analyse whether the irradiation affects the parameters that characterise dog sperm motility. Fresh dog sperm samples were divided into four groups and irradiated with a 655 nm continuous wave diode laser with varying doses: 0 (control), 4, 6 and 10 J/cm^2. At 0, 15 and 45 min following irradiation, pictures were taken of all the groups in order to study motility with computer-aided sperm analysis. Functional tests were also performed. Average path velocity, linear coefficient and beat cross frequency were statistically and significantly different when compared to the control. The functional tests also showed a significant difference. At these parameters, the 655 nm continuous wave diode laser improves the speed and linear coefficient of the sperm.

Kipshidze [1041] used HeNe laser on human corpus cavernosum smooth muscle cells in vitro. Laser induced an increase in the expression of NO and an elevation of cyclic guanosine monophosphate (cGMP). This substance is important in the process of smooth muscle relaxation in the corpus cavernosum and consequently for the erection. It is suggested that LPT could be used in a combination with pharmaceuticals, or as the sole therapy for patients with coronary artery disease or hypertension.

Animal studies

Cohen [596] reports an enhanced fertilisation rate of mouse spermatozoa in vitro using 633 nm laser light. The results suggest that the effect of 633 nm HeNe laser irradiation is mediated through the generation of hydrogen peroxide by the spermatozoa, and that this effect plays a significant role in the augmentation of the sperm cell's capacity to fertilise in vitro.

The aim of the study by Taha [1548] was to determine the quantitative and qualitative changes of the seminiferous epithelium after 830 nm laser radiation. The left testes of rats were daily exposed to laser light for 15 days; so that the cumulative doses used were 28.05 and 46.80 J/cm^2 in two experimental groups. Samples collected 24 hours after the last treatment were processed for light microscopy and transmission electron microscopy scrutiny. The number of germ cells, specially the pachytene spermatocytes and elongated spermatids, increased after 28.05 J/cm^2 laser radiation. Ultrastructural features of germ and Sertoli cells in this group were similar to that of the control; while laser irradiation at 46.80 J/cm^2 had a destructive effect on the seminiferous epithelium such as dissociation of immature spermatids and evident ultrastructural changes in them. The findings confirmed the existence of a biostimulatory threshold of applied laser energy and the importance of determining it for clinical applications. Moreover, it was revealed

The post surgery complication rate was 32% in the laser group and 63% in the control group.

Zhuk [1141] divided a number of patients with chronic tuberculosis into two groups. One group (group I, 174 patients) received chemotherapy and another (group II, 240 patients) chemotherapy and laser irradiation, 890 nm. Transcutaneous irradiation over the lung projection and skin irradiation of great blood vessels were used. Dose at skin varied between 0.002-0.05 J/cm^2, depending on the pulse repetition rate used. Within three months, sputum smear conversation/cavity closure was observed in 60/36% of the patients in treatment group II, and in 36/16% in group I. After six months, the percentages were 85/65 % in group II and 49/29% in group I.

Dube [1563] investigated the effect of nitrogen laser irradiation (337 nm) on viability of clinical isolates of Mycobacterium tuberculosis. Bacteria were exposed to a nitrogen laser (average power 2.0 mW) in vitro at a power density of 70 ± 0.7 W/m^2 for 0-30 min, and the cell viability was determined by a luciferase reporter phage assay. Immediately after laser exposure, all the clinical isolates investigated showed a dose-dependent decrease in cell viability. However, when the laser-exposed isolates were incubated in broth medium for three days, most of these showed a significant recovery from laser-induced damage. An addition of 5.0 g/ml acriflavine (a DNA repair inhibitor) to the incubation medium had no significant effect on recovery. This suggests that DNA damage may not be involved in the cell inactivation. Electron paramagnetic resonance studies using 5-doxyl strearic acid as a probe suggest alterations in lipid regions of the cell wall.

Further literature: [710, 965, 966, 1177, 1540, 1642]

4.1.57 Urology

LPT appears to be a promising therapy for male infertility and for inflammation in the genital organs.

Literature:
In vitro studies

In a study by Lubart [592], it was found that 780 nm laser light inhibits Ca^{2+} uptake by sperm mitochondria and enhances Ca^{2+} binding to sperm plasma membranes. The effect of light on Ca^{2+} uptake by plasma membrane vesicles in the absence of ATP was much greater than in the presence of ATP.

Lubart [1196] found that HeNe laser irradiation of human spermatozoa resulted in a significant increase in its egg-penetration ability. The effect appeared only in men with low sperm penetration rates. Using the electron paramagnetic resonance technique it was established that OH radicals are produced in irradiated spermatozoa.

Sato [580] found that LPT increases the mobility and speed of sperm in vitro.

Ocaña-Quero [683] compared the effects of HeNe laser, calcium and heparin with regard to the induction of the acrosome reaction and mortality

given once a week for five weeks, 2 J per trigger point. At the end of the trial, 10 of the 14 patients in the verum group were free from pain and 2 improved. At the one-year follow-up, 6 patients were still free from pain and 10 were back to the initial condition. In the placebo group, 1 patient was free from pain and 2 improved at six months. At the one-year follow-up, 1 was still free from pain and the other 13 were back to the initial state of pain. Consumption of analgesics was significantly reduced in the verum group at the end of the treatment period but was constant in the placebo group. If the patient had already received alcohol blocks, the treatment was less successful.

The objective of a study by Takamoto [1481] was to evaluate the efficacy of LPT in cases of trigeminal pain. Thirty patients were evaluated, male and female, who were using 400 mg to 1200 mg/day of carbamazepin to control the pain. The patients were treated with a diode laser of 830 nm wavelength, 40 mW, continouos emission, spot area 3 mm^2, with a total of 20 joules per weekly session. The LPT demonstrated moderate efficacy over the pain, allowing a reduction in the quantity of carbamezepin in most of the cases. The laser and drug treatments together enabled control of the pain using a smaller quantity of medicines.

Further literature: [191, 211, 218, 444, 452, 509, 517, 595, 635, 755, 757, 758, 762, 1057, 1070, 1111]

4.1.55 Thrombophlebitis

Literature:

In a study by Dudenko [567], a HeNe laser was used to treat thrombophlebitis. The laser produced a marked analgesic, desensitising, hypocoagulative and immunostimulating effect.

4.1.56 Tuberculosis

In a Cohrane Meta analysis of the available literature on the subject, Vlassov [1283] concludes that there is no support for any effect of LPT on tuberculosis. The studies analysed contain a wide variety of lasers, doses, therapeutical approaches and co-interventions. However, the exact parameters are seldom accounted for.

Literature:

Bhagwanani [715] has used nitrogen laser (337 nm) for the treatment of tuberculosis in patients resistant to traditional antibiotics. A needle is inserted into the lung and used as the carrier of the light. Ten minutes of irradiation is often enough for a clinical improvement in 90% of the patients. Altogether 60% of the patients showed an improvement on their X-rays.

Agaev [716] compared the effect of HeNe laser treatment in two groups of patients with chronic destructive pulmonary tuberculosis or postoperative broncopulmonary complications. A group of 50 patients had HeNe laser treatment and a non-irradiated group of 30 patients served as control.

4.1.53 Tonsillitis
"Laser peeling" of the tonsils has successfully been used at the hospital of Halmstad, Sweden, using a carbon dioxide laser. Children are able to eat without problems within 30 minutes after therapy. Considering the low depth of penetration (0.1-0.3 mm), this must partially be an example of therapeutic laser effects.

Literature:
In a pilot study, Petrek [524] used a HeNe laser to treat eight patients suffering from chronic tonsillitis. Three treatment sessions were given over a period of nine days. Shortly after the cessation of treatment, a significant increase of secretory immunoglobulin A in saliva was observed, followed by an increase of IgA serum levels after four weeks of follow-ups. These findings correlated well with the clinical improvement in seven out of the eight patients.

Hubacek [1036] irradiated each palatal tonsil with a HeNe laser, 0.6 J/cm^2 for one week and found an increase of T lymphocytes and plasmatic cells in the tonsils after therapy.

Further literature: [700, 701, 707]

4.1.54 Trigeminal neuralgia
There are no entirely effective treatment methods for this painful condition. Laser treatment comes with no guarantee of success, but bearing in mind that the method is painless and without side effects, it should be a more attractive initial choice than deep blockades and strong analgesics. Patients receiving LPT can often reduce their Carbamazepine dose. All three laser types can be used.

Both extraoral and intraoral trigger points and pain points are irradiated. A total of 2-3 J per standard point (standard points are the various foramina, such as the infraorbital, supraorbital, mental, mandibular, palatinum major, and incisivum) is an appropriate initial dosage. Pain points can be given 3-4 J. The course of the main nerve is then irradiated extra- or intraorally. When irradiating through bone, as with the n. mandibularis inferior, the dose must be increased by a factor of three to compensate for loss of penetration. A pain reaction is not unusual and should be interpreted as a positive sign. Patients should be warned about its likelihood beforehand. Treat twice a week initially and then allow a longer period between treatments. Treatment should not be interrupted if and when the pain disappears, but should continue at longer and longer intervals.

Literature:
Eckerdal [452, 595] used 830 nm laser light at 30 mW in a double-blind study of the effect of LPT on trigeminal neuralgia. A positive effect was evident. It is necessary to find the pertinent trigger points/zones and to include the II branch of the trigeminal nerve in the treatment. Treatment was

Therapy

9. Training in how to normalise abnormal head/neck posture ("vulture neck"), and training in how to relax masticatory, neck and shoulder muscles.

10. Training of autostretching of the suboccipital muscles (the rectus capitis posterior minor and major muscles and the obliquus capitis superior muscles), the upper and middle trapezius muscles and the levator scapulae muscles. LPT of tender areas in these muscles is also recommended.

11. Examination of occlusal function and presence of active interferences, followed by adjustment through selective grinding. The examination should preferably be performed with the patient in an upright position. Interferences in the central occlusion and in the retruded position are eliminated. Patient feedback is useful. Once the patient has experienced the positive feeling of having the occlusion improved, he/she will become quite aware of even minute interferences. It is typical to find a tender lateral pterygoid on one side and the "high" tooth on the contra-lateral side.

12. Information about the necessity of adjusting the patient's life style (stress).

13. Laser treatment of tender areas in the jaw and neck muscles, 5-15 J per point depending on the size and location of the muscle. Two to three sessions per week acc. to the evolution of improvement, with GaAlAs or GaAs laser.

14. Bite splint in selected cases.

15. Stop all intakes of analgesics in patients with bruxing habits. The use of analgesics can in many cases cause the patient to press the teeth even harder.

Common dental occlusal backgrounds:

16. The patient is clenching/bruxing on active shining facets of the front teeth, forcing the TMJ:s backwards in the fossa. This initiates a nociceptive reflex from the lateral pterygoid, trying to move the TMJ:s forwards.

17. Cross bite (sliding areas preventing central occlusion and balanced TMJ position).

18. Patients having had extractions of premolars for orthodontic reasons.

19. Crowns or bridges are a little bit too high. This may have been already on the initial crown or as a later effect, due to the fact that the abrasion rate of the material of the crown is less than that of the natural teeth.

Somatosensory tinnitus examination and therapy

Anamnesis

1 Does the patient experience a feeling of fatigue in the jaws, difficulties in mouth opening, sensations of tension in the jaws/neck, hypersensitive or tender teeth, clenching of tongue/jaws, tendency for general stress, or waking up at night due to tinnitus?

2 Can the patient manipulate his/her tinnitus through movements of the jaw and neck? Usual movements evoking this phenomenon are: opening the mouth wide, protrusion and side movements of the mandible, flexion/extension and side rotation of the upper cervical joints.

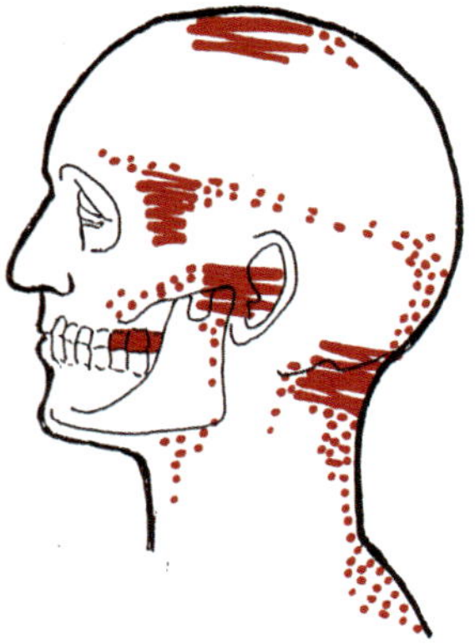

3 Can the patient manipulate his/her tinnitus by putting pressure/stimulation in the areas of the sensory innervation of the trigeminal nerve? Usual areas evoking this phenomenon are putting pressure on tragus, over the cheek, jaw or temple and the stylomandibular ligament, but also gazing with the eyes.

4 Are there other symptoms related to tension: pain in the jaws, face, neck, and headache?

Figure 4.20 The predominant tender areas.
Courtesy: Assar Bjorne

Status

5 Observation of hypertrophic masticatory muscles and possible abnormal posture of the head/neck ("Vulture neck", C7). The physiotherapist will frequently find tender areas in the upper trapezius.

6 Palpation of the masticatory muscles (the lateral pterygoid muscle in particular), the TMJ, and the suboccipital muscles.

7 Range of movement of the mandible and neck.

8 Active shining bruxing facets as signs of active bruxism.

The aim of a study by Tullberg [1890] was to investigate the presence of symptoms and signs of temporomandibular disorders (TMD) in patients with tinnitus, and to evaluate the effect of TMD treatment on tinnitus in a long-term perspective in comparison with a control group of patients on a waiting list. One hundred twenty patients with tinnitus were subjected to a clinical examination of the masticatory system and whether they had coexisting TMD to TMD treatment. Ninety-six patients had TMD, most frequently localized myalgia. Seventy-three of these completed the treatment and responded to a questionnaire two years later. Fifty patients with tinnitus who were on the waiting list served as a control group. Eighty percent of the patients had signs of TMD, most commonly myofascial pain. Forty-three percent of the patients reported that their tinnitus was improved at the two-year follow-up, 39% that it was unchanged, and 17% that it was impaired compared to before the treatment. Twelve percent of the subjects in the control group reported that their tinnitus was improved compared to two years previously, 32% that it was unchanged, and 56% that it was impaired. The difference between groups was significant. In conclusion, these results showed that TMD symptoms and signs are frequent in patients with tinnitus and that TMD treatment has a good effect on tinnitus in a long-term perspective, especially in patients with fluctuating tinnitus.

The suboccipital muscles should also be palpated, since these muscles and the masticatory muscles are closely functionally connected. In fact, the mandible and the upper cervical joint (C0/C1) constitute an integrated motor system. This area is often tender to palpation. The patient should be made aware of his/her posture and taught to perform stretching exercises. Attention should be given to the posture of the patient, and tenderness and protrusion of C7 ("vulture neck") should be observed and corrected. Tenderness in the suboccipital and/or C7 is often related to vertigo.

Tinnitus patients have a higher incidence of TMD problems [1488, 1722, 1723, 1724], so the participation of a dentist in the therapy is important.

The therapy outlined below brings new hope to a large group of "intractable" patients. It outlines the traditional therapy created by Bjorne, with the recent (year 2000) successful addition of LPT. Patients suffering from somatosensory tinnitus often live in a therapeutic "void". Many medical doctors are not aware of this connection and most dentists alike. And the patient is not likely to inform the dentist, believing that the condition has nothing to do with dentistry. A first step on the road is to include questions about tinnitus into the standard anamnestic questionaire.

sudden sensorineural hearing loss and muscular (TMD - Temporo-Mandibular Disorders) conditions, as reported by Axelsson [1633].

The percentage of patients with a muscular origin for their tinnitus/vertigo is not known but seems to be large. A differential diagnosis is therefore important before any therapy is applied; whether laser or traditional therapies. If this is not done, studies of the effect of transmeatal LPT become a gamble. The outcome would rather be related to the type of tinnitus dominating in the verum group than the actual effect of the therapy. An interdisciplinary co-operation between the ENT physician, a physiotherapist and a dentist is ideal.

Meniere's disease is a condition first described by the French physician Ménière in 1861. It is a clinical entity consisting of vertigo, fluctuating hearing loss and tinnitus. Few medical conditions have been so thoroughly studied and described, yet lacking an effective therapy. Tinnitus, however, is not necessarily associated with Meniere; it is often an isolated condition. But the treatment of somatosensory Meniere and somatosensory tinnitus is very similar. We will therefore, in the following text, simplify the terms and speak only about "tinnitus".

Muscular tension is a key element in somatosensory tinnitus. The role of the laser is to create an immediate reduction of muscle pain through consecutive relaxation. Thus, this intervention will make all the following therapy faster and more successful. Somatosensory tinnitus has been difficult to treat and is often passed by without a diagnosis. The combination of LPT in the traditional therapy of temporomandibular disorders (TMD) and cervical spine disorders (CSD) has been reported to be a more successful way of helping these patients, compared to traditional therapies. However, it is not to be expected that all symptoms will subdue rapidly. The skill of the dentist, the co-operation of the patient and the concomitant physiotherapy are all important factors. Many patients will not be completely relieved of symptoms, but the majority will experience a great reduction of their problems.

According to Bjorne [1263] and Estola-Partanen [1267], the treatment of somatosensory tinnitus reduces the severity of tinnitus more than the incidence. The three-year follow-up study by Bjorne [1263] showed simultaneous decreases in the intensities of vertigo, non-whirling dizziness, tinnitus, feeling of fullness in the ear, pain in the face and jaws, pain in the neck and shoulders, and headache that were both longitudinal and highly significant. Significant reductions in the frequency of vertigo, non-whirling dizziness and headache were also reported by the patients as well as a complete disappearance of pain located in the vertex area. A significant relief of TMD symptoms and a decrease in nervousness were also achieved. It must be underlined that the success in the study [1263] reflects the outcome of the therapy before the author started to use LPT as an additional method. The addition of LPT has then further improved the progress in this category of patients. Frequently, these patients can notice a change in the character of their tinnitus when the lateral pterygoid muscle is irradiated.

loudness, duration and degree of annoyance of tinnitus, was accepted to represent an improvement. The loudness, duration and degree of annoyance of tinnitus were improved, respectively, in up to 48.8, 57.7 and 55.5% of the patients in the active laser group. No significant improvement was observed in the placebo laser group.

The objectives of a study by Rhee [1919] were: 1: To investigate preventive effects of LPT on gentamicin-induced vestibular ototoxicity. 2: To evaluate the effectiveness of LPT in the treatment of tinnitus. Twenty guinea pigs were divided into control and laser groups. Vestibular ototoxicity was induced by intratympanic injection of gentamicin into the left ear. LPT was irradiated into the left ear canal of the animals in the laser group. Vestibular function of the animals was evaluated with vertical and off-vertical axis rotation testing. 2: Forty patients with tinnitus were treated with ginkgo biloba orally and randomly divided into control and laser groups. In a clinical study, twenty patients of the laser group received 80.4 J/cm^2 of a 830 nm laser, three times per week for four weeks, via transmeatal irradiation. Tinnitus was evaluated by visual analogue scale (VAS) and tinnitus handicap inventory (THI). Results: 1. Preventive effect of LLL to gentamicin induced vestibular ototoxicity was demonstrated by preventing reduction of gain in a slow harmonic acceleration test and modulation in the off-vertical axis rotation test. 2. Eleven out of twenty laser group patients have shown significant improvement in VAS and THI compared to those in the control group. Conclusions are: 1. LPT therapy may have a preventive effect on vestibular ototoxicity. 2. LPT therapy in combination with ginkgo biloba seems to be worth trying on patients with tinnitus.

In the clinical study by Cuda [1923], 47 patients suffering from tinnitus, mean age 56 years, were divided into two groups. One group received 5 mW red laser and the other group placebo laser, 20 minutes per day for four months. After the active period, 16 patients in the laser group had a 60% improvement on the Tinnitus Handicap Inventory VAS scale, which was significantly different from the patients in the placebo group.

Fridberger [1884] writes: "Light produces force when interacting with matter. Such radiation pressure may be used to accelerate small objects along the beam path of a laser. Here, we demonstrate that a moderately powerful laser can deliver enough force to locally stimulate the hearing organ, in the absence of conventional sound. Damped mechanical oscillations are observed following brief laser pulses, implying that the organ of Corti is locally resonant. This new method will be helpful for probing the mechanical properties of the hearing organ, which have crucial importance for the ear's ability to detect sound."

Further literature: [874, 1174, 1227, 1228, 1599, 1883]

All the above studies assume that tinnitus and vertigo are always inner ear problems. However, these conditions frequently have a muscular origin ("somatosensory tinnitus"). There also seems to be a correlation between

gical access. The fibre is fixed in place and was not in direct contact with cochlear structures. Stimulation threshold was measured as 0.018+/-0.003 J/cm^2. Laser radiation could be increased by 30-40 dB until drastic changes were seen in cochlear function. Cochlear response amplitudes to optical radiation were stable over extended stimulation times. The experiments showed that it is possible to stimulate the auditory nerve with optical radiation. No neural damage could be detected even after hours of continual stimulation. It may be argued that optical radiation stimulates outer or inner hair cells. However, the results from experiments with deafened animals support the view that auditory neurons are stimulated directly. If hair cells were involved in optical stimulation of auditory neurons, the optical CAP amplitude should have decreased drastically concurrent with the increase in acoustic thresholds. Moreover, it was possible to optically evoke CAPs after hair cells were destroyed by neomycin injection in the chronic deafened animals.

Twenty patients with unilateral Ménière's Disease (MD) were included in a study [1861]; all presented with uncontrolled vertigo. The patients were randomly divided into two groups: In group 1, the patients received LPT 20 min a day with a 5 mW red laser for six months, while group 2 received 16 mg βhistine twice a day for six months. According to American Academy of Otolaryngology-Head and Neck Surgery (AAO-HNS) guidelines, the main outcome for vertigo control was considered to be the number of spells per month in a six-month period before treatment compared with the same parameters during six months of therapy. The duration of spells expressed in minutes was also considered. Moreover, a hearing test was performed before and after therapy and results were reported as the pure tone average of 500-, 1000-, 2000-, and 3000 Hz frequencies. All results were valued at baseline, and after three and six months of therapy. Compared to baseline, the number and duration of spells were significantly reduced in both groups; statistical significance was detected for the three-month control in both groups. Betahistine seems to work faster in spell reduction. Audiometric examination did not show a statistically significant difference between the two groups. In the experience of the researchers, LPT seems to prevent vertigo spells in MD, although results indicate that it works slower than betahistine. Dose-dependent therapeutic effects could explain the last result. The authors speculate that increased blood flow in the inner ear is the main mechanism leading to the therapeutic results.

The objective in a study by Gungor [1885] was to evaluate the effectiveness of 5 mW laser irradiation in the treatment of chronic tinnitus in a prospective, randomised, double-blind study. This investigation included 66 ears in 45 patients with chronic unilateral or bilateral tinnitus. A 5 mW laser with a wavelength of 650 nm, or placebo laser, was applied transmeatally for 15 minutes, once daily for a week. A questionnaire was administered which asked patients to score their symptoms on a five-point scale, before and two weeks after laser irradiation. A decrease of one scale point, regarding the

Eight of the ten treated tinnitus patients also suffering from chronic hyperacusis claimed they had improvements on hyperacusis levels. Based upon that a prospective, unblinded, uncontrolled, clinical trial was planned and conducted. ROS and hyperacusis pain thresholds were measured. The patients were treated twice a week with a combination of therapeutic laser, rTMS and the control the and adjustment ROS. A magnetic field of a maximum of 100 µT was oriented behind the outer ear, in the area of the mastoid bone. ROS were measured and controlled by administrating different antioxidants. Every treatment session 177-504 J of laser light of two different wavelengths was administrated towards the inner ear via meatus acusticus. The improvements were significantly better in the verum group than in a placebo group where 40% of the patients were expected to get a positive treatment effect. The patients in the long-term follow-up group received significantly greater improvements than the patients in the short-term follow-up group.

A pilot study was performed by Gable [1224] on three individuals who were suffering from Chronic Otitis Externa, "Swimmer's ear" or "Tropical Ear", which had been unresponsive to conservative medical management for a minimum period of three months. Each patient was classed as chronic and referred by a medical practitioner for LPT. Each patient was irradiated over a two to six week period with a progressively increasing energy of 15 to 30 Joules via the single source of the ear canal using a 100 mW probe. Allowing for beam divergence within the confined canal, reflection and inverse square spread from the emission source to the tympanic membrane; these factors would roughly balance, equating to an approximate energy density dose of 15-30 J/cm^2. The individual patient's existing medical regime was continued unchanged. Each patient showed full condition resolution for a minimum period of one month post discharge. Two of the patients were swimmers, one competitive at state level. In both cases it enabled the individuals to return to swimming within one to three weeks of treatment commencing, and to remain in the water during the completion of the treatment period through to full resolution and post discharge follow-up at one month. On a six-month follow-up of one patient, a 9-year-old boy with grommets and a life history of ongoing ear infections, had remained infection free for the first time for a period longer than six weeks. A secondary effect was a reduction of motion sickness, indicating that the LPT had also affected the cochlear and vestibular apparatus.

Acute in vivo experiments using gerbils were conducted by Izzo [1749] to record optically evoked compound action potentials (CAPs) from the cochlea. Optical radiation evokes CAPs in normal hearing animals and in deafened animals, in which cochleae lack outer and inner hair cells. The optical source was a Ho:YAG laser, with a wavelength of 2120 nm, pulse duration of 250 microseconds, operating at 2 Hz. The laser output was coupled to a low-OH 100-mm-diameter optical fibre. The optical fibre was inserted at the basal turn of the cochlea, approximated to the round window membrane and visually oriented toward the modiolus as allowed by the sur-

have therapeutic benefits for patients with high-frequency sensorineural hearing loss.

In a further study, Wenzel [1797] writes: The cochlea is the mammalian organ of hearing. Its predominant vibratory element, the basilar membrane, is tonotopically tuned, based on the spatial variation of its mass and stiffness. The constituent collagen fibers of the basilar membrane affect its stiffness. Laser irradiation can induce collagen remodeling and deposition in various tissues. We tested whether similar effects could be induced within the basilar membrane. Trypan blue was perfused into the scala tympani of anesthetized mice to stain the basilar membrane. We then irradiated the cochleas with a 694 nm pulsed ruby laser at 15 or 180 J/cm². The mice were sacrificed 14 to 16 days later and collagen organization was studied. Polarization microscopy revealed that laser irradiation increased the birefringence within the basilar membrane in a dose-dependent manner. Electron microscopy demonstrated an increase in the density of collagen fibers and the deposition of new fibrils between collagen fibers after laser irradiation. As an assessment of hearing, auditory brainstem response (ABR) thresholds were found to increase moderately after 15 J/cm² and substantially after 180 J/cm². Our results demonstrate that collagen remodeling and new collagen deposition occurs within the basilar membrane after laser irradiation in a similar fashion to that found in other tissues.

The hearing performance with conventional hearing aids and cochlear implants is dramatically reduced in noisy environments and for sounds more complex than speech (e. g. music), partially due to the lack of localized sensorineural activation across different frequency regions with these devices. Laser light can be focused in a controlled manner and may provide more localized activation of the inner ear, the cochlea. Wenzel [2098] sought to assess whether visible light with parameters that could induce an optoacoustic effect (532 nm, 10-ns pulses) would activate the cochlea. Auditory brainstem responses (ABRs) were recorded preoperatively in anesthetized guinea pigs to confirm normal hearing. After opening the bulla, a 50-mum core-diameter optical fiber was positioned in the round window niche and directed toward the basilar membrane. Optically induced ABRs (OABRs), similar in shape to those of acoustic stimulation, were elicited with single pulses. The OABR peaks increased with energy level (0.6 to 23 mJ/pulse) and remained consistent even after 30 minutes of continuous stimulation at 13 mJ, indicating minimal or no stimulation-induced damage within the cochlea. These findings demonstrate that visible light can effectively and reliably activate the cochlea without any apparent damage.

A few other indications in otorhinolaryngology have been treated with lasers, even with intravenous irradiation. [688, 689, 690, 1095, 1096].

The objective of the study by Zazzio [1622] was to investigate if LPT in combination with pulsed electromagnetic field therapy/repetitive transcranial magnetic stimulation (rTMS) and the control of Reactive Oxygen Specimen (ROS) would lead to positive treatment results for hyperacusis patients.

bilobae preparations (73%) or Betahistadine (39%) and also had physical therapy, mainly directed at the neck vertebrae. LPT was performed with a 300 mW GaAlAs laser, 75 J/cm^2 into the ear and 135 J/cm^2 behind the ear. The outcome was: no more tinnitus 26%, more than 50% relief 43%, less than 50% relief 15%, no effect 16%. In addition, a group of 31 patients were selected for a double blind study where the same therapy as above was performed, but one group received placebo laser. At six months the outcome was as follows, with laser/no laser: no more tinnitus 25.8%/0.0%, more than 50% relief 35.5%/25.8%, less than 50% relief 19.4%/48.4%, no effect 19.4%/25.8%.

Hahn [1310] examined 120 patients with an average tinnitus duration of 10 years. The patients underwent pure-tone audiometry, speech audiometry and objective audiometry tests. The intensity and frequency of tinnitus were also determined. EGb 761 was administered three weeks before the start of LPT. The patients underwent 10 sessions of LPT, each lasting 10 minutes. An improvement in tinnitus was audiometrically confirmed in 50.8% of the patients; 10 dB in 18, 20 dB in 22, 30 dB in 10, 40 dB in 6 and 50 dB in 5 patients.

Rogowski [1094] divided a group of 32 tinnitus patients into one group receiving LPT and one receiving a placebo procedure. The 890 nm laser irradiation, 3000 Hz, was performed via the meatus with a maximum dose of 2,3 J/cm^2, and via the mastoid with a maximum dose of 0,028 J/cm^2. Ten daily sessions were given. The effect was evaluated through VAS. Transiently evoked otoacoustic emissions (TEOAE) were measured before, during and after therapy. No significant difference between laser and placebo was found in annoyance or loudness of the tinnitus and in changes of TEOAE amplitude. These results indicate that there is no relationship between the effect of low-power laser and changes in cochlear micromechanics **at these very low doses.**

LPT of the cochlea has been shown to modify the collagen organisation within the cochlea and also in the basilar membrane. Wenzel [1434] excised four guinea pig cochleae. These were stained with trypan blue. Two were irradiated with a 600 nm pulsed dye laser and two were used as controls. Collagen organization was visualized using a polarisation microscopy. Laser irradiation reduced the birefringence within the basilar membrane as well as within other stained collagen-containing structures. Larger reductions in birefringence were measured when more laser pulses were given. The effects were similar across all turns of each cochlea. Laser irradiation causes immediate alterations in collagen organization within the cochlea that can be visualized with a polarisation microscopy. These alterations may affect cochlear tuning. As would be expected, increased basilar membrane stiffness shifted the resonant frequency towards higher frequencies. Doubling basilar membrane stiffness raised the resonant frequency by a factor of 1.5 (from 1 to 1.5 kHz at the apex and from 20 to 30 kHz at the base). Doses were 5-30 J/cm^2. The author writes that it is conceivable that this technique may

Wilden [474, 1089] has pioneered a different method with a considerably increased dose. A set consisting of one visible laser and three powerful GaAlAs lasers is used, covering a large area over and around the ear in the non-contact mode. Doses between 3000 and 5000 J are given each session. Laser is applied as a monotherapy. More than 800 patients have been treated with this concept and positive effects are reported even for vertigo. Recent injuries in "the disco generation" are more easily treated than long-term chronic conditions. In a separate study [1090], Wilden reports improved hearing capacity in these patients, as evaluated by audiometry.

Tauber [1091] has performed an ex-vivo laser penetration study. Based on these findings, it was possible to calculate the energy needed to obtain a dose of 4 J/cm^2 in the cochlea itself. Irradiation via the mastoid showed values 103 to 105 times smaller (depending on wavelength) than irradiation through the tympanic membrane.

The above feasibility study presented a laser application system enabling dose-controlled transmeatal cochlear laser-irradiation (TCL). It was followed by preliminary clinical results in patients with chronic cochlear tinnitus [1092]. The laser TCL-system, consisting of four diode lasers (635 nm - 830 nm) and a new specific head-set applicator, was developed on the basis of dosimetric data from the former light-dosimetric study. In a preliminary clinical study, the TCL-system was applied to 35 patients with chronic tinnitus and sensorineural hearing loss. The chronic symptoms persisted after standard therapeutic procedures for at least six months, while retrocochlear or middle-ear pathologies have been ruled out. The patients were randomised and received five single diode laser treatments (635nm, 7.8 mW CW, n=17 and 830 nm, 20 mW CW, n=18) of 4 J/cm^2 at the site of the supposed maximal cochlear injury. For evaluation of laser-induced effects, complete otolaryngologic examinations with audiometry, tinnitus masking and matching, and a tinnitus-self-assessment were performed before, during and after the laser irradiation. The first clinical use of the TCL-system has been well tolerated without side-effects and produced no observable damage to the external, middle or inner ear. After a follow-up period of six months tinnitus loudness was attenuated in 13 of 35 irradiated patients, while 2 of 35 patients reported their tinnitus as totally absent. Hearing threshold levels and middle ear function remained unchanged.

Prochazka [1093] has evaluated the effect of combined Egb 761 Ginkgo infusion and laser in a blind study. A total of 37 patients were divided into three groups. One group was given Egb 761 only, one Egb761 and placebo laser, and one Egb761 and real laser, 830 nm. The results in the three groups were as follows: no effect 29/26/19, less than 50% relief 44/48/29, more than 50% relief 18/26/36, no more tinnitus 9/0/26. Irradiation was performed over the mastoid and over the meatus acousticus, twice a week, 8-10 sessions.

In an extended study over three years, Prochazka [1263] evaluated the effect of laser in a group of 200 patients. These patients were taking gingko

applied at a distance of one cm above the mastoid. The non-contact mode reduces penetration considerably and the mastoid is not ideal for reaching the inner ear.

Plath [306] treated 40 tinnitus patients with 50 mg ginkgo biloba; 20 patients received sham laser irradiation, 20 real laser. A HeNe laser with 12 mW output and a GaAs laser with five laser diodes, each with an average power output of 15 mW, were used; the irradiation procedure being approximately the same as for Partheniadis-Stumpf. In this study, however, 50% of the patients reported a reduction of the tinnitus by more than 10 dB, as compared with 5% in the control group, in both self-assessment and audiometric findings.

A similar study has been performed by von Wedel [1087]. One hundred fifty-five patients were treated with ginkgo infusion (5 ml Syxyl D3) and laser. The outcome was negative. **No information about the type of laser, treatment technique or dosage is given, making an evaluation impossible. However, in a book by Stennert, published by Louis Calero, Cologne, Germany, we have found the following: Laser parameters were HeNe 12 mW, GaAs five diodes, each of 30 W peak power. Average output at 1200 Hz 5.4 mW, 8.1 mW at 1800 Hz. Total dose at 1200 Hz 2.59 J, 3.88 J at 1800 Hz, power density for HeNe 17.4 mW/cm^2. Treatment via the mastoid at a distance of 2 cm from the skin. Total irradiation time per session eight minutes, 3 sessions per week, total number of sessions 12. Total dose of GaAs 77.64 J (at skin). HeNe has no possibility of reaching the cochlea via the mastoid and can be overlooked, except for a possible systemic effect.**

Shiomi [686] has investigated the effect of infrared laser applied directly into the meatus acousticus, 21 J, once a week for 10 weeks. The result of this non-controlled study is as follows: 26% of the patients reported improved duration, 58% reduced loudness, and 55% reported a general reduction in annoyance.

The same author [687] has also examined the effect of light on the cochlea using guinea pigs. Direct laser irradiation was administered to the cochlea through the round window. The amplitude of CAP was reduced to 53-83% immediately after the onset of irradiation. The amplitude then returned to the original level. The results of this investigation suggest that LPT might lessen tinnitus by suppressing the abnormal excitation of the eighth nerve of the organ of Corti.

More or less the same parameters were used in a controlled study by Mirtz [1088], but in this case there was no significant effect.

Nakashima [1266] treated 68 ears in 68 patients with tinnitus. A 60 mW laser was applied for six minutes (21.6 J), once a week for four weeks in a double-blind study. There was no significant difference between the two groups, which is not surprising considering the few sessions and the low energy applied. **No differential diagnosis between somatosensory and other causes of tinnitus was performed.**

4.1.52 Tinnitus, vertigo, Ménière´s disease

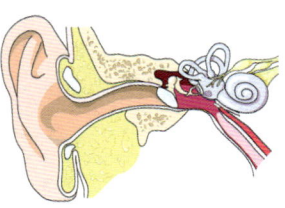

A new and promising indication for LPT is tinnitus. This supposed inner ear condition seems to be a growing problem in our noisy, modern society, and the number of persons suffering from tinnitus seems to be increasing. Traditional treatments for tinnitus include psychological support or various masking procedures. Acupuncture and ginko extracts have been tried with limited success. LPT alone offers a new and promising treatment modality. Irradiation is given partly through the meatus, partly behind the ear; provided the problem really is located in the inner ear. Since the bone behind the ear is very compact, high power densities and prolonged treatment times are necessary to reach a sufficient dose in the inner ear when irradiating through the bone. The dose at target depends on wavelength, power density, the distance between the laser eye and tissue, and the contact or pressure technique used. When irradiating through the meatus, the distance from the ear drum and the direction of the beam are important. The main objective is to obtain a reasonable dose at target, but since the variation in the mentioned parameters is so great, the discussion about the optimal therapy becomes rather confusing. Applying high energies (Joules) does not automatically mean that the dose at target (J/cm^2) is high. The laser should not give any unpleasant sensations of heat or pressure in the ear. If doing so, the power density should be reduced. This can easily be done by just distancing the probe a centimeter or so from the ear, unless the beam is collimated.

A closer look at the literature will reveal many studies using low to very low doses. Further, some studies do not give enough information even to make an estimation of the dose possibly used.

Literature:

Witt [1084] is one of the pioneers in this field, but to the knowledge of the authors, his results have not been published in any peer-review journals. Witt combines infusion of Gingko biloba (Egb 761, 17.5 mg dry extract per 5 ml ampoule) and laser. This may be a favourable combination, but an evaluation of the contribution of the laser is not possible. More than 500 patients have been treated since 1989 and Witt claims that more than 60% of the patients have attained a considerable or total relief. The laser used is a combination of a HeNe laser with a 12 mW output and a GaAs laser with five laser diodes, each with an average power output of 15 mW. **Treatment technique is not stated but is supposed to be via the mastoid.**

Swoboda [1085] did not find any significant effect of gingko/laser. However, the ginkgo infusion used was at a homeopathic level (D3 = 1:1000 dilution), according to Witt.

Partheniadis-Stumpf [1086] also failed to find any effect from the combined ginkgo (6 ml Tebonin) infusion and laser. However, the laser was

at those same intervals; (3) a significant decrease in disability of arm, shoulder, and hand questionnaire (DASH) scores at the end of 8 wk of treatment, and at 16 wk posttreatment; and (4) a significant decrease in health-assessment questionnaire (HAQ) scores at the end of 4 wk and 8 wk of treatment. There was some improvement in range of motion, but this did not reach statistical significance.

In a feasability study by Tumilty [1987], 20 patients were randomized into an active laser group or a placebo group; all patients, therapists, and investigators were blinded to allocation. All patients were given a 12-week eccentric exercise program and irradiated three times per week for 4 wk with either an active or placebo laser at standardized points over the affected tendons. Irradiation parameters in the active treatment group were: 810 nm, 100 mW, applied to six points on the tendon for 30 s, with a total dose of 3 J per point and 18 J per session. Outcome measures used were the VISA-A questionnaire, pain, and isokinetic strength. Patients were measured before treatment and at 4 and 12 wk. Within groups, there were significant improvements at 4 and 12 wk for all outcome measures, except eccentric strength for the placebo group at 4 wk.

The aim of the analysis of Tumilty [2110] was to assess the clinical effectiveness of LPT in the treatment of tendinopathy. Secondary objectives were to determine the relevance of irradiation parameters to outcomes, and the validity of current dosage recommendations for the treatment of tendinopathy. The following databases were searched from inception to 1(st) August 2008: MEDLINE, PubMed, CINAHL, AMED, EMBASE, All EBM reviews, PEDro, SCOPUS. Controlled clinical trials evaluating LPT as a primary intervention for any tendinopathy were included in the review. Methodological quality was classified as: high (>/=6 out of 10 on the PEDro scale) or low (<6) to grade the strength of evidence. Accuracy and clinical appropriateness of treatment parameters were assessed using established recommendations and guidelines. Twenty-five controlled clinical trials met the inclusion criteria. There were conflicting findings from multiple trials: 12 showed positive effects and 13 were inconclusive or showed no effect. Dosages used in the 12 positive studies would support the existence of an effective dosage window that closely resembled current recommended guidelines. In two instances where pooling of data was possible, LPT showed a positive effect size; in studies of lateral epicondylitis that scored >/=6 on the PEDro scale, participants' grip strength was 9.59 kg higher than that of the control group; for participants with Achilles tendinopathy, the effect was 13.6 mm less pain on a 100 mm visual analogue scale. Conclusion: LPT can potentially be effective in treating tendinopathy when recommended dosages are used. The 12 positive studies provide strong evidence that positive outcomes are associated with the use of current dosage recommendations for the treatment of tendinopathy.

(Also see chapter 4.1.19 "Epicondylitis" on page 230.)
Further literature: [195, 242, 736, 737, 1961]

same exercise protocol was given for the same time period. Patients were evaluated according to the parameters of pain, palpation sensitivity, algometric sensitivity, and shoulder joint range of motion before and after treatment. Analysis of measurement results within each group showed a significant post treatment improvement for some active and passive movements in both groups, and also for algometric sensitivity in Group I. Post treatment palpation sensitivity values showed improvement in 17 patients (85%) for Group I and in 6 patients (30%) for Group II. A comparison between the two groups showed superior results in Group I for the parameters of passive extension and palpation sensitivity, but no significant difference for the other parameters. **This study has been criticized by Bjordal [1740] for lack of parameter control. The given dose of 2.98 J/cm^2 is probably anything between 0.3 and 0.7 J/cm^2. WALT recommendation for muskoloskeletal pain is a minimum of 2 J/cm^2 per point for 904 nm.**

In the study by Stergioulas (180 seconds per point), a total of 52 recreational athletes with chronic Achilles tendinopathy symptoms were randomized to groups receiving either Eccentric Exercises (EE) + LPT or EE + placebo LPT over 8 weeks in a blinded manner. LPT (820 nm, 30 mW) was administered in 12 sessions by irradiating six points along the Achilles tendon with a power density of 60 mW/cm^2 and a total dose of 5.4 J per session. The results of the intention-to-treat analysis for the primary outcome, pain intensity during physical activity on the 100-mm visual analog scale, were significantly lower in the LPT group than in the placebo LPT group, with 53.6 mm versus 71.5 mm at 4 weeks, 37.3 mm versus 62.8 mm at 8 weeks, and 33.0 mm versus 53.0 mm at 12 weeks after randomization. Secondary outcomes of morning stiffness, active dorsiflexion, palpation tenderness, and crepitation showed the same pattern in favor of the LPT group. LPT, with the parameters used in this study, accelerates clinical recovery from chronic Achilles tendinopathy when added to an EE regimen. For the LPT group, the results at 4 weeks were similar to the placebo LPT group's results after 12 weeks. An important feature of this study is the low power density and long irradiation time used to target the inflammation rather than the pain.

In another study by Stergioulas [1878], 63 patients with a frozen shoulder condition were randomly assigned to one of two groups. In the active laser group (n=31), patients were treated with a 810 nm laser with a continuous output of 60 mW, applied to 8 points on the shoulder for 30 sec each, for a total dose of 1.8 J per point and 14.4 J per session. In the placebo group (n=32), patients received placebo laser treatment. During 8 wk of treatment, the patients in each group received 12 sessions of laser or placebo, 2 sessions per week (for weeks 1-4), and 1 session per week (for weeks 5-8). Relative to the placebo group, the active laser group had: (1) a significant decrease in overall, night, and activity pain scores at the end of 4 wk and 8 wk of treatment, and at the end of 8 wk additional follow-up (16 wk post-randomization); (2) a significant decrease in shoulder pain and disability index (SPADI) scores and Croft shoulder disability questionnaire scores

further analysis. Real Time PCR was employed to evaluate COX-1 and COX-2 expression in tendons. PGE2 production was measured by commercial ELISA kits. A low level of COX-1 RNA expression was attained after collagenase injection. On the other hand, a high and significant level of COX-2 expression in tendon tissue, occurring two hours after collagenase injection, was observed. Although COX-2 expression was much more pronounced than COX-1 in tendon tissue, we could observe that Prostaglandin E2 production was about the same (no significant difference) as a product of COX1 and COX-2. LPT was unable to produce any modification on PGE2 production derived from COX-1 enzyme. However, it was quite effective in reducing PGE2 production derived from COX-2 isoform. We could observe that 1 Joule and 3 Joules of energy significantly reduced PGE2 production in the tendon tissue, while 6 Joules presented no difference when compared to the collagenase group. The infrared laser radiation operating with a wavelength of 810 nm was effective in reducing important inflammatory markers in rat tendons, thus becoming a promising tool for treating tendon disorders.

Clinical studies

Strupinska [821] treated 50 patients with Achilles injuries and 50 patients with external epicondyalgia. The patients were irradiated with GaAs laser separately or together with HeNe laser. The result of the therapy was based on patient interviews and examinations, as well as on the Laitinen pain questionnaire. The results proved an analgesic effect.

Seven patients with bilateral Achilles tendinitis (14 tendons) who had aggravated symptoms by pain-inducing activities, were included in a study by Bjordal [1461]. A total of 1.8 Joules for each of three points along the Achilles tendon with a 904nm infrared laser or a placebo laser were administered to either Achilles tendons in a random order to which patients and therapist were blinded. Inflammation was examined by invasive microdialysis for measuring the concentration of the inflammatory marker PGE$_2$ in the peritendinous tissue, ultrasound with Doppler measurement of peri- and intratendinous blood flow, and pressure pain algometry. PGE$_2$ levels were significantly reduced at 60, 75, and 90 minutes after active laser compared both to pretreatment levels and to placebo. Changes in pressure pain threshold (PPT) were significantly different between groups. PPT increased by a mean value of 0.19 kg/cm^2 after treatment in the active laser group, while pressure pain threshold was reduced by -0.20 kg/cm^2 after placebo.

In a clinical study by Bingöl [1623], 40 shoulder pain patients were randomly assigned to either Group I (n = 20, laser treatment) or Group II (n = 20, control). In Group I, patients were given laser treatment and an exercise protocol for 10 sessions over a two-week period. Laser was applied over tuberculum majus and minus, bicipital groove, and anterior and posterior faces of the capsule, regardless of the existence of sensitivity, for 1 min at each location at each session with a pulse repetition rate of 2000 Hz using a GaAs diode laser, 2.98 J/cm^2 per point. In Group II, placebo laser and the

The best organization and aggregation of the collagen bundles were shown by the animals of group A, followed by the animals of group C and B, and finally, the animals of group D. All wavelengths and fluences used in this study were efficient at accelerating the healing process of Achilles tendon post-tenotomy, particularly the 685 nm laser irradiation, at 3 J/cm^2. It suggests the existence of wavelength tissue specificity and dose dependency.

Ng [1879] investigated the effects of different intensities of therapeutic laser and running exercise, and their combined effects on the repair of Achilles tendons in rats. 36 Sprague-Dawley rats that received surgical hemitransection of their right Achilles tendon were tested. Three laser dosages (4 J/cm^2, 1 J/cm^2 and 0 J/cm^2) and three running periods (30 min, 15 min, and 0 min) resulting in nine different dosages and time groups were studied with four rats in each group. The treatments were given on alternate days starting on day 5 post-injury. On day 22, the tendons were tested for load-relaxation, stiffness, and ultimate strength. There was a significant effect of laser on normalized load-relaxation; the rats receiving 4 J/cm^2 had less load-relaxation than those receiving no laser treatment. Results of stiffness testing revealed a significant effect, and rats that ran for 30 min had more stiffness than those that did not run. For ultimate strength, due to a significant interaction, the two factors were analyzed separately, and the results showed that for rats receiving no LPT, those that had run for 15 min and 30 min had more strength than those that did not run. In conclusion, both LPT and running were found to hasten Achilles tendon repair. In general, the rats that received higher dosages of laser energy (4 J/cm^2) and ran for longer periods (30 min) performed better than those that received lower dosages of laser energy and ran for shorter periods.

In another study, Ng [2018] found that a combination of certain herbs and LPT had a better effect than either of them separately.

A study by Delbari [1873] sought to investigate whether or not LPT with a helium-neon laser would increase fibril diameter of transected medial collateral ligament (MCL) in rats. Thirty rats received surgical transections to their right MCL, and five were assigned as the control group. After surgery, the rats were divided into three groups: group 1 (n= 0) received LPT with a HeNe laser and 0.01 J/cm^2 fluence per day, group 2 (n=10) received LPT with 1.2 J/cm^2 fluence per day, and group 3 (sham-exposed group; n=10) received daily placebo laser with the laser equipment turned off, while the control group received neither surgery nor LPT. Transmission electron microscope (TEM) examination was performed on days 12 and 21 after surgery and dimension and density of ligament fibrils were measured. On day 12, the fibril dimension of group 2 and their density were higher than those of groups 1 and 3.

In a study by Marcos [2042], rats weighing about 250 g were used. After anaesthesia, local collagenase injection was performed. The animals were sacrificed by CO_2 inhalation at different times. After the removal of skin and connective tissue, Achilles tendons were removed and processed for

used. The groups were further divided into four subgroups with 8 animals in each, receiving InGaAlP laser, 660 nm, treatment at (1) a mean output of 10 mW, or (2) 40 mW during 10 sec, (3) a sham subgroup, and (4) a non-treatment subgroup. Each animal was subjected to a lesion of the Achilles tendon by dropping a 186 g weight from a 20 cm height over the tendon. Treatment was initiated six hours post-injury for all the groups. Blood vessels were coloured with India ink injection and examined in a video microscope. Laser exposure promoted an increase in blood vessel count when compared to controls. The 40 mW group showed early neovascularization, with the greatest number of microvessels after three laser applications. The 10 mW subgroup showed angiogenesis activity around the same time as the sham laser group did, but the net number of vessels was significantly higher in the former than in the controls. After seven irradiations, the subgroup receiving 40 mW experienced a drop in microvessel numbers, but it was still higher than in the control groups.

A study by Fillipin [1708] investigated the effects of LPT on oxidative stress and fibrosis in an experimental model of Achilles tendon injury induced by a single impact trauma. Rats were randomly divided into four groups (n=8): control, trauma, trauma+laser for 14 days, and trauma+laser for 21 days. Achilles tendon traumatism was produced by dropping a load with an impact kinetic energy of 0.544 J. A GaAs laser of 45 mW average power was used, 5 J/cm^2 dosage, for a duration of 35 seconds, continuously. Studies were carried out on day 21. Histology showed a loss of normal architecture, with inflammatory reaction, angiogenesis, vasodilatation, and extracellular matrix formation after trauma. This was accompanied by a significant increase in collagen concentration when compared to the control group. Oxidative stress was also significantly increased in the trauma group. Administration of laser for 14 or 21 days markedly alleviated histological abnormalities, reduced collagen concentration and prevented oxidative stress. Superoxide dismutase activity was significantly increased by laser treatment over control values.

The objective of a study by Carrinho [1801] was to evaluate the effects of 685 nm and 830 nm laser irradiations at different fluences on the healing process of Achilles tendon of mice after tenotomy. Forty-eight male mice were divided into six experimental groups: Group A, tenomized animals, treated with 685 nm laser, at the dosage of 3 J/cm^2; group B, tenomized animals, treated with 685 nm laser, at the dosage of 10 J/cm^2; group C, tenomized animals, treated with 830 nm laser, at the dosage of 3 J/cm^2; group D, tenomized animals, treated with 830 nm laser, at the dosage of 10 J/cm^2; group E, injured control (placebo treatment); and group F, non-injured standard control. Animals were killed on day 13 post-tenotomy, and their tendons were surgically removed for a quantitative analysis using polarization microscopy, with the purpose of measuring collagen fibers organization through the birefringence (optical retardation, OR). All treated groups showed higher values of OR when compared to the injured control group.

lating collagen synthesis in the tendon gap, and enhancing the late remodeling of fibrous peritendonous adhesion.

Enwemeka [124] cut and sutured the Achilles tendons of twenty rabbits. Six of these rabbits were treated locally with HeNe, seven with GaAs laser. The other seven served as a control. After 14 days, the tensile strength of the tendons was checked. The mean value in the HeNe group was 251, in the GaAs group 233, and in the control group 154.

Early mechanical loading and LPT have been shown to promote tendon healing. Reddy [725] combined these two parameters, using HeNe laser on rabbit achilles tendons. The findings indicate that the combination of LPT and early mechanical loading of tendons increase collagen production, with marginal biomechanical effects on repaired tendons.

Reddy [546] tenectomised and repaired the Achilles tendons in rabbits. The limbs were immobilised and treated with 1 J/cm^2 of HeNe light for 14 days. Control animals received sham laser treatment. The collagen content in the treated tendons was significantly higher than in the control group. Extraction of collagen from the regenerating tissues revealed that the laser-treated tendons yielded significantly higher concentrations of neutral salt soluble and insoluble collagen than control tendons.

Parizotto [653] tenectomised the Achilles tendons in 32 rats and resutured the skin. After 24 hours, HeNe laser was applied daily for 10 days. Doses of 0.5, 5 and 50 J/cm^2 were used. HeNe laser enhanced the intra- and intermolecular hydrogen bonding in the collagen molecules. The treated tendons were more organised than controls.

The study by Elwakil [1747] was conducted to evaluate the role of HeNe laser on the healing process of surgically repaired Achilles tendons. Thirty unilateral Achilles tendons of 30 rabbits were transected and immediately repaired. Operated Achilles tendons were randomly divided into two equal groups. Tendons in group A were subjected to HeNe laser, while tendons in group B served as a control group. Laser irradiation was carried out; continuous wave at 1 J/cm^2. It was done on a daily basis, transcutaneously, by using computerized scanning software starting from the 1st to the 5th postoperative day, then continued after removal of the casts until the 14th postoperative day. Two weeks later, the repaired Achilles tendons were histopathologically and biomechanically evaluated. The histopathological findings suggest a favourable qualitative pattern of the newly synthesized collagen of the regenerating tendons after the laser stimulation. The biomechanical results support the same favourable findings from the functional point of view as denoted by the better biomechanical properties of the regenerating tendons after HeNe laser with a statistical significance in most of the biomechanical parameters. HeNe laser irradiation produced a great improvement after surgical repair of ruptured and injured tendons for a better functional outcome.

Salate [1624] divided 96 rats into three groups subject to treatment during three, five and seven days post-lesion. In each group, 32 animals were

Daily sessions for 5-6 days are needed to reduce inflammation, 8-10 days to increase collagen production. Steroids should be avoided when LPT is used [1462, 1463].

Dosage per point is adapted to the distance between skin and tendon (depth), and the number of points is adapted to the area of the inflammation. According to measurements performed by Bjordal, the various tendon locations have different characteristics that affect the determination of the dose. The figures below represent:

Indication	Tendon depth to target tendon	Tendon thickness	Area to treat
Plantar fasciitis	10.0 - 12.0 mm	3.0 - 4.0 mm	0.1 - 0.8 cm^2
Achilles tendinitis	1.5 - 3.0 mm	4.5 - 6.0 mm	0.5 - 2.0 cm^2
Patellar tendinitis	2.5 - 4.0 mm	5.5 - 8.0 mm	1.0 - 4.0 cm^2
Epicondylitis	1.5 - 2.5 mm	2.0 - 4.0 mm	0.09 - 0.3 cm^2
Rotatorcuff	5.0 - 10.0 mm	5.5 - 8.0 mm	0.5 - 1.5 cm^2

Table 4.2 Tendinitis/Bursitis different characteristics

Literature:
Animal studies

In a tendon healing experiment, Xu [781] used 50 white Leghorn hens. A total of 10 were randomly assigned as a normal control group; the other 40 were used in the study. After anaesthetising, one half of the profundus tendons of the second and third toe on both sides of the feet were cut. Postoperatively, the hens moved freely in the cages. One foot was randomly chosen to belong to the treatment group, the other foot served as an unirradiated control group. The injured tendons in the treatment group were irradiated for twenty minutes daily with a HeNe laser at a constant power density of 12.74 mW/cm^2, the first exposure taking place 24 hours after the operation. The longest course of treatment was 3 weeks. The control group was not irradiated. On day 3 day and at weeks 1, 2, 3 and 5 after surgery, 8 hens were sacrificed and their tendons were examined. The experimental results: (1) active, passive flexion and tendon gliding functional recovery were significantly better in the treatment group ($p < 0.01$); (2) width and thickness of the tendon at the cut site were significantly smaller in the treatment group ($p < 0.01$); (3) degrees of tendon adhesions were significantly lighter in the treatment group ($p < 0.05$). The experimental results demonstrate that HeNe laser radiation had significant effects on anti-inflammation, detumescence, progressive hematoma absorbing, inhibiting tendon extrinsic healing, reducing tendon adhesions, improving tendon intrinsic healing, i.e., stimulating epitenon and endotenon cell proliferation and migration into the gap, stimu-

Igarashi [2023] studied the effect of LPT on the development of synapses in the radiatum layer and the lacunosum-molecular layer of field CA3 of the neonatal rat hippocampus. Neonatal rats were irradiated with a laser (830 nm, 60 mW) at two points located above the hippocampi for 15 s, respectively, twice per day from birth (day 1) to day 5. The mean body weights of the laser-irradiated animals were found to be lower than those of the control animals, the deficit on day 20 being 22.6%. Moreover, the density of synaptic junctions stained by ethanolic phosphotungstic acid per unit area of the radiatum layer and the lacunosum-molecular layer of the neonatal rat hippocampus was significantly reduced on day 20. It was suggested that the low-power diode laser irradiation affected the development of synapses in the neonatal rat brain.

The aim of a study by Karabegovic [2057] was to determine the effects of LPT and to correlate with electrotherapy (TENS, stabile galvanization) in subjects after stroke. The researchers analyzed 70 subjects after stroke with pain in shoulder and oedema of a paralyzed hand. The examinees were divided in two groups of 35, and they were treated during 2006 and 2007. Experimental group (EG) had a treatment with LPT, while the control group (CG) was treated with electrotherapy. Both groups had kinesis therapy and ice massage. All patients were examined on the admission and discharge by using the VAS, DASH, Barthel index and FIM. The pain intensity in shoulder was significantly reduced in EG, swelling is lowered in EG. Barthel index in both groups was significantly higher. DASH was significantly improved after LPT in EG. EG had a higher level of independence. LPT used on EG shows significantly better results in reducing pain, swelling, disability and improvement of independence.

Further literature: [1589, 1590, 1804, 1257, 1935]

4.1.51 Tendinopathies

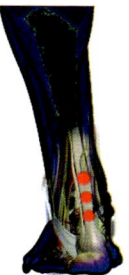

Bjordal [732] has analysed the literature regarding the treatment of shoulder tendinitis/bursitis and concludes: "The methodological quality of the LPT-trials of shoulder tendinitis/bursitis is similar to or higher than in trials with medical interventions for shoulder tendinitis/bursitis. Total sample size of high quality LPT-trials is similar to or higher than total sample size of high quality NSAID-trials or steroid injection-trials on the same diagnosis. The four LPT-trials should serve as a valid platform for drawing conclusions on clinical effects of LPT." Bjordal further concludes: "There is consistent evidence of clinical effects of LPT in all four shoulder trials, as the results are in favour of active LPT with confidence intervals not including zero. The trials with fewest treatment sessions per week had the lowest success rate. Best clinical effects were seen in patients with short duration of symptoms (less than one month)."

the active treatment group had successful outcomes than controls as measured by the change in mean NIHSS score from baseline to 90 days and the full mRS ("shift in Rankin"). Mortality rates and serious adverse events did not differ significantly. This study indicates that infrared LPT has shown to be initially safe and effective in the treatment of ischemic stroke in humans when initiated within 24 hours of stroke onset.

Irradiation of the brain is a general caveat because the balance between stimulating and inhibiting effects is not well known. The above studies suggest an important indication for LPT on brain tissue, but since the brain is a very complex organ, nothing can be taken for granted apart from upholding the general safety aspect. The researchers below have been looking at the effects of irradiation of brain tissue:

The aim of a study by Ahmed [2021] was to investigate the effects of three different intensities of infrared diode laser radiation on amino acid neurotransmitters in the cortex and hippocampus of rat brains. Lasers are known to induce different neurological effects such as pain relief, anesthesia, and neurosuppressive effects; however, the precise mechanisms of these effects are not clearly elucidated. Amino acid neurotransmitters (glutamate, aspartate, glutamine, gamma-aminobutyric acid [GABA], glycine, and taurine) play vital roles in the central nervous system (CNS). The shaved scalp of each rat was exposed to different intensities of infrared laser energy (500, 190, and 90 mW) and then the rats were sacrificed after 1 h, 7 d, and 14 d of daily laser irradiation. The control groups were exposed to the same conditions but without exposure to laser. The concentrations of amino acid neurotransmitters were measured by high-performance liquid chromatography (HPLC). The rats subjected to 500 mW of laser irradiation had a significant decrease in glutamate, aspartate, and taurine in the cortex, and a significant decrease in hippocampal GABA. In the cortices of rats exposed to 190 mW of laser irradiation, increases in aspartate accompanied by a decrease in glutamine were observed. In the hippocampus, other changes were seen. The rats irradiated with 90 mW showed a decrease in cortical glutamate, aspartate, and glutamine, and an increase in glycine, while in the hippocampus an increase in glutamate, aspartate, and GABA were recorded. It is concluded that daily laser irradiation at 90 mW produced the most pronounced inhibitory effect in the cortex after 7 d. This finding may explain the reported neurosuppressive effect of infrared laser energy on axonal conduction of hippocampal and cortical tissues of rat brains.

In a study by Shen-Zheng [2022], low power lasers were guided by optic fibers into the rat caudate nucleus or frontal cortex during conditioned avoidance response (CAR) training. The changes in striatal monoamine and amino acid concentrations were subsequently determined. Of six training groups tested, only the experimental group with helium-neon laser radiation to the caudate nucleus exhibited the formation of CAR and an increase of unconditioned leg contractions. The striatal concentrations of dopamine (DA) and norepinephrine (NE) were increased simultaneously in the group.

Nitric oxide (NO) has been shown to be neurotoxic while transforming growth factor-β 1 (TGF-β-1) and it is neuroprotective in the stroke model. The study by Leung [1707] investigated the effects of LPT on nitric oxide synthase (NOS) and TGF-β-1 activities after cerebral ischemia and reperfusion injury. Cerebral ischemia was induced for one hour in male adult rats by a unilateral occlusion of the middle cerebral artery. Laser irradiation was then applied to the cerebrum at different time intervals (1, 5 or 10 minutes). The wavelength of the laser was 660 nm, 8.8 mW, 2.64 J/cm², 10 kHz. The activity of NOS and the expression of TGF-β-1 were evaluated in groups with different time intervals of laser irradiation. After ischemia, the NOS activity increased gradually from day three, became significantly higher from day four to six, but returned to the normal level after day seven. The activity and expression of the three isoforms of NOS were significantly suppressed to different extents after laser irradiation. In addition, laser irradiation was shown to trigger the expression of TGF-β-1.

Oron [1756] performed two sets of experiments. Stroke was induced in rats by (1) permanent occlusion of the middle cerebral artery through a craniotomy, or (2) insertion of a filament. After induction of stroke, a battery of neurological and functional tests (neurological score, adhesive removal) were performed. At 4 and 24 hours post stroke, a GaAs diode laser was used transcranially to illuminate the hemisphere contra lateral of the stroke at a power density of 7.5 mW/cm². In both models of stroke, laser significantly reduced neurological deficits when applied 24 hours post stroke. Application of the laser at 4 hours post stroke did not affect the neurological outcome of the stroke-induced rats as compared with controls. There was no statistically significant difference in the stroke lesion area between control and laser-irradiated rats. The number of newly formed neuronal cells, assessed by double immunoreactivity to bromodeoxyuridine and tubulin isotype III as well as migrating cells (doublecortin immunoactivity), was significantly elevated in the subventricular zone of the hemisphere ipsilateral to the induction of stroke when treated by laser. These data suggest that a non-invasive intervention of laser issued 24 hours after acute stroke may provide a significant functional benefit with an underlying mechanism possibly being the induction of neurogenesis.

LPT was tested by Lampl [1807] for the ability to improve 90-day outcomes in ischemic stroke patients treated within 24 hours from stroke onset. This was a prospective, intention-to-treat, multicenter, international, double-blind trial involving 120 ischemic stroke treated patients, randomized 2:1 ratio, with 79 patients in the active treatment group and 41 in the sham (placebo) control group. Only patients with baseline stroke severity measured by NIHSS scores of 7 to 22 were included. Patients who received tissue plasminogen activator were excluded. Time of treatment ranged from 2 to 24 hours. More patients (70%) in the active treatment group had successful outcomes than did controls (51%). Similarly, more patients (59%) had successful outcomes than did controls (44%) as measured on day 90. Also, more patients in

Transcranial near-infrared laser therapy (TLT) is currently under investigation in a pivotal clinical trial that excludes thrombolytic therapy. To determine if combining tissue plasminogen activator (tPA; Alteplase) and TLT is safe, this study assessed the safety profile of TLT administered alone and in combination with Alteplase. The purpose of a study by Lapchak [2002] was to determine if the combination of TLT and thrombolysis should be investigated further in a human clinical trial. The researchers determined whether postembolization treatment with TLT in the absence or presence of tPA would affect measures of hemorrhage or survival after large clot embolism-induced strokes in rabbits. TLT did not significantly alter hemorrhage incidence after embolization, but there was a trend for a modest reduction of hemorrhage volume (by 65%) in the TLT-treated group compared with controls. Intravenous administration of tPA, using an optimized dosing regimen, significantly increased hemorrhage incidence by 160%. The tPA-induced increase in hemorrhage incidence was not significantly affected by TLT, although there was a 30% decrease in hemorrhage incidence in combination-treated rabbits. There was no effect of TLT on the hemorrhage volume measured in tPA-treated rabbits and no effect of any treatment on the 24-hour survival rate. In the embolism model, TLT administration did not affect the tPA-induced increase in hemorrhage incidence. TLT may be administered safely either alone or in combination with tPA because neither treatment affected hemorrhage incidence or volume. These results support the study of TLT in combination with Alteplase in patients with stroke.

The next study by this group was not quite as successful. A double-blind, randomized study by Zivin [2057] compared TLT treatment to sham control. Patients receiving tissue plasminogen activator and patients with evidence of hemorrhagic infarct were excluded. The primary efficacy end point was a favorable 90-day score of 0 to 2 assessed by the modified Rankin Scale. Other 90-day end points included the overall shift in modified Rankin Scale and assessments of change in the National Institutes of Health Stroke Scale score. The authors randomized 660 patients: 331 received LPT and 327 received sham; 120 in the LPT group achieved favorable outcome versus 101 in the sham group. Comparable results were seen for the other outcome measures. Although no prespecified test achieved significance, a post hoc analysis of patients with a baseline National Institutes of Health Stroke Scale score of <16 showed a favorable outcome at 90 days on the primary end point. Mortality rates and serious adverse events did not differ between groups with 17.5% and 17.4% mortality, 37.8% and 41.8% serious adverse events for LPT and sham, respectively. In conclusion, LPT within 24 hours from stroke onset demonstrated safety but did not meet formal statistical significance for efficacy. However, all predefined analyses showed a favorable trend, consistent with the previous clinical trial (NEST-1). Both studies indicate that mortality and adverse event rates were not adversely affected by LPT.

4.1.50 Stroke - irradiation of the brain

Is it safe to irradiate the brain? Part of the answer is given in the study by Ilic [1590]:

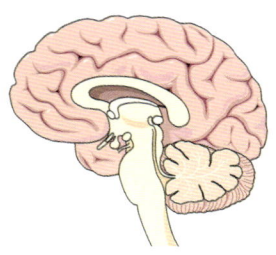

"The aim of the present study was to investigate the possible short- and long-term adverse neurological effects of LPT given at different power densities, frequencies, and modalities on the intact rat brain. One hundred and eighteen rats were used in the study. Diode laser (808 nm) was used to deliver power densities of 7.5, 75, and 750 mW/cm^2 transcranially to the brain cortex of mature rats, in either continuous wave (CW) or pulse (Pu) modes. Multiple doses of 7.5 mW/cm^2 were also applied. Standard neurological examination of the rats was performed during the follow-up periods after laser irradiation. Histology was performed at light and electron microscopy levels. Both the scores from standard neurological tests and the histopathological examination indicated that there was no long-term difference between lasertreated and control groups up to 70 days post-treatment. The only rats showing an adverse neurological effect were those in the 750 mW/cm^2 (about 100-fold optimal dose), CW mode group. In Pu mode, there was much less heating, and no tissue damage was noted. Long-term safety tests lasting 30 and 70 days at optimal 10× and 100× doses, as well as at multiple doses at the same power densities, indicate that the tested laser energy doses are safe under this treatment regime. Neurological deficits and histopathological damage to 750 mW/cm^2 CW laser irradiation are attributed to thermal damage and not due to tissue-photon interactions."

A fascinating possibility is suggested in the following studies:

In a study by Lapchak [1427], the rabbit small clot embolic stroke model (RSCEM) was used to assess whether laser treatment (7.5 or 25 $mW/J/cm^2$) altered clinical rating scores (behaviour) when given to rabbits starting 1 to 24 hours post embolisation. Behavioural analysis was conducted from 24 hours to 21 days after embolisation, allowing for the determination of the effective stroke dose (P50) or clot amount (mg) that produces neurological deficits in 50% of the rabbits. Using the RSCEM, a treatment is considered beneficial if it significantly increases the P50 compared with the control group. In the present study, the P50 value for controls were 0.97+/-0.19 mg to 1.10+/-0.17 mg; this was increased by 100% to 195% if laser treatment was initiated up to 6 hours, but not 24 hours, post embolisation (P50=1.23+/-0.15 mg). Laser treatment also produced a durable effect that was measurable 21 days after embolisation. Laser treatment (25 $mW/J/cm^2$) did not affect the physiological variables that were measured. This study shows that laser treatment improved behavioural performance if initiated within 6 hours of an embolic stroke and that the effect of laser treatment is durable.

studies have confirmed that the application of LPT could affect the cellular process. However, little is known about the effects of LPT on BMSCs. The aim of a study by Zhang [2009] was designed to investigate the influence of LPT at different energy densities on BMSCs proliferation, secretion and myogenic differentiation. BMSCs were harvested from fresh rat bone marrow and exposed to a 635 nm diode laser (60 mW; 0, 0.5, 1.0, 2.0, or 5.0 J/cm^2). The lactate dehydrogenase (LDH) release was used to assess the cytotoxicity of LPT at different energy densities. Cell proliferation was evaluated by using 3-(4, 5-dimethylithiazol-2-yl)-2, 5-diphenyl tetrazolium bromide (MTT) and 5-bromo-2'-deoxyuridine (BrdU) assays. Production of vascular endothelial growth factor (VEGF) and nerve growth factor (NGF) were measured by enzyme-linked immunosorbent assay (ELISA). Myogenic differentiation, induced by 5-azacytidine (5-aza), was assessed by using immunocytochemical staining for the expression of sarcomeric alpha-actin and desmin. Cytotoxicity assay showed no significant difference between the non-irradiated group and the irradiated groups. LPT significantly stimulated BMSCs proliferation and 0.5 J/cm^2 was found to be an optimal energy density. VEGF and NGF were identified and LPT at 5.0 J/cm^2 significantly stimulated the secretion. After 5-aza induction, myogenic differentiation was observed in all groups, LPT at 5.0 J/cm^2 dramatically facilitated the differentiation. LPT may provide a novel approach for the preconditioning of BMSCs in vitro prior to transplantation.

The aim of a study by Huo [2056] was designed to investigate the influence of LPT at different energy densities on bone marrow derived mesenchymal stem cells (BMSCs) proliferation, secretion and myogenic differentiation. BMSCs were harvested from rat fresh bone marrow and exposed to a 635 nm diode laser (60 mW; 0, 0.5, 1.0, 2.0, or 5.0 J/cm^2). The lactate dehydrogenase (LDH) release was used to assess the cytotoxicity of LPT at different energy densities. Cell proliferation was evaluated by using 3-(4, 5-dimethylithiazol-2-yl)-2, 5-diphenyl tetrazolium bromide (MTT) and 5-bromo-2'-deoxyuridine (BrdU) assay. Production of vascular endothelial growth factor (VEGF) and nerve growth factor (NGF) were measured by enzyme-linked immunosorbent assay (ELISA). Myogenic differentiation, induced by 5-azacytidine (5-aza), was assessed by using immunocytochemical staining for the expression of sarcomeric alpha-actin and desmin. Cytotoxicity assay showed no significant difference between the non-irradiated group and irradiated groups. LPT significantly stimulated BMSCs proliferation and 0.5 J/cm^2 was found to be an optimal energy density. VEGF and NGF were identified and LPT at 5.0 J/cm^2 significantly stimulated the secretion. After 5-aza induction, myogenic differentiation was observed in all groups and LPT at 5.0 J/cm^2 dramatically facilitated the differentiation. In conclusion, LPT stimulates proliferation, increases growth factors secretion and facilitates myogenic differentiation of BMSCs.

cells, measured by optical density, resulted in statistically significant increases in values compared to non-irradiated cells at both time points. Western blot analysis and immunocytochemical labeling indicated an increase in the expression of stem cell marker β1-integrin after irradiation. These results indicate that cm^2 of laser irradiation can positively affect human adipose stem cells by increasing cellular viability, proliferation, and expression of β1-integrin.

The aim of the study by Tuby [1809] was to investigate the effect of LPT on the proliferation of mesenchymal stem cells (MSCs) and cardiac stem cells (CSCs). Isolation of MSCs and CSCs was performed. The cells were cultured and laser irradiation was applied at energy densities of 1 and 3 J/cm^2. The number of MSCs and CSCs up to two and four weeks respectively, post-LPT, demonstrated a significant increase in the laser-treated cultures as compared to the control. These results may have an important impact on regenerative medicine.

Souza [1718] divided 60 amputated worms into three study groups: a control group, and two other groups submitted to daily 1 and 3 min long laser treatment sections at approximately 910 W/m^2 power density. A 685 nm laser with 35 mW optical power was used. Samples were sent for histological analysis on the 4th, the 7th and the 15th day after amputation. A remarkable increase in stem cells counts for the 4th day of regeneration was observed when the regenerating worms were stimulated by the laser radiation.

Abramovitch-Gottlib [1810] irradiated mesenchymal stem cells (MSCs) seeded on three dimensional (3D) coralline (Porites lutea) biomatrices with laser irradiation. The consequent phenotype modulation and development of MSCs towards ossified tissue were studied in this combined 3D biomatrix/LPT system and in a control group, which was similarly grown, but not treated by LPT. The irradiated and non irradiated MSC were tested on days 1-7, 10, 14, 21 and 28 of culturing via analysis of cellular distribution on matrices (trypan blue), calcium incorporation to newly formed tissue (alizarin red), bone nodule formation (von Kossa), fat aggregates formation (oil red O), alkaline phosphatase (ALP) activity, scanning electron microscopy (SEM) and electron dispersive spectrometry (EDS). The results obtained from the irradiated samples showed enhanced tissue formation, appearance of phosphorous peaks and calcium and phosphate incorporation to newly formed tissue. Moreover, in irradiated samples, ALP activity was significantly enhanced in early stages and notably reduced in late stages of culturing. These findings of cell and tissue parameters up to 28 days of culturing revealed higher ossification levels in irradiated samples compared with the control group. The authors suggest that both the surface properties of the 3D crystalline biomatrices and the LLLI have biostimulatory effects on the conversion of MSCs into bone-forming cells and on the induction of ex-vivo ossification.

Bone marrow derived mesenchymal stem cells (BMSCs) have shown to be an appealing source for cell therapy and tissue engineering. Previous

ice, compression, elevation), the second group (n=16) was treated with the RICE method plus placebo laser, and the third group (n=15) was treated with the RICE method plus a 820 nm GaA1As diode laser with a radiant power output of 40 mW at 16 Hz. Before the treatment and 24, 48, and 72 h later, the volume of the oedema was measured. The group treated with the RICE plus a 820 nm GaA1As diode laser presented a statistically significant reduction in the volume of the oedema after 24 h.

Further literature: [74, 122, 123, 281, 298, 299, 431, 709, 734, 735, 739, 1242]

4.1.49 Stem cells

Stem cells are characterized by the ability to renew themselves through mitotic cell division and differentiating into a diverse range of specialized cell types. Using stem cells in medicine has a very promising potential and a lot of research is directed into this field. It can be taken for granted that stem cells will react to laser irradiation, just as all other cells. By finding the optimal parameters, LPT could become a very valuable tool in boosting stem cell viability and proliferation.

Literature:

The aim of an in vitro study by Eduardo [1895] was to evaluate the potential effect of laser irradiation (660 nm) on human dental pulp stem cell (hDPSC) proliferation. Cells cultured under nutritional deficit (10% FBS) were either irradiated or left untreated (control) using two different power settings (20 mW/6 seconds to 40 mW/3 seconds). Cell growth was indirectly assessed by measuring the cell mitochondrial activity through the MTT reduction-based cytotoxicity assay. The group irradiated with the 20 mW setting presented significantly higher MTT activity at 72 hours than the other two groups (negative control -10% FBS- and lased 40 mW with 3-second exposure time). After 24 hours of the first irradiation, cultures grown under nutritional deficit (10% FBS) and irradiated presented significantly higher viable cells than the non-irradiated cultures grown under the same nutritional conditions. Under the conditions of this study it was possible to conclude that the cell strain hDPSC responds positively to laser phototherapy by improving the cell growth when cultured under nutritional deficit conditions. Thus, the association of laser phototherapy and hDPSC cells could be of importance for future tissue engineering and regenerative medicine.

The study by Mvula [1808] investigated the effect of LPT on primary cultures of adult human adipose derived stem cells using a 635 nm diode laser, at 5 J/cm^2 with a power output of 50.2 mW and a power density of 5.5 mW/cm^2. Cellular morphology did not appear to change after irradiation. Using the trypan blue exclusion test, the cellular viability of irradiated cells increased by 1% at 24 h and 1.6% at 48 h but was not statistically significant. However, the increase of cellular viability as measured by ATP luminescence was statistically significant at 48 h. Proliferation of irradiated

A study by Bayat [1638] sought to investigate whether or not LPT with a helium-neon laser increased biomechanical parameters of transected medial collateral ligament (MCL) in rats. Thirty rats received surgical transection to their right MCL, and five were assigned as the control group. After surgery, the rats were divided into three groups: group 1 (n=10) received laser with 0.01 J/cm^2 energy density per day, group 2 (n=10) received laser with 1.2 J/cm^2 energy density per day, and group 3 (sham exposed group; n=10) received daily placebo laser, while the control group received neither surgery nor laser. Biomechanical tests were performed on day 12 and 21 days after surgery. The data was analyzed by one-way analysis of variance. The ultimate tensile strength (UTS) of group 2 on day 12 was significantly higher than that of groups 1 and 3. Furthermore, the UTS and energy absorption of the control (uninjured) group were significantly higher than those of the other groups.

Clinical studies

Glinkowski [503] compared two groups of patients with sprained ankles. One group was treated conservatively with plaster casts for two weeks; the other received GaAs 3.6 J/cm^2 for one week. The results observed with plaster casts after two weeks were achieved within one week with LPT.

In three Danish studies by Axelsen [547], Darre [548] and Nissen [535], there were no effects seen on sprained ankles, achilles tendinitis, or medial tibial stress syndrome, using 830 nm, 30-40 mW. The laser type and dose may not be suitable for these indications. The dose in [547] is very low. Winther [549] was also unsuccessful until switching to GaAs for tendinitis. De Bie failed to obtain positive results in ankle sprain treatments. GaAs of either 0.5 J/cm^2 or 5 J/cm^2, or placebo, were used. However, only a very small area (1 cm^2) was treated.

Simunovic [957] confirms the positive effect of LPT in sports injuries in a double-blind multi centre study using a combination of GaAlAs and HeNe laser.

Ohshiro [961] selected six Japanese sumo wrestlers and treated their symptoms. LPT resulted in an alleviation of their symptoms and an increased win rate.

al-Shenqiti [1319] performed a double-blind, randomised study in 60 patients suffering from rotator cuff symptoms. Trigger points associated with this condition were treated with a 820 nm laser of 100 mW, modulated at 5000 Hz, dose 32 J/cm^2. On the whole 12 treatment sessions were given over four weeks. The outcome measures were pain, range of movement, functional activities and pressure pain threshold. Outcome measures were carried out pre- and post treatment, then three months later at follow-up. All outcome measures were considerably improved as compared to the control group.

Stergioulas [1492] randomly selected 47 soccer players with second degree ankle sprains. They were divided into the following groups: The first group (n=16) was treated with the conventional initial treatment (RICE: rest,

4.1.48 Sports injuries

The use of lasers in sports medicine is widespread. Top-level sportsmen and women often suffer from injuries, and it is vital the injuries heal quickly, so that the individual can resume training. Sports injuries have the "advantage" that the subject often knows when the injury occurred and where it is situated. The subjects also often have experience of how long it takes for a particular injury to heal. It is therefore easy to "calibrate" the effect of the laser. A rule of thumb is that a sports injury heals almost twice as fast if the healing process is stimulated by LPT. A common problem is that the subjective discomfort in the injured area soon disappears and the individual wants to return to training immediately. It is essential that the injured area be allowed to rest and that training be resumed gradually. Treatment should not be interrupted just because pain is gone. This is only the first sign of recovery.

LPT on chronic pain conditions can increase the pain level initially. This reaction is absent when treating acute injuries. Acute injuries can actually receive higher doses than chronic cases without side effects. Common conditions such as delayed onset muscle soreness and periostitis react very favourably to LPT. Therapy should be started as soon as possible after training or competition. In some instances, therapy before training/competition is useful. There is a strong incentive for the professional athlete to use LPT. Acc. to Swedish horse racing rules, LPT is not allowed during a period of 96 hours before a race.

Oedema is a common element in sports injuries. If there are a number of injured places, the patient should be treated according to Ohshiro's "proximal priority principle". This means that the proximal injury is treated first, the distal last. If the distal injury is treated first, lymph accumulation increases because the proximal injury prevents drainage. The result in such a case could be increased pain.

GaAs lasers with multiprobes give the shortest treatment times and have the widest range of indications. A GaAlAs laser is good for superficial and more limited injuries. However, the recent advent of high-powered GaAlAs lasers (500 mW or more) has widened the range of their indications. The handy format of medium-powered GaAlAs lasers makes them very useful for ambulatory work. (See chapter 4.1.51 "Tendinopathies" on page 322.)

Literature:
Animal studies

Weiss [276] and Bibikova [277] observed improved muscle regeneration as a result of the use of HeNe and GaAs lasers in experiments on rats and batrachians (a kind of frog), respectively.

Fung [1302] transsected the medial collateral ligaments in 24 rats. Of these, 16 animals were treated with a single dose of a 660 nm laser, and 8 served as control. The ligaments were mechanically tested at three or six weeks post operation. It is suggested that ultimate tensile strength and stiffnes can be improved by LPT.

gastrocnemius muscle. Cell influx and edema were evaluated at 3 or 24h after venom injection. Mice were irradiated at the site of injury by a 685nm laser with a dose of $4.2 J/cm^2$. A therapy that combines LPT and antivenom was also studied. B. jararacussu venom caused a significant edema formation 3 and 24h after its injection, and a prominent leukocyte infiltrate composed predominantly of neutrophils at 24h after venom inoculation. LPT significantly reduced edema formation by 53% and 64% at 3 and 24h, respectively, and resulted in a reduction of neutrophils accumulation. The combined therapy showed to be more efficient than each therapy acting separately. In conclusion, LPT significantly reduced the edema and leukocyte influx into the envenomed muscle, suggesting that LPT should be considered as a potentially therapeutic approach for the treatment of the local effects of Bothrops species.

In another study by Barbosa [2061] myonecrosis was induced in mice by injection of 0.6 mg/kg of B. jararacussu venom in the right gastrocnemius muscle and was evaluated at 3 or 24 h after venom injection. The site of venom administration was irradiated for 29 s with 685 nm at a dose of $4.2 J/cm^2$. Intravenous anti venom (AV) therapy (0.5 mL dose) was administered at different times: 30 min before venom injection or 0, 1, or 3 h afterward. Both AV therapy and LPT treatments were duplicated in mice groups killed at 3 or 24 h. B. jararacussu venom caused a significant myonecrotic effect 3 and 24 h after venom injection. LPT significantly reduced myonecrosis by 83.5% at 24 h but not at 3 h, and AV therapy alone was ineffective for reducing myonecrosis at 3 and 24 h. Only LPT significantly reduced myonecrosis of the envenomed muscle, suggesting that LPT is a potentially therapeutic approach for treating the local effects of B. jararacussu venom.

In a study by Doin-Silva [1998], the tibialis anterior muscle of rats was injected with snake venom, diluted in 0.9% saline solution or saline solution alone. Sixty minutes after venom injection, HeNe treatment was administered at three incident energy densities: dose 1, a single exposure of $3.5 J/cm^2$; dose 2, three exposures of $3.5 J/cm^2$, dose 3, a single exposure of $10.5 J/cm^2$. Muscle function was assessed through twitch tension recordings, whereas muscle damage was evaluated through histopathologic analysis, morphometry of the area of tissue affected and creatine kinase (CK) serum levels, and compared to unirradiated muscles. Laser application at the dose of $3.5 J/cm^2$ reduced the area of injury by 64%, decreased the neuromuscular blockade (NMB) by 62% and reduced CK levels by 58%, when compared to unirradiated controls. Dose 2 showed a lesser benefit than dose 1, and dose 3 was ineffective in preventing the venom's effects. Measurements of the absorbance of unirradiated and irradiated venom solution showed no difference in absorption spectra. In addition, no difference in the intensity of partial NMB in nerve-muscle preparation was shown by unirradiated and irradiated venom. The results indicate that the laser light did not alter venom toxicity.

Further literature: [1484]

transcutaneously with 16 mW of HeNe laser light for 20 days (high doses) over the operated area. The 7 dogs in the control group became paralysed as expected. The 10 dogs that underwent the same operation but were immediately treated with a laser were able to stand after 7-9 weeks, and could walk a few steps after 9-12 weeks. The histological picture obtained from the dogs 21 days post operation showed no rejection and no prominent scar tissue at the site of contact between the spinal cord tissue and the transplanted nerve. Moreover, new axons and blood vessels originating in the spinal tissue extended into the graft. These were seen only in the laser treated group and not in the control group, in which scar tissue had developed at the site of transection.

The study by Shamir [1182] evaluated the therapeutic effect of LPT on peripheral nerve regeneration after complete transection and direct anastomosis of the rat sciatic nerve. Thirteen out of twenty-four rats received postoperative LPT, 780 nm, applied transcutaneously, 30 min daily for 21 consecutive days, to corresponding segments of the spinal cord and to the injured sciatic nerve. Positive somatosensory evoked responses were found in 69.2% of the irradiated rats, as compared to 18.2% of the non-irradiated rats. Immunohistochemical staining in the laser-treated group showed an increased total number of axons and a better functioning regeneration process, due to an increased number of large-diameter axons compared to the non-irradiated control group.

Further literature: see "Nerve regeneration".

4.1.47 Snake bites

New indications for LPT are being discovered continuously. LPT as an adjunct treatment modality to reduce tissue breakdown after snake bites is just one of them.

Literature:

In a study by Dourado [1327], the venom of the bothrops moojeni snake was injected into the gastrocnemius of mice to mimic the effect of snakebites. Traditional therapies for this snakebite have proven rather ineffective. Three groups were tested: A=saline, B=venom, and C=venom+ laser. Two sessions of HeNe laser at 4 J/cm^2 for 1 min 32 s were administered and the animals were sacrificed at 24 h, and on days 3 and 7, respectively. The analysis showed myonecrosis with inflammation and an extensive area of degenerated fibres. In the laser group there was, by day 3, an incipient number of regenerating fibres. Laser accelerated the fagocytosis of fibre remnants and recovery of the tissue, decreasing the oedema and increasing regeneration.

The article by Barbosa [1814] reports the effect of LPT on the edema formation and leukocyte influx caused by Bothrops jararacussu snake venom as an alternative treatment for Bothrops snakebites. The inflammatory reaction was induced by an injection of 0.6mg/kg of B. jararacussu venom in the

on the skin and 4 J/cm² intraorally over the bottom of the sinus. The oedema of the mucosa was reduced.

Kruchinina [541] examined the effect of HeNe LPT in young patients with sinuitis through conjunctival biomicroscopy. LPT produced a positive effect on microcirculation. The primary effects were on vessel permeability (decrease of oedema) and red blood cell aggregation. The best results were obtained in acute cases.

Further literature: [340, 466, 534, 541, 542, 543, 555, 886, 1036, 1155]

4.1.46 Spinal cord injuries

Spinal cord injuries can, in seconds, change the life of a person from being fit to becoming crippled with the prospect of spending the rest of his/her life in a wheel chair. The actual injury normally has very small potential for healing. It is therefore a bit surprising that the potential of LPT has met with so little interest. The LPT should preferably be one of the first therapies used, in order to improve the healing capacity of the nerves.

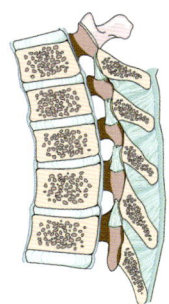

Literature:
Animal studies

The purpose of an experiment by Shi [839] was to elucidate the influence of the HeNe laser on the regeneration of peripheral nerves. Forty-four rabbits were used in the experiment. The animals were divided into 4, 8, 12, 16 week groups according to the observation period. Six animals were used in each irradiated group, and five rabbits were used in the control group during each observation period. Regeneration of the axons and myelinic sheaths, the latent rate of the common peroneal nerve, the condition of the anterior tibial muscle and the toe expansion test were all observed systematically in both groups. The experimental results were: A few thin regenerated axons were seen at 4 weeks in the irradiated group, while in the control group it could be not be observed until the 8th week. A low amplitude latent rate of the common peroneal nerve was determined at the peroneal side of the anterior tibial muscle in a few animals at 4 weeks in the irradiated group, but it was not observed in the control group until weeks 12 -16. The regeneration of the myeline sheath was evident in the irradiated group. At 16 weeks postoperatively, the toe expansion test was normal in the irradiated group, while in the control group it was the same as seen at 12 weeks after operation in the irradiated group.

Rochkind [561] and his group subjected 17 dogs to laminectomy and transection of the spinal cord at TH12-L1. An autograft of the left sciatic nerve was then implanted into the injured area. Neurorrhaphy was performed on the right sciatic nerve. Altogether 7 dogs did not receive any additional treatment and served as a control. The other 10 were treated

4.1.45 Sinuitis

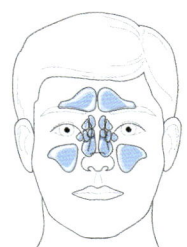

Patients suffering from maxillary sinuitis or allergic rhinitis can have difficulty breathing through the nose during dental treatment. A total of 4-6 J is given intraorally over the bottom of the sinus at three to four points on the buccal and palatal side in contact mode. The sinus opening inside the nose is irradiated in a non-contact mode, 2-3 J. The projections of the ethmoidal and frontal sinuses are also irradiated, if involved.

Intra-cavitary irradiation is reported by Plushnikov [513]. The cavity is irradiated with HeNe through a lightguide inserted into the cavity by a puncture needle.

Acute sinuitis responds more quickly to treatment than chronic. During extraoral treatment, the eyes should be protected by asking the patient to close them. Protective glasses may be obstructive.

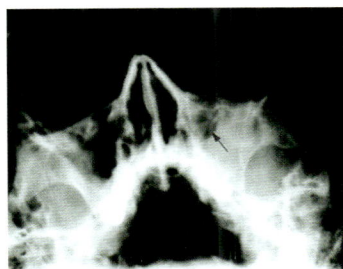 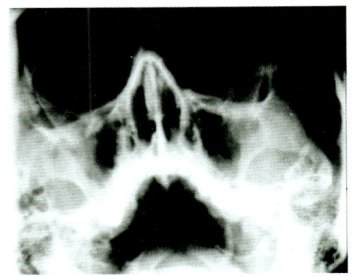

Figure 4.19 Sinuitis maxillaris before and after GaAlAs LPT.
Courtesy: M. Hacarova and J. Hubacek
http://www.sld.cu/galerias/pdf/sitios/rehabilitacion-fis/laser_y_sinusitis.pdf

Literature:

Moustsen [103] conducted a double-blind test using a 30 mW GaAlAs laser on a group of 60 patients. Two extraoral points on each side of the nose were irradiated, 3 J each, during three treatments. No significant results were achieved on the sinuitis.

Roshal [104], on the other hand, treated two groups of 227 and 120 children with allergic rhinitis. HeNe laser light was administered directly on the mucosa, via fibre optics, with excellent results. The positive results of this study were confirmed by tomography and direct inspection. Although this study does not report on sinuitis, it shows the importance of reaching the inflamed mucosa with the irradiation.

Kaiser [507] used HeNe laser in a double-blind study of acute maxillary sinuitis. Thirty patients participated in each group; 7 J/cm^2 was given

complications of diabetes because it can alter the carbohydrate and lipid metabolism of rats with diabetes.

Clinical studies

The first study of salivary stimulation was published in 1987 by Fructuoso [500]. Using a GaAs laser, 6 J/cm^2, in a double-blind study, a significant improvement of the salivary production of the parotid gland was achieved. Treatment was given three times a week for three weeks, followed by one week of rest and repeated sessions, with a total number of 25 sessions.

Nagasawa [106] treated patients with Sjögren's syndrome with a GaAlAs laser (20 mW) intraorally, five minutes per treatment. Approximately 15 to 20 treatment sessions were administered. After this treatment period, the patients' parotid gland function returned for an extended period.

Kats [279] treated 88 patients with sialoadenitis with HeNe laser. The treatment led to a quicker decline in inflammation and pain, higher salivation, longer discomfort-free periods, and an improvement of the gland structure.

Arao [1110] reports that the salivation in two patients with xerostomia could be stimulated with LPT.

A clinical case study reports on dry mouth symptoms in a patient with Sjögren's syndrome (SS) who was treated with LPT by Simões [2119]. A 60-year-old woman diagnosed with SS was referred to the laboratory for lasers in dentistry to treat her severe xerostomia. A diode laser (780 nm, 3.8 J/cm2, 15 mW) was used to irradiate the parotid, submandibular, and sublingual glands, three times per week, for a period of 8 months. The salivary flow rate and xerostomia symptoms were measured before, during, and after LPT. Dry mouth symptoms improved during LPT. After LPT, the parotid salivary gland pain and swelling were no longer present. Treatment with LPT was an effective method to improve the quality of life of this patient with SS.

The aim of a study by Simões [2120] was to verify how LPT used for oral mucositis could influence xerostomia symptoms and hyposalivation of patients undergiong RT. Patients were divided into two groups: 12 individuals receiving three laser irradiations per week (G1) and 10 patients receiving one laser irradiation per week (G2). A diode laser (660 nm, 6 J/cm(2), 0.24 J, 40 mW) was used until completely healing of the lesions or the end of the RT. At the first and last laser sessions, whole resting and stimulated saliva were collected, and questionnaires were administered. According to Wilcoxon and Student statistical test, xerostomia for G1 was lower than for G2, and salivary flow rate was no different before and after RT, except for stimulated collection of G2, which was lower. These results suggest that LPT can be beneficial as an auxiliary therapy for hypofunction of salivary glands.

higher than that in the non-irradiated group on days 5 and 7, and the difference was statistically significant. Greater expression of heat shock protein (HSP)25 and bcl-2 was seen on days 1 and 3 in the irradiated group. Assay of the released amylase showed no significant difference statistically between the irradiated group and the non-irradiated group. Trypan blue exclusion assay revealed that there was no difference in the ratio of dead to live cells between the irradiated and the non-irradiated groups. These results suggest that laser irradiation promotes cell proliferation and expression of anti-apoptosis proteins in Par-C10 cells, but it does not significantly affect amylase secretion or induce rapid cell death in isolated acinar cells from rat parotid glands.

The aim of another study by Simões [2121] was to evaluate the effect of laser irradiation on the amylase and the antioxidant enzyme activities, as well as on the total protein concentration of submandibular glands (SMG) of diabetic and non-diabetic rats. Ninety-six female rats were divided into eight groups: D0, D5, D10, and D20 (diabetic animals), and C0, C5, C10, and C20 (non-diabetic animals), respectively. Diabetes was induced by administering streptozotocin and confirmed later by the glycemia results. Twenty-nine days after diabetes induction, the SMG of groups D5 and C5, D10 and C10, and D20 and C20 were irradiated with 5, 10, and 20 J/cm^2, respectively. A diode laser (660 nm/100 mW) was used. On the day after irradiation, the rats were euthanized and the SMG were removed. Catalase, peroxidase, and amylase activities, as well as protein concentration, were assayed. Results: Diabetic rats without irradiation (D0) showed higher catalase activity when compared to C0 (0.16 +/- 0.05 and 0.07 +/- 0.01 U/mg protein, respectively). However, laser irradiction of 5, 10, and 20 J/cm^2 reduced the catalase activity of diabetic groups (D5 and D20) to non-diabetic values. In conclusion, laser irradiation decreased catalase activity in diabetic rats' SMG.

The objective of yet another study by Simões [2122] was to evaluate the effect of LPT on the glycemic state and the histological and ionic parameters of the parotid and submandibular glands in rats with diabetes. One hundred twenty female rats were divided into eight groups. Diabetes was induced by administration of streptozotocin and confirmed later according to results of glycemia testing. Twenty-nine days after the induction, the parotid and submandibular glands of the rats were irradiated with 5, 10, and 20 J/cm2 using a laser diode (660 nm/100 mW) without diabetes: C5, C10, and C20; with diabetes: D5, D10, and D20, respectively). On the following day, the rats were euthanized, and blood glucose determined. Histological and ionic analyses were performed. Rats with diabetes without irradiation (D0) showed lipid droplets accumulation in the parotid gland, but accumulation decreased after 5, 10, and 20 J/cm^2 of laser irradiation. A decrease in fasting glycemia level from 358.97+/-56.70 to 278.33+/-87.98 mg/dL for D5 and from 409.50+/-124.41 to 231.80+/-120.18 mg/dL for D20 was also observed. In conclusion, LPT could be explored as an auxiliary therapy for control of

the striated salivary ducts and in the intercalated ducts were less pronounced. Interestingly, the 760 Hz group exhibited stimulated mitosis, while the 190 Hz group was no different from the control group. **The report does not make clear whether the GaAs laser was pulse-train regulated (i.e. gave the same average power, regardless of pulse repetition rate), and the difference in response may thus be related to dosage.**

Plavnik [1109, 1493] found that HeNe LPT could elicit an acceleration of soluble proteins in hamster submandibular glands as a result of trophic cell stimulus.

The study by Simões [1796] aimed to investigate whether infrared LPT increased salivary flow rate and altered pH value, protein concentration, and peroxidase and amylase activities in saliva of rats. Wistar rats were used and divided into three groups. Experimental groups (A and B) had their parotid, submandibular and sublingual glands submitted to a diode laser, 808 nm wavelength, on two consecutive days. The doses were 4 and 8 J/cm^2, respectively. A red guide light was used to visualize the irradiated area. Group C was irradiated only with a red pilot beam and served as a control group. The saliva samples were collected after each irradiation step (first and second day of collection) and one week after the first irradiation (seventh day). Statistical analysis was performed, and differences were observed according to different days of salivary collection. The results showed that the salivary flow rate for groups A and B was higher on the seventh day when compared to the data obtained for the first day.

The aim of a study by Simões [1838] was to evaluate the effects of infrared LPT on tissues of the submandibular gland (SMG) and parotid gland (PG). Wistar rats were randomly divided into experimental (A and B) and control (C) groups. 808 nm in continuous wave mode was applied to the PG, SMG and sublingual gland in the experimental groups on two consecutive days. The doses were 4 J/cm^2 and 8 J/cm^2, and total energy was 7 J and 14 J, respectively. The power output (500 mW) and power density (277 mW/cm^2) were the same for both experimental groups. In order to visualize the area irradiated by the infrared laser, the authors used a red pilot beam (650 nm) with 3 mW maximum power for the experimental groups. For the control group, the red pilot beam was the only device used. The SMG and PG were removed after 1 week of the first irradiation. Total protein concentration, amylase, peroxidase, catalase and lactate dehydrogenase assays were performed, as well as histological analysis. Statistical tests revealed significant increase in the total protein concentration for groups A and B in the parotid glands.

Onizawa [1824] investigated cell response, including cell proliferation and expression of heat stress protein and bcl-2, to clarify the influence of GaAlAs laser irradiation on Par-C10 cells derived from the acinar cells of rat parotid glands. Furthermore, the author also investigated amylase release and cell death from irradiation in acinar cells from rat parotid glands. The number of Par-C10 cells in the laser-irradiated groups was

unilateral plantar fasciitis were enrolled in a randomized, double-blind, placebo-controlled trial, but 25 participants completed the therapeutic protocol. The contralateral asymptomatic fascia was used as control. After enrolment, symptomatic individuals were randomly assigned to receive LPT, or identical placebo, for 6 weeks. Ultrasonography was performed at baseline and after completion of therapy. The subjective subcalcaneal pain was recorded at baseline and after treatment on a visual analogue scale (VAS). After LPT, plantar fascia thickness in both groups showed significant change over the experimental period and there was a difference (before treatment and after treatment) in plantar fascia thickness between the two groups. However, plantar fascia thickness was insignificant (mean 3.627 +/- 0.977 mm) when compared with that in the placebo group (mean 4.380 +/- 1.0042 mm). Pain estimation on the visual analogue scale had improved significantly in all test situations (after night rest, daily activities) after LPT when compared with that of the placebo group. Additionally, when the difference in pain scores was compared between the two groups, the change was statistically significant. In summary, while ultrasound imaging is able to depict the morphologic changes related to plantar fasciitis, 904 nm gallium-arsenide (GaAs) infrared laser may contribute to healing and pain reduction in plantar fasciitis.

Further literature: [626]

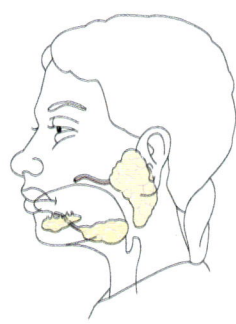

4.1.44 Salivary glands

Sjögren's syndrome is an RA-related condition characterised by low saliva and tear secretion, among other things. The treatment of Sjögren's syndrome with lasers is still in the experimental stage, although preliminary results show that the salivary glands do react quickly to local treatment. It has not yet been made clear whether LPT has a long-standing effect. All three wavelengths (HeNe, GaAlAs, GaAs) have been shown to stimulate the salivary glands.

Literature:
Animal studies

Takeda [113] examined the effects of a GaAs laser on the submandibular salivary glands of rats. The rats were divided into three groups: a control group, a group treated with GaAs laser irradiation at 760 pulses per second, and a group treated with GaAs laser irradiation at 190 pulses per second. The glands were uncovered and irradiated, after which they were sutured. The effects were studied histologically 1 hour and 24 hours after irradiation. Increased mitosis in the duct epithelium was observed in one laser group. The greatest increase was in the granular salivary ducts, while the effects in

genesis is still unknown and, as a consequence, there is no satisfactory treatment so far. Seven patients affected by burning sensation were selected in a pilot study by Kato [2047]. A laser emitting at 790 nm was used in this study. The time of irradiation was calculated based on the fluence of 6 J/cm2, output power of 120 mW. Energy was delivered by scanning the mucosal surface keeping the probe in contact with the tissue. The treatment was performed once a week for three consecutive weeks. Burning intensity was recorded through a visual analog scale (VAS) before, at the end of the treatment and in a six-week follow-up. The mean VAS value decreased significantly from the beginning to the end of laser therapy. After the laser irradiation, a mean reduction of 80.3% was obtained. There was no statistical difference between the end of the treatment and the six-week follow-up. Under the investigated parameters, infrared LPT was effective in the reduction of the BMS symptoms and it was able to maintain the improvement achieved for six weeks.

Further literature: [222, 443, 1045, 1055, 1261, 1445, 1570, 1630]

4.1.43 Plantar fasciitis

Plantar fasciitis can be successfully treated with LPT. Infrared light is needed in view of the dense skin and the depth of the target (10-12 mm). A good knowledge of the anatomy is essential, since the area of the tendon defect is less than 1 cm^2. A total of 6-10 J over the tendon insertion, followed by 3-4 J per cm along the arch of the foot, is a reasonable dosage. Three to six sessions may be needed, depending on the initial condition of the patient.

Literature:

Basford [1028] treated 32 patients with plantar fasciitis during 12 sessions. The origin of the plantar fascia was given 1 J of 830 nm laser (30 mW) and the medial border of the fascia was swept with a total dose of 2 J. The outcome was negative, quite possibly due to the low dosage.

Hronková [949] irradiated the place of maximum pain with a 200 mW, 870 nm laser, energy density 9 J/cm^2, 10 sessions every other day. Sixty-one patients had this therapy while fifty-two patients had a non-active placebo laser. In the laser group, 64% had a complete remission of pain, 26% experienced an improvement, and in 10% this therapy brought no effect at all. In the placebo group, 18% reported a full remission of pain, 42% reported an improvement and 40% felt no effect. In a separate study, ultrasound was used for 60 patients - 1 W/cm^2 applied for 5 minutes, 10 applications. All in all 50% of the patients had a complete remission of pain, 16.6% were improved and 33.3% reported no effect. Eight of the patients who had not experienced any effect from ultrasound were given LPT, no earlier than two weeks after ending the ultrasound treatment. Six of these patients evaluated their treatment as successful while the additional LPT had no effect in two patients.

The aim of a study by Kiritsi [2118] was to investigate the effect of LPT on plantar fasciitis documented by the ultrasonographic appearance of the aponeurosis and by patients' pain scores. Thirty individuals with diagnosis of

1999 to December 2002. Laser irradiation was applied for three minutes either every day or every other day for a total of 10 times. A semi-conductor laser with a wavelength of 830 nm and a power of 1 W was used. Evaluations were performed before and after the series of 10 exposures to laser irradiation. The evaluation included the measurement of pain using the visual analog scale (VAS) and serum prostaglandin E_2 (pg/mL). The analgesic effects were observed in 67 of 83 cases. The VAS scores for the effective cases decreased after the irradiation series from 8.5 +/- 0.2, to 2.8 +/- 0.2. The post-irradiation PGE_2 levels were lower than the pre-irradiation PGE_2 levels in the effective cases, which were 5.8 +/- 0.3 and 7.1 +/- 0.4 pg/mL, respectively. The post irradiation PGE_2 levels for the effective cases were lower than those for the ineffective cases, which were 5.8 +/- 0.3 and 7.3 +/- 0.9 pg/mL, respectively.

This study by Chow [1478, 1702] was undertaken to test the efficacy of a 300 mW, 830 nm laser in a prospective double-blind, randomised, placebo-controlled trial in patients with chronic neck pain. Ninety patients were enrolled. Laser was applied using the contact method over tender areas in the neck musculature, twice a week for 7 weeks. The primary outcome measure was change in a 10 cm Visual Analogue Scale for pain. Other measures used included a Self-Reported Improvement in pain, measured by a VAS, Short-Form 36 Quality-of-Life Questionnaire, Northwick Park Neck Pain Questionnaire, Neck Pain and Disability Scale and the McGill Pain Questionnaire. Measurements were taken at baseline, at the end of 7 weeks of treatment and at 12 weeks from baseline. Patients in the treated group experienced a mean self reported improvement of 48.5% compared with 3.99% in the placebo group.

Chow [2126] searched computerised databases comparing efficacy of LPT using any wavelength with placebo or with active control in acute or chronic neck pain. Effect size for the primary outcome, pain intensity, was defined as a pooled estimate of mean difference in change in mm on 100 mm visual analogue scale. The research group identified 16 randomised controlled trials including a total of 820 patients. In acute neck pain, results of two trials showed a relative risk (RR) of 1.69 (95% CI 1.22-2.33) for pain improvement of LPT versus placebo. Five trials of chronic neck pain reporting categorical data showed an RR for pain improvement of 4.05 (2.74-5.98) of LPT. Patients in 11 trials reporting changes in visual analogue scale had pain intensity reduced by 19.86 mm (10.04-29.68). Seven trials provided follow-up data for 1-22 weeks after completion of treatment, with short-term pain relief persisting in the medium term with a reduction of 22.07 mm (17.42-26.72). Side-effects from LPT were mild and not different from those of placebo. It was show that LPT reduces pain immediately after treatment in acute neck pain and up to 22 weeks after completion of treatment in patients with chronic neck pain.

Burning mouth syndrome (BMS) is a chronic disease that causes a burning sensation on an otherwise clinically normal oral mucosa. Its patho-

performed on 12 of these subjects and sham irradiation on the other 12, at the left maxillary third molar area. Far-field STEP latencies and amplitudes were recorded; at baseline, immediately after intervention, 10 and 20 minutes after intervention. In the irradiated group an immediate average STEP amplitude decrease from baseline of 60% occurred, with a further reduction to 65 and 72% at the 10 and 20 minute intervals. No significant changes occurred in the sham irradiation group and no change in latencies was observed in either group.

The aim of the study by Schuhfried [1717] was to examine the effects of helium-neon laser irradiation on the mechanical (pressure algometry) and electrical (1 ms monophasic square-wave pulses, 50 Hz) pain threshold. Thirty-two pain-free subjects were randomly assigned to either the experimental group (helium-neon laser stimulation: 5 mW, 10 min) or the placebo group (sham stimulation). Laser or sham stimulation and pain threshold ascertainment were carried out on the dorsal aspect of the forearm area. The contra lateral arm served as an untreated control. The groups were compared with each other and with the control arm. No significant differences were found between the laser stimulation and the sham stimulation in changes of either the mechanical or the electrical pain threshold. There were no changes in the mechanical pain threshold through laser stimulation and sham stimulation with respect to the untreated contra lateral arm. After laser stimulation, electrical pain threshold was significantly higher in the treated arm than in the untreated contra lateral arm, because this threshold decreased in the contra lateral arm. This was not the case in sham treatment.

A prospective, double-blind, randomized, and controlled trial was conducted by Gür [1433] in patients with chronic myofascial pain syndrome (MPS) in the neck to evaluate the effects of infrared 904 nm Gallium-Arsenide LPT on clinical issues and quality of life (QoL).: The study group consisted of 60 MPS patients. Patients were randomly assigned to two treatment groups: Group I (actual laser; 30 patients) and Group II (placebo laser; 30 patients). LPT continued daily for 2 weeks except weekends. Follow-up measures were evaluated at baseline, and at week 2, 3 and 12. All patients were evaluated with respect to pain at rest, pain at movement, number of trigger points (TP), the Neck Pain and Disability Visual Analog Scale (NPAD), Beck Depression Inventory (BDI), and the Nottingham Health Profile (NHP). In the active laser group, statistically significant improvements were detected in all outcome measures compared with baseline, while in the placebo laser group, significant improvements were detected in only pain score at rest at 1 week after the end of treatment. The score for self-assessed improvement of pain was significantly different between the active and placebo laser groups (63 vs. 19%). This study revealed that short-period application of LPT is effective in pain relief and in the improvement of functional ability and QoL in patients with MPS.

The subjects of the investigation by Mizutani [1276] consisted of 83 female patients that were treated during the two-year period from January

Bradley [436] treated 100 cases of painful oral conditions with a GaAlAs laser. A good improvement was achieved in nearly 60%.

In a double-blind study, Cieslar [626] treated a group of 522 patients suffering from various overloading syndromes of the motional system. One group was given sham irradiation, one 904 nm, another 850 nm, and yet another 633 nm laser irradiation. The diagnoses were epicondylitis humeri (1), periarthritis humeroscapularis (2), periarthritis genu (3), and aponeurosis-sitis plantaris (4). Distinct pain relief was generally obtained after five to seven sessions. Regression of swelling and increased mobility were obtained after 10-20 irradiations. The best results were obtained in epicondylitis (87%), followed by (2), (3), and (4), the latter 61%. Indications (3) and (4) required more sessions than (1) and (2). The results obtained were significantly better by comparison with the control group, although the high percentage of improvement in the control group (39%) indicates that laser also is a strong placebo tool. There was no significant difference between the three wavelengths.

Ceccherrelli [315] used a GaAs laser in a double-blind study on cervical myofascial pain. The patients were submitted to 12 sessions on alternate days, total dose per session 5 J. During each session, the four most painful muscular trigger points and five bilateral homometameric acupuncture points were irradiated. Pain relief was statistically significant both at the end of the treatment period and at a three-month follow-up examination.

Toya [255] performed a two-centre double-blind study on a group of 115 patients. The groups were: extremity joint pain, cervical pain and lumbar pain. A 830 nm 60 mW laser was used in the contact mode. All in all 82% of those in the laser group reported effective pain relief, compared to 42% in the sham treatment group.

Maricic [56] tested a GaAs laser on 53 dental patients with various pain conditions. The diagnoses included pain after extraction, neuralgia, solitary aphta, decubitus ulcer, dentitio dificilis and hyperaemic pulp. The average number of treatment sessions was 3.4 and each session took between 3 and 10 minutes. Full relief from pain was achieved in 69.8% of the cases, an obvious improvement in 20.7%, and some improvement in 9.4%. No patient reported a total lack of pain relief.

Taguchi [189] examined the effects of GaAlAs 780 nm on a group of 124 outpatients with various pain conditions. Treatment was administered one to three times a week for an average of seven weeks. The study was conducted double-blind. A high level of pain relief was achieved in 45 out of 63 members of the experimental group, and in 8 out of 61 of the control group. Thermography was carried out 92 times on 20 different patients. An increase in the skin's microcirculation was observed after LPT.

Nelson [1251] studied the effect on somatosensory trigeminal evoked potentials (STEP) and latencies by intraoral laser irradiation of the maxillary nerve. After electrical input at the left infraorbital foramen on 24 experimentally blinded, pain-free subjects, HeNe laser (1.7 mW, 50 Hz, 0.1 J) was

This reference is obviously not a matter of a double-blind study or a controlled experiment, and the dropout rate is high, but the size of the group is such that the study should be taken seriously. Shiroto later [217] evaluated an extended patient group of 7700 patients and arrived at the same results. Recently, Shiroto published the results from 8844 patients and the results are consistent. The most recent publication on this long-term study is [1446].

Zhong [303] and Choi [496] have also demonstrated the role of endogenous opiate-like peptides and serotonin in laser acupuncture anaesthesia.

Mizokami [54] studied the effects of GaAlAs laser on pain conditions at a neurosurgical clinic. The number of cases where the result of treatment was "excellent" or "good" among patients with occipital neuralgia was 81%, among patients with pain in arms/shoulders/neck 79%, and for patients with pain in the back 50%.

Irradiation of the stellate ganglion can be used as an additional treatment in pain patients. Hashimoto and Kemmutso [691, 692] have shown that even irradiation of the stellate ganglion alone can have an effect on pain. In a double-blind study, patients with postherpetic neuralgia were treated with either a 150 mW GaAlAs, a 60 mW GaAlAs or a placebo laser. VAS pain scores and regional skin temperature were affected by laser, but there was no change in the placebo group. The pain reduction was dose dependent. It is suggested that laser irradiation of the stellate ganglion is a good alternative to traditional blocks.

Phantom pain after amputation is a severe problem. Taguchi [663] reports that LPT has been the most effective way of releasing the phantom pain of an amputee.

In a double-blind study by Mohktar [161], experimental pain was induced in human volunteers. The pain was similar to that of an acute fracture. This type of pain is unresponsive to 900 mg of paracetamol or 600 mg of aspirin. A GaAlAs laser, however, did have a significant pain reducing effect.

Hansen [55] treated 40 patients with various chronic oro-facial pain conditions. The majority of the patients (38 female, 2 male) suffered from dysaesthesia ("burning mouth syndrome"). The patients had had their symptoms for approximately five years and were resistant to therapy. The effect was measured on a visual analogue scale (VAS) and by measuring 5-HIAA in urine. No positive effect was observed. **It is interesting to note that the authors themselves state the origin of "burning mouth" as multifactor, psychosomatic or psychogenic. Thus, there would be no actual injury to the tissue, and laser, like any other modality, would have no effect. The negative 5-HIAA measurement may indeed confirm the inappropriate inclusion parameters in this study.**

Eckerdal [595] used 830 nm, 30 mW laser light for atypical facial pain. At the end of the trial, 76% of the patients were pain-free, and at the one-year check-up 44%, were free from pain.

To better understand the mechanisms of therapeutic lasers for treating human myofascial trigger points, Chen [1997] designed a blinded controlled study of the effects of a therapeutic laser on the prevalence of endplate noise (EPN) recorded from the myofascial trigger spot (MTrS) of rabbit skeletal muscle. In eight rabbits, one MTrS in each biceps femoris muscle was irradiated with a 660 nm at 9 J/cm^2. The contralateral side of the muscle was treated with a sham laser. Each rabbit received six treatments. The immediate and cumulative effects were assessed by the prevalence of EPN with electromyographic (EMG) recordings after the first and last treatments. Compared with pretreatment values, the percentages of EPN prevalence in the experimental side after the first and last treatments were significantly reduced. The change in EPN prevalence in the experimental side was significantly greater than in the control side immediately after the first and last treatments. However, no significant differences were noted between the first and last treatments. It seems that laser irradiction may inhibit the irritability of an MTrS in rabbit skeletal muscle. This effect may be a possible mechanism for myofascial pain relief with LPT.

Hagiwara [1999] investigated whether pre-irradiation of blood by LPT enhances peripheral endogenous opioid analgesia. The effect of LPT pretreatment of blood on peripheral endogenous opioid analgesia was evaluated in a rat model of inflammation. Additionally, the effect of LPT on opioid production was also investigated in vitro in rat blood cells. The expression of the ß-endorphin precursors, proopiomelanocortin and corticotrophin releasing factor, were investigated by a reverse transcription polymerase chain reaction. LPT pretreatment produced an analgesic effect in inflamed peripheral tissue, which was transiently antagonized by naloxone. Correspondingly, ß-endorphin precursor mRNA expression increased with LPT, both in vivo and in vitro. These findings suggest that LPT pretreatment of blood induces analgesia in rats by enhancing peripheral endogenous opioid production, in addition to previously reported mechanisms.

Clinical studies

Laakso [253] wanted to study the possible relationship between LPT and opiods. In a double-blind study, 56 patients with chronic pain conditions were treated with a GaAlAs laser 820 nm, a 25 mW, InGaAlP laser 670 nm, 10 mW, and a LED 660 nm, 9.5 mW. ACTH and ß-endorphin levels were significantly elevated in the LPT groups but not in the LED group. Responses were dependent on dose and wavelength. The cumulative effect of LPT was confirmed.

Shiroto [53] carried out a retrospective interview-based study of patients who had received pain-relieving treatment with GaAlAs laser light. Of the 3635 patients treated over a period of 46 months, 82.8% regarded the treatment as effective. Of the 1300 patients who received more than 10 treatment applications, 76% regarded the treatment as effective. One single application could relieve pain for nine hours (15.5%) to three days (83.5%).

study of the effect of the laser on the sensitization increase of nociceptors. A HeNe laser of 2.5 J/cm^2 was used for irradiation. The researchers found that HeNe stimulation increased the pain threshold by a factor between 68% and 95% depending on the injected drug. They also observed a 54% reduction on the volume increase of the edema when it was irradiated. The analgesic effect seems to involve hyperalgesic mediators instead of peripheral opioid receptors.

Wedlock [1017] sought to establish dose dependency and time course for effects of cranial laser irradiation in two rodent models of pain. These were the hot plate and tail flick tests, which are both widely used to quantify analgesic drug effects. The laser used was GaAlAs, average power output 100 mW, pulse repetition rate 5 kHz. Irradiation was applied to shaved heads of rats above the midbrain. In the first experiment, four groups of 10 rats received doses of 0, 6, 12, 18, and 24 J/cm^2 in random order prior to hot plate testing either immediately, 30 min, 1 h or 24 h post laser. The second study employed three groups of 10 rats receiving 0, 12, and 18 J/cm^2 in random order prior to tail flick testing at the three shorter times above. Latency to lick hind paws on the hot plate was highly significantly prolonged by laser treatment across all doses and time periods. There was a clear dose dependency for immediate observations, but at 24 h 18 J/cm^2 was the most effective dose. Laser treatment also delayed tail flick responses at both doses and for all time periods, but 12 and 18 J/cm^2 doses were similar in efficacy.

In the study by Sato [1512], GaAlAs (830 nm, 40 mW) was used for the treatment of many kinds of pain. The mechanism of action of the laser irradiation for analgesia was studied in anesthetized rats. The effect of laser irradiation of the saphenous nerve was studied by recording neuronal activity at the L4 dorsal root filaments after the injection of a chemical irritant, turpentine. Laser irradiation inhibited both the asynchronous firing that was induced by turpentine and increased part of the slow components of the action potentials. Thus, the laser irradiation selectively inhibited nociceptive signals at peripheral nerves.

The aim of the study by Pozza [1993] was to evaluate the analgesic effect of laser therapy on healthy tissue of mice. Forty-five animals were divided into three groups of fifteen each: A: infrared laser irradiation (830 nm), B: red laser irradiation (660 nm), and C: sham irradiation with the laser unit off. After laser application, the mice remained immobilized by injecting 30 microl of 2% formalin into the plantar pad of the irradiated hind paw. The time that the mouse kept the hind paw lifted was measured with 5 minute intervals for 30 minutes. Results showed statistically significant differences comparing the control group with the infrared laser group at 5, 20, 25 and 30 accumulated minutes, and with the red laser group at all time points. The analysis of partial times, for each 5 minutes, showed statistically significant differences between the control and the laser groups up to 20 minutes. Thus, laser irradiation had an analgesic effect and red laser had the best results.

injection of 1-NAME blocked the analgesic effect obtained by 904 nm irradiation of rat skulls.

The purpose of a study by Aimbire [1560] was to investigate the effect of LPT on rat trachea hyperreactivity (RTHR), bronchoalveolar lavage (BAL) and lung neutrophils influx after Gram-negative bacteria lipopolysacharide (LPS) intravenous injections. The RTHR, BAL and lung neutrophils influx were measured over different intervals of time (90 min, 6 h, 24 h and 48 h). The energy density (ED) that produced an anti-inflammatory effect was 2.5 J/cm^2, reducing the maximal contractile response and the sensibility of trachea rings to methacholine after LPS. The same ED produced an anti-inflammatory effect on BAL and lung neutrophils influx. The Celecoxib COX-2 inhibitor reduced RTHR and the number of cells in BAL and lung neutrophils influx of rats treated with LPS. Celecoxib and laser reduced the PGE$_2$ and TXA2 levels in the BAL of LPS-treated rats. These results demonstrate that 685 nm LPT produced anti-inflammatory effects on RTHR, BAL and lung neutrophils influx in association with inhibition of COX-2-derived metabolites.

The purpose of another study by Albertini [1580] was to investigate the effect of LPT on the acute inflammatory process. Male rats were used. Paw oedema was induced by a sub-plantar injection of carrageenan, the paw volume was measured before and one, two, three and four hours after the injection, using a hydroplethysmometer. To investigate the mechanism action of the GaAlAs laser on inflammatory oedema, parallel studies were performed using adrenalectomised rats or rats treated with sodium diclofenac. Different laser irradiation protocols were employed for specific energy densities (EDs), exposure times and repetition rates. The rats were irradiated with laser for 80 s each hour. The EDs that produced an anti-inflammatory effect were 1 and 2.5 J/cm^2, reducing the oedema by 27% and 45.4%, respectively. The ED of 2.5 J/cm^2 produced anti-inflammatory effects similar to those produced by the cyclooxygenase inhibitor sodium diclofenac at a dose of 1 mg/kg. In adrenalectomised animals, the laser irradiation failed to inhibit the oedema. These results suggest that low-power laser irradiation possibly exerts its anti-inflammatory effects by stimulating the release of adrenal corticosteroid hormones.

The aim of the study by Ferreira [1733] was to evaluate the analgesic effect of the LPT with a HeNe laser on acute inflammatory pain, verifying the contribution of the peripheral opioid receptors and the action of LPT on the hyperalgesia produced by the release of hyperalgesic mediators of inflammation. Male rats were used. Three complementary experiments were done: (1) The inflammatory reaction was induced by the injection of carrageenin into one of the hind paws. Pain threshold and volume increase of the edema were measured by a pressure gauge and plethysmography, respectively. (2) The involvement of peripheral opioid receptors on the analgesic effect of the laser was evaluated by simultaneous injections of carrageenin and naloxone into one hind paw. (3). Hyperalgesia was induced by injecting PGE$_2$ for the

Animal studies

Montesinos [40] studied the blood concentration of various amino acids in rats after direct laser irradiation of the pituitary gland. The mean value in the control group was 4.57 µg/ml. In the laser group treated with HeNe, the mean level after day one was 47, day three 24, and day five 53. By day seven it had dropped to 0.8 and by day fifteen it had risen again to 24, then dropped once more to 22 by day twenty-one. In the GaAs group, the level was 44 after three days and 21 after seven days. Both lasers were thus effective but worked in different ways. The peptides studied build leukoencephalins and metencephalins, which affect the apprehension of pain.

Honmura [188], however, has conducted experiments which indicate that the pain-relieving effect of LPT is not only opiod-related. By injecting a substance which causes pain in the paws of rats (in accordance with a well-known experimental model), it was found that the analgesic effect was just as good whether indomethacin or LPT was used. In one group, a single dose of GaAlAs eliminated pain for 24 hours. Naloxone is a substance that counteracts the effects of opiates. When it was used, the effect of LPT was reduced but not eliminated. This experiment indicates that there are other possible explanations behind LPT's analgesic effects.

Katsuyama [662] studied the effect of 830 nm laser in a rat model of neuropathic pain. The left side's sciatic nerves of two groups of rats were ligated loosely to produce a neuropathic pain. The latency of the foot withdrawal reflex to noxious heat stimuli was measured before the ligation, immediately after laser/placebo radiation, and on day 14 after ligation. The laser group received 72 J through the dermis. This group showed a significant reduction in the left foot's withdrawal reflex immediately after irradiation and on day 14, the right foot remaining unchanged. Placebo irradiation did not change the latency either in the ligated group or in the non-ligated rats.

Giuliani [1515] used a red diode laser of 3 mW in experimental pain in rats. Acute inflammation was induced by an intraplantar injection of carrageenan, chronic inflammation was induced by a complete Freund's adjuvant (CFA), and neuropathic pain was produced by a sciatic nerve chronic constriction injury (CCI). In this study, laser was effective in reducing edema and hyperalgesia in acute and chronic inflammation if administered at the points usually selected for acupuncture. Moreover, spontaneous pain and thermal hyperalgesia were reduced in CCI rats treated with vLPT. In conclusion; laser reduced edema and induced analgesia in experimental plantar pain in rats. The author suggests that the enkephalin mRNA level was strongly upregulated in the external layers of the dorsal horn of the spinal cord in CFA and CCI animals, and that laser further increased the mRNA level in single neurons.

In an animal study by Mrowiec [432], it is suggested that nitric oxide is involved in the mechanism of low-power laser-induced analgesia. The

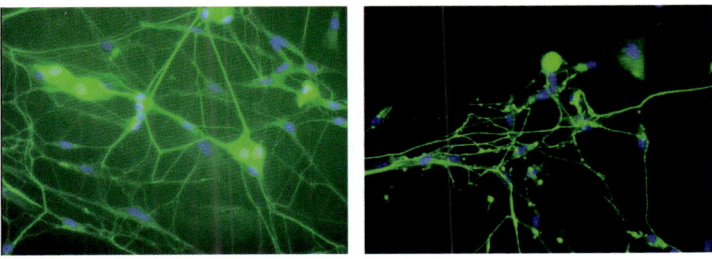

Figure 4.17 Formation of varicosities after 830 nm irradiation.
Courtesy: Roberta Chow

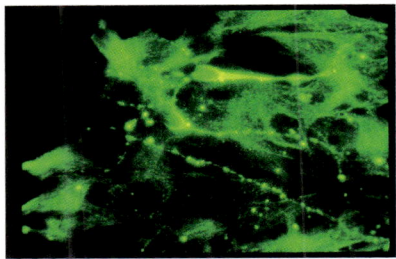

Figure 4.18 The same phenomenon observed with Nd:YAG laser.
Courtesy: Ambrose Chan

The study by Hagiwara [2000] investigated whether LPT may enhance peripheral endogenous opioid analgesia. The effect of LPT on opioid analgesia and production was evaluated in vivo in a rat model of inflammation as well as in vitro in Jurkat cells, a human T-cell leukemia cell line. mRNA expression of the β-endorphin precursors proopiomelanocortin and corticotrophin releasing factor was assessed by a reverse transcription polymerase chain reaction. LPT produced an analgesic effect in inflamed peripheral tissue which was transiently antagonised by naloxone. β-endorphin precursor mRNA expression increased with LPT, both in vivo and in vitro. This study demonstrates that LPT produces analgesic effects in a rat model of peripheral inflammation. The researchers also revealed an additional mechanism of LPT-mediated analgesia via enhancement of peripheral endogenous opioids. These findings suggest that LPT induces analgesia in rats by enhancing peripheral endogenous opioid production in addition to previously reported mechanisms.

the right upper lip of the test animals (n = 9) immediately after 10 min of Er:YAG laser irradiation (energy: 0.1 J/cm^2 per pulse at 10 Hz). Control animals (n = 9) were restrained for 10 min without laser application. The nociceptive response, i.e. the amount of time the rats spent rubbing the formalin injected area, was measured by an investigator blind to whether the animals had been laser irradiated or not. On laser irradiated rats, significantly less nociceptive behavior was observed only during the late phase (12-39 min) of the test. This result is similar to that reported for non-steroid antiinflammatory drugs (NSAIDs) and other peripherally acting antiinflammatory agents.

In a Meta analysis of the literature [872], there was a highly significant outcome for this kind of treatment of pain. The possible mechanisms and clinical effects found in randomized placebo controlled studies are presented in a review article by Bjordal [1681].

Literature:
In vitro studies

Chow [1784] reports the formation of 830 nm laser-induced, reversible axonal varicosities, using immunostaining with β-tubulin, in small and medium diameter, TRPV-1 positive, cultured rat DRG neurons. Laser also induced a progressive and statistically significant decrease in MMP in mitochondria in and between static axonal varicosities. In cell bodies of the neuron, the decrease in MMP was also statistically significant, but the decrease occurred more slowly. Importantly we also report for the first time that 830 nm laser blocked fast axonal flow, imaged in real time using confocal laser microscopy and JC-1 as mitotracker. Control neurons in parallel cultures remained unaffected with no varicosity formation and no change in MMP. Mitochondrial movement was continuous and measured along the axons at a rate of 0.8 microm/s (range 0.5-2 microm/s), consistent with fast axonal flow. Photoacceptors in the mitochondrial membrane absorb laser and mediate the transduction of laser energy into electrochemical changes, initiating a secondary cascade of intracellular events. In neurons, this results in a decrease in MMP with a concurrent decrease in available ATP required for nerve function, including maintenance of microtubules and molecular motors, dyneins and kinesins, responsible for fast axonal flow. Laser-induced neural blockade is a consequence of such changes and provides a mechanism for a neural basis of laser-induced pain relief. The repeated application of laser in a clinical setting modulates nociception and reduces pain.

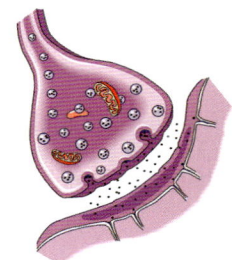

4.1.42 Pain

"Pain" could be the heading of almost any chapter in medicine. No step forward is appreciated more by the patients than the reduction of pain! The old exhortation "nil nocere" meshes well with the principles of LPT - lasers can prevent and reduce pain, as can be seen from much of the text above. A positive aspect of laser treatment is that pain can be alleviated as early as during the treatment session itself.

Large dosages are often required to achieve an immediate effect on acute pain since the pain relieving effect appears to be a matter of inhibition rather than of stimulation [1784]. A case of alveolitis can, for example, require as much as 20 J of GaAs laser light just to alleviate the pain. Less pronounced pain, such as a herpes sore or a decubital wound can require 3-4 J to achieve full relief from the symptoms. There is reason to believe that the large dosages used to alleviate severe pain also entail overdoses in the biostimulating range. The choice here is simple, however, and pain should be given priority. But care must be taken not to always give pain full priority. High doses over a knee, for instance, will soon reduce pain, but the stimulation of the chondrocytes may at the same time be inhibited. So the fine tuning can sometimes be delicate. Nonetheless, lowering the pain in an early phase can, on the other hand, allow the patient to go back to exercising, which in itself is positive.

Several mechanisms behind the pain relieving effect of LPT have been put forward, among them that the laser acts by inhibiting cyclooxygenase, interrupting the conversion of arachidonic acid into prostaglandin and also increases the production of β-endorphin [872].

Pain can be more than just suffering for the patient. It can also be an obstacle to any kind of treatment, for instance in dental surgery. A painful sore means that soft tissue anaesthetic is required to enable the dentist to manipulate the patient's lips and cheeks. Pain from the maxillary joint means that the patient cannot open his mouth sufficiently for an adequate occlusal adjustment to be performed, and it may not even be possible to take an imprint for a bite splint. Pain in the neck and back can make it difficult for a patient to lie down. In all these cases, reducing pain means that one can go straight ahead with normal therapy. Pain is often part of a vicious circle where the pain itself prevents the patient from exercise, thus aggravating the existing damage. When lasers are used for wound healing, one of the first observed effects is the reduction of pain. This is an observation not recorded in animal wound healing studies.

Laser is not only able to reduce pain sensations after injury; it can also be used preoperatively to reduce the expected pain reaction. In the study by Zeredo [1588], the researchers tested the possible antinociceptive effect of laser irradiation when applied to normal tissue before the onset of a painful stimulus. Male rats were used. A 1.5% formalin solution was injected into

powers lasting 60, 30, or 15 seconds. HSP-70 immunoreactivity was neither detected in control eyes nor outside the irradiated zones of treated eyes. Transpupillary laser irradiation lasting 15, 30, or 60 seconds induces a hyperexpression of HSP on choroidal layers.

A total of 203 patients (90 men and 113 women; mean age 63.4 ±5.3 y) with beginning ("dry") or advanced ("wet") forms of AMD (n=348 eyes) were included in a study by Ivandic [1850]. Altogether 193 (mean age 64. ± 4.3 y; n=328 eyes) with cataracts (n=182 eyes) or without cataracts (n =146 eyes) were treated four times using LPT (twice per week). A laser diode (780 nm, 7.5 mW, continuous emission) was used for transconjunctival irradiation of the macula for 40 sec (0.3 J/cm^2) resulting in a total dose of 1.2 J/cm^2. All in all 10 patients (n =20 eyes) with AMD received mock treatment and served as controls. Visual acuity was measured at each visit. LPT significantly improved visual acuity in 162/182 (95%) of eyes with cataracts and in 142/146 (97%) of eyes without cataracts. The prevalence of metamorphopsia, scotoma, and dyschromatopsia was reduced. In patients with wet AMD, the edema improved and the bleeding was reduced. The improved vision was maintained for 3-36 months after treatment. Visual acuity in the control group remained unchanged. No adverse effects were observed in those undergoing therapy. Monthly injections of ranibizumab into the eye has given promising results but the method is very expensive and invasive. In relation to this situation, the above study deserves attention.

Ivandic [2109] further investigated the potential use of LPT as a diagnostic tool for identifying hypertensive eyes at risk of glaucoma. The study of a case series included 123 healthy subjects with normal vision. The intraocular pressure (IOP) was determined before (baseline) and 30 min after a 30-sec irradiation of the limbus area with laser light (780 nm; 7.5 mW; 292 Hz modulation). Baseline IOP was >21 mm Hg in 44 of 211 eyes (20.9%), consistent with ocular hypertension. LPT decreased the mean IOP by 6.2 mm Hg in these eyes. The remaining 167 eyes (79.1%) exhibited a normo-tensive IOP <or=21 mm Hg. LPT reduced the mean IOP by 2.9 mm Hg in these eyes, but there were different response patterns: 1) the IOP did not change (27.0%); 2) the IOP was reduced by the same extent in both eyes (32.3%); 3) initial IOP differences between left and right eyes became level and the absolute IOP was reduced to a lower level that was identical in both eyes (18.0%); and 4) the initial difference in IOP between the left and right eye persisted despite LILI (22.7%). In conclusion, LPT lowers IOP, even in normotensive eyes. This effect may be useful to determine the individual physiological IOP and to diagnose latent ocular hypertension in eyes with presumably normotensive IOP.

Further literature: [571, 600, 601, 602, 603, 622, 1217]

shown by an earlier normalisation of the content of lipid peroxidation products and activity of superoxide dismutase.

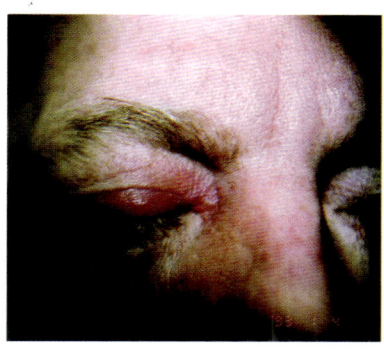 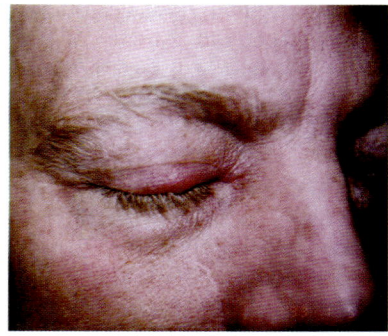

Figure 4.16 Stye day one and two, following HeNe LPT.

A review of Russian LPT studies in ophthalmology is presented by Pankov [1122]. The first studies appeared as early as 1976. HeNe lasers of a low output are used; some examples of which are 0.25 mW/cm and 0.05 mW/cm. Some indications treated are amotio retinae, functional amblyopia, post-traumatic iridocyclitis, endothelial-epithelial dystrophy, burn accidents, acute inflammatory and allergic diseases of the cornea, conjunctiva, iris and ciliary body. HeNe laser has also been shown to increase the lymphocirculation of the eye.

The study by Desmettre [1819] was performed with exposures shorter than 60 seconds to assess a choroidal heat shock protein hyperexpression after transpupillary thermotherapy (TTT). Male pigmented rabbits were anesthetized and TTT was performed on their right eyes with a 810 nm laser (spot size: 1.3 mm). Three exposure durations (60, 30, or 15 seconds) were used with three ranges of power for each duration ("high," "mild," or "low"). A series of laser impacts were delivered to the posterior pole of the retina. Left eyes were used as controls. Twenty-four hours after laser irradiation, the animals were killed and a histological study was performed on chorioretinal layers. Tissue samples were fixed in formalin and embedded in paraffin. A monoclonal antibody was used to detect Hsp70 immunoreactivity followed by a biotinylated goat anti-mouse antibody revealed by the avidin-biotin complex and the AEC chromogen. Retinal structures were further identified by HES coloration. During the experiments, the laser spots were not visible except for the strongest "high" powers for each exposure duration, where whitening was discernable at the end of the laser exposures. A strong HSP70 immunoreactivity was detected in choroidal, non-pigmented cells for laser exposures lasting 60, 30, or 15 seconds with "mild" laser powers. On the contrary, rare HSP hyperexpression was detected with "high" or "low" laser

close to the eye and the beam is highly divergent, the light will not be focused onto a small point, even if the eye is open. Therefore, the risk in this case is small, and even negligible. We therefore recommend a visible beam in this context. High-powered non-visible beams should only be used by a qualified therapist.

Treating a stye on the eyelid, for instance, is quite effective. Maeno [129] reported as early as 1989 that HeNe was effective in treating keratoconjunctivitis.

Literature:

Belkin and Schwartz [599] have presented a thorough review of the literature on LPT in ophthalmology. The majority of the studies are from Russia. The conclusion of the review is "that many studies must be looked at with skepticism because of lack of statistical evaluation, adequate inclusion and exclusion criteria, masking procedures etc. Nevertheless, the basic science experiments described in the earlier parts of the review and the demonstrable bioeffects of low-energy irradiation measured in various body systems leave us no option but to conclude that low-energy laser irradiation does exert some effects on ocular tissues in health and disease, and that these effects exhibit definite dose-response curves. Energy concentrations less than 1 J/cm^2 are generally ineffective and those over 5 J/cm^2 can be injurious. The precise dosage, however, depends on the specific laser/tissue combination. The clinical reports surveyed here are thus not theoretically impossible, but will have to be reconfirmed".

Eliseeva [654] has used intravenous irradiation in the therapy of ophthalmic problems.

In a report by Inkova [903], 82 patients with severe post-traumatic uveitis (eye inflammation), which could not be treated by traditional anti-inflammatory therapy, were exposed to LPT. The patients were divided into three groups: infrared laser exposure semiconductor pulsed laser, intravenous exposure of the blood to a He-Ne laser, and both treatments combined. The treatment efficacy was monitored by measuring lipid per-oxides and superoxide dismutase in the lacrimal fluid. The treatment proved to be effective. The best results were attained by applying both methods of exposure, as

postoperatively and all patients were given the Washington rehabilitation program until the end of the 12th week. In Group II (20 digits in 12 patients), the same treatment protocol was given, but the laser instrument was switched off during applications. The results of the study showed a significant improvement in the laser-treated group only for the parameter of edema reduction; the difference between the two groups was non-significant for pain reduction, hand grip strength, and functional evaluation performed according to the Strickland and Buck-Gramcko systems using total active motion and fingertip-to distal palmar crease distance parameters. The significant improvement obtained in edema reduction both immediately and 12 weeks after supplementary GaAs laser application in our study has been interpreted as an important contribution to the rehabilitation of human flexor tendon injuries, because edema is known to have a detrimental effect on functional recovery during both early and late stages of tendon healing. However, this study failed to show a significant positive effect of supplementary GaAs laser application on the other functional parameters.

The aim of a study by Markovic [1911] was to compare the effectiveness of LPT and dexamethasone after surgical removal of impacted lower third molars under local anaesthesia. There were 120 healthy patients divided into four groups of 30 patients each. Group 1 received LPT irradiation immediately after operation (4 J/cm^2, 50 mW, 637 nm); group 2 also received an intramuscular injection of 4 mg dexamethasone into the internal pterygoid muscle; group 3 received LPT irradiation supplemented by systemic dexamethasone 4 mg i.m. in the deltoid region, followed by 4 mg of dexamethasone intraorally six hours postoperatively; and the 4th (control) group received only the usual postoperative recommendations (cold packs, soft diet, etc.). Laser irradiation with local use of dexamethasone (group 2) resulted in a statistically significant reduction of postoperative edema in comparison to the other groups. No adverse effects of the procedure or medication were observed.

Further literature: [222, 485, 664, 769, 1696]

4.1.41 Ophthalmic problems

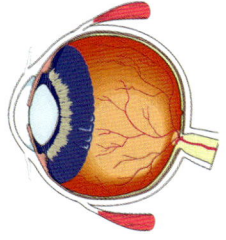

Treatment of the eye with LPT has been controversial, stemming from the early days of LPT and the hard-to-kill misconception that lasers in the low-milliwatt range could damage the eye. Patient and operator were recommended to use protective goggles even when treating a foot, using a laser of a couple of milliwatts.

Treating the unprotected eye is still the sole province of specialists. However, any reasonably trained person can carry out eye treatment through the eyelid. Closing the eye comes naturally when it is treated with a visible beam such as a HeNe laser. When a collimated invisible laser is used, one must make sure that the patient keeps his eyes closed. If the treatment probe is

and myeloperoxide activity (MPO) at 24 h after injury. The HI for the control group was 4.0. Celecoxib, laser, and dexamethasone all induced significantly lower HI than in the control animals at 2.5, 1.8 and 1.5, respectively. Dexamethasone, but not celecoxib, induced a slightly, but significantly lower HI than laser (p = 0.04). MPO activity was significantly decreased at 1.6 in groups receiving celecoxib at 0.87, dexamethasone at 0.50, and laser at 0.7 when compared to the control group, but there were no significant differences between any of the active treatments. In conclusion, LPT at a dose of 2.6 J/cm^2 induces a reduction of HI levels and MPO activity in hemorrhagic injury, which is not significantly different from that obtained by celecoxib. Dexamethasone is slightly more effective than LPT in reducing HI, but not MPO activity

Clinical studies

Røynesdal [93] studied the effects of GaAlAs in the surgical removal of impacted wisdom teeth. 6 J was administered before and after the operation. The same person operated on 25 people with bilaterally impacted wisdom teeth. The study showed that laser with these parameters had no effect on oedema, trismus or pain alleviation as compared with placebo laser. **The dose appears to be too low.**

Piller [928] has since 1993 treated over 700 patients with chronic secondary arm and leg lymphoedemas with GaAs scanning. LPT had no effect on any parameter on normal arms and legs. In the affected arms there was a significant reduction of volume, average 233 ml. There was also a significant effect on the level of fibrotically indurated tissues in the lymphatic territories of the upper arm and forearm. Average volume reduction in legs was 199 ml, which was not statistically significant. However, as with the arms, there were significant reductions in the level of free extra cellular fluids in the whole limb, and reductions in the level of fibrotic induration in the lymphatic territories of the lower posterior leg and the upper anterior leg. These results correlated strongly with the patients' subjective indications of feelings of tension, heaviness and aching.

Carati [1337] performed a randomised, double-blind study on the effect of GaAs laser on postmastectomy lymphoedema. There was no immediate effect of the irradiation, but at the one and three month follow-up after two cycles of laser treatment, about 30% of the patients had a clinically significant reduction of the arm volume and there was a significant softening of the tissue. Treatment did not appear to improve range of movement of the affected arm.

Similar, but not quite as positive results are reported by Kaviani [1692], using 890 nm, 1.5 J/cm^2 over the arm and axillary areas.

The study by Ozkan [1431]was performed in a total of 25 patients with 41 digital flexor tendon injuries in five anatomical zones. In Group I (21 digits in 13 patients), whirlpool and infrared GaAs diode laser with a pulse repetition rate of 100 Hz. was applied between the 8th and 21st day

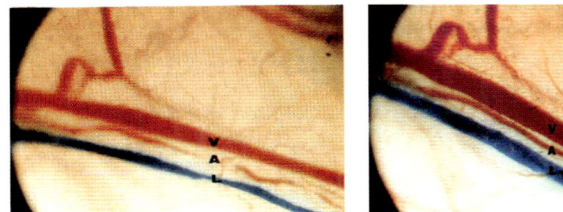

Figure 4.15 Vein, artery and lymph vessels before and after LPT.
Courtesy: Pierre Lievens

Honmura [96] studied the effects of a GaAlAs laser on experimentally produced inflammation in rats. In all cases in the laser group, the degree of inflammation was reduced by 20-30%. LPT also reduced the extent of the oedema in the acute inflammation phase. LPT was effective if administered within two hours after the inflammation-causing substance was given to the rats; if it was administered later, a poorer effect on the oedema was observed. In a comparison using the inflammation-reducing substance indomethacin, LPT was better in one experimental model, not so good in another, but effective in both cases. LPT also impeded the vessels' permeability in cases of acute inflammation and thereby reduced the acute oedema.

Prokofeva [1217] evaluated the doses of infrared laser exposure on the structure of the eye in rabbit experiments, and the potentials of such lasers in ophthalmology were assessed. Wavelength was 890 nm and doses varied from 0.0001 to 1.0 J/cm^2, corresponding to an exposure duration of 0.3 seconds to 45 min. Experiments were carried out on 20 animals. The right eyes were exposed, and the left ones were used as controls. An increase of intraocular pressure was recorded at a dose of 0.1 J/cm^2 (4.5 min) and higher. Morphological examination showed dilatated, well filled and newly formed vessels in the ciliary body and iris, as well as oedema and a destruction of the external layers of the retina. Exposure to a dose of 0.05 J/cm^2 and lower did not lead to the destruction of any ocular structures or to an increase of intraocular pressure. The maximal dose causing no side effects for the organ of vision was established at 0.05 J/cm^2.

The aim of a study by Aimbire [1800] was to investigate if LPT can modulate formation of hemorrhagic lesions induced by immune complex, since there is a lack of information on LPT effects in hemorrhagic injuries of high perfusion organs, and the relative efficacy of LPT compared to anti-inflammatory drugs. A controlled animal study was undertaken with 49 rats, randomly divided into seven groups. Bovine serum albumin i.v. was injected through the trachea to induce an immune complex lung injury. The study compared the effect of irradiation by a 650 nm laser with doses of 2.6 J/cm^2 to celecoxib, dexamethasone, and control groups for hemorrhagic index (HI)

cell proliferation significantly increased after exposure to a range of doses at 780 and 904 nm irradiation. MDA-MB-435S and Bre80hTERT cell lines showed negligible effects after one exposure from all three wavelengths, and no dose response relationships were noted. MCF-7 cells irradiated with 780 nm laser demonstrated an increasing dose response relationship after one exposure and a decreasing dose response relationship after three exposures. The MCF-7 cells irradiated with 904 nm laser demonstrated a decreasing dose response relationship after two and three exposures. Despite certain doses of laser increasing MCF-7 cell proliferation, multiple exposures had no effect or a decreasing effect on dose response relationships. Before a definitive conclusion can be made regarding the safety of LPT for post-mastectomy lymphoedema, further in vivo research must be conducted.

Animal studies

Labajos [300] noted that the flow of water and electrolytes through the intestinal wall was retarded by LPT, 1 J/cm^2.

Lievens [92, 298] studied the effects of GaAs laser light on the vasomotricity of the lymphatic system. The everted skin of mice was observed microscopically under a cold light source. The lymph vessels were visualised by an injection of a physiological dye. The vessels did not dilate after laser treatment if the tissue had not been subjected to trauma, but did dilate as a result of laser treatment when in an oedematous condition.

In another study of the regeneration of the lymphatic system, Lievens [299] used a combined GaAs/HeNe laser. A median incision along the linea alba was made on 600 white mice. The skin was turned back and pinned on a cork plate. The lymph vessels were visualised by means of an injection of Patent V Blue into an inguinal lymph node. There were 100 animals in the laser group and 500 in the control group. The results were as follows:

1.   Adhesion of the wound to the underlying tissue was present in 100% of the animals in the control group after day 4. The adhesion gradually disappeared after day 10. Adhesion hardly ever occurred in the laser group.
2.   The regeneration of the veins was faster in the laser group.
3.   In the control group, the lymphatic vessels regenerated through a network of small vessels. In the laser group, the lymph vessels regenerated into their original shape. Regeneration was much quicker in the laser group, in particular during the initial healing stage.
4.   The network-regenerated vessels in the non-irradiated group were very permeable. This increased permeability could be seen in 50% of the cases even after six months. The vessels in the laser group showed hardly any increased permeability after the first few days.

4.1.40 Oedema

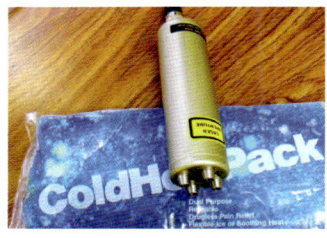

A more or less pronounced oedema always appears after a surgical intervention. The anti-oedematous effect is based on a dilatation of lymphatic vessels and a reduction in the permeability of blood vessels. Large doses are required if the oedema is already established - even 1-2 J/cm^2 with a GaAs laser or 10-15 J/cm^2 with a GaAlAs laser are on the low side after an operation. An established oedema may or may not be filled with blood, and haemoglobin is one of the most powerful chromophores in the organism. Penetration of the cases containing blood is therefore shallow, particularly with a HeNe laser.

Laser energy has a regenerative effect on lymphatic vessels, as it also has on veins. As can be seen in [92] and [299] below, LPT can probably not be used as an oedematic prophylaxis ahead of operation unless the oedema is already present before the operation.

When treating peripheral oedemas, the proximal sites of the body should always be irradiated first. Opening the blood flow at a peripheral site could be followed by a circulatory obstruction at the proximal site, thus causing pain.

Literature:
In vitro studies

Kiyoizumi [95] reported that a GaAlAs laser has two different effects on oedema. The laser stimulated the synthesis of PGI$_2$ (prostacyclin), which has a strong vasodilating effect, and counteracted the aggregation of platelets. The accumulation of PGI$_2$ in the tissue reduced the oedema tendency. Laser light was also shown to counteract the occurrence of fibrin networks, which were studied with radioactive iodine. Kiyoizumi's clinical experience of skin transplants is that LPT reduces oedema.

The aim of an investigation by Powell [2639] was to compare the cell proliferative effects of a range of doses of LPT at wavelengths of 780, 830 and 904 nm on human breast and immortalised human mammary epithelial cell lines in vitro. LPT is used in the clinical treatment of post-mastectomy lymphoedema, despite safety information being limited and circumstantial. This research was the first step in systematically developing guidelines for the safe clinical use of LPT in the management of post-mastectomy lymphoedema. Human breast adenocarcinoma (MCF-7), human breast ductal carcinoma (MDA-MB-435S), and immortalised human mammary epithelial (SVCT and Bre80hTERT) cell lines were irradiated with a single exposure of laser at 0.5, 1, 2, 3, 4, 10 and 12 J/cm^2 (780 nm) and at 0.5, 1, 2, 3, 4, 10 and 15 J/cm^2 (830 and 904 nm). MCF-7 cells were further irradiated with two and three exposures of all three laser wavelengths. XTT colorimetric assays were utilized to assess cell proliferation 24 hours after irradiation. SVCT

significant clinical improvement. She was off work for 5 months and soon after was fired. After this has become an antidepressant consumer and after a nervous breakdown in December 2008 the other side of the face (left) was paralysed. Medical treatments: is currently on anti-depressant (clonazepan), takes medication for high blood pressure (propanolol) and for thyroid hormone replacement (T4).

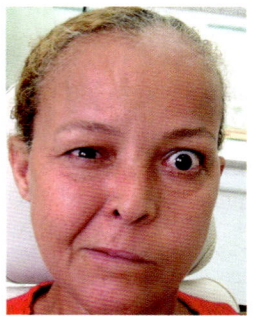 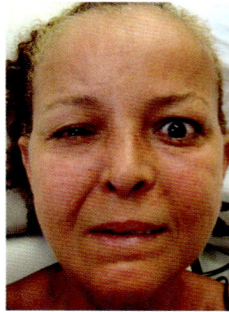 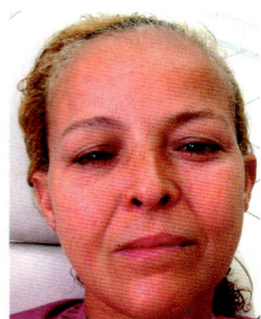

Figure 4.13   Laser treatment of bilateral facial paralysis

Laser treatment:
Spot area: 0,028 cm² (2 mm away from the target) or 0,0028 cm² in contact. Power output: 100 mW, 660 nm and 810 nm, energy: from 2 J to 3.4 J, energy density: from 70 J/cm² to 120 J/cm² Time of irradiation per point: 20 s to 34 s. Number of points: 30 per face. Distance between points: 1,5 to 2,5 cm. Number of sessions: 15 (7 sessions once a week, February and March), 2 session in May, 1 June, 3 August, 1 September, 1 November.

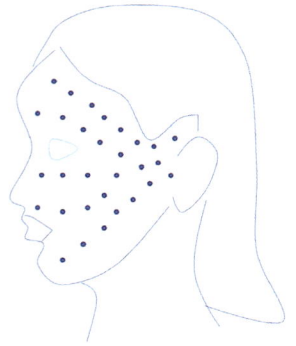

Figure 4.14   Face irradiation points

received LPT or a combination of LPT and SGB showed a similar picture of recovery from paralysis, in contrast to the group which received SGB only. The group that received only LPT also showed a better initial improvement.

Rochkind [1867] conducted a clinical pilot study to prospectively investigate the effectiveness of laser irradiation (780 nm) in the treatment of patients suffering from incomplete peripheral nerve and brachial plexus injuries for six months up to several years. Injury to a major nerve trunk frequently results in considerable disability associated with loss of sensory and motor functions. Spontaneous recovery of long-term severe incomplete peripheral nerve injury is often unsatisfactory. A randomized, double-blind, placebo-controlled trial was performed on 18 patients who were randomly assigned to placebo (non-active light: diffused LED lamp) or laser irradiation (wavelength, 780 nm; power, 250 mW). Twenty-one consecutive daily sessions of laser or placebo irradiation were applied transcutaneously for three hours to the injured peripheral nerve (energy density 450 J/cm^2) and for two hours to the corresponding segments of the spinal cord (energy density 300 J/cm^2). Clinical and electrophysiological assessments were done at baseline, at the end of the 21 days of treatment, and three and six months thereafter. The laser-irradiated and placebo groups were in clinically similar conditions at baseline. The analysis of motor function during the six-month follow-up period compared to baseline showed a statistically significant improvement in the laser-treated group compared to the placebo group. No statistically significant difference was found in sensory function. Electrophysiological analysis also showed a statistically significant improvement in recruitment of voluntary muscle activity in the laser-irradiated group compared to the placebo group.

Further literature: [375, 218, 493, 646, 933, 1038, 1113, 1469, 1669, 1670]

The following case comes from Daiane Thais Meneguzzo, Coordinator of Laser at São Leopoldo Mandic Dentistry School, Campinas, SP, Brazil.
Female, 48 years old.
Diagnosis: bilateral facial paralysis right side (2006) and left side (December 2008).
Probable causes:
  right side - thermal shock (she worked with solder components of cell phones)
  left side - vascular problem caused by high blood pressure after a nervous breakdown
Familiar history: aunt, nephew and sister have had facial paralysis.
Lesions history: In 2006 she worked with welding equipment and mobile phones one day she realized her face swollen, her eye was odd. The next day her face was paralysed, searched a hospital and was prescribed Meticorten (1 box, 20 days), Benerva (30 days) and Propranolol (to control high blood pressure). She did 6 months of physical therapy (25 min once a week) without

showed the best outcome. The laser was a 150 mW GaAlAs laser and the LPT was performed over the area of paralysis (36 J per session), the stylomastoid foramen (10.8 J) and the stellate ganglion (63.7 J). The number of sessions in the laser group ranged from 21 to 66, 5-12 weeks. In the combination group, success was achieved within 14-31 sessions, 3-10 weeks.

Paolini [960] treated 40 patients with Bell's paralysis. One group received only prednison (corticosteroid) 60 mg/day. The other group was treated with GaAs laser on points along the nerve, followed by an array of GaAs/HeNe five days a week for three weeks, then every second day, 30 sessions in all. The outcome in the laser group was significantly better than in the pharmacological group.

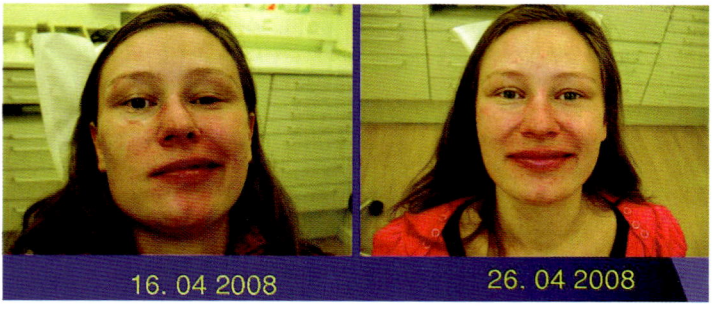

Figure 4.12 Ideopathic parasthesia after delivery resolved by LPT. Courtesy: Per Hugo Kristensen

Brugnera [970] treated two groups of patients with lesions to the inferior alveolar and mental nerves. The laser used was a 830 nm 40 mW, spot size 3 mm². All paraesthesias were due to surgical interventions. The first group was identified as immediate and was treated within 2-15 days after the injury. In this group, 72.7% achieved absolute recovery, 18.3% a relative improvement and 9% did not respond to treatment. In the latter group, the history of injury was 30-365 days. In this group, only 27.7% reached an absolute improvement.

Bernal [156] presented six years of experience of patients with facial paralysis on whom HeNe and GaAs lasers had been used. If the laser treatment was begun within two days of the occurrence of the injury, treatment with LPT was successful in 100% of cases and a maximum of 15 treatment sessions were required. If the patient was treated later, Meticorten (40 mg/day) was administered for seven days as a supplement. Up to 30 doses could be administered to the latter group. The degree of healing in this latter group varied, but complete rehabilitation was achieved by some of the patients.

Murakami [186] treated 52 people with idiopathic facial paralysis or Bell's paralysis; 26 were treated with stellate ganglion block (SGB), 11 received 830 nm LPT and 15 a combination of the two. The patients who

a total of seven sessions delivered immediately before surgery; at 6 and 24 hours after surgery; and on postoperative days 2, 3, 4 and 7. The clinical neurosensory test and VAS were completed just before each of the treatment sessions and on days 14 and 28 by one examiner. When the results of the patients treated with LPT were compared with published values for neurosensory recovery after orthognathic surgery, there was a significant acceleration in the time, as well as in the magnitude, of neurosensory return. Brush stroke directional discrimination approached normal values by 14 days, whereas 2-point discrimination and contact detection showed significant improvement on day 14 and returned to near-normal values by two months. The results of thermal discrimination and pinprick nociception revealed few neurosensory deficits; however, those patients who were affected showed a slower recovery trend and remained neurosensory-deficient for up to two months. The VAS analysis revealed a rapidly progressive improvement in subjective assessment, showing a 50% deficit on day 2 and only a 15% subjective deficit at two months.

The paper by Ozen [1635] reports on the effects of LPT in four patients with longstanding sensory nerve impairment following mandibular third molar surgery. Four female patients had complaints of paresthesia and dysesthesia of the lip, chin and gingiva, and buccal regions. Each patient had undergone mandibular third molar surgery at least one year earlier. The unit had a contact probe with a laser beam diameter of 0.5 cm. The system delivers a 70 mW output that emits a wavelength of 830 nm. The irradiance used was 6.0 J per treatment site, which was delivered by applying the laser for approximately 90 seconds. Each patient received a total of 20 laser treatment sessions. The patients were treated at 2-day intervals, three times a week until all sessions were completed. The laser probe was applied directly to the treatment sites. The patients experienced no sensation when the laser treatments were being carried out. The treatment time per point was 90 seconds. Thus, one treatment session, consisting of five treatment sites, took approximately eight minutes. The treatment sites were as follows: extraorally: the lower lip, chin and the region of mental foramen; intraorally: the mental foramen region, buccally in the region of the apicies of the first molar, and lingually in the region of the mandibular foramen. Clinical neurosensory tests (the brush stroke directional discrimination test, 2-point discrimination test, and a subjective assessment of neurosensory function using a visual analog scale) were used before and after treatment, and the responses were plotted over time. When the neurosensory assessment scores after treatment with LPT were compared with the baseline values prior to treatment, there was a significant acceleration in the time course, as well as in the magnitude, of neurosensory return. The VAS analysis revealed progressive improvement over time.

Yamada [1054] has compared corticosteroids, LPT and a combination of the two in a study comprising seven patients in each group. The effect of LPT was comparable to that of corticosteroids but the combined therapy

Patient with facial paresis following an ear operation 15 years ago. The second photo shows the situation after two laser sessions per week for one month.

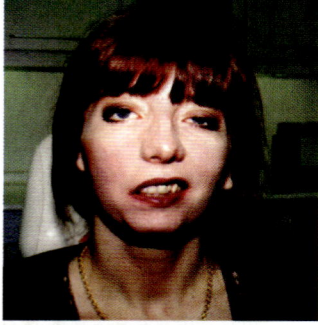

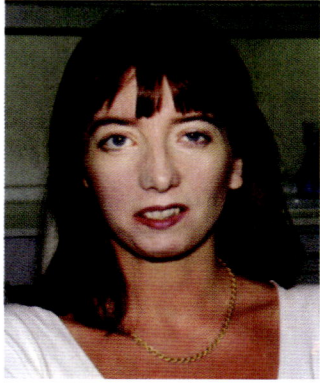

Figure 4.11 Long standing facial paresis after four session of LPT.

Courtesy: Per Hugo Kristensen

Clinical studies

The studies by Khullar [361, 900, 901, 902, 939, 1037] on the effects of LPT on long-standing paraesthesiae in the orofacial region found, in summary:

- A course of 20 LPT treatment sessions using a GaAlAs laser (820 nm) on an area of long-standing paraesthesiae in the orofacial region induced an objectively evaluated significant improvement in fine mechanosensory perception and a decrease in the area of paraesthesiae.

- The significant improvement in mechanosensory perception was also perceived as a subjective improvement by the patients.

- A course of 20 LPT treatment sessions with a GaAlAs laser (=820 nm) induced no change in thermoperception in an area of paraesthesiae.

- Daily LPT treatment over a 28 day period with a GaAlAs laser accelerated motor nerve reinnervation as assessed by a return of motor function subsequent to a standardised axonotmesis injury in the rat sciatic nerve.

- Treatment with a GaAlAs laser (820 nm) enhanced sensory reinnervation of peripheral target tissues subsequent to an IAN axotomy injury in the rat model. The findings are demonstrated immunohisto-chemically by the presence of CGRP positive neurones

A study by Miloro [899] examined the potential benefit of perioperative and short-term postoperative LPT on objective and subjective neurosensory recovery after bilateral sagittal split osteotomy surgery. Six consecutive patients undergoing bilateral sagittal split osteotomy procedures were enrolled in this prospective study. A complete preoperative clinical neurosensory test, consisting of brush stroke directional discrimination, 2-point discrimination, contact detection, pin prick nociception, and thermal discrimination, was performed on each patient; and a subjective assessment of neurosensory function was made by using a visual analogue scale (VAS). The protocol for LPT treatment consisted of 6 J per point along the distribution of the inferior alveolar nerve at four sites for

tional recovery were assessed. The laser treated groups had a significantly longer average axon growth and a higher total axon number in both the contusion and hemisection models compared to the control groups. In both models, the laser groups showed a significant functional improvement compared to the control groups.

The aim of a study by Ribeiro [2007] was to evaluate the action of an anti-COX-2 selective drug (celecoxib) on bone repair associated with LPT. A total of 64 rats underwent surgical bone defects in their tibias, being randomly distributed into four groups: Group 1) negative control; Group 2) animals treated with celecoxib; Group 3) animals treated with LPT, and Group 4) animals treated with celecoxib and LPT. The animals were killed after 48 h, and 7, 14 and 21 days. The tibias were removed for morphological, morphometric and immunohistochemistry analysis for COX-2. Statistically significant differences were observed in the quality of bone repair and quantity of formed bone between groups 3 and 4 on day 14 after surgery. COX-2 immunoreactivity was more intense in bone cells in the intermediate periods evaluated in the laser-exposed groups. Taken together, such results suggest that LPT is able to improve bone repair in the tibia of rats as a result of an upregulation of the cyclooxygenase-2 expression in bone cells.

The aim of a study by dos Reis [2008] was to analyze the influence of 660 nm laser light on the myelin sheath and functional recovery of the sciatic nerve in rats. The sciatic nerves of 12 Wistar rats were subjected to injury through neurotmesis and epineural anastomosis, and the animals were divided into two groups: group 1 was the control, and group 2 underwent LPT. After the injury, a 660 nm, 4 J/cm^2, 26.3 mW laser with a beam area of 0.63 cm2 was administered to three equidistant points on the injury for 20 consecutive days. In the control group, the mean area of the myelin impairment was 0.51 on day 21 after the operation, whereas this value was 1.31 in the LPT group. Comparison of the sciatic functional index (SFI) showed that there was no significant difference between the pre-lesion value in the laser therapy group and the control group. The use of 660 nm LPT provided significant changes to the morphometrically assessed area of the myelin sheath, but it did not culminate in any positive results for the functional recovery of the sciatic nerve in the rats after injury caused by neurotmesis.

A pilot double-blind randomized study by Rochkind [1867] evaluated the efficacy of 780 nm laser phototherapy on the acceleration of axonal growth and regeneration after peripheral nerve reconstruction by polyglycolic acid (PGA) neurotube. The right sciatic nerve was transected, and a 0.5 cm nerve segment was removed in 20 rats. A neurotube was placed between the proximal and the distal parts of the nerve for reconnection of the nerve defect. Altogether 10 of 20 rats received post-operative, transcutaneous, 200 mW, 780 nm laser irradiation for 14 consecutive days to the corresponding segments of the spinal cord (15 min) and to the reconstructed nerve (15 min). At three months after surgery, positive somato-sensory evoked responses were found in 70% of the irradiated rats, compared to 30% of the non-irradiated rats. The Sciatic Functional Index in the irradiated group was higher than in the non-irradiated group. Morphologically, the nerves were completely reconnected in both groups, but the laser-treated group showed an increased total number of myelinated axons.

The purpose of a study by Chen [2003] was to determine whether low-power pulsed laser irradiation could affect the regeneration of a 10-mm gap in the rat sciatic nerve created between the proximal and distal nerve stumps, which were sutured into silicone rubber tubes. After eight weeks of recovery, pulsed laser-irradiated groups at frequencies of 5 kHz and 20 kHz both had significantly lower success percentages of regeneration (50% and 44%, respectively) compared to sham-irradiated controls (100%). In addition, qualitative and quantitative histology of the regenerated nerves revealed a less mature ultrastructural organization with a smaller cross-sectional area and a lower number of myelinated axons in both pulsed laser-irradiated groups than in the controls. These results suggest that superpulsed laser irradiation could elicit suppressing effects on neural growth.

However, the conclusion in the above study has been questioned by Tunér [2004]. The references used by Chen are all from studies using continuous lasers. In a paper by Rochkind [2005], several wavelengths were compared, even 980 nm, and all had some effect, except for 904 nm. So it is probably not the wavelength per se but the superpulsing mode that makes the difference. GaAs is known to require a much lower dosage than continuous lasers [8]. The correct conclusion would be that the wavelength and doses used were inhibitory. Apart from a questionable conclusion, the study by Chen is valuable.

Spinal cord injury (SCI) is a severe central nervous system trauma with no restorative therapies. Previously, Anders [1898] demonstrated that LPT improves axonal regeneration and functional recovery in a dorsal hemisection rodent SCI model. Weight-drop contusion SCI rodent models are widely used since this model is comparable to human SCI. The comparative effectiveness of laser on these two SCI models was studied. The light treated groups were transcutaneously irradiated at the injury site with a 810 nm diode laser (150mW output power, 1,589 J/cm^2) for 14 consecutive days. All rats were euthanized 3 weeks after injury. Axonal regeneration and func-

expression revealed a significant increase in brain derived neurotrophic factor (BDNF), glial derived neurotrophic factor (GDNF), and collagen expression in the 0.2 J/cm^2 group in comparison to the non-irradiated and 68 J/cm^2 groups. OEC proliferation was also found to significantly increase in both light treated groups in comparison to the control group. These results demonstrate that low and high dosages of LPT alter OEC activity, including an upregulation of a number of neurotrophic growth factors and extracellular matrix proteins known to support neurite outgrowth.

A persistent increase in calcitonin gene-related peptide (CGRP) immunoreactivity in motoneurons may serve as an indicator for regeneration after peripheral nerve injury. Snyder [1719] examined the effects of laser treatment (633 nm) on axotomy-induced changes in alpha-CGRP mRNA and long-term neuronal survival in facial motoneurons. A quantitative reverse transcriptase-polymerase chain reaction (RT-PCR) assay for alpha-CGRP mRNA was used to detect changes in the response to axotomy and laser irradiation. Cell counts of neurons in injured and non-injured facial motor nuclei of laser-treated and non-treated rats were done to estimate neuronal survival. A 10-fold increase in mRNA for alpha-CGRP on day 11 post-transection and an almost 3-fold increase in neuronal survival at six to nine months post-transection were found in 633 nm light treated rats. These findings demonstrate that 633 nm laser light upregulates CGRP mRNA and support the theory that laser irradiation increases the rate of regeneration, target reinnervation, and neuronal survival of the axotomised neuron.

In a study by Ihsan [1866], 24 adult male rabbits were randomly assigned to two equal groups (control and laser-treated). General anesthesia was administered intramuscularly, and an exploration of the peroneal nerve was done in the lateral aspect of the left leg. Complete section of the nerve was performed, which was followed by suturing of the neural sheath (epineurium). Irradiation was carried out directly after the operation and for 10 consecutive days. The laser used was a diode with a wavelength of 901 nm (pulsed) and a power of 10 mW. It was a square-shaped window type (16 cm^2), and its energy was applied by direct contact of the instrument's window to the site of the operation. Three rabbits from each group were sacrificed at the end of weeks two, four, six and eight, and specimens were collected from the site of nerve suturing and sent for histopathological examination. Two important factors were examined via histopathology: diameter of the nerve fibers and individual internodal length. Compared to the control group, significant variations in regeneration were observed, including thicker nerve fibers, more regular myelin layers, and clearer nodes of Ranvier with an absence of short nodes in the treated group. Variations between the two groups for diameter were significant for the second week, highly significant for the fourth and sixth week, respectively, and very highly significant for the 8th week. Variations between the two groups for internodal length were highly significant for the second and fourth week and very highly significant for the sixth and eighth week.

regarding the amplitude, area, or duration and conduction velocity of CMAP for each applied dose (0.31, 2.48 and 19 J/cm^2) on the irradiated (right) side and the control (left) side, or between irradiated groups. There were no qualitative differences 21 days after injury in the morphological pattern of the regenerated nerve fibres in either irradiated (0.31, 2.48 and 19 J/cm^2) or control nerves when evaluated by light microscopy.

In a rat experiment by Byrnes [1222, 1527], the spinal cord was hemisected at vertebral level T9. The light from a 810 nm, 150 mW laser was applied immediately after hemisection and daily for 14 days, with a dosage of 1.589 J/cm^2. Control rats received identical treatment, but without laser. The results indicate that LPT initially blocks cell invasion and activation of the injured spinal cord. Once LPT ceases 14 days post-injury (the time point at which lesioned axons are reported to begin to sprout), there is a rebound increase in non-inflammatory cell invasion and activation that is visible 16 days post-injury. These alterations in the spinal cord environment may contribute to the ability of lesioned axons to regenerate following injury.

The objective of a study by Gigo-Benato [1562] was to investigate the effects of postoperative lasertherapy on nerve regeneration after end-to-side neurorrhaphy, an innovative technique for peripheral nerve repair. After complete transection, the left median nerve was repaired by end-to-side neurorrhaphy on the ulnar donor nerve. The animals were then divided into four groups: one placebo group, and three laser-treated groups that received LPT three times a week for 3 weeks starting on the first postoperative day. Three different types of laser emission were used: continuous (808 nm), pulsed (905 nm), and a combination of the two. Functional testing was carried out every 2 weeks after surgery by means of the grasping test. At the time of withdrawal 16 weeks postoperative, muscle mass recovery was assessed by weighing the muscles innervated by the median nerve. Finally, the repaired nerves were withdrawn, embedded in resin and analyzed by light and electron microscopy. Results showed that laser biostimulation induces: (1) a statistically significant faster recovery of the lesioned function; (2) a statistically significant faster recovery of muscle mass; (3) a statistically significant faster myelination of the regenerated nerve fibres. From comparison of the three different types of laser emissions, it turned out that the best functional outcome was obtained by means of pulsed-continuous-combined laser biostimulation.

Both LPT and olfactory ensheathing cells (OECs) transplantation improve recovery following spinal cord injury. However, neither the combination of these two therapies nor the effect of light on OECs have been reported. The purpose of a study by Byrnes [1587] was to determine the effect of light on OEC activity in vitro. OECs were purified from adult rat olfactory bulbs and exposed to 810 nm light (150 mW; 0.2 or 68 J/cm^2). After 7-21 days in vitro, cells underwent immunocytochemistry or RNA extraction and RT-PCR. Analysis of immunolabeling revealed a significant decrease in fibronectin expression in the cultures receiving 68 J/cm^2. Analysis of gene

ated rats. Immunohistochemical staining in the laser-treated group showed an increased total number of axons and better quality of the regeneration process, due to an increased number of large-diameter axons compared to the non-irradiated control group.

In the study by Shin [1500] the authors verified the therapeutic effect on neuronal regeneration by finding elevated immunoreactivities (IRs) of growth-associated protein-43 (GAP-43), which is upregulated during neuronal regeneration. Twenty rats received a standardised crush injury of the sciatic nerve, mimicking the clinical situations accompanying partial axonotmesis. The injured nerve received calculated LPT immediately after injury and for four consecutive days thereafter. The walking movements of the animals were scored using the sciatic functional index (SFI). In the laser treated rats, the SFI level was higher in the laser treated animals at three to four weeks while the SFIs of the laser treated and untreated rats reached normal levels at five weeks after surgery. In an immunocytochemical study, although GAP-43 IRs increased both in the untreated control and the laser treated groups after injury, the number of GAP-43 IR nerve fibers was much more increased in the laser group than those in the control group. The elevated numbers of GAP-43 IR nerve fibers reached a peak three weeks after injury, and then declined in both the untreated control and the laser groups at five weeks, with no differences in the numbers of GAP-43 IR nerve fibers of the two groups at this stage. This immunocytochemical study using a GAP-43 antibody study shows for the first time that laser has an effect on the early stages of the nerve recovery process following sciatic nerve injury.

Bagis [1565] evaluated the electrophysiological and histopathological effects of gallium arsenide (904 nm) laser irradiation on the intact skin injured rat sciatic nerve. Twenty-four male rats were divided into three groups (n=8 each) and the sciatic nerve situated at a level approximately one-third of the length of the femur was crushed bilaterally with an aneursym clip for half a second. A gallium arsenide laser (wavelength 904 nm, pulse duration 220 ns, peak power per pulse 27 W, spot size 0.28 cm^2, pulse repetition rate 16, 128 and 1000 Hz; total applied energy density of 0.31, 2.48 and 19 J/cm^2) was applied to the right sciatic nerve for 15 min daily at the same time on 7 consecutive days. The same procedure was performed on the left sciatic nerve on the same animal, but without radiation emission, and this was accepted as a control. Compound muscle action potentials (CMAP) were recorded from the right and left sides in all three groups before surgery, immediately after the injury was inflicted, at the 24th hour and on the 14th and 21st day in all rats. The rats were sacrificed 21 days after injury. The sciatic nerves of the operated parts were harvested from the right and left sides. Histopathological evaluation was performed by light microscopy. Statistical evaluation was done using analysis of variance for two factors (right and left sides), repeated-measures (CMAP variables within groups), and the Tukey-Kramer Honestly Significant Difference test (CMAP variables between laser groups). No statistically significant difference was found

was performed using both light and electron microscopy. With a trauma to the nerve, both the amplitude of the compound motor action potential and the nerve conduction velocity decreased significantly compared to the pre-trauma state. Morphologically, the numbers of myelinated axons and degenerated axons decreased and increased, respectively, compared with the control. Typical aspects were an onion skin-type lamellation, fragmentation, edematous swelling and rarefaction in the myelin sheath. All these parameters recovered almost to the level of the pre-trauma state with laser irradiation, in direct proportion to the time spent for treatment.

Walker [89] and Tsai [90] achieved results which indicate that the central nervous system is photosensitive. Wu [187] conducted Walker's experiment again on a larger scale, but was unable to confirm the results.

Rochkind [32] has carried out extensive studies on the effects of HeNe laser light on nerve damage. In one experiment, the sciatic nerves of rats were exposed and crushed in a standardised fashion. After suturing, HeNe laser light was administered transcutaneously. The effects were monitored at intervals of 1 to 360 days. In the experimental group, action potential was at a high level, while in the control group (no laser treatment) it was very low. This effect was only achieved if the laser treatment was administered immediately after the injury - when it was given 3 and 7 days afterwards, there was no difference as compared to the control group.

In another rodent study [1131], the sciatic nerves in rats were crushed in a standardised fashion and HeNe laser irradiation was performed directly after suturing. The irradiation was performed over the corresponding segment of the spinal cord and not over the crushed area. LPT was performed for 30 minutes daily for 21 consecutive days. The electrophysiological activity of the injured nerves (compound muscle action potentials – CMAPs) was found to be approximatively 90% of the normal precrush value, and remained so for a long time. In the control group, the CMAPs dropped to about 20% on day 21 and showed the first signs of slow recovery 30 days after surgery.

Anders [387] found that laser irradiation with certain wavelengths alters the rate of regeneration of the rat facial nerve. The facial nerve of rats was crushed unilaterally and transcutaneously irradiated with a laser beam directed at the area of the crush injury daily for seven, eight or nine days. The wavelengths examined were 361, 457, 514, 633, 720 and 1064 nm. Power ranged from 8.5 to 40 mW, length of irradiation from 13 to 120 minutes. The most effective wavelength was 633 nm and 45.9 J.

The double-blind randomised study by Shamir [1182] evaluated the effect of LPT on peripheral nerve regeneration after complete transection and direct anastomosis of the rat sciatic nerve. All in all 13 of 24 rats received postoperative LPT, 780 nm, applied transcutaneously, 30 min daily for 21 consecutive days, to corresponding segments of the spinal cord and to the injured sciatic nerve. Positive somatosensory evoked responses were found in 69.2% of the irradiated rats compared to 18.2% of the non-irradi-

cesses of the neuron isolated from the cell body by a separator. The action potentials elicited by bradykinin (BK) in the cell body were reversibly suppressed by the irradiation of laser light. The laser irradiation may block the conduction of nociceptive signals in primary afferent neurons.

The aim of a study by Oron [1872] was to investigate whether GaAs laser irradiation can enhance adenosine triphosphate (ATP) production in normal human neural progenitor (NHNP) cells in culture. NHNP cells were grown in tissue cultures and treated by a GaAs laser (808 nm, 50 mW/cm^2, 0.05 J/cm^2), and ATP was determined 10 min after laser application. The quantity of ATP in laser-treated cells was 7513 ± 970 units, which was significantly higher than in the non-treated cells which comprised 3808 ± 539 ATP units. Laser application to NHNP cells significantly increases ATP production in these cells.

Previously, Anders [2040] reported that 810 nm light was the optimal wavelength in the differentiation of normal human neural progenitor cells (NHNPC). Various combinations of dosimetry and power density for 810 nm were evaluated using in vitro NHNPC. NHNPC were placed into one of three treatment groups, two slides per group: 1) Control (no factors, no light); 2) Factors (no light); and 3) 810 nm Light Treated (spot size 0.78cm2). The 810 nm Light Treated group consisted of four subgroups: 1) 0.01 J/cm^2 dose: 1, 5 and 19 mW/cm2; 2) 0.05 J/cm^2 dose: 1, 5, 15, 19, 25, and 50 mW/cm2; 3) 0.2 J/cm^2 dose: 1, 5, 15, 19, 25, and 50 mW/cm2; and 4) 1 J/cm^2 dose: 1, 5, 15, 19, 25, and 50 mW/cm2. NHNPC were treated for three consecutive days and the cells were killed on day seven with 4% paraformaldehyde. Images of 20 random neurospheres per group were captured digitally and assayed for differentiation by determining neurite numbers and length. The total neurite length for all neurites per neurosphere was determined and averaged per group. The data was analyzed using one way ANOVA with Tukey Post tests. Based on this data, the total neurite length per neurosphere increased as power densities (19-50 mW/cm2) and dosages (0.05-1J/cm^2) increased. A low power density (1-15 mW/cm2) did not have an effect on the total neurite length. These data suggest that there is not one optimal combination of dose and power density, but rather an optimal window of effective combinations of dose and power density for a given wavelength. The same combinations of dosimetry and power density are currently being evaluated for other wavelengths (both continuous wave and pulsed).

Animal studies

The aim of a study by Bae [1489] was to determine if GaAs laser treatment stimulates the regeneration process of damaged nerves. A standardized crush to the sciatic nerve was applied to cause extensive axonal degeneration. After this procedure, low-power infrared laser irradiation was administered transcutaneously to the injured sciatic nerve, three minutes daily to each of four treatment groups for one, three, five and seven weeks, respectively. A nerve conduction study was done, and a morphological assessment

4.1.39 Nerve regeneration and function
The regeneration of damaged nerves is one of the most promising indications for LPT. Studies on Bell´s palsy are difficult to evaluate, bearing in mind the high spontaneous remission rate. However, the rapid pain relief is a good verification of the laser effect. The swelling and the neuritis in the bony fallopian canal is believed to be influenced. This intrabony region is the major target for LPT in this indication. The suspected association with herpes viruses also supports the use of LPT. See also 4.1.47 Trigeminal neuralgia.

Literature:
In vitro studies:
van Breugel [353] investigated HeNe laser irradiation effects on proliferation and laminin production of rat Schwann cells in vitro. Schwann cell (SwC) proliferation is an essential part of Wallerian degeneration after nerve damage, and thus a prerequisite for regeneration. HeNe irradiation in vitro showed a dose-related stimulation of SwC proliferation. Laminin production was not affected.

Mulligan [354] investigated the effect of HeNe laser irradiation on neurite elongation in vitro. Doses around 1.5 J/cm^2 were given to a rat neuronal clonal cell line for 5, 15, 30, 45 and 60 minutes. Neurite outgrowth was greater than that in the control for all groups, but only the 15 and 30 minute groups were statistically different from the control values.

Wollman [537] irradiated foetal brain cells in vitro using a HeNe laser. One single dose enhanced the appearance of brain cells around the treated aggregates. Two and three doses were correlated with 97% and 142% increases respectively. Rhodamine-labelled antibodies bound to receptors on cells indicated a massive neurite sprouting and an outgrowth of migrating brain cells in culture.

In a study by Rochkind [1236], embryonal spinal cord nerve cells dissociated from rat fetuses, cultured in biodegradable microcarriers and embedded in hyaluronic acid, were implanted in the completely transsected spinal cords of 24 adult rats. Altogether 15 rats underwent 14 days of consecutive laser irradiation (780 nm, 250 mW, 30 minutes daily), while 7 rats received the same treatment but without laser. Out of the 15 laser treated rats, 11 showed different degrees of active leg movements and gait performance compared to 4 of the 9 rats with implantation alone. In a control group of 7 rats with no therapy after the transsection of the spinal cord, 6 remained completely paralysed. Intensive axonal sprouting occurred in the laser group. In the control group, the transsected area contained proliferating fibroblasts and blood capillaries only.

In a study by Jimbo [835], the effects of GaAlAs (830 nm, 16.2 mW) laser irradiation on the distal portion of the processes of cultured murine dorsal root ganglion (DRG) neurons associated with C-fibers was studied by patch-clamp whole-cell recording of membrane potentials at the cell body. The chemical as well as the laser light stimulation were limited to the pro-

4.1.38 Nerve conduction

Literature:

Wakabayashi [190] demonstrated that C-fibres play a part in the analgesic effect of LPT. A small hole was drilled in the mandibular incisor of a rat through which a probe made contact with the dental pulp. The incisor was stimulated electrically and the subsequent action potential was registered through a probe from the ipsilateral trigeminal caudal neurons. A 830 nm laser was used to irradiate the incisor's cervical surface. The rate of firing discharges and the number of spikes evoked in the caudal neurons before and after laser treatment were compared. LPT suppressed the late discharges in the response of the caudal neurons which were evoked by excitatory inputs from C-fibre afferents, but did not suppress the early discharges evoked by inputs from A-delta-fibre afferents. This indicates that GaAlAs irradiation inhibited the excitation of unmyelinated fibres of the pulp without affecting fine myelinated fibres. It is suggested that LPT has a suppressive effect on injured tissue by blocking the depolarisation of the afferent C-fibres.

Ohno [719] demonstrated that laser irradiation suppresses the excitation of the unmyelinated C-fibres in the afferent sensory pathway. Substance P in the rat spinal dorsal root ganglion was measured after electrical stimulation of the sciatic nerve.

The involvement of afferent unmyelinated A-delta fibres in LPT pain attenuation has been demonstrated by Kasai [488]. High threshold evoked responses were reduced by 9% to 19% during low-power laser irradiation in experimental animals. The data in this study suggest that low-power laser acts as a reversible direct suppressor of neuronal activity

In a study by Tsuchiya [519], a GaAlAs laser reduced the action potentials in the dorsal roots elicited from the saphenous nerve of a rat. The amplitude of slower conduction parts of action potentials (velocity <12 m/s) was suppressed. The suppression was time-dependent. After three minutes of irradiation, the slowest velocity group (<1.3 m/s) was totally diminished and the 1.3-12 m/s group was reduced by 12-67%. In contrast, faster components (>12 m/s) were unaffected.

Balaban [650] concludes that HeNe laser does not affect silent neurons. However, when the spontaneously active neurons, generating spikes every 7-10 minutes, were irradiated in between their spontaneous spikes, the depolarisation of membrane and the generation of action potentials occurred as a function of light intensity.

Walsh [977] irradiated the skin overlying the human right superficial radial nerve in healthy individuals at three points (1.2 J per point, energy density 9.55 J/cm^2, 830 nm, 50 mW). Antidromic action potentials were recorded from the nerve prior to irradiation and at 5, 10 and 15 minutes after irradiation. There were no differences between the placebo laser group, the control group or the active laser groups regarding negative peak latency or skin temperature. Pulsing at 8, 12 or 73 Hz made no difference.

the increase was only 2.7 repetitions (+/- 2.9) (p = 0.0001). At the second session, blood lactate levels increased from a pre-exercise mean of 2.4 mmol/L to 3.6 mmol/L in the placebo group, and to 3.8 mmol/L in the active LPT group after exercise, but this difference between groups was not statistically significant. It is concluded that LPT appears to delay the onset of muscle fatigue and exhaustion by a local mechanism in spite of increased blood lactate levels.

A review article on photoengineering of tissue repair in skeletal and cardiac muscles is written by Oron [1682].

Further reading: chapter 4.1.47 "Snake bites" on page 311, chapter 4.1.15 "Delayed onset muscular soreness (DOMS)" on page 218.

Further literature: [356, 533, 587, 616, 702, 916, 1327]

4.1.37 Mycosis
Literature:

Paracoccidioidomycosis (PCM) is the most prevalent human mycosis in Latin America. The infection is thought to take place firstly in the lungs and then possibly disseminate to other organs and tissues. Treatment by currently available antifungals is lengthy, the drugs may have undesirable side effects, and some are costly. Occasional resistant strains of Paracoccidioides brasiliensis, the causative agent of PCM, have been reported. Therefore, the search for more efficient treatments or adjuvant therapies has to be continued. In the work by Ferreira [1848], the author evaluated the effects of HeNe laser irradiation on cutaneous inflammatory lesions caused by the inoculation of $5 \times 10^6/0.1$ ml yeasts cells into the back footpad of Balb/c mice. HeNe irradiation (3 mW, 3 J/cm^2) was applied on days seven, eight and nine post-infection, and histological and immunohistochemical analyses were done. Unirradiated animals were used as controls. The results showed that laser-treated mice presented a reduction of footpad edema, faster cutaneous wound healing, confluent granuloma, diffuse- and more loosely distributed immunolabeling of TNF-alpha, enhanced labeling of IFN-gamma and any P. brasiliensis form detected, whereas multiple viable fungi were seen in diffuse widespread granulomas obtained from non-treated mice foot-pads. Fungi that was harvested from laser-treated animals presented no capability of growth in vitro as compared to those obtained from non-treated mice. The authors conclude that HeNe laser irradiation was able to inhibit the progress of inflammatory local reaction produced by P. brasiliensis infection and influence local cytokines production. It is suggested that this treatment modality can be a useful coadjuvant tool to be combined with antifungal agents in the treatment of PCM ulcerations.

Further literature: [1909]

sections were stained with hematoxylin and eosin and used for quantitative morphological analysis, in which the number of leukocytes and fibroblasts were counted over an area of 4480 mum2. Quantitative data showed that the number of both polymorphonuclear and mononuclear leukocytes in the inflammatory infiltrate at the injury site was smaller in the ILI(1), ILI(2), and ILI(4) subgroups compared with their respective control subgroups (IN(1), IN(2), and IN(4)) for sessions one, two and four, respectively. On the other hand, the number of fibroblasts increased after the fourth treatment session. With regard to the regeneration of muscle fibers following injury, only after the fourth treatment session was it possible to find muscle precursor cells such as myoblasts and some myotubes in the ILI(4) subgroup. Thus, in the acute inflammatory phase, the laser treatment was found to have anti-inflammatory effects, reducing the number of leukocytes at the injury site and accelerating the regeneration of connective tissue.

The sciatic nerve-gastrocnemius muscles of 35 frogs were prepared in an experiment by Komatsu [1941]. In Experiment 1, continuous stimulation for gastrocnemius contraction was delivered to the sciatic nerve (10 minutes); the experimental group simultaneously received LPT. In Experiment 2, two sets of stimulation and cessation (2 minutes each) were repeated after the initial stimulation period (2 minutes); the experimental group received LPT during the resting period. In Experiment 1, 60 mW significantly facilitated an attenuation of AMP and maintained a smaller prolongation of CP, whereas 100 mW significantly influenced a retardation of AMP attenuation and LAT prolongation. In Experiment 2, 100 mW significantly influenced AMP attenuation and LAT prolongation by retardation; almost no effects were obtained in the case of 60 mW. These results suggest that 808 nm LPT influences both synaptic signal transmission at the neuromuscular junction and excitation-contraction coupling in the muscle fibers, but not the relaxation process. The authors conclude that LPT at relatively high doses can influence muscles by retarding AMP attenuation and LAT prolongation.

Leal Junior [2006] investigated if the development of skeletal muscle fatigue during repeated voluntary biceps contractions could be attenuated by LPT. Twelve male professional volleyball players were entered into a randomized double-blind placebo-controlled trial for two sessions (on day one and day eight) at a one-week interval, with both groups performing as many voluntary biceps contractions as possible, with a load of 75% of the maximal voluntary contraction force (MVC). At the second session on day eight, the groups were either given LPT (655 nm) of 5 J at an energy density of 500 J/cm^2 administered to each of four points along the middle of the biceps muscle belly, or placebo LPT in the same manner immediately before the exercise session. The number of muscle contractions with 75% of MVC was counted by a blinded observer and the blood lactate concentration was measured. Compared to the first session (on day one), the mean number of repetitions increased significantly by 8.5 repetitions (+/- 1.9) in the active LPT group at the second session (on day eight), while in the placebo LPT group

creatine phosphokinase activity and lower activity of acid phosphatase in the laser-treated muscles, relative to the injured non-irradiated ones. The content of antioxidants and heat shock proteins was also higher in the laser-treated muscles, relative to that of injured non-irradiated muscles. The present study describes for the first time the ability of LPT to significantly prevent degeneration following ischemia/reperfusion injury in skeletal muscles, probably by induction of synthesis of antioxidants and other cytoprotective proteins, such as hsp-70i. The elevation of antioxidants was also evident in intact muscles following laser irradiation. The above phenomenon may also be of clinical relevance in scheduled surgery or microsurgery requiring extended tourniquet applications to skeletal muscles followed by reperfusion.

The purpose of the study by Rizzi [1731] was to investigate the effects of LPT on nuclear factor kappa B (NF-kappaB) activation and inducible nitric oxide synthase (iNOS) expression in an experimental model of muscle trauma. The injury to the gastrocnemius muscle in the rat was produced by a single impact blunt trauma. A GaAs laser, 45 mW, and 5 J/cm^2 was applied for 35 seconds continuously. Histological abnormalities with an increase in collagen concentration, and oxidative stress, were observed after trauma. This was accompanied by activation of NF-kappaB and upregulation of iNOS expression, whereas protein concentration of I kappa B alpha decreased. These effects were blocked by LPT. The associated reduction of iNOS overexpression and collagen production suggest that the NF-kappaB pathway may be a signalling route involved in the pathogenesis of muscle trauma.

The purpose of a study by Prado [1732] was to develop an experimental model to be used in the study of low LPT on viability of random skin flaps in rats. The sample was 24 rats. The random skin flap measured 10 x 4 cm and a plastic sheet was interposed between the flap and donor site. Group 1 (control) underwent sham irradiation. Group 2 was submitted to laser irradiation with a diode laser (830 nm). The animals were submitted to LPT with a 36 J/cm^2 energy density (72 seconds) immediately after surgery and on four subsequent days. The probe was usually held in contact with the skin flap surface on a point at 2.5 cm cranial from the flap base. On the seventh postoperative day, the percentage of necrotic area was measured and calculated. Group 1 reached an average necrotic area of 48.86%, Group 2 - 23.14%.

A study by Cressoni [2012] aimed to investigate the effects of LPT on muscle regeneration. For this purpose, the anterior tibialis muscle of 48 male Wistar rats received treatment (785 nm) after a surgically-induced injury. The animals were randomized into four groups: uninjured rats (UN); uninjured and laser-irradiated rats (ULI); injured rats (IN); and injured and laser-irradiated rats (ILI). The direct contact laser treatment started 24 h after surgery. A laser emitting 75 mW of continuous power at 785 nm was used for irradiation. The laser probe was placed at three treatment points to deliver 0.9 J per point, for a total dose of 2.7 J per treatment session. The animals were euthanized after treatment sessions one, two and four. Mounted

injured area is exposed to GaAs-laser irradiation, following injury to the tibialis anterior muscle of mice.

In a study by Amaral [665], 15 mice received a single muscular injection of myotoxin in the tibialis anterior muscle of both legs. One group received HeNe laser irradiation with a dose of 2.6 J/cm^2, another 8.4 J/cm^2 and a third 25 J/cm^2 on one leg, while the other was sham irradiated. The 2.6 J group showed a significant difference, with evidence of a greater concentration of mitochondria in the treated muscle, whereas the higher doses did not produce this effect. The laser treated mice showed an increase of the cross-section area of the muscle fibres.

Popova [147] studied the effects of a HeNe laser on the healing of muscle tissue after irradiation with 10 Gy X-ray. The muscle tissue of rats was removed, irradiated with X-rays and re-transplanted. Improved healing compared with the control group was observed whether laser light was administered before or after the transplant.

Weiss [276] and Bibikova [277], in experiments on rats and toads respectively, observed improved muscle regeneration as a result of the use of HeNe and GaAs lasers.

Oliveira [1186] failed to find such regeneration in a rodent experiment using GaAs, 1.5 mW, with 3 or 10 J/cm^2 daily irradiations over intact skin. Although there was no effect on the muscular regeneration, the body weight of the mice was increased in the 10 J/cm^2 group.

Buliakova [570] found that HeNe laser indeed accelerated the regenerative process in crosscut gastrocnemius muscles of adult guinea pigs. However, the regenerating muscle tissue did not connect the two muscle stumps; a narrow connective tissue scar being formed instead. The same experiment on rats was more successful, so it is likely that the regenerative ability of LPT depends on the species' peculiarities.

Ramos [1477] treated four groups of rats with HeNe laser. The constriction potential of the anterior tibial muscle was recorded. Only animals with atrophic muscles showed any effect of the therapy.

The aim of a study by Avni [1601] was to investigate the effect of LPT on ischemic-reperfusion (I-R) injury in the gastrocnemius muscles of rats. Ischemic injury in skeletal muscles is initiated during hypoxia and aggravated by reoxygenation during blood reperfusion and accumulation of cytotoxic reactive oxygen superoxides. The injury was induced in the gastrocnemius muscles of 106 rats by complete occlusion of the blood supply for three hours, followed by reperfusion. Another group of intact rats served to investigate the effect of LPT on intact non-ischemic muscles. Creatine phosphokinase, acid phosphatase, and heat shock protein were determined seven days after I-R injury and antioxidant levels two hours after reperfusion. Laser irradiation (GaAlAs, 810 nm) was applied to the muscles immediately and one hour following blood supply occlusion. It was found that laser irradiation markedly protects skeletal muscles from degeneration following acute I-R injury. This was evident by a significantly higher content of

4.1.35 Mucositis
(See chapter 4.1.9 "Cancer" on page 190.)

4.1.36 Muscle regeneration
LPT has the ability to stimulate muscular regeneration in areas of trauma, even in cases of snake bites. The therapy can also improve muscular strength [1468] and reduce muscular fatigue.

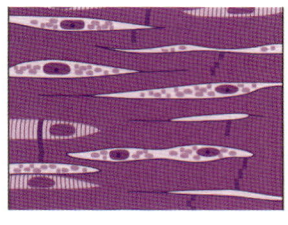

Literature:
In vitro studies
    Schwartz [626] found a transient elevation of intracellular calcium in the myotubes immediately after irradiation, using HeNe laser light at 3-10 J/cm^2. These findings suggest the hypothesis that transient changes in calcium may accelerate the release of cytokines from the myotubes.

    Shefer [1243] has demonstrated that HeNe laser can stimulate cell cycle entry and the accumulation of satellite cells around isolated single fibres, grown under serum-free conditions. It is demonstrated that LPT promotes the survival of muscle fibres and their adjacent cells, as well as cultured myogenic cells, under serum-free conditions that normally lead to apoptosis.

Animal studies
    Lievens [521] summarises a study on the effects of LPT on muscle regeneration as follows: The effect of GaAs, 904 nm, laser irradiation on the process of skeletal muscle regeneration after simple injuries to the tibialis anterior muscle of mice is studied histologically and statistically. The right-hand side injured zones in the experimental mice were subjected to one direct nuclear magnetic resonance technique laser irradiation for three minutes daily, starting on the first day post injury. The left-hand side injuries were left untreated and served as a control. Morphometric analysis was performed on histological sections of injured areas on days 7 and 18 post injury. On day 7 post injury, mononucleated cells populated most of the injured area. Thereafter, their proportion decreased gradually but more rapidly in the laser-irradiated muscles than in those on the control side. The early myotubes were evident in the control side, while they were less evident in the experimental side. The injured area was populated by myotubes in the experimental muscles, while they were less evident in the control side. On day 18 post injury, the process of muscle regeneration was almost completed in the laser-irradiated muscles. In the untreated muscles, myotubes still populated a large part of the injured zone, and there were less regenerated myofibres. It is concluded that the process of muscle regeneration is promoted when the

Patients with stage II and III arterial ischemia in the feet were studied. LPT at 890 nm increased microcirculation.

The pilot study by Al-Awami [1200] was performed to evaluate the efficacy of LPT as a new non-drug, non-invasive treatment for patients with primary and secondary Raynaud's disease. Altogether 40 patients (29 female, 11 male, mean age 51 years) with active primary (28%) and secondary (72%) Raynaud's phenomenon received 10 sessions of LPT distant irradiation during the winter months. Assessments of subjective and objective parameters were performed at baseline one week after the last session and three months later. Variations of subjective parameters, such as the number of daily acute episodes and the severity of discomfort, were assessed by a coloured visual analogue scale. A standardised cold challenge test using computed thermography of continuous temperature recordings by means of infrared telethermography was used to assess the digital blood flow. A significant improvement was noticed clinically and thermographically after six weeks and three months, respectively.

The effect of LPT on Raynaud's disease has also been investigated by Hirschl [1265]. Absolute and relative frequency and intensity of vasospastic attacks during three weeks of either LPT or placebo, and the results of infrared thermography before onset and at the end of both therapy sequences, were evaluated in 15 patients with primary Raynaud's phenomenon. The frequency of attacks was not significantly affected, but the intensity of the attacks was reduced. The mean temperature gradient after cold exposure was reduced after irradiation, but the number of fingers showing prolonged rewarming was unaffected.

Silveira [1907] did not find any change in vessel dilatation after LPT on excised hypertrophic human gingiva, but as the authors suspect, there was no time for such changes since the excised samples were formaline-fixed immediately after irradiation and excision.

For additional studies on microcirculation, see chapter 4.1.17 "Diabetes" on page 223.

Further literature: [145, 308, 1015, 1075, 1082, 1442, 1464, 1472, 1482, 1486, 1592, 2013]

4.1.34 Morbus Sluder
Literature:

Mb Sluder is a painful condition originating in the spheno-palatinal ganglion. Parascandalo [1071] used a GaAs laser on three patients for 12 sessions, irradiating the maxillary nerve apertures. Total pain relief was obtained after five sessions, difficulties in swallowing improved after three sessions, reduction of high tear flow after several sessions. Full recovery after nine sessions.

Further literature: [1070]

flowmetry method itself has a potential of influencing the outcome in both groups.

Schaffer [904] explored the effect of a diode laser (780 nm) on normal skin tissue. Time-dependent contrast enhancement was determined by magnetic resonance imaging (MRI). In the examinations, six healthy volunteers were irradiated on their right planta pedis (sole of foot) with 5 J/cm² at a power density of 100 mW/cm². T1-weighted magnetic resonance imaging was used to quantify the time-dependent local accumulation of Gadolinium-DPTA; its actual content in the local current blood volume, as well as its distribution to the extracellular space. Images were obtained before and after the application of laser light. When laser light was applied, the signal to noise ratio increased by more than 0.35 ± 0.15 (range 0.23-0.63) after irradiation according to contrast-enhanced MRT. According to the authors: "it can be observed that after biomodulation with light of low energy and low power, wound healing improves and pain is reduced. This effect might be explained by an increased blood flow in this area. Therefore, the use of this kind of laser treatment might improve the outcome of other therapeutic modalities such as tumour ionising radiation therapy and local chemotherapy".

Schindl [145] treated three cases of Bürger's Disease, which is characterised by reduced microcirculation in the extremities. In practice, this always leads to amputation, often up to and past the knee/elbow. The illness has a very poor prognosis, and patients suffer from acute ischaemic pain. The three patients in the study refused to undergo further amputations and discharged themselves from hospital at their own risk. They remained on antibiotics during the entire treatment, but other than that, HeNe laser light was the only treatment they received. All three patients avoided further amputations, began healing and could return to work. The intense pain also disappeared. Bearing in mind these encouraging results, HeNe laser should be tested more on diabetics, in whom peripheral circulation can fall, rendering amputation necessary.

In a case report by Sasaki [913], a patient with thromboangitis obliterans (Bürger's disease) was treated with a 60 mW, 830 nm laser and a defocused 20 W, Nd:YAG laser. Ulcers were remarkably improved. Agonising pain and ischemia were relieved. In the MRA findings, sudden arterial obliteration disappeared. In the thermographical findings, skin temperature increased to normal.

Schindl [674] treated a chronic radiation ulcer with HeNe laser, 30 J/cm². A video measuring system was used to determine the number of dermal vessels in the ulcer before and after the laser treatment. After seven irradiations, the ulcer had healed completely. Light microscopy in combination with the video measuring system showed a significant increase in the number of dermal capillaries after laser treatment.

Koslov [566] used laser dopplerography, TV capillaroscopy, and polarography of transcutaneous oxygen tension to study microcirculation.

sels were coloured by an India ink injection and were examined in a video microscope. Laser exposure promoted an increase in blood vessel count when compared to controls. The 40-mW group showed early neovascularization, with the greatest number of microvessels after three laser applications. The 10-mW subgroup showed angiogenesis activity around the same time as the sham laser group did, but the net number of vessels was significantly higher in the former than in the controls. After seven irradiations, the subgroup receiving 40 mW experienced a drop in microvessel numbers, but it was still higher than in the control groups.

The aim of a study by Corazza [1865] was to compare the angiogenic effects of laser and light-emitting diode (LED) illumination on wounds induced in rats, with varying fluences. The LED is an alternative light source that accelerates wound healing, and its efficiency concerning the angiogenic effect was compared to LPT. The experimental model consisted of a circular wound inflicted on the quadriceps of 120 rats, using a 15-mm-diameter "punch." Animals were divided randomly into five groups: two groups of laser, with dosages of 5 and 20 J/cm^2, respectively, two groups of LED, also with dosages of 5 and 20 J/cm^2, and a control group. Six hours after wound infliction, the treated groups received the diverse applications accordingly and were irradiated every 24 h. Angiogenesis was studied through histomorphometry on days 3, 7, 14 and 21 after the wounds were inflicted. On days 3, 7 and 14, the proliferation of blood vessels in all irradiated groups was superior in comparison to those of the control group. Treatment with a fluence of 5 J/cm^2 was better than for the group treated with 20 J/cm^2 on day 21. Red LPT and LED demonstrated expressive results in angiogenesis. Light coherence was shown not to be essential to angiogenesis under these circumstances.

The study by Ribeiro [1899] was carried out to evaluate the effects of LPT, 660 nm, in rat's burned skin with two different dose regimens by histomorphometry. The number of new blood vessels was quantified by appropriate software. The findings suggest that laser may accelerate angiogenesis compared to the control group, but no significant differences were observed between laser groups using fractionated or single doses during the entire experimental period.

Clinical studies

Podelinskaia [571] used a computer-aided analytical system of TV images to study the microcirculation in the anterior segment of the eye. Exposure to 890 nm LPT had a favourable impact on blood aggregation.

Saito [630] studied the effect of GaAlAs laser on the blood flow of 15 healthy male subjects. The upper side of the foot was irradiated for one minute (60 mW). Laser speckle flowmetry was performed at the start of irradiation, as well as 30 and 60 minutes post irradiation. During the period of irradiation, blood flow was reduced significantly but increased immediately after the treatment, remaining at this level for 60 minutes. The laser speckle

and 72 h postoperatively from the animals of both groups, control and treated. Rapid increases in the level of adenosine, GH, and FGF occurred. The F/C ratio and capillary diameter peaked at 12-16 h, after which their levels declined gradually, reaching normal values 72 h after irradiation in the treated group. Numerous collateral blood vessels proliferated the area, with marked increases in the diameters of the original blood vessels.

Maegawa [1030] used a 30 mW GaAlAs laser to irradiate the rat's mesenteric microcirculation in vivo, with a power density of 38.2 mW/mm^2. The irradiation caused a potent dilatation in the irradiated arteriole, which led to a marked increase in the arteriolar blood flow. The irradiation also caused a power-dependent decrease in $[Ca^{2+}]$ in the vascular smooth muscle cells.

Núñez [1441] performed a rodent study where an injury was provoked in 15 rats and blood flow was measured periodically over a period of 21 days. Control groups were established to evaluate Laser Doppler Flowmetry and HeNe laser effects on microcirculation. A 1 J/cm^2 dose was utilized, with a 6 mW/cm^2 irradiance. The results demonstrated flow alterations provoked by lesion, and an inflammatory response. There were no statistical differences between groups. The results did not show a significant effect on microcirculation with this HeNe dose.

The influence of HeNe laser radiation on the formation of new blood vessels in the bone marrow compartment of a regenerating area of the mid-cortical diaphysis of the tibiae of young adult rats was studied by Garavello [1544]. A small hole was surgically made with a dentistry burr in the tibia and the injured area received a daily LPT over 7 or 14 days transcutaneously starting 24 h after surgery. Incident energy density dosages of 31.5 and 94.5 J/cm^2 were applied during the period of the tibia wound healing being investigated. Light microscopic examinations of histological sections of the injured area and quantifications of the newly-formed blood vessels were undertaken. LPT accelerated the deposition of bone matrix and histological characteristics compatible with an active recovery of the injured tissue. HeNe LPT significantly increased the number of blood vessels after 7 days of irradiation at an energy density of 94.5 J/cm^2, but significantly decreased the number of vessels in the 14- day irradiated tibiae, independent of the dosage. These effects were attributed to laser treatment, since no significant increase in blood vessel numbers was detected between 8 and 15 non-irradiated control tibiae.

Salate [1624] divided ninety-six rats into three groups subject to treatment for 3, 5, and 7 days post-lesion. Thirty-two animals were used in each group. The groups were further divided into four subgroups with eight animals in each, receiving InGaAlP laser, 660 nm, treatment at (1) a mean output of 10 mW, or (2) 40 mW during 10 sec, (3) a sham subgroup, and (4) a non-treatment subgroup. Each animal was subjected to a lesion of the Achilles tendon by dropping a 186-g weight from a 20-cm height over the tendon. Treatment was initiated six hours post-injury for all the groups. Blood ves-

In an animal study by Kobayashi [666] the effect of GaAlAs laser on the blood flow in flaps was studied through laser speckle flowgraphy (LSF). Forty rats were divided into four groups. Two groups had random pattern flaps, two had axillary pattern flaps with the dominant vessels intact. Flaps were raised and peripheral blood flow assessed through LSF. Laser irradiation was performed in two groups, either directly on the dominant vessel or at one point on the distal part of the flap. The blood flow directly after irradiation was higher than before irradiation. On day five, there was a clear difference between the irradiated and the non-irradiated flaps. The flaps irradiated at the dominant vessels had a slightly better outcome than those irradiated at the centre of the flap.

In the experiment performed by Pinfildi [1603], 48 rats were used, weighed and divided into four groups with 12 rats each. A skin flap was performed, measuring 10 x 4 cm, with a plastic sheet interposed between the flap and the donor site. Group 1 (control) underwent sham irradiation with HeNe laser. Group 2 was submitted to laser irradiation, using the punctual contact technique on the skin flap surface. Group 3 was submitted to laser irradiation surrounding the skin flap, and Group 4 was submitted to laser irradiation both on the skin flap surface and around it. The experimental groups were submitted to HeNe laser irradiation with a 3 J/cm^2 energy density immediately after surgery and for four subsequent days. The percentage of necrotic area in the four groups was calculated on the seventh post-operative day, through a paper-template method. Group 1 reached an average necrotic area of 48.86%; Group 2, 38.67%; Group 3, 35.34%; and Group 4, 22.61%.

Studies by Bibikova [667, 587] conclude that during skeletal muscle regeneration in the toad, HeNe laser irradiation markedly promotes the process of neoformation of blood vessels and young myofibres in the injured zone.

Thirty-four adult rabbits were used in a study by Ihsan [1720]. Two of the rabbits were considered 0-h reading group while the rest were divided into two equal groups, with 16 rabbits each: control and those treated with laser. Each rabbit underwent two surgical operations; the medial aspect of each thigh was slit, the skin incised and the femoral artery exposed and ligated. The site of the operation in the treated group was irradiated directly following the operation and for three days thereafter, one session daily for 10 min/session. The laser system used was a GaAs laser with a wavelength of 904 nm and a power output of 10 mW. Blood samples collected from the femoral artery above the site of the ligation were sent for examination with high-performance liquid chromatography (HPLC) to determine the levels of adenosine, growth hormone (GH) and fibroblast growth factor (FGF). Tissue specimens collected from the site of the operation, consisting of the artery and its surrounding muscle fibres, were sent for histopathological examination to determine the fibre/capillary (F/C) ratio and capillary diameter. Blood samples and tissue specimens were collected at 4, 8, 12, 16, 20, 24, 48

effects of VEGF applications. Thoracic aortal rings were prepared from Sabra rats. Samples from group 1 served as control, group 2 samples were incubated with VEGF, group 3 samples were irradiated with laser (660 nm, 20 mW) in a drop (10 /l) of the medium for 10 min, and group 4 samples were incubated with VEGF and received 10 min of laser irradiation. The stained samples were photographed by a camera connected to a microscope. Laser irradiation activated the process of angiogenesis. In the control group (without VEGF or laser irradiation), angiogenesis of new vessels was not detected. Laser irradiation, however, promoted angiogenesis. The area covered by new vessels was 1,9±0,29 mm^2 and the maximal length of vessels was 0,75 ± 0,10 mm. No statistical difference was discovered between laser irradiation and VEGF application. After a combined influence of VEGF and laser light irradiation, the area covered by new vessels was 6,98 ± 0,88 mm^2 and the maximal length of vessels was 1,7 ± 0,23 mm.

The aim of a study by Tuby [1730] was to investigate the effect of LPT on the expression of vascular endothelial growth factor (VEGF) and inducible nitric oxide synthase (iNOS). Myocardial infarction was induced by occlusion of the left descending artery in 87 rats. Laser was applied to intact and post-infarction hearts. VEGF, iNOS, and angiogenesis were determined. Both the laser-irradiated rat hearts post-infarction and the intact hearts demonstrated a significant increase in VEGF and iNOS expression compared to non-laser-irradiated hearts. LPT also caused a significant elevation in angiogenesis

The possible molecular mechanism of HeNe laser irradiation on endothelial cells was proposed in the study by Chen [1845]. HeNe laser was used to stimulate human umbilical vein endothelial cell (HUVEC), and its effect on cell proliferation, nitric oxide secretion, and cell migration was determined. Irradiation enhanced endothelial nitric oxidase synthase (eNOS) protein expression, and irradiation of less than 0.26 J/cm^2 enhanced eNOS gene expression in HUVEC. The cell migration ability promoted HUVEC when irradiated with 0.26 J/cm^2. This agreed with the vinculin protein expression induced by irradiation. In addition, the angiogenesis was promoted. The induced eNOS expression was inhibited by LY294002, indicating that the effect of laser on EC could be attributed to the up-regulation of eNOS expression through the PI3K pathway at the cellular and molecular levels as a result of the HeNe laser. The study has shown that LPT increased endothelial cell proliferation, migration, NO secretion, and identified that activation of the PI3K/Akt pathway was a critical step in elevating the eNOS expression upon LPT.

Animal studies

Kubota [479] used the laser speckle flowgraphy to measure the microcirculation in rodent flaps. The blood flow rate was reduced immediately following one minute of irradiation at 830 nm. Thirty minutes later, the flap perfusion was greater than in the control flap.

active LPT; group B (182 patients) was treated only with nimesulide; and group C (182 patients) was treated with nimesulide and placebo LPT. LPT was applied behind the involved spine segment using a stationary skin-contact method. Patients were treated 5 times weekly, for a total of 15 treatments, with the following parameters: wavelength 904 nm; PRR 5000 Hz; 100 mW average power; power density of 20 mW/cm^2 and dose of 3 J/cm^2; treatment time 150 sec at whole doses of 12 J/cm^2. The outcomes were pain intensity measured with a visual analog scale (VAS); lumbar movement, with a modified Schober test; pain disability, with Oswestry disability score; and quality of life, with a 12-item short-form health survey questionnaire (SF-12). Subjects were evaluated before and after treatment. Statistical analyses were done with SPSS 11.5. Statistically significant differences were found in all outcomes measured, but were larger in group A than in B and C. The results in group C were better than in group B. The results of this study show better improvement in acute LBP treated with LPT used as additional therapy.

Further literature: [621, 956, 1061, 1304]

4.1.33 Microcirculation

Improving the microcirculation in tissue is one of the most important aspects of LPT. The self-healing capacity of the body will improve considerably if more blood is circulating in the tissue. Improved microcirculation in the region will also enhance the uptake of concomitant pharmaceutical agents.

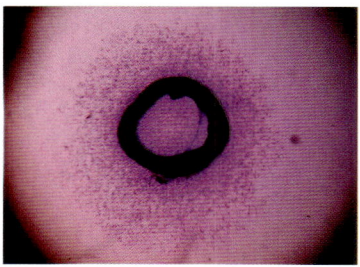 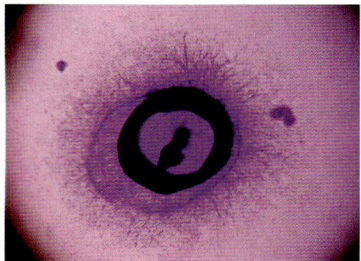

Figure 4.10 Rat aortas without (left) and with LPT (right). Note formation of new microvessels.

Courtesy: Levon Gasparyan.

Literature:
In vitro studies

Vascular endothelial growth factor (VEGF) is one of the most important growth factors for endothelium. VEGF induces angiogenesis and endothelial cell proliferation and it plays an important role in regulating vasculogenesis. The aim of a study by Gasparyan [1626] was to investigate the influence of red laser light on angiogenesis in vitro, and to compare with the

intervertebral disk herniation. The effect of laser irradiation was compared to TENS and Katoprofen. The most striking feature of the LPT was that the pain relief was more long lasting than the other therapies.

A study by Djavid [1849] was a randomised trial with concealed allocation, blinded assessors and intention-to-treat analysis. Sixty-one patients with low back pain for at least 12 weeks participated. One group received LPT alone, one received LPT and exercise, and a third group received placebo LPT and exercise. LPT was performed twice a week for 6 weeks. Outcomes were pain severity measured using a 10-cm visual analogue scale, lumbar range of motion measured by the Schober Test and maximum active flexion, extension and lateral flexion, and disability measured by the Oswestry Disability Index on admission to the study, after 6 weeks of intervention, and after another 6 weeks without intervention. There was no greater effect of LPT compared with exercise for any outcome, at either 6 or 12 weeks. There was also no greater effect of LPT plus exercise compared with exercise for any outcome at 6 weeks. However, in the LPT plus exercise group pain had reduced by 1.8 cm, lumbar range of movement increased by 0.9 cm on the Schober Test and by 15 deg of active flexion, and disability reduced by 9.4 points (more than in the exercise group at 12 weeks). In chronic low back pain, LPT combined with exercise seems to be more beneficial than exercise alone in the long term.

In a recent Cochrane analysis [1787]of the effect of LPT on low back pain the authors write: "Six RCTs with reasonable quality were included in the review. All of them were published in English. There is some evidence of pain relief with LPT, compared to sham therapy for subacute and chronic low-back pain. These effects were only observed at short-term and intermediate-term follow-ups. Long-term follow-ups were not reported. There was no difference between LPT and comparison groups for pain-related disability. There is insufficient evidence to determine the effectiveness of LPT on antero-posterior lumbar range of motion compared to control group in short-term follow-up. The relapse rate in the LPT group was significantly lower than in the control group at six months follow-up period according to the findings of two trials. No side effects were reported. However, we conclude that there are insufficient data to draw firm conclusions. There is a need for further methodologically rigorous RCTs to evaluate the effects of LPT compared to other treatments, different lengths of treatment, different wavelengths and different dosages. Comparison of different LPT treatments will be more reasonable if dose calculation methods are harmonized."

The aim ofa study by Konstantinovic [2124] was to investigate the clinical effects of LPT in patients with acute low back pain (LBP) with radiculopathy.Acute LBP with radiculopathy is associated with pain and disability and the important pathogenic role of inflammation. LPT has shown significant anti-inflammatory effects in many studies. A randomized, double-blind, placebo-controlled trial was performed on 546 patients. Group A (182 patients) was treated with nimesulide 200 mg/day and additionally with

4.1.32 Low back pain

This is certainly a difficult problem to treat, and LPT is by no means a panacea. It has, however, proven to be a valuable option in the hands of physiotherapists and chiropractors. High doses of infrared are essential. Relative lack of success in published studies is probably due to low dosages. WALT dosage recommendation per session for low back pain is a minimum of 8 J per point, 40 J in totalt for GaAlAs. For GaAs, the minimum is 4 J per point, not less than 10 J in total.

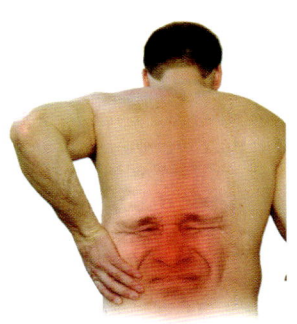

Literature:

Gruszka [551] used a GaAs laser in a group of 15 patients with one or more protruded lumbar disc herniations. Previous physical therapy had improved symptoms but CAT scans had not changed. A total of 9 J/cm² was given on 20 to 25 points. These points were on the lumbar spine and on points of referred radicular pain. Treatment was administered three to five times a week for four months. Before and after treatment, the patients' pain, gait, EMG, and CAT scan were evaluated. All patients were free from pain at the end of the treatment. Gait and neurological signs improved in all patients. EMGs improved and CAT scans showed less protrusion of the herniated discs.

Tasaki [125] treated 18 patients with low back pain with a GaAlAs laser at 30-80 mW. The sessions lasted 2-10 minutes and led to full pain relief. Pain relief took six to eight hours to take effect among the patients who did not experience it immediately.

Basford [1062] performed a double-blind, placebo-controlled, randomized clinical trial on patients with low back pain. Sixty-three ambulatory men and women between the ages of 18 and 70 years with symptomatic non-radiating low back pain of more than 30 days' duration and normal neurological examination results participated. Subjects were bloc randomised into two groups by a computer-generated schedule. All underwent irradiation for 90 seconds at eight symmetric points along the lumbosacral spine three times a week for four weeks by a masked therapist. The Nd:YAG laser emitted 542 mW/cm². The subject's perception of benefits gained, level of function as assessed by the Oswestry Disability Questionnaire, and lumbar mobility were evaluated. The treated group had a time-dependent improvement in two of the three outcome measures: perception of benefits and level of function. These results were most marked at the midpoint evaluation and end of treatment, but tended to lessen at the one-month follow-up. Lumbar mobility did not differ between the groups at any time.

In another clinical study by Zati [1537], a high power defocused Nd:YAG laser was used in patients suffering from low back pain caused by

nation. On day seven, the combined therapy demonstrated a significantly higher analgesic effect.

Seven patients with bilateral Achilles tendinitis (14 tendons), who had aggravated symptoms caused by pain-inducing activities, were included in a study by Bjordal [1461]. A total of 1.8 Joules for each of three points along the Achilles tendon with a 904nm infrared laser or placebo laser were administered to the Achilles tendons in a random order to which patients and therapist were blinded. Inflammation was examined by invasive microdialysis for measuring the concentration of the inflammatory marker PGE_2 in the peritendinous tissue, ultrasound with Doppler measurement of peri- and intratendinous blood flow, and pressure pain algometry. PGE_2 levels were significantly reduced at 60, 75, and 90 minutes after active laser compared both to pretreatment levels and to placebo. Changes in pressure pain threshold (PPT) differed significantly between groups. PPT increased by a mean value of 0.19 kg/cm^2 after treatment in the active laser group, while pressure pain threshold was reduced by -0.20 kg/cm^2 after placebo.

Markovic [1911] found that LPT enhanced the effect of intramuscular DEX after third molar extractions.

4.1.29 Inner ear conditions
(See chapter 4.1.52 "Tinnitus, vertigo, Ménière's disease" on page 330.)

4.1.30 Laryngitis
Although the literature is scarce, there is clinical experience of treating actors with temporary overloading of their voices. Suggested IR dosage is 4 J on five to six sites over the projection of the larynx.

Literature:

Hubacek [1036] reports positive results from treating laryngitis, using transcutaneous irradiation.

4.1.31 Lichen
LPT has a good effect on the subjective symptoms of lichen conditions, and it is a supportive method to conventional lichen treatment.

Literature:
[697, 724, 972]

tion of either total or differential leukocyte influx, exudation, total protein, NO, IL-6, MCP-1, IL-10, and TNF-alpha, in a dose-dependent manner. Under these conditions, laser treatment with 2.1 J was more effective than with 0.9 and 4.2 J.

Castano [1840] tested LPT on rats that had zymosan injected into their knee joints to induce inflammatory arthritis. The author compared illumination regimens consisting of a high and a low fluence (3 and 30 J/cm^2), delivered at a high and a low irradiance (5 and 50 mW/cm^2) using 810 nm laser light daily for five days, with a positive control of conventional corticosteroid (dexamethasone) therapy. Illumination with 810 nm laser was highly effective at reducing swelling (almost as good as dexamethasone), and a longer illumination time (10 or 100 minutes compared to 1 minute) was more important in determining effectiveness than either the total fluence delivered or the irradiance. LPT induced reduction of joint swelling correlated to a reduction in the inflammatory marker serum prostaglandin $E_2(PGE_2)$.

The aim of a work by Meneguzzo [2034] was to investigate the effects of infrared 810nm on the acute inflammatory process by the irradiation of lymph nodes, using the classical model of carrageenan-induced rat paw edema. Thirty mice were randomly divided into five groups. The inflammatory induction was performed in all groups by a sub-plantar injection of carrageenan (1mg/paw). The paw volume was measured before and 1, 2, 3, 4 and 6 hours after the injection using a plethysmometer. Myeloperoxidase (MPO) activity was analyzed as a specific marker of neutrophil accumulation at the inflammatory site. The control group did not receive any treatment (GC); GD group received sodium diclofenac (1mg/kg) 30 minutes before the carrageenan injection; GP group received laser irradiation directly on the paw (1 Joule, 100mW, 10 sec) 1 and 2 hours after the carrageenan injection; GLY group received laser irradiation (1 Joule, 100mW, 10 sec) on the inguinal lymph nodes; GP+LY group received laser irradiation on both paw and lymph nodes 1 and 2 hours after the carrageenan injection. MPO activity was similar in the sodium diclofenac as well as in the GP and GLY groups, but significantly lower than the GC and GP + LY groups. Paw edema was significantly inhibited in GP and GD groups when compared to the other groups. Interestingly, the GP+LY groups presented the biggest edema, even bigger than in the control group. LPT showed an anti-inflammatory effect when the irradiation was performed on the site of lesion or at the correlated lymph nodes, but showed a pro-inflammatory effect when both paw and lymph nodes were irradiated during the acute inflammatory process.

Clinical studies

Konstantinovic [554] compared the effect of corticosteroid infiltration, LPT (GaAs 1 J/cm^2) and laser plus corticosteroid infiltration in combi-

red (830 nm) laser energy, respectively. The animals were killed at 12, 36, and 72 h after the procedure and on day seven. Microscopic analysis revealed a significant vascular activation of irradiated sites during the first 36 h. Only group B showed decreases in the intensity of polymorphonuclear infiltrates and edema. Group D showed a higher degree of organization and maturation of collagen fibers than the other groups at 72 h. The animals in group C showed the best healing pattern on day seven. The anti-inflammatory action of Meloxicam was confirmed by the results obtained in this research. The quantification of interleukin-1ß mRNA by real-time polymerase chain reaction (PCR) did not show any reduction in the inflammatory process in the irradiated groups when compared to the other groups.

A study by Correa [1875] was designed to study the effect of a GaAs laser, 4 mW, on inflammatory cell migration in lipopolysaccharide (LPS)-induced peritonitis in mice. Sixty male mice were randomly divided into five groups, and one group was given an intraperitoneal sterile saline injection. In the remaining four groups, peritonitis was induced by an intraperitoneal LPS injection. Animals in three of the LPS groups were irradiated at a single point over the peritoneum with doses of 3 J/cm^2, 7.5 J/cm^2, and 15 J/cm^2, respectively. The fourth group injected with LPS was an LPS-control group. At 6 hours after injection the groups irradiated with doses of 3 J/cm^2 and 7.5 J/cm^2 had a reduced number of neutrophil cells in the peritoneal cavity compared with the LPS-control group, and there were significant differences in the number of neutrophils in the peritoneal cavity between the LPS-control group and the groups irradiated with doses of 3 J/cm^2 (42%) and 7.5 J/cm^2 (70%). In the group irradiated with 15 J/cm^2, neutrophil cell counts were lower than, but not significantly different from, LPS controls (38%). At 24 hours after injection, both neutrophil and total leukocyte cell counts were lower in all the irradiated groups than in the LPS controls. The 3J/cm^2 exposure group showed the best results at 24 hours, with reductions of 77% in neutrophil and 49% in leukocyte counts.

A sample of 48 female Wistar rats were divided into control and experiential groups by Boschi [1940]. An inflammation was induced by carrageenan (0.2 ml) being injected into the pleural cavity. At 1, 2, and 3 hours after induction a 20 mW, 660 nm laser was used in the four laser groups, with different doses and treatment patterns. One group received a single dose of 2.1 J while the other three groups received a total energy of 0.9, 2.1, and 4.2 J. Four hours later the exudate volume, total and differential leukocytes, protein concentration, NO, IL-6, IL-10, TNF-alpha, and MCP-1 were measured from the aspirated liquid. All the treatment patterns and quantity of energy studied showed a significant reduction of the exudate volume. Using an energy output of 0.9 J only NO, IL-6, MCP-1 and IL-10 were significantly reduced. On the other hand, higher energies (2.1 and 4.2 J) significantly reduced all variables independent of the treatment pattern. The neutrophil migration has a direct correlation to the TNF-alpha and NO concentration. Thus, 660 nm induced an anti-inflammatory effect characterized by inhibi-

Gene expression of the cytokines was measured using reverse transcriptase-polymerase chain reaction (RT-PCR) technique. The gene expression of IL-1ß and IFN-gamma was significantly inhibited in the test groups while the gene expression of PDGF and TGF-ß was significantly increased. The case and control groups did not differ significantly in the gene expression of TNF-alpha and bFGF. These findings suggest that HeNe laser irradiation decreases the amount of inflammation and accelerates the wound healing process by changing the expression of genes responsible for the production of inflammatory cytokines.

In the work by Bortone [1826], the author evaluated if LPT alters the kinin receptor's mRNA expression in carrageenan-induced rat paw edema. Experimental groups were designed as followed: A1 (Control-saline), A2 (Carrageenan-only), A3 (Carrageenan+laser 660 nm) and A4 (Carrageenan+laser 684 nm). Edema was measured by a plethysmometer. Subplantar tissue was collected for the quantification of the kinin receptor's mRNA by Real time-PCR. LPT of both 660 and 684 nm wavelengths administrated 1 h after the carrageenan injection was able to promote a reduction of the edema produced by carrageenan. In the A2 group, B1 receptor expression presented a significant increase when compared to the control group. Kinin B1 receptor mRNA expression significantly decreased after LPT of both 660 or 684 nm. Kinin B2 receptor mRNA expression also diminished after both laser irradiations. The results suggest that the expressions of both kinin receptors are modulated by LPT, possibly contributing to its anti-inflammatory effect.

The aim of the study by Lopes-Martins [1619] was to investigate the effect of LPT, 650 nm, on acute inflammatory pleurisy. A classical experimental model of pleurisy was used in a sample of 40 Balb male mice, randomly divided into five groups. Inflammation was induced by carrageenan (0.5 mg/cavity) administered by intrathoracic injections. Four groups received the inflammatory agent, and one received injections of sterile saline solution. At the first, second and third hour after injections, irradiation was performed using the same power (2.5 mW), but with different irradiation times. The energy densities at each of the three treatment sessions were 0 J/cm^2 (placebo), 3 J/cm^2, 7.5J/cm^2, and 15 J/cm^2, respectively. Total and differential cell analysis at the fourth hour after induction of pleurisy showed a significant reduction of inflammatory cell migration for all groups treated with active laser. However, four hours after injection, the most significant reduction of leukocyte cell migration was seen in the 7.5 J/cm^2 group. The greatest reduction of inflammatory cells was registered for neutrophils.

A study by Viegas [1868] evaluated the action of LPT on the modulation of inflammatory reactions during wound healing in comparison with Meloxicam. Standardized circular wounds were made on the backs of 64 Wistar rats. The animals were divided into four groups according to the selected postoperative therapies: group A, control; group B, administration of Meloxicam; and groups C and D irradiation with red (685 nm) and infra-

of the GaAlAs laser on inflammatory oedema, parallel studies were performed using adrenalectomised rats or rats treated with sodium diclofenac. Different laser irradiation protocols were employed for specific energy densities (EDs), exposure times and repetition rates. The rats were irradiated with laser for 80 s each hour. The EDs that produced an anti-inflammatory effect were 1 and 2.5 J/cm^2, reducing the oedema by 27% and 45.4%, respectively. The ED of 2.5 J/cm^2 produced anti-inflammatory effects similar to those produced by the cyclooxygenase inhibitor sodium diclofenac at a dose of 1 mg/kg. In adrenalectomised animals, the laser irradiation failed to inhibit the oedema. These results suggest that low power laser irradiation possibly exerts its anti-inflammatory effects by stimulating the release of adrenal corticosteroid hormones.

The aim of the study by Ferreira [1733] was to evaluate the analgesic effect of the LPT with a HeNe laser on acute inflammatory pain, verifying the contribution of the peripheral opioid receptors and the action of LPT on the hyperalgesia produced by the release of hyperalgesic mediators of inflammation. Male rats were used. Three complementary experiments were done. (1) The inflammatory reaction was induced by injecting carrageenin into one of the hind paws. Pain threshold and volume increase of the edema were measured by a pressure gauge and plethysmography, respectively. (2) The involvement of peripheral opioid receptors on the analgesic effect of the laser was evaluated by simultaneous injections of carrageenin and naloxone into one hind paw. (3). Hyperalgesia was induced by injecting PGE_2 for the study of the effect of the laser on the sensitization increase of nociceptors. A HeNe laser of 2.5 J/cm^2 was used for irradiation. The researchers found that HeNe stimulation increased the pain threshold by a factor of 68% to 95% depending on the injected drug. They also observed a 54% reduction in the volume increase of the edema after being irradiated. The analgesic effect seems to involve hyperalgesic mediators instead of peripheral opioid receptors.

Interleukin 1β (IL-1β), tumor necrotic factor-alpha (TNF-alpha), and interferon-gamma (IFN-gamma) play important roles in inflammation, while platelet-derived growth factor (PDGF), transforming growth factor-β (TGF-β) and blood-derived fibroblast growth factor (bFGF) are the most important growth factors of periodontal tissues. The aim of a study by Safavi [1891] was to investigate the effect of HeNe laser on the gene expression of these mediators in rats' gingiva and mucosal tissues. Twenty male Wistar rats were randomly assigned to four groups (A(24), A(48), B(24), B(48)) in which A(24) and A(48) were cases and B(24) and B(48) were controls. An incision was made on gingiva and mucosa of the labial surface of the rats' mandibular incisors. Group A(24) was irradiated twice with 24-hour intervals, while the inflamed tissues of group A(48) were irradiated three times with continuous HeNe laser at a dose of 7.5 J/cm^2 for 300 s. An energy of 5.1 J was given to the 68 mm2 irradiation zone. Rats were killed 30 min after the last irradiation of case and control groups, then an excisional biopsy was performed.

Literature:
Animal studies

Aimbire [1815] studied the effect of LPT on lung permeability and the IL-1ß level in LPS-induced pulmonary inflammation. Rats were divided into 12 groups (n = 7 for each group). Lung permeability was measured by quantifying extravasated albumin concentration in lung homogenate, inflammatory cells influx was determined by myeloperoxidase activity, IL-1ß in BAL was determined by ELISA and IL-1ß mRNA expression in trachea was evaluated by RT-PCR. The rats were irradiated on the skin over the upper bronchus at the site of tracheotomy after LPS. LPT attenuated lung permeability. In addition, there was a reduced neutrophil influx, myeloperoxidase activity and both IL-1ß in BAL and IL-1ß mRNA expressions in trachea obtained from animals subjected to LPS-induced inflammation showed a reduction. In conclusion, LPT reduced the lung permeability by a mechanism in which the IL-1ß seems to have an important role.

Aimbire [1800] further reports on the effect of 660 nm laser on mRNA levels of neutrophils anti-apoptotic factors in lipopolysaccharide (LPS)-induced lung inflammation. Mice were divided into eight groups (n=7 for each group) and irradiated with an energy dosage of 7.5 J/cm^2. The Bcl-xL and A1 mRNA levels in neutrophils were evaluated by Real Time-PCR (RT-PCR). The animals were irradiated after exposure time of LPS. LPT and an inhibitor of NF-kappaB nuclear translocation (BMS 205820) attenuated the mRNA levels of Bcl-xL and A1 mRNA in lung neutrophils obtained from mice subjected to LPS-induced inflammation. LPT reduced the levels of anti-apoptotic factors in LPS inflamed mice lung neutrophils by an action mechanism in which the NF-kappaB seems to be involved. The purpose of a study by Aimbire [1560] was to investigate the effect of LPT on rat trachea hyperreactivity (RTHR), bronchoalveolar lavage (BAL) and lung neutrophils influx after Gram-negative bacterial lipopolysacharide (LPS) intravenous injections. The RTHR, BAL and lung neutrophils influx were measured over different intervals of time (90 min, 6 h, 24 h and 48 h). The energy density (ED) that produced an anti-inflammatory effect was 2.5 J/cm^2, reducing the maximal contractile response and the sensibility of trachea rings to methacholine after LPS. The same ED produced an anti-inflammatory effect on BAL and lung neutrophils influx. The Celecoxib COX-2 inhibitor reduced RTHR and the number of cells in BAL and lung neutrophils influx of rats treated with LPS. Celecoxib and laser reduced the PGE$_2$ and TXA2 levels in the BAL of LPS-treated rats. These results demonstrate that 685 nm LPT produced anti-inflammatory effects on RTHR, BAL and lung neutrophils influx in association with inhibition of COX-2-derived metabolites.

The purpose of another study by Albertini [1580] was to investigate the effect of LPT on the acute inflammatory process. Male rats were used. Paw oedema was induced by a sub-plantar injection of carrageenan, the paw volume was measured before and one, two, three and four hours after the injection, using a hydroplethysmometer. To investigate the action mechanism

assessed by histopathology using polarized light and ultrastructural assessments by transmission electron microscopy. Changes seen in polymorphonuclear inflammatory cells, edema, mononuclear cells, and collagen fiber deposition were semi-quantitatively evaluated. The laser-treated group demonstrated an increased collagen content and a better arrangement of the extracellular matrix. Fibroblasts in these tissues increased in number and were more synthetically active. In the dexamethasone group, the collagen was shown to be non-homogenous and disorganized, with a scarcity of fibroblasts. In the group treated with both types of therapy, fibroblasts were more common and they exhibited vigorous rough endoplasmic reticulum, but they had less collagen production compared to those seen in the laser group. Thus, LPT alone accelerated post-surgical tissue repair and reduced edema and the polymorphonuclear infiltrate, even in the presence of dexamethasone.

It might therefore be prudent to avoid a combination of steroids and laser, if this is clinically feasible. There seems to be no negative effects from the combination of the two but a reduction of the total effect of laser. Since steroids in many clinical situations have undesired side effects, LPT could be a good alternative. This is confirmed in a study by Lopes-Martins [1456]. In this study, the classical experimental mice-model of carrageenan-induced pleurisy was used to investigate if the anti-inflammatory effect of LPT could be blocked by the steroid agent mifepristone. For the intervention group, mifepristone was injected into the pleural cavity an hour prior to the carrageenan injection. Pleurisy was then induced by an intrathoracic injection of carrageenan (0.5mg/cavity), or LPS from E. coli (250 mg/ cavity) in mice. Laser irradiation (650 nm) was then carried out three times with hourly intervals on the skin at the injection site for both groups. Laser was administered with a previously established optimal accumulated dose of 7.5 J/cm^2. While laser after four hours effectively reduced inflammation almost to pre-injection levels of neutrophil cell counts, the anti-inflammatory effect was blocked after pre-injection of mifepristone.

Meloxicam is an NSAID which significantly decreases symptoms of pain, function, and stiffness in patients, with a low incidence of gastrointestinal side effects. Meloxicam has been shown, especially at its low therapeutic dose, to selectively inhibit COX-2 over COX-1. LPT has been shown to have an effect equivalent to Meloxicam [1868].

Some studies showing a reduction of PGE_2 are [243,357,582,718,1008,1276,1461,1560,1800]. Reduction of IL1-ß [188, 370, 1314, 1815, 1891].

Research indicates that lower intensity and longer exposure are favorable when treating inflammation [1821,1840]. Higher intensities and shorter time spans will be more effective against pain itself, but in many instances the long term result will be better if the inflammation (causing the pain) is the main target of the therapy.

Below is a summary of some of the most interesting studies in this field.

useful targeted gene expressions, whereas DEX randomly altered many gene expressions, including the unwanted genes for anti-inflammation. Dexomethasone is a steroid known for having a long range of serious side effects. Thus, genome based gene expression monitored by the Gene Chip system together with a signal pathway based database provide unprecedented access to elucidate the mechanism of the biostimulatory effects of LPT.

Yamada [1054] has compared corticosteroids, LPT and a combination of the two in a study comprising seven patients in each group. The effect of LPT was comparable to that of corticosteroids, but the combined therapy showed the best outcome. The laser was a 150 mW GaAlAs laser and the LPT was performed over the area of paralysis (36 J per session), the stylomastoid foramen (10.8 J) and the stellate ganglion (63.7 J). The number of sessions in the laser group ranged from 21 to 66 for 5-12 weeks. In the combined therapy group, success was achieved within 14-31 sessions, after 3-10 weeks.

Steroids are frequently used to treat inflammation. Some studies report a reduced effect of LPT in the presence of steroids, while others have found positive results of LPT even in the presence of steroids. However, steroids are known to delay wound healing through a reduction of leukocyte migration and a suppression of interleukins, while LPT is known to stimulate wound healing. In a study by Pessoa [1455], 48 rats were used, and after the execution of a wound on the dorsal region of each animal, they were divided into four groups (n = 12), receiving the following treatments: G1 (control), wounds and animals received no treatment; G2, wounds were treated with laser; G3, animals received an intraperitoneal injection of sodium phosphate of dexametasone, dosage 2 mg/kg of body weight; G4, animals received steroids and wounds were treated with laser. The laser emission device used was a 904 nm unit, in a contact mode, with 2.75 mW gated with 2.900 Hz during 120 sec. After a period of 3, 7 and 14 days, the animals were sacrificed. The results showed that the wounds treated with steroid had a delay in healing, while laser accelerated the wound healing process. Additionally, wounds treated with laser in the animals also treated with steroids, presented a differentiated healing process with a larger collagen deposition as well as a decrease in both the inflammatory infiltrated and in the delay on the wound healing process. Laser accelerated healing, delayed by the steroids, acting as a biostimulative coadjutant agent, balancing the undesirable effects of the steroids on the tissue's healing process. The effect of LPT is almost as potent as dexametasone [1840], but, again, without side effects.

Reis [1904] investigated the role of extracellular matrix elements and cells during the wound healing phases following the use of LPT and anti-inflammatory drugs. Thirty-two rats were submitted to a wound inflicted by a 6-mm-diameter punch. The animals were divided into four groups: sham treated, those treated with the GaAlAs laser (4 J/cm^2, 9 mW, 670 nm), those treated with dexamethasone (2 mg/kg), and those treated with both LPT and dexamethasone. After three and five days, the cutaneous wounds were

latory effects when applied on the thymus projection area. The rise in IL-2 and Hsp70 production related to a short-term effect of laser application may be reversed after repeating the laser treatment.

Mikhailov [982] reports on the use of 890 nm laser treatment of the autoimmune thyroiditis. Forty-two patients were given 10 applications at 2.4 J/cm^2. The irradiated areas were the thymus projection zones (area of the sternum at a level of the second edge), vascular junction (left axillary area) and thyroid gland. A control group of a similar size was given L-thyroxin, 100 mg/day. The clinical effect in all laser patients was a decreased feeling of squeezing in the area of the thyroid gland, and a decrease of the facial oedema. The gland became softer palpatively and its size was reduced according to the ultrasound examination. The number of patients catching a cold during the winter decreased. The immunoregulatory index (Th/Ts) normalised from 7.5 to 4.2%. The laser effect was still noticeable in 78% of the patients 4 months after treatment. This index was only slightly changed in the control group.

Further literature: [645]

4.1.28 Inflammation

The effect of LPT on inflammation is covered in many chapters of this book. The anti-inflammatory effect of LPT has been widely studied. LPT seems to have a similar effect to steriods and NSAIDs, but without the severe side effects of these very common pharmaceuticals.

Recently, the understanding of the mechanism at work has been improved by using genetic technology. This technology has also to a certain extent explained why there are so few side effects of LPT. In an effort to clarify the molecular based mechanism of the anti-inflammatory effects of laser irradiation, Abiko [1860] used a rheumatoid arthritis (RA) rat model with human rheumatoid synoviocytes (MH-7) challenged with IL-1, treated with laser or dexamethasone (DEX), monitored by gene expressions and analyzed by the signal pathway database. RA rats were generated by the immunization of type-II collagen, after which foot paws and knee joints became significantly swollen. The animals were laser treated and the swelling rates measured. MH-7 was challenged with IL-1ß and gene expression levels monitored, using the Affymetrix Gene Chip system, and the signal pathway database analyzed using the Ingenuity Pathway Analysis (IPA) tool. LPT significantly reduced swellings in the rats' foot paws and knee joints and made it possible for them to walk on their hind legs. LPT altered many gene expressions of cytokines, chemokines, growth factors and signal transduction factors in IL-ß induced MH-7. IPA revealed that LPT as well as DEX kept the MH7A at a normal state to suppress mRNA levels of IL-8, IL-1ß, CXC1, NFkB1 and FGF13, which were enhanced by IL-1ß treatment. However, certain gene expression of inflammatory factors were reduced by LPT, but were enhanced by DEX. LPT reduced inflammatory factors through altering signal pathways by gene expression levels. Interestingly, LPT altered

power laser irradiation can modulate immune responses depending on the immunological status of the organism."

In a study by Inoue [405], a 830 nm laser has been shown to suppress the tuberculin reaction in a well-known immunological test for the evaluation of cellular immunity in vivo.

Funk [565, 731] has shown that HeNe laser affects cytokine production in human peripheral blood mononuclear cells in vitro.

The leukocyte stimulating effects of HeNe have been described by Klebanov [1006, 1007] and Mester [23].

Katsuyama [662] has found a suppressive effect of diode laser irradiation on picryl contact sensitivity in a rat model. The thickness of the right ear was used as an indicator of the immune response to various doses of 830 nm laser irradiation. LPT suppressed the cutaneous inflammation due to picryl contact sensitivity in an exposure-time dependent manner, and this suppressive effect was restricted to within the irradiation site.

Yu [590] used an argon pumped dye laser at a wavelength of 630 nm to study the effect of LPT on the immune system. Rats with experimentally induced sepsis (cecal ligation) received LPT, 5 J/cm^2. On day 60, the survival rate was 79% in the laser group and 42% in the control group. Ex vivo lymphocyte proliferation was 180 in the laser group and 130 in the control group. Enhanced lymphocyte ATP synthesis was observed in the laser group.

To study the possible side effects of laser immunotherapy, Novoselova [1768] monitored the productions of cytokines, nitric oxide (NO), and heat shock protein 70 (Hsp70) in mice subjected to a periodic laser exposure for one month. Helium-neon laser radiation with the power of 0.2 mW/cm^2 and a wavelength of 632.8 nm was applied on two different mouse skin surfaces, i.e. a thymus projection area or a hind limb. Healthy NMRI male mice were irradiated repeatedly with laser light for one minute with 48-h intervals for 30 days. The animals were divided into three groups of 25 mice. The first and the second group were exposed to laser light on the thymus and hind limb area, respectively. The third sham-irradiated group served as a control. Early and prolonged effects of laser radiation on the levels of NO (by Griess assay), Hsp70 (by Western blot assay), tumor necrosis factors (TNF-alpha and TNF-β) (by cytotoxic assay using L929 cells as targets), and interleukin-2 (IL-2) (by ELISA assay) were determined. The dynamics of immune responses to low-power laser light intensity was shown to be dependent on two factors, i.e. the cumulative dose and the localization of the irradiated surface. Moreover, various populations of cells demonstrated different sensitivity to laser radiation, with T cells being more responsive among examined cell populations. Low-intensity laser light induced an immune cell activity when the exposure duration did not exceed 10 days, while a more prolonged period of treatment generated more severe changes in the immune system, up to immunosuppression. The treatment of the thymus zone resulted in more pronounced changes in the cytokine production as well as in NO and Hsp70 synthesis. Low-power laser irradiation showed more effective immunomodu-

Literature:

Takaduma [373] reports the effects of LPT on the immune system: "The human immune system acts as a defence mechanism against exogenous or indigenous potentially harmful bodies, such as bacteria and viruses. The major histocompatibility complex (MHC class I and class II antigens) form key elements of legitimate body components, and the organisation of MHC molecules allows T-lymphocytes to distinguish between legitimate and foreign bodies. On detection of a foreign component, T-cells activate the necessary pathways for destruction of the foreign body. Occasionally however the system breaks down and the result is a disease of an autoimmune nature. Both visible light and infrared LPT have been shown to act on immune system cells in a number of ways, activating the irradiated cells to a higher level of activity. Infrared LPT has been shown to increase both the phagocytic and chemotactic activity of human leukocytes in vitro, for example. This is an example of photobiological activation. Photobiological cell-specific destruction is also possible using doses of low incident laser energy on cells which have been photosensitised for the specific wavelength of the laser, such as in photodynamic therapy (PDT) for superficial cancers. LPT has also been shown to act directly and selectively on the autoimmune system, restoring immunocompetence to cells. Although much more research needs to be done, there are enough experimental and clinical data to show that the laser, and LPT in particular, has a possibly exciting role both in immunobiological therapy for diseases of the immune system, and to activate and boost the normal reaction of the immune system components."

Kólarová [655] reports that doses of 5 to 10 J/cm^2 induced a significant increase of the phagocytic activity of leukocytes in vitro.

Duan [1163] has demonstrated a respiratory burst in bovine neutrophils after HeNe irradiation.

Schindl [581] describes an experiment on the immune modulating effect of a HeNe laser as follows: "Escherichia coli endotoxin preimmunized rabbits were used to determine the influence of transcutaneously applied low-power laser light on differential blood count and rectal temperature. After three initial immunizations, animals were either boostered with 5 ng/kg of endotoxin or injected with pyrogen-free saline and subsequently underwent irradiation using two different wavelengths of red laser light and sham irradiation respectively. The differential blood count of laser-treated animals was characterised by significantly higher lymphocyte values and lower neutrophil values at twenty hours (boostered rabbits) and twenty-three hours (non-boostered rabbits) after irradiation. Differential blood cell counts returned to baseline levels within 23 hours in the boostered animals, whereas in the non-boostered rabbits lymphocytes showed a tendency to further increase. Recording of rectal temperature revealed a further rise after laser application, changes being of greater magnitude and longer duration in the non-boostered animals. These results seem to indicate that a single low-

group. The nested polymerase chain reaction (PCR) method was used to detect HSV-1, EBV-1, and HCMV. Bacteria was identified by 16S rRNA-based PCR. HSV-1, HCMV, and EBV-1 were detected in 86.7%, 46.7%, and 33.3% of the AgP group, respectively; in 40.0%, 50.0%, and 46.7% of the CP group, respectively; in 53.3%, 40.0%, and 20.0% of the G group, respectively; and in 20.0%, 56.7%, and 0.0% of the C group, respectively. A. actinomycetemcomitans was detected significantly more often in the AgP group compared to the other groups ($P < 0.005$). P. gingivalis and T. forsythia were identified more frequently in AgP and CP groups, and AgP, CP, and G groups had higher frequencies of P. intermedia compared to the C group. In Brazilian patients, HSV-1 and EBV-1, rather than HCMV, were more frequently associated with CP and AgP. The impact of LPT in periodontal therapy can possibly and partly be an anti-viral effect.

Foyaca-Sibat [2033] studied the effect of LPT in 46 cases of HIV related post neuralgia in different age-groups (21 to 61 years) and with a varying duration of the illness ranging from 3 months to 3 1/2 years in the present investigation. The affected areas were irradiated from a distance of 5 cm using the probe of a GaAs laser, 12x70 watts peak power, at a PRR of 1000 Hz, each area being exposed for a time period of five minutes and six seconds. In each case, the laser therapy was given for 15 consecutive days and the effect of the therapy was evaluated after the 5th, 10th, and 15th laser application during the treatment with the help of a visual analogue scale (VAS). Patients started responding to the therapy after an average of 2.58 laser applications and VAS steadily decreased as the therapy progressed. After completion of therapy, 37 (80.4%) out of 46 cases showed excellent relief, and the remaining 9 (19%) cases showed partial relief, which could be due to multiple factors like prolonged duration of illness, involvement of ophthalmic division of trigeminal nerve and formation of scarring and keloids. No side effects were observed either during the treatment or in the follow-up period of 10 weeks.

The use of LPT to suppress infections caused by Herpes simplex viruses 1 and 2 was evaluated by Ferreira [2059], after one to five applications. A gradual reduction in replication of Herpes simplex viruses 1 and 2 was observed, with 68.4% and 57.3% inhibition, respectively, after five applications.

Further literature: [43, 61, 222, 628, 822, 1043, 1892, 1942, 1943]

4.1.27 Immune system modulation

The general aspect of immune modulation is one of the most important aspects of LPT. Systemic effects are always obtained since any irradiation involves the circulatory system.

Hachenberger [60] reports the results of treating 93 patients with a HeNe laser. Pain disappeared quickly and healing occurred within three days. In no case did the herpes reappear at the same site, and relapses were less frequent.

Michels [416] summarizes eight years of experience in treating herpes simplex with HeNe laser light; 582 cases of HSV1, and 34 cases of HSV2. Healing was fast and without side-effects. By and large 10% of the cases suffered relapses in loco, but all were patients with immune deficiency or a strong allergic background.

An important aspect of LPT of HSV1 has been described by Schindl [908], namely the possibility of treating patients with recurrent herpes attacks even during the symptom-free period. Fifty patients with recurrent perioral herpes simplex infections (at least once a month for more than six months) were treated with 690 nm, 80 mW laser, energy density 48 J/cm^2, in a double-blind study. Patients received daily irradiations for 2 weeks, 10 sessions in all. The treatment was given during a recurrence-free period and the irradiation was given at the site of the original herpes simplex infection. If both lips were involved, both upper and lower lips were treated. Patients were monitored for 52 weeks. The mean recurrence-free interval in the laser group was 37.5 weeks (range; 2-52 weeks), and in the placebo group 3 weeks (range 1-20 weeks). No side effects were noted.

Almeida-Lopes [1531] has shown that HSV-1 can be treated advantageously by irradiation of the involved lymph nodes. Microbes in wounds can be stimulated or suppressed by different wavelengths and doses [1496]. Therefore, irradiating the lymph nodes eliminates this potentially negative effect.

Guerra [1420] compared laser with traditional therapies in a group of 116 patients. Patients in the laser group received GaAlAs 670 nm, 1.2 J per blister in the prodromal stage and 2.4 J in the crust and secondarily infected stages, plus 1 J at the C2-C3 vertebras. All in all 116 patients in the HSV1 group received LPT while the rest received traditional therapy, such as Acyclovir cream or pills and palliative therapies. One of the dentists was responsible for the diagnosis, treatment and evaluation, respectively, to allow for a semi-blinded procedure. Patients were controlled daily during the first week to monitor healing, and monthly for one year to check for any recurrences. A very obvious effect of the LPT was found for both initial healing as well as for the number of recurrences.

A case-control study by Imbronito [2027] evaluated the presence of herpes simplex virus type I (HSV-1), Epstein-Barr virus type I (EBV-1), human cytomegalovirus (HCMV), Aggregatibacter actinomycetemcomitans (previously Actinobacillus actinomycetemcomitans), Porphyromonas gingivalis, Prevotella intermedia, and Tannerella forsythia (previously T. forsythensis) in patients with generalized AgP (AgP group), CP (CP group), or gingivitis (G group) and in healthy individuals (C group). Subgingival plaque samples were collected with paper points from 30 patients in each

effect was noted in the irradiated cells than in the control cells, more evident at 4 J. The two cell lines were incubated for seven days, frozen, and the released viruses inoculated in a new culture. An absence of cytopathic effect was noted in the cells infected with viruses derived from the cultures that received 12 J initially.

In an in vitro study by Hubacek [1036], HeNe laser had a cytopathogenous effect on HSV1 from 0.45 J/cm². On increasing the dose to 6 J/cm², no antiviral effect was noted.

In a study by Perrin [1009] it was observed that, in the ear experimental model of HSV latency, repeated exposure to infrared laser radiation of cervical ganglia following HSV inoculation appears to specifically hinder the establishment of virus latency in mice.

In an in vitro experiment by Eduardo [1893], epithelial cells and HSV-1 virus in culture were studied. Cells were irradiated with 660 or 780 nm using different dosages in four groups: 1) irradiation of non-infected epithelial cells, 2) epithelial cells irradiated prior to infection with the virus, 3) virus irradiated prior to infecting the epithelial cells, and 4) irradiation of HSV-1 infected cells. The irradiated epithelial cell growth was enhanced, but the only effect seen in cells infected with the virus was that the cell viability was prolonged if irradiated prior to infection. Thus, prolongation of cell survival may be one of the mechanisms at work.

Clinical studies

Landthaler [239] used a krypton laser (with a wavelength of 647 nm) to treat recurrent herpes simplex in loco, zoster, and postherpetic neuralgia. Treatment consisted of 50 mW, at 90 seconds per cm², each area 3 cm². Patients with recurrent HSV had symptom-free periods between outbreaks of 30 ± 19 days. After daily treatment sessions for 10 days, the average period between outbreaks was 73 ± 50 days. Seven of nine patients with herpes labialis experienced significant improvement, while only one of three with herpes glutealis improved. Two of four patients with acute zoster were freed from discomfort. Five of eight with postherpetic neuralgia experienced alleviation of pain or total pain relief.

Vélez-González [360] treated 60 patients suffering from herpes simplex in the oral (HSV1) or genital (HSV2) area. Three groups in each category received (I) 200 mg Acyclovir orally plus placebo laser, (II) placebo Acyclovir and HeNe laser light at 8 J/cm², or (III) Acyclovir and HeNe, in a randomised, double-blind study. Relapses on the lips and face were significantly reduced in the group treated with HeNe laser plus Acyclovir, as compared with the groups treated with Acyclovir or HeNe only. The number of relapses per year before and after treatment was 5.2/2.8 for group I, 7.83/1.16 for group II, and 7.28/1.28 for group III. There was no significant difference between the latter groups. However, healing time was shorter in the group that received a combination of treatments. The effects on the HSV2 groups were low for all 3 treatment modalities.

Picture on top shows typical labial HSV-1, three days after outbreak. GaAlAs 6 J applied with an immediate. Note crust formation.

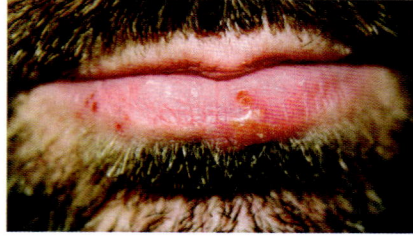

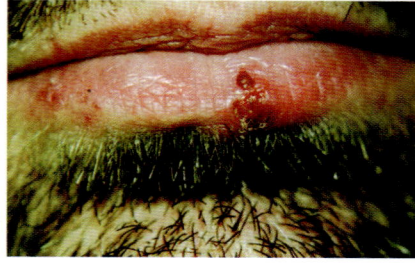

Figure 4.9 HSV-1 on day 1 and 2.

The results of treatment depend on the stage of the virus cycle in which the treatment begins. Patients often describe how the virus has a "favourite place", and experienced patients know where and when the blisters will appear, even before anything is visible. The use of a laser produces the best results in this prodromal stage, and may even prevent the attack. It also seems that a herpes sore is reluctant to return to a place where it has been treated before.

The later in the attack we treat, the poorer the results. However, even in the later stages of an attack, we can offer tangible (or perhaps even total) relief from the symptoms and an acceleration of the healing process. The dosage is determined by the patient. When obvious relief has been provided, we can stop treatment. If the attack is somewhat advanced before we can begin to treat it, the treatment should be repeated one to three times - an appropriate dosage is 4-6 J per sore.

If the herpes attacks are treated every time they manifest themselves, it appears that they return at longer and longer intervals [908]. It could be the case that LPT has a short-term effect on symptoms and a long-term effect on the onset of the virus per se.

HSV2 (genital) has been treated in two studies, but with a rather poor outcome. The poor result in HSV2 patients is a bit surprising, considering the excellent effect of LPT on HSV1 and varicella zoster.

Literature:
In vitro studies

Gilioli [102] studied the effects of GaAs on herpes simplex virus in vitro. It was found that the viral plaque was stimulated by laser light. The stimulating effect was greater for HSV-1 than for HSV-2. The anti-viral effect in vivo presumably depends on an immune-stimulating effect.

Tardivo [358] observed the behaviour of cells infected with HSV under a GaAs laser, 30 mW. Doses of 4 and 12 J were given. A lesser cytopathic

jective improvement. Patients also answered questionnaires assessing hair growth throughout the study. Neither patients nor physicians conducting the study received any financial compensation. The results indicate that on average patients had a decrease in the number of vellus hairs, an increase in the number of terminal hairs, and an increase in shaft diameter. However, paired i-testing indicated that none of these changes was statistically significant. Also, blinded evaluation of global images did not support an improvement in hair density or caliber. The authors suggest that LPT may be a promising treatment option for patients who do not respond to either finasteride or minoxidil, and who do not want to undergo hair transplantation. This technology appears to work better for some people than for others. Factors predicting who will most benefit are yet to be determined.

Further literature: [332, 631, 1643, 1686, 1740]

4.1.26 Herpes simplex

Herpes simplex (HSV1) is commonly encountered in the practice of dentistry. As students in the seventies, we learned that it disappears by itself after two weeks, but if treated, it heals within 14 days. There are now more effective treatment methods, and best by far is LPT. The mechanisms are still not fully understood.

thought to be an autoimmune disease which is treated with different modalities with varying success. Laser treatment of different wavelengths has been used in the management of this problem.

There are basically three types of "hair laser". The first one looks like a hood hair dryer, and it used to contain a HeNe laser tube with a maximum output of 6 mW. Nowadays, a number of GaAlInP laser diodes are generally used, with a somewhat longer wavelength (670 nm) and a higher output. The laser light is distributed via hundreds of small fibre-optic conductors over the whole of the inside of the hood. One problem is that there is a loss of energy in any area with hair, even if the hair is thin. These "hood hair dryer lasers" seem to work in many cases, but no convincing documentation has been put forward.

The second kind of "hair laser" is a normal HeNe or GaAlInP laser probe. Since the probe is held in direct contact with the scalp, the dosage level reached locally is much higher than in the "laser hair dryer", but the application method requires more work. Nevertheless, it still requires many treatment sessions and there is no guarantee of a successful result.

The third piece of equipment looks like a combe and the GaAlInP light comes out of the ends of the combe [1644].

Linear polarized near-infrared light has also been used to treat alopecia areata [1686].

Literature:

Waiz [1706] studied the effect of 904 nm in the treatment of alopecia areata. Sixteen patients with 34 resistant patches that had not responded to different treatment modalities for alopecia areata were enrolled in the study. In patients with multiple patches, one patch was left as a control for comparison. Patients were treated on a four-session basis, once a week, with a 904 nm laser. A photograph was taken of each patient before and after treatment. The treated patients were 11 males and 5 females. Their ages ranged from 4 to 50 years and the duration of their condition had lasted from 12 months to 6 years. Regrowth of hair was observed in 32 patches while only 2 patches failed to show any response. No regrowth of hair was observed in the control patches. The regrowth of hair appeared as terminal hair in its original color in 29 patches while 3 patches appeared as a white villous hair. In patients who showed response, the response was detected as early as one week after the first session in 24 patients, while another 8 patients started to show response from the second session.

Avram [2063] investigated the efficacy of LPT in enhancing hair growth. Seven patients were exposed to LPT twice weekly for 20 minutes each time over a period of 3-6 months. Five patients were treated for a total of 3 months and two were treated for 6 months. Videomicroscopic images were taken at baseline, 3 months, and 6 months, and analyzed for changes in vellus hair counts, terminal hair counts, and shaft diameter. Both videomicroscopic and global images underwent blinded review for evidence of sub-

Literature:

Wong [120, 975, 984] treated 20 patients with migraine or symptoms resembling migraine with a GaAlAs laser. The pain disappeared after one to five minutes. The effect was reported to be contingent on dosage and choice of treatment point.

Two laser acupuncture papers [1569, 1827] report positive results.

Further literature: [1520]

4.1.24 Haemorrhoids

In the treatment of first and second-degree haemorrhoids, the HeNe laser is an effective, simple and harmless clinical procedure, representing an alternative to medication or surgery, according to Trelles [706]. Therapy is carried out at intervals of five days for a total of six treatment sessions. LPT was effective in pain alleviation from the first session, and the final result was excellent.

The aim of the report by Khorsand [2045] is to compare the effect of LPT and botox injections in the treatment of anal fissure. Altogether 26 patients with resistance to conventional treatment were allocated into two groups (n=13). The case group was injected with 40 units of botox to the anal sphincter. The control group received LPT with 650 nm, 30mW, 1 J/cm^2 plus 980 nm, 200 mW, 2.4 J/cm^2, for 5-10 sessions. The researcher visited the patients after two weeks. As for symptoms (pain, bleeding, itching, and spasms of the sphincter) there were no statistically significant differences between the two groups before and after the treatment. The statistical analysis showed a significant difference in the reduction of symptoms before and after treatment in both groups. People responding to conventional treatment are candidates for surgery. Injection of botox is a chemical sphinctrotomy. The present study showed that LPT can heal fissures as successfully as botox injections. Botulinum toxin metabolizes after three to six months and a repetition of treatment may be needed. LPT has an effect on wound healing, pain reduction as well as reducing sphincter tonicity, and the results may be more long-lasting than for botox.

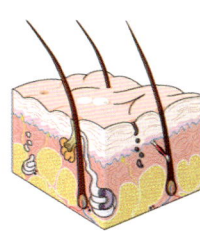

4.1.25 Hair loss

In one of Endre Mester's first experiments on rats [733], it was found that, on the shaved parts of the body, the coat grew back faster in areas that had been treated with a ruby laser. This led to a certain amount of interest in the possibilities of stimulating hair growth in humans. It is generally thought that the stimulation of hair growth with LPT is fictional, but this is only partly correct. One indication that seems to have acceptable results is LPT for alopecia areata. This is a rapid and complete loss of hair in one or several patches, usually on the scalp, affecting both males and females equally. It is

the intensity of pain was the same at the 1st and 10th minute after the application of plain light. In the laser group, the intensity of pain was smaller at the 1st and 10th minute after the application of LPT, this being statistically significant.

LPT has been used in parturient patients for postpartum mastitis and nipple soreness. However, previous studies have revealed hormonal and physiological effects of LPT on the lactation status. Therefore, Mokmeli [2069] selected 20 healthy women scheduled for cesarean section. They were randomly divided into two groups: a LPT group and a control group. LPT was delivered as follows: (1) irradiation with 980 nm (100 mW, 3.3 J/cm^2, total energy 60 J), and 650 nm (30 mW, 1.5 J/cm^2, total energy 27 J) to the incision line, and (2) intravenous laser irradiation at 2.5 mW and 650 nm for 15 min on three consecutive postoperative days. Except for LPT, all the therapeutic conditions in both groups were identical. Blood prolactin levels were measured in the groups on the third postoperative day, and tissue samples were taken from the wound margins for histological evaluation on the 10th postoperative day. Although there was a difference between blood prolactin levels in the two groups, the difference was not statistically significant. However, there was a statistically significant difference in the mean lymphocyte counts and number of vessel lumina, with higher numbers seen in the LPT group. LPT after cesarean section thus has no serious deleterious effects on lactation, and it helps to modulate metabolic processes and promotes wound healing post-surgery.

Further literature: [142, 633, 920, 1123, 1274]

4.1.23 Headache/Migraine

This very common complaint may have a variety of different causes. Myogenically conditioned headache responds well to GaAs and GaAlAs laser treatment administered to tender points and muscle attachments, 6-8 J per point. The practitioner should also take into account peripheral tender points in the neck and shoulders. The common correlation between myogenic headache and bruxism/clenching should be observed.

"Migraine" comes from the Greek "hemi crania", literally "half head". Even though not all migraines are single-sided, this is still a fairly good diagnosis. The cause of migraine is thought to relate to fast-acting dilation of cranial blood vessels. The treatment of migraine is based on irradiation of the occipital nerve paths. Furthermore, irradiation of the carotid arteries will stimulate the vascular system of the brainstem. This should be followed by local pain point irradiation. While migraine is a typical female condition, the Horton type of headache is a typical male vascular condition, which is also worth trying to treat with LPT.

A clear differential diagnosis is essential when treating "headaches".

Antipa [780] studied the effects of GaAs and HeNe laser irradiation, single or in combination, compared to placebo or conventional therapy on the recovery of 118 female patients with a diagnosis of chronic pelvic inflammatory disorders. LPT proved to be significantly more efficient than placebo or conventional therapy. The most efficient of all kinds of irradiation was the combination of GaAs and HeNe (laserpuncture and scanning).

Fibrotic masses in the breast secondary to fat necrosis or haematoma is a complication of breast reduction mammaplasty. The treatment commonly recommended for this condition is early surgical debridement of necrotic tissue from the entire area, which causes scarring. A case report by Nussbaum [909] describes the use of LPT for fibrotic lumps following reduction mammaplasty. The patient was a 46-year-old woman who had breast reduction surgery 80 days prior to referral for physical therapy. At the time of referral, the largest mass was 8.0 cm in diameter. The patient reported pain and said she was distressed about the breast disfigurement. Laser irradiation was initiated at an energy density of 20 J/cm^2 and with a pulse repetition rate of 5000 pulses per second. The laser settings were adjusted during the eight-month treatment period. The final dose was 50 J/cm^2. The mass was 33% of its original size after three sessions over the initial 11-day period. Pain relief was immediate. The rate of resolution decreased after the initial period. The patient had some tissue thickening at the time of discharge after six months of treatment.

Passeniouk [963] reports that LPT used in combination with chlorhexidine was more effective for vaginitis than daily 10 g metronidazole plus one initial dose of 150 mg fluconozole. LPT as well as conventional drug therapy were carried out for 10 consecutive days. The laser group consisted of 30 patients and the drug group of 20 patients.

LPT of mastitis has been successfully used on dairy cattle and Herzog [1002] reports good effects on 66 mothers, using 830 nm, 30 mW, 0.5-2 J per point. Kovalev [1003] reports positive results for this indication, using HeNe on 329 mothers. HeNe was more effective than 890 nm GaAs. Havlik [1039] also reports positive results when using GaAlAs for mastitis. On the other hand, Stoffel [1004] reports that HeNe 25 mW had no effect on bovine mastitis. **However, the irradiation area of 7.5 cm in diameter produces a very low energy density.**

Dotsenko [1005] and Skobelkin [1272] have used defocused carbon dioxide laser successfully for human lactation mastitis.

The objective of a study by Posso [1298] was to investigate the analgesic action of LPT on nipple pain during breastfeeding. Forty women in the immediate puerperium were studied. The patients were divided into two groups: Control group - application of plain light on the nipple for 40 seconds; Laser group - application of InGaAlP with the wavelength of 685 nm, a power of 100 mW and a fluence of 4 J/cm^2 on the nipple for 40 seconds. The intensity of pain was measured before and on the 1st and 10th minute after LPT application, using a Visual Analogical Scale. In the control group,

was assessed according to the Fibromyalgia Impact Questionnaire (FIQ). In the laser group, patients were treated at each tender point daily for two weeks, except weekends, each point being approximately 2 cm^2. The same unit was used for the placebo treatment group, for which no laser beam was emitted. Patients in the amitriptyline group took 10 mg daily at bedtime throughout the eight weeks. A significant difference was observed in clinical parameters for pain intensity, morning stiffness and fatigue in favour of the laser group. A significant difference was observed in morning stiffness, FIQ and depression in the amitriptyline group compared to the placebo group after therapy. Additionally, a significant difference was also observed in depression scores in the amitriptyline group in comparison to the laser group after therapy. This study suggests that both amitriptyline and laser therapies are effective on clinical symptoms and QOL in fibromyalgia, and that GaAs LPT is a safe and effective treatment of fibromyalgia cases. Furthermore, the study suggests that the GaAs LPT can be used as a monotherapy or as a supplementary treatment to other therapeutic procedures.

Further literature: [333]

4.1.22 Gynaecologic indications

In a still unpublished Swedish study on menstrual pain, 85% of the women reported pain relief from LPT. At the six-month control, the pain was back to baseline, indicating that the effect is transient. The authors also have excellent experience of treating Post Menstrual Stress. Here is an untapped therapeutic arsenal waiting for further exploration.

Literature:

Takac [143] treated women suffering from menstrual pain with a GaAs laser. He administered 20 J over each ovary and over the uterus respectively, distributing the radiation over an area of about 3 x 15 cm^2. He treated the women every day from the 12th day of the cycle up to menstruation. Of 12 patients, 10 were entirely or partially free of pain and experienced greater regularity in their menstrual cycles. A closer examination of the two who did not react showed microcysts on the ovaries.

For menstrual cramps, Ohshiro [978] recommends contact irradiation over the abdominal wall. It is also reported that delivery pain has been relieved through GaAlAs irradiation over the mouth of the cervix.

Another study by Ohshiro [1102] suggests the possibility of treating female infertility with LPT.

Kovács [341] has successfully used a HeNe laser clinically to treat ectopium of the portio uteri. Havlik [1039] also reports this.

Kosilov [651] treated 120 young female patients with neurogenic hyperreflexic bladder dysfunctions. HeNe irradiation on the projection of the bladder combined with irradiation of biologically active points were more effective than conventional treatment.

Clinical examination revealed swollen, bleeding and crusted lips and diffuse intraoral ulcerative lesions. At the beginning of the treatment, the patient showed a great improvement in all oral symptoms. At the end of the first laser irradiation, the patient was able to eat gelatin, through a syringe, with his father's assistance. On the second day, the crusts were dryer and lesions on the tongue had decreased. The condition was completely healed within 10 sessions.

4.1.21 Fibrositis/fibromyalgia

The origin of fibrositis is not known, and there is at present no effective treatment to offer this large group of mainly female patients. LPT is unlikely to cure a fibrositis patient. However, LPT does have a good pain relieving effect and will improve the quality of life of these patients. If the painful areas are treated, there is a rapid alleviation of pain. Repeated treatment further reduces pain, and sessions can soon be held at longer intervals. A suitable initial dose to test the patient's general reaction is 6-8 J per painful point. Superpulsed GaAs- and high powered GaAlAs lasers have proved to be quite useful in treating these patients, since they provide the higher kind of power densities important in pain therapy.

Literature:

Longo [636] treated 846 patients with fibromyositic rheumatism during a 15-year period. Diodes and carbon dioxide lasers were used. About two-thirds of the patients benefited from the treatment with regard to local pain, hypomobility, and phlogosis.

Thorsen [703] could not find any effect of GaAlAs laser on localised fibromyalgia in the neck and shoulder regions. The laser had a power of 30 mW and each treated point received 0.9 J and a maximum of 9 J per treatment. **This is, however, a low dose and power density for this indication.**

A randomised, single-blind, placebo controlled study was conducted by Gür [1226] to evaluate the efficacy of GaAs LPT in 40 female patients with fibromyalgia. The treatment was carried out daily for two weeks, weekends excepted. At the end of the therapy, there was a significant difference between the two groups for parameters such as pain, muscle spasm, morning stiffness and tender points.

The purpose of another study by Gür [1281] was to examine the effectiveness of LPT and low-dose amitriptyline therapy, and to investigate effects of these therapy modalities on clinical symptoms and quality of life (QOL) in patients with fibromyalgia. Seventy-five patients with fibromyalgia were randomly allocated to active (GaAs) laser (25 patients), placebo laser (25 patients) and amitriptyline therapy (25 patients). All groups were evaluated to establish the reduction of pain, number of tender points, skin fold tenderness, morning stiffness, sleep disturbance, muscular spasm, and fatigue. Depression was evaluated by a psychiatrist according to the Hamilton Depression Rate Scale and DSM IV criteria. Quality of life of the patients

low-up period, (2) a significant decrease in pain at palpation and pain on isometric testing after eight weeks of treatment and at the eighth week follow-up, (3) a significant decrease in pain during a middle finger test at the end of eight weeks of treatment and at the end of the follow-up period, (4) a significant decrease in pain during grip strength testing after eight weeks of treatment and at the eighth week follow-up, (5) a significant increase in the wrist range of motion at the eighth week follow-up, (6) an increase in grip strength after eight weeks of treatment and at the eighth week follow-up, and (7) a significant increase in the weight-test after eight weeks of treatment and at the eighth week follow-up. The results suggested that the combination of laser with plyometric exercises was a more effective treatment than placebo laser combined with the same plyometric exercises at the end of the treatment, as well as at the follow-up.

Further literature: [821, 1055, 1167]

4.1.20 Erythema multiforme major

Erythema multiforme minor is a self limiting condition, believed to be triggered by HSV viruses. It generally resolves within a week. Erythema myltiforme major, also called Stevens Johnson syndrome (SJS) is a progressive, fulminating, severe variety of the erythema multiforme major, with extensive mucocutaneous epithelial necrosis. It is a potentially life-threatening mucocutaneous drug reaction with systemic symptoms and signs with significant morbidity and mortality. Oral stomatitis has been associated with SJS and as caused by extensive keratinocyte apoptosis.

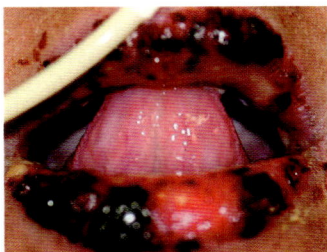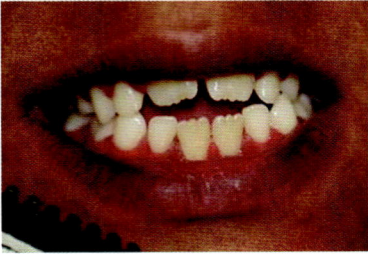

Figure 4.8 Young boy suffering from erythema multiforme major, unable to eat and in pain. Able to eat after few LPT sessions and completely healed at 10th session.
Courtesy: Alyne Simões.

Literature:

Simões [2091] reports on the resolution of SJS in a young man. After five days of hospitalisation, the LPT was initiated. As the patient was not able to drink or eat any solid food, a tube was used for his nutrition. He was also unable to speak, swallow or open the mouth and reported severe pain.

used a lateral counterforce brace for three weeks, US plus hot pack in the ultrasound group, and laser plus hot pack in the LPT group. In addition, all patients were given progressive stretching and strengthening exercise programs. Grip strength and pain severity were evaluated by visual analog scale (VAS) at baseline, at the second week of treatment, and at the sixth week of treatment. VAS improved significantly in all groups after the treatment and in the ultrasound and laser groups at the sixth week. Grip strength of the affected hand increased only in the laser group after treatment, but was not changed at the sixth week. There were no significant differences between the groups on VAS and grip strength at baseline and at follow-up assessments. The results show that, in patients with lateral epicondylitis, a brace has a shorter beneficial effect than US and LPT in reducing pain, and that LPT is more effective than the brace and US treatment in improving grip strength.

The aim of a study by Lam [1862] was to evaluate the effectiveness of 904 nm LPT in the management of lateral epicondylitis. Thirty-nine patients with lateral epicondylitis were randomly assigned to receive either active laser with an energy dose of 0.275 J per tender point (laser group) or sham irradiation (placebo group) for a total of nine sessions. The outcome measures were mechanical pain threshold, maximum grip strength, level of pain at maximum grip strength as measured by the Visual Analogue Scale and the subjective rating of physical function with Disabilities of the Arm, Shoulder and Hand (DASH) questionnaire. Significantly greater improvements were shown in all outcome measures in the laser group compared to the placebo group, except in the two subsections of DASH. This study revealed that LPT in addition to exercise is effective in relieving pain, and in improving the grip strength as well as the subjective rating of physical function of patients with lateral epicondylitis.

A study by Stergioulas [1874] was undertaken to compare the effectiveness of a protocol of laser combined with plyometric exercises, and a protocol of placebo laser in combination with the same exercise program, in the treatment of tennis elbow. Fifty patients who had tennis elbow participated in the study and were randomised into two groups. Group A (n=25) was treated with a 904 nm GaAs laser, pulse repetition rate of 50 Hz, average power 40 mW and energy density 2.4 J/cm^2, plus plyometric exercises, and group B (n=25), which received placebo laser plus the same plyometric exercises. During eight weeks of treatment, the patients of the two groups received 12 sessions of laser or placebo, two sessions per week (weeks one to four), and one session per week (weeks five to eight). Pain at rest, at palpation on the lateral epicondyle, during resisted wrist extension, middle finger test, and strength testing were evaluated using Visual Analogue Scales. The grip strength, the range of motion and a weight test were also evaluated. Parameters were determined before the treatment, at the end of the eight-week-course of treatment (week 8), and eight weeks after the end of treatment. In relation to group B, group A had (1) a significant decrease in pain at rest at the end of the eight-week-long treatment, and at the end of the fol-

patients who had much or slight improvement was 87%. There was no significant difference between the three wavelengths used.

Konstantinovic [554] compared the effect of corticosteroid infiltration, LPT (GaAs 1 J/cm²) and laser plus corticosteroid infiltration in combination. On day 7, the combined therapy demonstrated a significantly higher analgesic effect.

Nd:YAG (1064 nm) laser was used in a study by Basford [656]. Seven sites on the most symptomatic extremity were irradiated, three times a week for four weeks. There was no significant improvement. Total delivered energy was 220 Joules, but due to a large spot size (4.9 cm²) the dose expressed in J/cm² was only 0.542.

In a review of the literature on shoulder tendinitis/bursitis and lateral epicondylalgia, Bjordal [732] summarises: "The methodological quality of the four LPT trials for lateral epicondylalgia is slightly higher than the five best trials with steroid injections for lateral epicondylalgia. Total sample size of high quality LPT trials is about two-thirds of the total sample of high quality steroid injections trials on the same diagnosis. The four LPT trials should serve as a valid platform for making conclusions on clinical effects of LPT for lateral epicondylalgia. Inadequate treatment procedures or poor methodological quality were found in the three trials that reported no significant effects of LPT. Evidence of clinical effects from LPT was found at all four lateral epicondylalgia trials using acceptable methods. The results in these trials were significantly in favour of active LPT with confidence intervals not including zero. The trial with fewest treatments per week had the lowest success rate. Best clinical effects were seen in patients with short duration of symptoms (less than a month)."

Bjordal has also summarised data from the literature regarding the treatment of tendinitis:
- A synthesis of doses from 4 laboratory trials on inflamed collagen-producing cell cultures gives the following dose for optimal reduction of tendon tissue inflammation: Dose: 3-8 J/cm², Intensity: 5-21 mW/cm².
- A synthesis of 10 laboratory trials investigating collagen proliferation gives the following optimal dose for stimulation of tendon regeneration: Dose: 0.2-4 J/cm². Intensity: 2-10 mW/cm².
- For the treatment of tendinitis, an optimal suggested dosage at target location will be: Dose: 0.2-4 J/cm². Intensity: 2-10 mW/cm².
- Treatment should be applied daily for at least five days to reduce inflammation, and for at least 10 days to increase collagen production.

The aims of the study by Oken [1825] were to evaluate the effects of LPT and to compare these with the effects of brace or ultrasound (US) treatment in tennis elbow. The study design used was a prospective and randomized, controlled, single-blind trial. Fifty-eight outpatients with lateral epicondylitis were included in the trial. The patients were divided into three groups: 1) brace group-brace plus exercise, 2) ultrasound group-US plus exercise, and 3) laser group-LPT plus exercise. Patients in the brace group

ous reviews which failed to assess treatment procedures, wavelengths and optimal doses."

Trigger points can be given 4-6 J per point, but the intensity over the actual epicondyle, being superficial, should be much lower.

Literature:

Some early studies were negative [230, 231], but in these cases acupuncture points and/or local points and very low doses were used. The same authors [208] later achieved promising results using local points at 3.6 J per point, but in non-contact mode. Positive findings were also reported in the early literature by Gudmundsen [242].

More recent studies using higher doses in combination with trigger points have yielded more favourable results. In a two-centre study, Simunovic [607] treated 324 patients, 50 with epicondylitis ulnaris and 274 with epicondylitis radialis. All in all 32% of the patients were acute and 68% chronic cases. All patients had previously been treated with various methods such as TENS, ultrasound, drugs and surgery. The patients were divided into three treatment groups. One received 830 nm laser light on trigger points only, the second was treated only with a scanner, and the third group received a combined treatment. The third group was the most successful. In the three groups together, complete relief of pain and restored functional ability were achieved in 82% of the acute patients and in 66% of the chronic cases. One centre had more powerful lasers available. Though the same doses were used at both centres, this latter group was slightly more successful. Another 41 patients with bilateral problems were selected for a crossover study. Minimal dose in unilateral cases was 20 J, which could be increased step-by-step up to 60 J.

Simunovic [1134] has also compared laser and visible incoherent polarised light in the treatment of epicondylitis, given over 12 sessions. Altogether 40% of the patients in the laser group obtained 100% pain relief. In the non-coherent group, there was a maximal pain relief of 70%.

The negative outcome in the study by Krasheninnkoff [1188] might be explained by the rather high dosage applied for this superficial condition (13.2 J/cm^2). The high drop-out rate of 25% also compromises this study. Too high a dose is also a possible reason for the negative outcome of the study by Papadopuolos [1189] – 30 J/cm^2.

Terashima [126] treated 23 patients with lateral humeral epicondylitis and 40 patients with de Quervain's disease with GaAlAs laser. In the epicondylitis group, movement pains and soreness were positively affected in 61% of the cases, and in 70% of the cases in the de Quervain group. Movement pains were eradicated in 13% of all cases.

Cieslar [627] treated 182 patients with epicondylitis humeri in a double-blind study. After 5-7 sessions, distinct pain relief was obtained, and after 10-15 sessions movement pains and palpation had disappeared. Three different wavelengths were used (904, 850, and 633). The percentage of

4.1.19 Epicondylitis

Epicondylitis is known to be a difficult-to-treat condition. LPT has in the past often been used as a "last resort", and has thus been tried on the most difficult cases. But LPT should be one of the first treatment modalities to be used, preferrably in combination with traditional therapies. All wavelengths can be used, since the condition is superficial in the epicondylar area, but in our experience GaAs seems to work best. Trigger points in the shoulder and arm, if any, should also be laser treated, and there are more such trigger points on the lateral side than on the medial side. The possibility of an entrapment between C5-6 should also be considered.

As always, the success rate depends on suitable doses and methods of application. In the literature, as will be seen below, the outcome of LPT for epicondylitis appears to be hard to predict. But, as always, it is a matter of using reasonable parameters. We therefore quote the entire abstract of the review by Bjordal [1925], which is a typical illustration of the difficulties in finding the correct parameters and of evaluating the literature without being aware of these: "Recent reviews have indicated that low level level laser therapy (LLLT) is ineffective in lateral elbow tendinopathy (LET) without assessing validity of treatment procedures and doses or the influence of prior steroid injections. Systematic review with meta-analysis, with primary outcome measures of pain relief and/or global improvement and subgroup analyses of methodological quality, wavelengths and treatment procedures. 18 randomised placebo-controlled trials (RCTs) were identified with 13 RCTs (730 patients) meeting the criteria for meta-analysis. 12 RCTs satisfied half or more of the methodological criteria. Publication bias was detected by Egger's graphical test, which showed a negative direction of bias. Ten of the trials included patients with poor prognosis caused by failed steroid injections or other treatment failures, or long symptom duration or severe baseline pain. The weighted mean difference (WMD) for pain relief was 10.2 mm [95% CI: 3.0 to 17.5] and the RR for global improvement was 1.36 [1.16 to 1.60]. Trials which targeted acupuncture points reported negative results, as did trials with wavelengths 820, 830 and 1064 nm. In a subgroup of five trials with 904 nm lasers and one trial with 632 nm wavelength where the lateral elbow tendon insertions were directly irradiated, WMD for pain relief was 17.2 mm [95% CI: 8.5 to 25.9] and 14.0 mm [95% CI: 7.4 to 20.6] respectively, while RR for global pain improvement was only reported for 904 nm at 1.53 [95% CI: 1.28 to 1.83]. Doses in this subgroup ranged between 0.5 and 7.2 Joules. Secondary outcome measures of painfree grip strength, pain pressure threshold, sick leave and follow-up data from 3 to 8 weeks after the end of treatment, showed consistently significant results in favour of the same LPT subgroup. No serious side-effects were reported. LPT administered with optimal doses of 904 nm and possibly 632 nm wavelengths directly to the lateral elbow tendon insertions, seem to offer short-term pain relief and less disability in LET, both alone and in conjunction with an exercise regimen. This finding contradicts the conclusions of previ-

sity? The scientific value of this study is therefore small but the impact on Canadian health policies probably greater. The Medline information about laser parameters is non-existent, and all that remains for Medline readers is a seemingly negative study.

Kazemi-Khoo [1726] treated seven type 2 diabetic patients with grades II and III diabetic foot ulcers with LPT. The mean duration of diabetes was 10.5 years and the ulcers were present from an average of 6.5 months before treatment. The mean value for glycosylated hemoglobin was 8.14 mg/dl (range: 6-12.2), and foot blood flow in the Doppler ultra-sonography was normal. The author used LPT through local irradiation of the ulcer bed with 660 nm; power: 25 mW; 0.6-1 J/cm^2 and ulcer margins with 980 nm; power: 200 mW; 4-6 J/cm^2, along with intravenous laser irradiation with 650 nm; power: 1.5 mW for 15-20 min, in addition to laser acupuncture with infrared laser (1 J/cm^2) for LI-11, LI-6, SP-6, PC-6, ST-36 and GB-34 points. Sessions were every other day for 10-15 sessions, and then continued twice weekly until complete recovery was achieved. After approximately 19 sessions complete recovery was achieved in all cases, and there were no relapses or other problems with ulcers after approximately 6 months (range: 2-10 months) of follow-ups. With this treatment regimen, there were no side-effects reported by the patients.

In a study by Kazemi-Kho [2048], 10 diabetic type 2 patients received 7-12 sessions of intravenous blue light laser, 450 nm, 2.5 mW. Serum blood sugar (BS) was measured before and after treatment. Mean BS level before treatment was 333.8 mg mean value and mean BS level after treatment were 210.5. Serum blood sugar decreased significantly.

Further literature: [477, 526, 1080, 1179, 1185, 1203, 1275, 1277, 1493]

4.1.18 Duodenal/gastric ulcer

HeNe laser treatment of duodenal ulcers using a gastroscope has been reported in at least 25 Russian studies. With the arrival of successful pharmaceutical treatment, these findings may no longer be as attractive as previously, but still demonstrate the healing effect of HeNe on mucosa.

Literature:

Garkavoy [339] treated 622 patients with gastric and duodenal ulcers with a HeNe laser through a gastroscope. The treatment was administered with a power of 12 mW for three to five minutes a session. The healing rate of duodenal ulcers was 91% and of gastric ulcers 93% by the end of the eighth week.

Karu [1795] reports that even non-coherent red light can be used for this superficial condition and the results were the same for coherent and non-coherent light.

reduced the catalase activity of diabetic groups (D5 and D20) to non-diabetic values. In conclusion, laser irradiation decreased catalase activity in diabetic rats' SMG.

The objective of another study by Simões [2122] was to evaluate the effect of LPT on the glycemic state and the histological and ionic parameters of the parotid and submandibular glands in rats with diabetes. One hundred twenty female rats were divided into eight groups. Diabetes was induced by administration of streptozotocin and confirmed later according to results of glycemia testing. Twenty-nine days after the induction, the parotid and submandibular glands of the rats were irradiated with 5, 10, and 20 J/cm2 using a laser diode (660 nm/100 mW) without diabetes: C5, C10, and C20; with diabetes: D5, D10, and D20, respectively). On the following day, the rats were euthanized, and blood glucose determined. Histological and ionic analyses were performed. Rats with diabetes without irradiation (D0) showed lipid droplets accumulation in the parotid gland, but accumulation decreased after 5, 10, and 20 J/cm2 of laserirradiation. A decrease in fasting glycemia level from 358.97+/-56.70 to 278.33+/-87.98 mg/dL for D5 and from 409.50+/-124.41 to 231.80+/-120.18 mg/dL for D20 was also observed. In conclusion, LPT could be explored as an auxiliary therapy for control of complications of diabetes because it can alter the carbohydrate and lipid metabolism of rats with diabetes.

Clinical studies

In a double-blind placebo-controlled study, Schindl [552] applied a single dose of 30 J/cm^2 of HeNe light to 15 patients with diabetic microangiopathy. Following a single transcutaneous irradiation, a statistically significant rise in skin temperature was recorded through infrared thermography. In the sham irradiated group, there was a small but significant drop in temperature.

Grubnik [527] used HeNe laser irradiation in a group of patients with diabetic gangrene. During the amputation of the lower limb, intravenous HeNe was given. Percutaneous irradiation was applied after the operation. LPT improved healing as compared to a group of similar size where no laser was applied.

In a study by Landau [658], 50 patients with chronic diabetes foot ulcers were treated with topical hyperbaric oxygen alone (15 patients), or in combination with LPT. Altogether 43 of the patients were cured of ulcers.

Zinman [1430] conducted a randomized, double-masked, sham therapy-controlled clinical trial in 50 patients with painful diabetic sensorimotor polyneuropathy. There was a positive trend, but the measured effect was not statistically significant. **Unfortunately, this study cannot be evaluated since the documentation of the actual LPT is poor. The only information given about these essential facts is "The LILT device had a wavelength of 905 nm and an average power of 0-60 mW. All LILT treatments were for 5 min per site." Which output was used? Pulse repetition rate? Dose? Power den-**

tes was slower than on control rats without diabetes. LPT at appropriate treatment parameters can enhance the wound healing on diabetic rats. The optimum wavelength in this study was 633 nm, and the optimum incident dose 10 J/cm^2.

In a study by Mirzaei [1877], diabetes was induced in rats by streptozotocin 30 days after its injection. Two sets of skin samples were extracted under sterile conditions. Fibroblasts that were extruded from the samples were proliferated in vitro, and another set of samples were cultured as organ culture. A 24-well culture medium containing Dulbecco's modified minimum essential medium was supplemented by 12% fetal bovine serum. There were five laser-treated and five sham-exposed groups. A HeNe laser was used, and 0.9-4 J/cm^2 energy densities were applied four times to each organ culture and cell culture. The organ cultures were analyzed by light microscopy and transmission electron microscopy examinations. Statistical analysis revealed that 4J/cm^2 irradiation significantly increased the fibroblast numbers compared to the sham-exposed cultures.

In a study by Al-Anzari [2038], Streptozotocin was applied for diabetes induction. An oval full-thickness skin wound was created aseptically with a scalpel in 51 diabetic rats on the shaved back of the animals. The study was performed using 532, 633 nm, 810 nm and 980 nm lasers. Incident doses of 5, 10, 20 and 30 J/cm^2 and a treatment schedule of three sessions per week were used in the experiments. The rats treated were restrained in a Plexiglas cage without anesthesia during the laser irradiation period. The control group also received the same manipulation, excluding the laser exposure. The wound area on all rats was measured and plotted on a slope chart. The slope values (mm2/day) and the percentage of relative wound healing were computed in the study. The percentage of relative wound healing were 30.64 at 532 nm, 50.41 at 633 nm, 20.1 at 810 nm, and 21.19 at 980 nm. There were significant differences in the mean slope value of wound healing on diabetic rats between treatment and control groups.

The aim of a study by Simões [2121] was to evaluate the effect of laser irradiation on the amylase and the antioxidant enzyme activities, as well as on the total protein concentration of submandibular glands (SMG) of diabetic and non-diabetic rats. Ninety-six female rats were divided into eight groups: D0, D5, D10, and D20 (diabetic animals), and C0, C5, C10, and C20 (non-diabetic animals), respectively. Diabetes was induced by administering streptozotocin and confirmed later by the glycemia results. Twenty-nine days after diabetes induction, the SMG of groups D5 and C5, D10 and C10, and D20 and C20 were irradiated with 5, 10, and 20 J/cm^2 , respectively. A diode laser (660 nm/100 mW) was used. On the day after irradiation, the rats were euthanized and the SMG were removed. Catalase, peroxidase, and amylase activities, as well as protein concentration, were assayed. Results: Diabetic rats without irradiation (D0) showed higher catalase activity when compared to C0 (0.16 +/- 0.05 and 0.07 +/- 0.01 U/mg protein, respectively). However, laser irradiation of 5, 10, and 20 J/cm2

content, granulation tissue formation and collagen deposition as compared with the control group.

In a wound healing study on diabetic rats by Reddy [657], the following conclusions were made: 1) the GaAs LPT had no apparent systemic effect on the wound of the side opposite the treated side, and 2) laser photostimulation decreased the healing time for full thickness skin wounds in diabetic animals but had no effect on the biomechanical properties of the tissue once the wound had healed.

Byrnes [1455] used 632 nm laser to establish the effect of laser on cutaneous wounds in diabetic and non-diabetic mice. An initial series of experiments were done to establish optimal treatment parameters for the aforementioned model. Following the creation of bilateral full-thickness skin wounds, non-diabetic Sand Rats were treated with laser of differing dosages. Wound healing was assessed according to wound closure and histological characteristics of healing. Optimal treatment parameters were then used to treat type 2 diabetic Sand Rats, while a diabetic control group received no irradiation. In order to elucidate the mechanism behind an improvement in wound healing, the expression of basic fibroblast growth factor (bFGF) was assessed. Significant improvement in wound healing histology and wound closure were found following treatment with 4 J/cm^2 (16 mW, 250-sec treatments for four consecutive days). The 4 J/cm^2 dosage significantly improved histology and closure of wounds in the diabetic group in comparison to the non-irradiated diabetic group. Quantitative analysis of bFGF expression at 36 h post-injury revealed a threefold increase in the diabetic and non-diabetic Sand Rats after LPT.

In a study by al-Watban [1863], the effects of wound healing acceleration on diabetic rats were determined and compared using different laser wavelengths and incident doses. Male Sprague-Dawley rats were used. Streptozotocin was applied for diabetes induction. An oval full-thickness skin wound was created aseptically with a scalpel in 51 diabetic rats and six non-diabetic rats on the shaved back of the animals. The study was performed using 532, 633, 810, and 980 nm diode lasers. Incident doses of 5, 10, 20, and 30 J/cm^2 and treatment schedule of three times/week were used in the experiments. The wound area on all rats was measured and plotted on a slope chart. The slope values (mm2/day), the percentage of relative wound healing, and the percentage of wound healing acceleration were computed in the study. Mean slope values were 6.0871 in the non-diabetic control group, and 3.636 in the diabetic control rats. The percentages of wound healing acceleration were 15.23, 18.06, 19.54, and 20.39 with 532-nm laser, 33.53, 38.44, 32.05, and 16.45 with 633 nm laser, 15.72, 14.94, 9.62, and 7.76 with 810 nm laser, and 12.80, 16.32, 13.79, and 7.74 with 980 nm laser, using incident doses of 5, 10, 20, and 30 J/cm^2, respectively. There were significant differences in the mean slope value of wound healing on diabetic rats between control groups and treatment groups when using 532, 633, 810, and 980 nm lasers. In conclusion, the wound healing on control rats with diabe-

plete closure and an increased apoptosis. All cells irradiated with 16 J/cm^2 at all three wavelengths showed incomplete wound closure, an increased apoptosis, and a decreased bFGF expression. This study showed that diabetic-wounded cells respond in a dose- and wavelength-dependent manner to laser light. Cells responded best when irradiated with a fluence of 5 J/cm^2 at a wavelength of 632.8 nm.

The next study by Houreld [1927] aimed at determining the effect on cellular proliferation, migration, and cytokine interleukin-6 expression in diabetic and diabetic wounded fibroblast cells (WS1) post-laser irradiation. Diabetic and diabetic wounded WS1 cells were irradiated at 632.8 nm (23 mW) with 5 J/cm^2 or 16 J/cm^2. IL-6 level, cellular proliferation (neutral red assay), and morphology were then determined. Diabetic cells irradiated with 5 J/cm^2 showed no significant changes, while diabetic wounded cells showed an increase in IL-6 level, proliferation, and migration. On the other hand, diabetic and diabetic wounded cells irradiated with 16 cm^2 showed a significant decrease in proliferation and evidence of cellular damage, and wounded cells showed no migration. This study showed that phototherapy at the correct fluence level stimulates IL-6 expression, proliferation, and cellular migration in diabetic wounded cells.

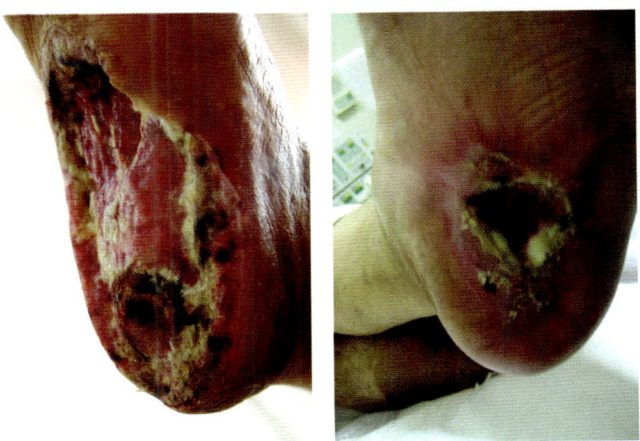

Figure 4.7 Diabetic foot ulcer before and at late stage of combined laser therapy.
Courtesy: Nooshafarin Kazemi-kho.

Animal studies

Yu [528] used an argon pumped dye laser at a wavelength of 630 nm, 20 mW/cm^2, to treat experimental wounds in diabetic mice. Histological evaluations showed that LPT improved wound epithelialisation, cellular

Normal human skin fibroblast cells (WS1) were used to simulate a wounded diabetic model. The effect of LPT (632.8 nm, 5 and 16 J/cm^2 once a day on two non-consecutive days) was determined by analysis of cell morphology, cytotoxicity, apoptosis, and DNA damage. Cells exposed to 5 J/cm^2 showed a higher rate of migration than cells exposed to 16 J/cm^2, and there was complete wound closure by day four. Exposure of WS1 cells to 5 J/cm^2 on two non-consecutive days did not induce additional cytotoxicity or genetic damage, whereas exposure to 16 J/cm^2 did. There was a significant increase in apoptosis in exposed cells as compared to unexposed cells. Based on cellular morphology, exposure to 5 J/cm^2 was stimulatory to cellular migration, whereas exposure to 16 J/cm^2 was inhibitory. Exposure to 16 J/cm^2 induced genetic damage on WS1 cells when exposed to a HeNe laser in vitro, whereas exposure to 5 J/cm^2 did not induce any additional damage.

Another study by Houreld [1871] investigated the effectiveness of helium-neon laser irradiation at increasing intervals on diabetic-induced wounded human skin fibroblast cells (WS1) at a morphological, cellular, and molecular level. The controversies over light therapy can be explained by the differing exposure regimens and models used. No therapeutic window for dosimetry and mechanism of action has been determined at the level of individual cell types, particularly in diabetic cells in vitro. WS1 cells were used to simulate an in vitro wounded diabetic model. The effect of the frequency of HeNe irradiation at a fluence of 5 J/cm^2 was determined by analysis of cell morphology, viability, cytotoxicity, and DNA damage. Cells were irradiated using three different protocols: they were irradiated at 30 min only; irradiated twice at 30 min and at 24 h; or irradiated twice at 30 min and at 72 h post-wound induction. A single exposure to 5 J/cm^2 30 min post-wound induction increased cellular damage. Irradiation of cells at 30 min and at 24 h post-wound induction decreased cellular viability, cytotoxicity, and DNA damage. However, complete wound closure, as well as an increase in viability and a decrease in cytotoxicity and DNA damage, occurred when cells were irradiated at 30 min and at 72 h post-wound induction. Thus, wounded diabetic WS1 cells irradiated with 5 J/cm^2 showed increased cellular repair when irradiated with an adequate amount of time between irradiations, allowing time for cellular response mechanisms to take effect. Therefore, the irradiation interval was shown to play an important role in wound healing in vitro and should be taken into account.

A following study by Houreld [1926] aimed at determining which dose and wavelength would better induce healing in vitro. Diabetic-induced wounded fibroblasts were irradiated with 5 or 16 J/cm^2 at 632.8, 830, or 1064 nm. Cellular morphology, viability (Trypan blue and apoptosis), and proliferation (basic fibroblast growth factor) were then determined. Cells irradiated with 5 J/cm^2 at 632.8 nm showed complete wound closure and an increase in viability and basic fibroblast growth factor (bFGF) expression. Cells irradiated at 830 nm showed incomplete wound closure and an increase in bFGF expression. Cells irradiated at 1064 nm showed incom-

4.1.17 Diabetes

In some previous research literature, diabetes can be found as a contra indication for LPT. On the contrary, LPT can be used to an advantage! The circulatory problems of diabetic patients are a great challenge. Schindl [478, 552] early on demonstrated the effectiveness of HeNe laser treatment on limbs with circulatory disorders. Non-healing wounds in diabetic patients are an excellent indication for LPT, and many amputations can be avoided. Genetically diabetic rats have become a standard for wound healing experiments with lasers, and the results from these animal experiments are more relevant than the studies performed on healthy animals. So far there is no evidence that LPT can be used to treat the intrinsic diabetic factors, however, used for the microcirculatory secondary complications, LPT is an excellent option in combination with conventional methods. A lot of pain and amputations could be eliminated if LPT was to become a standardised method.

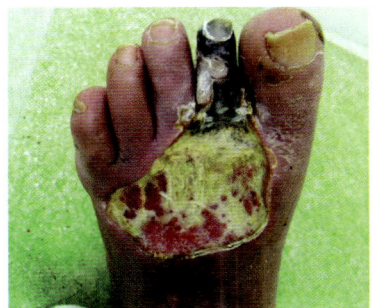
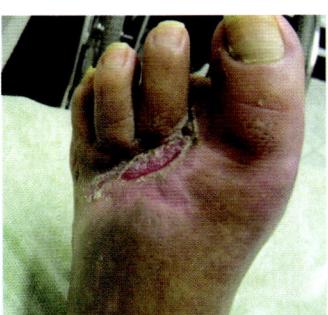

Figure 4.6 Healing of diabetic necroses after amputation.
Courtesy: Nooshafarin Kazemi-kho

Literature:
In vitro studies

Schindl [1136] presents a study aimed at evaluating the possible protective effect of LPT against high glucose-induced delay in proliferation of human endothelial cells. Human umbilical vein endothelial cells were cultured with either standard or elevated concentrations of glucose and were irradiated with a 670 nm diode laser. Irradiation was performed every other day for one week. Cell proliferation was evaluated on days two, four and seven. The results demonstrated a dose-dependent protective effect of laser irradiation on high glucose-induced reduction of cell counts on day seven. These data provide further evidence of the beneficial effects of LPT on patients with diabetic microangiopathy.

The aim of the investigation by Houreld [1864] was to assess morphological, cellular, and molecular effects of exposing wounded diabetic fibroblast cells to He-Ne (632.8 nm) laser irradiation at two different doses.

cross-over study. Young male volleyball players (n = 8) were enrolled and asked to perform three Wingate cycle tests after 4 x 30 sec LPT or LEDT pretreatment of the rectus femoris muscle with either (1) an active LEDT cluster-probe (660/850 nm, 10/30 mW), (2) a placebo cluster-probe with no output, and (3) a single-diode 810-nm 200-mW laser. The active LEDT group had significantly decreased post-exercise creatine kinase (CK) levels compared to the placebo cluster group and the active single-diode laser group. None of the pre-exercise LPT or LEDT protocols enhanced performance on the Wingate tests or reduced post-exercise blood lactate levels. However, a non-significant tendency toward lower post-exercise blood lactate levels in the treated groups should be explored further. Conclusion: In this experimental set-up, only the active LEDT probe decreased post-exercise CK levels after the Wingate cycle test.

Further literature: [1699, 1745]

4.1.16 Depression, psychosomatic problems

Using light to treat seasonal depression is a controversial but yet widely used method. Whether or not coherent light would add any specific advantage is not yet known.

Literature:

From a large population of over 5000 chronic pain patients during a 70 month period, Shiroto [844] chose 1800 seriously affected patients to participate in an elective written questionnaire, in addition to the usual oral pain removal assessment session. The longer-term, more chronically affected patients, because of the nature and history of their complaint, tend to exhibit less of a placebo effect than less-affected chronic, subacute or acute pain patients. The laser used was a GaAlAs diode system, 60 mW output, 830 nm, continuous wave, and was used in the contact pressure technique. The questionnaire contained a set of questions on psychological effects following LPT, in addition to the usual pain removal questions. The questionnaire was sent by post four weeks after the final treatment session. A total of 752 patients responded. On the whole, 67.7% of the respondents reported an improvement in general well-being, 60.2% reported increased physical energy, and 56.4% reported improved sleep. Another 47.5% and 41.5% reported increased emotional stability and improved mental vigour, respectively.

The results indicate that, in addition to its effective removal of pain (76%), LPT has a strong systemic psychosomatic effect, which is possibly not attributable to the placebo effect, in the longer-term chronic pain patient.

The authors believe that the mechanism here may be the same as in BLT (Bright Light Treatment) of seasonal depressions; *See chapter 11.1.6 "Bright Light Phototherapy" on page 541.*

ments for such conditions. Ramos [2043] investigated the effects of LPT (810 nm) in rat-induced skeletal muscle strain. Male wistar rats were anaesthetized with halothane prior to the induction of muscle strain. Previous studies have determined that a force equal to 130% of the body weight corresponds to approximately 80% of the ultimate rupture force of the muscle tendon unit. In all animals, the right leg received a controlled strain injury while the left leg served as control. A small weight corresponding to 150 % of the total body weight was attached to the right leg in an appropriate apparatus and left to induce muscle strain twice for 20 minutes with 3 minute intervals. Walking index, C-reactive protein, creatine kinase, vascular extravasation and histological analysis of the Tibial muscle were performed after 6, 12 and 24 hours of lesion induction. LPT in an energy dependent manner markedly or even completely reduced the Walking Index, leading to a better quality of movement. C-reactive protein production was completely inhibited by laser treatment, even more than observed with Sodium Diclofenac inhibition (positive control). Creative Kinase activity was also significantly reduced by laser irradiations. In conclusion, LPT operating in 810 nm markedly reduced inflammation and muscle damage after experimental muscle strain, leading to a highly significant enhancement of walking activity.

The aim of a study by Sussai [2051] was to investigate the effects of LPT on a decrease in creatine kinase (CK) levels and cell apoptosis. Twenty male Wistar rats were randomly divided into two equal groups: group 1 (control), resistance swimming; group 2 (LPT), resistance swimming with LPT. They were subjected to a single application of InGaAlP laser immediately following the exercise for 40 s at an output power of 100 mW, wavelength 660 nm and 133.3 J/cm^2. The groups were subdivided according to sample collection time: 24 h and 48 h. CK was measured before and both 24 h and 48 h after the test. Samples of the gastrocnemius muscle were processed to determine the presence of apoptosis using terminal deoxynucleotidyl transferase (TdT)-mediated deoxyuridine triphosphate (dUTP) nick end labeling. There was a significant difference in CK levels between groups as well as between the 24 h and 48 h levels in the control group, whereas there was no significant intra-group difference in the LPT group at the same evaluation times. In the LPT group there were 66.3 +/- 13.2 apoptotic cells after 24 h and 39.0 +/- 6.8 apoptotic cells after 48 h. The results suggest that LPT influences the metabolic profile of animals subjected to fatigue by lowering serum levels of CK. This demonstrates that LPT can act as a preventive tool against cell apoptosis experienced during high-intensity physical exercise.

There is anecdotal evidence that LPT may affect the development of muscular fatigue, minor muscle damage, and recovery after heavy exercises. Although manufacturers claim that cluster probes (LEDT) maybe more effective than single-diode lasers in clinical settings, there is a lack of head-to-head comparisons in controlled trials. The study by Junior [2052] was designed to compare the effect of single-diode LPT and cluster LEDT before heavy exercise. This was a randomized, placebo-controlled, double-blind

However, some effects on DOMS from LED therapy were found in a study by Douris [1888] as measured using the Visual Analog Scale (VAS), McGill Pain Questionnaire, Resting Angle (RANG), and girth measurements. This was a randomized double-blind controlled study with 27 subjects (18-35 years of age) assigned to one of three groups. The experimental group received 8 J/cm^2 of phototherapy each day for five consecutive days using super luminous diodes with wavelengths of 880 and visible diodes of 660 nm at three standardized sites over the musculotendinous junction of the bicep. The sham group received identical treatment from a dummy cluster. The controls did not receive treatment. The study was completed over five consecutive days: on day one baseline measurements of RANG and upper arm girths were recorded prior to DOMS induction. On days two to five, RANG, girth, and pain were assessed using VAS and the McGill Pain Questionnaire. The experimental group exhibited a significant decrease in pain associated with DOMS compared to the control and sham groups based upon the VAS at the 48-h period. The McGill Pain Questionnaire showed a significant difference in pain scores at the 48-h period between the experimental and the sham groups. There were no significant differences from day to day and between the groups with respect to girth and RANG.

Lopes-Martins [1676] investigated if 655 nm laser irradiation can reduce muscular fatigue during tetanic contractions in rats. Thirty-two male rats were divided in four groups receiving laser doses of 0 (control group), 0.5, 1.0 and 2.5 J/cm^2. Irradiation lasted 32, 80 and 160 seconds respectively with a fixed power density of 31.25 mW/cm^2. The total energy doses were 0.08, 0.2 and 0.4 Joules respectively. Electrical stimulation induced 6 tetanic muscle contractions in the tibial anterior muscle. Contractions were stopped when the muscle force fell to 50% of the initial value for each contraction (T50%). There was no significant difference between the 2.5 J/cm^2 laser-irradiated group and the control group in mean T50%-values. Laser-irradiated groups 0.5 J/cm^2 and 1.0 J/cm^2 had significantly longer T50% values than the control group. The relative peak force for the sixth contraction in the laser irradiated groups were significantly higher at 92.2 % for 0.5 J/cm^2, 83.2 % for 1.0 J/cm^2 and 82.9 % for 2.5 J/cm^2 respectively, than for the control group, which had its peak force at 50%. Laser groups receiving 0.5 J/cm^2 and 1.0 J/cm^2 showed significant increases in mean performed work compared both to the control group and their first contraction values. Groups receiving laser irradiation with doses of 1 and 2.5 J/cm^2 also showed significantly lower levels of Creatine Kinase in plasma than the non-irradiated control group.

Muscle strains and other musculoskeletal disorders (MSDs) are a leading cause of work absenteeism and are among the most common and often disabling injuries in athletes. Muscle pain, spasms, swelling, and inflammation are symptomatic of strains. NSAIDs are probably the mainstay of drug treatments for acute musculoskeletal conditions; however, their well known side effects and low efficacy highlights the necessity of new treat-

and LED:s [1674, 1675] failed to obtain any results, while the most recent one [1888] did find an effect from LED:s only. A laser-only animal study seems to confirm that the effect is dose dependent [1676].

Literature:

A double-blind, placebo-controlled study by Craig [1674] using male subjects (n=60) was conducted to investigate the efficacy of three different frequencies of combined LED/ LPT (CLILT) in alleviating the signs and symptoms of delayed-onset muscle soreness (DOMS). After screening for relevant pathologies, recent analgesic or steroid drug usage, current pain, diabetes, or current involvement in regular weight-training activities, subjects were randomly allocated to one of five experimental groups: Control, Placebo, or 2.5 Hz, 5 Hz, or 20 Hz CLILT groups (660-950 nm; 31.7 J/cm^2; pulsed at the given frequencies for a duration of 12 min; n=12 all groups). Once baseline measurements were obtained, DOMS was induced in the non-dominant arm, which was exercised in a standardised fashion until exhaustion, using repeated eccentric contractions of the elbow flexors. The procedure was repeated twice more to ensure that exhaustion was achieved, after which the subjects were treated according to group allocation. In the CLILT/placebo groups, the treatment head was applied directly to the affected arm at the level of the musculotendinous junction. Subjects returned on two consecutive days for further treatment and assessment. The range of variables used to assess DOMS included range of movement, mechanical pain threshold/tenderness and pain. Measurements were taken before and after treatment on each day, except for the McGill Pain questionnaire, which was completed at the end of the study. Analysis of results using repeated measures and one-factor analysis of variance with relevant post-hoc tests showed significant changes in ranges of movement, accompanied by increases in subjective pain and tenderness for all groups over time; however, such analysis failed to show any significant differences between the groups on any specific day.

In a later study with different light parameters, Craig [1675] used 36 subjects (18 M: 18 F) who were randomly allocated, under double-blind conditions, to one of three experimental conditions: Control, Placebo, and CLILT (660-950 nm; 11 J/cm^2; pulsed at 73 Hz). DOMS was induced in a standardised fashion in the non-dominant elbow flexors using repeated eccentric contractions until exhaustion was reached. Subjects returned on five consecutive days, and two days during the following week, for treatment according to group placement and assessments of outcome variables, including range of motion, pain, and tenderness. While analysis of results using repeated measures and one factor ANOVA with post-hoc tests showed significant changes in all variables over time as a result of the induction procedure, there were no significant differences observed between groups.

Vinck [1698] treated DOMS with a 950 nm LED, 160 mW, 3.2 J/cm^2 and did not find any statistically significant effects.

The same authors [613] also examined the effect of a GaAs laser on venous ulcers. The parameters stated in the report are: "The wavelength was 904 nm, average output 4 mW, peak power 10 W, pulse repetition rate 3800 Hz and duration 180 ns, and divergence 70 mrad. Energy density was 1.96 J/cm^2."

- First of all, the stated energy density must obviously be wrong as the treatment time was said to be 10 minutes per patient regardless of wound size. Wound size in the laser group was in the range 4-52 cm^2 (average 12 cm^2).
- Secondly, from the stated parameters, it is easy to calculate the average output power of the laser to be 6.84 mW, which in 10 minutes would give a total energy level of 4.1 J. For the smallest wound, this would mean 1 J/cm^2, and for the largest, 0.079 J/cm^2. The stated figure of 1.96 J/cm^2 cannot be correct. And, since each ulcer received a different dosage (ranging, for GaAs, from rather high to very low), doubt is cast on the whole report. Further, according to the manufacturer of the laser, a pulse repetition rate of 3800 Hz is not available in any of their equipment.

The two studies above have been used in a Cochrane literature review. In all, four randomised studies were found, two positive and two negative. With the shortcomings of the two studies above in mind, such an evaluation has little substance. (See chapter 13.2 "The Cochrane LPT analyses – can they be improved?" on page 604.)

A single blind randomised study on stage III pressure ulcers has been presented by Lucas [943] using a 904 nm multi array with 12 diodes of 8 mW each. An energy density of 1 J/cm^2 was obtained. The same array was used for all ulcers, regardless of size. There was no statistical difference between the laser group and the control group.

In a study by Telfer [776], LPT was used to treat chronic leg ulcers. Seven patients with 11 leg ulcers were referred to LPT by plastic surgeons. They had a history of ulceration ranging from 3 - 50 years, and five of the patients had breakdowns of previous skin grafts. Laser treatment was administered with 660 nm, 4-6 J/cm^2 and 880 nm, 4 - 8 J/cm^2. The patients were treated three to five times per week, 25 - 30 times per course. Three patients underwent two courses of LPT with a three week interval. All patients experienced pain relief after 5 - 10 treatment sessions and decreased the amount of analgesics used. All ulcers in six patients were completely healed, and two ulcers in a seventh patient decreased in size by 75%.

Further literature: [829, 934]

4.1.15 Delayed onset muscular soreness (DOMS)

DOMS is a constant follower of athletic training and several efforts have been made to reduce DOMS with light treatment. In our own experience, GaAs applied immediately after training has a good effect, but there is no scientific documentation. Two clinical studies using a combination of laser

the female group. There was a partial response in 8% and a poor response in 16% of the patients. LPT was used parallel to traditional treatment.

In a study extended over six years, Soriano [678] treated 231 patients with venous leg ulcers. The exclusion criteria were diabetes, arterial disease, vasculitis, congestive heart failure and an inability to follow-up after six months. Altogether 122 of 154 patients in the laser group and 46 of 77 patients in the control group (traditional treatment only) completed the study. Wounds were all of Size Rate 4 or larger (diameter major + diameter minor). A 40 mW GaAs laser at 10 000 Hz was used. The laser was applied with the point technique at 3 J/cm^2 per point around the border and onto the bed of the ulcer in a non-contact mode. Three sessions a week were performed for four months, or until the ulcer was completely healed. The results were evaluated either as complete healing, partial healing (more than 50%) or non-healing (less than 50%). In the laser group there was a 70% healing rate and a 14% rate of partial healing. In the control group 26%, of the patients had complete healing and 22% partial healing. In the laser group, only 19% of the ulcers of great size (>16) healed completely, and if the wound was more than one year old the rate of complete healing was 40%. Wounds with an oedema failed to heal with the parameters used.

A total of 55 patients with long lasting chronic venous ulcers, suffering for more than six months without improvement, were treated with LPT by Lichtenstein [677, 1095]. Altogether 42 patients were treated with HeNe laser, and 13 with a 780 nm GaAlAs laser. The follow-up ranged from six months to six years. Wound closure was achieved after 7 to 40 treatments in most of the patients. Complete healing was achieved in 47 patients and moderate improvement in 4 patients. LPT was used parallel to traditional treatment.

Georgadze [558] treated 351 patients with persistent wounds and trophic ulcers in an outpatient clinic. Complete epithelialisation occurred in 236 patients.

Santoianni [560], however, found no effect of HeNe laser at 1 or 4 J/cm^2 on venous leg ulcers, as compared to a control group receiving only antiseptic local compresses.

In a study by Lundeberg and Malm [612], a 6 mW HeNe laser was used to treat leg ulcers, the stated dose being 4 J/cm^2. The area of the ulcers varied from 3 cm^2 to 32 cm^2, and to achieve the stated dose the period of therapy would thus have had to vary from 33 minutes to 6 hours per session. **The method by which the dose was calculated is therefore questionable. No indication is given of the method of treatment. If a scanning laser with an unexpanded beam was used, the power density would have been about 0.15 W/cm^2. If the beam was expanded to a diameter capable of illuminating the whole area of the ulcer at once, the power density when treating the largest ulcer would have been about 0.00019 W/cm^2, which is close to the level of moonlight when the moon is full. Unless all the parameters are accounted for, it is impossible to evaluate this study.**

nificant differences). However, animals in group C demonstrated a wound closure of 36.3 +/- 4.8%.

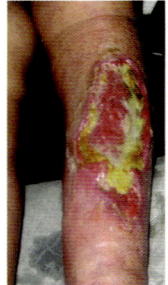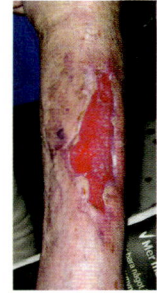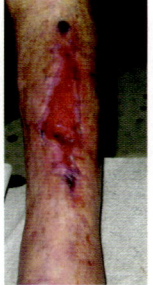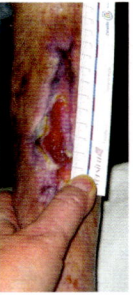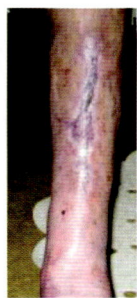

Figure 4.5 Woman of 80 years developing this leg ulcer during hospitalisation after hip fracture. 16 weekly laser sessions cured the wound completely. Pain and oedema disappeared after two sessions.
Courtesy: Ewa Waerner.

Clinical studies

Skoric [553] administered 1 J/cm² twice a week for seven weeks to ten patients with ulcus cruris. Complete epithelialisation was obtained in four patients, and in all other patients the ulcers became smaller (minimal 4%, maximal 52%).

Bihari [13] treated three groups of patients with crural ulcers, each group consisting of five patients. Group 1 received HeNe laser light, group 2 HeNe and GaAs in combination, and group 3 non-coherent unpolarised red light. Groups 1 and 2 showed excellent healing, with group 2 showing slightly better results than group 1. Healing in group 3 was poor. The study was double-blind.

Lievens [352] treated 10 patients aged 65-90 years, all with crural ulcers. In combination with classic treatment, they received GaAs laser light daily for three months. There was a statistically significant reduction in pain, wound surface, and inflammatory symptoms.

Sugrue [556] used infrared laser irradiation in a group of 12 patients with chronic venous ulcers unresponsive to conservative measures. The ulcers were treated for 12 weeks. Two ulcers healed completely and there was a 27% reduction in the other ulcers, 44% in the entire group. The most dramatic effect of LPT was the reduction of ulcer pain, from 7.5 to 3.5 on a VAS scale.

Soriano [559] treated 25 patients, average age 67 years, with therapy-resistant leg ulcers. GaAs laser light at 3 J/cm² was administered three days a week for a maximum of 16 weeks. The average treatment time was 10 weeks. 76% of the patients were completely healed, with the best results in

4.1.13 Cerebral palsy
Literature:
Asagai [660] reports on the use of GaAlAs (100 mW) laser treatment in a group of 1000 patients with cerebral palsy. The laser reduced muscle spasms and increased the mobility of the muscles. Although the duration of the LPT effect was limited to one to several hours, it can be applied in conjunction with conventional functional therapies, thereby enhancing the effects of the latter.

4.1.14 Crural and venous ulcers
Bedsores are common among bedridden patients. This condition is difficult to treat since the actual insult returns shortly after any therapy. HeNe (over the open wound) and GaAs (over the skin areas) have been shown to be valuable in the combined treatment of crural ulcers. Treatment is time-consuming, so scanners are useful. However, point treatment should be given around the dermal periphery of the wound in combination with full-wound scanning. Power output on the open wound should be lower than on the skin. In addition to the irradiation over the open wound and over the wound periphery, a large area surrounding the wound should also be irradiated since the pathology is not solely located in the visible wound area.

Literature:
Animal studies
Rakcheev [557] carried out an animal study on 60 guinea pigs and 110 rabbits using HeNe laser on experimental trophic ulcers. Due to the positive effects achieved at 0.75 J/cm^2, a successful clinical study was performed on 56 humans.

The ability of pressure ulcers to heal after the removal of the pressure has been demonstrated by Lanzafame [1447]. Pressure ulcers were created in mice by placing the dorsal skin between two round ceramic magnetic plates for three 12-h cycles. Animals were divided into three groups (n = 9 per group) for daily light therapy, 830 nm, 5.0 J/cm^2 on days 3-13 post ulceration in both groups A and B. A special heat-exchange device was applied in group B to maintain a constant temperature at the skin surface (30 degrees C). Group C served as controls, being irradiated with 5.0 J/cm^2 using an incandescent light source. Temperature of the skin surface, and temperature alterations during treatment, were monitored. The wound area was measured and the rate and time taken to complete healing were noted. The maximum temperature change during therapy was 2.0 +/- 0.64 degrees C in group A, 0.2 +/- 0.2 degrees C in Group B, and 3.54 degrees C +/- 0.72 in group C. Complete wound closure occurred at 18 +/- 4 days in groups A and B and 25 +/- 6 days in group C. The percentage of the wound closure on day 14 was 75. 4 +/- 7.2% and 77.7 +/- 5.6% for groups A and B, respectively (non-sig-

early stages and notably reduced in late stages of culturing. These findings of cell and tissue parameters up to 28 days of culturing revealed higher ossification levels in irradiated samples compared with the control group. The authors suggest that both the surface properties of the 3D crystalline biomatrices and the LPT have biostimulatory effects on the conversion of MSCs into bone-forming cells and on the induction of ex-vivo ossification.

Thus far, attempts to supplement damaged host muscles with donor satellite cells by means of myoblast transplantation therapy have been mostly unsuccessful due to massive and rapid loss of donor cells within a few hours after transplantation. The study by Shefer [1813] aimed at following the effects of LPT on the fate of implanted myoblasts. Primary myogenic cells, harvested from male rat skeletal muscles, were irradiated with low energy laser, seeded on a biodegradable scaffold and expanded in vitro. The scaffold containing cells was transplanted into partially excised muscles of host female rats. Donor cells were identified in the host muscle tissue, using Y-chromosome in situ hybridization. In this study, it was shown that laser irradiated donor primary myogenic cells not only survive, but also fuse with host myoblasts to form a host-donor syncytium. The data shows that the use of LPT as a non-surgical tool, is a promising means to enhance both the survival and functionality of transplanted primary myogenic cells.

The long term effects of LPT can involve mechanisms connected with activation of migration of stem cells towards damaged areas. Migration of stem cells was tested by Gasparyan [1627] under the influence of laser light alone, as well as in cases of combined influences of light and stromal cell-derived factor-1 alpha (SDF-1 alpha). This cytokine plays an important role in stem cell homing. Group 1 cells were the control, group 2 cells received red laser light irradiation, group 3 cells had IR laser light irradiation, group 4 cells were treated with SDF-1 alpha, group 5 cells were irradiated with red laser light in addition to SDF-1 alpha, and group 6 cells with IR laser light and SDF-1 alpha. The migrated cell count was 1496,5±409 (100%) in the control group. Red and IR laser light increased migration activity of stem cells up to 1892±283 (126%) and 2255,5±510 (151%) respectively. Influence of SDF-1 alpha was more significant than the effects of light irradiation alone: 3365,5±489 (225%). Combined effects of light irradiation and SDF-1 were significantly stronger: 5813±1199 (388%) for SDF-1 alpha and red laser light, and 6391,5±540 (427%) for SDF-1 alpha and IR laser light.

Souza [1718] divided 60 amputated worms into three study groups: a control group, and two other groups submitted to daily one and three minute long laser treatment sessions at approximately a 910 W/m2 power density. A 685 nm laser with 35 mW optical power was used. Samples were sent to histological analysis on the 4th, the 7th and the 15th day after amputation. A remarkable increase in stem cell counts for the 4th day of regeneration was observed when the regenerating worms were stimulated by the laser radiation.

Further reading: chapter 4.1.49 "Stem cells" on page 315.

4.1.12 Cell transplants

Much attention has recently been given to the use of stem cells and primary cells for cell transplantation. These cells do not differ from any other cells when it comes to the ability to respond to laser irradiation. Thus, LPT could be a valuable tool in maintaining the vitality of such cell cultures before being applied to a donor site.

Literature:

The study by Mvula [1808] investigated the effect of LPT on primary cultures of adult human adipose derived stem cells using a 635 nm diode laser, at 5 J/cm^2 with a power output of 50.2 mW and a power density of 5.5 mW/cm^2. Cellular morphology did not appear to change after irradiation. Using the trypan blue exclusion test, the cellular viability of irradiated cells increased by 1% at 24 h and 1.6% at 48 h but was not statistically significant. However, the increase of cellular viability as measured by ATP luminescence was statistically significant at 48 h. Proliferation of irradiated cells, measured by optical density, resulted in statistically significant increases in values compared to non-irradiated cells at both time points. Western blot analysis and immunocytochemical labeling indicated an increase in the expression of stem cell marker 1-integrin after irradiation. These results indicate that 5 J/cm^2 of laser irradiation can positively affect human adipose stem cells by increasing cellular viability, proliferation, and expression of β1-integrin.

The aim of the study by Tuby [1809] was to investigate the effect of LPT on the proliferation of mesenchymal stem cells (MSCs) and cardiac stem cells (CSCs). Isolation of MSCs and CSCs was performed. The cells were cultured and laser irradiation was applied at energy densities of 1 and 3 J/cm^2. The number of MSCs and CSCs up to two and four weeks post-LPT demonstrated a significant increase in the laser-treated cultures as compared to the control. These results may have an important impact on regenerative medicine.

Abramovitch-Gottlib [1810] irradiated mesenchymal stem cells (MSCs) seeded on three dimensional (3D) coralline (Porites lutea) biomatrices with laser irradiation. The consequent phenotype modulation and development of MSCs towards ossified tissue was studied in this combined 3D biomatrix/LPT system and in a control group, which was similarly grown, but not treated by LPT. The irradiated and non-irradiated MSC were tested on days 1-7, 10, 14, 21 and 28 of culturing via analysis of cellular distribution on matrices (trypan blue), calcium incorporation to newly formed tissue (alizarin red), bone nodule formation, fat aggregates formation, alkaline phosphatase (ALP) activity, scanning electron microscopy (SEM) and electron dispersive spectrometry (EDS). The results obtained from the irradiated samples showed enhanced tissue formation, appearance of phosphorous peaks and calcium and phosphate incorporation to newly formed tissue. Moreover, in irradiated samples, ALP activity was significantly enhanced in

irradiation. There were no significant changes in group B, except for changes in the clinical symptoms.

Chang [2020] placed an 830 nm laser directly above the transverse carpal ligament, which is between the pisiform and navicular bones of the tested patients, to determine the therapeutic effect of LPT. Thirty-six patients with mild to moderate degrees of CTS were randomly divided into two groups. The laser group received laser treatment (10 Hz, 50% duty cycle, 60 mW, 9.7 J/cm^2), and the placebo group received sham laser treatment. Both groups received treatment for two weeks consisting of a 10 min laser irradiation session each day, five days a week. The therapeutic effects were assessed on symptoms and functional changes, and with nerve conduction studies (NCS), grip strength assessment, and with a visual analogue scale (VAS), soon after treatment and at the two-week follow-up. Before treatment, there were no significant differences between the two groups for all assessments. The VAS scores were significantly lower in the laser group than in the placebo group after treatment and at the follow-up. After two weeks of treatment, no significant differences were found in grip strengths or for symptoms and functional assessments. However, there were statistically significant differences in these variables at the two-week follow-up. Regarding the findings of NCS, there was no statistically significant difference between groups after treatment and at the two-week follow-up. No side effects were noted.

Two laser acupuncture studies report favourable outcome [1677, 1678].

A study by Yagci [2060] aimed to compare the short-term efficacy of splinting (S) and splinting plus low-level laser (SLPT) in mild or moderate idiopathic carpal tunnel syndrome (CTS) with a prospective, randomized controlled study. The patients with unilateral, mild, or moderate idiopathic CTS who experienced symptoms over 3 months were included in the study. The SLPT group received ten sessions of laser therapy and splinting while S group was given only splints. The patients were evaluated at the baseline and after 3 months of the treatment. Forty-five patients with CTS completed the study. Twenty-four patients were in S and 21 patients were in SLPT group. In the third-month control, SLPT group had significant improvements on both clinical and NCS parameters (median motor nerve distal latency, median sensory nerve conduction velocities, BQ symptom severity scale, and BQ functional capacity scale) while S group had only symptomatic healing (BQ symptom severity scale). The grip strength of splinting group was decreased significantly. According to clinical response criteria, in SLPT group, five patients had full and 12 had partial recovery; four patients had no change or worsened. In S group, one patient had full and 17 partial recovery; six patients had no change or worsened.

Further literature: [661, 1152]

In a double-blind trial by Irvine [1426], 15 CTS patients, 34 to 67 years of age, were randomly assigned to either a control group (n = 8) or a treatment group (n =7). Both groups were treated three times per week for five weeks. Those in the treatment group received 860 nm GaAlAs laser at a dosage of 6 J/cm^2 over the carpal tunnel, whereas those in the control group were treated with sham laser. The primary outcome measure was the Levine Carpal Tunnel Syndrome Questionnaire, and the secondary outcome measures were electrophysiological data and the Purdue pegboard test. All patients completed the study without adverse effects. There was a significant symptomatic improvement in both the control (P= 0.034) and treatment (P =0.043) groups. However, there was no significant difference in any of the outcome measures between the two groups. Note that 6 J/cm^2 was applied, not 6 J per point.

Another negative low-dose study is that of Bakhtiary [1679], who used 830 nm, 1.8 J per point on five points along the median nerve and the wrist.

The study by Elwakil [1794] was conducted to evaluate the effectiveness of LPT for CTS in comparison to the standard open carpal tunnel release surgery. Out of 54 patients, 60 symptomatic hands suffering from CTS were divided into two equal groups. Group A, was subjected to Helium Neon laser, whereas group B was treated by the open approach for carpal tunnel release. The patients were evaluated clinically and by nerve conduction studies (NCSs) about six months after the treatment. LPT showed overall significant results but at a lower level in relation to surgery. LPT showed significant outcomes in all parameters of subjective complaints except for muscle weakness. Moreover, LPT showed significant results in all parameters of objective findings except for thenar atrophy. However, NCSs expressed the same statistical significance after the treatment by both modalities

Ekim [1841] reports that laser at 1.5 J per point was no more efficient than placebo, which underlines the importance of being within the therapeutic window.

The study by Shooshtari [1996] evaluated the effects of LPT through nerve conduction measurements and clinical signs and symptoms. A total of 80 patients were included. Diagnosis of CTS was based on both clinical examination and electromyographic (EMG) findings. Patients were randomly assigned into two groups. Test group (group A) underwent laser therapy (9-11 J/cm^2) over the carpal tunnel area. Control group (group B) received sham laser therapy. Pain, hand grip strength, median proximal sensory and motor latencies, and transcarpal median sensory nerve conduction (SNCV) were recorded. After fifteen sessions of irradiation (five times per week), parameters were recorded again and clinical symptoms were measured in both groups. Pain was evaluated by VAS; day-night. Hand grip was measured by Jamar dynometer.There was a significant improvement in clinical symptoms and hand grip in group A. Proximal median sensory latency, distal median motor latency and median sensory latencies were significantly decreased. Transcarpal median SNCV increased significantly after laser

Literature:

Weintraub [538] investigated whether repeated laser light exposure directed at the median nerve could reverse the symptoms and electro-physiological latencies in CTS. The study covered 30 hands displaying moderate to severe CTS. A low power, continuous GaAlAs laser was percutaneously applied at 33 second intervals to five points along the median nerve delivering 9 J/point without discomfort or heat sensations. A complete resolution of pre-treatment symptoms and abnormal physical findings was achieved in 77% of the cases. Nocturnal complaints were the earliest symptom to disappear, followed by tingling, stiffness and weakness. Normalisation of distal latency was achieved in 11% with a further tendency towards improvement in 23.4%. Work status was maintained with no new interventions, and after completion of the treatment trial 11 patients resumed previously impossible activities.

Wong [539] observed that CTS patients have poor posture. Upon palpation, they experience pain and tenderness at the spinous processes C5-T1 and the medial angle of the scapula. In 35 such patients, treatment was focused primarily on the posterior neck area and not the wrists and hands. A 100 mW GaAlAs laser was used and directed at the tips of the aforementioned spinous processes, 12-30 J/point. The laser rapidly alleviated pain and tingling in the arms, hands and fingers.

Roig [893] treated 20 patients with carpal tunnel syndrome with a GaAs/HeNe laser, 3.6 J/cm^2. Altogether 20 consecutive sessions, each lasting for 10 minutes, were given. At the end of treatment the outcome for pain and paraesthesia was: complete remission 7 patients, partial remission 8, no improvement 5. As for loss of muscle strength the outcome was: complete recovery 10 patients, partial recovery 5, no improvement 5.

Yu [192] treated car assembly-line workers with good results using a 100 mW GaAlAs laser.

Padua [937] compared the effect of a 830 nm three-diode LPT on primary carpal tunnel syndrome in 17 patients. Neurophysiological parameters and a patient questionnaire were used to evaluate the outcome. Immediately after therapy and 15 days post-therapy there was a positive effect, but at the follow-ups in month 2 and 12, almost all parameters had progressively returned to the pre-treatment pattern and were similar to those of an untreated group.

In the study by *Rappl [1282]*, 72 hands with CTS treated by laser (15 sessions/30 min, over a period of five weeks) were evaluated by a double-blind, randomised study. ENG and VAS (visual analogous scale) were performed prior to and after therapy (830 nm, 400 mW) with an energy of 3 J per point focused on the carpal tunnel, as well as on trigger and acupuncture points. In 38 cases, a red light pen was used. Follow-ups ranged from 8 to 12 months. ENG and VAS improved in 66%, was unchanged in 8% and got worse in 26% of the patients in the laser group after a 12 month period. No improvement was recorded in the control group.

essary. For instance, carpal tunnel symptoms caused by pseudoradicular irritation from the C5-C6 region will not respond to irradiation over the carpal area. Patients could, on the other hand, be irradiated in this very area according to Wong [539]. If venous compression in the axilla is the cause of the symptoms, local irradiation over the compressed area in combination with exercise will then be successful. If the carpal area has become very fibrotic, surgery is the only alternative. Under such conditions, LPT will only give a transient pain release and a reduction of the oedema. Complete remission of the symptoms will only be achieved in the earlier phases of the syndrome and in combination with exercise and a change in the working conditions.

A reasonable energy output over the area is 6-8 J per point. Negative studies have used lower energies. As for many other conditions, the diversity of success in reports on LPT on carpal tunnel syndrome may also depend on the inclusion criteria, i.e. the stage of the condition. The success rate of studies is closely related to the dosage. WALT recommendations for 780-830 nm is a minimum of 6 J per point, 2-3 points, and for a GaAs a minimum of 2 J per point (www.walt.nu).

LPT of CTS was the first indication to receive an approval by the Food and Drug Administration (FDA) in the USA. This approval is limited to "adjunct use" for obtaining temporary relief of pain associated with CTS. The study [1712] which formed the base of this approval has not been published, but is available on-line.

In conclusion, LPT is an effective treatment modality for mild and moderate carpal tunnel syndrome, provided adequate dosage is applied and differential diagnosis is correct.

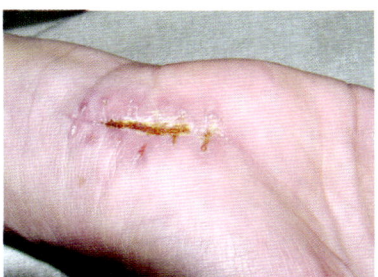 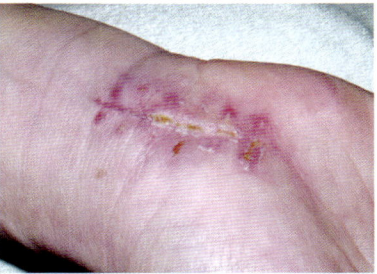

Figure 4.4 35 years old diabetic patient patient operated for carpal tunnel syndrome. First photo after removal of sutures, next after one week of LPT.

Courtesy: Chrisse Bäckström.

Shoji [1476] has successfully laser treated acute dihiscence in cardiac patients where the saphenous vein has been used in myocardia revascularisation surgery. 655 nm 4 J/cm^2 was applied punctually around the wound.

Chavantes [1480] writes that in the western world cardiovascular disease is the causa mortis leader. There has been a significant increase in the rate of chronic pathologies such as Diabetes mellitus, Obesity, Hypertension. These illnesses are aggravating factors for heart disease, which tend to elevate the morbidity-mortality after conventional risky surgery. The aim in this study was to prevent wound dehiscence and/or incision infection post-surgery, which still represents a therapeutical challenge in the medical field. 112 patients underwent two different protocols to open heart surgery. Laser was applied every third day (two sessions). The Laser Group presented five times less incidence of dehiscence than the Control Group, which stayed twice as long as in-patients. Laser also revealed a decrease of complications, especially dehiscence to one-third compared with placebo. The laser group showed early pain reduction, better healing processes and shorter recovery time.

In a study by Kazemi-kho [2044], 30 cases with two or three coronary vessel occlusions (2VD/3VD) underwent LPT post-CABG, and 32 patients acted as a control group. A diode laser (810 nm, 500 mw) was used as LPT protocol for three successive days post-CABG. Repeated measurements of blood cell count (CBC) and cardiac damage markers (CPK, CPK-MB, LDH) accomplished before CABG and through five days of LPT post-operatively were carried out 1 and 12 hours after daily laser irradiation. Mean age of participants was 57.27±11.88 years; and male-to-female ratio was 3/1. Mean cardiac ejection fraction was 49.62±9.04% before and 47.04±7.49% after CABG surgery. Serum CPK-MB level decreased significantly in the LPT group in comparison to the placebo controls during 12 hours of post-laser irradiation measurements. None of the other parameters measured, including BS, CPK, LDH and blood leukocytes, lymphocytes and neutrophiles counts were affected by the laser irradiation during the measurement period. It is concluded that laser irradiation after CABG surgery could lower the cardiac cellular damage and help cardiac tissue repair to occur faster post-operatively.

Further literature: [408, 426, 905, 952, 991, 992, 993, 1124, 1125, 1198, 1199]

4.1.11 Carpal tunnel syndrome

Repetitive stress movements cause the Carpal Tunnel Syndrome (CTS), which is a debilitating condition resulting in many problems for employers and employees in industrial and office environments.

LPT is a valuable adjuvant treatment modality for this group of patients. The main effect is believed to be reduction of oedema and improved microcirculation in the affected area, since the venous blood flow impairment seems to be the first stage in CTS. However, a correct diagnosis is nec-

grammable manner and with uniform intensity. Two pilot LP procedures carried out are described below. The patients were diagnosed before treatment and followed up three and six months after the LP procedure with non invasive tests. After six months, a control angiography was also performed. The procedures were well tolerated. In both cases, the follow-up examinations showed no evidence of restenosis. No negative side effects were observed after two procedures.

Based on the results of these previous experiments proving the beneficial effects of laser light on the activity of vascular and inflammatory cells, Derkacz [1636] continued to use LPT to prevent restenosis. Irradiation was performed in 41 patients after stent implantation or balloon angioplasty. Illumination power of 100 mW and an energy dose equal to 9 J/cm^2 was used. Patients were monitored for major adverse cardiac events (MACE) after 30 days and six months. At six months, angiography as a control was performed to assess the influence of LP on the restenosis rate. Results: The angiographic follow-up (n = 30) revealed restenosis in 9% and 25% of patients after stent implantation and balloon angioplasty, respectively. The MACE rate was 4.5% and 12.5% in stent and balloon-treated patients, respectively. Laser phototherapy gives very promising results in restenosis prevention, especially after stent implantation.

Infrared irradiation of the skin applied to the projections of the heart and its reflexogenic areas is also reported by other authors to be successful. There are many Russian reports on intravascular HeNe irradiation as a treatment modality for patients with heart infarction or other ischemic heart diseases. Reported effects include reduced need of nitroglycerine tablets, decreased number of angina attacks, alleviation of pain, suppression of lipid peroxidation, promotion of antioxidant protection of erythrocyte membranes, reduction of fibrinogen levels, normalization of antithrombin-III, reduction of arrhythmic deaths as of a two-year check-up, reduction of the activities of the hypophyseoadrenocortical and aldosteron-renin-angiotensin systems. Three to five sessions of 30-40 minutes are frequently used.

Carvalho [1470] analysed forty patients after sternotomy and divided them into two groups. Control Group: submitted to a conventional therapeutic hospital scheme, and Laser Group: GaAlAs laser irradiation after the surgical incision. The laser was a continuous diode with a wavelength of 655 nm; dose 8 J/cm^2; surrounding the surgery incision and starting from the first 12 hours of Post-Operative (PO), third PO and sixth PO. A VAS scale was used in order to analyse the pain related to the wound. The investigators observed in the 3rd PO an average of 4,5 of pain intensity in the Control Group, and 2,8 in the Laser Group. In the sixth PO, an average of 4,1 in the Control Group, and 2,7 in the Laser Group were measured. Morphological analysis of repaired nerves showed that laser accelerated the regeneration process of nerve fibers.

with non-irradiated rats. In the CAM model, a slight inhibition of angiogenesis up to two days post irradiation, and a significant enhancement of angiogenesis in the laser-irradiated foci as compared with the non-irradiated control spots, were evident. The laser irradiation caused a 1.8-fold significant increase in the rate of proliferation in endothelial cells in culture compared to non-irradiated cells.

The aim of a study by Tuby [1730] was to investigate the effect of LPT on the expression of vascular endothelial growth factor (VEGF) and inducible nitric oxide synthase (iNOS). Myocardial infarction was induced by occlusion of the left descending artery in 87 rats. Laser was applied to intact and post-infarction. VEGF, iNOS, and angiogenesis were determined. Both the laser-irradiated rat hearts post-infarction and the intact hearts demonstrated a significant increase in VEGF and iNOS expression compared to non-laser-irradiated hearts. LPT also caused a significant elevation in angiogenesis.

Whittaker [1912] reports: In vitro, fibroblasts were irradiated for one minute twice a day for four days (5 mW; 780 nm). In addition, one day after infarction, rats were randomly assigned to 5 or 10 mW transdermal irradiation twice a day for four days or to sham treatment. One week after infarction, we measured the remodeling parameters; cavity volume, infarct thickness, and vascular structure, and the healing parameters; collagen content and inflammation. Laser-treated fibroblasts occupied a larger area than controls. Hearts receiving the 10 mW treatment had smaller volumes than sham-treated hearts. Laser treatment reduced infarct thinning and preserved the arterial lumen area; however, collagen did not increase and inflammation was inhibited. In conclusion, LPT attenuated infarct-associated remodeling. In contrast to expectations from the in vitro study, these effects were not a result of enhanced healing.

Clinical studies

Lee [752] successfully used LPT for the relief of cervicothoracic pain syndromes.

De Scheerder [968] has used HeNe laser as an adjunct in coronary stent implantation. The preliminary findings suggest that LPT results in a decrease of in-stent restenosis when used during primary stenting. A long term evaluation is published [1636].

According to Derkacz [1545], the main problem after percutaneous coronary intervention (PCI) is restenosis affecting the site where dilatation is performed. In order to minimize its occurrence, the method of intravascular laser photostimulation (LP) with low power irradiation has been developed. The procedure is carried out during PCI. A special setup was prepared for intravascular photostimulation with a 808 nm wavelength laser diode and a special diffuser, delivering the laser light into the coronary artery. The construction of the device makes it possible to irradiate the coronary artery in the place of previously performed dilatation in a satisfactory and pro-

Itoh [723] has demonstrated that HeNe laser has a protective effect on the type of damage to the erythrocytes caused by heart-lung machines.

Animal studies

Kipshidze [717] reports that a single endoluminal irradiation with HeNe (1.8 J) prevents restenosis after balloon angioplasty in an atherosclerotic rabbit model.

Kipshidze [344] reports further promising results in the treatment of acute myocardial infarction by guiding HeNe laser light into the heart cavity.

Oron [1097] found that 803 nm LPT reduced the formation of scar tissue following experimentally induced ischemic myocardial infarction in rats and dogs. Following the induction of the infarction, the dogs (24 in the experimental group, 24 in the control group) received laser irradiation epicardially with a dose of 1.08 J/cm^2. At five to six weeks postop., the dogs were sacrificed and infarction size was determined by TTC staining and histology. The infarct size in the laser group was reduced by 52% as compared to the control group. Catalase enzymatic activity (antioxidant marker) was higher in the laser group. The results were confirmed in a separate study of 83 rats. In this experiment, the left ventricular dilatation was also reduced by 50-60% in the laser group.

Yaakov [1197] has studied the effect of 804 nm laser on the interstitial scarring in the hearts of rats subjected to experimental heart hypertrophy. The rats were injected with isoproternol (ISO), a substance known to induce hypertrophy without a marked mortality rate in the rat's heart. A careful dosage analysis was performed, resulting in a measured power of 5 mW near the heart, and a power density of 4.5 mW/cm^2 on the myocardium. ISO treatment resulted in an 11% increase in hypertrophy, which was not altered by laser irradiation. However, a 57% reduction in interstitial scarring in the myocardium was evident in laser-irradiated rats as compared to non-irradiated rats.

Drugova [1714] studied the effects of low-intensity red light (HeNe or broadband) on lipid peroxidation in isolated rat hearts in the postischemic period. It was established that both laser and wideband luminescent irradiation applied during reperfusion reduced the content of lipid peroxidation products in tissues to a near-control level. Acc. to the authors of the study, the effect is possibly associated with reactivation of antioxidant enzymes.

The effect of HeNe irradiation on the process of angiogenesis in the infarcted rat heart and in the chick chorioallantoic membrane (CAM), as well as the proliferation of endothelial cells in tissue cultures, were investigated by Mirsky [1591]. Formation of new blood vessels in the infarcted rat heart was monitored by counting proliferating endothelial cells in blood vessels. In the CAM model, defined areas were either laser-irradiated or non-irradiated and blood vessel density was recorded in each site in the CAM at various time intervals. Laser irradiation caused a 3.1-fold significant increase in newly formed blood vessels 6 days post infarction, as compared

major component of arteriosclerotic diseases, including aneurysm. Macrophage recruitment and secretion of pro-inflammatory cytokines and the vasodilator, nitric oxide (NO), are central to most immune responses in the arterial wall. The present study [1944] was designed to determine the effect of LPT on cytokine gene expression and secretion, as well as the gene expression of inducible nitric oxide synthase (iNOS) and NO production in lipopolysaccharide (LPS)-stimulated macrophages. Murine monocyte/macrophages were irradiated with a 780 nm (2 mW/cm^2, 2.2 J/cm^2) during stimulation with LPS (0, 0.1, and 1 microg/ml). Gene expression of chemokines, cytokines, and iNOS were assessed by RT-PCR. Secretion of interleukin (IL)-1β and monocyte chemotactic protein (MCP)-1 and NO were assessed by ELISA and the Griess reaction, respectively. LPT reduced gene expression of MCP-1, IL-1, IL-10, IL-1β, and IL-6 when cells were stimulated by 1 microg/ml LPS. LPT reduced LPS-induced secretion of MCP-1 over non-irradiated cells by 17+/-5% and 13+/-5% at 12 hours (0.1 and 1 microg/ml LPS), and reduced IL-1β by 22+/-5% and 25+/-9% at 24 hours (0.1 and 1 microg/ml LPS). However, LPT increased NO secretion after 12 hours. These properties of LPT, with its effects on smooth muscle cells reported previously, may be of profound therapeutic relevance for arterial diseases such as aneurysm, where inflammatory processes and a weakening of the matrix structure of the arterial wall are major pathologic components.

Another study by Gavish [1945] was designed to determine the effects of LPT on arterial SMC proliferation, inflammatory markers, and matrix proteins. Porcine primary aortic SMCs were irradiated with a 780 nm laser (1 and 2 J/cm^2). Trypan blue exclusion assay, immunofluorescent staining for collagen I and III, Sircol assay, gelatin zymography, and RT-PCR were used to monitor proliferation, collagen trihelix formation, collagen synthesis, matrix metalloproteinase-2 (MMP-2) activity, and gene expression of MMP-1, MMP-2, tissue inhibitor of MMP-1 (TIMP-1), TIMP-2, and IL-1β, respectively. LPT increased SMC proliferation by 16 and 22% (1 and 2 J/cm^2, respectively) compared to non-irradiated cells. Immediately after LPT, trihelices of collagen I and III appeared as perinuclear fluorescent rings. Collagen synthesis was increased twofold (two days after LPT: 14.3+/-3.5 microg, non-irradiated control: 6.6+/-0.7 microg, and TGF-β stimulated control: 7.1+/-1.2 microg), MMP-2 activity after LPT was augmented (over non-irradiated control) by 66+/-18% (2 J/cm^2), and MMP-1 gene expression upregulated. However, TIMP-2 was upregulated, and MMP-2 gene expression downregulated. IL-1β gene expression was reduced. In conclusion, LPT stimulates SMC proliferation, stimulates collagen synthesis, modulates the equilibrium between regulatory matrix remodeling enzymes, and inhibits pro-inflammatory IL-1β gene expression. These findings may be of therapeutic relevance for arterial diseases such as aneurysm, where SMC depletion, weakened extracellular matrix, and an increase in pro-inflammatory markers are major pathologic components.

In a recent review article Zimin [2125] writes: Although low-power visible (VIS) and near infrared (nIR) radiation emitted from lasers, photodiodes, and other sources does not cause neoplastic transformation of the tissue, these phototherapeutic techniques are looked at with a great deal of caution for fear of their stimulatory effect on tumour growth. This apprehension arises in the first place from the reports on the possibility that the proliferative activity of tumour cells may increase after their in vitro exposure to light. Much less is known that these phototherapeutic modalities have been successfully used for the prevention and management of complications developing after surgery, chemo- and radiotherapy. The objective of the present review is to summarize the results of applications of low-power visible and near infrared radiation for the treatment of patients with oncological diseases during the last 20-25 years. It should be emphasized that 2-4 year-long follow-up observations have not revealed any increase in the frequency of tumour recurrence and metastasis.

Further literature: [2, 3, 47, 371, 564, 978, 979, 980, 1072, 1073, 1076, 1133, 1176, 1483, 1485, 1728]

4.1.10 Cardiac conditions

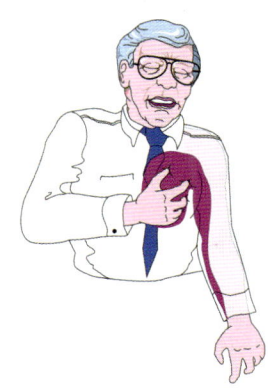

A number of studies report on the use of LPT in cardiac surgery. LTP appears to be able to reduce the risk of aneurysm, reduce the necrotic area after infarction, protect damage to erythrocytes in heart-lung machines, reduce the incidence of wound dehiscence after open heart surgery, and reduce complications after stent operations. The cardiac area is easily accesible using fibre optics. The scientific support for the use of LPT for wound healing after cardiac surgery is strong, whereas the use of intraoperatory LPT still needs more clinical research. It appears, though, to have great potential.

Literature:
In vitro studies:
Kipshidze [1124] reports that HeNe laser can influence the vascular endothelian growth factor and proliferaration of human endothelial cells in vitro. These data may have significant importance, leading to the establishment of new methods for endoluminal postangioplasty vascular repair and myocardial photoangiogenesis.

Gavish et al. have shown that LPT (780 nm) increases the aortic smooth muscle cell proliferation and matrix protein secretion and modulates the activity and expression of matrix metalloproteinases. Inflammation is a

developed OM. Patients received intervention for 5 days. The LPT group was treated with 830 nm, 100 mW, 4 J/cm^2, and the placebo group underwent sham treatment. The grade of OM was clinically assessed by the National Cancer Institute, Common Toxicity Criteria scale. Twenty-one patients developed OM and were evaluable for analysis; 18 (86%) patients had a diagnosis of leukemia or lymphoma and 3 (14%) had solid tumors. The mean age was 8.2 (+/-3.1) years. Nine patients were randomized in the laser group and 12 in the placebo-control group. Once OM was diagnosed, the patients had daily OM grading assessments before laser or sham application and thereafter until complete healing of the lesions. On day 7 after OM diagnosis, 1/9 of patients remained with lesions in laser group and 9/12 of patients in the placebo-control group. In the laser group, the mean of OM duration was 5.8+/-2 days and in the placebo group was 8.9+/-2.4 days.

The aim of a study by Simões [2120] was to verify how LPT used for oral mucositis could influence xerostomia symptoms and hyposalivation of patients undergiong RT. Patients were divided into two groups: 12 individuals receiving three laser irradiations per week (G1) and 10 patients receiving one laser irradiation per week (G2). A diode laser (660 nm, 6 J/cm(2), 0.24 J, 40 mW) was used until completely healing of the lesions or the end of the RT. At the first and last laser sessions, whole resting and stimulated saliva were collected, and questionnaires were administered. According to Wilcoxon and Student statistical test, xerostomia for G1 was lower than for G2, and salivary flow rate was no different before and after RT, except for stimulated collection of G2, which was lower. These results suggest that LPT can be beneficial as an auxiliary therapy for hypofunction of salivary glands.

In a review of the literature, Bjordal [2094] comes to the following conclusion:
1. There is moderate evidence of a dose-dependent LPT effect which is significantly better than placebo in relieving pain and severity of oral mucositis.
2. The use of J/cm^2 causes confusion and should be substituted with energy doses in Joules. Wavelengths of 632-685 nm and 810-830 nm should be preferred.
3. Optimal procedures should cover all of the oral lesions with irradiation exceeding 30 seconds/1-4 Joules per point, placed 1-2 cm apart. Treament sessions should be performed 3-5 days per week before, or during chemotherapy.

A literature review [2115] revealed 33 potentially relevant papers. Of these, nine studies were reviews and six studies were case studies, while another three were animal studies. Three controlled studies were excluded for lack of randomization, while one study lacked a placebo-control group. The final sample consisted of 11 randomized placebo-controlled trials published from 1997 until 2009 with a total of 415 patients. The analysed papers confirm that there is moderate to strong scientific evidence for the use of LPT to treat mucositis.

tis of grade 0 when compared with the placebo group, and 18% presented grade 1. In group 2, 27% had no mucositis and did not require therapy. In group 3, the patients experienced a marked pain relief (as assessed by a visual analogue scale), and a decrease in the severity of mucositis, even when they had severe granulocytopenia.

In a study by Jaguar [1986], 24 patients received prophylactic laser therapy (L+ group). The applications started from the beginning of the conditioning regimen up to day +2. The oral assessment was performed daily until day +30. This group was compared with historical controls, namely 25 patients, who did not receive laser therapy (L- group). All patients developed some grade of mucositis. However, the L- group presented initial mucositis by 4.36 days, whereas the L+ group presented it in 6.12 days. The maximum mucositis occurred between day +2 and day +6 with healing by day +25 in the L- group, and between day +2 and day +7 with healing by day +14 for the L+ group. Laser therapy also reduced the time of oral pain from 5.64 to 2.45 days and decreased the consumption of morphine.

The study by Nes [1985] was performed as a clinical test with a sample consisting of 13 adult patients receiving oncology treatment. The patients were treated during a five-day period, and the pain was measured before and after each laser application. A 830 nm 250 mW laser was used. The energy given was 35 J/cm^2. There was a 67% decrease in the daily average experience of pain felt before and after each treatment, confirming that LPT can relieve pain among patients who have developed mucositis. The low number of COM patients at the hospital did not allow a control group to be included in the study, and therefore the results contain a potential placebo effect.

The study by Zanin [2037] included a total of 84 patients, divided into two groups: group (L): 43 patients with laser, group (C): 41 patients without laser. Area of irradiated tissue was considered as $1 cm^2$ per application point, in a contact mode. Irradiated regions were: three points in the jugal mucosa, three points in the internal mucosa of the inferior lip, three points on the soft palate, two points on the palatine folds, two points on the sublingual caruncles and five points on the tongue. Applications were given twice weekly, before or after radiotherapy sessions. Statistically significant differences were observed between the two studied groups (NCI scale). Patients in group (L) usually did not present OM. However, all patients in group (C) presented OM levels I to III. Patients in group (C) presented growing indexes of pain from the first week of Rt treatment. Patients in group (L) reported absence of pain during the whole radiotherapy treatment. LPT was effective in preventing and treating severe oral effects induced by radio and chemotherapy, controlling inflammation, maintaining mucosal integrity, bringing more comfort to patients, thus improving their quality of life.

A placebo-controlled randomized trial was carried out by Kuhn [2101], using LPT or placebo (sham treatment). Children and adolescents with cancer receiving chemotherapy or hematopoietic stem-cell transplantation between October 2005 and May 2006 were eligible as soon as they

radiotherapy (after six weeks), mean pain score and mucositis grade were significantly lower in the study group compared to the control group.

Migliorati [1195] used 780 nm 60 mW, 2 J/cm² in a group of 11 patients receiving high-dose chemotherapy and could confirm the pain relieving effect of LPT for this indication.

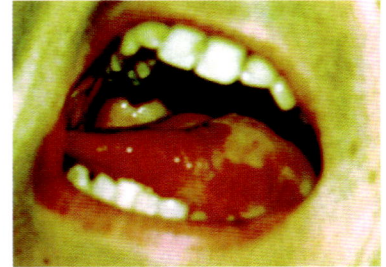

Figure 4.3 Typical mucositis
Courtesy: René-Jean Bensadoun

da Cuhna [1334] compared the effect of visible and infrared laser in patients who were undergoing radiotherapy. With 15 patients in each group, the effects of the two wavelengths were almost identical.

A study by Balakirev [1212] suggests that the application of LPT makes it possible to reduce the time needed for the management of radiation injuries and chemotherapy complications in paediatric patients 1.5-2-fold. It was shown that exposure to LPT caused mononuclear levels of donors' blood to rise, which in turn led to a release, in higher concentrations, of IL-1 and FNO cytokins, which are major factors of the immune response development.

A study by Durnov [1213] outlines the outcomes of treatment for complications associated with chemo- and radiation therapy in children with malignant neoplasms by using laser radiation. The use of this therapy may reduce the duration of the treatment of these complications by 1.5-2 times. The use of therapeutic laser radiation in the treatment of other complications that are common in paediatric oncological care is briefly described.

In a study by Arora [1823], 24 hospitalized patients with oral cancer, scheduled to undergo radiotherapy were enrolled in the study and assigned to laser (Group I)/control group (Group II). They were treated using HeNe laser (10 mW, 1.8 J/cm²). Patients were subjected to treatment using a laser scanner for eight days and were subsequently treated using a laser probe at six anatomic sites in the oral cavity for five minutes each. The patients were evaluated on each day of treatment for pain severity (NRS), functional impairment (FIS), and oral mucositis (RTOG) and were followed until the end of cancer treatment. Statistical analysis was done using SPSS version 10. LPT applied prophylactically during radiotherapy could reduce the severity of oral mucositis, severity of pain, and functional impairment.

In a study by Abramoff [1472] patients undergoing chemotherapy (22 cycles) without mucositis were randomized into a group receiving prophylactic laser irradiation (group 1), and a group receiving placebo light treatment (group 2). Patients who already presented mucositis were placed in a group receiving irradiation for therapeutic purposes (group 3, with 10 cycles of chemotherapy). Serum granulocyte levels were taken and compared to the progression of mucositis. In group 1, most patients (73%) presented mucosi-

nization (WHO) scale. In the LPT group, 94.7% of the patients had an OM grade (WHO) lower than or equal to grade 2, including 63.2% with grade 0 and 1, whereas in the control group, 31.5% of the patients had an OM grade lower than or equal to grade 2 . Remarkably, the hazard ratio (HR) for grades 2, 3 and 4 OM was 0.41, and for grades 3 and 4 it was 0.07. By using OMAS to calculate the ulcerous area, 5.3% of the laser group presented ulcers from 9.1 /cm^2 to 18 cm^2, whereas 73.6% of the control group presented ulcers from 9.1 cm^2 to 18 cm^2.

It is interesting to compare the relatively modest result in the Schubert study to the results in the studies by Bensadoun and Antunes. Bensadoun used HeNe 2 J/cm^2, which was also the dose in the Schubert study. However, we believe that red diodes need higher dosage than HeNe, because of the short coherence length of the diodes. This assumption seems to be confirmed by Antunes, also using a red diode but at double the Bensadoun dose and with better results. [See ref. 1634]

A study by Cruz [1746] assessed the use of therapeutic laser in the prevention or reduction of the severity of oral mucositis. A randomized clinical trial was carried out. Patients from 3 to 18 years of age treated with chemotherapy or hematopoietic stem-cell transplantation were eligible. The intervention group received laser application (780 nm, 60 mW, 4 J//cm^2) for 5 days following the start of chemotherapy: Sixty patients were included for analysis; thirty-nine were males, 35 (58%) patients had a diagnosis of leukemia or lymphoma, and 25 had solid tumors. Twenty-nine patients were randomized in the laser group and 31 in the control group. On day 1, no patients presented mucositis. On day 8, out of the 20 patients who had developed mucositis, 13 of them were from the laser group and 7 from the control group. On day 15, a total of 24 patients had developed mucositis, 13 of them were from the laser group and 11 from the control group. There was no significant difference between groups concerning the grades of mucositis on day 8 or on day 15.

Although the dose of 4 J/cm^2 appears to be within the therapeutic window, it is not. The energy per point was only 0.18 J. The seemingly reasonable dose is achieved by using a very thin fibre.

In a study by Arun Maiya [1727], patients with carcinoma of the oral cavity with stages II-IV, being uniformly treated with a curative total tumour dose of 66 Gy in 33 fractions over six weeks, were selected for the study. The patients were divided based on computer generated randomisation into laser (study group) and control groups, with 25 patients in each group. Both study and control groups were comparable in terms of the site of the lesion, the stage of the cancer and the histology. The study group's patients were treated with HeNe laser, output of 10mW, and the control group's patients were given oral analgesics, local application of anaesthetics, 0.9% saline and povidine wash during the course of radiotherapy. All patients tolerated the laser treatment without any adverse effects or reactions. The result showed a significant difference in pain and mucositis between the two groups. At the end of

reduce discomfort to a great extent, and administering LPT prophylactically before the treatment could also alleviate the problems.

Cowen [575] used a HeNe laser in the prevention of oral mucositis in patients undergoing bone marrow transplant in a double-blind randomized trial. Significant reduction of the radiation-induced oral mucositis was reported using a 60 mW HeNe laser.

Barasch [611] treated 20 patients subjected to bone marrow transplantation and receiving mucositis-inducing medications. One side of the mouth received HeNe laser irradiation, the other one sham irradiation. Oral mucositis and pain scores were significantly lower for the treated side compared with the untreated side.

In a double-blind phase III study by Bensadoun [929], 30 patients were about to receive radiotherapy for head and neck neoplasms. With conventional fractionation (2 Gy/day, 5 fractions per week), mucositis becomes evident in the third week of irradiation and progresses to confluent mucositis. The severity of mucositis is a major problem in head and neck radiotherapy. In this study, patients in the laser group received HeNe laser irradiation daily (Monday to Friday) during the seven weeks of radiotherapy, prior to each fraction. Nine points in the oropharyngeal area were irradiated, 2 J/cm^2. Except for the first week of treatment, daily grade of mucositis was higher in the non-laser group, the difference being statistically significant for weeks four, five, six and seven. In particular, the number of weeks in which patients had grade 3 mucositis was reduced. Pain was also reduced in the laser group and the ability to swallow improved.

The phase III randomized double-blind placebo-controlled study by Schubert [1805] was designed to compare the ability of 2 different GaAlAs lasers (650 nm and 780 nm) to prevent oral mucositis in HCT patients conditioned with chemotherapy or chemoradiotherapy. A total of 70 patients were enrolled and randomized into one of three treatment groups: 650 nm laser, 780 nm laser, or placebo. All active laser treatment patients received daily direct laser treatment to the lower labial mucosa, right and left buccal mucosa, lateral and ventral surfaces of the tongue, and floor of the mouth with energy densities of 2 J/cm^2. Study treatment began on the first day of conditioning and continued through the day +2 post HCT. Mucositis and oral pain were measured on days 0, 4, 7, 11, 14, 18, and 21 post HCT. The 650 nm wavelength reduced the severity of oral mucositis and pain scores, whereas the 780 nm laser group was less effective. LPT was well-tolerated and no adverse events were noted.

Antunes [1782] investigated the clinical effects of LPT on the prevention and reduction of severity of conditioning-induced oral mucositis (OM) for hematopoietic stem cell transplantation (HSCT). Altogether 38 patients who underwent autologous (AT) or allogeneic (AL) HSCT were randomized into groups. A laser at 660 nm, 50 mW, and 4 J/cm^2, measured at the fiberoptic end with 0.196 /cm^2 of section area was used. The evaluation of OM was done using the Oral Assessment Scale (OMAS) and the World Health Orga-

spot size 3 mm2. Cryotherapy was done positioning ice packs in the hamster mucosa 5 min before 5-FU infusion and 10 min afterwards. To study the healing of mucositis, the left pouch mucosa of each hamster in the TLG received laser irradiation on the injured area. Irradiation parameters were kept the same as mentioned above. The control hamsters in the TCG did not receive any treatment. The mucositis degree and the animal's body mass were evaluated. An assessment of blood vessels was made based on immunohistochemical staining. The CG animals lost 15.16% of their initial body mass while the LG animals lost 8.97% during the first five days. The laser treated animals had a better clinical outcome with a faster healing, and more granulation tissue. The quantity of blood vessels in both the LG and CG were higher than in healthy mucosa. Regarding the therapeutic analysis, the severity of the mucositis in the TLG was always lower than in the TCG. TLG presented a higher organization of the granulation tissue, parallel collagen fibrils, and an increased angiogenesis.

Clinical studies

Skobelkin [2] compared the effect of HeNe and infrared 890 nm irradiation in 60 oncologic patients. The irradiation was delivered during the immediate preoperative period. Parameters analysed were cell components of the blood: behaviour of T-lymphocyte fractions and immunoglobulin activity. The total immunoresponse increased following LPT, with no visible increase in the tumoral remnant size. The 890 nm laser was more effective.

Podolskaya [366] has used HeNe lasers on post-radiation reactions and injuries in lip skin and mucous membranes (post-radiation heilitis). The method has been more successful than previously used medical treatments. There were no complications in the laser group, while the traditionally treated group had several allergic reactions and reoperations. The pace of epithelialisation was 7 mm/week in the HeNe group, as compared with 4.1 mm/week in the control group.

In a study by Schaffer [907], three women with painful mastitis from irradiation after breast cancer with ionising radiation, and a male with a radiation ulcer, were treated with GaAlAs laser 780 nm, 5 J/cm^2. The healing of the ulcers was controlled using MRI measurement before and after treatment. In all patients, a complete clinical remission was noted following LPT. The results were confirmed by a decrease in inflammatory changes as depicted in MRI imaging.

The same indication is reported by Schindl [967]. Three patients with radiation ulcers following breast cancer therapy were treated with HeNe laser, 30 J/cm^2, three times weekly. At the 36-month control, no patient showed any recurrence of the radiation ulcers or neoplasm.

Pourreau-Schneider [46] used a HeNe laser to reduce the oral side-effects of fluorouracil. The drug causes painful mucositis, which in turn causes eating problems. The mucositis dictates the limit for the dosage of fluorouracil (dose limiting factor). The use of a HeNe laser was shown to

60, which was applied in a single dose of 3000 cGy on the femur. The laser groups received seven applications with a 48-h interval in four points per session of $DE = 4$ J/cm^2, $P = 40$ mW, $t = 100$ sec, with a beam diameter of 0.04 cm^2. All animals were killed six weeks after radiotherapy. Clinical examination revealed cutaneous erosions on experimental groups (II, III, and IV) starting at the sixth week after radiotherapy. The radiographic findings showed higher bone density in groups II and IV compared to the control group. The results further showed an increase of bone marrow cells, and number of osteocytes and Haversian canals in experimental groups II and IV. Further findings disclosed an increase of osteoblastic activity in groups II, III, and IV. LPT on bone tissue in rats presented a positive biostimulative effect, especially when applied before or four weeks after radiotherapy. However, the use of laser in the parameters above should be used with caution due to epithelial erosions.

The aim of a study by Desmons [1924] was to investigate the effect of laser preconditioning on the re-vascularisation of X-ray irradiated bone. A bone chamber was implanted onto the calvaria of rabbits to study the vascularisation process. Digital pictures were taken of the vascular plexus at the target bone site using a modified digital camera. Vascular density (VD) was determined using image processing. It was defined as the ratio of blood vessel pixels to the total number of pixels in the region of interest. Laser preconditioning was performed with a diode laser (810 nm, 2 W, 3 seconds, 48 J/cm^2, 4 mm). A 12-week follow-up study was performed on 20 rabbits divided into four groups: No 1: control group (n = 5), No 2: laser irradiation alone (n = 5), No 3: X-ray radiation (18.75 Gy) alone (n = 5), No 4: laser preconditioning 24 hours prior to X-ray radiation (n = 5). Vascular density remained stable during the 12-week follow up for group No 1. No significant difference was observed between laser irradiation group (No 2) and control group (No 1). The angiolytic action of X-ray radiation was confirmed in groups 3 and 4, which were statistically different from group 1. However, the decrease of the vascularisation was limited in group 4, highlighting a different evolution between group 3 and 4. These results were confirmed by histological analysis. The bone chamber is an effective reproducible method for the longitudinal analysis of the dynamics of vascularisation. These findings have shown that laser preconditioning is capable of preserving vascularisation in an X-ray irradiated bone site, thus suggesting a novel approach for promoting the healing of bone tissue in which the vascular supply has been damaged.

França [1990] divided a group of hamsters into four groups: preventive cryotherapy, preventive laser, therapeutic laser and therapeutic control group. Mucositis was induced in hamsters by an intraperitoneal injection of 5-fluorouracil (5-FU) and superficial scratching. All preventive treatment was performed on the right cheek pouch mucosa. The left pouch mucosa was used for a spontaneous development of mucositis and did not receive any preventive therapy. Laser parameters were: 660 nm, 30 mW, 1.2 J/cm^2, 40 s,

gether 26 rats with implanted Walker carcinosarcoma, 75 with cancer of the mammary glands (implanted) and 188 animals with spontaneous cancer of the mammary glands were used in the study. LPT promoted dystrophic and necrotic changes in the tumoral nodes.

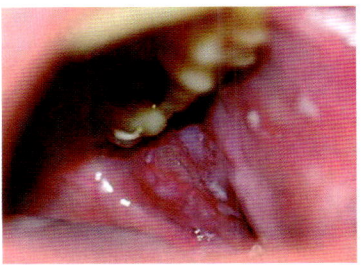 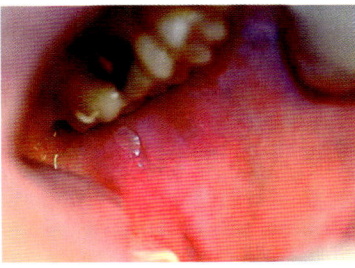

Figure 4.2 Mucositis at day 1 of treatment and at day 6
Courtesy: Alyne Simões

Humzah [286] has used GaAs in cases of neoplastic ulceration with some response.

In a study by Lara [1783], 44 rats were treated with fluorouracil and, in order to mimic the clinical effect of chronic irritation, the palatal mucosa was irritated by superficial scratching with an 18-gauge needle. When all of the rats presented oral ulcers of mucositis, they were randomly allocated to one of three groups: group I was treated with laser (GaAlAs), group II was treated with topical dexamethasone, and group III was not treated. Excisional biopsies of the palatal mucosa were then performed, and the rats were killed. Tissue sections were stained with haematoxylin and eosin for morphological analyses, and with toluidine blue for mast-cell counts. Group I specimens showed higher prevalence of ulcers, bacterial biofilm, necrosis and vascularisation, while group II specimens showed higher prevalence of granulation tissue formation. There were no significant statistical differences in the numbers of mast cells and epithelial thickness between groups. For the present model of mucositis, rats with palatal mucositis treated with laser showed characteristics compatible with the ulcerative phase of oral mucositis, and rats treated with topical dexamethasone showed characteristics compatible with the healing phase of mucositis. Topical dexamethasone was more efficient in the treatment of rats' oral mucositis than the laser.

The aim of the study by da Cunha [1812] was to investigate the effect of LPT (780 nm) on bone tissue submitted to ionizing radiation. Twenty-two Wistar rats were randomly divided into four groups: group I, control (n = 4), submitted only to radiotherapy; group II, laser treatment starting one day prior to radiotherapy (n = 6); group III, laser treatment starting immediately after radiotherapy (n = 6); group IV, laser treatment starting four weeks after radiotherapy (n = 6). The source of ionizing radiation used was Cobalt

activity in the osteoblast line was increased after 830 nm laser irradiation at 10 J/cm^2, whereas ALP activity in the osteosarcoma line was not altered, regardless of laser wavelength or intensity. Based on the conditions of this study, the authors conclude that each cell line responds differently to specific wavelength and dose combinations.

The aim of an investigation by Powell [2039] was to compare the cell proliferative effects of a range of doses of LPT at wavelengths of 780, 830 and 904 nm on human breasts and immortalised human mammary epithelial cell lines in vitro. LPT is used in the clinical treatment of post-mastectomy lymphoedema, despite safety information being limited and circumstantial. This research was the first step in systematically developing guidelines for the safe clinical use of LPT in the management of post-mastectomy lymphoedema. Human breast adenocarcinoma (MCF-7), human breast ductal carcinoma (MDA-MB-435S) and immortalised human mammary epithelial (SVCT and Bre80hTERT) cell lines were irradiated with a single exposure of laser at 0.5, 1, 2, 3, 4, 10 and 12 J/cm^2 (780 nm) and 0.5, 1, 2, 3, 4, 10 and 15 J/cm2 (830 and 904 nm). MCF-7 cells were further irradiated with two and three exposures of all three laser wavelengths. XTT colorimetric assays were utilized to assess cell proliferation 24 hours after irradiation. SVCT cell proliferation significantly increased after exposure to a range of doses at 780 and 904 nm irradiation. MDA-MB-435S and Bre80hTERT cell lines showed negligible effects from one exposure of all three wavelengths and no dose response relationships were noted. MCF-7 cells irradiated with 780 nm laser demonstrated an increasing dose response relationship after one exposure and a decreasing dose response relationship after three exposures. The MCF-7 cells irradiated with 904 nm laser demonstrated a decreasing dose response relationship after two and three exposures. Despite certain doses of laser increasing MCF-7 cell proliferation, multiple exposures had no effect, or a decreasing effect, on dose response relationships. Acc. to the authors, before a definitive conclusion can be made regarding the safety of LPT for post-mastectomy lymphoedema, further in vivo research must be conducted.

Animal studies

In a study by Pavlova [774], the main goal was to establish the capability of laser to oppose the free radical oxidative chain reactions inherent in the effects of radiation. Adequate doses of laser were shown to produce positive effects upon the metabolism similar to those of pharmacologic radioprotectors.

A study by Korolev [1214] showed that exposure of rat adrenals 30 days after radiation (1 Gy) to infrared laser radiation arrested the development of ultrastructural disorders in the cells of the hypothalamus and the parathyroid gland, and enhanced subcellular manifestations of adaptation and rehabilitation processes.

Mikhailov [3] states that an 890 nm diode laser produces a tumorostatic effect at minimal power, while higher doses produce other effects. Alto-

effect to induce the checkpoint mechanisms, which are normally responsible for altering cell cycle progression.

The aim of this study by Mognato [1454] was to investigate the effects of different wavelengths and doses of laser radiation on in vitro cell proliferation. Two human cancer cell lines, HeLa (epithelial adenocarcinoma) and TK6 (lymphoblast) were used. Attention was focused on the combination of the two laser emissions, as it could have a synergic effect greater than the single emissions applied separately. A laser device was used for cell irradiation with a continuous wave diode (808 nm), a pulsed wave diode (905 nm), and a combination of wave diodes (808 nm + 905 nm), in the dose range of 1-60 J/cm^2. The effect of the combined 808-905 nm laser irradiation was slightly superior to that achieved with either laser alone in HeLa cells. TK6 cellular proliferation was not found to be significantly affected by any of the energy levels and the varying exposure doses investigated. These results are a confirmation of previous [1399] observations carried out on human cells, where only the proliferation of slowly growing cell populations appeared to be stimulated by laser light. HeLa cells grow slower than TK6 cells. The fact that laser stimulates slowly growing cells better than fast growing cells (cancer) may be an important aspect of LPT.

Effects of combined exposure to a 633 nm laser and gamma-radiation, and laser and protons with the energy of 150 MeV, on the survivabilty of mice fibroblast cells C3H10T1/2 were compared in a study by Voskanian [1811]. Cell suspension was distributed in 2-ml plastic vials with 1 cm in diameter. The time interval between two exposures in a combination was no more than 60 s. Immediately after exposure, a required quantity of cells was inoculated in special vials for survivability assessment. Based on results of the experiment, preliminary and repeated laser treatment was favourable to the survivability of fibroblast cells subjected to gamma- or proton irradiation (dose variation factor was within 1.3 to 2.2). Simultaneous exposure of C3H10T1/2 cells to the laser and proton beams also increased their survivability. The radioprotective effect of the HeNe laser on fibroblasts earlier exposed to ionizing radiation is of chief interest, as most of the present-day radioprotectors are effective only if introduced into the organism prior to exposure.

The aim of a study by Renno [1869] was to investigate the effects of 670, 780 and 830 nm laser irradiation on cell proliferation of normal primary osteoblast (MC3T3) and malignant osteosarcoma (MG63) cell lines in vitro. Neonatal murine calvarial osteoblastic and human osteosarcoma cell lines were studied. A single laser irradiation was performed at three different wavelengths, at the energies of 0.5, 1, 5, and 10 J/cm^2. Twenty-four hours after laser irradiation, cell proliferation and alkaline phosphatase assays were assessed. Osteoblast proliferation increased significantly after 830 nm laser irradiation (at 10 J/cm^2), but decreased after 780 nm laser irradiation (at 1, 5, and 10 J/cm^2). Osteosarcoma cell proliferation increased significantly after 670 nm (at 5 J/cm^2) and 780 nm laser irradiation (at 1, 5, and 10 J/cm^2), but not after 830 nm laser irradiation. Alkaline phosphatase (ALP)

beam cross section 1 mm at local light doses between 0.04 and 4.8 J/cm^2). For 670 nm, significant differences in the proliferation were observed between the two concentrations of FBS and between irradiated cultures and controls. Although the results were not significant, 635 nm irradiated cells also proliferated more than non-irradiated ones. This occurred under both conditions of nutrition. It was concluded, that irradiation with 670 nm laser light applied at doses between 0.04 and 4.8 J/cm^2 could significantly increase proliferation of laryngeal cancer cells.

Tamachi [44] has studied the uptake of 5Fluorouracil (5FU) in various experiments using rats. Laboratory rats that received 6 J/cm^2 of HeNe showed a greater uptake of 5FU than those that were given 5FU only.

Konchugova [214] studied whether LPT, under experimental conditions, could be used to increase cyclophosphamide-developed immune suppression. The experiment suggests that LPT can be used to reduce the therapeutic dosage and its consequent negative side effects.

Ulrich [489] summarises a rodent experiment: 1) Single doses of 830 nm light (1J and 100 J/cm^2) do not stimulate or inhibit growth of rhabdomyosarcomas R1H. 2) Fractionated treatment of R1H tumours with 15 or 1500 J/cm^2 for three weeks does not alter the growth kinetics in comparison to untreated controls. 3) Histological findings showed an increase of tumour necrosis after fractionated irradiation with 1500 J/cm^2.

The aim of a study by Kreisler [1567] was to investigate the effect of 809 nm laser irradiation on the proliferation rate of human larynx carcinoma cells in vitro. Epithelial tumor cells were obtained from a laryngeal carcinoma and cultured under standard conditions. For laser treatment the cells were spread on 96-well tissue culture plates. Sixty-six cell cultures were irradiated with an 809 nm GaAlAs laser. Another 66 served as controls. Power output was 10 mW (CW) and the time of exposure 75-300 s per well, corresponding to an energy fluence of 1.96-7.84 J/cm^2. Subsequent to laser treatment, the cultures were incubated for 72 h. The irradiated cells revealed a considerably higher proliferation activity. The differences were highly significant up to 72 h after irradiation.

Joyce [1016] has investigated the potential ability of LPT to induce an adaptive response against the damaging effects of ionising radiation in Indian muntjac fibroblasts. LPT at 660, but not 820 nm, at 11.5 and 23.0 J/cm^2, induced an apparent adaptive response in the form of a reduction in the frequency of radiation-induced chromosome aberrations, but not in cell survival. There was also a trend towards a reduction in the level of single-stranded and double-stranded DNA breaks induced by ionising radiation when cells were preconditioned with LPT. However, this did not contribute to the reduced chromosome aberration frequency. Further analysis revealed that the reduced aberration frequency was caused by a laser-induced extension of G2 delay. The adaptive response was therefore the result of cell cycle modulation by LPT at a wavelength where there is no known DNA damaging

malignant cells. Furthermore, LPT in general would be impossible to use if the condition would be a thorough cancer examination before each treatment.

The following studies approach several aspects of oncology; the actual *in vitro* effect on malignant cells, some clinical observations, the radioprotective effect of LPT and the therapeutic effect on the side effects of chemo- and radiotherapy (mucositis). The conclusion is that there is strong scientific support for the use of LPT as a protective and therapeutic method for patients scheduled for chemo- och radiotherapy.

78-year-old patient treated for oropharyngeal carcinoma with external radiotherapy. Acute grade 3 dermatitis at 60 Gy (5 x 2 Gy per week). The same patient after three sessions of HeNe irradiation, 25 mW, 4 J/cm^2 in scanning mode.

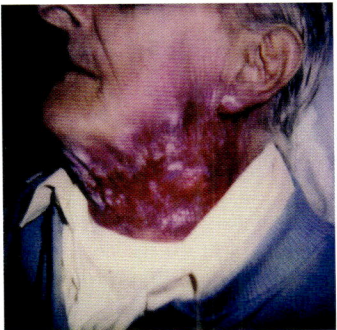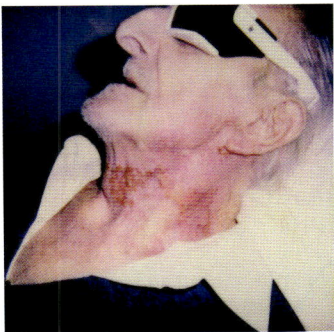

Figure 4.1 Radiation-induced dermatitis before and after HeNe therapy.
Courtesy: René-Jean Bensadoun

Literature:
In vitro studies

Schaffer [594] irradiated four cell cultures with 805 nm laser light with fluences between 0 and 20 J/cm^2. The cell types were (1) murine skeletal myotubes, (2) normal urothelial cells, (3) human squamous carcinoma cells of the gingival mucosa, and (4) urothelial carcinoma cells. The mitotic index of 1, 2, and 4 increased at a fluence of 4 J/cm^2, whereas a fluence of 20 J/cm^2 resulted in a slight decrease. The no. 3 cell culture showed a decrease of the mitotic index at both fluences. No differences could be observed if the power density was varied between 10 mW/cm^2 and 150 mW/cm^2.

The aim of a study by Pinheiro [1211] was to assess the effect of 635 nm and 670 nm laser irradiation on H.Ep.2 cells in vitro using MTT. It was decided to evaluate the effect of increased doses of laser light on these cells. The cells were obtained from SCC of the larynx. The cultures were kept either at 5% or 10% of FBS. Twenty-four hours after transplantation, the cells were irradiated with laser light (5 mW diode lasers; 635 and 670 nm;

4.1.9 Cancer

As explained previously, LPT does not cause cancer. There are, on the contrary, some indications that cancer tumours in their initial stage can be positively influenced (i.e. to the patient's benefit) by LPT. The mechanism at work here is thought to be the general stimulation of the immune system. In the same way as bacteria and viruses, cancer cells can be stimulated *in vitro* [594] but generally not *in vivo* due to the presence of the immune system.

LPT has also been shown to ease the symptoms of cancer patients who have received chemo- and/or radiation therapy resulting in oral side-effects (mucositis). This is an example of the use of LPT in oncology where the cancer itself is not treated, but rather the side effects of the cancer therapy [907,967]. LPT can also, to advantage, be given as a palliative measure to cancer patients in the terminal stage. Mucositis occurs in about 40% of patients receiving chemotherapy, in 80% of those receiving bone marrow transplants and in 100% of those receiving radiotherapy to the head and neck, if the oral cavity is in the irradiated field. Younger patients have a higher incidence of oral complications than older patients receiving similar oncologic treatment [1472]. The type of intraoral local point irradiation now practiced is rather time consuming but compared to the cost of extra days of hospitalisation cost effective - the suffering of the patients not even being considered.

The radioprotective effect of laser light was discovered very early. In a paper from 1966 by McGuff [1856], human adenocarcinomas were implanted in the cheek pouch of hamsters. Roentgen radiation of 1000 r was found to be inhibitory to the tumor growth. Ruby laser irradiation of 214 J proved to have an even better effect. In a following experiment, roentgen and laser energies were reduced to 50% and given at the same time. This proved to further improve the outcome of the therapy, providing a synergistic effect. McGuff et al performed several studies during 1965-1966 [1853-1859] with very interesting effects on various tumors. Different energies were used but, unfortunately, the authors have not been specific about optimal doses, only dose ranges. Although published in well-known scientific journals, these observations seem to have fallen into oblivion.

Recent and ongoing research [986,1081] has shown that low doses of irradiation, ionising as well as non-ionising, can protect the cells if the low-dose irradiation is given prior to radiation therapy [1016,1214,1773,1778,1811,1812]. This radioprotective ability of LPT deserves further attention in oncology.

It should, again, be underlined that cancer therapy is the sole concern of the specialist. Patients with known malignancies in an area otherwise suitable for LPT should not be treated with LPT by anyone but the specialist. A concern sometimes raised is that we cannot be certain that there is no unknown malignancy in the area selected for LPT. The answer is that the immune stimulation is likely to override the possible stimulation of the

plete after six months, with or without laser. Early comparisons would be more appropriate in order to determine the possible effect of LPT.

González [1552] reports that 26 ortognathic surgery patients were operated by one and the same surgeon and with laser applied to the right side only. The irradiation was carried out postop for 10 sessions. At four and eight weeks postop, biopsies were taken in five patients and sent for blinded histological evaluation. At six weeks, X-rays confirmed a better bone condensation on the irradiated side. The biopsies showed higher fibroblastic activity, dense collagenisation and less inflammation on the irradiated side.

Necrosis of the jawbone has been described in association with systemic bisphosphonate therapy with drugs including zoledronic acid, pamidronate, and alendronate. The extent and clinical characteristics of bisphosphonate-associated osteonecrosis (BON) of the jaw are extremely variable, and range from the presence of fistulae in the oral mucosa or orofacial tissues, to large exposed areas of necrotic bone within the oral cavity. Clinical signs and symptoms commonly reported include pain, swelling, the presence of pus, loose teeth, ill-fitting dentures, and paresthesias of the inferior alveolar nerve when the necrosis affects the mandible. Fractures have also been reported. The treatment of BON of the jaw is still controversial since no therapy has proven to be efficacious as shown by the literature on the subject. In a study by Vescovi [2014], researchers report results achieved in 28 patients affected by BON of the jaw, and who received treatment by the Nd:YAG laser alone, or in combination with conventional medical or surgical treatments. Clinical variables such as severity of symptoms, presence of pus, and closure of mucosal flaps before and after therapy were evaluated to establish the effectiveness of laser irradiation. The 28 patients with BON were subdivided into four groups: 8 patients were treated with medical therapy only (antibiotics with or without antimycotics and/or antiseptic rinses), 6 patients were treated with medical and surgical therapy (necrotic bone removal and bone curettage), 6 patients were treated with medical therapy associated with laser biostimulation, and 8 patients were treated with medical therapy associated with both surgical therapy and laser biostimulation. Of the 14 patients who underwent laser biostimulation, 9 reported complete clinical success (no pain, symptoms of infection, or exposed bone or draining fistulas), and 3 improved their symptomatology only, with follow-ups between months four and seven. While the results reported in this study are not conclusive, they indicate that LPT has potential to improve management of BON.

A review of the literature on laser bone stimulation has been published by Barber [1253], Pinheiro [1920] and Bashardoust Tajali [1889].

Further literature: [213, 258, 413, 414, 430, 437, 438, 439, 440, 466, 484, 516, 642, 962, 1117, 1194, 1238, 1299, 1301, 1309, 1331, 1465, 1764, 1843, 1994]

Further reading: chapter 5.3.12 "Implantology" on page 411.

were greater in rabbits that were given LPT. Crystallinity and the chemical composition of the bone at the distraction osteogenesis site were similar to the that of the control group. The results showed that LPT had a positive effect on the biomodulation of newly formed bone.

The objective of a study by Kazem Shakouri [2054] was to evaluate the effect of LPT on fracture healing. Thirty rabbits were subjected to tibial bone open osteotomies that were stabilized with external fixators. The animals were divided into two study groups: laser group and control group. Callus development and bone mineral density were quantitatively evaluated by CT; the animals were then killed and the fractures were assessed for biomechanical properties. The results demonstrated that the increasing rate of bone mineral density was higher in the laser (L) group than in the control (C) group. CT at 5 weeks revealed a mean callus density of 297 Hounsfield units (HU) for the control group and 691 HU for the L group, which was statistically significant. In the L group, the mean recorded fracture tension was 190.5 N and 359.3 N for healed and intact bones, respectively, which was statistically significant. The result of the study showed that the use of laser could enhance callus development in the early stage of the healing process, with doubtful improvement in biomechanical properties of the healing bone.

Murine bone marrow cells, which contain both osteoblast and osteoclast progenitors, were cultured and induced to differentiate in the absence or in the presence of LPT in a study by Bouvet-Gerbettaz [2055]. Laser exposition parameters were determined using a power meter and consisted in an 808 nm light in CW mode, with an energy density of 4 J/cm^2 administered three times a week. Cell proliferation and differentiation were assessed after specific staining and microscopic analysis of the cultures after various times, as well as by quantitative RT-PCR analysis of a panel of osteoblast and osteoclast markers after nucleic acid extraction. The use of a power meter revealed that the power emitted by the optical fiber of the laser device was markedly reduced compared to the displayed power. This allowed to adjust the LPT parameters to a final energy density exposure of 4 J/cm^2. In these conditions, proliferation of bone marrow mesenchymal stem cells as well as osteoclast or osteoblast differentiation of the corresponding progenitors were found similar in control and LPT conditions. Using the present experimental protocol, the authors concluded that an 808 nm wavelength infrared LPT does not alter murine bone progenitor cell proliferation and differentiation. **Moreover these results confirm the necessary use of a power meter to fix LPT protocol parameters.**

Clinical studies

In a clinical study by Kucerová [1042], the bone density after tooth extraction was measured by digital X-ray. The images taken immediately after extraction and six months later were compared between laser and non-laser patients. There was no difference between these patients at six months. **This is hardly surprising, since the remodeling of bone is more or less com-**

A study by Pinheiro [1881] assessed histologically the effect of laser on the repair of surgical defects created in the femurs of treated and non-treated Wistar rats with bone morphogenetic proteins (BMPs) and organic bovine bone graft. A total of 48 adult male Wistar rats were divided into four randomized groups: group 1 (controls, n=12); group 2 (laser, n=12); group 3 (BMPs + organic bovine bone graft + GBR, n=12); and group 4 (BMPs + organic bovine bone graft + GBR + laser, n=12). The irradiated groups received seven irradiations every 48 h, the first immediately after the surgical procedure. Laser (830 nm, 40 mW, CW, 0.6 mm) consisted of a total of 16 J/cm^2 per session at four points (4 J/cm^2 each) equally spaced around the periphery of the defect. The animals were sacrificed after 15, 21, and 30 days, and the specimens were routinely embedded in wax and stained with hematoxylin and eosin and Sirius red stains and analyzed under light microscopy. The results showed histological evidence of increased deposition of collagen fibers (on days 15 and 21), as well as an increased amount of well-organized bone trabeculi at the end of the experimental period (day 30) in irradiated animals compared to non-irradiated controls.

The aim of the paper by Almeida-Lopes [2036] was to search for the best application fluency and emission mode, using an infrared laser in the repair of bone defects in the rat tibia. Thus, the histological quality of the neoformed bone was evaluated by analysis using common optic microscopy and polarized light. Application parameters: 100 mW, 830 nm, laser beam diameter = 0,06 nm, CW and 10 Hz, three sessions with 72 h intervals, energies and respective fluencies: 2J =70 J/cm^2, 4J =140 J/cm^2, 6J =210 J/cm^2, 8J =160 J/cm^2, 10 =200 J/cm^2. Conclusions: Laser therapy has increased and sped up the time bone repairing process (in the initial period of 10 days). This laser effect showed to be dose-dependent with the presence of an effective therapeutic window presenting biostimulation of the bone tissue between a total energy of 4J and 8 J for both emission modes. The use of the laser with 10 J of energy generated, characterized by the bioinhibition of the tissues (in the initial period of 10 days). This inhibition took place at the exact irradiation spot.

A study by Hübler [2053] evaluated the effect of LPT on the chemical composition, crystallinity and crystalline structure of bone at the site of distraction osteogenesis. Five rabbits were subjected to distraction osteogenesis (latency=3 days; rate and frequency=0.7 mm/day for 7 days; consolidation=10 days), and three were given LPT with 830 nm, 40 mW): 10 J/cm^2 dose per spot, applied directly to the distraction osteogenesis site during the consolidation stage at 48 h intervals. Samples were harvested at the end of the consolidation stage. X-ray fluorescence and X-ray diffraction were used to analyze chemical composition, crystallinity and crystalline structure of bone at the distraction osteogenesis site. The analysis of chemical composition and calcium and phosphorus ratios revealed greater mineralization in the LPT group. Diffractograms showed that the crystalline structure of the samples was similar to that of hydroxyapatites. Crystallinity percentages

with the following parameters: 15 mW, exposition time of 17 sec, 0.025 cm^2 irradiated area, and energy density of 10 J/cm^2. Square full-thickness skin samples (18 mm each side, including both injured and non-injured tissues) were obtained 4, 7, and 15 days after surgery and analyzed by qualitative and quantitative histological methods. Quantitative histopathological analysis confirmed the results of the qualitative analysis through histological microscope slides. When comparing tissue components (inflammatory cells, vessels and fibroblast/area), the authors found that treated animals had a less intense inflammatory process than controls.

Because bone healing at the graft site is similar to that of a fracture repair, the purpose of the study by da Silva [1762] was to evaluate the effects of laser irradiation on the repair of rat skull defects treated with autogenous bone graft. A defect measuring 3 mm in diameter was produced in the left parietal bone and filled with an autogenous bone graft obtained from the right parietal bone. The animals were divided into three groups of 20 rats each: non-irradiated control, irradiated with 5.1 J/cm^2, and irradiated with 10.2 J/cm^2. The laser (2.4 mW, 735 nm, 3.4 x 10 W/cm, 3 mm spot size) was applied three times per week for four weeks. A greater volume of newly formed bone was observed in the irradiated group treated with 10.2 J/cm^2. In both irradiated groups, a greater volume of newly formed bone occurred only in the first two weeks.

The purpose of a study by Liu [1876] was to demonstrate the biological effects of LPT on tibial fractures, using radiographic, histological and bone density examinations. A total of 14 white rabbits with surgically induced mid-tibial osteotomies were included in the study; 7 were assigned to a group receiving LPT (LPT-A) and the remaining 7 served as a sham-treated control group (LPT-C). A 830 nm laser and a sham laser (a similar design without laser diodes) were used for the study. Continuous irradiation with a total energy density of 40 J/cm^2 and a power of 200 mW/cm^2 was directly delivered to the skin for 50 seconds at four points along the tibial fracture site. Treatment commenced immediately postsurgery and continued once daily for four weeks. Radiographic findings revealed no statistically significant fracture callus thickness difference between the LPT-A and LPT-C groups. However, the fractures in the LPT-A group showed less callus thickness than those in LPT-C group three weeks after treatment. The average tibial volume was 14.5 mL in the LPT-A group, and 11.25 mL in the LPT-C group. The average contralateral normal tibial volume was 7.1 mL. Microscopic changes at 4 weeks revealed an average grade of 5.5 and 5.0 for the LPT-A group and the LPT-C group, respectively. The bone mineral density (BMD) as ascertained using a grey scale (graded from 0 to 256) showed darker coloration in the LPT-A group (138) than in the LPT-C group (125). The study suggests that LPT may accelerate the process of fracture repair or cause increases in callus volume and BMD, especially in the early stages of absorbing the hematoma and bone remodeling.

trol group. Notably, in the association between laser and bisphosphonate, the trabecular bone volume was significantly greater in vertebrae L2 and T13 and similar to that in the sham-operated control group. It was concluded that the laser therapy combined with bisphosphonate treatment was the best method for reversing vertebral osteopenia caused by the ovariectomy.

The aim of a study by Matsumoto [1922] was to analyze the role of cyclo-oxygenase-2 following bone repair in rats submitted to LPT. A total of 48 rats underwent surgery to inflict bone defects in their tibias after being randomly distributed into two groups: negative control, and a laser exposed group, i.e., the animals were treated with LPT by means of gallium arsenide laser at 16 J/cm^2. The animals were killed after 48 h, 7 days, 14 days, or 21 days. The tibias were removed for morphological, morphometric, and immunohistochemistry analysis for cyclo-oxygenase-2. Statistical significant differences were observed in the quality of bone repair and quantity of formed bone between groups 14 days after surgery. In the same way, cyclo-oxygenase-2 immunoreactivity was more intense in bone cells for intermediate periods evaluated in the laser exposed group. Taken together, such results suggest that LPT is able to improve bone repair in the tibia of rats 14 days after surgery as a result of an up-regulation for cyclo-oxygenase-2 expression in bone cells.

A study by Liriani-Galvao [1645] aimed to compare the consequences of LPT and low-intensity pulsed ultrasound (LIPUS) on bone repair. Many studies have assessed the effects of LPT and LIPUS on bone repair, but a comparison of them is rare. Male Wistar rats (n=8) with tibial bone osteotomy were used. One group had the osteotomized limb treated with LPT (780 nm, 30 mW, 112.5 J/cm^2) and the second group with LIPUS (1.5 MHz, 30 mW/cm^2), both for 12 sessions (five times per week); a third group was the control. After 20 days, rats were sacrificed and had their tibias submitted to a bending test or histomorphometric analysis. In the bending test, maximum load at failure of the LPT group was significantly higher. Bone histomorphometry revealed a significant increase in osteoblast number and surface, and osteoid volume in the LPT group, and a significant increase in eroded and osteoclast surfaces in the LIPUS group. In conclusion LIPUS enhanced bone repair by promoting bone resorption in the osteotomy area, while LPT accelerated this process through bone formation.

The aim of a study by Rabelo [1887] was to compare the effect of LPT on the wound healing process in non-diabetic and diabetic rats. Among the clinical symptoms caused by diabetes mellitus, a delay in wound healing is a potential risk for patients. It is suggested that LPT can improve wound healing. The tissue used for this study was extracted from animals suffering from diabetes, which was induced by Streptozotocin, and from non-diabetic rats. Animals were divided into two groups of 25 rats each (treated and control) and further subdivided into two groups: diabetic (n=15) and non-diabetic (n=10). A full-thickness skin wound was made on the dorsum area, with a round 8-mm holepunch. The treated group was irradiated by a HeNe laser

intermediate zones in the regenerated bone, at all time periods. The formation of a complete inferior border occurred sooner in the treatment group than in the controls.

The aim of a study by Renno [1760] was to investigate the effects of 830 nm, used in two doses, on femora of osteopenic rats. Sixty female animals, divided into six groups, were used: sham-operated control (SC), osteopenic control (OC), sham-operated irradiated at a dose of 120 J/cm^2 (I120), osteopenic irradiated at a dose of 120 J/cm^2 (O120), sham-operated irradiated at a dose of 60 J/cm^2 (I60), and osteopenic irradiated at a dose of 60 J/cm^2 (O60). Animals were 90 days old when operated. Laser irradiation was initiated eight weeks after operation, and it was performed three times a week for two months. Femora were submitted to a biomechanical test and to a physical properties evaluation. Maximal load of O120 did not show any difference when compared with SC and I120, but it was higher than the O60 group. Wet weight, dry weight, and bone volume of O60 and O120 did not show any difference when compared with SC. The results of the study indicate that laser phototherapy had stimulatory effects on femora of osteopenic rats, mainly at the dose of 120 J/cm^2

Osteoporosis affects 30% of postmenopausal women, and it has been recognized as a major public health problem. Based on the stimulatory effects of LPT on proliferation of bone cells found in the study above, Renno [1761] hypothesized that LPT would be efficient in preventing bone mass loss in ovariectomied (OVX) rats. Forty female rats were divided into four groups: sham-operated control (SC), OVX control (OC), sham-operated irradiated at a dose of 120 J/cm^2 (I120), and OVX irradiated at a dose of 120 J/cm^2 (O120). Animals were operated at the age of 90 days. Laser irradiation was initiated one day after the operation and was performed three times a week for two months. Femora were submitted to a biomechanical test and a physical properties evaluation. Maximal load of O120 was higher than in control groups. Wet weight, dry weight, and bone volume of O120 did not show any difference when compared with SC. The results of this study indicate that LPT was able to prevent bone loss after OVX in rats.

The purpose of a study by Diniz [1918] was to verify the effect of laser therapy in combination with bisphosphonate on osteopenic bone structure. The 35 Wistar female rats used were divided into five groups: (1) sham-operated rats (control), (2) ovariectomized (OVX'd) rats with osteopenia, (3) OVX'd rats with osteopenia treated with laser, (4) OVX'd rats with osteopenia treated with bisphosphonate, and (5) OVX'd rats with osteopenia treated with bisphosphonate and laser. Groups 3 and 5 were given daily 6 mg doses of bisphosphonate orally. Groups 4 and 5 underwent irradiation with 830 nm, 50 mW and 4 J/cm^2 on the femoral neck and vertebral segments (T13-L2). Both treatments were performed over an 8-week period. Rats from the osteopenic control and the osteopenic + laser groups presented marked osteopenia. In the osteopenic + bisphosphonate group, the trabecular bone volume in vertebra L2 was significantly greater than in the osteopenic con-

There was a significant difference between group C and control but not between A and control.

Nicola [1262][1566] studied the activity in bone cells after 660 nm laser irradiation, close to the site of the bone injury. The femurs of 48 rats were perforated (24 in the irradiated group and 24 in the control group) and the irradiated group was treated with a GaAlInP laser of 660 nm, 10 J/cm^2 of radiant exposure on the 2nd, 4th, 6th and 8th day after surgery (DAS). The researchers carried out histomorphometry analysis of the bone. It was found that activity was higher in the irradiated group than in the control group: (a) bone volume at 5 DAS; (b) osteoblast surface at 15 DAS; (c) mineral apposition rate at 15 and 25 DAS; (d) osteoclast surface at 5 DAS and 25 DAS; and (e) eroded surface. It is concluded that this type of irradiation increases the activity in bone cells (resorption and formation) around the site of the repair without changing the bone structure.

In a study by Ghoreyshian [1631], 24 adult male rabbits underwent left mandibular body corticotomy. After 5 days of latency, an external distraction device was activated at a rate of 0.5 mm / day for 10 days. Seven doses of a GaAs laser of 200 mW power (3 J/cm^2 per point) were directed at the corticotomy site of 12 rabbits for a total time of 30 seconds every other day while the control group received no laser irradiation. The distraction sites were evaluated by SEM and histological examinations during the 10th, 20th and 40th day of the consolidation phase. Histological examination revealed that new bone formation in 10 days of consolidation in the laser and control groups did not significantly differ, but SEM examinations showed more calcified and even a smoother surface of spongy bone. GaAs laser seems to be able to improve the process of calcification and bone remodelling in early stages of distraction osteogenesis rather than in later stages.

The purpose of a study by Miloro [1735] was to determine whether LPT application during distraction osteogenesis could accelerate bone regeneration and decrease the length of the consolidation phase and thereby reduce potential patient morbidity. Nine adult rabbits underwent bilateral mandibular corticotomies and placement of unidirectional distraction devices. Each rabbit served as its own internal control. After a latency of 1 day, distraction progressed bilaterally at 1 mm per day for 10 days. Immediately after each device's activation, the experimental side, chosen randomly, was treated with LPT of 6.0 J × 6 transmucosal sites in the area of the distraction gap. Radiographs were taken presurgically, immediately postsurgically, and weekly until sacrifice, and the bone was analyzed using a semiquantitative 4-point scale. Three animals each were sacrificed two, four and six weeks post distraction, and each hemi-mandible was prepared for histological examination in a blinded fashion. Ten mm of distraction was achieved in each rabbit bilaterally. Radiographically, the Bone Healing Score was higher for the laser-treated group at all time periods. Histologically, the area of new bone trabeculation and ossification was more advanced for the laser-treated group, with less intervening fibrovascular

tion test revealed preservation of articular cartilage stiffness with 3.9 and 5.8 W/cm² therapy. LPT may possibly prevent biomechanical changes by immobilisation.

The influence of HeNe laser radiation on the formation of new blood vessels in the bone marrow compartment of a regenerating area of the mid-cortical diaphysis of the tibiae of young adult rats was studied by Garavello [1544]. A small hole was surgically made with a dentistry burr in the tibia and the injured area received a daily LPT over 7 or 14 days transcutaneously starting 24 h after surgery. Incident energy density dosages of 31.5 and 94.5 J/cm² were applied during the period of the tibia wound healing investigated. Light microscopic examination of histological sections of the injured area and quantification of the newly-formed blood vessels were undertaken. LPT accelerated the deposition of bone matrix and histological characteristics compatible with an active recovery of the injured tissue. HeNe LPT significantly increased the number of blood vessels after 7 days of irradiation at an energy density of 94.5 J/cm², but significantly decreased the number of vessels in the 14- day irradiated tibiae, independent of the dosage. These effects were attributed to laser treatment, since no significant increase in blood vessel number was detected between 8 and 15 non-irradiated control tibiae.

The aim of the work by Lizarelli [914] was to evaluate histometrically the effect of irradiation with 790 nm laser in the chronology of alveolar repair of rats. Groups of five animals had their upper right incisors extracted under anaesthesia and the mucous sutured; three groups received 1.5 J/cm² of irradiation immediately after the extraction with laser sweeping over the operated area. After that, the animals were sacrificed 7, 14 and 21 days after the dental extraction. The material was decalcified and processed for inclusion in paraffin. Longitudinal sections of seven micrometers in the alveolus were made and stained with HE and the percentage of the bone tissue was assessed. The results show that LPT produced acceleration in osseous formation (10%) in some periods. The influence of laser irradiation on the healing process is more significant when the laser light can be applied just after the tissue trauma. Cells with a lower than normal pH, where the redox state is shifted in the reduced direction, are considered to be more sensitive to the stimulative effect of light than those in which the respective parameters are optimal or near optimal. The proposed redox-regulation mechanism may present a fundamental explanation of some of the clinical effects of irradiation. A consequence of this is that the difference between the groups after 7 days is more significant than between the other groups.

Pinheiro [1128] evaluated morphometrically the amount of newly formed bone after 830 nm laser irradiation of surgical wounds created in the femur of rats. A total of 48 rats were divided into four groups with 12 animals in each group. Group A received 4.8 J/cm² transcutaneously, three times a week, and sacrificed after 28 days. Group C received only three sessions and was sacrificed after 7 days. Group B and D served as control.

of 1.2 to 1.4 compared to the control group. Irradiation in the later period (days four to six) was not effective, neither was a single irradiation.

Pyczek [832] studied the effect of low power laser light on the haematopoietic system of rats and also on the basic haematological parameters. A 5 mW HeNe and an 80 mW GaAs laser were used. Intact skin on the hind legs of rats was exposed over a section of the femur. Peripheral blood analysis was carried out before and after the experiments. These indicated that GaAs laser light induced a decrease in bone marrow mastocytes and peripheral blood basophils with an increase in the number of eosinophils. An increase in mitotic activity in the bone marrow was observed in the exposed groups of animals. No significant changes in Hb, Ht, erythrocyte or reticulocyte levels in the peripheral blood were noted, nor was there an increase in megakaryocyte emperipolesis.

The results of a rat study by Ozawa [1011] suggest that laser irradiation may play two principal roles in stimulating bone formation. One is stimulation of cellular proliferation, especially proliferation of nodule-forming cells of osteoblast lineage, and the other is stimulation of cellular differentiation, especially to committed precursors, resulting in an increase in the number of more differentiated osteoblastic cells and an increase in bone formation. The two processes can only be stimulated through laser irradiation of immature cells.

Atomic Force Microscopy (AFM) and Scanning Electron Microscopy (SEM) were used in the study by Cruz-Höfling [1326] to quantify bone morphology during post-injury ossification in rat tibiae and characterise the differences induced by laser compared with the naturally occurring regenerative process. A 1.5 diameter hole was made surgically in the tibia and two different doses of laser were applied for 7 or 14 consecutive days, starting 24 hrs after lesion. The collagen fibre lamellar organisation in the matrix, typical of mature bone, was promoted by the HeNe laser at doses of either 31.5 J/cm^2 or 94.5 J/cm^2

Gordjestani [1271] failed to find any stimulatory effect of bone regeneration in a rat experiment. Even though this study was well designed, the dose was high. The artificially created bony defects in the parietal bone were irradiated through the rat fur every day for 28 consecutive days with a dose of 20 J/cm^2 and a power density of 33.3 mW/cm^2. The laser used was a GaAs laser and it is generally recognised that dosages with this type of laser should be kept lower than for GaAlAs.

Akai [466] studied the influence of 810 nm laser on bone and cartilage during joint immobilisation of rats' knee models. The hind limbs of 42 young rats were operated on in order to immobilise the knee joint. They were assigned to three groups one week after operation; irradiance 3.9 W/cm^2, 5.8 W/cm^2, and sham treatment. After six sessions of treatment for another two weeks both hind legs were prepared for 1) indentation of the articular surface of the knee (stiffness and loss tangent), and for 2) dual energy X-ray absorptiometry (bone mineral density) of the focused regions. The indenta-

tinely processed. The light microscopic analysis was performed by an experienced pathologist. In the groups where the laser was used during surgery on the surgical bed (G2/G4), bone remodeling was both quantitatively and qualitatively more evident when compared to subjects of groups G1 and G3.

Nagasawa [107] has also studied the effects of an argon laser (514 nm) used at an output level appropriate for LPT. Periapical lesions, which despite conventional endodontics had shown no sign of starting to heal two months after the start of root treatment, were treated with an argon laser (100-400 mW) directly in the root canal. In some cases, the healing process began after a single treatment.

Trelles [108] studied the effects of a HeNe laser on bone fractures (of the tibia) in mice. The administered dose to one point was 2.4 J. The fracture was treated every other day for three weeks. The healing process was studied under an electron microscope. From a histological point of view, the laser group exhibited better healing characteristics than the control group, which was not treated with a laser. The laser group also showed increased vascularisation and faster formation of bone tissue with a tighter mesh of trabeculae. The control group showed poorer vascularisation and more cartilage tissue.

David [942] failed to verify these findings using 0, 2 or 4 J every other day for two to six weeks.

Luger [536] subjected 50 rats to tibial bone fracture with internal fixation. A total of 25 animals were treated with a HeNe laser, 35 mW transcutaneously 30 minutes daily for two weeks. The other 25 animals served as the control. After four weeks the maximal load at failure (MLF), the structural stiffness of the tibia (SST), and the extension maximal load (EML) were measured. The MLF and the SST were found to be significantly elevated, whereas the EML was reduced. Four non-unions were found in the control group, none in the irradiated group.

Lomnitski [179] studied reparative osteogenesis in 105 rabbits. The healing of drilled cavity defects in the mandibles stimulated with HeNe laser light of various powers was monitored using a histological method, and the distinctive reparative effects of the laser light were evaluated.

Yaakobi [87] made holes in the tibias of rats. HeNe laser irradiation on days 5 and 6 post-injury increased calcium accumulation twofold compared to control. Osteoblastic activity increased, too, as reflected by alkaline phosphatase activity.

Horowitz [473] performed calvarial trepanations in 18 rats. HeNe laser light was applied every day for two weeks. Through infrared spectroscopy the following parameters were found to have improved compared with the control group: 1) amount of mineralisation, 2) factor of conformation, 3) protein to lipid ratio, 4) structural stage.

Saito [569] expanded the midpalatal suture in rats. A 100 mW GaAlAs laser was used to influence bone regeneration. Irradiation during the two first postoperative days was effective, accelerating regeneration by a factor

Sirius red and analyzed by light microscopy. There was histological evidence of improved collagen fiber deposition at early stages of the healing; an increased amount of well-organized bone trabeculae at the end of the experimental period on irradiated animals.

The aim of a study by Gerbi [1471] was to evaluate the effectiveness of a GaAlAs laser (830 nm, 40 mW, CW) in the repair of bone defects (3 mm^2) submitted to organic and inorganic bovine bone graft implantation in the femur of rats (42 animals). The sample was divided into five groups: Group I (control, 6 animals); Group II (Organic Bone graft, 9 animals); Group III (Organic Bone + Laser, 9 animals); Group IV (Anorganic Bone Graft, 9 animals); Group V (Anorganic Bone Graft + Laser, 9 animals). The irradiated groups received seven irradiations every 48 hours, the first immediately after the surgical procedure. The dosimetry was of 16 J/cm^2 per session, divided in four points of 4 J/cm^2. The sacrifice periods were of 15, 21 and 30 days. The obtained results demonstrated that an improved and faster bone repair could be observed in the irradiated groups, evidenced by the largest concentration of collagen fibres in the period of 15 and 21 days and for a larger bone formation and a well organized bone trabeculae at the end of the period (day 30), when compared with the control group. Both biomaterials favoured bone neoformation inside the defect

Another paper by Gerbi [1620] is part of an ongoing series of works in which biomaterials (bone morphogenetic proteins) are used in association with LPT. Forty-eight adult male Wistar rats were divided into four randomized groups: group I (control, n = 12); group II (LPT, n = 12); group III (BMPs + organic bovine bone graft, n = 12); and group IV (BMPs + organic bovine bone graft + LPT, n = 12). The irradiated groups received seven irradiations every 48 h, beginning immediately after the surgical procedure. The laser therapy (830 nm, 40 mW CW, spot size = 0.6 mm) consisted of 16 J/cm^2 per session divided equally over four points (4 J/cm^2 each) around the defect. The subjects were sacrificed after 15, 21, and 30 days, and the specimens were routinely embedded in wax, stained with hematoxylin and eosin and sirius red, and analyzed under light microscopy. The results showed histological evidence of increased deposition of collagen fibers (on days 15 and 21), as well as an increased amount of well-organized bone trabeculae at the end of the experimental period (30 days) in the irradiated animals versus the non-irradiated controls.

The aim of a study by Weber [1615] was to histologically assess the effect of 830 nm laser on the healing of bone defects associated with autologous bone graft. Sixty male rats were divided into four groups: G1 (control); G2 (laser on the surgical bed); G3 (laser on the graft) and G4 (laser on both the graft and the surgical bed). The dose per session was that of 10 J/cm^2, and it was applied to the surgical bed (G2/G4) and on the bone graft (G3/G4). Irradiation was carried out at every other day for 15 days (830 nm, 50 mW, 10 J/cm^2). The dose was fractioned into four points. The animals were sacrificed 15, 21 and 30 days after surgery; specimens were taken and rou-

and mitochondria distributed throughout the cytoplasm were observed 72 h following proliferation. Such changes led to an in vitro proliferation process, as confirmed by the MTT assay. In conclusion, LPT showed itself capable of altering mitochondrial activity and the population of OFCOL II cells.

Animal studies

Nagasawa [106] describes two experiments on bone regeneration. In the first experiment, holes of 1 mm diameter were drilled in the femurs of 36 rats. The rats were divided into six groups of six. Before suturing, the holes in the femurs of five of the groups were irradiated with one type of laser light per group (Nd:YAG, GaAlAs, HeNe, CO2, KrF excimer 248 nm). The sixth group was the control and was not treated with a laser. After ten days, the wound area was studied under a microscope. Some osteoclasts were visible in the untreated group, but few samples were spongy and there were few trabeculae. In the Nd:YAG group, active spongy formation could be observed, with visible trabeculae. Similar formations were observed in the GaAlAs and HeNe groups. In the group treated with a carbon dioxide laser, delayed healing was observed, while the excimer laser group showed signs of necrosis. All rats received a 100 J/cm^2 dosage, except the excimer group, in which the dosage was 2 J/cm^2.

The other experiment involved the use of BMP (bone morphogenetic protein). This is a bioactive substance, which participates in bone formation. It exists in osteoblasts and can be stored in an inactive form. Small pellets were made from calf collagen and impregnated with extracted BMP. The dry weight of the pellets was 8 mg. Pellets of this kind were implanted under the skin on the backs of rats. Six rats were treated with 100 J/cm^2 of GaAlAs laser, and six with 50 J/cm^2 of HeNe laser, after the implantation, but before the wound was sutured. A control group of six rats was not treated. After three weeks, all the pellets were removed and weighed, measured and analysed with respect to their content of Ca and P. The average dry weight of the control group's pellets was 11.6 mg, while it was 14.24 mg for the GaAlAs group, and 13.98 mg for the HeNe group. The Ca levels were 0.86 mg (control group), 1.28 mg (GaAlAs), and 1.0 mg (HeNe). The P levels were 1.04, 1.24, and 1.22 respectively. Nagasawa suggested the following explanation of the results: in addition to stimulating BMP, LPT also causes undifferentiated mesenchymal cells to change into osteoblasts, by means of which the osteogenetic activity increases.

The study by Márquez Martínez [2016] assessed histologically the effect of LPT on the repair of surgical defects on the femur of rats filled with lyophilized bovine bone. The animals were divided into three groups: group I (control); group II (graft); group III (graft + LPT). The animals in the irradiated groups received 16 J/cm^2 per session divided into four points around the defect receiving the first irradiation immediately after surgery and repeated every 48 h for two weeks. Animal death occurred 15, 21, and 30 days after surgery. The specimens were routinely processed and stained with H/E and

and colorimetric MTT assay 24 and 48 h after the second irradiation. A significant 31-58% increase in cell survival (MTT assay) and higher cell count in the once-irradiated as compared to non-irradiated cells were monitored. Differentiation and maturation of the cells was followed by osteogenic markers: alkaline phosphatase (ALP), osteopontin (OP), and bone sialoprotein (BSP). A two-fold enhancement of ALP activity and expressions of OP and BSP were much higher in the irradiated cells compared to non-irradiated osteoblasts.

The aim of another in vitro study by Stein [2014] was to investigate the initial effect of LPT on growth and differentiation of human osteoblast-like cells. SaOS-2 cells were irradiated with laser doses of 1 J/cm^2 and 2 J/cm^2 using a laser with 670 nm wavelength and an output power of 400 mW. Untreated cells were used as controls. At 24 h, 48 h and 72 h post-irradiation, cells were collected and assayed for viability of attached cells and specific alkaline phosphatase activity. In addition, mRNA expression levels of osteopontin and collagen type I were assessed using semi-quantitative RT-PCR. Over the observation period, cell viability, alkaline phosphatase activity and the expression of osteopontin and collagen type I mRNA were slightly enhanced in cells irradiated with 1 J/cm^2 compared with untreated control cells. Increasing the laser dose to 2 J/cm^2 reduced cell viability during the first 48 h and resulted in persistently lower alkaline phosphatase activity compared with the other two groups. The expression of osteopontin and collagen type I mRNA slightly decreased with time in untreated controls and cells irradiated with 1 J/cm^2, but their expression was increased by treatment with 2 J/cm^2 after 72 h. These results indicate that LPT has a biostimulatory effect on human osteoblast-like cells during the first 72 h after irradiation.

The influence of laser radiation on human osteoarthrotically changed chondrocytes was investigated by Bauman [1846] using various wavelengths, power densities and dependences on the exposure time in order to confirm the positive results obtained in an animal experiment. It was manifested that, if there was a specific parameter constellation (2 W; 16 W/cm^2; 60 s; 120 J), an enhanced matrix synthesis (cartilage material from 36 patients) could be achieved. The proof succeeded by applying the radioisotope marking method (3H-proline). Interestingly enough, it turned out that the application of too high a power density but constant energy density resulted in a reduced matrix synthesis rate (reduction of 28%).

Pires Oliveira [1908] irradiated osteoblastic cell cultures (OFCOL II) with 830 nm; 50 mW; 3 J/cm^2; 600 microm diameter optical fiber, and divided into two groups: group 1: irradiated cells, and group 2: non-irradiated cells. Irradiation occurred at 24-h intervals for a total of three days. After each interval, the cells were marked with Mito Tracker Orange dye to assess the biostimulatory effect on mitochondrial activity and cell proliferation using an MTT assay. Intense grouping of mitochondria in the perinuclear region was observed at 24 h and 48 h following irradiation. Changes from a filamentous to a granular appearance in mitochondrial morphology

cultivated cells were irradiated once only or once a day for 21 days at various energy doses (10.8-108 J/cm^2 per day). The total area of mineralised bone nodules on day 21 was evaluated. DNA content, alkaline phosphatase activity (ALP), and the amount of extracellular collagen were also measured. LPT significantly increased the number and the total area of bone nodules in a dose-dependent manner. Cell proliferation and ALP activity were higher in the early and middle culture periods, while the collagen content was higher in the middle and late periods as compared to controls. Calcium and phosphorus were both higher in the irradiation groups.

Hamajima [1564] investigated the stimulatory effect of laser irradiation on bone formation during the early proliferation stage of cultured osteoblastic cells. A mouse calvaria-derived osteoblastic cell line, MC3T3-E1, was utilised to perform a cDNA microarray hybridisation to identify genes that induced expression by laser at the early stage. Among those genes that showed at least a twofold increased expression, the osteoglycin/mimecan gene was upregulated 2.3-fold at two hours after laser irradiation. Osteoglycin is a small leucine-rich proteoglycan (SLRP) of the extracellular matrix which was previously called the osteoinductive factor. SLRP are abundantly contained in the bone matrix, cartilage cells and connective tissues, and are thought to regulate cell proliferation, differentiation and adhesion in close association with collagen and many other growth factors. The researchers investigated the time-related expression of this gene by laser, using a reverse transcription polymerase chain reaction (RT-PCR) method, and more precisely with a real-time PCR method, and found increases of 1.5-2-fold at two to four hours after laser treatment, compared with the non-irradiated controls. These results suggest that the increased expression of the osteoglycin gene by laser irradiation in the early proliferation stage of cultured osteoblastic cells may play an important role in the stimulation of bone formation in concert with matrix proteins and growth factors.

In the study by Ueda [1181], osteoblastic cells isolated from fetal rat calvariae were irradiated once with a low-power GaAlAs laser (830 nm, 500 mW) in two different irradiation modes; continuous irradiation (CI), and 1 Hz pulsed irradiation (PI). The authors then investigated the effects on cellular proliferation, bone nodule formation, alkaline phosphatase (ALP) activity, and ALP gene expression. Laser irradiation in both groups significantly stimulated cellular proliferation, bone nodule formation, ALP activity, and ALP gene expression, as compared with the non-irradiation group. Notably, PI markedly stimulated these factors when compared with the CI group. Since 1 Hz pulsed laser irradiation significantly stimulated bone formation in vitro, it is most likely that pulse frequency is an important factor affecting biological responses in bone formation.

In a study by Stein [1763], cultured osteoblast cells were irradiated using HeNe laser irradiation (632.8 nm; 10 mW). On the second and third day after seeding, the osteoblasts were exposed to laser irradiation. The effect of irradiation on osteoblast proliferation was quantified by cell count

subjects and cell cultures, and these are responsible for the great concentration of collagen fibres seen within irradiated bone.

Another important aspect to be observed are the effects of the laser light on the blood vessels. The vascular response to LPT is one of the possible mechanisms responsible for the positive clinical results observed following LPT. Vascularisation is an important and decisive factor for the healing of wounds and for the relief of the pain. Repeated irradiation is necessary to keep the process going; a single exposure is not enough. Three to four sessions per week for two consecutive weeks is an approximate schedule.

A promising area is the association of the LPT with biomaterials. It has been shown that combining the laser with both organic and inorganic bone grafts results in quicker healing of the bone. The use of BMPs further improve the results and complete harvesian systems can be seen as early as 14 days after wounding. Another promising area is the use of LPT to improve the results of autologous bone grafts. The aims of a report by Pinheiro [1920] were to report the state of the art with respect to photoengineering of bone repair using LPT. LPT has been reported to be an important tool in positive bone stimulation both in vivo and in vitro. These results indicate that photophysical and photochemical properties of some wavelengths are primarily responsible for the tissue responses. The use of correct and appropriate parameters has been shown to be effective in the promotion of a positive biomodulative effect in healing bone. A series of papers reporting the effects of laser therapy on bone cells and tissue, as well as new and promising developed protocols, have been presented. The results indicate that bone irradiated mostly with infrared (IR) wavelengths show increased osteoblastic proliferation, collagen deposition, and bone neoformation when compared to nonirradiated bone. Furthermore, the effect of laser therapy is more effective if the treatment is carried out at early stages when high cellular proliferation occurs. In conclusion, it is possible that the LPT effect on bone regeneration depends not only on the total dose of irradiation, but also on the irradiation time and the irradiation mode. The threshold parameter of energy density and intensity are biologically independent of one another. This independence accounts for the success and the failure of laser therapy achieved at low-energy density levels.

Literature:

In vitro studies

Yamada [414] irradiated cultured osteoblastic cells with a HeNe laser. The cell growth rate and DNA synthesis were increased only in the growing phase of culture. During long-term culture, calcium accumulation was enhanced by laser irradiation at 1 J/cm^2, with four sessions of irradiation resulting in a 46% increase compared to the control group. Alkaline phosphatase activity, however, was unchanged.

Ozawa [369] studied the effect of GaAlAs on bone formation in vitro. Osteoblast-like cells were isolated from rat calvariae of 21d rat fetuses. The

nous laser with a 630 nm, 2.5 mW power at the end of an intravenous fiber. Pulse rate, systolic, diastolic, and pulse pressures were measured before, after, and 15 minutes after the IVL. There was no statistically significant difference for pulse rate, systolic and diastolic blood pressure in normotensive group, however a significant difference was observed for pulse rate, systolic and diastolic blood pressure in pre-hypertensive group as for systolic and diastolic blood pressure in hypertensive group. In conclusion, IVL is an effective method for modifying factors to result in a reduction of arterial pressure. It can be combined with anti hypertensive drugs in pre-hypertensive and hypertensive patients as a modality of treatment; the method is also safe to use on normotensive patients.

Further literature: [574, 698, 971, 1166, 1215]

4.1.8 Bone and cartilage regeneration

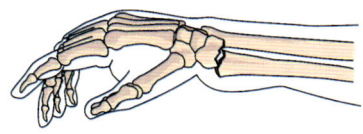

Bone loss may occur due to trauma, pathologies or following some surgical procedures. The regeneration of bone tissue is of central interest in relation to a great number of interventions. Wound healing is a complex process, which involves both local and systemic responses and bone healing is slower than that observed in soft tissues. Bone healing differs from the healing of soft tissues due to both the morphology and composition being slower than that of soft tissues and consists of consecutive phases, which differ depending upon the type and the intensity of the trauma and of the extension of the damage to the bone.

All laser wavelengths have been shown to influence bone regeneration, but, as always, the penetration of the different wavelengths must be taken into consideration. LPT has been found to accelerate cell proliferation optimally in the growing phase, when cells are considered as undifferentiated osteoprogenitor cells [1908].

The photobiological effect is a response to the absorption of a specific wavelength by a molecular photoreceptor. The magnitude of the biomodulative effect depends on the physiologic status of the cell at the irradiation time, and may explain why the biomodulative effect is not always detectable. A unique parameter in itself able to produce a photobiological response does not exist, but the conjugation of different parameters and its variations does. It still remains uncertain if bone stimulation by laser light is a general effect, or if the isolated stimulation of osteoblasts is possible.

It is known that the stimulant effect of laser light on bone occurs during the initial phase of proliferation of both fibroblasts and osteoblasts, as well as on initial differentiation of mesenchymal cells. Fibroblastic proliferation and its increased activity have been detected previously on irradiated

after 5 years in order to confirm the LPT proliferative effect. A 685 nm laser with 25 mW power was used as the source of irradiation. Cultures were exposed to energy densities of 0.1, 0.5, 1.0, 1.5, and 2.0 J/cm^2 before incubation (10 irradiated and 10 controls at each energy density group). A higher number of CFU was observed at the dose of 1.0 J/cm^2 (control 21.3 ± 8.5 × 105 cells, irradiated 40.1 ± 10.5 × 105 cells). No differences were observed in cultures exposed to doses of 0.1, 0.5, and 1.5 J/cm2. A decreased number of CFU was demonstrated in samples exposed to the dose of 2.0 J/cm^2 (control 21.4 ± 11.9×105 cells). PBPC samples cryopreserved for 5 years were thawed for CFU assays and exposed to a single dose of 1.0 J/cm^2; once again the exposed group showed a higher number of CFU (control 8.8 ± 7.8 × 105 cells, irradiated 18.1 ± 13.1 × 105 cells). Dependent upon the energy density, LPT elevates (1.0 J/cm^2) or decreases (2.0 J/cm^2) the potential of long-term cryopreserved PBPC for growth of CFU in vitro.

Further literature: [987, 1129, 1448]

4.1.7 Blood pressure

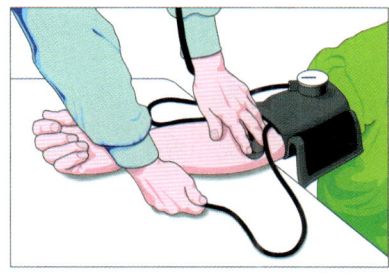

The literature here is meagre and no definite conclusions can be made. However, the hints in the literature below are interesting and deserve further attention. Blood pressure medication is one of the most profitable businesses in the pharmaceutical industry and certainly an important contribution to global health. Yet, non-pharmacological methods without side effects are sought after.

Literature:

Umeda [144] tested the effects of a GaAlAs laser on the control of blood pressure. Radiation was administered via the medulla oblongata. The results from a group of 30 patients suffering from hypertension were excellent in 20% of the cases, good in 37%, fairly good in 23%, and the treatment had no effect in 20%. In a control group of patients with normal blood pressure, no noteworthy results were achieved, except that those bordering on low blood pressure experienced a rise.

Velizhanina [698] used laser irradiation as monotherapy in 42 patients with early essential hypertension. Hypotensive and antioxidant effects of LPT plus its ability to decrease total peripheral resistance were more pronounced in patients with stage I hypertension.

Mokmeli [2046] allocated 125 patients according to their systolic blood pressure in 3 groups: 1. Normotensive (<120 mmHg, n=50), 2. Pre-hypertensive (120-139 mmHg n=50), 3. Hypertensive (stage I =140-159 mmHg, n=25). All the groups were treated for 30 minutes with an intrave-

prospective analysis included 50 patients treated during 2000, 2001 and 2002. Together with conservative treatment of present disease, these patients were treated with laser stimulation of acupuncture points for 10 days. During treatment changes of functional respiratory parameters were recorded. Results were compared with those in the control group. The control group consisted of the same number of patients and differed from the examination group only by not using laser stimulation. Patients with bronchial asthma showed a significant improvement of all estimated lung function parameters just 30 minutes after laser stimulation. Improvement achieved on the third and the tenth day of treatment was significantly higher in the examination group in comparison with the control group. Further investigation confirmed that improvement of measured lung function parameters was significantly higher in younger patients, in patients whose disease lasted shorter, as well as in women. Patients with asthma, who were treated every three months for a one-year period, displayed a significantly lower frequency and intensity of attacks. A 10-day course of laser stimulation of acupuncture points in patients with bronchial asthma improves both the lung function and gas exchange parameters. Positive effects of laser treatment in patients with bronchial asthma are achieved in a short time and they last long, for several weeks, even months. Successive laser stimulation in asthmatics prolongs periods of remission and decreases the severity of asthmatic attacks.

It is unknown if the decreased ability to relax airways smooth muscles in asthma and other inflammatory disorders, such as acute respiratory distress syndrome (ARDS), can be influenced LPT. In this context, the work by de Lima [2102] was developed in order to investigate if LPT could reduce dysfunction in inflamed bronchi smooth muscles (BSM) in rats. A controlled ex vivo study was developed where bronchi from Wistar rat were dissected and mounted in an organ bath apparatus with or without a TNF-alpha. LPT administered perpendicularly to a point in the middle of the dissected bronchi with a wavelength of 655 nm and a dose of 2.6 J/cm^2, partially decreased BSM hyperreactivity to cholinergic agonist, restored BSM relaxation to isoproterenol and reduced the TNF-alpha mRNA expression. An NF-kappaB antagonist (BMS205820) blocked the LPT effect on dysfunction in inflamed BSM. The results obtained in this work indicate that the LPT effect on alterations in responsiveness of airway smooth muscles observed in TNF-alpha-induced experimental acute lung inflammation seems to be dependent of NF-kappaB activation.

Further literature: [340, 710, 840, 1315, 1318, 1667, 1668]

4.1.6 Blood preservation

The aim of a study by do Nascimento [1738] was to investigate the effects of LPT at different energy densities (0.1-2.0 J/cm^2) on the capacity of long-term cryopreserved peripheral blood progenitor cell (PBPC) for growth of colony-forming units (CFU) in vitro. Cryopreserved PBPC samples were thawed after 3 years in order to demonstrate the positive effect of LPT and

smooth muscles are characteristic of asthma. A controlled animal study with rats randomly divided into groups was performed. The responsiveness of TSM and the cAMP accumulation were measured 24 h after incubation with TNF-alpha. Five minutes after incubation, the TSM were irradiated by a 655 nm GaAlAs laser with laser-doses of 2.6 J/cm^2 and mounted in an organ bath apparatus. Laser irradiation was able to restore the relaxing response of TSM to isoproterenol but not to forskolin after TNF-alpha incubation. Laser also restored the cAMP induced by isoproterenol. These results demonstrate that the laser irradiation increased the responsiveness of TSM and the accumulation of cAMP to isoproterenol, probably due to the inhibition of the TNF-alpha.

It has not been known if the decreased ability to relax airway smooth muscles in asthma and other inflammatory airway disorders can be influenced by therapeutic laser irradiation. To investigate if this modality could reduce impairment in inflamed trachea smooth muscles (TSM) in rats, Aimbire [1668] performed a controlled rat study, where trachea was dissected and mounted in an organ bath apparatus with or without a TNF-alpha solution. LPT was administered perpendicularly to a point in the middle of the dissected trachea with a wavelength of 655 nm and a dose of 2.6 J/cm^2. This irradiation partially restored TSM relaxation response to isoproterenol. Tension reduction was 47.0 % in the laser-irradiated group compared to 22.0% in the control group. Accumulation of cAMP was almost normalized after LPT at 22.3 pmol/mg compared to 17.6 pmol/mg in the non-irradiated control group.

The aim of another study by Aimbire [1560] was to investigate the effect of LPT on male rat trachea hyperreactivity (RTHR), bronchoalveolar lavage (BAL) and lung neutrophils influx after Gram-negative bacterial lipopolysacharide (LPS) intravenous injections. The RTHR, BAL and lung neutrophils influx were measured over different intervals of time (90 min, 6 h, 24 h and 48 h). The energy density (ED) that produced an anti-inflammatory effect was 2.5 J/cm^2, reducing the maximal contractile response and the sensibility of trachea rings to methacholine after LPS. The same ED produced an anti-inflammatory effect on BAL and lung neutrophils influx. The Celecoxib COX-2 inhibitor reduced RTHR and the number of cells in BAL and lung neutrophils influx of rats treated with LPS. Celecoxib and laser reduced the PGE$_2$ and TXA2 levels in the BAL of LPS-treated rats. These results demonstrate that 685 nm LPT produced anti-inflammatory effects on RTHR, BAL and lung neutrophils influx in association with inhibition of COX-2-derived metabolites.

Intravenous HeNe laser irradiation has been used to reduce symptoms in asthmatic patients [1032, 1033, 1035].

Laser acupuncture is reported to be successful in treating this condition. [118, 878, 879, 883]. One example is the investigation by Milojevic [1546] which was aimed at defining therapeutic effects of low power laser irradiation by stimulating acupuncture points or local treatment of asthma. A

groups was 810 nm laser, power 100 mW, in continuous mode. Fifteen laser sessions were applied transcutaneously on 5 knee points (6 J/point) per session. In addition, patients in both groups received a quadriceps strength program based on isometric exercises. A visual analogue scale (VAS) was used for pain evaluation in different situations, such as in standing, in knee flexion/extension, and when going up and down stairs. VAS pain scores were evaluated before, in the middle of, and after treatment. Results showed no significant differences between groups for all VAS scores or in the interaction with the sessions. The VAS score results showed a statistically significant pain reduction throughout all sessions. Interferential laser therapy is safe and effective in reducing knee pain. However, the results of the study indicate that it is not superior to the use of a single conventional laser.

In a study by Hegedus [2065] patients with mild or moderate KOA were randomized to receive either LPT or placebo LPT. Treatments were delivered twice a week over a period of 4 wk wth 830 nm, CW, 50 mW) in skin contact at a dose of 6 J/point. The placebo control group was treated with an ineffective probe (power 0.5 mW) of the same appearance. Before examinations and immediately, 2 wk, and 2 mo after completing the therapy, thermography was performed: joint flexion, circumference, and pressure sensitivity were measured; and the visual analogue scale was recorded. In the group treated with active LPT, a significant improvement was found in pain (before treatment [BT]: 5.75; 2 mo after treatment : 1.18); circumference (BT: 40.45; AT: 39.86); pressure sensitivity (BT: 2.33; AT: 0.77); and flexion (BT: 105.83; AT: 122.94). In the placebo group, changes in joint flexion and pain were not significant. Thermographic measurements showed at least a 0.5 degrees C increase in temperature-and thus an improvement in circulation compared to the initial values. In the placebo group, these changes did not occur.

Further literature: [98, 99, 100, 152, 193, 210, 325, 343, 434, 453, 605, 617, 738, 1019, 1020, 1026, 1027, 1055, 1060, 1133, 1139, 1150, 1166, 1172, 1308, 1313, 1419, 1449, 1532, 1680, 1799]

4.1.5 Asthma

Inflammation, increase of cytokine production and decreased relaxation capacity of airway smooth muscles are characteristic of asthma. LPT seems to have an ameliorating relaxing response of trachea smooth muscles exposed to TNF-alpha. The research literature available for treating asthma is thin on the clinical side, but we have here yet another example of an indication where there are only benefits to be gained by trying.

Literature:

The purpose of a study by Aimbire [1668] was to investigate the effect of LPT on the mechanism of TNF-alpha-induced alteration of adrenoceptor responsiveness in trachea smooth muscle (TSM) in male rats. Inflammation, increase of cytokine production and decreased relaxation capacity of airway

author concludes: "LPT is no better than placebo at reducing pain, morning stiffness, or improving functional status for OA-hand patients". **We believe this is a questionable conclusion since the study used only 0.12 J per finger joint, a previously untested wavelength and random pulsing. The discussion also fails to discuss the great differences in dosage and treatment techniques in the references [1683].**

In a double-blind study by Ortutay [609] on the effect of LPT on psoriatic arthritis using 820 nm light, seven out of eight patients in the treatment group showed improved clinical activity: increased range of movement, decreased joint stiffness and tenderness. In the placebo group, only two out of eight patients improved.

Treatment efficacy of physical agents in osteoarthritis of the knee (OAK) pain has been largely unknown, and a systematic review by Bjordal [1279] was aimed at assessing their short-term efficacies for pain relief. The authors performed a systematic review with meta-analysis of efficacy within 1-4 weeks and at follow-ups 1-12 weeks after the end of treatment. A total of 36 randomised placebo-controlled trials (RCTs) were identified with 2434 patients where 1391 patients received active treatment. Three or more out of five methodological criteria (Jadad scale) were satisfied by 33 trials. The patient sample had a mean age of 65.1 years and a mean baseline pain of 62.9 mm on a 100 mm visual analogue scale (VAS). Within 4 weeks of the commencement of treatment manual acupuncture, static magnets and ultrasound therapies did not offer statistically significant short-term pain relief over placebo. Pulsed electromagnetic fields offered a small reduction in pain of 6.9 mm [95% CI: 2.2 to 11.6] (n = 487). Transcutaneous electrical nerve stimulation (TENS, including interferential currents), electro-acupuncture (EA) and low level laser therapy (LPT) offered clinically relevant pain relieving effects of 18.8 mm [95% CI: 9.6 to 28.1] (n = 414), 21.9 mm [95% CI: 17.3 to 26.5] (n = 73) and 17.7 mm [95% CI: 8.1 to 27.3] (n = 343) on VAS respectively versus placebo control. In a subgroup analysis of trials with assumed optimal doses, short-term efficacy increased to 22.2 mm [95% CI: 18.1 to 26.3] for TENS, and 24.2 mm [95% CI: 17.3 to 31.3] for LPT on VAS. Follow-up data up to 12 weeks were sparse, but positive effects seemed to persist for at least 4 weeks after the course of LPT, EA and TENS treatment was stopped. In conclusion, TENS, EA and LPT administered with optimal doses in an intensive 2-4 week treatment regimen, seem to offer clinically relevant short-term pain relief for OAK.

The aim of a study by Montes-Molina [2064] was to evaluate the effectiveness of an interferential pattern generated by two identical and independent lasers in the relief of knee pain. A double-blind controlled clinical trial was performed on 152 patients with knee pain who were randomly assigned into two different groups. Group I patients (n=76) received interferential laser therapy generated by two identical laser probes located opposite each other on the knee joint. Group II patients (n=76) received one live probe in conventional laser therapy and one dummy probe. The device used in both

toid arthritis, enough for recommending the method for clinical purposes. **These two studies, however, lack a proper analysis of the dosages used, and the result of using a very low dosage in some studies confuses the true outcome of LPT studies. Further, the different wavelengths are "put into the same basket" although it is obvious that they have different effects.**

In another Meta analysis of the effect of LPT on osteoarthritis pain, Bjordal [588] summarises: "A literature search identified 88 randomised-controlled trials, of which 20 trials included patients with osteoarthritis and chronic joint disorders. Five trials were excluded for not irradiating the affected joint capsule. Two trials that reported significant results in favour of active laser were excluded from statistical pooling due to insufficient data presentation and lack of repeated laser irradiation. Of the remaining thirteen trials, five trials reported non-significant results. These five trials used treatment parameters outside our predefined optimal dose range, and their results were significantly poorer (p<0.001) than the results from eight trials giving treatment within the optimal dose range. For the 398 patients included in these eight trials, a pooled mean weighted difference of 42.9% (range 23-62) was registered in favour of active treatment. Adverse effects were few and mild, and unblinded follow-up observations suggested that pain reduction could last for more than one month. With the reservation of possible heterogeneity in the limited patient sample, location-specific doses of LPT appear to be effective in reducing pain from mild osteoarthritis." **This study underlines the importance of a proper dosage and subgroup analysis, an issue that has been largely overlooked by previous reviewers of LPT.**

In the study by Basirnia [1323], treatment was performed on 20 patients, ageing from 42 to 60 years. All patients had received conservative treatment with poor results. Laser device used for this treatment was a pulsed diode laser; 810 nm, once a day for five consecutive days, followed by a 2-day interval. There was a total of 12 sessions of laser application. Irradiation was performed on five periarticular tender points, each for two minutes. The treatment outcome (pain relief and functional ability) was observed and measured according to the following methods: 1) Numerical rating scales, 2) Self assessment by the patient, 3) Index of severity for osteoarthritis of the knee, 4) Analgesic requirements. Significant improvement in pain relief and quality of life was achieved in 70% of patients, compared to their previous status. There was no significant change in range of motion of the knee.

Brosseau [1528] examined efficacy of active GaAlAs (860 nm) versus sham-laser on finger joints and three superficial nerves. Randomly assigned OA-patients received three treatments per week for six weeks of laser (n = 42) or sham (n = 46). Pain relief, morning stiffness, and functional status did not significantly improve for laser versus placebo. No significant differences were found in finger range of motion, except carpometacarpal opposition (P = 0.011), grip strength and patient global assessment, which improved for active LPT participants (P = 0.041).The

Similar parameters but a different treatment schedule was used by Bülow [1025]. Each patient received 22.5 J per session in nine sessions over three weeks. Laser source was a GaAlAs laser of 25 mW. **Although reported as negative, a closer analysis of the data submitted reveals a significant short-term effect, which is masked in the text. When these masked facts are revealed, both Stelian and Bülow present a significant but short-term effect of LPT for these parameters.**

Haimovici [82] studied osteoarthritis in finger joints and found that both HeNe and GaAlAs improved all the parameters measured. In the same study, the effects of anti-inflammatory medication and laser were compared. The medication gave slightly better results than the laser, but the best effects of all were achieved when the two were used in combination. **This underlines the fact that laser should not be seen as a single form of therapy but as a valuable means of assistance.**

Obata [397] performed "Total Laser Irradiation" on 89 patients. This means that all active inflammatory joints were treated each session until pain relief was observed in all joints. The laser used was a 10 mW 780 nm unit. The erythrocyte sedimentation rate improved by more than 10 mm in 55% of the patients in the 20-session group. Lansbury's index improved by 10% in 47% of the cases. The serum immune-complex tended to decrease and the findings of synovial scintigraphy correlated well with the clinical effects.

Simunovic [955] reports that patients with osteoarthrosis of joints in the upper extremities had a 70% pain relief and improved function using local irradiation and irradiation of trigger points.

Lerner [826] used a HeNe laser on a group of 33 patients suffering from Mb Bechterew. Irradiation was given over the spine and joints for 20 sessions. A total of 20 patients received LPT in combination with 75-100 mg of indomethacin per day, while 13 patients received LPT alone due to indomethacin intolerance. Therapeutic efficacy was assessed according to a number of clinico-laboratory indices. The most marked effect was observed in the combination group. The use of LPT alone was comparable with using indomethacin at a daily dose of 75 mg.

The double blind study by Gladkova [1078] has a rather negative outcome. **However, since doses between 0.004-0.02 J/cm^2 were used, a negative outcome is to be expected.**

In a double-blind crossover study, Gärtner [199, 568] used GaAs and HeNe lasers to treat stage III-IV ankylosing spondylarthritis. Treatment was given for 20 to 30 minutes daily for five consecutive days each week for three weeks. Spinal ROM and laboratory tests including CRP and ESP showed no significant changes. However, pain score, morning stiffness and frequency of nocturnal awakening were significantly reduced. **With today's more powerful lasers, the results are likely to improve.**

In two Meta analyses of osteoarthritis and rheumatoid arthritis, Brosseau [1023, 1024, 1154] found a moderate but short term effect for rheuma-

LPT and also yielded better, or at least similar, results in most of the cases compared to classical anti-inflammatory therapy.

In the study by Rogvi-Hansen [1138] the outcome was negative, but the actual area of the articular capsule was not irradiated, although the indication studied was condromalacia patellae. This study used the treatment method implemented by Walker [38], irradiating the patella, the ipsilateral femoral nerve in the groin and the proximal part of the peroneal muscle. Walker used 1 mW HeNe, whereas this latter study used GaAs 17 mW. A 1 mW HeNe is unlikely to produce any results in a large joint such as the knee. **And, as suggested by the Latin name of the condition, the cartilage itself has to be irradiated, not only the secondary complications. Although one of these studies is positive, the protocol of both is questioned.**

In a clinical study comprising 224 patients, Glazewski [1079] found that "application of low-intensity laser irradiation enables us to shorten NSAIDs treatment duration, reduce dose size and obtain better therapeutic effects." Indications treated were i.a. rheumatoid arthritis, coxarthrosis, gonarthrosis and spondylosis. The lasers used were GaAs 890 nm in the range 3.6 - 7.4 mW, dose range 0.75 - 3.0 J/cm^2.

In the double blind study by Taghawinjad [335] the outcome in the verum group was no better than that of the placebo group. However, the laser used was a combined HeNe (4.4 mW) + GaAs (5 × 0.3 mW) held at a distance of 160 mm from the skin, and covering an area of 40 mm^2. **The power density in this set-up is very low and the penetration insufficient.**

Molina [334] compared two groups where one received ASA (acetylsalicylic acid) and the other ASA (four gram daily) plus LPT. During the initial double-blind phase, GaAs 6-8 J/cm^2 was applied to a total of 21 points in the hand. In an additional open phase, HeNe 6-10 J/cm^2 was administered. The ASA/LPT group responded more favourably to the therapy. GaAs appeared to be more successful than HeNe.

Soriano [331] reports good results in treating a group of 938 patients with osteoarthritis, using 904 nm, 6-10 J/cm^2. Acute conditions responded better than chronic conditions. The subgroups were: NSAID + LPT, massage/physiotherapy + LPT, and LPT only. The results in the three subgroups were practically identical. Chronic knee and hip pain had low scores (38%), others ranged from 84% to 100%.

Stelian [617] divided 50 patients with knee OA into three groups: one received 830 nm GaAlAs, one HeNe and one placebo laser. The infrared group was double blind whereas the HeNe group had to be an open study. The patients treated their knees twice daily for 10 days, a total of 22 J per day. GaAlAs and HeNe had approximately the same effect. The laser groups had significantly less pain at the end of the therapy and at checkups at 2-12 months. Their general well-being was measured with a Disability Index Questionnaire. This index was reduced by half in the laser groups but remained unchanged in the placebo group.

Johannsen [605] treated 22 patients with RA in a double-blind study. The two most painful MCP joints on the most affected hand were chosen for treatment, and 2.9 J of GaAlAs light was applied to four points. Treatment was offered three times a week for a month. None of the five parameters measured showed any effect of LPT.

Ortutay [518] used 1-4 J/cm^2 (830 nm) per joint with compression technique on a daily basis. Total dose per joint ranged between 25 and 40 J/cm^2. Total doses below a total of 25 J/cm^2 were ineffective, while 25-40 J/cm^2 was effective in all cases.

Amano [578] applied 790 nm 0.8 J to six points for six consecutive days on the lateral side of the knee in a group of 14 RA patients due to undergo arthroplasty. During operation, small samples of the synovial membrane were removed from the lateral and the medial non-irradiated area. Histological findings in the irradiated synovial membrane showed flattening of epithelial cells, decreased villous proliferation, narrowed vascular lumen, and less infiltration of inflammatory cells by comparison with the non-irradiated synovia.

Barberis [718] treated 12 patients with chronic rheumatoid arthritis stages II and III. One knee in each patient was selected and irradiated with HeNe, 8 J/cm^2, 11 points, 15 applications. Synovial tissue analysis showed that LPT reduced pre- and post-treatment levels of PGE$_2$.

Obata [185] studied the effect of GaAlAs on a group of patients with diagnosed rheumatoid arthritis. Thermography was used on the treated hand to check the possible correlation between pain relief and thermographic response. A VAS scale was used to assess the degree of pain relief. In 10 patients, the HST (highest skin temperature) decreased immediately after irradiation. Nine of these patients experienced significant pain relief. Eight patients had an increase of HST following irradiation and five of these experienced non-significant pain relief.

Palmgren [97] conducted a controlled double-blind study of the effects of GaAlAs on 35 patients with rheumatoid arthritis. Eight joints on the worst affected hand were treated with a laser 3.58 J/cm^2 or placebo laser. In the experimental group, grip strength and movement were improved and swelling decreased; pain and morning stiffness were reduced. Pain was also reduced in the placebo group, although less than in the experimental group, while other parameters stayed unchanged.

Antipa [775] has tried to establish the efficiency of LPT in various inflammatory and non-inflammatory rheumatic diseases over a five-year period. In the study, 514 patients with osteoarthrosis, 326 patients with non-articular rheumatism and 82 patients with inflammatory rheumatism were treated. Four different treatment procedures were used: 1) only GaAs; 2) both GaAs and HeNe; 3) placebo laser; and 4) classic anti-inflammatory therapy. The results were analysed using local objective improvements and the score obtained from a pain scale before and after treatment. It was concluded that LPT (especially HeNe with GaAs) is more efficient than placebo

scanner analyzer after Alcian blue (AB) stain. The densities of mucopolysaccharide induced after treatment in arthritic cartilage were compared and correlated with their histopathological changes. The density of mucopolysaccharide rose at the initial stage of induced arthritis, and decreased progressively in later stages. The densities of mucopolysaccharide in treated rats increased upon complete laser treatment more than in those of the controls, which is closely related with the improvement in histopathological findings, but conversely with the changes in arthritic severity. HeNe laser treatment will enhance the biosynthesis of arthritic cartilage and result in the improvement of arthritic histopathological changes.

Castano [1840] tested LPT on rats that had zymosan injected into their knee joints to induce inflammatory arthritis. The author compared illumination regimens consisting of a high and low fluence (3 and 30 J/cm^2), delivered at high and low irradiance (5 and 50 mW/cm^2) using 810 nm laser light daily for five days, with the positive control of conventional corticosteroid (dexamethasone) therapy. Illumination with a 810 nm laser was highly effective (almost as good as dexamethasone) at reducing swelling, and a longer illumination time (10 or 100 minutes compared to 1 minute) was more important in determining effectiveness than either the total fluence delivered or the irradiance. LPT induced reduction of joint swelling correlated with reduction in the inflammatory marker serum prostaglandin E_2 (PGE_2).

Clinical studies

The Hungarian experience of using LPT in rheumatoid arthritis has been summarised by Mester [894] as follows:

"Barabás [1018] irradiated the joints of rheumatoid arthritis (RA) patients. In the first open study the range of motion and circumference of the treated joints were measured, a Ritchie index was used as a semi-objective parameter, while subjective parameters as joint tenderness and pain on a visual analogous scale (VAS) were registered. Walking time was registered as a functional disability parameter. Laboratory activity parameters and the 99mTechnetium index were measured. The second part of the clinical study was double blind. Infrared (10 mW and 100 mW) lasers were used, versus dummy devices with the same appearance. The third part of the study was in vitro experiments. Synovial membranes of rheumatoid arthritis patients were irradiated. The DNA/RNA ratio of the RA group was compared to the control group. A significant difference was detected between the two groups. The fourth phase of the clinical studies was to detect the effects of laser irradiation in other rheumatic diseases: psoriatic arthritis, sacroileitis, osteoarthritis, entesopathy, tenosynovitis, bursitis calcarea, fibromyalgia, localised muscle spasm, periarthritis humeroscapularis etc. The different wavelengths (604, 630, 660, 670, 690, 750, 780, 790, 820, 830, 904, 1053, 1219 nm,) were compared (30 - 100 mW) with other physiotherapy modalities, such as ultrasound." The group size in the double blind study was 80 (50 laser, 30 placebo) and each finger joint received 1 J/cm^2 daily for 25 days.

there was slight irregularity of the articular surface and necrosis in the OA group, and serious cartilage damage, despite slight chondrocyte regeneration, in the 4-week control group. Conversely, the 4-week treatment group showed chondrocyte replacement, with sometimes close to normal articular cartilage on the articular surface. These results suggest that LPT was effective in the treatment of chemically-induced OA.

In a total of 45 rabbits, knee-joint arthrosis was induced in a study by Pfander [1741]. Depending on the post-operative survival time, the cartilage was investigated macroscopically, histologically and immunohistochemically (within a period of 10 days to 8 months). Thereafter, the influence of laser irradiation at a wavelength of 692.6 nm and energy densities of 1 and 4 J/cm^2 on the cartilage morphology seven days following the exposure was examined. After joint instability surgery it was found that the cartilage changes in the main stress area (MSA) and in regions outside the main stress area (ROMSA) progressed differently. Various qualitative and semi-quantitative changes were found for collagens I, II, IV and V, and for the glycoproteins fibronectin and tenascin. Immunohistochemically, there was a growing expression of collagen I in the apical layers, collagen II showed a stronger pericellular expression, and collagen IV showed, after an initial growth of the pericellular expression, a reduced territorial expression and a stronger apical-interterritorial expression in the osteoarthrotic cartilage. For fibronectin, the cellular expression turned out to grow in the ROMSA. In the MSA it decreased, but at the same time the interterritorial expression grew. For Tanascin, there was a decrease of the interterritorial expression in the radial zone while the pericellular and interterritorial expression of the apical layers of the osteoarthrotic cartilage grew. Lasing proved to significantly influence the osteoarthrotically changed cartilage when applied at an energy density of 1 J/cm^2, i.e., the morphological changes had not yet progressed to the extent the control group had. Both the chondrocyte density and the glucosaminoglycan content turned out to be higher. When lasing was applied at higher energy densities, no significant difference among the control groups was found. Thus, it could be demonstrated in vivo that an arthrotic process decelerates through the influence of laser light of low-energy densities.

In a study by Lin [1742], 72 rats with three different degrees of pain-induced OA over right knee joints were collected for helium-neon laser treatment. The severity of induced arthritis was measured by 99mTc bone scan and classified into three groups (I-III) by their radioactivity ratios (right to left knee joints). The rats in each group were further divided into study subgroups (Is, IIs, and IIIs) and control subgroups (Ic, IIc, and IIIc) randomly. The arthritic knees in the study subgroups received HeNe laser treatment, while those in the control groups received sham laser treatment. The changes of arthritic severity after treatment and at the follow-up two months later were measured. The histopathological changes were evaluated through light microscope after disarticulation of sections (H.E. stain), and the changes of mucopolysaccharide density in cartilage matrix were measured by Optimas

divided in two subgroups of six animals each. The AEG and CEG groups began to receive laser treatment 2 and 5 d after the induction of inflammation, respectively. Laser irradiation at 830 nm, 77 mW, power density 27.5 W/cm2 was applied daily for 7 d for either 0.12 sec or 0.32 sec, resulting in doses of 3.4 J/cm^2 and 8 J/cm^2, respectively. Body mass, joint perimeter, joint temperature, and the morphology of the SF were analyzed. There were no statistically significant differences between groups in the body mass, joint perimeter, and SF morphology. Laser irradiation with the selected parameters produced only a few subtle differences in the inflammatory signs and the SF. The lack of effects may have been due to the extremely short irradiation time.

The course of arthrosis was investigated by Gottlieb [1701] on an animal-experimental arthrosis model considering macroscopic aspects, and the proteoglycan and the glycosaminoglycan contents. Based on these parameters, the influence of a diode laser of 692.6 nm, 20 mW, on the progress of arthrosis was investigated. Thirty days following joint instability surgery another operation was carried out during which the femoral condyles were irradiated using different energy densities (1 or 4 J/cm^2). Seven days after the second operation, macroscopic findings were made and the proteoglycan content was established. Macroscopically, a progressively increasing severity of cartilage changes during the course of arthrosis was detected, and the proteoglycan content was found to decrease. The changes in the irradiated joints proved to be less severe, with the higher energy density having a greater positive influence of statistical significance.

The aim of a study by Cho [1425] was to determine whether LPT aided the recovery of damaged articular cartilage in joints with artificially induced osteoarthropathy (OA). OA was induced by injecting hydrogen peroxide (H_2O_2) into the articular spaces of both knees in rabbits, twice a week for four weeks. The induction of OA and the effect of LPT were evaluated by biochemical, radiological and histopathological analysis. Superoxide dismutase (SOD) activity increased about 40% in the OA group, as compared to the controls. Although SOD activity in the OA group was not significantly different from the 2-week groups, it was significantly different from the 4-week control and treatment groups. There was also a significant difference between the 4-week control and treatment groups. Simple radiographs and three-dimensional computed tomographs (3D CT) did not show detectable arthropathy in the OA group, nor any particular changes in the 2-week groups. In contrast, distinct erosions were seen in the distal articular cartilage of the femur, with irregularity of the articular surface, in the 4-week control group, while the erosions were reduced and arthropathy improved slightly in the 4-week treatment group. Generally, erosions formed on the articular surface in the OA group. In comparison, severe erosions damaged the articular cartilage in the 4-week control group, but not in the 2-week control and treatment groups. Regeneration of articular cartilage was seen in gross observations in the 4-week treatment group. Histopathologically,

of trachea rings to methacholine after LPS. The same ED produced an antiinflammatory effect on BAL and lung neutrophils influx. The Celecoxib COX-2 inhibitor reduced RTHR and the number of cells in BAL and lung neutrophils influx of rats treated with LPS. Celecoxib and laser reduced the PGE_2 and TXA2 levels in the BAL of LPS-treated rats. These results demonstrate that 685 nm LPT produced anti-inflammatory effects on RTHR, BAL and lung neutrophils influx in association with inhibition of COX-2-derived metabolites.

Guerino [1666] investigated the effects of HeNe laser irradiation on the inflammatory process induced in the articular cartilage of the right knee of guinea pigs. Through electron microscopy analysis it was possible to identify the induced arthritis in the articular cartilage and its modification after the laser treatment. The laser radiation promoted a reduction in the proliferation of the inflammatory cells in the damaged tissue and also induced the formation of cartilage bridges that tied the destroyed parts favouring the formation of a repaired tissue in the injured cartilage.

A study by Moriyama [1694] was designed to demonstrate that bioluminescence imaging (BLI) can be used as a new tool to evaluate the effects of LPT during in vivo inflammatory process. Here, the efficacy of LPT in modulating inducible nitric oxide synthase (iNOS) expression using different therapeutic wavelengths was determined using transgenic animals with the luciferase gene under control of the iNOS gene expression. Thirty transgenic mice were allocated randomly to one of four experimental groups treated with different wavelengths (635, 785, 808 and 905 nm) or a control group (non-treated). Inflammation was induced by intra-articular injection of zymosan A in both knee joints. Laser treatment (25 mW, 200 s, 5 J/cm^2 was applied to the knees 15 min after inflammation induction. Measurements of iNOS expression were performed at various times (0, 3, 5, 7, 9 and 24 h) by measuring the bioluminescence signal using a highly sensitive charge-coupled device (CCD) camera. The results showed a significant increase in BLI signal after irradiation with 635 nm laser when compared to the non-irradiated animals and the other laser treated groups, indicating wavelength dependence of LPT effects on iNOS expression during the inflammatory process, and thus demonstrating an action spectrum of iNOS gene expression following LPT in vivo that can be detected by BLI. Histological analysis was also performed and demonstrated the presence of fewer inflammatory cells in the synovial joints of mice irradiated with 635 nm compared with non-irradiated knee joints.

The purpose of a study by Sandoval [2067] was to evaluate the effects of LPT on the clinical signs of inflammation and the cellular composition of synovial fluid (SF) in the inflamed knee of the rabbit. Inflammation in the right knee of 36 rabbits was induced by intracapsular injection (0.2 mL) of Terebinthina commun (Tc). The animals were randomly assigned to three groups: acute experimental group (AEG), chronic experimental group (CEG), and control group (CG), which only received Tc. Each group was

The production of IL-1ß and TNF-alpha were reduced by 810 nm after treatment.

An extended explanation of the fundamental effect of LPT in general is presented by Hamblin [1897]. Red and near-IR light is thought to be primarily absorbed by cytochrome c oxidase, which is unit four in the mitochondrial respiratory chain. Since the recent discovery of mitochondrial nitric oxide synthase, it has been realized that nitric oxide produced in the mitochondria can inhibit respiration by binding to cytochrome c oxidase and competitively displacing oxygen, especially in stressed or hypoxic cells. Light absorption displaces or photodissociates the nitric oxide and thus allowed the cytochrome c oxidase to recover and cellular respiration to resume.

Animal studies

The anti-inflammatory effect of HeNe laser was observed by Campaña [1133]. Calcium pyrophosphate was injected into both joints of the lower limbs in rats, to mimic microcrystalline arthropaty (gout). The untreated group showed a strong diffuse inflammatory reaction for mono and polymorphonuclears with fibro and angioblastic proliferation, with edematous lax stroma. No inflammation was observed in the laser group. The experience of this research group is reviewed in [1680].

In an experiment in rats, Campaña [582] found that laser induced a similar reduction of PGE2 levels as NSAID in experimentally induced synovitis.

In the study by Lievens [1324] cartilage tissue of the ear of mice was used as an experimental set-up. It is clear that the elastic cartilage tissue of the ear is not totally comparable with the hyaline cartilage of articulations. For technical reasons, however, and because of the fact that the chondrocytes are comparable, it was decided to use mice ears in this experiment. A 0,4 mm hole was drilled in both ears on 30 mice. The right ear remained untreated, while the left ear was treated daily with GaAs laser for three minutes. Macroscopical as well as histological evaluations were performed on the cartilage regeneration of both ears. The results show that after one day post-surgery no differences were found between the irradiated and the non-irradiated group. After the second day, only in the irradiated group was there a clear activation of the perichondrium. After four days, there was a significant ingrowth of the perichondrium into the drill hole in the experimental group and there was only an active perichondrium zone in our control group.

The purpose of a study by Aimbire [1560] was to investigate the effect of LPT on rat trachea hyperreactivity (RTHR), bronchoalveolar lavage (BAL) and lung neutrophils influx after Gram-negative bacterial lipopolyssacharide (LPS) intravenous injection. The RTHR, BAL and lung neutrophils influx were measured over different intervals of time (90 min, 6 h, 24 h and 48 h). The energy density (ED) that produced an anti-inflammatory effect was 2.5 J/cm^2, reducing the maximal contractile response and the sensibility

on HIG-82 cell proliferation were affected by cAMP content, which is known to influence the cell cycle via inducing CKIs. LPT promoted HIG-82 synovial fibroblast proliferation and induced cytoplasmic localization of cyclin-dependent kinase inhibitor p15 (INK4B/CDKN2B). Moreover, the proliferation of HIG-82 synovial fibroblasts was reduced by cAMP, while cAMP inhibitor, SQ22536, induced p15 cytoplasmic localization and as a result, elevated synovial fibroblast proliferation was observed. In addition, the promotive effect of laser-induced HIG-82 synovial fibroblast proliferation was abolished by cAMP treatment. These findings suggest that cAMP may be involved in the effect of laser on synovial fibroblast proliferation. The researchers revealed the effect and molecular link involved in synovial fibroblast proliferation induced by 660 nm irradiation.

In an in vitro study on the effect on the synovial membrane, it was found that a total dose of 25 J/cm^2 had a stimulating effect, less so with 50 and even less with 100 J/cm^2, while 250 J/cm^2 had an inhibitive effect. A continued study of eight patients, using 100 J/cm^2 in total instead of 25 J/cm^2, confirmed this observation. The laser used was a Neodymium-Phosphate-Glass-laser, wavelength 1053 nm, energy 100 mJ per pulse.

In a study by Yamura [2066] synoviocytes from RA patients were treated with 810 nm radiation before or after addition of tumor necrosis factor-alpha (TNF-alpha). mRNA for TNF-alpha, interleukin IL-1β, IL-6, and IL-8 was measured after 30, 60, and 180 minutes using RT-PCR. Intracellular and extracellular protein levels for 12 cytokines/chemokines were measured at 4, 8, and 24 hours using multiplexed ELISA. Radiation at 810 nm (5 J/cm^2) given before or after TNF-alpha decreases the mRNA level of TNF-alpha and IL-1β in RA synoviocytes. This treatment using 25 J/cm^2 also decreases the intracellular levels of TNF-alpha, IL-1β, and IL-8 protein but did not affect the levels of seven other cytokines/chemokines. TNF-alpha-induced activation of NF-kappaB is not altered by 810 nm radiation using 25 J/cm^2 The authors conclude that the mechanism for relieving joint pain in RA by LPT may involve reducing the level of pro-inflammatory cytokines/chemokines produced by synoviocytes. This mechanism may be more general and underlie the beneficial effects of LPT on other inflammatory conditions.

Skinner [754] stimulated cultured human embryonic fibroblast cells with GaAs. Fibroblast procollagen production was monitored by the synthesis of {3H} hydroxyproline, and DNA replication was assessed by {3H} thymidine incorporation. Following laser treatment, controlled pepsin digestion measured the increase in cell biostimulation. Maximum increase of collagen production and cell biostimulation occurred after four episodes of LPT at 24-hour intervals.

Yamura [1896] studied the effect of 810 nm radiation on synoviocytes from rheumatoid arthritis (RA) joints. Cells were pre-exposed to TNF-alpha to mimic the inflammatory environment of a RA joint. The mRNA and protein levels of multiple cytokines were measured as a function of time after LPT.

vitro. The cartilage sample used for the biostimulation treatment was taken from the right knee of a 19-year-old patient. After the chondrocytes were isolated and suspended for cultivation, the cultures were incubated for 10 days. The culture was divided into four groups. Groups I, II, III were subject to biostimulation with the following laser parameters: 300 J, 1 W, 100 Hz pulse repetition rate, 10 min. exposure, 300 J, 1 W, 300 Hz pulse repetition rate, 10 min. exposure; and 300 J, 1 W, 500 Hz pulse repetition rate, 10 min. exposure, respectively. Group IV did not receive any treatment. The laser biostimulation was conducted for five consecutive days. The data showed good results in terms of cell viability and levels of Ca and Alkaline Phosphate in the groups treated with laser by comparison with the untreated group. The results obtained confirm previous positive in vitro results from the same authors, that the GaAlAs laser provides biostimulation without cell damage. The very high doses used complicate the conclusions from earlier studies.

Herman [151] used Nd:YAG in vitro on bovine articular cartilage. Irradiation could be shown to consistently up-regulate cartilage proteoglycan, collagen, noncollagen protein and DNA synthesis in the absence of histological or biochemical evidence of enhanced matrix catabolism. Laser-induced repair could be shown biochemically in an in vitro model system of enzymatically mediated cartilage matrix deposition.

In a study by Wong [1605] condrocyte proliferation following in vitro heating through different methods, including Nd:YAG laser, was demonstrated. The stimulation observed is attributed to the heat effect only. However, no evidence of chondrocyte DNA replication was observed in tissues heated by non-laser methods. Since the laser source of heating was the only one showing DNA replication, it is likely that the biostimulatory effect in the peripheral part of the laser beam contributed to this effect.

The influence of low-power (632.8 nm, 13 J/cm^2, three times a week) laser on 13-week immobilised articular cartilages was examined by using a rabbit knee model in a study by Bayat [1640]. The number of chondrocytes and the depth of articular cartilage of the experimental group were significantly higher than those of the sham irradiated group. Surface morphology of the sham-irradiated group had rough prominences, fibrillation and lacunae but the surface morphology of the experimental group had more similarities to the control group than to the sham irradiated group. There were marked differences between ultrastructure features of the control group and the experimental group in comparison with the sham irradiated group. Thus, laser irradiation on 13-week immobilised knee joints of rabbits neutralised the adverse effects of immobilisation on articular cartilage.

In a study by Taniguchi [2068] HIG-82 rabbit synovial fibroblasts were cultured, and laser irradiation (660 nm) was applied at the power density of 40 mW/cm^2 for 2 minutes, corresponding to laser fluence of 4.8 J/cm^2. The effect of laser irradiation on cell proliferation, cell cycle progression, and expression of cyclin-dependent kinase inhibitors (CKIs) were investigated. The researchers also examined whether the effects of laser irradiation

The table shows suggested optimal range of power density in mW/cm2 and dose in joule/cm2 for the most common joints for infrared GaAlAs (continuous) lasers with wavelength 820, 830 and Nd:YAG lasers with wavelength 1064 nm, infrared GaAs lasers with wavelength 904 nm, and HeNe lasers, respectively. The number of points will have to be adjusted acc. to the size of the joint in question.
Modified after Bjordal [588].

Literature:
In vitro studies
Palma has previously showed that HeNe laser light blocks the increment of Prostaglandin E1 (PGE1) and Bradykinine (B) in the Plasma Fibrinogen Level (PFL). In a new study [357], another substance related to the inflammatory process, Tromboxane (Tx), was studied. The experiment confirmed the total block of PGE1/B when HeNe was administered. However, the complex PGE1/B/Tx was only partially blocked.

The study by Gavish [1579] was designed to determine the influence of LPT on the kinetics of MMP stimulation and decay, specific cytokine gene expression, and subcellular localization of promyelocytic leukemia (PML) protein on HaCaT human keratinocytes: The cells were irradiated by a 780 nm titanium-sapphire (Ti-Sa) laser with 2 J/cm^2 energy density. MMP was monitored with Mitotracker, a mitochondrial voltage-sensitive fluorescent dye. Cytokine gene expression was carried out using semi-quantitative-reverse transcription polymerase chain reaction. Subcellular localization of PML protein, a cell-cycle checkpoint protein, was determined using immunofluorescent staining. The fluorescence intensity of MMP was increased immediately after the end of laser by 148 +/- 6% over control. Subsequently it decayed, reaching 51 +/- 14% of the control level within 200 minutes. This decay was characterized by an exponential curve with a lifetime of 79 +/- 36 minutes. Following irradiation, the expression of interleukin-1alpha, interleukin-6, and keratinocyte growth factor (KGF) genes were transiently upregulated; but the expression of the proinflammatory gene interleukin-1ß, was suppressed. The subnuclear distribution of PML was altered from discrete domains to its dispersed form within less than 1 hour after laser irradiation. These changes reflect a biostimulative boost that causes a shift of the cell from a quiescent to an activated stage in the cell cycle heralding proliferation and suppression of inflammation. Further characterization of MMP kinetics may provide a quantitative basis for assessment of the effect of laser irradiation in the clinical setting.

Indications of an effect on the metabolism of cartilage are found in studies by Akai [466], Ruiz Calatrava [1057] and van der Veen [1058]. These studies used dosages similar to those in fibroblast studies. Researchers using higher dosages failed to demonstrate a stimulative effect [1191].

The aim of a study by Morrone [898] was to verify the effects of LPT performed with GaAlAs (780 nm, 2500 mW) on human cartilage cells in

Norwegian research group has been highlighted by articles in several major newspapers across Europe and North America, and with more than 60 unique website-listings within two weeks after publication. The recent development is further moving the balance in disfavour of NSAIDs and coxibs, and may well be the end of the era where they served as reference treatment for osteoarthritis.

The current situation may pave the road for other risk-free alternatives such as LPT, which has appeared to provide clinically relevant changes in several randomised placebo-controlled trials. From the findings of a Norwegian Health Technology Assessment Report, LPT could potentially be at least twice as effective as NSAIDs, if applied with optimal dose and energy. Even though the number of laser trials are still smaller than for NSAIDs, the unequivocal scientific findings so far have earned LPT a top spot in levels of evidence and treatment recommendations for knee osteoarthritis issued by the Norwegian Drug Agency. LPT is also reimbursed in the physiotherapy program by the National Health Insurance Agency, and is one of the standard therapies for knee osteoarthritis pain in Norway. As with all laser applications, it is necessary to use the laser and dosimetry parameters within the therapeutic window.

In conclusion, LPT for arthritis is an excellent indication. Being a chronic condition, there are no methods that can cure OA or RA, treatment will have to be life long. The problem is that some medications will shorten the life of the patient it is supposed to help. LPT is safe and without the serious side effects of pharmaceuticals. Being a life-long therapy, it would ideally mean initial therapy by a trained therapist three to four times per year, and a suitable low powered home laser unit for maintaining the effect.

Location	820, 830, 1060 nm		904 nm		632 nm	
	Lowest power density in mW/cm^2	Dose per point in joules	Lowest power density in mW/cm^2	Dose per point in joules	Lowest power density in mW/cm^2	Dose per point in joules
Finger/toe	10	1–5	3	0.5-5	10	2–5
Knee	10	5–20	3	0.5-5	10	6–30
Lumbar spine	100	40–200	15	7.5-37.5	Not investigated	>30
TMJ	10	1–5	3	0.5-5	10–400	2-4

Table 4.1 Arthritis

GaAs appears to have the best effect on osteoarthritis, and the majority of the positive studies for this indication have used GaAs [588].

The importance of high energy per point is illustrated in the study by Tascioglu [1505]. This study design was randomised, placebo-controlled and single blinded. Sixty patients with knee OA, according to the American College of Rheumatology criteria, were included and randomly assigned to three treatment groups: active laser with a dosage of 3 J per painful point (15 J per session), active laser with a dosage of 1.5 J per painful point (7.5 J per session) and placebo laser treatment groups. A GaAlAs laser with a power output of 50 mW, 830 nm was used. The patients were treated 5 times weekly with 10 treatments in all. Compared to baseline, at week three and at month six, no significant improvement was observed within the groups. Similarly, no significant differences were found among the treatment groups at any time. Only painful points were irradiated whereas cartilage and synovia remained untreated. Irradiation of painful points is only of secondary importance in LPT, irradiation at the target area is more important.

A Meta analysis by Bjordal [1421,1798] on the effect of NSAIDs on knee osteoarthritis pain appears to become important for the recognition and future development of LPT. A research group summarises that nonsteroidal anti-inflammatory drugs (NSAIDs), including cyclo-oxygenase-2 inhibitors (coxibs), reduce short-term pain associated with knee osteoarthritis only slightly better than placebo, and long-term use of these agents should be avoided. Up for analysis were 23 placebo-controlled trials involving 10,845 patients, 7767 of whom received NSAID therapy and 3078 placebo therapy. All in all 21 of the NSAID-studies were funded by the pharmaceutical industry, and the results of 13 of these studies were inflated by patient selection bias as previous NSAID-users were excluded if they had not previously responded favourably to NSAID. Such an exclusion criterion for non-responders has never been seen in any controlled trial of LPT or other non-pharmacological therapies of osteoarthritis. In the remaining 10 unbiased NSAID-trials, the difference from placebo was only 5.9 mm on a 100 mm pain scale. This is far less than established data on differences that are considered minimally perceptible (9 mm) or clinically relevant (12 mm) for knee osteoarthritis patients. In addition, none of the trials found any effects beyond 13 weeks. This bleak support for long term use of NSAIDs is an excellent support for non-pharmaceutical methods, such as LPT.

Adverse effects of long term medication with NSAIDs, and particularly coxibs, have received much attention in the "Vioxx-scandal". Consequently, coxibs like Vioxx have been withdrawn, Prexige has been withheld from the market, and the whole group of coxibs are now under special observation by drug agencies in both Europe and the United States. In contrast to the virtually non-existent side effects of LPT, NSAID side effects cause an estimated 2000 deaths annually in Great Britain alone, due to the fact that half of the 8.5 million osteoarthritis patients in Britain take these drugs on a regular basis. The considerable international interest in the findings of the

tinue the treatment. The pain reaction in itself is unpleasant, but is actually an indication of a positive reaction to the treatment.

Prolonged treatment schedules are necessary with a total accumulated (all sessions) dose of no less than 25 J for a small joint such as a finger. Three to five sessions per week are recommended in the initial phase. Patients in the early stages are more likely to experience prolonged benefits from LPT [1100], whereas patients in the later stages will obtain a better quality of life but with more or less transient effects of LPT [1023]. However, in sharp contrast to pharmaceuticals [1059], there will be no other side effects than the potential initial pain reaction. About 90% of the prescribed NSAIDs in Canada are attributed to the treatment of arthritis [1140]. It has also been postulated that about one third of the arthritis budget has been used to handle side effects of NSAIDs. These figures support the use of a side-effect free method such as LPT. It would be ideal for an elderly chronic patient to have a suitable laser of his own, or one leased from the hospital.

LPT influences the synovial fluid and its membranes [63, 639,718,751,1018,1022] and the articular cartilage [151,550,898,1021]. The PGE_2 activity is also modified [243,1008] as well as interleukin 1-ß [188,370].

Since the whole organism is involved, irradiating one or several joints will only give temporary relief [293,1023]. To obtain true improvement of quality of life, all the joints involved should be treated in many consecutive sessions [397] and comparatively high energies must be used [585]. It is essential that the large and deep-lying joints be given a sufficient dosage. Such treatment is certainly time-consuming but the alternatives, on the other hand, are rather bleak. It is possible for the patients to treat themselves according to instructions, as suggested by Stelian [617].

Although all wavelengths will have some effect, there is a difference in the total outcome, with some wavelengths more effective than others, due to better penetration of infrared light in large joints. In a study by Giavelli [638], 406 patients with osteoarticular diseases were treated with various wavelengths. The results were as follows: In gonarthrosis patients, statistical analysis of the results showed no significant differences between CO_2 laser and GaAs laser treatments, but there were significant differences between CO_2 laser and HeNe laser treatments, and between GaAs laser and HeNe laser treatments. In lumbar arthrosis patients treated with a GaAs or HeNe laser, significant differences were found between the two laser treatments, and the combined sweeping plus point techniques appeared to have a positive trend relative to the sweeping method alone, especially in sciatic suffering. In the algodystrophy syndrome in hemiplegic patients, significant differences were found between CO_2 and HeNe laser treatments, between high and low CO_2 laser doses, and between a low CO_2 laser dose and a high HeNe laser dose. The differences above do not indicate that HeNe is less useful in LPT, only that the deep lying structures treated could not be sufficiently saturated by HeNe laser light alone.

Hematuria, indicating renal involvement, was noted in 18.75% of the non-laser treated children.
  Further literature: [350, 1052, 1205]

4.1.3 Arteriosclerosis

Two small studies are not an impressive foundation for a recommendation. But again, with no side effects reported, and traditional therapies not very successful, what is there to loose?

Literature:
  Laser treatment of arteriosclerosis (claudicatio intermittens) of the lower limbs has been described by Attia [964]. In the study, 20 patients with arteriosclerosis in the lower limbs were treated with HeNe 20 mW, 830 nm, 250 mW, applied transcutaneously to the lumbar region by a scanner for 30 minutes, six days a week for two months. The duration of the condition varied from one to eight months. Pain was relieved in 16 patients after three to seven applications of treatment. At the end of the therapy, 8 patients were able to walk 1500 metres without experiencing pain in the calf muscles. Three patients discontinued therapy for reasons not related to the therapy and one patient showed no improvement.
  Similar results are reported by Klimenko [1306].

4.1.4 Arthritis

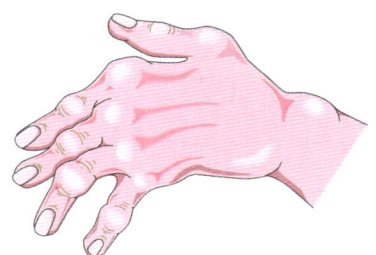

Arthritis is a wide indication, including diagnoses such as rheumatic arthritis (RA), osteoarthritis (OA), morbus Bechterew and psoriatic arthritis. It is unlikely that laser treatment will cure any of these conditions, as with any other medication, but the symptoms and the quality of life of the patients can often be improved considerably. In addition to pain relief, increased range of movement and reduced swelling can be achieved to some extent. A suitable dosage for a small joint such as a finger is from the lateral side 1-2 J, with GaAs always at a lower dose. For larger joints, a considerably higher dosage is needed. A knee, for instance, may need 15-25 J per session. Hip and shoulder arthritis require a high laser output, and a probe applied with strong pressure on suitable anatomical points, to achieve a sufficient dose to the target area. Only infrared will work on deep structures, while all wavelengths will work on small joints.

  Conditions of chronic pain may react with an increase in pain, which is why it is best to begin with a low dosage. This should be explained to the patient, so that the initial occurrence of pain is not used as a reason to discon-

treatment included pointing around loci for 5 minutes per point and locally lesion lighting 10 minutes per area, and a course consisted of at least six treatments with the program once a day. Then, the therapeutic trial was assessed after two courses of the aforementioned schedule were completed. The mixed remedy of both LPT with antibiotic formula produced better response, total effective rate 96.45 %, better than the sham placebo and single antibiotic control groups. Meanwhile, it also showed less scar formation and hypopigmentation or even less skin whitening than both control groups did.

Further literature: [62, 833]

4.1.2 Allergy

Allergy is yet another example of an indication with poor scientific backing. We still dare to recommend the use of LPT. Not only because it is safe, but because we have seen it work well. Allergy is an increasing problem worldwide and prolonged intake of pharmaceuticals is yet another problem to tackle. Relief from seasonal pollinosis is an excellent indication, especially if the patient can use a home care laser.

Literature:

Takeyoshi [1052] has treated patients suffering from allergic rhinitis with ganglion blocks. In a comparative study 20 patients had traditional stellate ganglion block (SGB) and 12 patients had laser irradiation over the stellate ganglion (SGL). GaAlAs lasers of 60 mW (10 minutes of irradiation) and 150 mW (7 minutes of irradiation) were used. The number of sessions was maximum 20 over a period of one month. 60% of the patients receiving SGB reported the outcome as "excellent" or "good" while 100% of the patients in the SGL group had this rating.

Ailioaie [981] and Tulebaev [555] report positive effects on allergic rhinitis using LPT.

Ailioaie [1204] reports promising results in the laser treatment of children's allergic purpura. This condition, of unknown aetiology, is characterised by migratory polyarthralgia or polyarthritis, abdominal pain, vasculitis of the small vessels and in the kidney. Conventional therapy consists of NSAIDs to control subjective problems, antibiotics when indicated and corticosteroids in acute phases. The prognosis for recovery is generally good, though symptoms frequently (25-50%) return over a period of several months. In the Ailioaie study, 31 children aged 2-16 years were divided into two groups (15/16) after clinical and laboratory tests. One group was given conventional therapy whereas the other was treated with a laser scanner of 670 nm (50 mW) and 830 nm (300 mW) nm in combination, 4-10 J/cm^2. Scanning was performed daily for 21 days. The clinical outcome was good in both groups but in the laser group the improvement was spectacular during the first 10 days and all final scores measured were better in the laser group.

generate any new knowledge. In these studies, the possible effects on the microbes are discussed; however, the important biostimulatory effect is not recognized by some of these authors. There is a lot of anecdotal reports on acne and therapeutic lasers but hardly anything published. Although the scientific evidence is poor, LPT for acne can be recommended, not only because it reduces the acute symptoms, but also because it reduces scarring.

Literature:

Simunovic [958] used a combination of GaAlAs point irradiation and HeNe scanning to treat acne and acne scars in a two-centre study on 80 patients. In the first therapy group, LPT was used as monotherapy and in the second it was used in combination with topical application of tetracycline. Both groups included acute as well as chronic cases. Mono therapy demonstrated relief of all local clinical symptoms. Used in combination with tetracycline, the healing process was accelerated and there was a decrease in tetracycline side effects and reduced occurrence of relapses. In all patients treated with LPT, scars were significantly prevented or reduced.

Seaton [1328] treated acne vulgaris using a low level pulsed dye laser. One single irradiation was given to 31 patients and sham irradiation to 10 patients. After 12 weeks, acne severity (measured by Leeds revised grading system) was reduced from 3.8 to 1.9 in the laser group and 3.6 to 3.5 in the sham group. Total lesion counts fell by 53% in laser patients and 9% in controls, and inflammatory lesion counts reduced by 49% in laser patients and 10% in controls. The most rapid improvements were seen in the first four weeks after treatment.

Webb [615] wanted to test the claim that LPT could prevent or improve previously created hypertrophic scar tissue. A 17 mW 660 nm laser diode was used at dosages of 2.4 or 4 J/cm^2. Two cell lines derived from hypertrophic scar tissue (HST) and normal dermal tissue explants (NDT) were irradiated and a cell count was taken. The irradiated hypertrophic cells exhibited significantly higher cell counts than control on days one to four for HST and days one to three for NDT.

A reduction of hypertrophic fibroblast proliferation following HeNe irradiation is reported by Shu [1705]. **Since fibroblast proliferation is enhanced by suitable doses of LPT, inhibitory high doses must be used to decrease established hypertrophic scars, while early irradiation at lower doses could reduce the risk of scarring.**

In a study by Hou [2041], 186 patients with severe acne were selected from the out-patient department in the hospital. The sex ratio was 1:1.5 (male:female), age ranging from 17-58 years old. Before treatment, all cases were scored according to a 4-point assessment schedule, and those with serious heart problems, chronic infectious disorders and long-term use of corticosterone drug were ruled out of the trial. A sham placebo and single antibiotic groups were carried out throughout the trial. The laser treatment parameters were 810 nm, power adjustable 5-1200 mW, 4-8 J/cm^2. Every

Medical and dental indications are often interrelated. In the following section, we have provided cross-references where the indication is applicable to both. Relatively little commentary is provided on the various indications. Instead we have selected some studies, letting their contents speak for themselves. We have included some indications for which the documentation is weak, in hopes of inspiring future research.

When doses in quoted *in vitro* studies are to be extrapolated for clinical use, several things must be remembered. Therefore, we have limited the text to quoting whatever is stated in the report. Indeed, we have the feeling that some authors have not understood the difference between "Joule" and "J/cm²". And keep in mind that a high value for J/cm^2 does not necessarily mean that the energy applied was high, maybe only that the fibre was thin. The best way of gaining information about suitable dosages for musculoskeletal conditions is to check the recommendations of the *World Association for Laser Therapy* found on www.walt.nu.

In the following text, we have included some personal comments in the scientific abstracts. These are marked in **bold** text.

4.1 Who and what can be treated?

It is not unusual for therapists to ask: "Can I treat this with LPT?" As soon as we hear the question "Can I treat ...", we can answer: "Yes"! LPT is a completely safe treatment as long as it is done with lasers up to a few hundred milliwatts. But we always point out the importance of having a reliable diagnosis - a diffuse pain can be due to cancer, ilius or ...

However, the correct question is not "Can I treat that?" but "Can that be treated?" It is not true that anyone successfully can treat anything; a combined knowledge of medicine and LPT is mandatory for good clinical results. With few exceptions, the worst thing that can happen is that nothing happens. In the following text, evaluations of the application of LPT for various indications will be given. These recommendations are mainly based upon the available scientific literature, but also upon our own experience and the experience of our broad network of therapists. Many indications for LPT are not yet "invented". Still, some of them are being used with success, even though no studies have been published. However, in this book we have restricted ourselves to those indications actually found in the literature, even though the scientific quality in some cases is low.

Since LPT works by stimulating the natural cellular processes, it is easy to imagine many new indications documented in the near future.

4.1.1 Acne
Acne is one of the oldest indications for LPT. HeNe laser has been used by beauticians for more than 25 years and has been reported to be effective in combination with traditional therapies such as dermabrasion. Recent studies using expensive dye lasers have had great media exposure, but do not really

Chapter 4
Medical indications

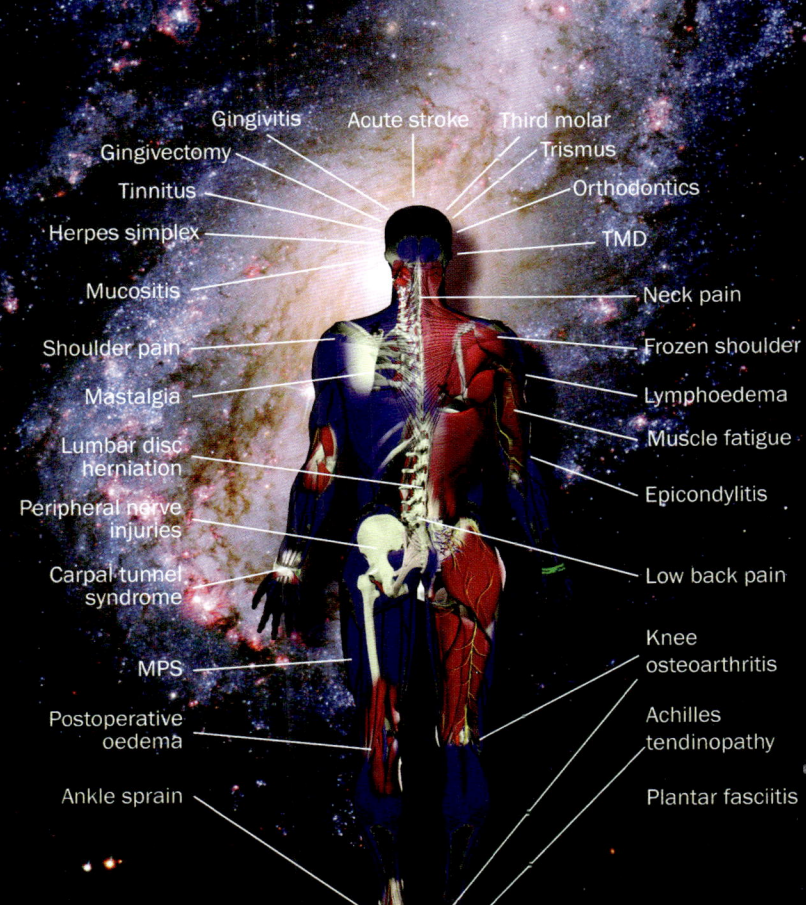

laser therapy. A more detailed survey was then addressed to these 215. 139 (63.1%) responded to this survey and were asked to grade five common electronic treatment methods (interferential therapy, pulsed electromagnetic energy, short-wave diathermy, ultrasound, and laser therapy). Laser therapy was considered the best method for the treatment of pain (by a small margin) and for wound healing (by far). Laser therapy was in third place for the treatment of oedema. However, it is likely that today's laser equipment, with its considerably higher power, may give laser therapy a higher ranking for oedema, and a much greater margin of victory for the treatment of pain. The predominant indications were (in order) wound healing, soft tissue damage, pain, and arthritic conditions. All of the laser therapy users were dissatisfied with the lack of independent and clinically oriented literature in the field. Most of them had acquired their knowledge from brochures and courses run by suppliers and manufacturers. Many were also dissatisfied with the conflicting advice given by various sales representatives.

Cambier [637] carried out a similar survey of physiotherapists in Flanders in 1996. Wounds and tendinitis seemed to be the indications of choice. The results were compared with those from Baxter's study and the two studies seem to match quite well.

In the Netherlands, about 10% of dentists (approximately 600) used laser therapy in 1995. In a study by Oudoff [465], 200 Dutch dentists were asked to fill in a standard questionnaire. All of the 92 respondents used a 830 nm 30 mW laser. The dentists were positive regarding the results of laser treatment after surgery and for mucosal lesions, periodontology, and muscular disorders. They were less positive about the long-term results for toothache and hypersensitive dentine.

In Hungary, more than 30% of the dentists and family doctors were using laser therapy in 1999 [870].

3.8.8 The funding of research

It is now and then suggested that manufacturers of laser therapy equipment should prove their claims by financing research. While quite a few of the manufacturers actually have used their scarce resources to do precisely that, it is not reasonable to expect much such funding. There is no patent on laser therapy equipment, so any valuable information found in research will be available to every manufacturer on the market. Funding pharmaceutical research is quite a different matter. Pills can be patented.

condylalgia. Next I was surprised to find that the evidence in favour of laser therapy was at the same level both in clinical effect and statistical power."

It is interesting to note that Bjordal [1456] has published a meta analysis on the effect of non-steroidal anti-inflammatory drugs, including cyclo-oxygenase-2 inhibitors in osteoarthritic knee pain in 2004. The negative outcome of this analysis had great media coverage. However, there was hardly any media coverage when the same group of evaluators presented scientific evidence enough to make laser treatment of osteoarthritic knee pain reimbursable and accepted as one out of three recommended therapies in Norway.

3.8.6 Confused?

Anyone who studies the literature carefully can become confused. Some wavelengths achieve the best effects on this and that, while others have poorer effects or none at all. Some doses lead to beneficial effects, but when the dose is increased, the effects wear off. If we treat a condition, some of the parameters we want to influence may be affected, but perhaps not all. If we administer treatment from a distance, we do not get the same effect as if we treat in contact or with pressure. Some frequencies produce effects on pain, others on oedema. What are we to believe? And what do we do to find the best dose, wavelength, etc.?

There is still much to learn in the field of laser therapy, and for the time being we must be satisfied with the knowledge that we have. This is often a combination of clinical experience with a degree of scientific foundation. The biological effects we produce can, in any case, be seen as an empirical mean value effect, and as long as this entails concrete and positive results we can be satisfied with this rather rigid treatment model. In the future, people are likely to think that we used laser light in a primitive fashion - but for the time being, we must content ourselves with the fact that laser therapy really works.

Is the use of laser therapy, then, only a job for trained scientists? Hardly! As usual, reality is rather more difficult than the producers of glossy brochures would have us believe, but in practice it is a lot easier than this book sometimes implies. Anyone with medical knowledge can successfully use laser therapy after an introductory course. You do not need to know everything to be a good therapist, but the more you learn the greater the success you will encounter in your day-to-day work.

3.8.7 Experience and attitudes

In the literature on the subject, a great deal of individual experience and approaches to laser therapy have been presented. One of the few attempts so far to compile the experience of a large group of professional practitioners was made by Baxter in 1990 [281]. Every physiotherapist in Northern Ireland received a written questionnaire inquiring into his or her experience with laser therapy. 397 of 533 responded, and 215 of these had experience of

3.8.5 How well documented?

A substantial body of scientific documentation is required for a new treatment method to be accepted by the medical community, which is of course positive. However, more than 30 years' clinical experience without any reports of significant side effects or injury should suffice for laser therapy not to inspire fears of unknown side effects. Over 2500 research reports are not that many in this context, but neither are they negligible. However, do we need to know everything before we begin to use a method, if we know for sure that it is not dangerous?

Let us make a comparison with the world's most widely used medicine: acetylsalicylic acid. It has been used for generations, as its pain-relieving and antipyretic properties could be easily observed. However, the theory that acetylsalicylic acid works by alleviating pain centres in the brain has been abandoned in recent years. It is now believed that it inhibits the production of some prostaglandins. It has also been discovered recently that the substance has a positive effect on vascular illnesses. In any event, empiricism has held sway here. We do not know exactly how laser therapy works either, but whoever decides to put it to the test in a clinical environment will soon see that it works.

We can compare laser therapy with a description of NSAID (non-steroidal anti-inflammatory drugs) in a medical book. This group of pharmaceuticals for the treatment of osteoarthritis is described as follows:

"NSAID has a beneficial effect on inflammation and reduces morning stiffness, and alleviates swelling and pain in the joints. In spite of this, there is no proof that the substances affect the course of the illness, or that they can prevent erosion of the cartilage and joints. The clinical effects of NSAID are usually obtained within a week. If no effect is noted, it can be worthwhile to try another substance within the NSAID group, as patients show individual sensitivity to closely related substances."

If we substitute "laser therapy" for "NSAID" and "laser" for "substance", those who work with biostimulation will recognise the situation.

"Laser therapy has a beneficial effect on inflammation and reduces morning stiffness, and alleviates swelling and pain in the joints. In spite of this, there is no proof that the laser therapy affects the course of the illness, or that it can prevent erosion of the cartilage and joints. The clinical effects of laser therapy are usually obtained within a week. If no effect is noted, it can be worthwhile to try another laser within the laser therapy group, as patients show individual sensitivity to different laser wavelengths."

Both the statements above are true and documented, but only one is generally accepted. It is interesting to quote the foreword of the Master Thesis by Bjordal [732]: "First I was surprised by the scant evidence in favour of NSAID or steroid injections in shoulder tendinitis/bursitis and lateral epi-

Institutional Review Board is a committee of laypersons from different professions. Such a committee can issue a permit to use an "investigational advice" like a therapeutic laser, provided the therapist produces satisfactory evidence of the efficacy and a simple design of the proposed study. Patients treated by laser therapy also have to sign a written consent to say that they accept being treated. At the beginning of 2002 three so-called 510(k) were issued by the FDA, clearing the use of laser therapy for a few indications. This has been followed by others, once the ice was broken.

The status of laser therapy in the United States is formulated on the web site of the FDA:

Biostimulation lasers, also called low level laser therapy (LLLT), cold lasers, soft lasers, or laser acupuncture devices, were cleared for marketing by FDA through the Premarket Notification/510(k) process as adjunctive devices for the temporary relief of pain. These clearances were based on the presentation of clinical data to support such claims. FDA will consider similar applications for these and other claims with the decision to require clinical data being made on an individual basis, taking into consideration both the device and the claim. Please note that FDA law and regulations contain provisions that permit limited distribution of unapproved devices for use in clinical investigations. There are numerous clinical investigations being conducted in this and other countries to determine safety and efficacy with these devices for the intended uses that are proposed.

Certain unapproved, nonsignificant risk Class III medical devices, including biostimulation lasers, may only be distributed in the U.S. to individual practitioners who have approval from an Institutional Review Board (IRB) for the investigational clinical use of the device, or to investigators participating in a study under an Investigational Device Exemption (IDE) approved by the Center for Devices and Radiological Health (CDRH), as specified in the Code of Federal Regulations (CFR), 21 CFR 812. Even with IRB approval, a sponsor must comply with IDE requirements such as monitoring investigations, maintaining records, making reports, and complying with prohibitions on promotion and commercialization of investigational devices. The investigators would have similar responsibilities, also covered in 21 CFR 812.

A few lasers have received FDA clearance, each one for a specific indication. Other laser manufacturers have used the old approach of several LED manufacturers, i.e. to have the laser approved for "heat therapy". The use of heat in the treatment of musculo-skeletal conditions is noncontroversial and therefore manufacturers of LEDs and lasers can apply for clearance from the FDA, not for biostimulation but for topical heat therapy. The clearance makes it possible for the manufacturers to sell their equipment, but not to make any medical claims of biostimulation. Thus, a "FDA approval" is a rather vague description of the scientific base of the equipment.

Laser therapy has been accepted in central and Eastern Europe and in Asia in an entirely different way. In Japan, where the medical authorities are known for being as strict as the FDA - if not stricter - the method has been accepted for selected indications and is in widespread use. The use of laser therapy as a medical modality was approved by the Japanese government in 1987 and the application in health insurance started in 1996. Laser therapy is reimbursed in Hungary, provided that the doctor has attended a training course and received a diploma. In Norway, laser therapy is reimbursed when used in physiotherapy. A meta analysis of the laser therapy literature for tendinitis was the basis when the Norwegian government accepted the therapy in 2001.

3.8.3 Does it have to be a laser?

A good point - does it have to be a laser? Could we use a normal torchlight instead? Of course we could, but we would not achieve the same biological effects as with a laser. It is known, see chapter 11.1 "Are the biostimulative effects laser specific?" on page 528, that all light affects the living organism, but in a number of studies in which the effects of light from various sources have been compared, the laser light is shown to give the strongest effect.

Polarised wide band light (i.e. incoherent but polarised light) will indeed have a fair effect on "naked" tissues such as open wounds and mucous membranes, and, of course, on tissue *in vitro*. This has been demonstrated in early studies by Mester [23], Kana [204] and Marín [498]. However, polarisation is lost very soon after the light enters the tissue [1192]. Thus, only superficial structures will react to polarised light. If you are interested in the details and more literature, you can read more in Chapter 11.

Literature:

The effect of HeNe and monochromatic red incoherent light on the protein and glycose metabolism in hamsters was studied by Onac [447]. Both light sources had a stimulative effect but the effect of incoherent light (peak at 618 nm) was lower.

3.8.4 FDA (Food and Drug Administration)

In a panel discussion at the 2nd Congress of the World Association for Laser Therapy in 1998 in Kansas City, USA, the authors of this book pointed out that there is a clear difference between the medical authorities in the USA and Europe: In the USA everything that is not approved by the medical authority (Food and Drug Administration - FDA) is forbidden, but in Europe everything that is not forbidden is allowed. This means that laser therapy has been used by clinicians in Europe all the time - and still is.

Recently, however, the FDA has started its own investigations on laser therapy on wound healing [953, 1222]. Although the use of laser therapy in the USA is restricted, there are still many practitioners who use it. However, in order to use it they must have what it called an "IRB approval". A local

For those who are well acquainted with the subject and follow research developments in publications and international conferences, it is easy to answer the questions posed above:

- Laser therapy works: on chronic ulcers, neuralgia, pain, oedema, inflammations and on several other indications.
- There is extensive international documentation.
- A great deal is already known about the mechanisms.

3.8.2 Why the controversy?

Despite the fact that so much has been done, many people have great difficulty in accepting that laser therapy can have a positive effect on various conditions. This skepticism stems from several factors, of which the following is a selection:

- Many critics have not bothered to examine the extensive documentation but have instead relied upon the daily press or grapevines.

- Laser therapy was first described in "Eastern Europe". People within the field of medicine are more used to Americans and Western Europeans making the most important breakthroughs, and during the Cold War there was great skepticism in the West about the standard of science in "Eastern Europe".

- Laser therapy was not approved for any indication by the Food and Drug Administration (FDA) in the USA until 2002.

- Because laser therapy does not involve risks, other than certain risks of eye injury, and does not have any side-effects or negative effects, and may therefore be used by personnel other than doctors/dentists, many persons find it difficult to believe that it can have any positive effect.

- Bogus "lasers" and laser instruments of deficient quality, which have led to little or no biological effect, have given laser therapy systems a bad reputation.

- The effects of treatment are not always evident in the short term, as they are after operations using scalpels or powerful lasers.

- It is indeed hard to accept the fact that one single therapeutic modality can have an effect on so many indications.

Furthermore,

- There are individuals who do not react well to laser therapy.

- It has taken a long time to find out how this, admittedly fairly weak, laser light, which does not provide any noticeable heat, can relieve pain and influence inflammations and infections, oedema, etc. It is only recently that we have begun to understand the mechanisms involved.

3.8.1 Does laser therapy really work?

So, does laser therapy really work, or is it a sophisticated placebo? If it works, what kind of problems is it useful for? Is there any proof? Have controlled, randomised, double blind studies been published in which significant medical benefits have been proved? And if so, what mechanisms are associated with these benefits?

The following quotations are worth considering:

1. "A hard judgement has been passed on low-level lasers, which have been said to have no effect. Yet isn't it rather strange that ineffective lasers to the tune of a couple of hundred million dollars have been sold over the space of a few years? And why are there so many who can describe how the laser has helped them find a new life without pain?

It seems to be difficult, in scientific studies, to demonstrate the biological effects of the low-level laser. This raises an irreverent thought: perhaps there is something wrong with the scientific methods, or even worse, that the research scientists are not sufficiently skilled? It is unacceptable to blame placebo effects and the fact that people are dissatisfied with public health care.

In any case: a committed research scientist who sticks his neck out and says that money spent on low-level laser treatment is money wasted is taking a big risk. He cannot expect to be believed by anyone who has been successfully treated with a laser. If he is conscious of his scientific standing, he would be better advised to adopt a more humble approach".

Sten Erik Jensen, editor of Medicinsk Teknik, No 1, 1990.

2. "The work with this thesis can be described as my first exciting journey into Physiotherapy Science, and I feel like a novice seeking adventure. At the end of this journey, the turbulent story of laser therapy reminds me of a fairytale by H. C. Andersen. It is named after the main character and called "The Ugly Duckling", which after some time turned out to be a beautiful swan. In science things are not always what they seem to be at first sight. I have learned that a touch of humbleness and an open mind are always needed in scientific work."

Jan M. Bjordal, Master Thesis in Physiotherapy Science, Division of Physiotherapy Science, University of Bergen, Norway, 1997.

Words worth considering! There are a number of other issues to be considered, such as the animal experiments conducted where healing has been observed - are these also placebo effects? What about the researchers who have demonstrated the medical effects of low-level lasers on cell cultures, laboratory animals, and in more than 100 double-blind studies on patients: have they lied about their results, and together decided to fool the whole world? Probably not.

6.4 J/cm^2 brought about significantly increased strength. The difference in collagen concentration, however, did not reach a significant level.

There are several positive studies on tensile strength. Braverman [50], Lyons [462], and Riendeau [68] used HeNe, while Enwemeka [463] used GaAs and Stadler [954] GaAlAs.

3.7.5 Other objective methods

Other examples of objective methods are measurements of nerve conduction velocity, nerve action potential, chemiluminescence of blood, the study of vascularisation by means of a microscope [35], and the secretion of metabolites.

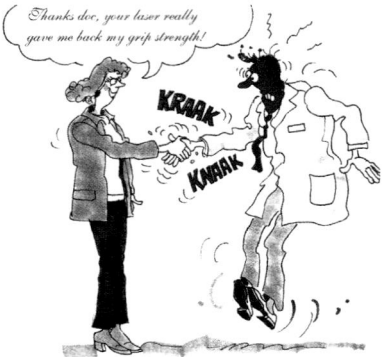

3.8 "Is laser therapy effective?"

Why do we put this question here, when you already have read more than 100 pages and are convinced? Well after all the information given in these first 100 pages, with objective test methods and all, it is natural that you are convinced. But there are many people, still, that are not and we believe it is valuable to know this part of the "history". This can also support you with some arguments for discussions with "non-believers".

Many people wonder whether laser therapy really works or is simply a sophisticated form of placebo. This skepticism comes mostly from doctors, and has spread via certain media to dentists and veterinary surgeons. Many other professionals - nurses, physiotherapists, chiropractors, and masseurs, for example - have tested lasers and generally been pleasantly surprised by the results.

Unfortunately, it is not unusual that professionals in high medical positions, without knowledge or own experience of laser therapy, tell the media: "Laser therapy has no effect!" or "Laser therapy is humbug!"

Makihara [1769] reports that his results suggested that low-level laser irradiation had a long-lasting effect on facial cutaneous tissues. Nine healthy subjects underwent irradiation using the continuous wave setting of a CO_2 laser with a power output of 1.0 W. The laser tip was positioned 10 cm above the skin over the right TMJ area for 10 min. The actual fluence on the facial surface was 7.64 J/cm^2. Variation of the facial temperature was evaluated by using thermography. The facial temperature 10 min after stopping irradiation was higher than that after 10 min of irradiation applied to the opposite side. The warmer area was found not only over the TMJ area but also over the temporal area, forehead area, and eyelid area on both sides.

Further literature: [126, 232, 189, 478, 495, 1208, 1246, 1249, 1659, 2065].

3.7.2 Magnetic resonance imaging

This is another objective method of quantifying the effect of laser therapy tissue repair.

Schaffer [904] explored the effect of a diode laser (780 nm) on normal skin tissue. Time-dependent contrast enhancement was determined by magnetic resonance imaging (MRI). In the examinations, six healthy volunteers were irradiated on their right planta pedis (sole of foot) with 5 J/cm^2 at a power density of 100 mW/cm^2. T1-weighted magnetic resonance imaging was used to quantify the time-dependent local accumulation of Gadolinium-DPTA, its actual content in the local current blood volume as well as its distribution to the extracellular space. Images were obtained before and after the application of laser light. When laser light was applied, the signal to noise ratio increased by an average of 0.35 (range 0.23-0.63) after irradiation according to contrast-enhanced MRT. According to the authors, it can be observed that, after biomodulation with light of low energy and low power, wound healing improves and pain is reduced. This effect might be explained by an increased blood flow in this area. Therefore, the use of this kind of laser treatment might improve the outcome of other therapeutic modalities such as tumour ionising radiation therapy and local chemotherapy.

3.7.3 High resolution digitised ultrasound B-scan

This is yet another method of objectively measuring the effect of laser therapy in wound healing, described by Dyson [923].

3.7.4 Tensile strength

Asencio-Arana [148] examined the strength and collagen concentration of high-risk anastomosis in the colons of rats after endoscopic irradiation with HeNe laser. The results showed that repeated irradiation (1.9 J/cm^2) with HeNe laser light increased the tensile strength of the anastomosis by almost 100% by the fourth day after the operation. An equivalent experiment with

3.7 How to measure effects of laser therapy

In many "alternative medical therapies", the effects are measured by asking the patient before and after "How do you feel?", and if, after therapy, the patient says "Much better!", the therapy is considered effective. In the case of laser therapy, several biological treatment effects can be studied by means of objective detection methods rather than subjective evaluations.

3.7.1 Thermography

One such method is thermography. With this technique, the temperature distribution on a surface is presented as a picture in which the different temperatures are shown in different colours (a "colour-coded" image). Thus, a change in blood flow can be detected second-by-second and minute-by-minute after a laser exposure.(See thermograpy pictures on page 282-283.)

Literature:

Kamikawa [319] used three different types of laser in a group of pain patients. Apart from irradiating the painful area, distant acupuncture points were used. The three lasers were: Nd:YAG of maximum 200 mW, GaAlAs 10 mW, and GaAs 10 mW. The laser beam focus was 1 mm^2. The thermographs showed a remarkable circulatory increment, extending in a wide area around the irradiated spots. Heat production in the irradiated spots disappeared soon after therapy, but the circulatory increment lasted for a while and pain was relieved. In a patient with Raynaud's disease, recordings were made at different room temperatures. At a room temperature of about 18 degrees, vascular response was easily evoked by laser therapy. At a room temperature of around 14 degrees, peripheral vasodilatation reluctantly appeared under prolonged irradiation. Fingers were used to illustrate the effect. Stimulatory effects could only be seen in the irradiated fingers. When a 150 mW Nd:YAG was used for three minutes on a spot, the temperature elevation was 3 degrees. The effect lasted for a few hours. This patient was given forty treatments, and his symptoms were reduced the following winter without further treatment.

Bradley [117] used thermography to examine the difference between the effect of needles and a GaAs laser on acupuncture points. Both needle and laser acupuncture produced an area of raised thermal emission at the site of stimulation. The effect was somewhat slower when initiated by a laser (2-4 minutes) than with needles (immediate).

Obata [185] studied the effect of 30 mW GaAlAs on a group of patients with diagnosed rheumatoid arthritis. Thermography was used on the irradiated hand to check the possible correlation between pain relief and thermographic response. A VAS scale was used to assess the degree of pain relief. Patients reacting with an immediate decrease in temperature had the best pain relief.

observed at 100 W/m² in the recA- strain, some protection appeared to be there at 2 W/m². Mechanistic studies carried out on these strains at the two irradiances suggest that, whereas the protection observed at 100 W/m² is mediated by singlet oxygen that observed at 2 W/m² is not. Further, the fact that protection at 100 W/m² was observed only in recA proficient strains suggests that it may arise due to the induction of DNA repair processes controlled by the recA gene. The latter may arise due to the oxidative stress produced by singlet oxygen generated by He-Ne laser irradiation. In contrast, the protection observed at 2 W/m² appears to be independent of the DNA repair proficiency of the strain.

Kohli [1775] observed that pre-irradiation with a helium-neon laser induces protection against UVC radiation in wild-type E. coli strain K12AB1157. The magnitude of protection was found to depend on the helium-neon laser irradiance, exposure time and period of incubation between helium-neon laser exposure and subsequent UVC irradiation. The optimum values for dose, irradiance and interval between the two exposures were found to be 7 kJ/m², 100 W/m² and 1 h, respectively. The possible involvement of singlet oxygen in the helium-neon laser-induced protection is also discussed.

A study was made by Voskanian [1776] of the combined effect of laser radiation (helium-neon laser) and X-rays on bacteriae of different genotypes. The sensitivity of cells to X-rays was decreased by pre- and post-irradiation with laser. In the latter case, the radio-modifying effect of laser was more pronounced.

The combined effect of 532 nm laser radiation and alpha-particles on survival of Escherichia coli (AB 1157) was investigated by Voskanian [1777]. The sensitivity of cells to alpha-particles was decreased by pre- and post-irradiation with laser.

In an experiment by Karu [1778] monolayer of HeLa cells, at the stationary phase of growth, exposed to He-Ne laser radiation (632.8 nm; 100 J/m²) either 5 min or 60 min prior to gamma irradiation (0.1-10 Gy; 6.75 Gy/min), or 5 min after irradiation has been investigated. With a 5-min interval between irradiation sessions (both sequences) the survival curves are virtually the same as those for gamma-irradiated cells only. With He-Ne laser radiation delivered 60 min before gamma irradiation with doses exceeding 5 Gy, a fraction of radioresistant cells is identified whose D0 is almost twice as high as D0 of basic cell mass (3.6 and 1.7 Gy respectively. The survival curve becomes a two-component one. A hypothesis is proposed that HeNe laser radiation activates, in some cells, the processes that promote the repair of radiation

Further literature: [1081]

To investigate the cellular mechanisms by near-infra-red laser on the nervous system, Mochizuki-Oda [2020] examined the effect of 830 nm laser irradiation on the energy metabolism of the rat brain. The laser was applied for 15 min with an irradiance of 4.8 W/cm². Tissue adenosine triphosphate (ATP) content of the irradiated area in the cerebral cortex was 19% higher than that of the non-treated area, whereas the adenosine diphosphate (ADP) content showed no significant difference. Laser irradiation at another wavelength (652 nm) had no effect on either ATP or ADP contents. The temperature of the tissue was increased by 4.4-4.7 degrees C during the irradiation of both wavelengths. These results suggest that the increase in tissue ATP content did not result from the thermal effect, but from a specific effect of the laser operated at the 830 nm wavelength.

3.6.9 Protection against radiation injury

Podolskaya [366] has used HeNe laser on post-radiation reactions and injuries in lip skin and mucous membranes (post-radiation heilitis). The method has been more successful than previously used medical treatments. There were no complications in the laser group, while the traditionally treated group had several allergic reactions and re-operations. The pace of epithelialisation was 7 mm/week in the HeNe group, as compared to 4.1 mm/week in the control group.

Popova [147] studied the effects of HeNe laser light on the healing of muscle tissue after irradiation with 10 Gy roentgen. The muscle tissue of rats was removed, irradiated with X-rays and re-transplanted. Improved healing compared with the control group was observed whether laser light was administered before or after the transplant.

Literature:

The effect of HeNe laser pre-irradiation on UVA (343 nm)-induced DNA damage in the human B-lymphoblast cell line NC37 was investigated by Dube [1773], using the comet assay. HeNe laser pre-irradiation was observed to result in a dose-dependent decrease in UVA-induced DNA damage. This effect was also found to be dependent on the incubation period between HeNe laser pre-irradiation and the UVA exposure. Whereas the control cells with a higher DNA damage point to an initial ability of faster repair, both the control and the HeNe laser pre-irradiated cells subsequently show the same rate of DNA repair. The results suggest that HeNe laser irradiation protect the cells from UVA-induced DNA damage primarily through an influence on processes that prevent an initial DNA damage.

HeNe laser pre-irradiation-induced protection against UVC damage was investigated in wild-type E. coli K12 strain AB1157 and its isogenic DNA repair mutant strains. At a dose of 7 kJ/m2, pre-irradiation was observed by Kohli [1774] to induce protection in recA proficient strains (AB1157 and uvrA(-) AB1886) at both the irradiances investigated (2 and 100 W/m2). However, at the same dose (7 kJ/m2), while no protection was

of cultured lymphocytes of the Molt-4 cell line were irradiated with 904 nm, pulsed mode, 6 kHz PRR, with an average emission power of 10 mW for 60 min. A Spectra Physics M404 power meter was used to measure light intensity. Controls were treated similarly but not irradiated. The amount of ATP was measured by the luciferin-luciferase bioluminescent assay. The amount of ATP in irradiated cell cultures was 10.79 +/- 0.15 microg/L and in non-irradiated cell cultures it was 8.81 +/- 0.13 microg/L. The average percentage increase of irradiated versus control cell cultures was about 22.4% +/- 0.56% SD. This significant increase is probably due to laser irradiation; it cannot be attributed to any thermal effect, as the temperature during irradiation was maintained at 37.0 degrees +/- 0.5 degrees C. Thus the therapeutic effects of the biostimulating power of this type of laser are identified and its indications may be expanded.

A study by Stadler [2090] investigated the change in local skin temperature in black and white mice during irradiation at 830 nm. Groups of mice (n = 12 in each group) were lightly anesthetized. The dorsum was shaved and a 1.0 x 0.5 cm spot was marked in the same location on each subject. Animals wereirradiated with a diode laser (CW, 830 nm, 36 mW output at 5 cm distance). Fluences of 0.0-5.0 J/cm^2 were delivered. Skin surface temperature was monitored by a thermal camera. Two thermocouples were placed 1 mm below the skin surface at the site of light exposure. Temperature increased with increasing fluences of exposure. CW irradiation at 830 nm and 5.0 J/cm^2 fluence thus induces a small temperature increase at the surface and at 1 mm in depth. The smaller effects seen in white mice might be due in part to reflection. This suggests that the thermal effects of irradiation at 830 nm are unlikely to explain the LPT effect. However skin color should be considered, particularly at higher fluences.

In a study by Lanzafame [2089] pressure ulcers were created in mice by placing the dorsal skin between two round ceramic magnetic plates for three 12-h cycles. Animals were divided into three groups (n = 9) for daily light therapy (830 nm, CW, 5.0 J/cm^2) on days 3-13 post ulceration in both groups A and B. A special heat-exchange device was applied in Group B to maintain a constant temperature at the skin surface (30 degrees C). Group C served as controls, with irradiation at 5.0 J/cm^2 using an incandescent light source. Temperature of the skin surface, and temperature alterations during treatment were monitored. The wound area was measured and the rate and time to complete healing were noted. The maximum temperature change during therapy was 2.0 +/- 0.64 degrees C in Group A, 0.2 +/- 0.2 degrees C in Group B and 3.54 degrees C +/- 0.72 in Group C. Complete wound closure occurred at 18 +/- 4 days in Groups A and B and 25 +/- 6 days in Group C. The percentage of the wound closure at 14 days was 75. 4 +/- 7.2% and 77.7 +/- 5.6% for Groups A and B, respectively (NS differences). However, animals in Group C demonstrated a wound closure of 36.3 +/- 4.8%. These results demonstrate that the salutary effects of LPT on wound healing are temperature independent in this model.

eration twofold [355]. It may be concluded that stimulative dose ranges do not seem to lead to any histopathological cell changes.

The aim of th study by Fontana [1716] was to evaluate temperature variation induced by a diode laser in periodontal repair. The temperature variation induced by a 810 nm diode laser was investigated in an in vitro study, varying the soft tissue thickness, and in an in vivo study for soft periodontal and bone tissues. The laser powers used were 600 mW, 800 mW, 1.0 W, and 1.2 W, and the light was delivered by a 300-microm fiber. The laser parameters and irradiation time used did not induce a temperature variation high enough to cause thermal irreversible damage to the periodontal tissues investigated.

The aim of a study by Ilic [1590] was to investigate the possible short- and long-term adverse neurological effects of LPT given at different power densities, frequencies, and modalities on the intact rat brain. One hundred and eighteen rats were used in the study. Diode laser (808 nm) was used to deliver power densities of 7.5, 75, and 750 mW/cm^2 transcranially to the brain cortex of mature rats, in either continuous wave (CW) or pulse (Pu) modes. Multiple doses of 7.5 mW/cm^2 were also applied. Standard neurological examination of the rats was performed during the follow-up periods after laser irradiation. Histology was performed at light and electron microscopy levels. Both the scores from standard neurological tests and the histopathological examination indicated that there was no long-term difference between lasertreated and control groups up to 70 days post-treatment. The only rats showing an adverse neurological effect were those in the 750 mW/cm^2 (about 100-fold optimal dose), CW mode group. In Pu mode, there was much less heating, and no tissue damage was noted. Long-term safety tests lasting 30 and 70 days at optimal $10\times$ and $100\times$ doses, as well as at multiple doses at the same power densities, indicate that the tested laser energy doses are safe under this treatment regime. Neurological deficits and histopathological damage to 750 mW/cm^2 CW laser irradiation are attributed to thermal damage and not due to tissue-photon interactions.

3.6.8 Is it only an effect of temperature?
Heating pads and lights are used a lot and the beneficial effect is uncontroversial. It has been claimed that the effects of LPT are just an effect of the increased tissue temperature. With the very low outputs used in the 80s and 90s this explanation appears to be rather amateurish. Modern therapeutic lasers can be considerably more potent and indeed an increase of 1 or 2 centigrades in the superficial areas can be measured. This may be beneficial or not, but the small elevation of the temperature is not the basis of the medical effects.

Literature:

A study by Benedicenti [1955] investigated whether diode pulsed laser irradiation enhances ATP production in lymphocytes. Aliquots of an extract

3.6.7 Do high doses of laser therapy damage tissue?

Reasonable doses given in the course of laser therapy have proved to cause no macroscopic or microscopic damage to tissues. However, there has been concern about the new "high-power" laser therapy systems capable of emitting 100 – 1000 mW and more from a point source. Could GaAlAs applied to a single small spot for 3 minutes cause macroscopic damage? If not, what about 30 minutes? And what about elevation of tissue temperature? Let us have a look at some interesting experiments.

Literature:

Sasaki's [232] study was designed to evaluate concerns about possible damage to tissue following high doses of laser therapy. A 60 mW 830 nm laser was used (spot size 0.3 cm^2, power density 0.2 W/cm^2) on rat skin and subcutaneous tissue. One group received 3 minutes on one single spot per animal (36 J/cm^2), one group 30 minutes on one single spot (360 J/cm^2), and one untreated group served as control. Macroscopic and microscopic evaluations were carried out and photographic records taken. Tissue temperature was also recorded using digitised thermography. Skin temperature in the irradiated areas rose by 1.1 °C over the first 4 minutes of irradiation and then remained constant during the remainder of the 30-minute irradiation period. Macroscopically, there were no visible signs of alteration of skin colour or texture. Histology revealed no difference in the epidermal, dermal or subdermal tissue architecture in the control specimens or in those irradiated for 3-minute or 30-minute periods.

Calderhead [245] conducted a similar experiment, evaluating possible photothermal damage to articular membranous tissue following extended exposure to a 830 nm 60 mW laser. Two groups of rats received an incident energy of 108 J on a single joint, one group through the capsule and the other group with the capsule dissected away to allow direct exposure. A third group of animals served as control. No damage was visible microscopically, and no difference was found in the histology of the control specimens or in the indirectly or directly irradiated synovial membrane specimens.

Yoshida [1600] used GaAlAs at powers ranging from 300 to 700 mW, irradiating the stellate ganglion in rats. Exposure times ranged from 10 to 20 minutes. A slight oedema appeared 24 hours after the fifth irradiation at 700 mW. In other groups no pathological changes in the ganglion or in the immediately surrounding tissues were seen.

These three reports indicate that laser therapy does not cause damage to tissue, even when very high doses are given. Bear in mind, however, that these doses were given to healthy tissues and that only structural components in the tissues were studied.

Shefer [181] subjected rate skeletal muscle cells in vitro to HeNe laser at 180 mW/cm^2 (dose not stated). At four days post irradiation there were no histopathological changes as compared to non irradiated control cells. The same dose had previously been demonstrated to enhance satellite cell prolif-

In spite of the low risk associated with the irradiation of cancerous areas, any such area should be avoided when performing laser therapy. Only specialists should treat cancer, regardless of the type of therapy.

3.6.3 Cytogenetic effects?

In a study by Chio [456], human lymphocytes were irradiated by argon laser, HeNe laser or GaAlAs laser light in various doses. With an argon laser, there was a dose-related cytostatic effect between 30 and 300 J/cm^2. Mitosis was inhibited above 240 J/cm^2, and there was an increase in chromosome and chromatid breaks above 180 J/cm^2. As for the other two lasers, there was no significant increase in the frequency of chromosome aberrations. Doses of 0.5-1.5 J/cm^2 (GaAlAs) and 1-4 J/cm^2 (HeNe) increased mitotic activity.

3.6.4 A false picture of health

It is sometimes the case that pain disappears very quickly after a treatment session. It is then essential for the damaged tissue (e.g. an inflamed tendon) that caused the pain not to be overloaded. It is vital to inform the patient that such a false picture of health may emerge, and that the patient himself or herself is responsible for avoiding any stress to the injury. Even if the pain disappears and laser therapy shortens the healing time, the tissue must be given proper time to recover.

3.6.5 Tiredness

One "risk" associated with laser therapy is that the patient may experience extreme tiredness. This is probably due to release of metabolites, but sometimes also to the fact that the treatment eases long-standing pain. This relief allows the patient to catch up on the rest that the pain prevented him or her from getting. There are examples of trotting horses that were completely knocked out for two days after laser therapy treatment but then went back to competing as usual.

3.6.6 Pain reaction

A patient may sometimes experience pain the day after treatment. This is particularly common after the treatment of chronic complaints. It occurs because an injury is "made acute" when the process of healing starts. It is usually not a matter of an overdose. The patient should be informed of the risk of a pain reaction, that it is of a short-term nature and a positive sign. The patient may otherwise think it is some kind of "laser damage".

Except for the treatment of open wounds the risk of overdose on an individual level is actually low. Individual sensitivity should be taken into account.

to lower wavelengths used. The less transparent the tissue, the better the coagulating effect and the control of injuries in the surrounding tissue. A "surgical" diode laser in this range is an excllent biostimulator and some manufacturers have added a control switch, lowering the output into a traditional power output of therapeutic lasers.

Literature:
[1788-1792]

3.6 Risks and side effects

There are, of course, two sides to every story. What risks and side effects are associated with laser therapy? (We are naturally inclined to think along those lines.) We must first make it clear that the radiation we are dealing with here is visible light or infrared radiation and nothing more. The purity of the light does not in itself entail any risk - it is as dangerous as the pure tone of a flute compared with any pandemonium of the same volume.

3.6.1 The importance of a correct diagnose

Let us assume that a young person has got a pain in his knee. The knee is treated a number of times over a couple of months. Finally he is investigated by a specialist who finds a tumour in his knee. The doctor's question is: "Why haven't you come here before?"

This is not an actual case. But we give the example to illustrate the importance of obtaining a proper diagnosis before assuming that the pain is not due to cancer. It is important that the laser treatment does not cause a delay in the treatment of cancer and other serious diseases!

3.6.2 Cancer

Can laser therapy cause cancer? The answer is no. (See chapter 1.1.7 "Can electromagnetic radiation cause cancer?" on page 5.) No mutational effects have been observed resulting from light with wavelengths in the red or infrared range in doses used within laser therapy.

But what happens if I treat someone who has cancer and is unaware of it? Can the cancer's growth be stimulated? Well, the effects of laser therapy on cancer cells *in vitro* have been studied, and it was observed that they could be stimulated by laser light. However, with respect to a cancer *in vivo*, the situation is rather different. Experiments on rats have shown that small tumours treated with laser therapy may recede and completely disappear, although laser treatment had no effect on tumours over a certain size [9]. The local immune system is probably stimulated more than the tumour. See also [1, 2, 3].

The situation is the same for bacteria and virus in culture. Laser light in certain doses stimulates these, while a bacterial or viral infection *in vivo* is cured much faster after the right treatment with laser therapy.

"High power semiconductor lasers" on page 42.) Now, more and more ruby lasers are sold worldwide.

We wish to remind readers that it was with the ruby laser that the biostimulative effects were discovered by Mester's group in Hungary. The ruby laser is quite a good laser for laser therapy, but very expensive. However, if you already have one - use it for herpes, zoster, ulcers, scars, sinuitis etc! Penetration is better than light from a HeNe-laser. If you test it, you can see that in a dark room the light pulse goes through your hand.

But before starting, it is important to set the energy density at a setting which will not burn the patient. For example, if the pulse energy (the ruby laser is always pulsed) is 5 joules, we recommend that you use a surface of at least 5 cm^2, giving an energy density of 1 J/cm^2 when the pulse hits the surface to be treated. This means that for each laser pulse fired, each cm^2 will receive a dose of 1 J/cm^2 and 3 shots on the same surface will give a total treatment dose of 3 J/cm^2.

3.5.4 Laser therapy with Er:YAG lasers

Although these lasers have been introduced into biostimulation only recently, there is evidence of the pain relieving effect of Er:YAG lasers. This was first demonstrated in the treatment of hypersensitive dentine. Most researchers have looked at the morphological changes of the dentinal tubuli and overlooked the actualy pain relieving effect.

Literature:

In the study by Zeredo [1588] the researchers tested the possible antinociceptive effect of laser irradiation when applied to a normal tissue before the onset of a painful stimulus. Male rats were used. A 1.5% formalin solution was injected into the right upper lip of the test animals (n = 9) immediately after 10 min of low-power Er:YAG laser irradiation (energy: 0.1 J/cm^2 per pulse at 10 Hz). Control animals (n = 9) were restrained for 10 min without laser application. The nociceptive response, i.e., the amount of time the rats spent rubbing the formalin injected area, was measured by an investigator blind to whether the animals had been laser irradiated or not. On laser irradiated rats, significantly less nociceptive behavior was observed only during the late phase (12-39 min) of the test. This result is similar to that reported for nonsteroid antiinflammatory drugs (NSAIDs) and other peripherally acting antiinflammatory agents.

Further literature: [1311, 1606, 1646]

3.5.5 Laser therapy with surgical diode lasers

High powered GaAlAs lasers are increasingly popular in dental "surgery" due to their rather small size and comparatively low price. A typical output is 1 W. Indications are minor surgery such as pocket debridement, incisions, gingival contouring, clearing of implants, perimiplantitis, removal of vascular lesions. 980 nm is a common wavelength and could probably be preferred

Nd:YAG lasers should be aware that there is more to this type of laser than the instruction manual would have us believe.

Aphtous ulcers can be successfully treated with Nd:YAG. The energy suggested in the literature is much higher than when therapeutic lasers are used but the treatment can generally be performed without anaesthesia.

Literature:

Abergel [8] has shown that collagen can not only be stimulated by means of different doses, but that it can also be regulated, that is, both inhibited (keloids) and promoted (healing). Abergel [150] has also demonstrated a stimulating effect on human skin fibroblasts as a result of the use of Nd:YAG laser therapy.

Goldman [152] conducted a controlled study of 30 patients with rheumatoid arthritis. He found significant effects of Nd:YAG laser therapy on pain and stiffness.

Kaneko [218] has reported effects of 50 mW Nd:YAG treatment on pain relief from dry socket, paraesthesia of the lower jaw, trigeminal neuralgia, wounds on the tongue and mucous membrane, as well as pain related to TMJ disorders.

Kawamura [202] used Nd:YAG to study the effects of laser therapy on periodontal wound healing. Epithelial down-growth after a flap operation was reduced by laser therapy.

Basford [1062] performed a double-blind, placebo-controlled, randomized clinical trial on patients with low back pain. Sixty-three ambulatory men and women between the ages of 18 and 70 years with symptomatic non-radiating low back pain of more than 30 days' duration and normal neurologic examination results. Subjects were bloc randomised into two groups with a computer-generated schedule. All underwent irradiation for 90 seconds at eight symmetric points along the lumbosacral spine three times a week for 4 weeks by a masked therapist. The Nd:YAG laser emitted 542 mW/cm^2. Subject's perception of benefit, level of function, as assessed by the Oswestry Disability Questionnaire, and lumbar mobility were evaluated. The treated group had a time-dependent improvement in two of the three outcome measures: perception of benefit and level of function. These results were most marked at the midpoint evaluation and end of treatment but tended to lessen at the 1-month follow-up Lumbar mobility did not differ between the groups at any time.

Further literature: [63, 150, 151, 160, 219, 220, 243, 248, 312, 402, 610, 656, 830, 831].

3.5.3 Laser therapy with ruby lasers

The first laser of them all - the ruby laser - had almost disappeared from the world laser market when it was found that strong ruby laser pulses could be used to remove hair growth permanently. (See chapter 1.4.8 "Ruby laser" on page 41 and chapter 1.4.9 "Alexandrite" on page 42 as well as chapter 1.4.10

belief of some individuals that the depth of penetration is high because of the high output power of the laser, or because it is a class 4 instrument (i.e. only for doctors, dentists and veterinarians).

Literature:

Longo [174] compared a CO_2-laser with a GaAs laser in the treatment of acute lumbago in a double-blind study. 3 J/cm^2 was administered to both experimental groups, while a third group received sham irradiation. The two experimental groups had similar results, but the GaAs group was slightly more improved.

Galletti [307] compared the effect of a CO_2-laser and a GaAlAs laser (830 nm) on the healing of surgical wounds in the external femoral condylus of the right hind-limb knee of 12 pigs. The CO_2-laser dose was 1.5 J/cm^2 and the GaAlAs laser dose was 0.5 J/cm^2. The result was approximately the same for both laser types, but significantly better than the controls. Effects were noted down to 4 cm.

Tsai [579] irradiated a radial defect in the avascular zone of rabbit menisci. Energy densities of 50 and 100 J/cm^2 of CO_2 laser were used. A marked increase in fibrochondrocytic proliferation and regeneration of collagen fibres was demonstrated in the 100 J group.

Giavelli [638] found similar results from CO_2- and GaAs-laser when treating gonarthrosis.

Gao [823] has cured 367 persons with facial acne by using direct high-power CO_2-laser irradiation combined with low-power CO_2-laser additional therapy. The cure rate is close to 100%. It was shown that this therapeutic approach is simple. There are no scars after healing.

Nicola [824] presents the results of five years' experience in the application of CO_2 low power laser therapy treating chronic pharyngitis. 85 patients with non-specific chronic pharyngitis were elected to be treated: Group I, 40 patients, predominance of hyperaemic aspect; and Group II, 45 patients, predominance of hypertrophied aspect. Both groups were treated for eight to ten sessions. It was concluded that this method is very suitable for the treatment of chronic pharyngitis, a very common and disturbing symptom for a great number of ear, nose, and throat patients, which still lacks an effective form of therapy.

Further literature: [94, 142, 166, 173, 196, 197, 200, 236, 237, 258, 280, 296, 747, 974, 1772]

3.5.2 Laser therapy with Nd:YAG lasers

The Nd:YAG laser can also have a biostimulating effect if the dose and power density is chosen within the limits of the lasers's therapeutic window. Positive influences on bone regeneration and secondary dentine formation are just two of the effects documented [106, 202]. However, vendors of Nd:YAG systems are often unwilling to discuss the biostimulating functions of this laser because of the controversial nature of laser therapy. Owners of

plete healing the skin was normal, with no recurrence *in situ* after three years. Interestingly enough, lesions not irradiated but close to the treated site also disappeared.

At Uppsala Academic Hospital, a CO_2-laser has been tested successfully for biostimulative treatment of epicondylitis. This method is also called EDL (Emitted Defocused Laser-light). It should be noted, however, that carbon dioxide lasers are not used as surgical lasers in this context; their incident energy and power density are set within the laser therapy range by spreading out the beam over such a large surface that the laser does not cause burning.

Another surprising effect of the CO_2-laser that has been demonstrated is "laser peeling", a skin treatment for wrinkles. To our knowledge, this was first presented by Abergel [51] in 1989 and in a follow-up [62] in 1992. Some years later, Chernoff [294, 295] performed over 50 exfoliations to smooth out perioral, lip, and periorbital wrinkles and scars. The thermal damage depth was between 75 and 150 µm. The result is surprisingly good and much better than what can be achieved with chemical peeling and mechanical dermabrasion. The mechanism is in part biostimulation.

Kaplan [422], one of the pioneers of CO_2-laser surgery, attributes the excellent healing and lower postoperative pain experienced with CO_2-laser surgery compared to conventional surgery to the simultaneous laser therapy effect. Laser surgery and laser therapy, Kaplan argues, should be regarded as two sides of the same coin.

The CO_2-laser can also be used as an acupuncture tool. Stimulation of acupuncture points has been carried out both with biostimulating power densities (e.g. 100 mW/cm^2) and burning/coagulating/evaporating power densities. Some clinics maintain that carbon dioxide lasers give better results on acupuncture points than HeNe lasers. As the carbon dioxide laser's beam cannot penetrate more than around 0.5 mm into tissue [296], (See chapter 11.1.5 "How deep does light penetrate into tissue?" on page 539), the effects must be due to the influence of the laser energy on the cells encountered, so that signal substances are released and then circulate in the organism. This indirectly confirms the hypothesis that conventional laser therapy has both a local effect in the area treated by laser light, and a systemic effect through the release of metabolites. It is well known that these kinds of secondary effects also occur at the traditional wavelengths of 633, 830, and 904 nm.

One advantage of the carbon dioxide laser is its high power density, which can be achieved over wide areas, thus leading to shorter treatment periods. Another advantage is that the patients also feel the heat (can even be painful) which influences the placeboeffect. (See chapter 9.2.9 "HeLa cells" on page 501.) The disadvantage, for the foreseeable future, will be the cost of the apparatus. Prices vary between US$ 15 000 and US$ 30 000 for equipment with similar qualities.

The fact that this form of laser therapy has, despite the cost, become popular with some doctors and veterinary surgeons is probably due to the

In the study by Zan-Bar [2092] sperm of ram and tilapia were irradiated with various light sources (400-800 nm white light, 660 nm red light, 360 nm blue light, 294 nm UV), and their motility and fertility rates were measured. The amount of ROS generated by irradiation was estimated using electron paramagnetic resonance (EPR) technique. Sperm taken from tilapia showed higher motility and fertility following red and white light irradiation. In contrast, the motility and fertility of ram sperm were slightly increased only by red light. A negative effect on motility and fertility of sperm of both species was obtained following irradiation with UV and blue light. The amount of ROS produced in irradiated tilapia sperm was much higher than that of ram sperm. The results show that different wavelengths differentially affect tilapia and ram sperm motility and fertilization. The difference in response to the various light sources might be explained by the different amounts of ROS formation by ram and tilapia, which are in agreement with the physiology of fertilization appropriate to each of these species. Based on these results, it is suggested that in vitro fertilization in mammals should be performed in darkness or at least under red light.

3.4.6 In vitro/in vivo

Many experiments have been performed *in vitro*. As always, the interpretation of these experiments must be made with caution. We have already discussed the consequences of the "nakedness" of cells in the *in vitro* situation. Therefore, doses used in such studies are difficult to extrapolate into a clinical situation. Furthermore, we must remember that a reaction seen or not seen in an *in vitro* experiment reflects the effect of laser therapy on a single isolated cell. In the clinic, there is no single cell effect. Every cell in the body is influenced by a very complex and multipath cascade of processes at each particular moment.

3.5 Laser Therapy with high output lasers

3.5.1 Laser therapy with carbon dioxide lasers

Laser therapy is a relatively new area for carbon dioxide lasers, although papers on the subject were published as early as the mid-eighties. There are several examples of researchers using a carbon dioxide laser without realising the biostimulative effect. Some Swedish studies during the 90's illustrate this fact:

At Malmö General Hospital 506 women were treated for cellular changes in the cervix of the uterus. The tissue was removed by means of a carbon dioxide laser. Before surgery 69% of the patients had papilloma virus. After surgery only 16% of these women had any detectable papilloma viruses. This is a clear example of biostimulation with a CO_2-laser.

At the University Hospital in Lund a carbon dioxide laser was tested on psoriasis. After superficial burning, the lesion disappeared and after com-

groups 1 and 2 showed significant improvement when compared to non-irradiated animals of the same group.

van den Brande [508] used laser doppler flowmetry to study the microcirculatory flow at the anteromedial surface of the lower leg during and after a 10-minute HeNe + GaAs application. In healthy volunteers, no change in microcirculatory flow was noted, although there was a marked increase in vasomotor activity. In vascular patients, the skin flux increased by a factor of 2.3.

Yamada [510] exposed osteoblastic cells to HeNe irradiation. No significant change was observed in the lines where the cells were in the confluent state. However, in the lines of cells in the sparse state, DNA incorporation increased 32% compared to control.

In a study by Lubart [592], it was found that the effect of a 780 nm laser on Ca^{2+} uptake by plasma membrane vesicles in the absence of ATP was much greater than in the presence of ATP.

3.4.5 The importance of ambient light

In the clinic the ambient light is not very important but when LPT is performed, the ambient light should be reasonably reduced, not to interfere with the therapeutic light. For the *in vitro* situation, the importance of regulating the ambient light is indeed important and may be more complex than first suggested.

Literature:

The effect of laser light may be partly or completely reduced by broad-spectrum light. There are few studies that investigate the benefit or detriment of combining laser irradiation with broad-spectrum or IR light. In a study by Hawkins [2087] wounded human skin fibroblasts were irradiated with a dose of 5 J/cm^2 using a HeNe laser, a diode laser, or a Nd:YAG laser in the dark, in the light, or in IR. Changes in cell proliferation were evaluated using optical density at 540 nm, alkaline phosphatase (ALP) enzyme activity, cytokine expression, and basic fibroblast growth factor (bFGF) expression. The optical density and ALP enzyme activity indicate that 5 J/cm^2 using 1064 nm in the light is more effective in increasing cell proliferation or cell growth than 830 nm in the light, but not as effective as 632.8 nm in the light. bFGF expression shows that the response of wounded cells exposed to 5 J/cm^2 in IR light is far less than the biological response of wounded cells exposed to 5 J/cm^2 in the dark or light. The results indicate that wounded cells exposed to 5 J/cm^2 using 632.8 nm in the dark results in a greater increase in IL-6 when compared to cells exposed to 5 J/cm^2 in the light or in IR. Results indicate that 5 J/cm^2 (using 632.8 nm in the dark or 830 nm in the light) is the most effective dose to stimulate cell proliferation, which may ultimately accelerate or improve the rate of wound healing.

In the literature, it is accepted that the first step following visible light irradiation is the formation of ROS by endogenous cellular photosensitizers.

the pulse repetition rate of the light and were mainly measurable during the growth phase of the infection, i.e. during a certain immunological status of the organism. All the wavelengths tested were effective, but 660 nm was the most effective. A pulse repetition rate of 5000 Hz was most effective. 16 Hz was ineffective.

Karu [512] summarises an experiment on the effect of monochromatic visible light sources on cells: "One can draw two conclusions from experiments with the combined action of light and redox chemicals. First, there is a strong dependence of the irradiation effect on the cell redox state at the moment of irradiation. The cellular response is weak or absent when the redox potential is optimal or near optimal and stronger when shifted. This explains why the magnitudes of cellular responses can differ markedly and sometimes be non-existent. The second conclusion is that an alteration of the redox state toward oxidation is correlated with stimulation, whereas reduction correlates with inhibition. Cells with lower than normal pH, where the redox state is shifted in the reduced direction, are considered to be more sensitive to the stimulative action of light than those with the respective parameters being optimal or near optimal. This circumstance explains the possible variations in observed magnitudes of low-power laser effects. Light action on the redox state of a cell via the respiratory chain also explains the diversity of low-power laser effects."

Ryabykh and Karu [448] went on to measure the CL in a number of healthy donors. 820 nm irradiation had no effect. However, CL was influenced by laser irradiation in patients with acute respiratory illness, blast cells in patients with haemoblastoses (820 nm) and patients with colon cancer (pulsed HeNe laser had effect - CW had no effect).

Severtsev [457] studied whether or not HeNe laser light could improve the ability of the lymphocytes to change their immunogenicity. In three blood donors out of five there was a threefold stimulation and in two cases there was no change. It is very likely that the immunological statuses of the five donors were different.

Brill [417] summarises an experiment involving HeNe irradiation of giant chromosomes: "Biologic effects of low power laser radiation depend both on the irradiation dose and on the temporal presentation of the dose. In prolonged continuous low power laser irradiation a peculiar adaptation of the biosystem is observed manifested by the disappearance of changes typical to the action of lower doses. Response of the genetic apparatus to the photo action depends on the initial functional state of chromosomes' loci. Resulting photoeffects may be manifested both by activation and inhibition of definite genome regions. There are chromosome regions particularly sensitive to HeNe laser action."

Kotani [501] irradiated experimental wounds in three groups of rats: 1) animals with induced diabetes mellitus, 2) animals treated with the fibroblast and collagen inhibitor Doxorubicin, and 3) healthy animals. Group 3 did not heal significantly better than non-irradiated controls. However,

the transmitted radiation measured. The intensity of laser radiation reduced by 66% after being transmitted through a 0.784 mm sample of human abdominal tissue. In this study most laser radiation was absorbed within the first 1 mm of skin.
   Further literature: [429, 1215, 2094]

3.4.3 Laser light irradiation through clothes

It has been suggested that patients can be treated with their clothes on. Taking the great absorption in skin in mind, this appears to be a bad idea, especially if the therapy is performed from some distance and with red light. A non-published experiement by the authors of this book revealed that 20 mW 660 nm laser light was reduced 100% by a thin black T-shirt, while 3 mW remained after passing a white cotton shirt.

3.4.4 The importance of the tissue and cell condition

Clinical and experimental experience shows that laser therapy has its greatest effects on cells/tissue/organs affected by a generally deteriorated condition, such as in patients suffering from some type of functional disorder, infection or injury to tissue. The light energy seems to produce the greatest benefit where it is most needed. On the other hand, experimentally induced inflammation in otherwise healthy people seems not to react quite as strongly to laser therapy [42]. One can assume that these individuals have good immune systems.

   It is reasonable to conclude that some of the contradictory results reported in the literature actually stem from the fact that the above parameters have not been considered.

Literature:

Steinlechner [4] used HeNe and GaAs lasers to stimulate keratinocyte cultures. The conclusion was that laser therapy indeed stimulates keratinocyte proliferation. However, it was found that the cultures growing in a "poor" environment - 1% fetal calf serum (FCS) - were stimulated more by laser therapy than the cultures growing in a better environment - 5% FCS.

Yamamoto [604] made a similar observation. Human fibroblasts were irradiated, using two cultures. One culture was kept in a serum-starved medium and one in an FCS-containing medium. Enhanced laser effect was consistently observed in the serum-starved medium (50%) but not in the FCS medium.

Karu [180] has made an interesting observation with respect to the effects of different laser wavelengths on the chemiluminescence of human blood. Chemiluminescence (CL) is a sensitive tool used within clinical differential diagnostics to measure changes in oxidative cell metabolism. Spontaneous CL of blood from a healthy young woman was tested during a period when she happened to suffer from a cold virus on two occasions. It was evident that the effects of laser light were dependent on both the wavelength and

Literature:

Byrnes [1527] made ex vivo and in vivo spectrophotometric and power transmission analyses before performing a study on the regeneration and functional recovery after spinal cord injury in rats. Optimum penetration was found between 770 and 850 nm. With 150 mW of 810 nm 6% of the power (9 mW) remained at the area of the ventral side of the spinal cord.

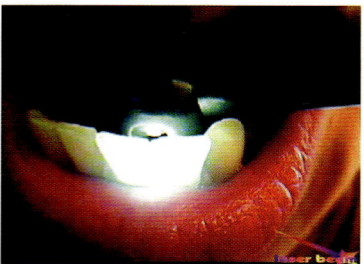

Figure 3.13 830 nm through teeth photographed with IR-camera.
Courtesy: Aldo Brugnera Jr.

Enwemeka [1770] studied the depth of penetration and the magnitude of attenuation of 632.8nm and 904nm light in skin, muscle, tendon, and cartilagenous tissues of live anaesthetized rabbits. Tissue specimens were dissected, prepared, and their thicknesses measured. Then, each wavelength of light was applied. Simultaneously, a power meter was used to detect and measure the amount of light transmitted through each tissue. All measurements were made in the dark to minimize interference from extraneous light sources. To determine the influence of pulse rate on beam attenuation, the 632.8nm light was used at two predetermined settings of the machine; continuous mode and 100 pulses per second (pps), at an on:off ratio of 1:1. Similarly, the 904 nm infra-red light was applied using two predetermined machine settings: 292 pps and 2,336 pps. Multiple regression analysis of the data obtained showed significant positive correlations between tissue thickness and light attenuation ($p < .001$). Collectively, our findings warrant the conclusions that: (1) The calf muscles of the New Zealand white rabbit attenuates light in direct proportion to its thickness. In this tissue, light attenuation is not significantly affected by the overlying skin, a finding which may be applicable to other muscles. (2) The depth of penetration of a 632.8nm and 904nm light is not related to the average power of the light source. The depth of penetration is the same notwithstanding the average power of the light source. (3) Compared to the 904 nm wavelength, 632.8 nm light is attenuated more by muscle tissue, suggesting that is is absorbed more readily than the 904 nm wavelength or conversely that the 904 nm wavelength penetrates more. Thus, wavelength plays a critical role in the depth of penetration of light.

Mathematical simulations and estimates from the literature suggest that the depth of penetration of laser radiation using wavelengths from 630 nm up to 1100 nm may be up to 50 mm. The aim of a study by Esnouf [2093] was to directly measure the penetration depth of a Low Level Laser in human tissue. Human abdominal skin samples up to 0.784mm thickness were harvested by dermatome following abdominoplasty procedures. These samples were irradiated by an 850 nm, 100 mW, 24 kHz, 0.28 mm diameter probe and

pendicular to the surface of the skull delivers >10⁴ photons per second to the cochlea.

Another factor is reflection. We can here differentiate between surface reflection and backscatter reflection. If treatment is done with a distance between the aperture of the probe and the tissue, the total loss due to reflection is 10-20%. When treating in contact with the tissue the reflection loss can be reduced by 80%.

3.4.2.2 Tissue compression

A factor of importance here is the compressive removal of blood in the target tissue. When you press lightly with a laser probe against skin, the blood flows to the sides, so that the tissue right in front of the probe (and some distance into the tissue) is fairly empty of blood. As the haemoglobin in the blood is responsible for most of the absorption, this mechanical removal of blood greatly increases the depth of penetration of the laser light. In the case of tissue compression, other types of cells than the blood cells will absorb a larger part of the light energy.

3.4.2.3 How deep does the light penetrate?

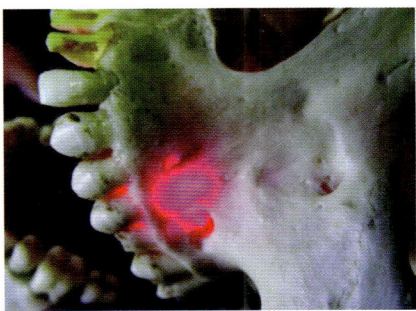

Figure 3.12   30 mW laser through dry bone

There is no exact limit with respect to the penetration of the light. The light gets weaker and weaker the further from the surface it penetrates. There is, however, a limit at which the light intensity is so low that no biological light effect can be registered. This limit, where the effect ceases, is called the greatest active depth.

N.B.: We are now talking about the direct effect of laser light on cells and not biological effects due to systemic effects from laser therapy.

For example: a HeNe laser with an output power of 3.5 mW has a greatest active depth of 6-8 mm depending on the type of tissue involved. A HeNe laser with an output of 7 mW has a greatest active depth of 8-10 mm. A GaAlAs probe of considerable strength has a penetration of 3.5 cm with a 5.4 cm (radius 2.7 cm) lateral spread [429]. A GaAs laser has a greatest active depth of between 20 and 30 mm (sometimes up to 40 mm), depending on its peak pulse output (around a thousand times greater than its average output power). If you are working in direct contact with the skin and press the probe against the skin, then the greatest active depth will be achieved.

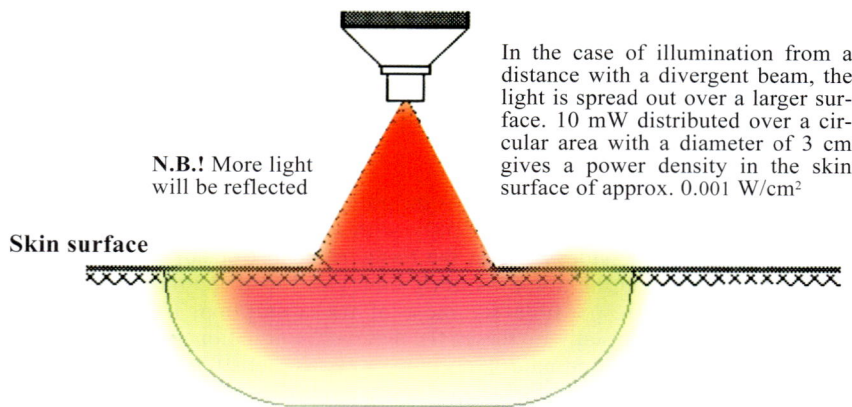

In the case of illumination from a distance with a divergent beam, the light is spread out over a larger surface. 10 mW distributed over a circular area with a diameter of 3 cm gives a power density in the skin surface of approx. 0.001 W/cm².

N.B.! More light will be reflected

Skin surface

The light penetrating into the tissue will, in this case, get a more shallow but wider distribution than in the case above.

Figure 3.11 Depth of penetration, distance

3.4.2.1 Factors that reduce penetration

Different tissue types absorb light to different degrees. Dirty skin and dark skin reduce penetration. Unpigmented caucasian skin, absorbs about 5% of the incident energy. Adipose tissue is more transparent [1215] than muscle tissue. Highly vascularised tissue (such as muscle tissue) absorbs more than less vascularised. Haemangiomas tissue contains much haemoglobin and thus needs higher doses.

It is worth noting that laser light also can penetrate bone [26]. Bone absorbs usually not more light than muscles, and there are differences between different types of bone. It is a common misconception that bone is stopping light as it does ultrasound. But it is not hardness that is important in this case (thick glass!) but a materials' absorption coefficient. If you have a HeNe or InGaAlP laser, let the red laser beam hit one of you teeth - you will see that it penetrates well. It can also be done with common laser pointer.

Oron (Tel Aviv University, 1996) measured the penetration of 660, 780 and 830 nm lasers through flat bone (skull or medial part of tibia of rat, 0.6-0.7 mm) and thick bone (femur of rat, 3 mm). The remaining power measured after penetration was 21%, 23%, and 14% for flat bone and 4.5% for thick bone. Denser bone, such as the bone overlapping the inner ear in humans, would reduce penetration even more. However, it can be estimated that a 100 mW source, 820 nm wavelength, placed in contact with and per-

ter, treatment technique, and so on, will determine the actual effective depth of penetration for any given laser.

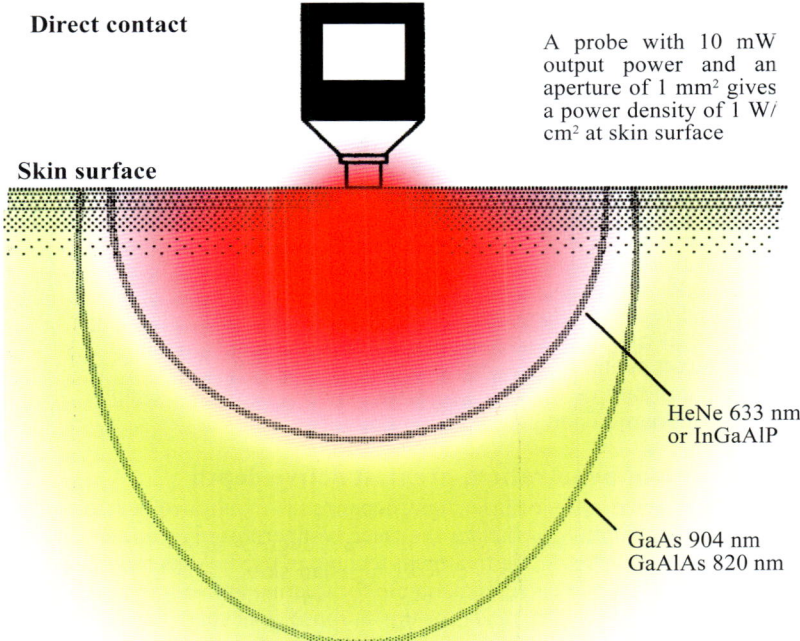

Direct contact

A probe with 10 mW output power and an aperture of 1 mm² gives a power density of 1 W/cm² at skin surface

Skin surface

HeNe 633 nm or InGaAlP

GaAs 904 nm
GaAlAs 820 nm

The light from the laser distributes in the tissue like a ball or an egg independently if the incoming beam is parallel or divergent. This is, however, dependent on the wavelengths of the light. Short wavelengths give a smaller but fairly round ball, whilst longer wavelengths give a more egg shaped light distribution.

Figure 3.10 Depth of penetration, direct contact

3.4 Other considerations

3.4.1 What about collimation?

The light from a laser diode is always divergent, usually with a fan shaped beam with an angle of divergence of around 30-90 degrees and perpendicular with an angle of divergence of 5-10 degrees when it is emitted from the semiconductor crystal. If a collimating lens is placed in front of the diode, the light's parallelity can be highly increased, more or less reaching the same parallelity as the beam of a HeNe laser. This is called collimation. The beam from a laser pointer is hence collimated this way. Parallel beams are only advantageous when treating from a distance, since the light is kept together and hits a small surface. This means that we can irradiate from a distance and still achieve a high power density on a small area. If there is no collimation, this can be compensated for by holding the probe closer to the tissue. When light, parallel or not, hits the tissue, it immediately spreads unrestrainedly [429]. Light is spread downwards into the tissue, roughly in the form of a hemisphere like a Ping-Pong ball cut in half, (see Figure 3.10 "Depth of penetration, direct contact" on page 119.) So for treatment involving tissue contact, the parallelity of the beam is of no significance. (See chapter 3.4.2.2 "Tissue compression" on page 121.)

3.4.2 Depth of penetration, greatest active depth

The depth of penetration of laser light depends, as mentioned previously, on the light's wavelength, on whether the laser is superpulsed or not, and on the output power; but also on the treatment technique used. A laser designed for the treatment of humans is rarely suitable for treating animals with fur. There are, in fact, lasers specially made for this purpose. The special design feature here is that the laser diode(s) obtrude from the treatment probe rather like the teeth on a comb. By delving between the animal's hairs, the laser aperture comes into contact with the skin and more light from the laser is "forced" into the tissue.

A rough guide to effective penetration depths of continuous wave & modulated continuous wave lasers (all other parameters being equal) would look roughly like:

Visible Red (630-700 nm): 0.5-1 cm
Near-Infrared (700-800 nm): 2-3 cm
Near Infrared (800-960 nm): 3-5 cm
Near Infrared (970-990 nm): 1-2 cm
Near Infrared (990-1200 nm): 4-5 cm

Further, other factors such as power density, tissue type, tissue temperature, tissue condition, probe/applicator design, operating mode of the laser emit-

skin of the injection site for both groups. Laser therapy was administered with a previously established optimal accumulated dose of 7.5 J/cm^2. While laser therapylaser therapy after 4 hours effectively reduced inflammation almost to pre-injection levels of neutrophil cell counts (1.11_10 (6), [95% CI: 0.41-1.82]), the anti-inflammatory effect was blocked after pre-injection of mifepristone (5.94_10(6), [95% CI: 4.83-7.04]). The implications of these findings are that steroid therapy should be avoided in conjunction with laser therapy, and that clinical studies violating this precaution, should be excluded from reviews and meta-analyses of laser therapy.

The aim of the study by Pessoa [1462] was to evaluate the effect of laser therapy on the wound healing process in the presence of steroids. Forty-eight rats were used, and after execution of a wound on the dorsal region of each animal, they were divided into 4 groups (n = 12), receiving the following treatments: G1 (control), wounds and animals received no treatment; G2, wounds were treated with laser therapy; G3, animals received an intraperitoneal injection of steroid dosage (2 mg/kg of body weight); G4, animals received steroid and wounds were treated with laser therapy. The laser emission device used was a 904 nm unit, in a contact mode, with 2.75 mW, 2.900 Hz, during 120 sec (33 J/cm^2). After 3, 7, and 14 days the animals were sacrificed and the parts sent to histological processing. The results have shown that the wounds treated with cortisone had a delay in healing, while laser therapy accelerated the wound healing process. Also, wounds treated with laser in the animals treated with steroid presented a differentiated healing process with a larger collagen deposition and also a decrease in both the inflammatory infiltration and the delay on the wound healing process. laser therapy accelerated healing, caused by the steroid, acting as a biostimulative coadjutant agent, balancing the undesirable effects of cortisone on the tissue healing process.

Fujihara [1550] irradiated rat calvaria osteoblast cells with 780 nm, 3 J/cm^2. The cells were grown in nutritional deficit. The anti-inflammatory agent dexamethasone was added to some cultures. The laser irradiated cultures showed faster cell growth, probably by promoting faster cell adhesion. The presence of the steroidal anti-inflammatory agent impaired cell adhesion and growth. This process, however, was reduced by the laser irradiation.

Yang Li [1135] has observed that animals in wound healing studies frequently have reacted with a negative response if anesthetics such as ketamine and ether have been used. It is speculated that there is some reagent competing against laser for the same receptor in the fibroblast..

the latter block the membrane channels and antennae pigment receptors that laser therapy relies upon. The degree of reduction and total effect is variable and determined by blood levels of the chemical and individual cell receptability. Similar actions on the cell membrane and the receptor site and bonds are caused by beta blockers, calcium channel antagonists and several of the cardiac and neurological medications. These effects have till now not often been considered in research work and are significant when a meta-analysis of the literature is made and such medications is factored in. In this case many of the 'negative studies' on laser therapy are found to not have screened and excluded for the potential of pharmaceutical counter effects. In contrast, specific chemicals are found to be positive agents for laser therapy that will increase the biostimulative effect by preparing the cell receptors and membrane to be capable of a maximal effect. This facilitatory action of laser therapy acceptors is demonstrated by Plenosol, that is photoreceptive at 660 nm, whilst ubiquinon- ferrum- and copper-based local substances that can be subcutaneously infused are 810 nm and 904 nm receptive. Clinically, the total effect is that of a two-stage process that uses a combination of local injection or cutaneously absorbed substances that can be administered or applied and then irradiated with the specific wavelength. It is also demonstrated that the use of Procaine as the local anaesthetic of choice facilitates the passage of specific photo acceptor substances into the affected tissue effectively acting as a 'taxi' whilst serving its primary purpose of local anaesthetic management. The conclusion is that, where possible, medication should be excluded or included if the maximal effect of laser therapy is to be achieved. Where research is initiated to determine the effect of laser therapy, the presence of such chemicals must be considered, then noted and factored into the statistical analysis.

Literature:

Lopes-Martins [1463] writes: Interventions with anti-inflammatory actions such as steroids and nonsteroid anti-inflammatory drugs are frequently used in the treatment of rheumatic and musculoskeletal pain. Recent studies from our and other research groups have shown that low level laser therapy also has an anti-inflammatory effect. Clinical studies have produced less homogeneous results, and non-optimal laser therapy dosage has been identified as a key factor for this. However, poor clinical results may also be caused by pharmacological co-interventions that block the antiinflammatory effect of laser therapy. In the present study, we used the classical experimental mice-model of carrageenan-induced pleurisy, to investigate if the anti-inflammatory effect of low power laser therapy could be blocked by the steroid agent mifepristone. For the intervention group, mifepristone was injected into the pleural cavity an hour prior to the carrageenan injection. Pleurisy was then induced by an intrathoracic injection of carrageenan (0.5mg/cavity), or LPS from E. coli (250 ng/ cavity) in mice. Laser irradiation (650 nm) was then carried out three times with hourly intervals at the

the outcome of the healing was better if they were used alone. This is not the result in the two following studies:

Demir [1490] performed a randomised controlled study investigating the effects of ultrasound and laser treatments on wound healing in rats. The duration of the inflammatory phase decreased with both laser and ultrasound treatments; however, laser was more effective than ultrasound, with more significant results. The proliferation phase showed, for both treatments, an increase in the level of hydroxyproline and the number of fibroblasts, as well as stimulation of the collagen synthesis and the composition. Laser treatment was again more effective than ultrasound. The wound breaking strength was significantly higher with both treatments, and no statistically significant difference emerged between the laser and ultrasound groups, although laser treatment provided a much greater increase in the wound breaking strength than ultrasound. Both treatments had beneficial effects on the inflammatory, proliferation, and maturation phases of wound healing. Both could be used successfully for decubitus ulcers and chronic wounds, in conjunction with conventional therapies such as debridement and daily wound caring. However, laser treatment was more effective than ultrasound in the first two phases of wound healing.

In another study by Demir [1491] 84 healthy male rats were divided into three groups consisting of 28 rats, the left Achilles tendons were used as treatment and the right Achilles tendons as controls. The right and left Achilles tendons of rats were traumatised longitudinally. The treatment was started on post injury day one. The US treatment was applied with a power of 0.5 W/cm^2, a pulse repetition rate of 1 MHz, continuously, 5 minutes daily. A GaAs laser was applied with a 904 nm wavelength, 6 mW average power, 1 J/cm^2 dosage, 16 Hz pulse repetition rate, for 1 minute duration. Although US, L, and combined US + L treatments increased tendon healing biochemically and biomechanically more than the control groups, no statistically significant difference was found between them. Also the researchers did not find significantly more cumulative positive effects of combined treatment.

3.3.5 Interaction with medication

It is demonstrated that laser therapy will interact with pharmaceuticals, such as steroids and NSAIDs. This is still an untapped field of knowledge where much work remains to be done. An interaction with pharmaceuticals could possibly explain why some patients react well to laser therapy whilst others are impervious. One of the first attempts to investigate this problem was done by Meersman [1278]. It was hypothesised a positive and a negative interaction between laser therapy and pharmaceuticals. The pilot research work on Achilles tendinopathy management demonstrated that various chemicals commonly used will interfere positively or negatively with laser therapy and would be a logical explanation for the intermittent and often varied results. The biostimulatory action of laser therapy is countered by the presence of NSAIDs and steroids that are non-acceptors of laser therapy, as

3.3.3.2.6 Irradiation of lymph nodes
Whenever there is a local infection, the recommendation is to irradiate the local lymph nodes to boost the immune system [915]. Recent research by Almeida-Lopes [1470] also suggests that irradiation of lymph nodes in the facial area can reduce pain conditions and oedema. This mode of treatment is especially useful when the focal area is infected, since the laser would partly enhance the local microorganisms as well. In these cases, and in particular for immune depressive patients, a lymph drainage technique can be used. With knowledge of the lymphatic anatomy the lymph nodes involved in the inflammatory process can be irradiated in cases such as periocoronitis, herpes simplex, endodontic abscesses and avleolitis. Almeida-Lopes suggests a dose around 70 J/cm^2 with a two-day interval.

3.3.3.2.7 Irradiation of ganglions
Stellate ganglion blocks are reported to be an effective but invasive treatment of upper extremity pain. Irradiation with different light sources offers a non-invasive and safer alternative. Lasers have succesfully been used in several studies [186, 421, 423, 523, 685, 691, 692, 1053, 1054]. Linear polarised light was used in [1574, 1575, 1577, 1578]. In [1576], however, laser, linear polarised light as well as Xenon-ray irradiation were used, but all were ineffective.

Literature:
Takeyoshi [1052] has treated many patients suffering from allergic rhinitis with ganglion blocks. In a comparative study 20 patients had traditional stellate ganglion block (SGB) and 12 patients had laser irradiation over the stellate ganglion (SGL). GaAlAs lasers of 60 mW (10 minutes of irradiation) and 150 mW (7 minutes of irradiation) were used. The number of sessions were maximum 20 over a period of one month. 60% of the patients receiving SGB reported the outcome as "excellent" or "good" while 100% of the patients in the SGL group had this rating.

3.3.4 Combination treatment
In the clinical situation, laser therapy is often used in combination with other therapies. While this is not a good research set-up, it is very often advantageous in the clinic. Laser therapy will enhance the outcome of traditional therapies.

If heat is used in combination with laser therapy, the laser treatment should come first. Heat will increase the blood flow in the tissue, thus increasing the absorption of the light in blood. The opposite then applies to cryogenic therapy.

Ultrasound is very often used in physical therapy. One study [726] has compared the effect of ultrasound, laser therapy and the two modalities in combination. The results suggest that they may counteract one another, since

all groups at 0.5, 1, 1, 2, 4, 6, 8, 10, 12, 16, 20, 24, 36, 48 and 72 hours intervals after the injection of the antibiotic and sent for laboratory analysis using HPLC. The results of this study revealed a significant increase in the level of Ampicilline (ng/ml) in the treated group as compared with the control one. The increase in the level was significant as compared with the pretreatment time. The results obtained from this study are said to be attributed to the improvement of reheological properties of blood, and an increase in the capillaries, blood flow, in addition to reduced vascular resistance and vascular tone which lead to increase the motion and out flow of fluids from the interstitial spaces in to the lymphatic improvement of tissue trophic activity.

It is reported here by Mi [1767] that laser irradiation can reduce the Hbm contents in pig's erythrocytes, providing the explanation for the improvement of erythrocyte deformability. The decrease of the Hbm was proportional to the irradiation dose, but the relative change of Hbm was saturated around 35%. The 532 nm laser was more efficient at lowering Hbm than the 632.8 nm laser, consistent with the absorption spectrum of Hbm.

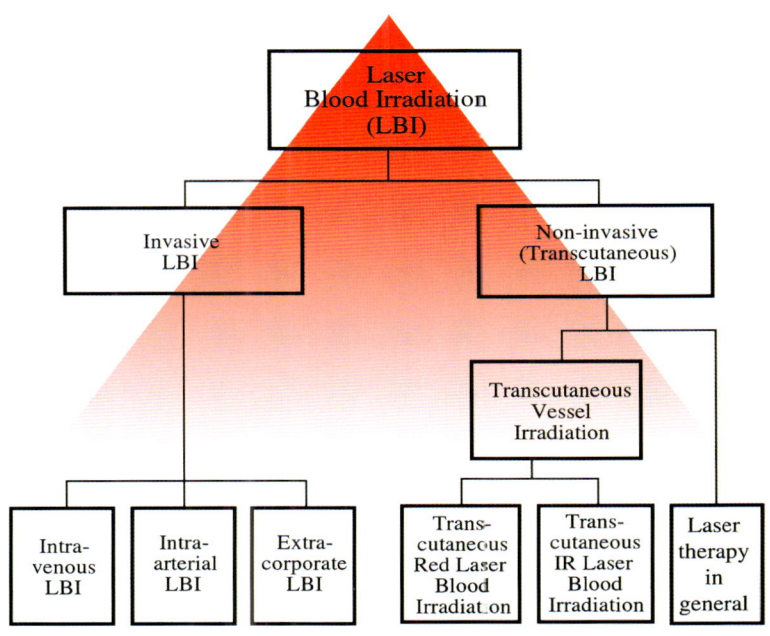

Figure 3.9 Methods of blood irradiation. Modified from Levon Gasparyan

tissue rose. The amount of drugs used was reduced and the duration of the hospitalisation decreased by an average of 7 days.

Koukoui [481] used the same procedure for this indication, but the blood was irradiated extracorporally.

The effects of laser therapy on the blood is considered to be a subject of great importance in elucidating the mechanisms of action between laser light and biological tissues. The study by Siposan [1325] investigates some in vitro effects of laser on some selected rheologic indices of human blood. After establishing whether or not damaging effects could appear due to laser irradiation of the blood, the author tried to find a new method for rejuvenating the blood preserved in haemonetics-type bags. Blood samples were obtained from adult regular donors (volunteers). HeNe laser and laser diodes were used as radiation sources, in a wide range of wavelengths, power densities, doses and other parameters of irradiation protocols. In the first series of experiments he established that laser therapy does not alter the fresh blood from healthy donors, for doses between 0 and 10 J/cm^3 and power densities between 30 and 180 mW/cm^3. In the second series of experiments he established that laser does have, in some specific conditions, a revitalising effect on the erythrocytes in preserved blood. It was concluded that laser irradiation of the preserved blood, following a selected protocol of irradiation, could be used as a new method to improve the performances of preservation: prolonging the period of storage and blood rejuvenation before transfusion.

Acc. to the study by Nascimento [1738] LPT elevates (1.0 J/cm^3) or decreases (2.0 J/cm^3) the potential of long-term cryopreserved peripheral blood progenitor cells for growth of colony-forming units in vitro.

Kirichuk [483] applied transcutaneous HeNe laser light to rats that had been exposed to pathological stress. It was shown that stress-induced platelet aggregation was reduced by 34% through the irradiation.

The work by Mehdi [1530] was designed to evaluate the effect of intravenously administered laser irradiation on the level of antibiotic in the blood. A locally constructed GaAs laser of 200 nsec pulse width, average power of 1 mW at 1 kHz pulse repetition rate was used. It had further an optical package containing a connector and optical fibre with fine canula fixed in its end. Twenty eight male adult New Zealand white rabbits were used in this study. They were divided into two groups (control & treated with the laser radiation). Each group was subdivided into two subgroups depending upon the manner of administration of the Ampicilline. The first subgroup was injected with 10 mg/kg B.W of Ampicilline at the time of irradiation while the other subgroup was given the Ampicilline in a shape of gelatine capsules, each one containing 10 mg/kg B.W, orally prior to the anaesthesia. Each animal underwent a surgical operation carried out on the medial aspect of the left thigh to expose the femoral vein. Blood of the animals of the treated group was irradiated by introducing the fine needle of the canula into the vein for 5 minutes. Samples of blood were collected from the animals of

diseases in the extremities, unstable angina, acute myocardial infarction, diabetic angiopathies, acute pneumonia, lung abscess, bronchial obstructive diseases of the lungs, drug resistant forms of schizophrenia, rheumatoid arthritis, acute calculous pyelonephritis, ischemic heart disease, circulatory encephalopathy, haemorrhagic shock, Tourette's syndrome, and OPH gestosis.

The use of lasers instead of UV light only started in the 70s (in the former Soviet Union). Laser Blood Irradiation (LBI) seemed to have effects similar to UV Blood Irradiation (UBI). Although LBI seemed to be slightly less effective than UBI, the great advantage was that LBI was easier to perform. HeNe laser could penetrate the skin, whereas UV light does not.

Several treatment methods have been used. The most common is irradiation with HeNe laser via a thin light-guide and an IV needle, which is then withdrawn. HeNe lasers of 1-10 mW are used (most frequently 1 mW) and duration of treatment varies from 30 to 60 minutes. Usually the cubital vein is used. In some cases an artery is used.

Another method is to irradiate the blood outside the body in plastic or quartz tubes. Only a small amount of the patient's blood is irradiated. This method is mainly used for UBI.

Transcutaneous irradiation is non-invasive and has several advantages, such as better patient acceptance, ease of application and lack of cross infection risks. Some researchers claim that 1 mW intravenous HeNe irradiation equals 20-30 mW transcutaneous irradiation. Intravenous irradiation is said to cause a sensation of warmth and sleepiness. This sensation is less obvious with transcutaneous irradiation [670]. LBI also seems to improve microcirculation, thus improving the uptake of pharmaceuticals. For transcutaneous irradiation, infrared lasers are used.

An interesting aspect of blood irradiation is the effect of normal sunshine. In the Nordic countries the solar power density varies from almost 0 in winter to 100 mW/cm^2 in the summer. Some of this energy comes in the infrared and can penetrate down to the aretrioles. One hour in the sun during a clear summer day thus would give a dose from penetrating light of roughly 0.05 W × 3600 seconds = 180 J/cm^2 of the bodily areas which are at a right angle to the incoming light. That area could be rather large, suppose 50 × 60 cm = 3000 cm^2. The biological effects of the sun are obvious, but they differ a lot from that of laser therapy. However, it has been demonstrated that the effects on cells from a laser can be eradicated if the cells later are subjected to broadband light (like the sunshine). So the question is - should patients avoid gross doses of sunlight after being treated by laser?

Literature:

Kipshidze [472] used HeNe irradiation in 900 patients with acute myocardial infarction. All patients were treated within four hours of the anginal attack. There was a painkilling effect as well as a limitation of the ischaemic area. Antioxidant blood activity and oxygen content of blood and

3.3.3.2.5 Blood irradiation

An interesting treatment technique has been used in Russia for many years. The patient's blood is irradiated in order to improve the immune system and the microcirculation. The irradiation can be done through the skin via a fibre leading directly into the blood stream or via a dialysis-like machine. Wavelengths used are 633 and 890 nm.

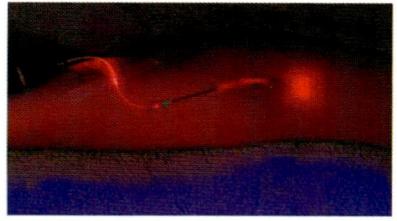

Figure 3.8 Laser blood irradiation.
Courtesy: Levon Gasparyan

Irradiating the blood is not a recent treatment modality [671]. In fact, as early as 1923 the US scientist Knott began to experiment with ways to irradiate the blood in order to destroy infectious organisms. In those days there were no lasers, so UV light was attempted. The works of Nobel Prize winner Ryberg Finsen spurred the idea.

This was a time when there were no antibiotics and scientists were trying every possibility in coping with infections. In initial experiments Knott irradiated the entire blood of experimentally infected dogs. He found that the irradiation cleared the blood of infection, but the dogs died in 5-7 days of profound depression and a progressive respiratory slowing and failure. This led Knott to experiment with irradiating different amounts of the blood of the dogs until he determined that the optimal approach was to irradiate 1.5-3 ml of blood for every pound of body weight (about 5% of the total blood) for about 10 seconds.

The first treatment of a human subject occurred in 1928. The patient was a woman moribund following septic abortion complicated by haemolytic streptococcus septicaemia. Treatment with UV blood irradiation rapidly returned her to normal health. Knott waited five years to make sure that the woman did not suffer from any subtle long-range effects before further treatment of a human subject was undertaken.

With the advent of antibiotics the idea of UV blood irradiation vanished. The new miracle therapy was used extensively, while the long term side effects and bacterial backlash were not yet discovered. Russian researchers [669] took a new look at the old idea in the 70s and since then the treatment has been extensively investigated in the laboratory and in the clinic.

Samoilova [482] names this "photohaemotherapy" or "photomodification" and states that it has been used for 17 years in Russia. There are reports of general effects on the immune system, including decrease of the blood viscosity, improvement of microcirculation, detoxification and oxygenation, normalisation of haemostatis, and activation of immune and proliferative processes. Some indications reported in the literature are: occlusive vascular

7. When performing regular laser therapy, many random acupuncture points are irradiated, nolens volens. Which are the consequences?

8. Moxa (heat) is used on acupuncture points but laser acupuncture is usually not a heat phenomenon. However, some therapists use carbon dioxide lasers for acupuncture and actually burn the acupuncture point.

9. Several therapists use different pulsing systems (Nogier, Baar etc), others use continuous irradiation. Is pulsing important and, if so, what scientific documentation is there? The Nogier pulse repetition rate list was "inherited" from electro acupuncture – is it relevant to use that in the pulsing of light?

Summing up, it is obvious that a multitude of parameters are used in laser acupuncture and that there is no real consensus on these. However, since laser acupuncture seems to be an acceptable alternative to needle acupuncture, this possibility merits further research. Laser acupuncture is pain free, sterile and can safely be used on infected individuals, persons with needle phobia and on infants.

3.3.3.2.2 Trigger points

It is generally clinically advantageous to combine local treatment with trigger point treatment. The reduction in pain on palpating very often coincides with pain reduction in the inflamed area. However, only irradiating the trigger points in not a good idea, all laser therapy should primarily be aimed at "the heart of the matter".

Further literature: [253, 302, 313, 315, 647, 670]

3.3.3.2.3 Spinal processes

Irradiation of the spinal processes corresponding to the area where the pain is located will reduce the pain. In the case of golf or tennis elbow, it may be a false golf or tennis elbow. It may be a nerve entrapment in the nerve passage leading into the spinal cord and laser treatment of C6 may reduce an oedema around the nerve and hence give pain relief.

Further literature: [540]

3.3.3.2.4 Dermatome

In cases of skin eruptions such as herpes zoster, the entire dermatome should be irradiated.

Further literature: [57]

fully produce opposite effects to the first experiment and effect a positive treatment. The 10 Hz condition produced a significant but transient reduction in pica measured by attempts at pica on a supervised walk shortly after each treatment. The subject was also easier to manage on walks, and appeared happier.

Further literature: [45, 111, 116, 118, 119, 175, 227, 876-891, 939]

Laser acupuncture – some thoughts by the amateur

In needle acupuncture there is always a sensory effect of the needle. This may or may not be of importance but it is a fact that the sensory input is absent in laser acupuncture. There is evidence enough to accept that laser acupuncture works, but there are even more questions involved in laser acpuncture that in needle acupuncture:

1. Is there a wavelength difference?

2. Which is the "correct" dose for an acupuncture point? Considering the difference in depth (for instance between ear acupuncture points and body acupuncture points) there should be a difference. The doses used in the literature differ a lot.

3. When an acupuncture point is irradiated, there is a large "light ball" surrounding the area of the light incidence. The energy of the beam is then greatest in the center of the beam, but how crucial is it to be on the exact anatomical spot?

4. When an acupuncture point is irradiated, a certain volume of blood is also affected. Is this significant?

5. The ideal acupuncture laser should have a very small aperture to be able to pinpoint the acupuncture point and to give a high energy density. But many therapists just use the laser that happens to be at hand and they all claim that their therapy is effective.

6. In auricular acupuncture several points will be affected whenever one selected point is irradiated, even if the laser has a very small aperture. This is not the case in needle acupuncture. What is the implication of this? Would a laser with e.g. green light (less penetration) be better?

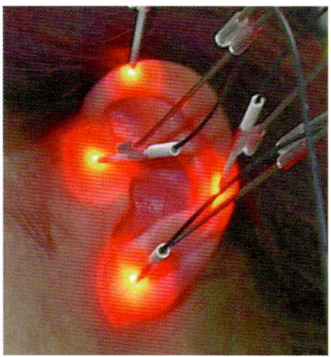

Figure 3.7 Laser needle auriculotherapy.
Courtesy: Michael Weber

A study by Litscher [1832] comprises scientific-theoretic fundamental investigations of laserneedle technology, a new and painless method of acupuncture stimulation. Laserneedles are not inserted in the skin, but are merely placed on the surface of the acupuncture point. The study documents the significant changes in peripheral microcirculation and surface temperature of the skin induced by laser, in 22 healthy volunteers. In addition, a randomised cross-over study to characterise the specific changes in cerebral blood flow velocity with laserneedle acupuncture is presented.

Several treatment modalities for children suffering from monosymptomatic nocturnal enuresis are available, but desmopressin is a well-established option. In the study by Radmayr [1836] forty children aged over 5 years presenting with primary nocturnal enuresis underwent a previous evaluation of their voiding function to assure normal voiding patterns and a high nighttime urine production. Then the children were randomized into two groups: group A children were treated with desmopressin alone, and group B children underwent laser acupuncture. All children were investigated after a minimum follow-up period of 6 month to evaluate the duration of the response. The children of both groups had an initial mean frequency of 5.5 wet nights per week. After a minimum follow-up period of 6 months reevaluation revealed a complete success rate of 75% in the desmopressin-treated group. Additional 10% of the children had a reduction of their wet nights of more than 50%. On the other hand, 6 months after laser acupuncture, 65% of the randomized children were completely dry. Another 10% had a reduction of the enuresis frequency of more than 50% per week. 20% of the children in the desmopressin-treated group did not respond at all as compared with 15% in the acupuncture-treated group. Statistical evaluation revealed no significant differences among the response rates in both groups. In comparison with pharmacological therapy using desmopressin, the study showed that laser acupuncture should be taken into account as an alternative, noninvasive, painless, cost-effective, and short-term therapy for children with primary nocturnal enuresis in case of a normal bladder function and high nighttime urine production. Success rates indicated no statistically significant differences between the well-established desmopressin therapy and the alternative laser acupuncture.

Read [1837] reports on a 28-year-old woman with acquired brain damage who suffered subsequent profound mental disability and an intense hyperphagic syndrome complete with life-threatening pica. She was the single subject of two consecutive experiments. In the first, Naltrexone, an orally administered opiate blocker, was given to reduce hyperphagia and distress, but was associated with even greater urgency when eating meals and a manifest increase in distress. While distress reduced to premedication levels on withdrawal of treatment, urgency of eating did not reduce so quickly. In the second experiment a laser acupuncture procedure was used at 2.5 Hz and 10 Hz for 10 days each with an intervening 10-day placebo condition to increase the availability of the subject's endogenous opiates, and thus hope-

fell from baseline by 16.1 points in the intervention group and by 6.8 points in the sham control group. The difference showed only a trend four weeks later, but was again significant after 12 weeks. Laser acupuncture was well tolerated with transient fatigue as the most common adverse effect.

The study by Siedentopf [1831] aimed to explore the central effect using laser acupuncture. The authors investigated the cerebral effects of laser acupuncture at both acupoints GB43 with functional magnetic resonance imaging (fMRI). As a control condition the laser was mounted at the same acupoints but without application of laser stimulation. The group results showed significant brain activations within the thalamus, nucleus subthalamicus, nucleus ruber, the brainstem, and the Brodmann areas 40 and 22 for the acupuncture condition. No significant brain activations were observed within the placebo condition. The activations we observed were laser acupuncture-specific and predominantly ipsilateral. This supports the assumption that acupuncture is mediated by meridians, since meridians do not cross to the other side.

The paper by Litscher [1833] presents an experimental double-blind study in acupuncture research in healthy volunteers using a new optical stimulation method. The authors investigated 18 healthy volunteers in a randomized controlled cross-over trial using functional multidirectional transcranial ultrasound Doppler sonography (fTCD; n = 17) and performed functional magnetic resonance imaging (fMRI) in one volunteer. Stimulation of vision-related acupoints resulted in an increase of mean blood flow velocity in the posterior cerebral artery measured by fTCD. Mean blood flow velocity in the middle cerebral artery decreased insignificantly. Significant changes of brain activity were demonstrated in the occipital and frontal gyrus by fMRI. Optical stimulation using properly adjusted laser needles has the advantage that the stimulation cannot be felt by the patient (painless and no tactile stimulation) and the operator may also be unaware of whether the stimulation system is active. Therefore true double-blind studies in acupuncture research can be performed.

The aim of a study by Siedentopf [1835] was to investigate the effect of laser acupuncture on cerebral activation. Using functional magnetic imaging (fMRI) cortical activations during laser acupuncture at the left foot (Bladder 67) and dummy acupuncture, were compared employing a block design in ten healthy male volunteers. All experiments were done on a 1.5 Tesla magnetic resonance scanner equipped with a circular polarized head coil. During laser acupuncture, we found activation in the cuneus corresponding to Brodmann Area (BA) 18 and the medial occipital gyrus (BA 19) of the ipsilateral visual cortex. Placebo stimulation did not show any activation. We could demonstrate that laser acupuncture of a specific acupoint, empirically related to ophthalmic disorders, leads to activation of visual brain areas, whereas placebo acupuncture does not. These results indicate that fMRI has the potential to elucidate effects of acupuncture on brain activity.

Patients were randomized to receive a course of 4 treatments over 4 weeks with either active or placebo laser. The primary outcome measure was a difference in numbers of headache days between baseline and the 4 months after randomization. Secondary outcome measures included a change in headache severity using a 10cm Visual Analogue Scale (VAS) for pain and a change in monthly hours with headache. Measurements were taken during 4 weeks before randomization (baseline), at weeks 1-4, 5-8, 9-12 and 13-16 from baseline. The mean number of headaches per month decreased significantly by 6.4 days in the treated group and by 1.0 days in the placebo group. Secondary outcome measures headache severity and monthly hours with headache decreased as well significantly at all time points compared to baseline and were as well significantly lower than those of the placebo group at all time points. It is concluded that laser acupuncture can provide a significant benefit for children with headache with active laser treatment being clearly more effective than placebo laser treatment.

In the study by Zeredo [1828] the authors tested the analgesic effects of high-intensity infrared laser for acupuncture-like stimulation. Twelve adult Sprague-Dawley rats weighing 230 to 250 g were randomly assigned to laser, needle, or restraint groups. Stimulation was directed to the meridian point Taixi (KI 3) for 10 min. For laser stimulation, a pulsed Er:YAG system was used. The laser settings were adjusted to provide a focal raise in the skin temperature to about 45 degrees C. The anti-nociceptive effect was evaluated by the tail-flick test. Both needling and laser stimulation significantly increased the tail-flick latency. Peak needling effect was observed immediately after treatment, while laser stimulation was effective both immediately and 45 min after treatment. High-intensity laser stimulation may be used alternatively or in combination with conventional acupuncture needling for pain relief.

In the work by Lihong [1829], 68 cases of acne vulgaris were randomly divided into a treatment group of 36 cases treated with HeNe laser auricular irradiation plus body acupuncture, and a control group of 32 cases treated with body acupuncture only. The results showed that the cure rate was 77.8% in the treatment group and 46.9% in the control group, indicating that HeNe laser auricular irradiation plus body acupuncture may exhibit better effects for acne vulgaris.

Quah-Smith [1830] performed a double-blind randomised controlled trial, conducted to test the efficacy of laser acupuncture in mild to moderate depression. Thirty patients with depression were randomised to receive either active or inactive laser treatment. The laser unit could be switched to one of two settings. One switch position delivered active laser acupuncture and the other was inactive (sham). In the active mode, 0.5 J was delivered to each of six to eight individually tailored acupuncture sites per visit. All patients were treated twice weekly for four weeks then weekly for a further four weeks. The patients and the acupuncturist were both blinded to conditions. At the end of the treatment period, Beck Depression Inventory scores

intensity was 1.3J (approximately 13 cm².). Ten sessions were given, three per week. The placebo group was treated in a similar way except that the output power of the equipment was set to zero. The outcome variables were headache intensity (VAS), duration of attacks, and number of days with a headache per month, by daily diary, assessed monthly to three months after treatment. There were significant differences between groups (P<0.001) in changes from baseline in months one, two and three, in median score for headache intensity (treatment group -5, -3 and -2, placebo group -1, 0 and 0), median duration of attacks (treatment group -6, -4 and -4, placebo group -1, 0 and 0 hours), and median number of days with headache per month (treatment group -15, -10 and -8, placebo group -2, 0 and 0).

Aigner [1700] used HeNe 5 mW, 0.075 J per point as an adjuvant treatment modality ina group of whiplash injured patients. There was no additional effect of the treatment.

The Cochrane collaboration [1524] has performed a literature analysis on the effect of acupuncture, acupressure, laser therapy or electrostimulation for smoking sessation. Quote: " ...on the extracted data in duplicate on the type of smokers recruited, the nature of the acupuncture and control procedures, the outcome measures, method of randomisation, and completeness of follow-up. We assessed abstinence from smoking at the earliest timepoint (before 6 weeks), at six months and at one year or more follow-up in patients smoking at baseline. We used the most rigorous definition of abstinence for each trial, and biochemically validated rates if available. Those lost to follow-up were counted as continuing to smoke. Where appropriate, we performed meta-analysis using a fixed effects model. MAIN We identified 22 studies. Acupuncture was not superior to sham acupuncture in smoking cessation at any time point. The odds ratio (OR) for early outcomes was 1.22 (95% confidence interval 0.99 to 1.49); the OR after 6 months was 1.50 (95% confidence interval 0.99 to 2.27) and after 12 months 1.08 (95% confidence interval 0.77 to 1.52). Similarly, when acupuncture was compared with other anti-smoking interventions, there were no differences in outcome at any time point. Acupuncture appeared to be superior to no intervention in the early results, but this difference was not sustained. The results with different acupuncture techniques do not show any one particular method (i.e. auricular acupuncture or non-auricular acupuncture) to be superior to control intervention. Based on the results of single studies, acupressure was found to be superior to advice; laser therapy and electrostimulation were not superior to sham forms of these therapies. There is no clear evidence that acupuncture, acupressure, laser therapy or electrostimulation are effective for smoking cessation."

Gottschling [1827] investigated whether laser acupuncture is efficacious in children with headache and if active laser treatment is superior to placebo laser treatment in a prospective, randomized, double-blind, placebo-controlled trial of low level laser acupuncture in 43 children) with headache (either migraine (22 patients) or tension type headache (21 patients)).

be effective in reducing the frequency of headache attacks. Acupuncture showed the best effectiveness over time.

Wozniak [1521] reports that laser acupuncture can reduce postmenstrual obesity. The study population consisted of 74 postmenopausal females with visceral obesity that was divided into two groups according to an employed 6-month slimming procedure. In the first group (n = 36) a low-calorie diet was applied, while women in the second group (n = 38) were on the same kind of diet, having additionally one cycle of laser acupuncture procedure at the same time. At baseline and at the end of the study, body weight, body mass index and waist-to-hip ratio were determined in all women. After 6 trial months both groups exhibited a statistically significant drop in body weight, body mass index and waist-to-hip ratio. The mean reduction of body weight, body mass index and waist-to-hip ratio was significantly higher in the second group of women (laser acupuncture plus low-calorie diet).

A double blind, placebo controlled, crossover study was performed by Gruber [1522] to investigate the possible protective effect of a single laser acupuncture treatment on cold dry air hyperventilation induced bronchoconstriction in 44 children and adolescents of mean age 11.9 years (range 7.5-16.7) with exercise induced asthma. Laser acupuncture was performed on real and placebo points in random order on two consecutive days. Lung function was measured before laser acupuncture, immediately after laser acupuncture (just before cold dry air challenge (CACh)), and 3 and 15 minutes after CACh. CACh consisted of a 4 minute isocapnic hyperventilation of -10 degrees C absolute dry air. Comparison of real acupuncture with placebo acupuncture showed no significant differences in the mean maximum CACh induced decrease in forced expiratory volume in 1 second (27.2 (18.2)% v 23.8 (16.2)%) and maximal expiratory flow at 25% remaining vital capacity (51.6 (20.8)% v 44.4 (22.3)%).

As recent studies demonstrated, acupuncture can elicit activity in specific brain areas. The study by Siedentopf [1559] aimed to explore further the central effect using laser acupuncture. The researchers investigated the cerebral effects of laser acupuncture at both acupoints GB43 with functional magnetic resonance imaging (fMRI). As a control condition the laser was mounted at the same acupoints but without application of laser stimulation. The group results showed significant brain activations within the thalamus, nucleus subthalamicus, nucleus ruber, the brainstem, and the Brodmann areas 40 and 22 for the acupuncture condition. No significant brain activations were observed within the placebo condition. The activations observed were laser acupuncture-specific and predominantly ipsilateral. This supports the assumption that acupuncture is mediated by meridians, since meridians do not cross to the other side.

Fifty patients with chronic tension-type headache were randomly allocated to treatment or placebo groups in the study by Ebneshahidi [1569]. Patients in the treatment group received laser acupuncture to LU7, LI4, GB14, and GB20 bilaterally. Points were irradiated for 43 seconds, and the

that the control cohort improvements may have been due to participants' belief that they were receiving active treatment from the stimulator.

The paper by Litscher [1518] presents an experimental double-blind study in laser acupuncture research in healthy volunteers, using a new optical stimulation method. 18 healthy volunteers (mean age +/- SD: 25.4 +/- 4.3 years; range: 21-30 years; 11 female, 7 male) were included in a randomized controlled cross-over trial using functional multidirectional transcranial ultrasound Doppler sonography (fTCD; n=17) and performed functional magnetic resonance imaging (fMRI) in one volunteer. Stimulation of vision-related acupoints resulted in an increase of mean blood flow velocity in the posterior cerebral artery measured by fTCD [before stimulation (mean +/- SE): 42.2 +/- 2.5; during stimulation: 44.2 +/- 2.6; after stimulation: 42.3 +/- 2.4 cm/s, n.s.]. Mean blood flow velocity in the middle cerebral artery decreased insignificantly. Significant changes of brain activity were demonstrated in the occipital and frontal gyrus by fMRI. Optical stimulation using properly adjusted laser needles has the advantage that the stimulation cannot be felt by the patient (painless and no tactile stimulation) and the operator may also be unaware of whether the stimulation system is active. Therefore true double-blind studies in acupuncture research can be performed.

In an experimental animal study Litscher [1519] investigated the effects of the new technique of laser needle stimulation (wavelength: 685 nm; energy density: 4.6 kJ/cm^2. per point; application duration: 20 min). The results revealed changes in microcirculatory parameters of the skin resulting in an increase in blood flow. However, the quality and intensity of the laser light did not induce micromorphological alterations in the skin.

In an open, randomized trial, Allais [1520] evaluated transcutaneous electrical nerve stimulation (TENS), infrared laser therapy and acupuncture in the treatment of transformed migraine, over a 4-month period free of prophylactic drugs. Sixty women suffering from transformed migraine were assigned, after a one month run-in period, to three different treatments: TENS (Group T; n=20), infrared laser therapy (Group L; n=20) or acupuncture (Group A; n=20). In each group the patients underwent ten sessions of treatment and monthly control visits. In Group T patients were treated for two weeks (5 days/week) simultaneously with three TENS units with different stimulation parameters (I: pulse rate = 80 Hz, pulse width = 120 micros; II: 120 Hz, 90 micros; III: 4 Hz, 200 micros). In Group L an infrared diode laser (27 mW, 904 nm) was applied every other day on tender scalp spots. In Group A acupuncture was carried out twice a week in the first two weeks and weekly in the next 6 weeks. A basic formula (LR3, SP6, LI4, GB20, GV20 and Ex-HN5) was always employed; additional points were selected according to each patient's symptomatology. The number of days with headache per month significantly decreased during treatment in all groups. The response in the groups differed over time, probably due to the different timing of applications of the three methods. TENS, laser therapy and acupuncture proved to

according to Nottingham Health Profile gave the superiority of the laser treatment. However, those differences among the groups were not observed at 6-month follow up.

Zalewska-Kaszubska [1517] reports that fifty-three alcoholics were treated with two types of laser stimulation in four sessions. Each session consisted of 20 consecutive daily helium-neon laser neck biostimulations and 10 auricular acupuncture treatments with argon laser (every 2nd day). The Beck Depression Inventory-Fast Screen (BDI-FS) was used to assess their frame of mind before the session and after 2 months of treatment. Moreover, beta-endorphin plasma concentration was estimated five times using the radioimmunoassay (RIA) method. Improvement in BDI-FS and increase in beta-endorphin level were observed. These results suggest that laser therapy may be useful as an adjunct treatment for alcoholism.

However, in a study by Trümpler [1834] inpatients undergoing alcohol withdrawal were randomly allocated to laser acupuncture (n = 17), needle acupuncture (n = 15) or sham laser stimulation (n = 16). Attempts were made to blind patients, therapists and outcome assessors, but this was not feasible for needle acupuncture. The duration of withdrawal symptoms (as assessed using a nurse-rated scale) was the primary outcome; the duration of sedative prescription was the secondary outcome. Patients randomized to laser and sham laser had identical withdrawal symptom durations (median 4 days). Patients randomized to needle stimulation had a shorter duration of withdrawal symptoms and tended to have a shorter duration of sedative use, but these differences diminished after adjustment for baseline differences. The data from this pilot trial do not suggest a relevant benefit of auricular laser acupuncture for alcohol withdrawal.

O'Reilly [1516] studied the effect of at-home laser acupuncture therapy. Interstitial cystitis (IC) is a debilitating condition which causes irritative bladder symptoms, pain and a decrease in health status. The pathophysiology is poorly understood so therapeutic options are diverse. Women meeting the National Institutes of Health National Institute for Diabetes and Digestive and Kidney Diseases criteria for IC were prospectively recruited and randomized to treatment (29) or placebo (27) cohorts in a double-blind trial. At home the patient performed laser therapy daily for 30 seconds over the SP6 acupuncture point for 12 weeks. Measures at baseline and at 84-day follow-up included the 7-day voiding diary, the Interstitial Cystitis Problem Index, Interstitial Cystitis Symptom Index and RAND 36-Item Health Survey questionnaires. There were no significant differences between the treatment and control cohorts on any of the measures. However, there was a significant decrease between baseline and 12-week follow-up in the amount voided, symptom problems and severity, and on all 8 SF-36 scales. There was no significant effect of fluid intake. This study demonstrated no difference between the active and sham device. However, it is interesting that treatment and control cohorts experienced similar improvements, suggesting

manifested immediately when using needles, and after 2-4 minutes with the laser. A comparison was also made of the effects of stimulation of a randomly chosen spot (instead of a known acupuncture point). The effects of stimulation of the acupuncture points were greater than those of the randomly chosen spots.

Kreczi [324] studied the analgesic effect of laser acupuncture in a single blind cross-over study. 21 patients suffering from radicular or pseudoradicular pain were given either laser or mock irradiation. Mean pain levels after laser treatment were significantly lower than after placebo treatment.

Smesny [445] compared the effect of needle and HeNe laser acupuncture. In a group of 112 patients with cervico-occipital headache, 50% were treated with needles and 50% with laser on identical points. Results in the two groups were equivalent (60% in both groups).

Hoffman [494] irradiated LI 4 in 5 subjects. The typical reaction was a temperature reduction of approximately 1 °C in the region of the fingers. Irradiation of placebo points failed to induce this reaction.

King [540] used HeNe laser in auricular therapy in 80 healthy volunteers, aged 18-39 years. 41 received laser therapy and 39 sham irradiation at appropriate acupuncture points in the left ear. Experimental pain threshold at the ipsilateral wrist was determined with an electrical stimulus immediately before and after treatment. The laser group demonstrated a significant increase in pain threshold after treatment, but the control group did not.

In a double blind, randomised, placebo controlled study by Schlager [892] the effectiveness of point P6 acupuncture on postoperative vomiting in children undergoing strabismus (eye) surgery was studied. A 10 mW 670 nm laser was used and the P6 point was irradiated for 30 seconds 15 minutes before anaesthesia and 15 minutes after arriving in the recovery room. In the laser group the incidence of vomiting was 25% and in the placebo group 85%.

These results are confirmed by Butkovic [1703] in a paediatric group scheduled for hernia repair, circumcision or orchidopexy. Laser acupuncture was equally effective as metoclopramide in preventing post operative vomiting.

Ilbuldu [1459] performed a placebo controlled, prospective, long-term follow up study with 60 patients who had trigger points in their upper trapezius muscles. The patients were divided into three groups randomly. Stretching exercises were taught to each group and they were asked to exercise at home. Treatment duration was 4 weeks. Placebo laser was applied to group 1, dry needling to group 2 and laser to group 3. HeNe laser was applied to three trigger points in the upper trapezius muscles on both sides. The patients were assessed before, post-treatment, and at 6 months after treatment for pain, cervical range of motion and functional status. The investigators observed a significant decrease in pain at rest, at activity, and increase in pain threshold in the laser group compared to other groups. Improvement

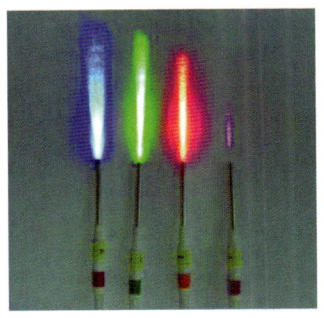

A new concept of laser acupuncture is the so-called "laser needles" [1519]. These are very thin fibres with an adhesive ring at the top. The adhesive ring can fix the laser fibre firmly to an acupuncture point. Since the fibre is thin, the power density over the point becomes considerable, even though output powers are in the 50 mW range. The system is equipped with several fibres and many acupuncture points can be treated simultaneously, making the situation more similar to the needle acupuncture situation. Further to that, single blind studies can now be performed, since the patient will not be aware whether the fibres are active or not.

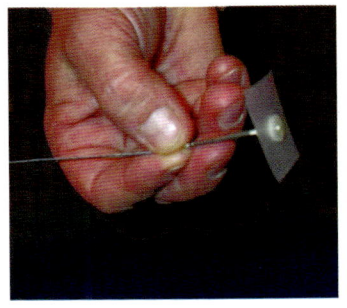

Even tough laser are the tools in laser acpuncture and many practitioners use a combination of local irradiation and laser acupuncture, such combination is not acceptable in a research procedure [1802]. The effects are different and one cannot be compared to the other.

Literature:

Zhao [115] studied the changes in metencephalin in rat brains after HeNe laser irradiation of the Zusanli point. During irradiation, the pain threshold rose, while levels of metencephalin and diencephalin were redu-ced.

Yamamoto [406] has compared the effect of needle acupuncture and laser acupuncture in a rat model, using 830 nm. A selected acupuncture point was irradiated for 90 minutes. The pain threshold was elevated and reached a maximum after 60-90 minutes. After the end of the irradiation, the pain threshold gradually returned to the previous level. The analgesic effect was antagonised by naloxene but a difference between laser and needle was found using dexamethasone.

Bradley [117] studied the effects of laser acupuncture by means of thermography. St 6 was chosen as the standard point. Four minutes of stimulation with a GaAs laser (5000 Hz, 5 mW) and 30 minutes of needle stimulation were compared on the same subject. The facial tissue response showed up thermographically on videotape. It was observed that both needles and laser therapy caused vasodilatation in the faciat region, both on the stimulated side and the opposite side. GaAs and needles produced the same results, but it took longer for GaAs stimulation to take effect. The effect was

1958 and 1965 and until 1971 experimented with acupressure on dental indications. Since 1971 he has worked with laser acupuncture, mainly as anaesthesia for extractions and minor operations. Zhou has developed an interesting technique that involves a small number of acupuncture points being subjected to high outputs. For extractions in the lower jaw, one single point is irradiated for five minutes with a HeNe laser (2-6 mW). The extraction starts immediately after, but the laser is held on the Hegu point (the thumb grip) during the whole process. Zhou also works with a CO_2-laser within the laser therapy range 0-100 mW, which he considers even more effective than the HeNe laser. His experience is that coagulation times are shorter with laser acupuncture than with normal anaesthetics and that subsequent discomfort is also reduced. Postoperative oedema and trismus are also less pronounced after laser acupuncture.

Bearing in mind that, since 1971, Zhou has performed over 10 000 tooth extractions with LAA (Laser Acupuncture Anaesthesia), the method cannot be dismissed as a placebo or something which only works on the Chinese - which was often the argument put forward before needle acupuncture was accepted in the West. LAA is not very well known amongst European authorities on acupuncture, despite the fact that Zhou, as early as 1984, published an account in English of his experience after the first 600 extractions.

The points in the upper jaw for extraction are Sibai and Quanliao, and for the lower jaw, Jiache. The Hegu grip is used during extractions from both the lower and the upper jaw. Yangbai, Yuyao, Yintang, Sibai, Quanliao, and Jiache are the main points used for minor maxillofacial operations. Zhou also uses a HeNe or carbon dioxide laser directly on the alveolus after an extraction. In the thousands of extractions performed with LAA and its subsequent local treatment, not a single case of alveolitis or postoperative bleeding has occurred. Sutures are very rarely needed.

Even though it was the Chinese who pioneered laser acupuncture, it was a Canadian - Friedrich Plog - who, quite early on, highlighted the usefulness of the HeNe laser in this context. He was already testing lasers instead of needles in 1973 [227].

The literature in this area is rather large but the actual mechnisms have not been well documented. Recent studies using fMRI and comparing the effects of laser and needle acupuncture, have contributed to a more objective confirmation of the observed clinical effects and confirming the the fact that acupuncture points actually can be influenced by laser light [1833, 1835]. Thus, laser acupuncture has ceased to be controversial.

given incident beam diameter; and 2) the transmittance at a particular wavelength increases asymptotically with incident beam diameter. For some skin tissues, the transmittance flattens at about 8 mm for 532 nm photons and approaches saturation at about 12 mm for all other colours. The results on pig skin are similar.

3.3.3.1.3 Treating inside the body

In some cases you may realize that the problem volume can not be reached through overlying skin, muscles, bone etc. A possible way to overcome this may be to use fibre optics or specialised probes to reach the place of a problem. Hence, the light can be brought into rectum, vagina, bladder, nose cavity etc by suitably designed probes. An optical fibre can be guided into blood vessels to treat angina etc. With an endoscope, ulcers in throat and stomach can be treated. A fibre can also be attached into a syringe needle, which can penetrate through lacerated muscles, emitting the light at its tip. Another, very simple method that has been used for problems in rectum and vagina, is to insert a test tube of glass or transparent plastic in order to expand the tissue and then to insert a laser probe inside the test tube. The light must then be properly spread or directed so that the right target is illuminated.

3.3.3.2 Systemic treatments

Systemic treatment means that we irradiate areas outside or far from the area where the patient would otherwise locate the problem. Examples of such treatment are treatment of acupuncture points and trigger points.

3.3.3.2.1 Acupuncture.

Acupuncture with lasers is an exciting phenomenon. A wide range of opportunities is open to a therapist with acupuncture training. The method is sterile and painless, and therefore highly acceptable to the patient and especially to children. Practitioners with little or no knowledge can use acupuncture with some success on a narrow range of indications. If well-known and uncontroversial points are used in laser acupuncture therapy, pain, tension, nausea, and anxiety can be influenced. Both laser acupuncture and conventional needle acupuncture affect the acupuncture points, but according to experienced therapists they do not always result in identical effects. They could be said to complement each other.

Lasers only cause a negligible rise in temperature in tissue [109, 170, 189, 1221], which is why laser acupuncture should not be confused with moxa treatment. Indeed, in some cases, even a small reduction in temperature has been reported [494]. Lasers seem to stimulate acupuncture points in a similar way to needles, although needles are more suitable for deep-lying points.

The pioneers of laser acupuncture come, unsurprisingly, from China. The oral surgeon Yo-Cheng Zhou worked with needle acupuncture between

- irradiating the blood
- irradiating lymph nodes

In these instances we irradiate areas outside or far from the area where the patient would otherwise locate the problem.

Direct and indirect treatment can be combined. In fact, even direct irradiation is a mode of indirect irradiation. The beam will always find blood, lymph and nerves, influencing the circulating metabolites. So every local treatment is also a systemic treatment but not vice versa.

3.3.3.1 Local treatment

This means that the laser light irradiates the affected area, e.g. a wound or an inflamed tendon. The treatment technique used depends on the depth of the tissue that you want to treat.

3.3.3.1.1 Shallow problems

1. Open wounds: The probe is held 1-2 cm from the wound. The depth of penetration is insignificant, which is of course the intention. Treat the periphery of the wound in skin contact. Give the open area of the wound a lower dose than the skin periphery.

2. Tissue lying close to the skin surface: Hold the probe in light contact with the skin.

3.3.3.1.2 Deeper problems

At medium depth: Press the probe against the skin. The deeper the tissue to be treated, the higher the pressure.

At great depth: Only the GaAs and high-powered GaAlAs laser can reach to these depths, but the therapist's knowledge of anatomy is also crucial. If the patient moves his/her arm/leg to various positions, an obstructing muscle mass can be moved aside to expose openings in deep muscle attachments. Pressing the probe firmly against the skin will also move the light closer to the target and decrease absorption through the ischemia caused by the pressure.

Literature:

For many skin treatments with light, it is important to have deep photon penetration into the skin. Because of absorption and scattering of photons by skin tissue, both the colour and the diameter of the incident beam affect the penetration depth of photons. In a study by Zhong-Quan [1748], the dependence of light transmission through human skin tissues (ear lobes and between the fingers) has been measured in-vivo at six wavelengths (532 nm, 632 nm, 675 nm, 810 nm, 911 nm, and 1064 nm). The same measurement was also made on pig skin in-vitro for comparison. It was observed that 1) the photons at 1064 nm penetrate deeper than the other colours studied for a

Alleviation resulted both from irradiation prior to chemotherapy and irradiation following the debut of symptoms. This effect is confirmed by Bensadoun [929].

In an in vitro study by Karu [1107] it was found that the cell-glass adhesion increased in a dose-dependent manner after irradiation. The addition of different antioxidants eliminated this effect. Pre-irradiation was found to decrease (or normalise to the control level) the suppressive effects of these chemicals.

Bibikova [587] found that the process of regeneration in degenerated muscles can be markedly enhanced if the muscle is irradiated with HeNe laser prior to the injury.

Pöntinen [1285] has been using laser pretreatment in patients scheduled for various surgical intervention. Laser therapy has been performed on the day before surgery and immediately before surgery. This therapy has improved the rehabilitation process through reduced postoperative pain and oedema.

In the study by Zeredo [1588] the researchers tested the possible antinociceptive effect of laser irradiation when applied to a normal tissue before the onset of a painful stimulus. Male rats were used. A 1.5% formalin solution was injected into the right upper lip of the test animals (n = 9) immediately after 10 min of low-power Er:YAG laser irradiation (energy: 0.1 J/cm^2 per pulse at 10 Hz). Control animals (n = 9) were restrained for 10 min without laser application. The nociceptive response, i.e., the amount of time the rats spent rubbing the formalin injected area, was measured by an investigator blind to whether the animals had been laser irradiated or not. On laser irradiated rats, significantly less nociceptive behavior was observed only during the late phase (12-39 min) of the test. This result is similar to that reported for nonsteroid antiinflammatory drugs (NSAIDs) and other peripherally acting antiinflammatory agents.

Further literature: [564]

3.3.3 Treatment method parameters

There are several ways of administrating the laser light:

A. Local treatment (produces primarily local effects). This means that the laser light irradiates the affected area, e.g. a wound or an inflamed tendon.

B. Systemic or indirect irradiation (produces primarily systemic effects)

Examples of indirect irradiation are:

- irradiating acupuncture points
- irradiating trigger points
- irradiating spinal processes
- irradiating the dermatome

He-Ne irradiation at a fluence of 5 J/cm^2. was determined by analysis of cell morphology, viability, cytotoxicity, and DNA damage. Cells were irradiated using three different protocols: they were irradiated at 30 min only; irradiated twice, at 30 min and at 24 h; or irradiated twice, at 30 min and at 72 h post-wound induction. A single exposure to 5 J/cm^2. 30 min post-wound induction increased cellular damage. Irradiation of cells at 30 min and at 24 h post-wound induction decreased cellular viability, cytotoxicity, and DNA damage. However, complete wound closure as well as an increase in viability and a decrease in cytotoxicity and DNA damage occurs when cells were irradiated at 30 min and at 72 h post-wound induction. Thus, wounded diabetic WS1 cells irradiated to 5 J/cm^2. showed increased cellular repair when irradiated with adequate time between irradiations, allowing time for cellular response mechanisms to take effect. Therefore, the irradiation interval was shown to play an important role in wound healing in vitro and should be taken into account.

3.3.2.3 Pre- or postoperative treatment?

Previously the predominant view was that there is nothing to gain by irradiating tissue pre-operatively. If the tissue is healthy, laser treatment has no effect. It may be time to reconsider the conventional wisdom, however, based on the results of several studies.

All irradiation, even of healthy tissue, activates a variety of processes, leading, for example, to the production of singlet oxygen. If no trauma exists or occurs later, these products disappear quickly and the normal state returns. If trauma occurs immediately after irradiation, however, the tissues' defence systems are in a more favourable state. If the tissue is already in poor condition prior to the operation (oedema, inflammation etc.), laser energy is even more beneficial pre-operatively.

Some conditions are cyclic and there are studies suggesting the possibility of treating these even in the inactive period. This has been demonstrated for herpes simplex [908] and asthma [1205].

Literature:

A study by Rosner [494] entailed crushing the optical nerve of rats. The object of the study was to investigate the capacity of the HeNe laser to delay or prevent nerve degeneration. Surprisingly, the effects were equally beneficial whether radiation was applied immediately before or immediately after the nerve was crushed.

In this study the tissue was intact before inflicting a trauma. In the following studies, the tissue was in a state of imbalance: Popova [147] removed muscle tissue from rats, irradiated it with X-rays, and then replanted the tissue. Improved healing was observed in those animals given laser therapy, prior to X-ray as well as after X-ray.

A study by Pourreau-Schneider [46] showed that mucositis associated with chemotherapy in cancer patients was alleviated by HeNe laser light.

Literature:

In the study by Ng [1508] sixteen rats were used, with 12 receiving surgical transection to their right MCL and 4 receiving a sham injury. Group 1 (n = 4) received a single dose of InGaAlP laser therapy (wavelength 660 nm, average power 8.8 mW, pulse 10 kHz, dosage 31.6 J/cm²) directly to their MCL during surgery. Group 2 (n = 4) received 9 doses of GaAlAs laser therapy applied transcutaneously on alternate days (wavelength 660 nm, average power 8.8 mW, pulse 10 kHz, dosage 3.5 J/cm²). The controls (Group 3, n = 4) received one session of placebo laser at the time of surgery, with the laser equipment shut down, while the sham injured Group 4 (n = 4) received no treatment. Biomechanical tests for structural stiffness, ultimate tensile strength (UTS), and load-relaxation were done at 3 weeks after injury. The stiffness and UTS data were normalised by expressing as a percentage of the left side of each animal before statistical analysis. The load-relaxation data did not show any differences between the groups. The normalized stiffness levels of Groups 2 (81.08+/-11.28%) and 4 (92.66+/-13.19%) were significantly higher than that of the control Group 3 (58.99+/-15.91%). The normalized UTS of Groups 2 (81.38+/-5.68%) and 4 (90.18+/-8.82%) were also significantly higher than that of the control (64.49+/-9.26%). Although, Group 1 had higher mean stiffness and UTS values than the control, no statistically significant difference was found between these two groups. Multiple laser therapy improves the normalized strength and stiffness of repairing rat MCLs at 3 weeks after injury. The multiple treatments seemed to be superior to a single treatment.

In the study by Carati [1337] post mastectomy oedema was treated with GaAs laser. One session of laser kept the oedema below the volume of that in the patients of the control group, whereas patients receiving two sessions showed a continuous improvement during a 3-months follow up.

The results of the cell study by Hawkins [1744] show that the correct energy density or fluence (J/cm²) and number of exposures can stimulate cellular responses of wounded fibroblasts and promote cell migration and cell proliferation by stimulating mitochondrial activity and maintaining viability without causing additional stress or damage to the wounded cells. Results further indicate that the cumulative effect of lower doses (2.5 or 5 J/cm²) determines the stimulatory effect, while multiple exposures at higher doses (16 J/cm²) result in an inhibitory effect with more damage.

A study by Houreld [1889] investigated the effectiveness of helium-neon laser irradiation at increasing intervals on diabetic-induced wounded human skin fibroblast cells (WS1) at a morphological, cellular, and molecular level. The controversies over light therapy can be explained by the differing exposure regimens and models used. No therapeutic window for dosimetry and mechanism of action has been determined at the level of individual cell types, particularly in diabetic cells in vitro. WS1 cells were used to simulate an in vitro wounded diabetic model. The effect of the frequency of

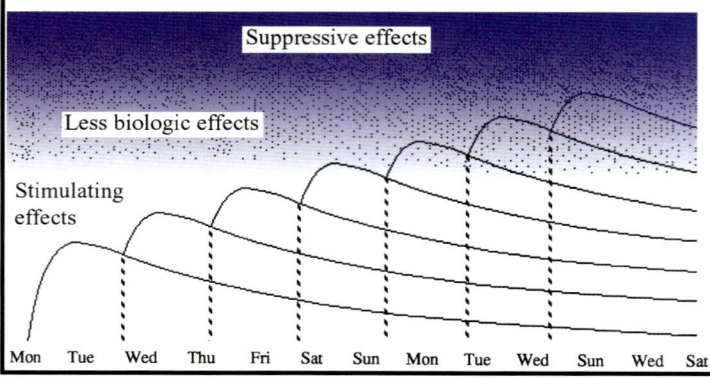

Figure 3.5 Cumulative dose

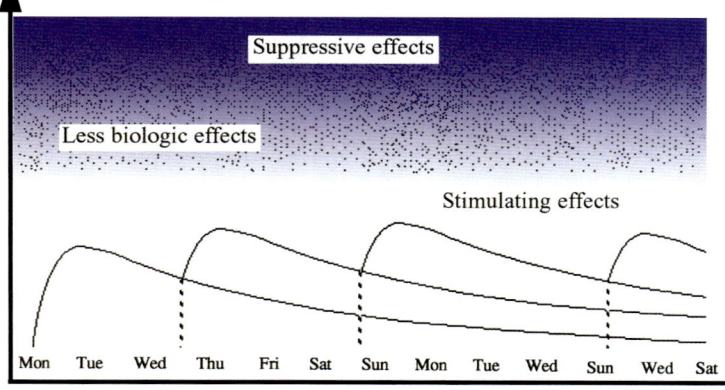

Figure 3.6 Shorter treatment intervals

be traced in blood and urine, that can reach disturbingly high levels when large areas are treated. It can also be a question of saturation.

3.3.2.2 Treatment intervals

Treatment intervals must be assessed for each individual case. Those expecting detailed advice on how to treat each particular case will be disappointed by what follows here. The same rules apply to laser treatment as to all other forms of medical treatment: the best results are achieved by the therapist who possesses sound medical knowledge, can listen to the patient and has a good intuition. As a general rule, however, it is better to use 3-4 treatments a week with moderate doses than using higher doses and few treatments.

Mester demonstrated that small doses with appropriate periods of time in-between are more effective than treatments that are very close. Abergel [8] has also demonstrated this on fibroblast cultures. Because laser therapy treatment has been shown to be cumulative (the dose from one treatment lasts some time, and what "remains" of the dose is added to the dose at the next treatment), it is vital that treatments are not too close together, so as to avoid a situation where the accumulated dose eventually ends up above the biostimulating range or even in the bio-inhibiting range, with consequently poorer results.

Acute problems are usually dealt with by a few treatments, which can be closely spaced. Acute herpes simplex or herpes zoster, for example, can be treated every day for a few days. Acute pain conditions can be given close treatment. Chronic complaints are usually best handled with more widely spaced treatment.

It has been shown to be beneficial to treat at closer intervals in the beginning (e.g. every other day or every third day for two weeks) and then at longer and longer intervals (e.g. once a week for a few weeks). Experience shows that it is not disadvantageous to temporarily suspend treatment after a number of introductory sessions. In some circumstances, this can actually be beneficial.

Another aspect is that you always have to take the patients' economy into account. If we haven't noted a clear reaction after 4-5 sessions, we may suggest that further therapy is to be postponed for some weeks (or even months), to see if there will be a "late reaction". Then we can "speed it up" with more sessions. This also convinces the patient that our primary aim is not the patients' "money", but the clinical results.

Joules; 56 mW constant power at 664 nm. The best results were achieved with 2 J. In the next experiment the energy was set at 2 J and the power used was either 28 or 56 mW. Best results were achieved with the higher power. Finally, the power of 56 mW and energy of 2 J were used either in continuous mode or at different pulse modes. The continuous mode provided the best stimulation and among the frequencies used the higher pulse frequencies presented the best results. These experiments elegantly demonstrate the importance of a correct amount of energy, that the energy density is important and that continuous mode is better than pulsed modes.

Al-Watban [1495] compared the wound healing effect of pulsed and continuous 635 nm laser. Continuous beam provide the best results, and the 100 Hz pulse repetition rate the best among the different frequencies used. And this pulse repetition rate happens to be the one closest to continuous among the frequencies used, which further underlines the superiority of the continuous beam for wound healing procedures.

The effect of pulsing is also studied by Ueda [1181]. Osteoblastic cells isolated from fetal rat calvariae were irradiated once with GaAlAs laser (830 nm, 500 mW) in two different irradiation modes; continuous irradiation (CI), and 1 Hz pulsed irradiation (PI). The author then investigated the effects on cellular proliferation, bone nodule formation, alkaline phosphatase (ALP) activity, and ALP gene expression. Laser irradiation in both groups significantly stimulated cellular proliferation, bone nodule formation, ALP activity, and ALP gene expression, as compared with the non-irradiation group. Notably, 1 Hz markedly stimulated these factors, when compared with the continuous group. In this study the lowest possible pulse mode was compared to continuous, and the possible effect of higher frequencies is not known.

Further literature: [773, 1158]

3.3.2 Patient parameters

Of course the laser parameters depend very much on what we are going to treat. For instance, if we are going to treat an ulcer, we choose other settings than if we are going to treat knee arthroses.

3.3.2.1 Treatment area

In order to calculate dose, power density and treatment time, it is necessary to know the treatment area. In the formulas for calculation, the treatment area must be expressed in cm^2 if the outcome is to be correct.

Also, it is of importance for deciding the dose to have a knowledge of the depth below skin surface of the site to be treated.

Practical experience indicates that it may be more beneficial to treat a smaller area more intensively and then treat nearby areas later, rather than treating a larger area over a longer period of time at a single session. This may well be related to the fact that certain substances are released, which can

The table applies only to truly pulsed lasers.

Local treatment		Laser acupuncture	
Diagnosis:	Frequency range:	Point type:	Frequency:
Pain, neuralgia	1-100 Hz	Endpoints	73 Hz
General stimulation	700 Hz	Source points	146 Hz
Oedema, swellings	1000 Hz	Sedation points	584 Hz
General stimulation	2500 Hz	Tonification points	1000 Hz
Inflammations	5000 Hz	Alarm points	2500 Hz
Infections	10 000 Hz	Beginning points	5000 Hz

Table 3.6 Pulse pulse repetition rates - laser acupuncture

The frequencies discussed here have nothing in common with the different pulse frequencies recommended for laser acupuncture.

There are GaAs lasers that automatically vary the pulse repetition rate during treatment, going from low to high and back. As can be seen from the above studies, it is not self-evident that this concept is beneficial.

Literature:

Mohktar [161] studied the pain-relieving effects of 16 Hz and 73 Hz frequencies, with otherwise unchanged parameters, in a double-blind study of experimental ischaemic pain. Significant effects were obtained, compared to the reference group, at 16 Hz but not at 73 Hz. The equipment used was a combined laser/LED array.

In another comparative double-blind study, also by Mohktar [162], nerve action potential was measured under irradiation at 73 Hz and 5000 Hz, under otherwise unchanged conditions. 73 Hz gave no significant effect when compared to the placebo group, whereas 5000 Hz did produce effects.

Kim [283] studied the effect of different GaAs pulses by irradiating 360 cultures of candida albicans with 5, 500, 1500, and 10 000 Hz. Significant differences were seen amongst the groups depending on the pulse type with which irradiation was given.

Martin [308] has shown that photobiological effects upon lower limb blood flow can be PRR-specific.

Fagnoni [509] had better results using 30 Hz rather than 70 Hz when treating patients suffering from trigeminal neuralgia.

El Sayed [529] compared the effect of GaAs at different frequencies on mast cell number and degranulation. All frequencies were effective compared to the sham irradiated groups, but only 20 Hz and 292 Hz, among the frequencies used, were significantly effective.

Almeida Lopes [1330] performed three interesting studies on fibroblasts. In the first study the fibroblasts were irradiated with 2, 5, 10 and 15

In short, pulsing probably has an effect but we know very little about it today. The general recommendation is therefore: use continuous unless you have a very good reason not to do so.

In a reveiw from 2003, Corral-Baqués [1260] writes:

We've gone through more than 150 papers in search of conclusive data to develop new treating parameters for skeletal muscle injury. We were especially concerned, among the different parameters, on the frequencies used. Of those papers, only 35 reported the used PRR, but just 25 of them specified all the parameters (fluence, radiance, spot, etc) and just 6 were done in vitro.

In order to make the most of the gathered information, we built charts of each wavelength and the different frequencies used depending on the pretended effect.

Focusing just on the 904 nm wavelength we've noticed:
- That most of the articles were previous to 1990 (a big fall not understandable when considering that up to 84% of the reviewed papers showed positive effects) with a big increase on papers dealing with the 820 nm.
- From the 26 papers found dealing with 904 nm, we've identified 29 different frequencies (no related among themselves, that is, not based on previous studies).
- From that table we can conclude that, to get an analgesic effect we need a PRR in the range from 4 Hz to 5120 Hz (that means any PRR is supposed to be useful).
- The same happens with the trophic effect, any PRR from 5 Hz to 10000 Hz is supposed to be equally effective.
- If we are to compare other parameters (power density, energy density, etc.) we will get to the same point: it's impossible to make any sense out of it.

ERGO: it's impossible to extract any conclusions as a starting point to start new researches in order to find more suitable working parameters.

So, for super pulsed lasers, there is not yet much literature providing advice on which PRR:s are suitable for what (as regards pulsing, see chapter 1.2.10 "Continuous and pulsed lasers" on page 16 and Figure 1.7 "Different types of pulsing" on page 19.)

Although the literature in this field has not yet made clear which frequencies are particularly suited to which treatments, the many users of laser therapy have still produced a large body of empirical material. The table below shows the frequencies that, on empirical grounds, are considered particularly suitable for certain types of problem. The column to the right shows the frequencies with which many acupuncturists consider various acupuncture points should be treated.

2. Even with a GaAs laser you still have to watch out when it comes to deciding a pulse repetition rate ("frequency"). Some GaAs laser will shift power along with the pulsing. If, for instance, the maximum average power is 10 mW and the highest pulse repetition rate is 10 000 Hz, then follows that using 1000 Hz reduces the power to 1 mW. And if 100 Hz is used, then the power drops further to 0.1 mW. Modern GaAs lasers can handle this problem and give the same average power over all pulse frequencies. But still, you have to select one particular pulse repetition rate and rely on anecdotal evidence.

3. Many *in vitro* studies have showed that different pulse frequencies give different effects. In such settings a particular isolated biological event is studied in cell monolayers. When irradiating such a complex target as a mammal, the situation is quite different. The selected pulse repetition rate may (or may not) work the way the laboratory study suggests, but several other biological effects may be negative at the same time or at least unknown.

4. Looking at the literature, it becomes clear that very few studies provide a rationale for the selected pulsing. The frequencies used seem to have been chosen at random or adopted from an older study, where the pulse repetition rate also was chosen at random. In a literature study on the effects of laser therapy on musculoskeletal pain Corral-Baqués [1260] identified 150 papers. Among these 35 reported the used pulse repetition rate and only 25 all the laser parameters used. Before the 90ies the dominating wavelength was 904 nm but after the 90ies many 808-830 nm lasers were used in a pulsing mode. More than 30 frequencies were used, switched and super pulsed. The only conclusion which can be made from this analysis is that no conclusion can be made.

5. Many laser manufacturers favour certain frequencies, particularly for switched mode. One favourite is 73 Hz, used already by Walker [38] in 1983. This pulse repetition rate is initially recommended for electrotherapy and there is no evidence for its use in light therapy. Other frequencies originate from the auriculo-therapy field and there possible advantages there have not been documented in laser therapy or any other light therapy.

6. When an effort is made to evaluate studies using pulsing, several questions arise. Was the output power the same for both frequencies? Or was the time of irradiation changed to compensate for the reduction of power? Was the laser well calibrated and the pulse mechanism quality verified? Too often the questions remain unanswered.

3.3.1.12 Pulsed or continuous light

As mentioned previously, a laser can work continuously (most typical for InGaAlP, HeNe, and GaAlAs lasers) or pulsed (the GaAs laser).

The GaAs laser (904 or 905 nm) is always superpulsed, with two possible consequences. Firstly, the pulsing of the laser light may interfere with other pulsing phenomena in the organism, and secondly, continuous/switched and superpulsed lasers may have different active depths. A superpulsed laser always penetrates deeper than a continuous or switched laser with the same wavelength and the same average output power. The extremely intense light flashes of the GaAs laser achieve greater light intensity extending deep into the tissue.

3.3.1.13 Pulse repetition rate (PRR)

Few aspects of laser therapy cause so much confusion as the concept of pulsing. So let us try to make it a bit easier.

1. It is important to understand the difference between "switching" and "super pulsing". Continuous lasers can be pulsed through mechanical or electronical devices. This means that the continuous beam is shut on and off. The power of the beam remains the same. If the "on-time" and the "off-time are the same, then the so called "duty cycle" is 50%. This means that the average laser power is 50% of the continuous wave power. If the laser is in the on mode during 90% of the cycle time, then the duty cycle is 90%, i.e. close to continuous. With 50% duty cycle the treatment time has to be doubled in order to achieve the same dose as with a continuous beam.

In some cases, the "on-time" is very short, which means that the duty cycle is very low. This is often called super pulsing. Characteristic for super pulsing is that the power in the peaks - peak power - is very high compared to the average power. Some semiconductor lasers, like the GaAs laser, can only be powered with very, very short but strong current pulses. The reason for this is that the GaAs chrystal needs a very high current density to lase. Typically a current of 25 - 100 ampere is fed through a 1 cubic millimeter chrystal and such current pulses have to be very, very short (no more than 200 ns) not to burn the chrystal. After such a current pulse, it needs a long time (typically more than 100 micro seconds) to cool down before the next pulse heats it again. This means that the duty cycle for a GaAs laser typically is in the order of 0.1% or less, which in turn means that the peak power usually is about 1000 times higher than the average power. For a GaAs laser with 10 mW average power and 0.1% duty cycle, the peak power is 10 watt.

The biological response to this type of pulsing is very likely different to a switched beam. Some manufacturers like to list the peak power only, to make the equipment look more powerful and impressing.

Treatment time for 50 cm² surface area with a GaAlAs laser. If the laser is pulsed, the average output power should be used. Treatment should be done with skin contact.

Depth	10 mw	25 mw	50 mw	100 mw	250 mw	500 mw
0.5 cm	25 min	10 min	5 min	2 min	1 min	30 sec
1 cm	50 min	20 min	10 min	5 min	2 min	1 min
2 cm	*)	40 min	20 min	10 min	4 min	2 min
3 cm	*)	*)	30 min	15 min	6 min	3 min
4 cm	*)	*)	40 min	20 min	8 min	4 min

Table 3.5 Treatment time with a GaAlAs laser

*) Unrealistic depth and time

As can be seen, table 3.5, shows longer treatment time for corresponding powers and depths, reflecting the higher doses needed for the GaAlAs laser compared to the GaAs laser.

Example 2: Another approach, which many people find easier, is to ascertain the time it takes for the laser to produce 1 joule. If the laser has an output power that is 40 mW, it takes 25 seconds to produce 1 joule (calculate it by dividing 1 by your laser's power output given in watt in this example $1/0.04 = 25$ sec). This means that if you radiate the area of 1 cm² for 25 seconds, you have given a dose of 1 J/cm².

The complexity of dosage is discussed elsewhere in this book. At this early stage we just want to underline the difference between irradiating with a laser of 10 mW for 100 seconds and a laser of 1000 mW for 1 second. Both will produce 1 joule, but the effect on cells is quite different. High power densities are useful for pain conditions, whereas lower power densities are better for wound healing. One difference is that the longer treatments times also mean more absorption by blood and consequent distant effects.

3.3.1.11 Dose per point

In the treatment of trigger points and acupuncture points the dose is often said to be a number of joules per "point" and it is assumed that a point is something small. We have defined a "point" as an area that is 5 mm in diameter (= 0.2 cm²) or less. This means that if we hit the skin with the light concentrated to this small area and administer 1 joule, we have given 1 J "per point", and in this "point" (= 0.2 cm²) the dose value is 5 J/cm².
This is also explained in chapter 10.10 "Dose per point" on page 522.

What parameters to use

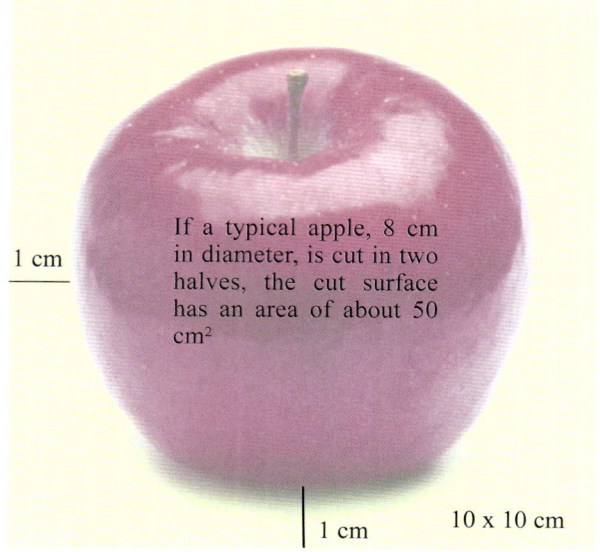

Figure 3.4 Apple ready reckoner

Treatment time for 50 cm² surface area with a GaAs-laser. The output powers are average powers. Treatment should be done with skin contact.

Depth	10 mW	25 mW	50 mW	100 mW	200 mW
0.5 cm	2.5 min	1 min	30 sec	15 sec	10 sec
1 cm	5 min	2 min	1 min	30 sec	15 sec
2 cm	10 min	4 min	2 min	1 min	30 sec
3 cm	15 min	6 min	3 min	1.5 min	45 sec
4 cm	20 min	8 min	4 min	2 min	1 min

Table 3.4 Treatment time with a GaAs-laser

at hand. If the problem to treat is situated at a depth **d** (where d = 0 to 4 cm), the following approximate formula can be used to find the treatment time:

$$t = \frac{D \times A}{P} \times (1 + d) \quad [\sec]$$

N.B. For this formula to work, the correct units to be used are: **P** must be given in watts (not milliwatts), **D** must be given in J/cm², **A** must be expressed in cm² and **d** in cm. The treatment time will then come out in seconds. Values 1 - 4 of the parameter **d** are only applicable to the deeper penetrating laser types (GaAs laser and GaAlAs lasers). For CO_2-, HeNe- and GaAlInP-lasers, use value d=0. Usually your laser power is given in milliwatts. If you want to use the formulas in this book, you must use the power expressed in watts. To convert from milliwatts to watts, you simply divide by 1000. E.g. 40 milliwatts (40 mW) becomes 0.040 watts (0.040 W). A simple rule can be: Use 3 decimals and your power will be seen as: 0.040 W for your 40 mW probe and 0.250 W for your 250 mW probe.

3.3.1.10 "Ready reckoner"

For most people, mathematical formulas have negative associations. For the common therapist it is, however, not necessary to use a calculator for every treatment. We have made the process easy. For the treatment of larger areas, such as back, neck, shoulders, arms, knees, etc., we use "apples". If you cut an apple in two halves, the cut surface has an area of about 50 cm². Supposing that you know what laser type you have and its output power, you simply use the tables on the following pages. Find your laser's output power and then enter the depth of the problem: Is it deep or superficial? The table will show you the treatment time in minutes per "apple" at different depths.

Example 1: To treat an area with the size of an apple and with a problem situated 3 cm underneath said surface, using a **GaAs-laser** probe with an average output power of 50 mW at the chosen treatment pulse repetition rate, you need a minimum of 3 minutes. If the area is larger than an apple – e.g. the size of 4 apples – treat 4 times 3 minutes as a minimum. Maximum treatment time: Choose twice the minimum value. Move the probe evenly over the surface.

to treat pain or achieve a more long-term effect. As stated before, specifying the "right" dose for a particular condition is not easy. Numerous parameters must be taken into account: wavelength and output, contact or non-contact with skin/mucous membrane, type of tissue, acute/chronic, how deep in the tissue you want to reach, the patient's general condition, the skin's pigmentation, etc. "The right dose" may sometimes be whatever the instrument is able to deliver.

Literature:

Abergel [8] investigated the effect of HeNe-laser light and GaAs-laser light on the connective tissue metabolism. In this comparison the author writes: "Similar stimulation of collagen production was also observed with GaAs-laser. With this laser a two- to threefold stimulation in two separate cell lines was achieved with energy densities that were considerably lower than those required for stimulation with HeNe-laser."

Bolton [419] irradiated human fibroblasts with a 50 mW GaAlAs laser. The proliferation of fibroblasts and the succinic dehydrogenase activity increased at doses of 2 J/cm^2, but both were inhibited at doses of 16 J/cm^2.

Igarashi [579] irradiated neonatal rats with a 830 nm laser, delivering 0.9 J twice daily from birth to day five at two points located above the hippocampus. The mean body weight of the irradiated animals on day 20 was 22% lower than that of the control animals. The density of synaptic junctions was also reduced in the irradiated animals as of day 20. (This may seem alarming, but don't worry! Suppose the weight of a newborn rat is 3 g. A newborn human weights around 3.000 g. Thus, the extrapolated dose would be 900 J. Another factor is the size of the neonathal rats; here we have millimeters when with human babies have centimeters, giving much higher power densities and local doses for the rat fetus). This study is an example of bioinhibition.

The inhibitive effect of high doses of laser energy has also been demonstrated by Gross [779]. The effect of HeNe laser light on the cell cycle and the growth of rat kidney epithelial cells was studied. Daily doses of 11.9 - 142 J/cm^2 significantly inhibited cell growth, while less than 4.7 J/cm^2 had no effect.

Other examples of stimulation and inhibitions are [1095, 1101]. (See Table 11.3 "Examples of different dose levels in vitro" on page 544.)

3.3.1.9 Calculation of treatment time for a desired dose

The most common situation in laser therapy is that we wish to administer a certain dose **D** to a specified area **A** with our laser, having an (average-) output power **P**, and we need to calculate the treatment time **t** for the laser probe

Indication	Laser type	Dose in J/cm^2
Open wound	HeNe InGaAlP GaAlAs GaAs CO_2	0.5-1.5 1-2 0.5-1.5 0.01-0.2 1-10
Wound periphery	HeNe InGaAlP GaAlAs GaAs CO_2	1-4 2-6 1-4 0.5-1 -
Superficial pain	HeNe InGaAlP GaAlAs GaAs CO_2	0.5-2 1-4 2-4 1-2 5-100
Deep lying pain	HeNe InGaAlP GaAlAs GaAs CO_2	- - 4-10 2-5 5-100

Table 3.3 Dose ranges for different lasers and indications

Doses for other lasers, like the Ruby laser and Nd:YAG lasers are not as well known. Mester's group used Ruby laser and indicated 1-2 J/cm^2. Doses for acupuncture points: See chapter 3.3.3.2.1 "Acupuncture." on page 97.

As can be seen above, it appears that lower doses are required with GaAs laser than with HeNe laser. This has been observed by e.g. Abergel [8]. In general, tissue tolerates higher "overdoses" of HeNe, InGaAlP and GaAlAs than of GaAs, which more quickly reaches an inhibiting level.

In the treatment of healthy, optimally working tissue, almost any dose can be used without noticeably macroscopic negative effects. This is e.g. the case in the use of surgical lasers cutting, evaporating and coagulating tissue, using very high power and energy densities. Right outside the destructive zone, very high levels of power density and dose occur, but this is not found to be negative.

When irradiating "naked cells", in an open wound, for example, the optimal dose is much lower than when irradiating through overlying skin. The dose and the treatment interval differ depending on whether the condition in the tissue is chronic or acute, but also on whether we primarily want

We often meet therapists who do not know what type of laser they are using. When asked, it is not unusual for them to respond "3B". Often they do not know what "dose" means, much less how to calculate one. Frequently, they have believed that the output power of the instrument was completely different from what it actually was.

One day we received a call from a clinic in Stockholm. They said there must be something wrong with their instrument; results were not good recently. It turned out to be a GaAs laser. The brochure stated that the average output power of the single probe (with one laser diode) was 20 mW, and the output of the multiprobe was 60 mW (with three laser diodes). Testing resulted in the following table

Pulse rep. rate	Single probe	Multiprobe
10 Hz	0.002 mW	0.02 mW
100 Hz	0.02 mW	0.25 mW
1000 Hz	0.20 mW	2.1 mW
10 000 Hz	1.81 mW	20 mW

Table 3.2 Output power dependent on pulse repetition rate

As can be seen, the output from the single probe was less than 10% of the stated nominal output at the highest pulse repetition rate. Neither the brochure nor the manual mentioned that the output power was dependent on the pulse repetition rate setting.

3.3.1.8 Dose ranges

Biostimulation has been reported in the literature with doses from as low as 0.001 J/cm^2 to 10 J/cm^2 and more. How is this possible? Can we just use any dose? Certainly not - this is where we have to start thinking! There is a great difference between irradiating naked cells in the laboratory and treating a deep lying pain condition! In fact, a "dose" is a very complicated issue. It is a matter of wavelength, power density, type of tissue, condition of the tissue, chronic or acute problem, pigmentation, treatment technique and so forth. However, there is certainly a "therapeutic dose window". Doses that are too low result in no or only a weak effect. If a dose above the highest one suitable is administered, weaker or no biological effects will result. With an even greater dose, the bio-suppressive range is entered (inhibiting effect result). This is most obvious in wound healing and stimulation of hair growth. (See Figure 10.6 "Arndt-Schulz law" on page 514.)

So which are the "correct" doses? You want to know - and we seem to be beating around the bush (for good reasons). The answer is: read this book carefully, think, and do the best you can with the laser you happen to have. Doses do not have to be "perfect" to produce a good biological response. Anyway, the table below gives you a rough view of suitable doses.

ond) where W stands for watt and s for second. The dose D is hence measured in joules per square centimetre (J/cm²) and is calculated as

$$D = \frac{P \times t}{A} \quad [\text{J/cm}^2]$$

where P is the laser's output power in watts, t is the treatment duration in seconds, and A is the area treated, given in cm². If the laser is pulsed, the average output power in watts should be used instead.

Choosing a variety of output powers and times, we can calculate the corresponding doses and present them in a table. The table below shows doses in J/cm², under various treatment durations, reached with lasers of different output power. Using a 20 mW GaAs single-probe laser or a 30 mW GaAlAs single-probe laser, for example, we can calculate, using the formula in the section on dose calculation below, that when treating an area of 1 cm² for a certain duration we achieve the dose (in joules) shown in the columns in the table.

Time/cm²	Output power from the laser						
	10 mW	30 mW	60 mW	120 mW	240 mW	500 mW	1000 mW
1 sec	0.01 J	0.03 J	0.06 J	0.12 J	0.24 J	0.5 J	1.0 J
3 sec	0.03 J	0.09 J	0.18 J	0.36 J	0.72 J	1.5 J	3.0 J
10 sec	0.1 J	0.3 J	0.6 J	1.2 J	2.4 J	5 J	10 J
30 sec	0.3 J	0.9 J	1.8 J	3.6 J	7.2 J	15 J	30 J
1 min	0.6 J	1.8 J	3.6 J	7.2 J	14 J	30 J	60 J
3 min	1.8 J	5.4 J	11 J	22 J	43 J	90 J	180 J
10 min	6.0 J	18 J	36 J	72 J	144 J	300 J	600 J

Dose to skin surface for different laser powers and exposure times per square centimeter area

Table 3.1 Dose to skin surface

N.B.! We have said it before; It is of the greatest importance that you know the output power of your laser! If you don't, you have no idea of the doses you give! It is not self-evident that the power of your laser is the same as when you bought it. Furthermore, the power specified in a brochure is frequently quite different from what you actually get out of your probe. The output should be measured from time to time! If you don't have a built-in power meter, you should check your laser with an external one regularly.

Trelles [458] found that the effects of HeNe laser light on mast cells were accomplished faster at 50 mW than at 4 mW, although all cell lines were irradiated with 2.4 J.
Further literature: [291]

3.3.1.5 Energy density

Energy density is the same as dose or fluence. The difference between power density and energy density is simply the time. As mentioned above, the power density is measured in watts per cm^2. The energy density is measured in watt-seconds per cm^2, which is the same as joules per cm^2. For calculation of energy density, see chapter 3.3.1.7 "Calculation of doses" on page 78.

Looking at a specific situation with laser light penetrating into tissue, we will have points and areas with high power density and other areas with low power density. If this distribution of light is held constant over a certain period, we will have an <u>energy</u> distribution that, in every point, is exactly proportional to said <u>power</u> distribution. If we keep the same situation going on for ten times as long, we have an energy density (i.e. dose) that is ten times higher in every point reached by the light. (See chapter 10.3 "Power density" on page 508 and chapter 10.7 "Energy density" on page 513.)

Just like the power density, the energy density is not constant - it has a two-dimensional distribution over a surface (this is also true of the area that is hit by the laser light when a treatment probe is held in skin contact) and has a three-dimensional distribution in the treated tissue volume.

3.3.1.6 Treatment dose

Treatment dose is the same as the energy density. We will in future mainly use the term dose. The dose is the most important treatment parameter. Dosage refers to the amount of energy per unit area brought to bear on tissue or cell culture. Dosage and treatment intervals can only be specified schematically. This is because the various laser wavelengths mean that different doses must be given, and treatment conditions likewise vary. People are receptive to laser treatment to varying degrees - some can "feel the laser right down to their toes", others are entirely impervious. It is appropriate to begin with a low dose for a new patient to ensure that you do not enter a biosuppressive dose range or trigger a pain response on the first treatment.

3.3.1.7 Calculation of doses

The dose is the amount of energy administered to a surface area of tissue. In the calculation we will measure area in cm^2. Energy can be measured in joules or calories (old measure). A joule is the same as a Ws (reads watt-sec-

3.3.1.2 Output power

Of course you should know what laser type you have as well as its wavelength. But it is just as important to know the output power of your instrument in order to calculate the right dose to administer. A significant advantage of a higher output power is that it takes less time to reach a given dose. This has a financial significance for the patient but is not a decisive factor in achieving good results. Dosage is the primary factor. Output power is, however, of great consequence in that a higher output power gives a higher power density, which very often is beneficial. Output power is also of some importance with respect to light penetration in tissue.

3.3.1.3 Average output power

When a laser works in pulsed mode, it is the laser's average output power that is significant in terms of dose calculation. (See Figure 1.7 "Different types of pulsing" on page 19.) If you do not know the average output power of your pulsed laser, you cannot calculate the dose to administer.

3.3.1.4 Power density

Power density is the same as the "intensity" of the light and is measured in watts or milliwatts per cm^2. Spreading the light over a large area gives a low intensity. As biostimulation is based on local effects, with the transport of various substances through cell membrane and tissue, power density should not be too low, even if the number of joules is high. Low power cannot entirely be compensated by increased time. Since the dose can easily become too high locally when the laser is held directly against the skin/mucous membrane, one must ensure that the treatment time is not too long when using point treatment. The power density (I) can be calculated as

$$I = \frac{P}{A} \quad [W/cm^2]$$

(See chapter 10.3 "Power density" on page 508.)

Literature:

van Breugel [228] studied the effects of HeNe laser light on human fibroblast cultures. Irradiation was administered on three consecutive days at various power densities with exposure times of between 30 seconds and 10 minutes. The laser output power varied between 0.55 and 5.98 mW. It was apparent that the most significant effects were obtained by laser output power below 2.91 mW, while 5.98 mW had no effect. The stimulative effects were strongest during irradiation periods between 30 seconds and 2 minutes. The study demonstrates that power density and exposure time are important parameters. Another conclusion is that power density is important in itself. Treating an area with 40 mW for 10 seconds is usually more beneficial than using 10 mW and 40 seconds, although the dose would be the same.

3.3 What parameters to use

For laser therapy systems, we know that the following parameters (among others) significantly affect treatment results: choice of laser wavelength, size of dose, level of power density, the laser's method of working, pulse repetition rate, depth of penetration, treatment methodology, treatment frequency and total number of treatments.

3.3.1 Laser parameters

There are basically two types of parameters – laser parameters and patient parameters. The laser parameters will sometimes have to be changed from patient to patient depending on the patient parameters.

3.3.1.1 Which wavelength?

It is important to use the right wavelength (i.e. laser type) for the right indications. Although it has not yet been possible to determine the "best" wavelength for each indication, the authors believe that the HeNe or InGaAlP laser (633-670 nm) is the best option for ulcers and nerve regeneration. Due to the poor penetration of light of this wavelength (up to one cm), other wavelengths must sometimes be used, although they may not be optimal.

In addition, we consider that the GaAs laser is a better choice for the treatment of deeper problems such as sports injuries and that it has a greater effect on postoperative pain and swelling than the shorter wavelength lasers. Further about this laser in chapter 11.1.5 "How deep does light penetrate into tissue?" on page 539.

GaAlAs lasers are usually the best choise for tendinitis but it can also be a good alternative for treating pain and oedema, and we have positive experience of treating chronic ulcers with this laser type. The high power density of modern GaAlAs lasers has also proved to be advantageous in physiotherapy.

It must be stressed that any wavelength, with a reasonable dose in the target area, will have a biological effect. If "the best" wavelength is not at hand, it is of course recommended to use other wavelengths. Probably, the correct dose may be just as important as the wavelength. However, that dose is sometimes not known or obtainable, e.g. due to the lack of penetration.

Karu [180] found, by measuring chemiluminescence, that the oxidative processes of blood cells were influenced by various laser wavelengths during the initial phase of acute viral respiratory illness. Of the four different wavelengths tested (660, 820, 880 and 950 nm), 660 nm was found to be the most effective. The dose range in this *in vitro* study was 0.1 - 1 J/cm^2.

Some studies have shown improved results when two wavelengths were combined. However, it could be asked whether the clinical results of these studies are sometimes just as much dependent on the combined doses as on the two different wavelengths.

and near-IR laser light with the parameters that were used in this study changed the biochemical behaviour of ATP molecules.

Previous studies using 670 nm light-emitting diode (LED) arrays suggest that cytochrome c oxidase, a photoacceptor in the NIR range, plays an important role in therapeutic photobiomodulation. If this is true, then an irreversible inhibitor of cytochrome c oxidase, potassium cyanide (KCN), should compete with LED and reduce its beneficial effects. This hypothesis was tested on primary cultured neurons in a study by Wong-Riley [1499]. LED treatment partially restored enzyme activity blocked by 10-100 micromol KCN. It significantly reduced neuronal cell death induced by 300 micromol KCN from 83.6 to 43.5%. However, at 1-100 mm KCN, the protective effects of LED decreased, and neuronal deaths increased. LED significantly restored neuronal ATP content only at 10 micromol KCN but not at higher concentrations of KCN tested. Pretreatment with LED enhanced efficacy of LED during exposure to 10 or 100 micromol KCN but did not restore enzyme activity to control levels. In contrast, LED was able to completely reverse the detrimental effect of tetrodotoxin, which only indirectly down-regulated enzyme levels. Among the wavelengths tested (670, 728, 770, 830, and 880 nm), the most effective ones (830 nm, 670 nm) paralleled the NIR absorption spectrum of oxidized cytochrome c oxidase, whereas the least effective wavelength, 728 nm, did not. The results are consistent the hypothesis that the mechanism of photobiomodulation involves the up-regulation of cytochrome c oxidase, leading to increased energy metabolism in neurons functionally inactivated by toxins.

In a search for chromophores responsible for photobiostimulation, endogenous porphyrins, mitochondrial and membranal cytochromes, and flavoproteins were found to be suitable candidates This is described in the review article by Lubart [1506]. The above-mentioned chromophores are photosensitizers that generate reactive oxygen species (ROS) following irradiation. As the cellular redox state has a key role in maintaining the viability of the cell, changes in ROS may play a significant role in cell activation. In the present review, we summarize evidence demonstrating that various ROS and antioxidants are produced following laser illumination. It was found that very little evidence for NO formation in illuminated non-vascular smooth muscle cells exists in the literature. The author suggests that the change in the cellular redox state, which plays a pivotal role in maintaining cellular activities, leads to photobiostimulative processes.

Further literature: [1451], [1452, 1525, 1526]

3.2.1 Photoreceptors
In order for the laser light to be absorbed, there must be receptors. Such receptors are well known in plants, but are there human light receptors other than those in the eyes and in the skin? The following is quoted from Enwemeka [1160]:

"We may have to step back in time in order to begin to understand the mechanisms involved. That low energy light particles can produce significant, and at times, life-supporting changes in various organisms, is not at all new. Our primordial ancestor, the purple bacteria, provides a vivid example. Found in abstemious habitats below that of plant life – e.g. the bottom of ponds and topsoil, depending on the species – the purple bacteria inevitably lives on a meagre amount of light. Only the reminder of light unharvested by plants penetrates to those depths. But with the carotenoids in its light-harvesting complexes absorbing light at 500 nm wavelength, and its bacteriochlorophyll absorbing at 800-850 nm, this life form is able to carry out complex life-supporting metabolic processes with relatively minimal light energy.

To date, more than three hundred photochemically reactive proteins, capable of harvesting low light energy, have been identified in both prokaryotic and eukaryotic organisms. Many more are being discovered yearly. In humans, the most commonly known photochemically active receptor proteins are rod and cone pigments in the eye. However, other human photoreceptors have been discovered in recent times. Examples are encephalopsins in the brain and pinopsin in the pineal gland. Given the discovery of photoreceptor proteins in the pineal gland, the hypothalamus, and other tissues of lower vertebrates, it is only a matter of time that it will become clear that other human tissues have photoreactive proteins as well". (See chapter 11.1.6 "Bright Light Phototherapy" on page 541.)

Literature:
Adenosine triphosphate (ATP) is an important molecule in biology because it stores chemical energy and releases it to the biochemical processes occurring in the cell. In the study by Amat [1533] the authors analysed the biochemical behaviour of ATP after irradiating it with 635 and 830 nm diode lasers. They analysed the luminescence peak, the reaction rate and the area under the luminescence curve at 2×10^{-9} mol/l of ATP in the luciferine-luciferase luminescence reaction before and after irradiating the molecule at several irradiances and radiant exposures. The absorption spectrum of ATP at 3×10^{-3} mol/l concentration was measured between 650 and 900 nm after laser irradiation at 635 nm (Argon-Dye) and 830 nm (diode laser). It was found significant differences in the measured parameters when ATP was irradiated with both wavelengths. The absorption spectra of non-irradiated and irradiated ATP showed a physical-chemical difference in the ATP molecule after irradiation with both lasers. It can concluded that visible

Inoue [405] has demonstrated that GaAlAs 780 nm laser irradiation suppressed the tuberculin reaction in sensitised guinea pigs. The suppression was seen not only on the irradiated side but also on the contralateral, non-irradiated side.

Schindl [350] induced the arthus phenomenon (an anaphylactic effect) in the corneas of 57 rabbits. The healing effect of a HeNe laser as compared to control was obvious. Consensual co-reaction could be observed in the contralateral non-irradiated eyes in the experimental group.

The above studies may explain why studies involving contralateral untreated control lesions on the same animal/patient have not always produced good or clear results. The non-irradiated "control" lesion in fact benefits from the treated lesion because of the systemic reaction just discussed.

This theory is supported by a study by Halevy [467]. Using a 780 nm 30 mW laser, 6 patients with cutaneous fissures located in the hands and feet were treated every 2-3 days. There were similar fissures on both sides of the body. On the irradiated side, 4 of the 6 fissures healed completely and in the remaining 2 there was a decrease of 40%. On the non-irradiated side, 3 healed completely and 1 healed partially.

Friedmann [513] draws the following conclusion: "Due to transmission of neural excitation and calcium waves, photobiomodulation is a systemic effect."

Villaplana [424] irradiated the anterior pituitary gland with HeNe laser through the surgically exposed lamina dura in two groups of rats (n = 30 per group). The calculated incident power at the gland was 2.75 mW. Population I Leydig cells of the central part of the rat testicles showed signs of increased but non-specific activity in the entire series of experimental animals as compared to sham-irradiated controls. Thus, laser therapy may have a systemic effect on testosterone production under these experimental conditions.

Hall [673] failed to find any systemic effect in a wound healing study in rats using GaAs. However, the parameters used did not enhance wound healing in the irradiated wound, so obviously there could be no systemic effect iun the first place.

Systemic effects, however, are not always found, even when there is an effect on the irradiated side. In a wound healing study on diabetic rats by Reddy [657] the following conclusions were reached: 1) the GaAs laser therapy had no apparent systemic effect on the wound on the opposite side of the treatment side; and 2) laser photostimulation decreased the healing time for full thickness skin wounds in diabetic animals, but had no effect on the biomechanical properties of the tissue once the wound was healed.

Further literature: [1456]

RNA in the cell nucleus [33], local effects on the immune system [34], increased new formation of capillaries by the release of growth factors [35], increased activity of leukocytes [36], transformation of fibroblasts to myofibroblasts [37], and a great number of other measured effects.

Secondly, there is a systemic effect, well illustrated through the use of CO_2-lasers as biostimulators. The wavelength of CO_2-lasers cannot penetrate the tissue for more than a fraction of a millimetre, so there is no other primary responding tissue than the outer part of the dermis. The stimulative effects found when using CO_2 are in many cases quite similar to those observed in treatment with the classic wavelengths. We can thus draw the following conclusions:
1. CO_2-lasers work through a secondary response; and
2. Deep light penetration is not a necessity per se in biostimulation, at least not for some of the biostimulative effects.

The possible reason for this is that cells in the tissue subjected to the light produce substances that then spread and circulate in blood vessels and the lymphatic system.

Literature:

In case of biostimulation with deeper penetrating laser wavelengths, the systemic effects are often due to treatment of blood cells, which in turn influence other cells, tissue and mechanisms in the system. This is illustrated by Zhuk [1141] who treated patients with chronic tuberculosis by treating the blood in a vein. The patients were divided into two groups, both getting conventional medical treatment but only one group getting laser treatment as well. The laser group showed significantly shorter recovery times. (See chapter 4.1.56 "Tuberculosis" on page 343.) Yet another illustration of the systemic effect is a report by Braverman [50]. In a study using experimental wounds, laboratory animals were treated with a HeNe or GaAs laser, or both in combination. The tensile strength of the newly healed wounds was greater in all the laser therapy groups than in the control group. There was also a group of animals on which two wounds were inflicted, only one of which was treated with laser. Even the untreated wound showed better results than in the control group. The authors of the report drew the following conclusion: "The laser irradiation can thus have released substances in the circulatory apparatus so that the tensile strength increased even in the wound on the opposite, untreated side."

The same observation has been made by Rochkind [39]. HeNe laser treatment on only the right-hand side of bilaterally inflicted skin wounds increased the healing process on both sides as compared to the control group. This also applied in the case of bilateral burn wounds.

In a crossover study, Airaksinen [302] treated patients with chronic neck and shoulder pain unilaterally with HeNe. The pressure pain threshold increased significantly on both the non-treated and the treated side, although the increase was larger on the treated side.

3.2 A few words on mechanisms

In this chapter we will only give a brief overview of the mechanisms behind successful laser therapy. A much more detailed description is given in chapter 11.

Treatment with laser therapy is not based on heat development but on photochemical and photobiological effects in cells and tissue. What happens when this relatively weak laser light encounters our cells?

Firstly, quite a lot happens locally, where the light hits (primary response). As mentioned above, it has been observed that if laser light is administered in the right dose, certain cell functions are stimulated, and this is particularly evident if the cell in question has an impaired function. (See chapter 3.4.4 "The importance of the tissue and cell condition" on page 123.)

As will be discussed in chapter 11, it is known that chromophores, in the form of e.g. porphyrins, play an important role. It is known that small amounts of singlet oxygen build up when tissue is irradiated with laser light [28]. Rochkind's and Lubart's group in Israel has demonstrated this [29] using the NMR technique (Nuclear Magnetic Resonance). Singlet oxygen is a "free radical" which itself influences the formation of ATP (adenosine triphosphate) [30, 140, 2019, 2020], which constitutes the cells' fuel and energy store.

Another recently suggested photoreceptor is NADPH oxidase [1336], which has been found to exist in non-blood cells. It possesses a flavoprotein which can be the target of light. Several chromophores are photosensitisers and generate reactive oxygen species (ROS) following irradiation. ROS, such as singlet oxygen, NO and H_2O_2 are cell destructive in large amounts but in small amounts they serve as "secondary messengers" in the cascade of events following laser irradiation. The influence of ROS has been demonstrated by irradiating fibroblasts and establishing the stimulative ratio of the laser light. The antioxidant catalase was then added to the Petri dish and new irradiation was performed. The previous stimulation did not appear. Catalase is a ROS scavenger and the inhibition of the ROS obviously blocked the stimulation.

It is also thought that nitric oxide can play an important role [432, 469]. Additionally, it has been observed that the calcium ion balance [31] in the cell is affected. The influence of laser light on the oxidative processes has been demonstrated by Karu [180] and others. Karu [512] suggests cytochrome a/a3, a respiratory chain component, as an important photoreceptor.Lilveria [1848] has, for instance showed that laser therapy significantly increased the activities of complexes II and IV (cytochrome c oxidase) but did not affect succinate dehydrogenase activity.

This leads in turn to a number of secondary effects (secondary responses) which have been studied and measured in various contexts: increased cell metabolism and collagen synthesis in fibroblasts [8], increased action potential of nerve cells [32], stimulation of the formation of DNA and

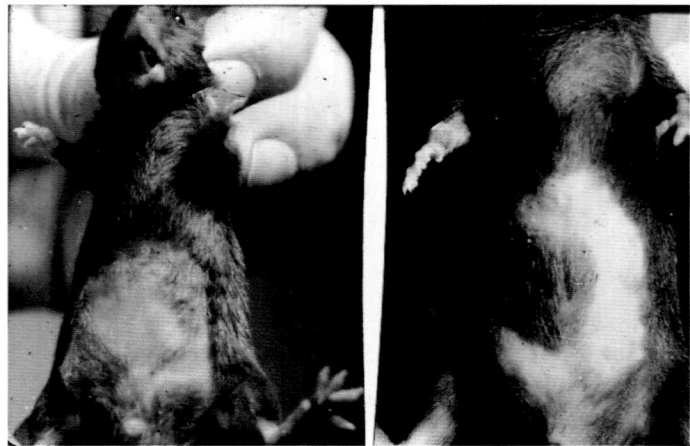

Figure 3.2 "The historic mice" I.
Courtesy: Andrew Mester

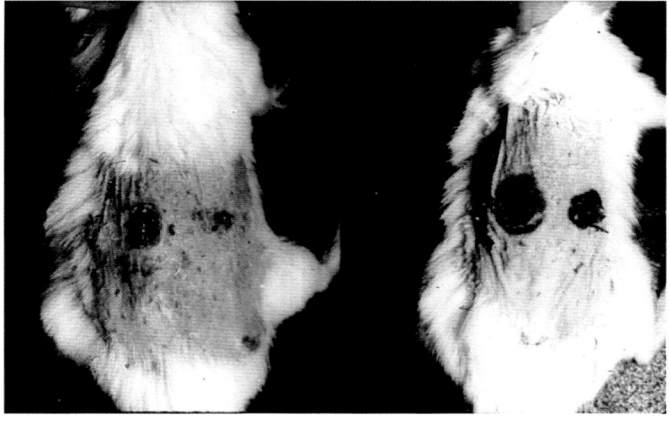

Figure 3.3 "The historic mice" II.
Courtesy: Andrew Mester

In this article it is no doubt a biostimulation effect that is referred to. This is, according to our knowledge, the first time this effect was reported, though it was not understood. The report refers to studies by McGuff [1853-1859] in which ruby and HeNe laser had been used in hamsters with experimental tumors.

In 1965 Laor [589] used 700-900 J with high power densities, causing high mortality among the laboratory rats. However, doses below 20 J rarely resulted in any microscopic changes. In the same year, Derr [28] published a report on the occurrence of free radicals in irradiated biological materials. In 1967, Carney [520], using a ruby laser, demonstrated an increase in collagen synthesis in skin wounds treated with power densities of 0.4 - 2.5 J/cm^2.

In 1966, (Orvosi Heitlap 1966, 107:1012, in Hungarian, abstract in English) Mester's group at the Semmelweiss hospital in Budapest published the first scientific report of the stimulatory effects of non-thermal ruby laser light (694 nm) on the skin of rats. (See figures on next page.) These pictures were published in [733, 734]. The following year, articles were published on the effects of lasers on wounds (see figure on next page) and leukocytes in culture [10]. Mester demonstrated that cells in culture and in tissue can be stimulated by a certain dose (input energy, measured in joules per cm^2 of skin) of laser light. Too low a dose has no or an insufficient effect. Too high a dose is also less effective, or has no effect at all, while a dose that is much too large can lead to inhibiting effects. A ruby laser was used. Along with Endre Mester, Viktor Injushin in Kazakhstan was researching early about the possible biological effects of low laser energies.

3.1 History

Initially, researchers' interest was focused on the use of lasers in surgery. Thus, rather high doses were used in early experiments.

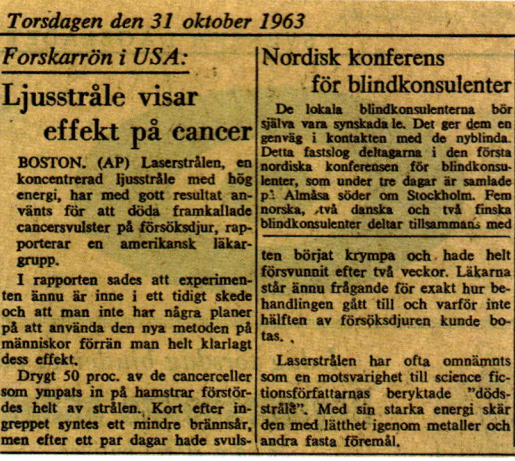

Figure 3.1 The Swedish daily Svenska Dagbladet, October 31st, 1963

Boston (AP). An American group of physicians report that laser light, a concentrated beam of light of high energy, has successfully been used to kill cancer tumours induced in laboratory animals. In the report it is stated that the experiment still is in an initial stage and that there are no plans to use it in humans until the effect is fully documented. Some 50% of the cancerous cells that had been implanted in hamsters were completely destroyed by the laser. Shortly after therapy, a minor burn was visible but within a few days the tumour had started to shrink and was completely gone in two weeks. The researchers still do not understand exactly how the therapy worked and why the other half of the experimental animals could not be cured. The laser beam has often been referred to as an equivalent of the feared "death beam" of science fiction. With its strong energy it easily cuts metals and other solid objects.